DATE DUE

Comprehensive Textbook
of AIDS Psychiatry

COMPREHENSIVE TEXTBOOK OF AIDS PSYCHIATRY

Edited by
Mary Ann Cohen
and
Jack M. Gorman

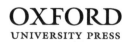

OXFORD
UNIVERSITY PRESS

2008

OXFORD
UNIVERSITY PRESS

Oxford University Press, Inc., publishes works that further
Oxford University's objective of excellence
in research, scholarship, and education.

Oxford New York

Auckland   Cape Town   Dar es Salaam   Hong Kong   Karachi
Kuala Lumpur   Madrid   Melbourne   Mexico City   Nairobi
New Delhi   Shanghai   Taipei   Toronto

With offices in

Argentina   Austria   Brazil   Chile   Czech Republic   France   Greece
Guatemala   Hungary   Italy   Japan Poland   Portugal   Singapore
South Korea   Switzerland   Thailand   Turkey   Ukraine   Vietnam

Library of Congress Cataloging-in-Publication Data
Comprehensive textbook of AIDS psychiatry / edited by Mary Ann Cohen and Jack M. Gorman.
p. cm.
Includes bibliographical references.
ISBN-13: 978-0-19-530435-0
1. AIDS (Disease)—Psychological aspects.   2. HIV infections—Psychological aspects.
3. AIDS (Disease)—Patients–Mental health.   4. HIV-positive persons—Mental health.
I. Cohen, Mary Ann, 1941-   II. Gorman, Jack M.
[DNLM: 1. HIV Infections–psychology.   2. HIV Infections—complications.   3. Mental Disorders—complications.
4. Mental Disorders—diagnosis.   5. Mental Disorders—therapy. WC 503.7 C7375 2008]
RC606.6.C662 2008
616.97'9206—dc22   2007003716

1 3 5 7 9 8 6 4 2
Printed in the United States of America
on acid-free paper

This book is dedicated to the courageous men, women, and children with HIV and AIDS, to their families, and to their loved ones. It is also dedicated to the devoted teams of HIV clinicians who provide care and support for persons with HIV and AIDS. I thank my family and friends for their support.
M.A.C.

With thanks to Lauren, Sara, Rachel, and Avi.
J.M.G.

Foreword

Despite all the medical advances we have made in the treatment of HIV infection, the psychiatric care of persons with HIV and AIDS has remained one of the most challenging aspects of medical care. Although the need for palliative care has decreased, it also remains an integral part of HIV care. In some ways, doctors in training are not as aware of what palliative care for those with HIV entails. The *Comprehensive Textbook of AIDS Psychiatry* offers the reader an enormous historical overview of HIV as well as a review of the most current management of all aspects of HIV/AIDS care with a strong emphasis on psychiatric manifestations.

One of the fundamental parts of a patient's initial medical history and physical encompasses the patient's sociobehavioral and psychiatric histories. Frequently the "medical" primary care provider overlooks the significance of these factors. Fortunately, congressional Ryan White acts have recognized the significance of mental health and have included funding to support mental health professionals and programs.

Mental health programs are a necessity to all comprehensive HIV clinics and should also be readily available for those seen in private practices.

Depression remains one of the most common psychiatric illnesses that plague those with HIV. HIV carries a tremendous stigma throughout the world. Patients need assistance with acceptance of their diagnosis and with disclosure of their HIV status to others. We need to be prepared to handle not only the needs of our patients but also those of our patients' support systems, whether they be partners, family, or friends. We have to understand all the factors that play into the acquisition of HIV disease and the subsequent management of their illness.

Frequently persons with HIV have underlying mental health issues and conditions. Whether it is substance use, mood disorders, or psychosis, individuals with these issues need evaluation by a skilled mental health specialist. Perhaps the most challenging issue to address is the etiology of the psychiatric manifestation. Was it preexisting but undiagnosed? Is it from HIV or could the therapies themselves be contributing? Are there other infectious or organic reasons for this behavior? In this textbook, the authors discuss the importance of thorough psychiatric and neuropsychological examinations. They thoughtfully divide this book into sections addressing all aspects of care.

In the first section, Psychiatric Relevance and Implications of AIDS Psychiatry, the history of AIDS psychiatry is reviewed with case vignettes that are familiar to all of us treating those with HIV. These cases remind me of so many patients I have seen through the years and instill appreciation that I have always had mental health specialists available to my patients. Additional chapters focus on how HIV itself, its effects on the immune system, and medications used to treat HIV contribute to psychiatric illness. They also provide a review of the prevalence of psychiatric disorders in persons with HIV and AIDS, along with a brief description of these conditions.

The second section, Comprehensive AIDS Psychiatric Assessment, is an impressive detailing of all the aspects of complete psychiatric and neuropsychiatric evaluations. It includes select questionnaires and recommendations for history taking.

The third section, Psychiatric Disorders and HIV Infection, covers the most commonly encountered mental health disorders—frankly, those I need the most help with in diagnosing and treating patients. What I think should be most obvious to treat is not always so easily addressed. I find that my HIV-infected patients have such complex lives that dealing with substance use, mood disorders, cognitive disorders, anxiety disorders, psychotic disorders, and/or personality disorders becomes increasingly challenging. As with patients having medical complications, HIV-infected persons do not follow the textbook rule of having one psychiatric disorder. This book acknowledges that our patients may have multiple disorders and that each caregiver needs to be diligent to evaluate a person for all aspects of neurological and psychiatric disorders, and all of these need care.

The fourth section, Unique Psychiatric Manifestations of HIV Infection, pays particular attention to those common occurrences that truly distress our patients yet do not have our complete understanding as to why they occur, such as insomnia and fatigue. The authors also discuss unique manifestations of dementia and the dynamics surrounding the suicidal patient. As stated in Chapter 18, "there is no treatment for suicide, only prevention." Although we all are

confronted with helping our patients face death and actively accepting death, suicide is a subject that frequently causes discomfort for both the messenger and the recipient. Having had a patient who did commit suicide, I recognize that there is no more powerful state of helplessness a clinician can face.

The fifth section, Neuropathologic Manifestations of HIV Infection, provides an in-depth review of cognitive impairment and neuropathies. The chapters discuss the neuropathogenesis followed by diagnostic and therapeutic interventions.

The sixth section, Psychiatric Aspects of Risk Behaviors, Prevention of HIV Transmission, and Adherence to Medical Care, underscores the importance that mental health plays in the overall management of HIV disease. The bottom line remains that if patients do not take their medications, the medications will not work. If life could only be that simple—by saying those magic words, our patients would be adherent to their treatment. These chapters illustrate the chaotic lives of our patients, address how mental health issues affect their insight and ability to take care of themselves, and suggest how to empower them to do so.

The seventh section, AIDS Psychiatry through the Life Cycle, addresses the three major phases of age that create anxiety for providers as well as patients. The transition from childhood to adolescence and young adulthood is anxiety provoking for most young persons. For children who were perinatally infected with HIV (vertical transmission), the transitions can be devastating. Their lives have been surrounded by loss. Many have seen their parents die, even grandparents. Others have been shuffled among foster homes. Their pediatrician has been their stable structure, and the fear of losing their surrogate parent is great. How does one transition to adult care? Another chapter deals with reproduction and discordant couples. Again, this issue plays a major role in our young, vertically infected teens and young adults as they try to lead normal lives and want to have their own families. This issue also affects thousands of young adults who have become infected through other means. Finally, with aging, all the issues that confront us as we get older are complicated by HIV.

The eighth section, AIDS Psychiatric Treatment and Psychotherapeutic Modalities, addresses therapeutic interventions, including spirituality, psychotherapy, and medical treatment. The authors discuss the roles of the support systems of social work and nursing in such interventions. They also detail the complexities of all the various classes of psychiatric medications and their drug interactions with commonly prescribed antiretroviral therapies.

The ninth section, AIDS Psychiatry and Comorbid Medical Conditions, provides an excellent overview of major coinfections and comorbidities. Discussed are not only conditions that may mimic or conceal psychiatric disorders but also the ways in which these other illnesses have an impact on mental health or even create mental distress, such as that seen with metabolic syndromes.

Finally, the last section, Ethical and Health Policy Aspects of AIDS Psychiatry, deals with those issues surrounding us as health care providers, such as burnout. Another helpful section is on managing ethical decisions and evaluating patients with impaired judgment. I am frequently confronted with patients who refuse therapies, and it remains unclear to me whether they are competent or whether their judgment is impaired. Where is that fine line between respecting one's wishes and giving patients the right to choose? These last chapters I found particularly intriguing.

At first glance, it may seem overly ambitious to cover all these topics in one book; however, the authors do achieve this goal. I cannot recall ever reading a textbook cover to cover by choice and actually finding myself engaged throughout. Psychiatric illness is a major component of routine medical care of those infected with HIV. As the title implies, this textbook offers a comprehensive review of the psychiatric aspects that all our patients face daily. Consequently, a mental health evaluation should not be a mere offer to all our HIV-infected patients, it is a medical necessity.

Judith A. Aberg, M.D.
Principal Investigator, AIDS Clinical Trials Unit
Director of HIV, Bellevue Hospital Center
Associate Professor of Medicine,
New York University School of Medicine

Foreword

The publication of the *Comprehensive Textbook of AIDS Psychiatry*, edited by two psychiatrists who have "been there" since the beginning of the epidemic, is a benchmark for the field — it has come of age.

The book begins with an important history of the disease. In the early 1980s, we were sure that infectious diseases were on their way to being eradicated. Then the first cases of a strange "wasting disease" appeared in New York and San Francisco. Frightening, mysterious, without known cause or cure, and without knowledge of the route of transmission, this disease instilled near-panic levels of fear among the public. The same fears existed in health care personnel. Society quickly stigmatized AIDS as it had done with all prior epidemics—from the plague, to tuberculosis, to cancer. The short course of three decades has resulted in the panic dissipating as information about cause and treatment emerged.

However, the stigma took another direction as we learned more about this disease. It appeared disproportionately in populations that carried their own complex and negative social connotations, gay men and substance abusers. Research was slowed by these biases, yet in three decades, treatment has turned a devastating disease into one with a chronic course in the industrialized world. The tragedy of our current world condition is that the places where most of these cases are occurring have little access to the known preventive measures and effective treatments that are now accepted practice in the United States. It will be a blot on the Western world when the history of this era is written on this pandemic, for the fiber of life was allowed to be destroyed in Africa while the resource-rich countries looked on.

It is crucial that the psychiatric and psychosocial manifestations of HIV/AIDS be widely understood by physicians and their teams who provide care for persons with HIV. The care of children is a critical component, especially in the developing world. The central nervous system sequelae of delirium and dementia are serious effects requiring management by those with a good knowledge of the psychiatry of medical illness.

The psychological issues of sadness, depression, anxiety, and coping with a disease that has no cure require thoughtful management. All the problems of a chronic illness, with its need for adherence to treatment and for social support, make this one of the chronic diseases of the twenty-first century that will require continued allocation of resources as the challenges of patients change as the disease evolves. The thoughtful explication of symptoms and signs of the common psychiatric disorders is a contribution to the literature on AIDS, written by our best authorities.

It is crucial that the psychiatric and psychosocial manifestations of HIV/AIDS be widely understood by physicians and their teams who care for these patients. The care of children is a critical component, especially in the developing world. The central nervous system sequelae of delirium and dementia are serious effects requiring management by those with a good knowledge of the psychiatry of medical illness. The psychological issues of sadness, depression, anxiety, and coping with a disease that has no cure require thoughtful management. All the problems of a chronic illness, with its need for adherence to treatment and for social support, make this one of the chronic diseases of the twenty-first century that will require continued allo-

cation of resources as the challenges of patients change as the disease evolves. The thoughtful explication of symptoms and signs of the common psychiatric disorders is a contribution to the literature on AIDS, written by our best authorities

Attention to the means of transmission of HIV by sexual contact and substance abuse–related behavior has made prevention as important as the treatment. Application of what we know today in the developing world will begin to change the devastation that has occurred in Africa.

This is truly a comprehensive review of the range of topics that are crucial to HIV/AIDS patient care. Policy issues and palliative care also have a place in this overview. I commend the editors and their contributors for preparing this important overview of the psychosocial and psychiatric sequelae of a pandemic that we thought could not happen in the "modern" world.

Jimmie Holland, MD
Wayne E. Chapman Chair in Psychiatric Oncology
Memorial Sloan Kettering Cancer Center and Professor of Psychiatry, Weill Medical College of Cornell University

Foreword

The Comprehensive Textbook of AIDS Psychiatry, edited by Mary Ann Cohen and Jack Gorman, is an impressive and important contribution to the field of HIV medicine. To say it is a comprehensive treatise is an understatement. It is unlikely to be equaled in its scope, consistency, authority, and practical value. The editors, who also contributed a substantial amount of the book's content, clearly set out to not only summarize the psychiatric presentation and management of HIV disease but to place these manifestations and management in the larger context of the patient and society and within our complex health care system. The editors are well positioned for this ambitious undertaking, having helped create models of comprehensive AIDS care beginning early in the epidemic. They have augmented their own expertise with an equally impressive list of contributors and have clearly succeeded in eliciting a consistency of tone and approach that increases the usability of this lengthy work.

This textbook sets the stage by reviewing the history of the epidemic and of early efforts of care coordination. The book covers many facets relevant to AIDS psychiatry with an organization that makes its rich content accessible. For example, separate chapters address sociocultural aspects of HIV, a biopsychosocial approach, neurophysiology, and psychoneuroimmunology. This allows the reader to view AIDS psychiatry from distinct but obviously complementary models of presentation that contribute to individualized management strategies. Similarly, the book in its organization allows a nuanced discussion of HIV effects on mood, personality, distress, anxiety, and cognition, each summarized by leading experts.

Another unique organizational approach to the book's broad agenda is the interaction between the life cycle and HIV psychiatry. Well-written chapters address issues of concern to the management of adolescents, young adults, and the elderly. Similarly, separate chapters summarize the roles of various health care professionals in HIV management, including psychiatry, social services, nursing, and spiritual advisors.

The Comprehensive Textbook of AIDS Psychiatry is a unique and immensely valuable work. It will be of true assistance, particularly in comprehensive HIV care centers where it is likely to be used by all components of the health care team. It is truly an impressive achievement.

Paul A. Volberding, M.D.
Chief of Medical Service, San Francisco Veterans
Affairs Medical Center
Professor and Vice Chair, Department
of Medicine
Codirector, Center for AIDS Research, University
of California San Francisco
Coeditor-in-Chief, *Journal of Acquired Immune
Deficiency Syndromes*

Contents

Contributors

NAOMI ADLER, B.A.
Center for AIDS Prevention Studies
University of California at San Francisco
San Francisco, CA

ASHER D. ALADJEM, M.D.
Clinical Associate Professor
Department of Psychiatry
New York University School of Medicine
New York, NY

CÉSAR A. ALFONSO, M.D.
Assistant Professor of Clinical Psychiatry
Department of Psychiatry
Columbia University College
    of Physicians and Surgeons
Attending Psychiatrist
Department of Psychiatry
Lenox Hill Hospital
New York, NY

ANDREW F. ANGELINO, M.D.
Assistant Professor
Department of Psychiatry and Behavioral Sciences
Johns Hopkins University School of Medicine
Clinical Director
Department of Psychiatry
Johns Hopkins Bayview Medical Center
Baltimore, MD

MICHAEL H. ANTONI, PH.D.
Director
Center for Psycho-Oncology Research
Professor, Department of Psychology
University of Miami
Coral Gables, FL

DAVID R. BANGSBERG, M.D., M.P.H.
Associate Professor of Medicine in Residence
Division of Infectious Diseases
San Francisco General AIDS Division

University of California at San Francisco
San Francisco, CA

SHARON M. BATISTA, M.D.
Psychiatry Resident Physician
Department of Psychiatry
Mount Sinai Hospital
New York, NY

ALAN BERKMAN, M.D.
Associate Professor
Department of Epidemiology and Sociomedical
  Sciences
Mailman School of Public Health
Columbia University
New York, NY

PHILIP A. BIALER, M.D.
Associate Professor of Clinical Psychiatry
Department of Psychiatry and Behavioral Sciences
Albert Einstein College of Medicine
Chief, Psychosomatic Medicine
Department of Psychiatry,
Beth Israel Medical Center
New York, NY

WILLIAM BREITBART, M.D.
Professor and Chief of Psychiatry Service
Department of Psychiatry and Behavioral Sciences
Memorial Sloan-Kettering Cancer Center
New York, NY

REBECCA W. BRENDEL, M.D., J.D.
Assistant Director
Forensic Fellowship Program
Law & Psychiatry Service
Massachusetts General Hospital
Instructor in Psychiatry
Harvard Medical School
Boston, MA

DESIREE BYRD, PH.D.
Assistant Professor
Department of Pathology
Assistant Professor
Department of Psychiatry
Mount Sinai School of Medicine
New York, NY

ADAM W. CARRICO, PH.D.
Postdoctoral Fellow

Department of Psychiatry
University of California at San Francisco
San Francisco, CA

DAVID CHAO, M.D.
Resident in Pediatrics
Children's Hospital of Philadelphia
Philadelphia, PA

HARVEY MAX CHOCHINOV, M.D., PH.D., F.R.C.P.C.
Canada Research Chair in Palliative Care Director
Manitoba Palliative Care Research Unit Professor
Department of Psychiatry
University of Manitoba Cancer Care
Winnipeg, Manitoba
Canada

MARY ANN COHEN, M.D.
Clinical Professor of Psychiatry
Department of Psychiatry
Mount Sinai School of Medicine
Attending Psychiatrist
Mount Sinai Hospital
New York, NY

FRANCINE COURNOS, M.D.
Professor of Clinical Psychiatry
Columbia University
Director
Washington Heights Community Service
New York State Psychiatric Institute
New York, NY

KELLY L. COZZA, M.D.
Staff Psychiatrist
Infectious Disease Service
Department of Medicine
Walter Reed Army Medical Center
Assistant Professor of Psychiatry
Uniformed Services University of Health Sciences

STEPHEN CRYSTAL, PH.D.
Research Professor II
Associate Institute Director for Health
Services Research
Director, Center for Health Services Research
  on Pharmacotherapy
Chronic Disease Management, and Outcomes
Chair, Division on Aging
Institute for Health

Rutgers University
New Brunswick, NJ

ANNA L. DICKERMAN, B.A.
Medical Student
New York University School of Medicine
New York, NY

JEFFREY DITZELL, D.O.
Clinical Instructor
Division of Alcoholism and Drug Abuse
New York University School of Medicine
New York, NY

KARIN DORELL, M.D.
Attending Psychiatrist
Department of Psychosomatic Medicine
St. Luke's Roosevelt Medical Center
New York, NY

STEPHEN J. FERRANDO, M.D.
Professor of Clinical Psychiatry
Attending Psychiatrist
Professor of Clinical Public Health
Weill Cornell Medical College
New York, NY

MARSHALL FORSTEIN, M.D.
Associate Professor
Department of Psychiatry
Harvard Medical School
Director of Adult Psychiatry Residency
  Training
Department of Psychiatry
The Cambridge Health Alliance
Boston, MA

ROBERT E. FULLILOVE, ED.D.
Associate Dean
Community and Minority Affairs
Professor of Clinical Sociomedical Sciences
Mailman School of Public Health
Columbia University
New York, NY

HOWARD E. GENDELMAN, M.D.
Professor and Chairman
Director
Center for Neurovirology and Neurodegenerative
  Disorders

University of Nebraska Medical Center
Omaha, NE

HAROLD W. GOFORTH, M.D.
Assistant Professor of Psychiatry and
  Behavioral Sciences
Department of Psychiatry and Behavioral Sciences
Liaison Psychiatrist to Infectious Diseases Clinic
Duke University Medical Center
Co-Director
Consulation-Liaison Psychiatry
Durham Veterans Affairs Medical Center
Duke University Medical Center
Durham, NC

MARIA FERNANDA GOMEZ, M.D.
Associate Professor of Clinical Psychiatry and
  Behavioral Sciences
Albert Einstein College of Medicine
Associate Director of Psychosomatic Medicine
Montefiore Medical Center
North Central Bronx Hospital
Bronx, NY

KARL GOODKIN, M.D., PH.D.
Associate Professor
Department of Psychiatry
University of Miami
Coral Gables, FL

JACK M. GORMAN, M.D.
Adjunct Professor
Department of Psychiatry
Mount Sinai School of Medicine
New York, NY

SILVIA HAFLIGER, M.D.
Assistant Clinical Professor of Psychiatry
Columbia University College of Physicians
  and Surgeons
Attending Psychiatrist
Center for Liver Disease and Transplantation
Columbia University
New York, NY

DANIEL B. HERMAN, D.S.W., M.S.
Associate Professor
Department of Epidemiology
Mailman School of Public Health
Columbia University

Research Scientist
New York State Psychiatric Institute
New York, NY

ROSALIND G. HOFFMAN, M.D.
Attending Psychiatrist
Department of Psychiatry
Consultation-Liaison Psychiatry Division
North Shore University Hospital
Manhasset, NY

ALICIA HURTADO, M.D.
Psychiatry Resident Physician
Department of General Psychiatry
Mount Sinai Hospital
New York, NY

HEIDI E. HUTTON, PH.D.
Assistant Professor
Department of Psychiatry and Behavioral Sciences
Senior Staff Psychologist
AIDS Psychiatry Service
Johns Hopkins University School of Medicine
Baltimore, MD

IRENA KADIU, B.S.
Graduate Student
Department of Pharmacology and Experimental
  Neuroscience
University of Nebraska Medical Center
Omaha, NE

SETH C. KALICHMAN, PH.D.
Professor
Department of Psychology
University of Connecticut
Storrs, CT

GEORGETTE KANMOGNE, PH.D., M.P.H.
Assistant Professor
Department of Pharmacology and Experimental
  Neuroscience
Senior Scientist
Center for Neurovirology and Neurodegenerative
  Disorders
University of Nebraska Medical Center
Omaha, NE

SAMI KHALIFE, M.D.
Clinical Fellow

Mood Disorder Research Unit
National Institute of Mental Health
Bethesda, MD

CARL KIRTON, R.N., M.A., A.P.R.N., B.C.
Adjunct Clinical Associate Professor
Department of Nursing
New York University
Administrative Director & Nurse Practitioner
HIV/AIDS Services
North General Hospital
New York, NY

MARY KLOTMAN, M.D.
Professor of Medicine/Infectious Diseases
Professor of Microbiology
Associate Professor of Gene and Cell Medicine
Mount Sinai School of Medicine
New York, NY

NORMAN B. LEVY, M.D.
Professor of Psychiatry
University of Southern California
Los Angeles, CA

JOSEPH Z. LUX, M.D.
Assistant Professor of Psychiatry
Department of Psychiatry
New York University School of Medicine
Attending Physician
Department of Psychiatry
Bellevue Hospital
New York, NY

CONSTANTINE G. LYKETSOS, M.D., M.H.S.
Elizabeth Plank Althouse Professor
Chairman
Department of Psychiatry
Johns Hopkins Bayview Medical Center
Vice Chairman
Department of Psychiatry and Behavioral
  Sciences
Johns Hopkins Hospital
Baltimore, MD

MARY ANN MALONE, L.C.S.W., M.S.W.
Licensed Clinical Social Worker
Department of Social Work
Mount Sinai Hospital
New York, NY

KAREN McKINNON, M.A.
Staff Associate
Department of Psychiatry
Director
HIV Mental Health Training
Columbia University College of Physicians
   and Surgeons
New York, NY

CHRISTINA S. MEADE, PH.D.
Research Fellow in Psychology
Department of Psychiatry
McLean Hospital
Harvard Medical School
Boston, MA

MICHAEL P. MULLEN, M.D.
Assistant Professor
Department of Medicine
Mount Sinai School of Medicine
New York, NY

JAMES MURROUGH, M.D.
Psychiatry Resident Physician
Department of General Psychiatry
Mount Sinai Hospital
New York, NY

MARY ALICE O'DOWD, M.D.
Professor of Clinical Psychiatry
Department of Psychiatry and Behavioral Science
Albert Einstein College of Medicine
Bronx, NY

MARYLAND PAO, M.D.
Deputy Clinical Director
National Institute of Mental Health
National Institutes of Health
Bethesda, MD

JESSICA ROBINSON PAPP, M.D.
Clinical Neurophysiology Fellow
Department of Neurology
Mount Sinai Medical Center
New York, NY

ASHLEY REYNOLDS, B.S.
Graduate Research Assistant
Department of Pharmacology and Experimental
   Neuroscience

University of Nebraska Medical Center
Omaha, NE

JULIO RIASCOS, M.D.
Resident
Department of Psychiatry
Elmhurst Hospital Center
Mount Sinai School of Medicine
New York, NY

ELIZABETH RYAN, PH.D., A.B.P.P.
Assistant Professor
Department of Psychiatry and Pathology
Mount Sinai School of Medicine
Clinical Neuropsychologist
Department of Psychiatry
Mount Sinai Medical Center
New York, NY

VIVIANA SIMON, M.D., PH.D.
Assistant Professor
Department of Medicine
Division of Infectious Diseases
Mount Sinai School of Medicine
New York, NY

DAVID M. SIMPSON, M.D.
Professor
Department of Neurology
Mount Sinai School of Medicine
Director
Clinical Neurophysiology Laboratories
   and Neuro-AIDS Research Program
Mount Sinai Hospital
New York, NY

JULIA L. SKAPIK, M.P.H.
M.D. Candidate
Johns Hopkins School of Medicine
Baltimore, MD

JOCELYN SOFFER, M.D.
Psychiatry Resident Physician
Department of General Psychiatry
Mount Sinai Hospital
New York, NY

DAVID M. STOFF, PH.D.
Program Chief
AIDS Research Training

HIV Health Disparities
HIV Neuropsychiatry
Division of AIDS
Health and Behavior Research
Center for Mental Health Research on AIDS
National Institute of Mental Health
Bethesda, MD

EZRA S. SUSSER, Dr.PH., M.D., M.P.H
Department Chair
Anna Cheskis Gelman and Murray Charles
   Gelman Professor of Epidemiology
Department of Epidemiology
Mailman School of Public Health
Department Head of Epidemiology
   of Brain Disorders
New York State Psychiatric Institute
New York, NY

ALEXANDER THOMPSON, M.D., M.B.A.
Acting Instructor
Department of Psychiatry and Behavioral Sciences
University of Washington
Seattle, WA

GLENN J. TREISMAN, M.D.
Associate Professor
Director of AIDS Psychiatry
Department of Psychiatry and Behavioral Sciences
Johns Hopkins University School of Medicine
Baltimore, MD

SAGAR A. VAIDYA, M.D., PH.D.
Resident Physician PGY-I
Internal Medicine/Pediatrics
Mount Sinai Hospital
New York, NY

JAMES T. WALKUP, PH.D., M.LITT., M.A.
Associate Professor
Department of Clinical Psychology
Graduate School of Applied and Professional
   Psychology
Institute for Health, Health Care Policy,
   and Aging Research
Rutgers University
New Brunswick, NJ

FRANCES WALLACH, M.D.
Associate Professor

Department of Infectious Disease
Mount Sinai Medical School
Medical Director, Jack Martin Fund Clinic
AIDS Center
Mount Sinai Medical Center
New York, NY

JEFFREY J. WEISS, PH.D.
Assistant Professor
Department of Psychiatry
Mount Sinai School of Medicine
Attending Psychologist
Department of Psychiatry
Mount Sinai Hospital
New York, NY

LORI WIENER, PH.D.
Coordinator
Pediatric Psychosocial Support and Research
   Program
Pediatric Oncology Branch, National Cancer
   Institute
Bethesda, MD

SCOTT G. WILLIAMS, M.D.
Resident
Department of Internal Medicine and Psychiatry
Walter Reed Army Medical Center
Washington, DC

JONATHAN A. WINSTON, M.D., M.S.
Associate Professor
Department of Medicine
Mount Sinai School of Medicine
Attending Physician
Mount Sinai Hospital
New York, NY

GARY H. WYNN, M.D.
Department of Psychiatry
Walter Reed Army Medical Center
Clinical Instructor
Uniformed Services University of Health Sciences
Bethesda, MD

LAWRENCE J. YOUNG, M.D.
Resident
Department of Psychiatry
Mount Sinai Medical Center
New York, NY

Part I

Psychiatric Relevance and
Implications of AIDS Psychiatry

Chapter 1

History of AIDS Psychiatry:
A Biopsychosocial Approach—
Paradigm and Paradox

Mary Ann Cohen

We shall assume that everyone is much more simply human than otherwise. . . . [M]an . . . as long as he is entitled to the term human personality, will be very much more like every other instance of human personality than he is like anything else in the world.
—H.S. Sullivan (1953)

THE HISTORY OF AIDS PSYCHIATRY

In 1981, previously healthy young men and women were being admitted with pneumonia and severe respiratory distress to the intensive care unit of our municipal academic medical center in New York City. They were dying of respiratory failure. The reason for these deaths was not clear. At about the same time, Michael Gottlieb, an immunologist in an academic medical center in Los Angeles, California, began to investigate the reasons for the occurrence of *Pneumocystis carinii* pneumonia (PCP) in five previously healthy young men. On June 5, 1981, his report of these cases was published in the *Morbidity and Mortality Weekly Report* (CDC, 1981a). Gottlieb's first patients were also described as having cytomegalovirus and candida infections.

As a result of the publication of this report, specialists in pulmonary medicine, internal medicine, and infectious disease at our hospital as well as other hospitals recognized that the young men and women were severely ill with PCP and this new disease and that in addition to intensive medical treatment, some would benefit from psychiatric consultations to help them to cope with this devastating illness.

In a more detailed article, published on December 10, 1981, in the *New England Journal of Medicine*, Gottlieb and colleagues (1981) linked an immune deficiency with this new cluster of infections. They presented evidence for an association of the illnesses PCP, candidiasis, and multiple viral infections and "a new acquired cellular immunodeficiency" with a decrease in CD4 T cells as a hallmark. Another article (Masur et al., 1981) described this "outbreak of community-acquired *Pneumocystis carinii* pneumonia" as a manifestation of an "immune deficiency." Over the next year, several other articles described the opportunistic infections and cancers that characterized this new syndrome of immune deficiency, including not only *Pneumocystis carinii* (now named *Pneumocystis jeroveci*) pneumonia but also cytomegalovirus retinitis, central nervous system toxoplasmosis, progressive multifocal

3

leukoencephalopathy, disseminated Kaposi's sarcoma, and central nervous system lymphoma. Initially, the immune deficiency was thought to occur only in gay men (CDC, 1981b), but later in 1981 and in 1982 it became clear that this acquired immune deficiency syndrome, or AIDS, as it came to be called in 1982 (CDC, 1982a), was transmitted by exchange of blood or body fluids through sexual contact, including heterosexual contact (CDC, 1983), sharing of needles or drug paraphernalia in intravenous drug use (CDC, 1982a), through transfusions of contaminated blood and blood products (CDC, 1982b), and through perinatal transmission (CDC, 1982c). When it became evident that this immune deficiency might itself have an infectious etiology and that it led to rapidly fatal complications, many staff members became fearful of the possibility of contagion. An "epidemic of fear" (Hunter, 1990) began to develop along with the AIDS epidemic. As a result, some persons with AIDS who were admitted to hospitals for medical care experienced difficulty getting their rooms cleaned, obtaining water or food, or even getting adequate medical attention.

At our hospital, initial psychiatric consultations for persons with AIDS were requested for depression, withdrawal, confusion, and treatment refusal. As the psychiatrist responding to these initial consultations, it was clear to me that the uncertainty about the etiology of the immune deficiency had resulted in palpable fear of contagion in staff. This fear was leading to distress and an increase in frequency of absences and requests for transfers away from the floors with the most AIDS admissions. These reactions in staff members seemed to heighten the sense of isolation and depression in patients.

Although the AIDS epidemic was first described in the medical literature in 1981, it was not until 1983 that the first articles were published about the psychosocial or psychiatric aspects of AIDS. The first article, written by Holtz and colleagues (1983), was essentially a plea for attention to the psychosocial aspects of AIDS. They stated that "noticeably absent in the flurry of publications about the current epidemic of acquired immune deficiency syndrome (AIDS) is reference to the psychosocial impact of this devastating new syndrome." The authors deplored ostracism of persons with AIDS by both their families and their medical systems of care. These authors were the first to describe the profound withdrawal from human contact as the "sheet sign" observed when persons with AIDS hid under their sheet and completely covered their faces. The first psychiatrist to address these issues was Stuart E. Nichols (1983). In his article in *Psychosomatics*, Nichols described the need for compassion, support, and understanding to address the fear, depression, and alienation experienced by patients. He also made recommendations for use of psychotherapy and group therapy as well as antidepressant medications to help persons with AIDS cope with intense feelings about this new illness that was still of undetermined etiology. Nichols stated: "Since AIDS apparently is a new disease, there is no specific psychiatric literature to which one can refer for guidance. One must be willing to attempt to provide competent and compassionate care in an area with more questions than answers." The earliest articles published in the first decade of AIDS psychiatry, from 1983 to 1993, were primarily descriptive observations, case reports, case series, and documentation and prevalence of psychiatric diagnoses associated with AIDS. They were written by sensitive and compassionate clinicians, some of whom openly expressed their outrage at ostracism and rejection of persons with HIV and AIDS by not only the community at large but also by the medical community. These clinicians also emphasized the need for compassion and for competent medical and psychiatric care. These early articles are summarized in Table 1.1.

In the 23 years (1983–2006) since AIDS psychiatry references first appeared in the medical literature, there have been 14,248 articles written (according to PubMed, accessed on March 19, 2007), in addition to a textbook (Fernandez and Ruiz, 2006), other books (Treisman et al., 2004), and numerous chapters. Most of the articles reflect a growing body of research in the area as well as the beginnings of an evidence base for the practice of AIDS psychiatry. Some of these articles provide evidence for the need for a comprehensive biopsychosocial approach to the care of persons with HIV and AIDS.

A BIOPSYCHOSOCIAL APPROACH TO HIV AND AIDS AND AIDSISM

In the summer of 1981, I responded to my first psychiatric consultation request for a 29-year-old man with AIDS. There was a tray of food on the floor outside his room. When I knocked on his door, I received a response and entered his room. I discovered that the floor of the room was very sticky and my shoes stuck to

TABLE 1.1. Early Literature of AIDS Psychiatry*

Year	Issues Addressed, Comments
1983	Psychosocial impact of AIDS–ostracism, the "sheet sign," and the need for psychiatric literature about AIDS (Holtz et al.)
1983	Psychiatric aspects of AIDS–need for psychiatric consultations and for group therapy; first article by a psychiatrist about AIDS psychiatry (Nichols)
1984	Psychiatric implications of AIDS–the first book about AIDS psychiatry (Nichols and Ostrow)
1984	Psychosocial aspects of AIDS–the first description of the biopsychosocial approach applied in the general care setting by Cohen (Deuchar)
1984a	AIDS anxiety in the "worried well" (Forstein)
1984b	Psychosocial impact of AIDS (Forstein)
1984	Case reports and treatment recommendations for persons with AIDS seen in psychiatric consultation (Barbuto)
1984	Psychiatric complications of AIDS (Nurnberg et al.)
1984	Neuropsychiatric complications of AIDS (Hoffman)
1984	Cryptococcal meningitis presenting as mania in AIDS (Thienhaus and Khosla)
1984	Description of a support group for persons with AIDS (Nichols)
1984	Psychiatric problems in patients with AIDS at New York Hospital (Perry and Tross)
1985	Findings in 13 of 40 persons with AIDS seen in psychiatric consultation (Dilley et al.)
1985	Description of psychiatric and psychosocial aspects of AIDS (Holland and Tross)
1986	A biopsychosocial approach to AIDS (Cohen and Weisman)
1986	Neuropsychiatric aspects of AIDS (Price and Forejt)
1987	Psychiatric aspects of AIDS (Faulstich)
1987	Dementia as the presenting or sole manifestation of HIV infection (Navia and Price)
1987	Psychiatric aspects of AIDS: a biopsychosocial approach–comprehensive chapter (Cohen)
1987	Stigmatization of AIDS patients by physicians (Kelly et al.)
1988	Discrimination against people with AIDS (Blendon and Donelan)
1988	First article on high prevalence of suicide among persons with AIDS (Marzuk et al.)
1989	AIDism, a new form of discrimination (Cohen)
1989	Anxiety and stigmatizing aspects of HIV infection (Fullilove)
1990	A biopsychosocial approach to the HIV epidemic (Cohen)
1990	Firesetting and HIV associated dementia (Cohen et al.)
1990	Suicidality and HIV testing (Perry et al.)
1992	Suicidality and HIV status (McKegney and O'Dowd)
1993	Manic syndrome early and late in the course of HIV (Lyketsos et al.)

*Listed here are descriptions of psychosocial and psychiatric aspects of AIDS with emphasis on discrimination. A sample of articles, chapters, and books published in the first decade of AIDS psychiatry (1983–1993) is given here.

it and made strange noises as I approached the bedside. The patient's head was covered with a sheet. When I introduced myself and began to speak to the patient, he gradually removed the sheet from his head. He was extremely cachectic, almost skeletal, and appeared much older than his stated age of 29 years. He spoke slowly and softly and related well. He had evidence of cognitive impairment, depression, and substance use disorder as well as multiple and complex medical illnesses. He was alienated from his family.

The "sticky-floor syndrome" joined the "sheet sign" as one of the early unique responses to the AIDS pandemic. The causes for the sticky floor were related to both staff and patient factors. The floor was sticky as a result of an accumulation of spilled food and beverages as well as body fluids that went unattended by fearful hospital maintenance staff. The patient was weak and had difficulty grasping and holding onto objects. There were frequent spills as a result. Ambulation was slow and difficult for him and he did not always make it to the bathroom on time. It was clear to me that only a hospital-wide, multidisciplinary program and education of every level of staff on all shifts would enable us to improve the care of persons with AIDS, diminish stigma and discrimination, and help to alleviate fear, anxiety, and stigma in our caregivers. In 1983, the infectious-disease director, a social worker, and I developed a multidisciplinary AIDS program at our hospital to provide coordinated and comprehensive care for persons with AIDS and to provide education for hospital staff as well as medical students and their faculty. This program was the first to be described in the literature as a response to the epidemic (Deuchar, 1984; Cohen and Weisman, 1986). Deuchar, a British medical student, took an elective on our service in 1983 and then wrote an article about the psychosocial aspects of AIDS in New York City. He described our program as a means of providing coordination of care and communication among the multiple subspecialties and disciplines involved in the care of persons with AIDS (Deuchar, 1984). He characterized our program exactly as we did, as a "comprehensive program" with a "bio-psycho-social approach" that "maintains a view that each individual is a member of a family and community and deserves a coordinated approach to medical care and treatment with dignity." He wrote: "The programme includes maintenance of a multidisciplinary treatment team, provision of ongoing psychological support for patients and families, and education and support for hospital staff. As such, it is clearly a good example of consultation-liaison psychiatry."

Many persons with AIDS were treated as lepers in the early years of the epidemic. Some found that they were shunned and ostracized. In some areas of the world, persons with AIDS were quarantined because of the irrational fears, discrimination, and stigma associated with this pandemic. Initially, in the United States, some persons who were diagnosed with AIDS were rejected by not only their communities but also families and friends. Some persons with AIDS lost their homes, some children and adolescents were excluded from classrooms, and some lost their jobs. In the early 1980s, a diagnosis of AIDS led to rejection by shelters for the homeless and nursing homes, long-term-care facilities, and facilities for the terminally ill. The attitudes of families, houses of worship, prison guards, employers, teachers, hospital staff, and funeral directors led to catastrophic stigma and discrimination. Persons with AIDS had difficulty finding support, obtaining health care, keeping a job, finding a home, and finding a chronic-care facility or even a place to die.

Discrimination against persons with AIDS was described (Cohen, 1989) as a new form of discrimination called "AIDSism." AIDSism is built on a foundation of homophobia, misogyny, addictophobia, and fears of contagion and death. Discrimination and stigma were recognized early in the AIDS psychiatry literature as contributing to psychological distress (Holtz et al., 1983; Nichols, 1983; Deuchar, 1984; Nichols, 1984; Holland and Tross, 1985; Cohen and Weisman, 1986; Blendon and Donelan, 1988; Cohen, 1989; Fullilove, 1989; Chesney et al., 1992) and have been explored

subsequently following the introduction of potent antiretroviral therapy (Herek et al., 2002; Parker and Aggleton, 2003; Brown et al., 2003; Kaplan et al., 2005).

Early in the epidemic, many physicians surveyed had negative attitudes toward persons with HIV and AIDS (Kelly et al., 1987; Thompson, 1987; Wormser and Joline, 1989). Although the medical profession has made great strides against discrimination and stigma and most physicians are "accustomed to caring for HIV-infected patients with concern and compassion" (Gottlieb, 2001), society as a whole has not kept up—not only globally but also in the United States. As recently as June 2006, a full quarter-century since the epidemic was first described, a child with AIDS was initially excluded from attending a New York sleep-away camp until his parents threatened legal action. In February 2006, an out-of-state psychiatry resident applied online to rent an apartment in New York City for the month of his elective on our AIDS psychiatry service. The renter e-mailed the resident to ask the subject of the elective. When the renter learned the subject of the elective, he informed the resident that he was a married man with a 3-year-old child. The renter refused to rent the apartment to the resident because he assumed that the resident was infected with HIV if he was taking an elective in AIDS psychiatry. AIDS stigma and AIDSism have implications not only for anguish in the individuals who experience them but also for health and public health. Stigma and AIDSism present a barrier to getting tested for HIV, to obtaining test results, to disclosing serostatus to intimate partners, to obtaining optimal medical care in a timely manner, and to engaging in safer sex practices.

Psychosomatic medicine psychiatrists who specialize in AIDS psychiatry as well as general psychiatrists and other mental health clinicians are in a unique position to work with primary HIV clinicians, infectious-disease specialists, and other physicians and health professionals to combat AIDS stigma and AIDSism.

AIDS PSYCHIATRY: PARADIGM AND PARADOX

AIDS Paradigms

For psychiatrists who work in psychosomatic medicine, AIDS and other manifestations of HIV infection may be thought of as a paradigm of a medical illness. AIDS is an illness similar to the other complex and severe medical illnesses that define the subspecialty. *Psychosomatic medicine*, the psychiatric aspects of complex and severe medical illness, was previously called "consultation-liaison psychiatry" and became a subspecialty of psychiatry in 2003. AIDS is a paradigm because it has elements of nearly every illness described in the *American Psychiatric Publishing Textbook of Psychosomatic Medicine* (Levenson, 2005). Persons with HIV and AIDS are also vulnerable to a multiplicity of other comorbid complex and severe medical illnesses including those related and unrelated to HIV infection. The concept of AIDS as paradigm is illustrated in Figure 1.1.

Lipowski (1967) provided a classification of commonly encountered problems in psychosomatic medicine. The original classification defined five commonly occurring diagnostic problems that lead to psychiatric referrals and included "psychosomatic" disorders as the fifth problem (the quotation marks appeared in the original article). Lipowski was dismissive of this category in his 1967 article and stated that the term "psychosomatic disorder" is a "misnomer with a vague meaning" and that it "haunts the consultant like a bad ghost from the past." Querques and Stern (2004)

suggest a modification of Lipowski's original classification. Querques and Stern substituted "comorbid medical and psychiatric conditions" for "psychosomatic" disorders for the fifth problem. With minor modifications, Lipowski's classification is relevant to AIDS psychiatric care. The five commonly encountered problems in AIDS psychiatry include psychiatric presentation of medical illness; psychiatric complications of medical illnesses or treatments; psychological response to medical illness or treatments; medical presentation of psychiatric illness or treatments; and comorbid medical and psychiatric illness.

Since the development of potent combination antiretroviral therapies, the life expectancy of persons with HIV has increased, and for persons who are adherent to care, the incidence of the opportunistic infections and cancers previously associated with AIDS has decreased (Huang et al., 2006). However, persons with psychiatric disorders may lack access to care because severe mental illness is associated with nonadherence to care. Untreated depression, substance dependence, cognitive impairment, posttraumatic stress disorder, or psychosis may impede ability to adhere to care. Persons with severe mental illness may have

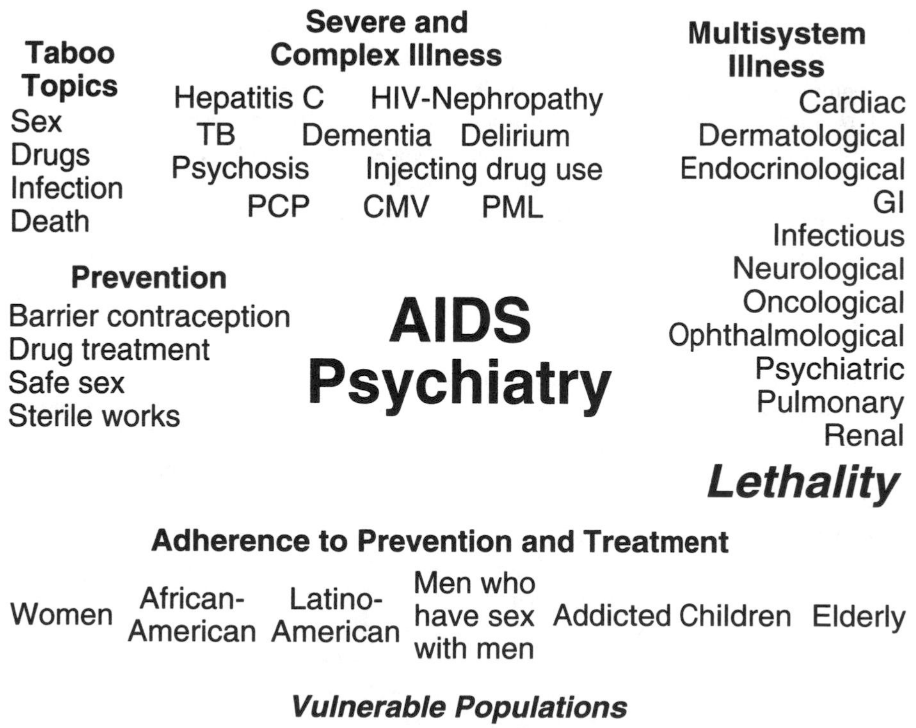

FIGURE 1.1. **AIDS psychiatry: a paradigm of psychosomatic medicine.**

difficulty getting to medical appointments, taking medications regularly, or obtaining laboratory tests and follow-up care. As a result, persons with AIDS and untreated psychiatric disorders may present with AIDS-related illnesses not usually encountered in developed countries since the advent of potent antiretrovirals or highly active antiretroviral therapy (HAART). In addition, among those persons who are adherent to care, there has been an increase in the prevalence of endocrine, pulmonary, cardiac, gastrointestinal, renal, and metabolic disorders, some of which may be comorbid and unrelated to HIV and AIDS while others may be related to HIV and AIDS or to its treatments. The life expectancy of persons with HIV and AIDS who are treated with potent antiretroviral therapy is now similar to that of the general population (Manfredi 2004a, 2004b). Among the 68,669 persons with AIDS who died in New York City from 1999 to 2004, the percentage of deaths from non-HIV-related causes increased significantly from 19.8% to 26.3% (Sackoff et al., 2006). Of these non-HIV-related deaths, 76% were related to substance use, cardiovascular disease, and cancer. Other causes of death included diabetes, suicide, homicide, and chronic renal disease. Sackoff and colleagues (2006) and Aberg (2006) recommend a paradigm shift in the care of persons with AIDS from a primary focus on HIV prevention and care to a more comprehensive approach to medical and mental health. The complexity and severity of the multiple medical and psychiatric illnesses prevalent in persons with HIV and AIDS are important in the psychiatric assessment and substantiate the need for a comprehensive and compassionate biopsychosocial approach that takes into account the full range of medical, psychiatric, social, and cultural factors and their synergistic implications relevant to patient care (Deuchar, 1984; Cohen and Weisman, 1986; Cohen, 1987; Cohen and Weisman, 1988; Cohen, 1992). The five commonly encountered problems in persons with HIV and AIDS are illustrated in the following vignettes.

ILLUSTRATIVE CASE VIGNETTES

Case Vignette 1.1: Inpatient Neurology Unit Psychiatric Consultation: Psychiatric Presentation of Medical Illness

Ms. A is a 41-year-old unemployed former school teacher with HIV and a CD4 of 806 who presented with

depression after admission for new-onset seizures and was found to have a right frontoparietal subarrachnoid hemorrhage. She also had end-stage renal disease due to polycystic kidney disease and was on hemodialysis. She had a history of pancreatic carcinoma treated with radiation therapy and chemotherapy. Ms. A was found to have mild dementia with anosognosia and mood disorder as a result of complex medical illnesses. She responded well to support.

Ms. A had a psychiatric presentation of her medical illnesses, including mood disorder with depressive features due to multiple medical illnesses, and dementia with anosognosia due to her subarrachnoid hemorrhage.

Case Vignette 1.2: Outpatient HIV Clinic Psychiatric Consultation: Psychiatric Complication of Medical Illness or Treatment

Ms. B is a 52-year-old unemployed former administrative assistant with HIV and a CD4 of 317. She also had ulcerative colitis, osteoarthritis, and hypertension. She presented with depression and suicidal ideation after being started on efavirenz, a nonnucleoside reverse transcriptase inhibitor. Ms. B was found to have posttraumatic stress disorder due to early childhood trauma and major depressive disorder, recurrent. She responded well to psychotherapy, antidepressants, and discontinuation of efavirenz as well as her other antiretroviral medications. She has been adherent to psychiatric and medical care and understands that she may need to resume antiretroviral therapy.

Ms. B had a psychiatric complication of her medical treatment that responded well to discontinuation of efavirenz and to treatment for depression and posttraumatic stress disorder.

Case Vignette 1.3: Outpatient HIV Clinic Psychiatric Consultation: Psychological Response to Medical Illness

Ms. C is a 31-year-old unemployed teacher's assistant with HIV and a CD4 of 1024 who presented with depression and anxiety. Ms. C felt isolated and alone because she was unable to disclose her diagnosis. She withdrew from friends, did not tell family members, and feared being seen attending the HIV clinic. Ms. C felt that she would never again be able to date anyone because she feared rejection if she disclosed her HIV serostatus.

In psychotherapy, she was able to work through her fears of rejection and to some extent was able to come to terms with the "embarrassment" about her diagnosis in psychotherapy. Ms. C returned to work and responded to suggestions to join an HIV-positive social group.

Ms. C had a psychological response to medical illness, to the stigma of HIV infection.

Case Vignette 1.4: Inpatient General Care Psychiatric Consultation: Medical Presentation of Psychiatric Illness

Mr. D is a 29-year-old unemployed actor and former Walt Disney World Donald Duck character who was admitted to medicine with weight loss, cough, night sweats, and fever and gave a history of PCP and AIDS. A psychiatric consultation was requested when his history of PCP and AIDS could not be verified and he refused HIV testing. He was living in New York City–supported housing for persons with AIDS and had fabricated his history to pursue his acting career in New York and obtain both housing and entitlements.

Mr. D was malingering with AIDS in order to obtain entitlements and housing to further his acting career by establishing a home and support in New York City (Cohen, 1992).

Case Vignette 1.5: Outpatient HIV Clinic Psychiatric Consultation: Comorbid Medical and Psychiatric Illness

Mr. E is a 58-year-old unemployed man with chronic obstructive pulmonary disease (oxygen-dependent), hepatitis C, and HIV with a CD4 count of 1384, who was referred for depression with suicidal ideation. Mr. E was found to have major depressive disorder, recurrent, and a history of opioid dependence in full sustained remission for 20 years. He responded well to long-term psychotherapy and antidepressants but became intermittently depressed and suicidal until he was able to find meaning in doing volunteer work in the radiology department, an area of the hospital where he had dreamed of working since he was a young child.

Mr. E had comorbid medical and psychiatric illness that responded to psychiatric care and meaning-centered psychotherapy.

BIOPSYCHOSOCIAL ASPECTS OF HIV AND AIDS

AIDS is a severe, chronic, multiorgan, multisystem illness with multiple and severe comorbid psychiatric and other medical illnesses. AIDS is also a prevalent illness that presents with psychiatric responses to illness, is associated with psychiatric illness because of the affinity of HIV for brain and neural tissue, and occurs with comorbid psychiatric illness as well as other medical illnesses. In many ways, AIDS and other manifestations of HIV infection can be seen as a paradigm of a complex and severe medical illness, the model of illnesses that comprise the field of psychosomatic medicine. There thus is a need for a biopsychosocial approach to the care of persons with HIV and AIDS. A summary of some of the factors involved in a biopsychosocial approach to AIDS can be found in Table 1.2.

Psychiatrists make ideal AIDS educators. General psychiatrists who work in the areas of inpatient and outpatient psychiatry settings, private offices, addiction psychiatry, geriatric psychiatry, child and adolescent psychiatry, correctional facilities, and long-term care facilities are all in a prime position to provide education, help prevent transmission of HIV, suggest or provide condoms and information about safe sex, and suggest or offer HIV testing to lead toward early diagnosis and treatment. Most psychiatrists take detailed sexual and drug histories and work with patients to help them change behaviors. The significance of taking a detailed sexual history was especially evident in a population-based study of men in New York City. This study revealed discordance between sexual behavior and self-reported sexual identity; nearly 10% of straight-identified men reported at least one sexual encounter with another man in the previous year (Pathela et al., 2006). Most psychiatrists form long-term, ongoing relationships with their patients and work with patients toward achieving gratification in long-term, intimate-partner relationships. All of these characteristics can be of major importance in primary prevention as well as early diagnosis and treatment of HIV infection.

Psychosomatic medicine clinicians or psychiatrists and AIDS psychiatrists are in a unique position to provide psychiatric care for persons with HIV, from the time of infection to the time of death and its aftermath, with provision of support for partners and families. However, AIDS psychiatrists rarely have the chance to provide care for their patients until they are diagnosed with HIV infection. Ruiz (2000) has provided

TABLE 1.2. A Biopsychosocial Approach to HIV and AIDS

Biological	Psychological	Social
Opportunistic Infections (Most Common)	**Diagnoses (Most Common)**	Alienation
		Stigma
Protozoal	Mood disorders	Poverty
Pnuemocystis jeroveki pneumonia	Major depressive disorder	Job loss
Toxoplasma gondii encephalitis	Mood disorder due to medical	Rejection
	condition with depression	Eviction
Bacterial	Mood disorder due to medical	
Mycobacterium avium intracellulare	condition with mania	
	Bipolar disorder	Losses
Viral	Cognitive disorders	Disparities
Cytomegalovirus disease	Dementia	AIDSism
	Delirium	Racism
Fungal	Substance use disorders	Ageism
Cryptococcal meningitis		
Esophageal candidiasis		
	Adjustment disorders	
Opportunistic cancers	Anxiety disorders	
	Posttraumatic stress disorder	
Kaposi's sarcoma	Bereavement	
Comorbid Medical Illnesses (Most Common)	*Symptoms*	
Chronic hepatitis C and liver disease	Depression	
Cardiac disease	Anxiety	
Cerebrovascular disease	Confusion	
Diabetes mellitus	Psychosis	
Lung disease	Suicidality	
Clostridium difficile colitis	Existential anxiety	
Neuropathy	Grief	
Renal disease		
Symptoms		
Pain		
Insomnia		
Fatigue		
Nausea		
Vomiting		
Diarrhea		
Wasting		
Pruritus		
Hiccups		
Incontinence		
Weakness		
Paresis and paralysis		

a description of the psychiatric care of one of his patients, extending from before his patient's diagnosis of HIV through the course of his illness and progression to AIDS to end-stage AIDS at the end of his life. Ruiz also documented his provision of support for the family after the death of the patient. AIDS psychiatrists can provide colocated psychiatric services, education and support for trainees, and support and leadership for the multidisciplinary teams of physicians, nurses, social workers, other health professionals, and staff. It is especially gratifying to work as part of a dedicated and compassionate team of clinicians who are providing comprehensive care for persons with HIV and AIDS.

HIV and AIDS also present us with paradoxes. One of the most tragic paradoxes of HIV is the disparity in access to care resulting from racial, political, and economic factors in many areas of the world as well as in certain areas of the United States and other industrialized nations. Another tragic paradox is the disparity in access to care among persons with psychiatric illness. In addition, age, intelligence, and level of education do not necessarily correlate with ability to adhere to risk reduction, safe sexual behavior, and medical care (Cochran and Mays, 1990; De Buono et al., 1990; MacDonald et al., 1990; Reinisch and Beasley, 1990). Among adolescents, who say "I can use a condom, I just don't" (Mustanski et al., 2006), as well as the elderly (Goodkin et al., 2003; Stoff et al., 2004; Karpiak et al., 2006), who may not feel a need for barrier contraception to prevent pregnancy and whose physicians may be uncomfortable discussing sexual activity, there are high rates of HIV infection. The process of care for persons with AIDS at the end of life is also paradoxical and there is a clear need for provision of care along a continuum that includes both palliative and curative care. This concept has been proposed but appears hard to implement. The need to overcome the "false dichotomy of curative vs. palliative care for late stage AIDS" has been suggested (Selwyn and Forstein, 2003).

AIDSISM AND THE MULTIPLE DISPARITIES OF HIV AND AIDS

AIDSism results from a multiplicity of prejudicial and discriminatory factors and is built on a foundation of racism, homophobia, ageism, addictophobia, misogyny, and discomfort with mental and medical illness, poverty, sexuality, infection, and death in many communities throughout the world as well as in the United States. AIDSism has contributed to disparities in the care of persons with HIV and AIDS.

Racial, Ethnic, and Socioeconomic Disparities

Racial, ethnic, and socioeconomic disparities have been observed and documented in all aspects of the United States health care system (Agency for Health Care Research and Quality, 2005a). The overall HIV death rate of African Americans was found to be 10.95 times higher than that of whites (Agency for Health Care Research and Quality, (2005b) and racial disparities have been shown to contribute to increased HIV incidence and inadequate access to medical and psychiatric care (CDC, 2006a). U.S. correctional facilities and urban drug epicenters may be seen as microcosms of discrimination. Correctional facilities may

also be instrumental in perpetuating the HIV epidemic both inside and outside of prison walls (Hammett et al., 2002; Blankenship et al., 2005; Golembeski and Fullilove, 2005; CDC, 2006b).

It would be difficult to calculate the true impact of these disparities on persons with HIV and AIDS. In addition to the incalculable distress, suffering, and anguish (Cohen et al., 2002), persons with AIDS have multiple comorbid medical and psychiatric illnesses, all of which are also found among those who experience disparities in care (Cohen et al., 1991; Cohen, 1996; Kolb et al., 2006).

Psychiatric Disparities

Psychiatric factors take on new relevance and meaning as we approach the end of the third decade of the AIDS pandemic. Persons with AIDS are living longer and healthier lives as a result of appropriate medical care and advances in antiretroviral therapy. However, in the United States and throughout the world, some men, women, and children with AIDS are unable to benefit from medical progress. Inadequate access to care results from a multiplicity of barriers, including economic, social, political, and psychiatric ones. Psychiatric disorders and distress play a significant role in the transmission of, exposure to, and infection with HIV (Cohen and Alfonso, 1994; Cohen and Alfonso, 1998; Blank et al., 2002). They are relevant to prevention, clinical care, and adherence throughout every aspect of illness from the initial risk behavior to death. They result in considerable suffering from diagnosis to end-stage illness (Cohen and Alfonso, 2004). Untreated psychiatric disorders can be exacerbated by HIV stigma to make persons with HIV and AIDS especially vulnerable to suicide (Marzuk et al., 1988; Perry et al., 1990; McKegney and O'Dowd, 1992; Alfonso and Cohen, 1997). Psychiatric treatment with individual (Cohen and Weisman, 1986; Cohen, 1987; Cohen and Alfonso, 1998; Cohen and Alfonso, 2004), group (Alfonso and Cohen, 1997), and family therapy can alleviate suffering, improve adherence, and prevent suicide.

CONCLUSION

AIDSism, stigma, discrimination, and fear, in conjunction with denial, omnipotence, and lack of awareness, complicate and perpetuate the HIV pandemic. The creation of supportive, nurturing, nonjudgmental health care environments can help combat AIDSism and provide comprehensive and compassionate care. AIDS psychiatrists and other mental health professionals need to be integrated closely into clinical, academic, and research aspects of HIV prevention and treatment. In order for persons with HIV and AIDS to live more comfortable lives, with preservation of independence and dignity, it is important to establish special nurturing, supportive, and loving health care environments. Such environments can enable persons with AIDS, their loved ones, and caregivers to meet the challenges of AIDS with optimism and dignity (Cohen and Alfonso, 2004).

References

Aberg JA (2006). The changing face of HIV care: common things really are common. *Ann Intern Med* 145:463–465.

Agency for Health Care Research and Quality (2005a). *National Healthcare Disparities Report, 2005.* Retrieved March 20, 2007, from http://www.ahrq.gov/qual/nhdr05/nhdr05.htm.

Agency for Healthcare Research and Quality, Rockville, MD (2005b). *National Healthcare Disparities Report, 2005.* Appendix D: Data Tables. Retrieved March 20, 2007, from http://www.ahrq.gov/qual/nhdr05/nhdr05.htm.

Alfonso CA, and Cohen MAA (1997). The role of group psychotherapy in the care of persons with AIDS. *J Am Acad Psychoanal* 25:623–638.

Blank MB, Mandell DS, Aiken L, and Hadley TR. (2002). Co-occurrence of HIV and serious mental illness among Medicaid recipients. *Psychiatr Serv* 53:868–873.

Blankenship KM, Smoyer AB, Bray SJ, and Mattocks K (2005). Black–white disparities in HIV/AIDS: the role of drug policy in the corrections system. *J Health Care Poor Underserved* 16:140–156.

Barbuto J (1984). Psychiatric care of seriously ill patients with acquired immune deficiency syndrome. In SE Nichols and DG Ostrow (eds.), *Psychiatric Implications of Acquired Immune Deficiency Syndrome.* Washington, DC: American Psychiatric Press.

Blendon RJ, and Donelan K (1988). Discrimination against people with AIDS: the public's perspective. *N Engl J Med* 319:1022–1026.

Brown L, Macintyre K, and Trujillo L (2003). Interventions to reduce HIV/AIDS stigma: what have we learned? *AIDS Educ Prev* 15:49–69.

[CDC] Centers for Disease Control and Prevention (1981a). *Pneumocystis* pneumonia—Los Angeles. *MMWR Morb Mortal Wkly Rep* 30:250–252.

[CDC] Centers for Disease Control and Prevention (1981b). Kapsosi's sarcoma and *Pneumocystis* pneumonia among homosexual men—New York City and California. *MMWR Morb Mortal Wkly Rep* 30:305–308.

[CDC] Centers for Disease Control and Prevention (1982a). Current trends on acquired immune deficiency syndrome (AIDS)-United States. *MMWR Morb Mortal Wkly Rep* 31:507–508, 513–514.

[CDC] Centers for Disease Control and Prevention (1982b). Possible transfusion-associated acquired immune deficiency syndrome (AIDS)—California. *MMWR Morb Mortal Wkly Rep* 31:652–654.

[CDC] Centers for Disease Control and Prevention (1982c). Unexplained immunodeficiency and opportunistic infections in infants—New York, New Jersey, California. *MMWR Morb Mortal Wkly Rep* 31:665–667.

[CDC] Centers for Disease Control and Prevention (1983). Immunodeficiency in female partners of males with acquired immune deficiency syndrome (AIDS)—New York. *MMWR Morb Mortal Wkly Rep* 31:697–698

[CDC] Centers for Disease Control and Prevention (2006a). Racial/ethnic disparities in diagnoses of HIV/AIDS—33 states, 2001–2004. *MMWR Morb Mortal Wkly Rep* 2006; 55:121–125.

[CDC] Centers for Disease Control and Prevention (2006b). HIV transmission among male inmates in a state prison system—Georgia, 1992–2005. *MMWR Morb Mortal Wkly Rep* 55:421–426.

Chesney MA, and Smith AW (1992). Critical delays in HIV testing and care: the potential role of stigma. *Am Behav Sci* 42:1162–1174.

Cochran SD, and Mays VM (1990). Sex, lies and HIV. *N Engl J Med* 22:774–775.

Cohen MA (1987). Psychiatric aspects of AIDS: A biopsychosocial approach. In GP Wormser, RE Stahl, and EJ Bottone (eds.), *AIDS Acquired Immune Deficiency Syndrome and Other Manifestations of HIV Infection.* Park Ridge, NJ: Noyes Publishers.

Cohen MA (1989). AIDSism, a new form of discrimination. *Am Med News*, January 20, 32:43.

Cohen MA (1992). Biopsychosocial aspects of the HIV epidemic. In GP Wormser (ed.), *AIDS and Other Manifestations of HIV Infection*, second edition (pp. 349–371). New York: Raven Press.

Cohen MAA (1996). Creating health care environments to meet patients' needs. *Curr Issues Public Health* 2:232–240.

Cohen MAA, and Alfonso CA (1994). Dissemination of HIV: how serious is it for women, medically and psychologically? *Ann N Y Acad Sci* 736:114–121.

Cohen MA, and Alfonso CA (1998). Psychiatric care and pain management in persons with HIV infection. In GP Wormser (ed.), *AIDS and Other Manifestations of HIV Infection*, third edition. Philadelphia: Lippincott-Raven.

Cohen MA, and Alfonso CA (2004). AIDS psychiatry: psychiatric and palliative care, and pain management. In GP Wormser (ed.), *AIDS and Other Manifestations of HIV Infection*, fourth edition (pp. 537–576). San Diego: Elsevier Academic Press.

Cohen MA, and Weisman H (1986). A biopsychosocial approach to AIDS. *Psychosomatics* 27:245–249.

Cohen MA, and Weisman HW (1988). A biopsychosocial approach to AIDS. In RP Galea, BF Lewis, and LA Baker (eds.), *AIDS and IV Drug Abusers*. Owings Mills, MD: National Health Publishing.

Cohen MA, Aladjem AD, Brenin D, and Ghazi M (1990). Firesetting by patients with the acquired immunodeficiency syndrome (AIDS). *Ann Intern Med* 112:386–387.

Cohen MAA, Aladjem AD, Horton A, Lima J, Palacios A, Hernandez L, and Mehta P (1991). How can we combat excess mortality in Harlem? A one-day survey of adult general care. *Int J Psychiatry Med* 21:369–378.

Cohen MA, Hoffman RG, Cromwell C, Schmeidler J, Ebrahim F, Carrera G, Endorf F, Alfonso CA, and Jacobson JM (2002). The prevalence of distress in persons with human immunodeficiency virus infection. *Psychosomatics* 43:10–15.

De Buono BA, Zinner SH, Daamen M, and McCormack WM (1990). Sexual behavior of college women in 1975, 1986 and 1989. *N Engl J Med* 322:821–825.

Deuchar N (1984). AIDS in New York City with particular reference to the psychosocial aspects. *Br J Psychiatry* 145:612–619.

Dilley JW, Ochitill HN, Perl M, and Volberding PA (1985). Findings in psychiatric consultation with patients with acquired immune deficiency syndrome. *Am J Psychiatry* 142:82–86.

Faulstich ME (1987). Psychiatric aspects of AIDS. *Am J Psychiatry* 144:551–556.

Fernandez F, and Ruiz P (2006). *Psychiatric Aspects of HIV/AIDS* (pp. 39–47). Philadelphia: Lippincott Williams & Wilkins.

Forstein M (1984a). AIDS anxiety in the worried well. In SE Nichols and DG Ostrow (eds.), *Psychiatric Implications of Acquired Immune Deficiency Syndrome* (pp. 77–82). Washington, DC: American Psychiatric Press.

Forstein M (1984b). The psychosocial impact of the acquired immunodeficiency syndrome. *Semin Oncol* 11:77–82.

Fullilove MT (1989). Anxiety and stigmatizing aspects of HIV infection. *J Clin Psychiatry* 50(Suppl.):5–8.

Golembeski C, and Fullilove RE (2005). Criminal (in)justice in the city and its associated health consequences. *Am J Public Health* 95:1701–1706.

Goodkin K, Heckman T, Siegel K, Linsk N, Khamis I, Lee D, Lecusay R, Poindexter CC, Mason SJ, Suarez P, Eisdorfer C (2003). "Putting a face" on HIV infection/AIDS in older adults: a psychosocial context. *J Aquir Immune Defic Syndr* 33(Suppl. 2):S171–S184.

Gottlieb MS (2001). AIDS—past and future. *N Engl J Med* 344:1788–1791.

Gottlieb MS, Schroff R, Schanker HM, Weisman JD, Fan PT, Wolf RA, and Saxon A (1981). *Pneumocystis carinii* pneumonia and mucosal candidiasis in previously healthy homosexual men: evidence of a new acquired cellular immunodeficiency. *N Engl J Med* 305:1425–1431.

Hammett TM, Harmon MP, and Rhodes W (2002). The burden of infectious disease among inmates of and releasees from US correctional facilities 1997. *Am J Public Health* 92:1789–1794.

Herek GM, Capitanio JP, and Widaman KF (2002). HIV-related stigma and knowledge in the United States: prevalence and trends, 1991–1999. *Am J Public Health* 92:371–377.

Hoffman RS (1984). Neuropsychiatric complications of AIDS. *Psychosomatics* 25:393–340.

Holland JC, and Tross S (1985). Psychosocial and neuropsychiatric sequelae of the acquired immunodeficiency syndrome and related disorders. *Ann Intern Med* 103:760–764.

Holtz H, Dobro J, Kapila R, Palinkas R, and Oleske J (1983). Psychosocial impact of acquired immunodeficiency syndrome. *JAMA* 250:167.

Huang L, Quartin A, Jones D, and Havlir DV (2006). Intensive care of patients with HIV infection. *N Engl J Med* 355:173–181.

Hunter ND (1990). Epidemic of fear: a survey of AIDS discrimination in the 1980s and policy recommendations for the 1990s. American Civil Liberties Union AIDS Project 1990. New York: ACLU.

Kaplan AH, Scheyett A, and Golin CE (2005). HIV and stigma: analysis and research program. *Curr HIV/AIDS Rep* 2:184–188.

Karpiak SE, Shippy RA, and Cantor MH (2006). *Research on Older Adults with HIV*. New York: AIDS Community Research Initiative of America, 2006.

Kelly JA, St. Lawrence JS, Smith S, Jr, Hood HV, and Cook DJ (1987). Stigmatization of AIDS patients by physicians. *Am J Public Health* 77:789–791.

Kolb B, Wallace AM, Hill D, Royce M (2006). Disparities in cancer care among racial and ethnic minorities. *Oncology* 20:1256–1261.

Levenson JL (2005). *American Psychiatric Publishing Textbook of Psychosomatic Medicine* (pp. 3–14). Washington, DC: American Psychiatric Publishing.

Lipowski ZJ (1967). Review of consultation psychiatry and psychosomatic medicine: II. Clinical aspects. *Psychosomat Med* 29:201–224.

Lyketsos CG, Hanson AL, Fishman M, Rosenblatt A, McHugh PR, and Treisman GJ (1993). Manic syndrome early and late in the course of HIV. *Am J Psychiatry* 150(2):326–327.

MacDonald NE, Wells GA, Fisher WA, Warren WK, King MA, Doherty JA, and Bowie WR. High-risk STD/HIV behavior among college students. *JAMA* 1990; 263:3155–3159.

Manfredi R (2004a). HIV infection and advanced age: emerging epidemiological, clinical and management issues. *Ageing Res Rev* 3:31–54.

Manfredi R (2004b). Impact of HIV infection and antiretroviral therapy in the older patient. *Expert Rev Anti Infect Ther* 2:821–824.

Marzuk PM, Tierney H, Tardiff K, Gross EM, Morgan EB, Hsu MA, and Mann JJ (1988). Increased risk of suicide in persons with AIDS. *JAMA* 259:1333–1337.

Masur H, Michelis MA, Greene JB, Onorato I, Stouwe RA, Holzman, Wormser G, Brettman L, Lange M, Murray HW, and Cunningham-Rundles S (1981). An outbreak of community-acquired *Pneumocystis carinii* pneumonia: initial manifestation of cellular immune dysfunction. *N Engl J Med* 305:1431–1438.

McKegney FP, and O'Dowd MA (1982). Suicidality and HIV status. *Am J Psychiatry* 149:396–398.

Mustanski B, Donenberg G, and Emerson E (2006). I can use a condom, I just don't: the importance of motivation to prevent HIV in adolescent seeking psychiatric care. *AIDS Behav* 10:753–762.

Navia BA, and Price RW (1987). The acquired immunodeficiency syndrome dementia as the presenting or sole manifestation of human immunodeficiency virus infection. *Arch Neurol* 44:65–69.

Nichols SE (1983). Psychiatric aspects of AIDS. *Psychosomatics* 24:1083–1089.

Nichols SE (1984). Social and support groups for patients with acquired immune deficiency syndrome. In SE Nichols and DG Ostrow (eds.), *Psychiatric Implications of Acquired Immune Deficiency Syndrome* (pp. 77–82). Washington, DC: American Psychiatric Press.

Nichols SE, and Ostrow DG (eds.) (1984). *Psychiatric Implications of Acquired Immune Deficiency Syndrome.* Washington, DC: American Psychiatric Press.

Nurnberg HG, Prudic J, Fiori M, and Freedman EP (1984). Psychopathology complicating acquired immune deficiency syndrome. *Am J Psychiatry* 141:95–96.

Parker R, and Aggleton P (2003). HIV and AIDS-related stigma and discrimination: a conceptual framework and implications for action. *Soc Sci Med* 57:13–24.

Pathela P, Hajat A, Schillinger J, Blank S, Sell R, and Mostashari F (2006). Discordance between sexual behavior and self-reported sexual identity: a population-based survey of New York City men. *Ann Intern Med* 145:416–425.

Perry SW, and Tross S (1984). Psychiatric problems of AIDS inpatients at the New York Hospital: preliminary report. *Public Health Rep* 99:200–205.

Perry S, Jacobsberg L, and Fishman B (1990). Suicidal ideation and HIV testing. *JAMA* 263:679–682.

Price WA, and Forejt J (1986). Neuropsychiatric aspects of AIDS: a case report. *Gen Hosp Psychiatry* 8:7–10.

Querques J, Stern TA (2004). Approach to Consultation Psychiatry: assessment strategies. In TA Stern, GL Fricchione, NH Cassem, MS Jellinek MS, and JF Rosenbaum (eds.), *Massachusetts General Hospital Handbook of General Hospital Psychiatry*, fifth edition (pp. 9–19). Philadelphia: Mosby.

Reinisch JM, and Beasley R (1990). America fails sex information test. In *The Kinsey Institute New Report on Sex: What You Must Know to Be Sexually Literate* (pp. 1–26). New York: St. Martin's Press.

Ruiz P (2000). Living and dying with HIV/AIDS: a psychosocial perspective. *Am J Psychiatry* 157:110–113.

Sackoff JE, Hanna DB, Pfeiffer MR, and Torian LV (2006). Causes of death among persons with AIDS in the era of highly active antiretroviral therapy: New York City. *Ann Intern Med* 145:397–406.

Selwyn PA, and Forstein M (2003). Overcoming the false dichotomy of curative vs. palliative care for late-stage AIDS. "Let me live the way I want to live until I can't." *JAMA* 290:806–814.

Stoff DM (2004). Mental health research in HIV/AIDS and aging: problems and prospects. *AIDS* 18(Suppl. 1): S3–S10.

Sullivan HS (1953). *The Interpersonal Theory of Psychiatry* (pp. 32–33). New York: WW Norton and Company.

Thienhaus OJ, and Khosla N (1984). Meningeal cryptococcosis misdiagnosed as a manic episode. *Am J Psychiatry* 141:1459–1460.

Thompson LM (1987). Dealing with AIDS and fear: would you accept cookies from an AIDS patient? *South Med J* 80:228–232.

Treisman GJ, and Angelino AF (2004). *The Psychiatry of AIDS: A Guide to Diagnosis and Treatment.* Baltimore: Johns Hopkins University Press.

Wormser GP, and Joline C (1989). Would you eat cookies prepared by an AIDS patient? Survey reveals harmful attitudes among professionals. *Postgrad Med* 86:174–184.

Chapter 2

HIV/AIDS at 25: History, Epidemiology, Clinical Manifestations, and Treatment

Sagar A. Vaidya, Mary Klotman, and Viviana Simon

Acquired immunodeficiency syndrome (AIDS) appeared 25 years ago and mystified doctors and scientists alike as it became one of the worst plagues in human history. Now an estimated 38.6 million children, women, and men are living worldwide with human immunodeficiency virus (HIV) infection (UNAIDS, 2006). While prevention options have expanded substantially, a cure or protective vaccine remain elusive. Antiretroviral combination treatments slow disease progression and have transformed AIDS from an inevitably fatal condition to a manageable, chronic illness.

ORIGIN AND HISTORY

Human immunodeficiency virus type 1 (HIV-1), the agent causing AIDS, is a lentivirus genetically closely related to SIVcpz found in chimpanzees (Keele et al., 2006). HIV-2 is less pathogenic than HIV-1 and likely originated from macaques and sooty mangabeys (Fig. 2.1). Analysis of the phylogenetic relationships between circulating human and simian immunodeficiency viruses (SIV) suggests that multiple, independent cross-species transmission events occurred between non-human primates and humans, resulting in the present circulating HIV-1 strains. The HIV strains that spread around the world belong predominantly to HIV-1 group M, whereas HIV-1 group N, HIV-1 group O, and HIV-2 have a more restricted geographic distribution (e.g., Western and Central Africa). HIV-1 group M comprises nine major clades that differ in frequency and global distribution: 50%–55% of all infections are due to subtype C (Thomson and Najera, 2005) (Fig. 2.1). In this text, use of the acronym *HIV* refers to HIV-1 unless otherwise specified.

Estimates suggest that HIV-1 was introduced into humans in the first decades of the past century but remained rare and unrecognized for several decades (Korber et al., 2000). The earliest time point that HIV infection could be documented retrospectively in humans is 1959 (Zhu et al., 1998). Case reports of opportunistic infections in people without clear reason

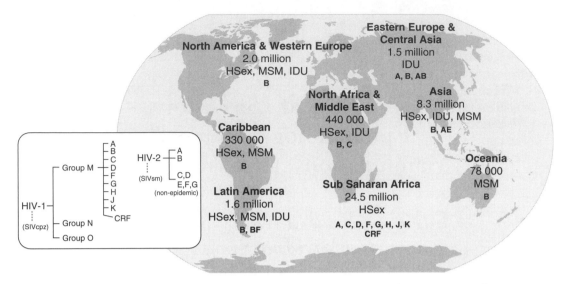

FIGURE 2.1. Global pandemic as defined by number of infected people, predominant route of transmission, and prevalent HIV subtypes (based on 2005 data published in UNAIDS, 2006). Heterosexual transmission is responsible for the vast majority of infections and HIV subtype C is the most prevalent worldwide. CRF, recombinant circulating forms; HSex, heterosexual transmission; IDU, intravenous drug use; MSM, men who have sex with men.

for immune suppression indicate sporadic occurrence throughout the 1950–1970s, with HIV-specific genetic materials being detected in retrospect in some of the preserved tissues (Zhu et al., 1998).

It was not until 1981 that HIV/AIDS first emerged as a public health issue, after a clustering of unusual opportunistic infections and cancers were reported in men who have sex with men in New York and San Francisco (CDC, 1981). It was hypothesized that the men were suffering from a common syndrome; a report from the Centers for Disease Control and Prevention (CDC) suggested that the disease might be caused by a sexually transmitted infectious agent (CDC, 1982a). The disease was initially associated with homosexual lifestyles, despite the fact that similar clinical cases were reported in injecting drug users, hemophiliacs, and newborns and infants receiving blood transfusions (CDC, 1982b). In 1982, the acronym "AIDS" was coined to describe this syndrome of unknown origin, which was associated with a variety of opportunistic infections and unusual tumors, in persons with the risk behaviors described above as well as in persons with hemophilia and in newborns who had received blood transfusions (CDC, 1982b). HIV, initially designated HTLV-III (human T-lymphotropic virus III) was isolated from AIDS patients in the follow-

ing years by several research groups (Barre-Sinoussi et al., 1983; Popovic et al., 1983; Barre-Sinoussi, 1996). Soon after, an HIV-1 antibody screening test was developed which allowed for the diagnosis of HIV prior to the development of clinically apparent end-stage immunodeficiency (Popovic et al., 1984; Sarngadharan et al., 1984). This was pivotal not only for gaining a better understanding of the extent of the epidemic and the course of infection, but most importantly for allowing screening of blood and blood products.

Screening for compounds with antiviral activity became possible when cell culture systems allowing viral propagation were established. The first drug approved for the treatment of HIV was azidothymidine (AZT), a nucleoside analogue, which was originally developed in 1964 for the treatment of cancers. Although AZT proved ineffective against neoplastic diseases, it was found to be a potent inhibitor of HIV. Its efficacy was such that the 1987 randomized, double-blinded clinical trial was stopped after only 6 months, as it was deemed unethical to deny AZT to all participants in light of excessive deaths in the placebo study arm (Fischl et al., 1987). Additional nucleoside/nucleotide analogues (reverse-transcriptase inhibitors, or NRTIs) with a similar mechanism of action targeting reverse transcription in the viral life cycle were

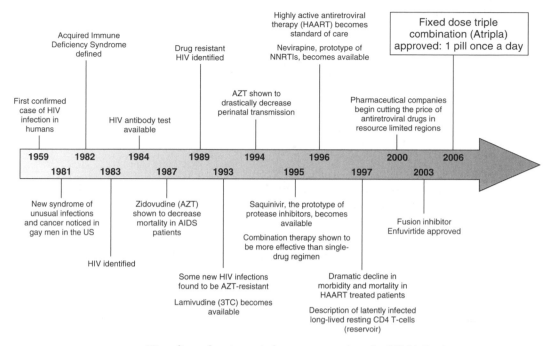

FIGURE 2.2. Time line of antiretroviral treatment options for HIV infection.

developed soon after. Combinations of two of these NRTIs were more effective in delaying disease progression and prolonging life in individuals with AIDS than was monotherapy (Staszewski, 1995), a result establishing multidrug regimens as the mainstay of therapy. It is now recognized that a three-drug regimen is more effective than dual therapy, which is considered obsolete. A second class of drugs, the nonnucleoside reverse transcriptase inhibitors (NNRTIs), that block the activity of the viral reverse transcriptase through direct binding to the enzyme were added to therapies beginning in 1996 (Spence et al., 1995). A new class of very potent drugs targeting the viral protease, the enzyme necessary for the production of infectious virions, became available in 1995 (Kitchen et al., 1995).

Combination triple-drug therapy known as HAART (highly active antiretroviral therapy) resulted in remarkable clinical success; HIV/AIDS has become a manageable chronic disease when there is access to these drugs (Hammer et al., 1997). Drug discovery continues to focus on defining new drug targets (e.g., viral integrase) as well as developing drugs with lower toxicity and more favorable pharmacokinetic profiles. Development of viral resistance to current drugs, associ-

ated toxicities, drug–drug interactions, and nonadherence to complex regimens continue to drive new drug development. The current objective for an optimal regime is a once-daily dosing with as few pills as possible, leading to profound suppression of viral replication with a favorable short- and long-term safety profile.

Aggressive public health campaigns have been successful in decreasing the rate of HIV transmission. Mother-to-child transmission was dramatically reduced by administration of single or a combination of antiretrovirals before and during delivery (Luzuriaga and Sullivan, 2005). Additional measures such as performance of caesarean delivery in some cases and the avoidance of breastfeeding have helped prevent maternal-to-fetal transmission, although the applications of all of these measures are challenging worldwide (McIntyre, 2006) . By the late 1990s, the number of AIDS deaths was found to be decreasing in the United States and other developed nations (see Fig. 2.2 for time line).

These milestones formed the base for the future scientific agenda aimed at preventing HIV infection and controlling viral replication in those already HIV infected.

EPIDEMIOLOGY

Since AIDS was first recognized in the early 1980s, there have been over 25 million deaths and 65 million individuals infected with the virus (CDC, 2006). The most recent estimates (2005) suggest that 64% of the 38.6 (33.4–46.0) million HIV-positive people world-wide live in sub-Saharan Africa (UNAIDS, 2006). The first decade of the pandemic was characterized by a restricted distribution of HIV infection in (a) indus-trialized countries where risk behaviors included un-protected sexual contact among men who have sex with men (MSM) and sharing of contaminated nee-dles and drug paraphernalia by injecting drug users, and (b) in central, east and West Africa and the Ca-ribbean where the virus spread in the general popu-lation through heterosexual transmission. The second decade witnessed the rapid spread of HIV to almost every part of the world along with increasing viral subtype diversity. There was an explosive increase of HIV in southern Africa, with prevalence rates of less than 1% in 1990 to over 20% by the end of the decade (UNAIDS, 2006). Now, in the third decade, sub-Saharan Africa remains the epicenter of the pandemic and accounts for more than 70% of all new HIV in-fections worldwide (UNAIDS, 2006). Heterosexual transmission continues to be the dominant route of transmission worldwide while injection drug use ac-counts for almost one-third of all new infections out-side of sub-Saharan Africa.

The number of sexually active young women in-fected with HIV is steadily increasing, the majority of whom live in southern Africa (UNAIDS, 2006). In-fection rates in this region are significantly higher in female adolescents than in their male counterparts; this discrepancy bears additional grave consequences for vertical transmission (UNAIDS, 2006). Women are recognized to be at increased risk due to the high-risk behavior of their male partners, such as injection drug use, commercial sex, or sex with other men, along with cultural barriers that often prohibit the use of proven protective measures such as condoms. In the United States, AIDS is a leading cause of death among African-American women aged 25–34 (Hodge, 2001).

In the United States there has been a recent (2001–2004) resurgence in HIV transmission by male-to-male sexual contact (men who have sex with men). This risk now accounts for up to 44% of new infections while heterosexual transmission accounts for 33% and intravenous drug use (IDU) for 7% (CDC, 2005).

Many newly reported cases of HIV infection are also attributable to immigrants from high-prevalence areas such as sub-Saharan Africa, who acquired the infection through heterosexual contact in their native countries (Kent, 2005).

PATHOBIOLOGY

The Virus and the Cell

The manipulation and hijacking of cellular processes is an essential viral survival strategy, since viruses rely on the cell machinery of the infected host for their replication. An impressive 8% of the human genome is composed of sequences of viral origin, suggesting that humans and viruses share a lengthy common history (Lander et al., 2001). Humans have evolved sophisticated defenses in the form of innate and ac-quired immunity (Stevenson, 2003). The HIV pan-demic illustrates that the virus has found efficient ways to evade innate and adapted immunity and to silence essential components of the intrinsic immune system (Simon et al., 2006).

Lentiviruses, which include HIV, are small, en-veloped retroviruses that package their genome in the form of two RNA copies. The name is due to the slow and chronic nature of diseases associated with these viruses. Like all retroviruses, they encode for a unique enzyme that allows the virus to reverse transcribe their (RNA) genome into DNA with subsequent insertion into the host chromosomes, thereby becoming an integral part of the cell's chromosomal DNA. Reverse transcription generates a swarm of related but distinct viral variants (known as viral quasi-species), since the viral enzyme reverse transcriptase (RT) is prone to error (Coffin, 1995). Every transcribed viral genome, therefore, differs from one another on average by one nucleotide. HIV replication in vivo is very dynamic, with more than 10 billion viruses being produced per day in an untreated, chronically infected patient (Coffin, 1996; Simon and Ho, 2003). The high rep-lication rate, together with the high error rate of re-verse transcription, is at the root of the extensive HIV sequence diversification that complicates treatment interventions and vaccine development.

HIV life cycle can be divided into early and late phases, with integration indicating the mid-point of infection and irreversibly rendering the cell infected. The virus enters the target cell through binding with a high-affinity interaction between its envelope gp120 protein and the CD4 receptor on the T cells, followed by gp120 interaction with a co-receptor, usually the chemokine receptors CCR5 or CXCR4. Once internalized, the viral core disassembles as proviral DNA is generated by the viral reverse transcriptase incorporated into the incoming core. The double-stranded proviral DNA ultimately integrates into the host genome. Host and viral factors drive transcription of viral proteins, which are assembled into new virions adjacent to the cell membrane. Immature viral particles are released from the infected cells in a noncytolytic manner. Lastly, infectious HIV-1 is generated when the viral Gag protein is cleaved by the viral enzyme protease (PR). Essential viral proteins, including the viral envelope, reverse transcriptase, protease, and integrase, have been major targets for the development of antiretroviral drugs (see Fig. 2.3).

The Virus and the Infected Patient

The hallmark of HIV infection is the slow depletion of naïve and memory CD4+ T lymphocytes; cell populations that are crucial for effective humoral and cellular immune responses. Expansion in CD8+ T-cell numbers and dysregulation of CD8+ T-cell functions are also seen throughout most of the disease.

Upon sexual transmission, HIV first replicates in the epithelium and the local lymphoid organs such as the draining lymph nodes. T lymphocytes, macrophages, and dendritic cells located in the lamina propria of the vaginal, cervical, and rectal epithelium are probably among the first infected target cells (Shat-

tock and Moore, 2003). Local amplification and migration of infected cells and/or virions throughout the body via the bloodstream leads to the very high levels of circulating virus in the plasma compartment associated with acute HIV-1 infection. According to experimental infections of rhesus macaques with SIV, viral dissemination occurs within days following exposure (Haase, 2005). Most infected humans develop HIV-specific CD8+ cytotoxic T lymphocytes (CTL) within 6 weeks of infection whereas seroconversion with HIV-specific antibodies is generally observed after 1–3 months (see Fig. 2.4).

The mounting of an HIV-specific immune response (e.g., CTL) is temporally correlated with a reduction in the peak of viremia, as determined by the quantity of viral RNA copies per ml of plasma, to a level that is maintained over years in the untreated individual. This association suggests that cell-mediated immunity plays a role in controlling replication, although this control is incomplete. The established level of viral RNA in the plasma, termed the *viral set point*, differs between patients and predicts disease progression (Mellors et al., 1997) Thus, CD8+-mediated cellular immune responses initially reduce viral replication, but the rapid selection of viral CTL escape mutants limits the long-term efficacy during chronic infection (Lichterfeld et al., 2005).

It is important to note that although symptoms may be mild in the first years of disease (so-called latent/dormant phase), HIV continuously replicates in the vast majority of those infected until the replacement of CD4+ cells cannot keep pace with the loss of these cells. The time from infection to the point when CD4+

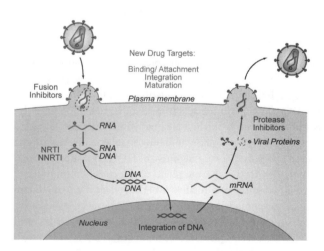

FIGURE 2.3. HIV life cycle. Antiretroviral drugs belong to three different classes. Fusion inhibitors prevent entry into the target cell. Reverse transcription is blocked by nucleoside analogues (NRTI) or nonnucleoside reverse transcriptase inhibitors (NNRTI). Proteolytic processing of the viral proteins is inhibited by protease inhibitors. The targets for future treatment interventions include binding and attachment, integration, and maturation inhibitors. Reproduced with permission from *Nature Reviews Microbiology*, Simon, V., and Ho, D. D., HIV-1 dynamics in vivo: implications for therapy. 1(3), 181–190, copyright 2003, Macmillan Magazines Ltd.

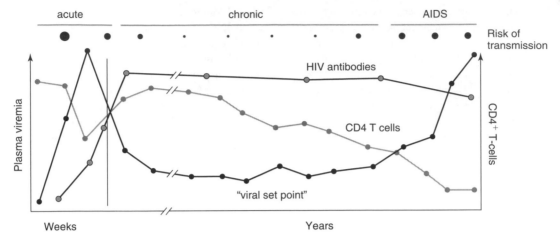

FIGURE 2.4. The natural course of HIV infection as depicted by the surrogate markers plasma viremia and CD4+ T-cell counts. Primary infection can be associated with clinical symptoms. During the first weeks of infection the risk of transmission is high, while HIV antibodies are still absent. Viremia stabilizes after the first month of infection, reaching an individual viral set point. Opportunistic diseases and certain HIV-associated malignancies define the stage of clinically apparent immunodeficiency (AIDS). Reproduced with permission from *Nature Reviews Microbiology*, Simon, V., and Ho, D. D., HIV-1 dynamics in vivo: implications for therapy. 1(3), 181–190, copyright 2003, Macmillan Magazines Ltd.

T cells fall below a critical circulating level needed to prevent opportunistic infections varies among individuals (e.g., 10 to 15 years). Genetic factors have been identified to account for some of the observed variation, including HLA haplotypes, and mutations in CCR5 co-receptor gene/promoter or co-receptor ligands (O'Brien and Nelson, 2004).

CLINICAL PRESENTATIONS

Diagnosis

Many commercially available kits allow the detection of HIV-specific antibodies. The recent availability of simple and rapid antibody detection systems should allow broader screening and earlier identification of infected individuals (MMWR, 2006). These serological tests fail to provide a reliable diagnosis in newborns and infants born to HIV-infected mothers who bear maternal antibodies and in the setting of acute infection when antibodies are still absent. In these clinical scenarios only the direct detection of viral nucleic acids establishes a diagnosis. The quantity of viral RNA circulating in the plasma (*viral load*) is a direct measurement of replication, whereas the proportion of CD4 helper cells indicates the degree of

immunodeficiency. Both parameters have been shown to predict disease progression in untreated individuals (Mellors et al., 1997).

Signs and Symptoms

The natural course of HIV infection can be divided into three phases: acute, chronic, and immunodeficiency stages (see Fig. 2.4). During primary infection, flu-like symptoms with rash and fever may occur (acute retroviral syndrome). The probability of transmission has been linked to the level of viral replication (Quinn et al., 2000). Since the plasma viral loads are highest during acute infection, in the late stages of HIV disease and during concurrent sexually transmitted infections, these are considered high-risk periods for transmission. Therefore, the risk of transmission may be high during relatively asymptomatic periods of infection. Newly infected individuals are often unaware of their serostatus and, thus, inadvertently may expose others to a very high risk of HIV acquisition.

In the chronic phase of infection, the number of absolute and relative CD4 T cells is maintained and eventually gradually decreases. However, patients are generally free of major symptoms until CD4+ T-cell depletion reaches a certain level (e.g., $<250/mm^3$)

and the immunodeficiency becomes clinically apparent. A variety of pathogens such as viruses, bacteria, fungi, or protozoa may cause opportunistic diseases. (Benson et al., 2005). Infections with *Pneumocystis carinii* (e.g., pneumonia), *Toxoplasma gondii* (e.g., cerebral manifestation), cytomegalovirus (e.g., generalized CMV, encephalitis), *Mycobacterium avium* complex, and neoplastic diseases such as Kaposi sarcoma and non-Hodgkin lymphoma were common AIDS-defining events in patients in North America and Europe during the pre-HAART era. In other geographic settings (e.g., sub-Saharan Africa) mycobacterium tuberculosis or wasting syndrome takes a more prominent role as an AIDS-defining disease.

Staging Systems

In the first decade of the pandemic, classifications systems (Walter Reed, CDC classification) served as important tools in predicting disease progression and initiating clinical interventions such as preemptive prophylactic treatments (e.g., *Pneumocystis carinii* prophylaxis). In the era of HAART, HIV/AIDS disease is staged on the basis of CDC classification from 1993, which combines CD4+ cell counts (categories 1–3) and clinical manifestation of certain opportunistic infections or tumors (CDC, 1993). Its relevance for daily management of the disease is somewhat reduced since the single most important determinant of disease progression, the level of virus replication as measured in the plasma, is not part of the classification. Additionally, HAART increases CD4+ T cells to near-normal levels, drastically reducing the risk of opportunistic infections. But backstaging from a more advanced CDC category is not a part of current staging. In resource-limited regions, infrastructure may not allow sophisticated laboratory testing and clinical symptoms are the only available criteria on which to base treatment decisions. The World Health Organization (WHO) has therefore developed a classification system based solely on clinical presentations (clinical stages 1–4) (WHO, 2006b).

BASIC PRINCIPLES OF TREATMENT

Antiretroviral Treatment

In the absence of a preventive vaccine or cure, prophylactic measures directed at preventing opportunis-

tic infections, and HAART are the best options to reduce morbidity and mortality. Widespread use of HAART in industrialized countries has transformed HIV infection into a treatable chronic disease. However, current drugs fail to eradicate HIV, and lifelong treatment with multiple active compounds is needed. HAART is expensive and requires regular clinical monitoring for side effects and treatment failures. Treatment of HIV is based on the simultaneous blocking of one or more steps in the viral life cycle with at least three different active agents.

Recent treatment guidelines for HAART initiation are largely based on the quantification of CD4+ T lymphocytes, the level of circulating virus in the plasma, and presence of clinical symptoms (DHHS, 2006; WHO, 2006a), as well as the patient's readiness to initiate and comply with what is presently considered lifelong therapy. Plasma viral load and CD4+ T-cell levels are used to determine the need for treatment and to monitor the virological success of the intervention.

Prophylactic Interventions against Opportunistic Infections

In addition, chemotherapeutic prophylaxis for *Pneumocystis carinii*, *Mycobacterium avium* complex, and *Toxoplasma gondii* (for antibody-positive patients) is recommended once CD4+ cell counts drop below a certain level (e.g., 200/mm^3 for *Pneumocystis carinii*). Secondary prophylaxis may prevent recurrence of an opportunistic manifestation such as *Cryptococcus neoformans* encephalitis or cerebral toxoplasmosis (DHHS, 2006). These interventions depend on an assessment of an individual's immune status, which currently is based largely on the stable measurement of CD4+ helper T cells. Most of the primary and secondary prophylaxis for opportunistic infections can be stopped in patients who have had sustained recovery of CD4+ cells in response to HAART (Benson et al., 2005).

Antiretroviral Drugs

Despite the tremendous successes in antiretroviral development, viral targets for treatment interventions are limited because of the development of resistance. Currently, U.S. Food and Drug Administration (FDA)-approved antiretroviral drugs target two viral enzymes: protease (PR) and reverse transcriptase (RT) and the transmembrane component (gp41) of the HIV envelope.

TABLE 2.1. Summary of Antiretroviral Drugs Currently FDA Approved for Combination Treatment of HIV Infection

Target	No. of Drugs	Name
Entry	1	Enfuvirtide
Protease	9	Fos-amprenavir, atazanavir, darunavir, indinavir, nelfinavir, ritonavir, saquinavir, tripanavir, lopinavir/ritonavir
Reverse transcriptase nucleoside	7	Abacavir, didanosine, emtricitabine, lamivudine, stavudine, zalcitabine, zidovudine
Nucleotide	1	Tenofovir
Nonnucleoside	3	Delaviridine, efavirenz, nevirapine
Fixed-dose combination tablets	5	Epzicom (abacavir/lamivudine); Combivir (zidovudine/lamivudine); Truvada (tenofovir/emitricitabine); Trizivir (abacavir/lamivudine/ziduvudine); Atripla (tenofovir/emtricitabine/efavirenz)

Table 2.1 lists the antiretroviral compounds and fixed-dose combination tablets approved by the FDA. The year 2006 will be the first in which licensing of some of the less effective drugs will be revoked (e.g., ddC) while more potent drugs such as darunavir, a protease inhibitor especially designed to inhibit resistant viruses, will emerge from the development pipeline. Enfuvirtide (T-20) is the first drug that targets viral entry (Tashima and Carpenter, 2003). By interfering with the gp41 region of the viral envelope, the fusion process stops and viral entry into the cell is prevented. However, the need to inject this drug subcutaneously twice daily along with an elaborate and expensive manufacturing process limits its widespread application. Its usage is generally reserved for treatment of antiretroviral-experienced patients in whom drug resistance limits therapeutic options.

Interference with viral entry is an attractive drug target, since de novo infection of target cells is prevented. In addition to fusion inhibitors with better pharmacokinetics and bioavailability, agents that block CD4 or co-receptor binding are under active preclinical and clinical development. The apparent immunological health and resistance to HIV infection of individuals with a homozygous deletion of a functional CCR5 as well as the slower disease progression in individuals heterozygous for this deletion has provided enthusiasm for a class of inhibitors directed at CCR5. Initial clinical studies demonstrate that blocking the human CCR5 co-receptors with small molecules results in profound inhibition of viral replica-

tion. The enthusiasm for this class of drugs has been dampened by concerns ranging from cardiac electrophysiological side effects and uncertain long-term toxicities to selection of preexisting, more pathogenic CXCR4 using viral variants (Weber et al., 2006).

Inhibitors that target the third viral enzyme, integrase, are currently in clinical trials. This drug target has proved challenging for the development of active compounds. Compounds under development profoundly inhibit viral replication in early human trials (DeJesus et al., 2006; Grinsztejn et al., 2006) and display activity against RTI and/or PI viral isolates resistant to reverse transcriptase and protease inhibitors (Reeves and Piefer, 2005). Nevertheless, advanced clinical trial testing will be needed to establish the safety profile and efficacy of these integrase inhibitors. Inhibitors of viral assembly and maturation that specifically interfere with the later viral life-cycle steps and result in production of immature viruses are currently being tested in early clinical trials (Reeves and Piefer, 2005).

HAART Principles

More than a decade ago, the high genetic variability combined with the high replication rate of HIV-1 provided the rational for combination antiretroviral therapy. The goal of antiretroviral treatment is to decrease morbidity and mortality associated with HIV-1 infection by completely suppressing viral replication in reservoirs throughout the body.

In most patients, a combination of three or more active drugs is required to achieve this goal. Effective treatment normalizes turnover rates of both CD4 and CD8 T-cell populations, although the CD4 population may remain low in some sites, particularly in gut-associated lymphoid tissue. Nevertheless, recovery of circulating CD4 T-cell levels correlates with effective immune reconstitution as indicated by a profound reduction in opportunistic infections and cancers in patients with stable CD4-cell recovery. Potent but well-tolerated drugs with prolonged bioavailability profiles and simplified regimens have improved the options for first- and second-line chemotherapeutic interventions. By combining several potent antiretroviral agents, viral replication can be suppressed to such low levels that the emergence of drug-resistant HIV-1 variants is significantly delayed. By doing so, CD4 T-lymphocyte numbers increase, leading to a degree of immune reconstitution sufficient to reverse clinically apparent immunodeficiency.

Findings on the early depletion of gut mucosal–associated CD4 cells and the limits of immune reconstitution provide arguments for beginning treatment early, preferably before critical populations of the immune system have been damaged and before viral quasi-species diversify. However, the timing of HAART initiation in asymptomatic patients with good CD4+ cell counts remains controversial for a number of reasons, including long-term drug toxicity of drugs leading to side effects that reduce quality of life, the complexity of dosing schedules, and prohibitive costs.

Limitations of Antiretroviral Treatment

The success of HAART is limited by virological, biological, and behavioral factors. The selection of viral variants with reduced drug susceptibility, the limited penetration of drugs in biological compartments (e.g., brain), presence of long-lived cells that harbor the virus, and short- and long-term toxicities are some of the obstacles that need to be overcome before a long-lasting cure becomes available. Furthermore, successful response to HAART requires rigorous individual adherence to a daily regimen for a very long time. Emergence of drug resistance limits the efficacy of HAART. HIV variants with reduced susceptibility to RTI and PI have a selective growth advantage in the presence of the specific inhibitor. In the absence of drug pressure (e.g., after discontinuation of treatment) the wild-type viruses often replicate more efficiently

and, being less resistant, generally outgrow the resistant quasi-species.

Some drug-resistant isolates, however, do in fact display replication capacities comparable to fully drug-susceptible HIV-1 strains (Simon and Ho, 2003). These multidrug-resistant (MDR) isolates have been observed to express a stable drug resistance over prolonged periods of time in the absence of selective drug pressure. This poses a risk for the individual as well as for public health, as transmission of drug-resistant viruses has now been demonstrated in regions of the world where HAART is widely prescribed.

On a cellular level, there are reservoirs in the body where the virus is integrated in the genome but the cell does not produce viral proteins or infectious virus. These reservoirs, however, can be induced to produce virus. These latent reservoirs may be quite longed-lived and remain a challenge for an ultimate cure (Blankson et al., 2002). Viral reservoirs comprise anatomical sanctuaries such as the central nervous system, the testis, and the kidney, as well as a small pool of circulating latently infected, long-lived memory T lymphocytes (Finzi et al., 1999; Blankson et al., 2002). These quiescent cell populations are inaccessible to current antiviral combination treatments that only work on active virus replication. Furthermore, they are not recognized by the immune system and therefore elude the goal of total eradication. A number of strategies are under active investigation to eradicate these pools. Intensification of combination treatments suggests that the potency of current regimens is insufficient to fully quench ongoing viral replication (Ramratnam et al., 2004). Attempts to purge the reservoirs by means of immunomodulatory substances (e.g., interleukin-2 or 7) or histone deacetylase-1 inhibitors (e.g., valproic acid) are currently under way; the clinical benefits of theses interventions remain unclear (Lehrman et al., 2005).

CONCLUSIONS

HAART has transformed HIV infection into a treatable disease. For the vast majority of infected people living in resource-limited regions, however, this transformation has not been completely realized. Knowledge of HIV-1 status remains essential for targeted prevention and early access to care. Life expectancy of persons with AIDS who do have access to care and adhere to therapeutic regimens now approaches that of the general population (Sackoff et al., 2006). Future challenges include the development of effective prevention strategies, providing HAART to resource-limited regions throughout the world, and strategies to address the long-term side-effect toxicities of antiretroviral therapy.

References

Barre-Sinoussi F (1996). HIV as the cause of AIDS. *Lancet* 348(9019):31–35.

Barre-Sinoussi F, Chermann JC, Rey F, Nugeyre MT, Chamaret S, Gruest J, Dauguet C, Axler-Blin C, Vezinet-Brun F, Rouzioux C, Rozenbaum W, and Montagnier L (1983). Isolation of a T-lymphotropic retrovirus from a patient at risk for acquired immune deficiency syndrome (AIDS). *Science* 220(4599): 868–871.

Benson CA, Kaplan JE, Masur H, Pau A, and Holmes KK (2005). Treating opportunistic infections among HIV-infected adults and adolescents: Recommendations from CDC, the National Institutes of Health, and the HIV Medicine Association/Infectious Diseases Society of America. *Clin Infect Dis* 40(Suppl. 3), 131–235.

Blankson JN, Persaud D, and Siliciano RF (2002). The challenge of viral reservoirs in HIV-1 infection. *Annu Rev Med* 53:557–593.

[CDC] Centers for Disease Control and Prevention (1981). *Pneumocystis* pneumonia—Los Angeles. *MMWR Morb Mortal Wkly Rep* 30(21):1–3.

[CDC] Centers for Disease Control and Prevention (1982a). A cluster of Kaposi's sarcoma and *Pneumocystis carinii* pneumonia among homosexual male residents of Los Angeles and Orange Counties, California. *MMWR Morb Mortal Wkly Rep* 31:305–307.

[CDC] Centers for Disease Control and Prevention (1982b). Update on acquired immune deficiency syndrome (AIDS)—United States. *MMWR Morb Mortal Wkly Rep* 31(37):507–508, 513–514.

[CDC] Centers for Disease Control and Prevention (1993). Centers for Disease Control and Prevention. 1993 revised classification system for HIV infection and expanded surveillance case definition for AIDS among adolescents and adults. *JAMA* 269(6):729–730.

[CDC] Centers for Disease Control and Prevention (2005). Trends in HIV/AIDS diagnoses—33 States, 2001–2004. *MMWR Morb Mortal Wkly Rep* 54(45): 1149–1153.

[CDC] Centers for Disease Control and Prevention (2006). The global HIV/AIDS pandemic, 2006. *MMWR Morb Mortal Wkly Rep* 55(31):841–844.

Coffin JM (1995). HIV population dynamics in vivo: implications for genetic variation, pathogenesis, and therapy. *Science* 267(5197):483–489.

Coffin JM (1996). HIV viral dynamics. *AIDS* 10(Suppl. 3):S75–S84.

DeJesus E, Berger D, Markowitz M, Cohen C, Hawkins T, Ruane P, Elion R, Farthing C, Cheng A, Kearney B, and Team A-S (2006). The HIV integrase inhibitor GS-9137 (JTK-303) exhibits potent antiviral activity in treatment-naïve and experienced patients. Presented at the 13th Conference on Retroviruses and Opportunistic Infections, Denver, 160LB.

[DHHS] U.S. Department of Health and Human Services (2006). U.S. Department of Health and Human Services, Panel on Clinical Practices for Treatment of HIV Infection. Guidelines for the use of antiretroviral agents in HIV-1-infected adults and adolescents. Washington, DC: U.S. Department of Health and Human Services. Retrieved March 16, 2007, from http://www.aidsinfo.nih.gov/ContentFiles/AdultandAdolescentGL.pdf.

Finzi D, Blankson J, Siliciano JD, Margolick JB, Chadwick K, Pierson T, Smith K, Lisziewicz J, Lori F, Flexner C, Quinn TC, Chaisson RE, Rosenberg E, Walker B, Gange S, Gallant J, and Siliciano RF (1999). Latent infection of CD4+ T cells provides a mechanism for lifelong persistence of HIV-1, even in patients on effective combination therapy. *Nat Med* 5(5):512–517.

Fischl MA, Richman DD, Grieco MH, Gottlieb MS, Volberding PA, Laskin OL, Leedom JM, Groopman JE, Mildvan D, Schooley RT, et al. (1987). The efficacy of azidothymidine (AZT) in the treatment of patients with AIDS and AIDS-related complex. A double-blind, placebo-controlled trial. *N Engl J Med* 317(4):185–191.

Grinsztejn B, Y, N B, Katlama C, J, G, A, L, Vittecoq D, Gonzalez C, Chen J, Isaacs R, and Team a t P S (2006). Potent antiretroviral effect of MK-0518, a novel HIV-1 integrase inhibitor, in patients with triple-class resistant virus. Presented at the 13th Conference on Retroviruses and Opportunistic Infections, Denver, 159LB.

Haase AT (2005). Perils at mucosal front lines for HIV and SIV and their hosts. *Nat Rev Immunol* 5(10):783–792.

Hammer SM, Squires KE, Hughes MD, Grimes JM, Demeter LM, Currier JS, Eron JJ, Jr, Feinberg JE, Balfour HH, Jr, Deyton LR, Chodakewitz JA, and Fischl MA (1997). A controlled trial of two nucleoside analogues plus indinavir in persons with human immunodeficiency virus infection and CD4 cell counts of 200 per cubic millimeter or less. AIDS Clinical Trials Group 320 Study Team. *N Engl J Med* 337(11):725–733.

Hodge CE (2001). HIV/AIDS: impact on the African American community. *Compend Contin Educ Dent* 22(3 Spec. No.):52–56.

Keele BF, Van Heuverswyn F, Li Y, Bailes E, Takehisa J, Santiago ML, Bibollet-Ruche F, Chen Y, Wain LV, Liegeois F, Loul S, Ngole EM, Bienvenue Y, Delaporte E, Brookfield JF, Sharp PM, Shaw GM, Peeters M, and Hahn BH (2006). Chimpanzee reservoirs of pandemic and nonpandemic HIV-1. *Science* 313(5786):523–526.

Kent (2005). Impact of foreign-born persons on HIV diagnosis rates among Blacks in King County, Washington. *AIDS Educ Prev* 17(6 Suppl B):60–67.

Kitchen VS, Skinner C, Ariyoshi K, Lane EA, Duncan IB, Burckhardt J, Burger HU, Bragman K, Pinching AJ, and Weber JN (1995). Safety and activity of saquinavir in HIV infection. *Lancet* 345(8955):952–955.

Korber B, Muldoon M, Theiler J, Gao F, Gupta R, Lapedes A, Hahn BH, Wolinsky S, and Bhattacharya T (2000). Timing the ancestor of the HIV-1 pandemic strains. *Science* 288(5472):1789–1796.

Lander ES, Linton LM, Birren B, Nusbaum C, Zody MC, Baldwin J, Devon K, Dewar K, Doyle M, FitzHugh W, Funke R, Gage D, Harris K, Heaford A, Howland J, Kann L, Lehoczky J, LeVine R, McEwan P, McKernan K, Meldrim J, Mesirov JP, Miranda C, Morris W, Naylor J, Raymond C, Rosetti M, Santos R, Sheridan A, Sougnez C, Stange-Thomann N, Stojanovic N, Subramanian A, Wyman D, Rogers J, Sulston J, Ainscough R, Beck S, Bentley D, Burton J, Clee C, Carter N, Coulson A, Deadman R, Deloukas P, Dunham A, Dunham I, Durbin R, French L, Grafham D, Gregory S, Hubbard T, Humphray S, Hunt A, Jones M, Lloyd C, McMurray A, Matthews L, Mercer S, Milne S, Mullikin JC, Mungall A, Plumb R, Ross M, Shownkeen R, Sims S, Waterston RH, Wilson RK, Hillier LW, McPherson JD, Marra MA, Mardis ER, Fulton LA, Chinwalla AT, Pepin KH, Gish WR, Chissoe SL, Wendl MC, Delehaunty KD, Miner TL, Delehaunty A, Kramer JB, Cook LL, Fulton RS, Johnson DL, Minx PJ, Clifton SW, Hawkins T, Branscomb E, Predki P, Richardson P, Wenning S, Slezak T, Doggett N, Cheng JF, Olsen A, Lucas S, Elkin C, Uberbacher E, Frazier M, Gibbs RA, Muzny DM, Scherer SE, Bouck JB, Sodergren EJ, Worley KC, Rives CM, Gorrell JH, Metzker ML, Naylor SL, Kucherlapati RS, Nelson DL, Weinstock GM, Sakaki Y, Fujiyama A, Hattori M, Yada T, Toyoda A, Itoh T, Kawagoe C, Watanabe H, Totoki Y, Taylor T, Weissenbach J, Heilig R, Saurin W, Artiguenave F, Brottier P, Bruls T, Pelletier E, Robert C, Wincker P, Smith DR, Doucette-Stamm L, Rubenfield M, Weinstock K, Lee HM, Dubois J, Rosenthal A, Platzer M, Nyakatura G, Taudien S, Rump A, Yang H, Yu J, Wang J, Huang G, Gu J, Hood L, Rowen L, Madan A, Qin S, Davis RW, Federspiel NA, Abola AP, Proctor MJ, Myers RM, Schmutz J, Dickson M, Grimwood J, Cox DR, Olson MV, Kaul R, Shimizu N, Kawasaki K, Minoshima S, Evans GA, Athanasiou M, Schultz R, Roe BA, Chen F, Pan H, Ramser J, Lehrach H, Reinhardt R, McCombie WR, de la Bastide M, Dedhia N, Blocker H, Hornischer K, Nordsiek G, Agarwala R, Aravind L, Bailey JA, Bateman A, Batzoglou S, Birney E, Bork P, Brown DG, Burge CB, Cerutti L, Chen HC, Church D, Clamp M, Copley RR, Doerks T, Eddy SR, Eichler EE, Furey TS,

Galagan J, Gilbert JG, Harmon C, Hayashizaki Y, Haussler D, Hermjakob H, Hokamp K, Jang W, Johnson LS, Jones TA, Kasif S, Kaspryzk A, Kennedy S, Kent WJ, Kitts P, Koonin EV, Korf I, Kulp D, Lancet D, Lowe TM, McLysaght A, Mikkelsen T, Moran JV, Mulder N, Pollara VJ, Ponting CP, Schuler G, Schultz J, Slater G, Smit AF, Stupka E, Szustakowski J, Thierry-Mieg D, Thierry-Mieg J, Wagner L, Wallis J, Wheeler R, Williams A, Wolf YI, Wolfe KH, Yang SP, Yeh RF, Collins F, Guyer MS, Peterson J, Felsenfeld A, Wetterstrand KA, Patrinos A, Morgan MJ, Szustakowki J, de Jong P, Catanese JJ, Osoegaw K, Shizuya H, Choi S, and Chen YJ (2001). Initial sequencing and analysis of the human genome. *Nature* 409(6822):860–921.

Lehrman G, Hogue IB, Palmer S, Jennings C, Spina CA, Wiegand A, Landay AL, Coombs RW, Richman DD, Mellors JW, Coffin JM, Bosch RJ, and Margolis DM (2005). Depletion of latent HIV-1 infection in vivo: a proof-of-concept study. *Lancet* 366(9485):549–555.

Lichterfeld M, Yu XG, Le Gall S, and Altfeld M (2005). Immunodominance of HIV-1-specific CD8+ T-cell responses in acute HIV-1 infection: at the crossroads of viral and host genetics. *Trends Immunol* 26(3):166–171.

Luzuriaga K, and Sullivan JL (2005). Prevention of mother-to-child transmission of HIV infection. *Clin Infect Dis* 40(3):466–467.

McIntyre J (2006). Strategies to prevent mother-to-child transmission of HIV. *Curr Opin Infect Dis* 19(1): 33–38.

Mellors JW, Munoz A, Giorgi JV, Margolick JB, Tassoni CJ, Gupta P, Kingsley LA, Todd JA, Saah AJ, Detels R, Phair JP, and Rinaldo CR, Jr (1997). Plasma viral load and CD4+ lymphocytes as prognostic markers of HIV-1 infection. *Ann Intern Med* 126(12):946–954.

[MMWR] Morbidity and Mortality Weekly Report (2006). Revised recommendations for HIV testing of adults, adolescents, and pregnant women in health-care settings. Vol. 55, No. RR–14.

O'Brien SJ, and Nelson GW (2004). Human genes that limit AIDS. *Nat Genet* 36(6):565–574.

Popovic M, Sarin PS, Robert-Gurroff M, Kalyanaraman VS, Mann D, Minowada J, and Gallo RC (1983). Isolation and transmission of human retrovirus (human T-cell leukemia virus). *Science* 219(4586): 856–859.

Popovic M, Sarngadharan MG, Read E, and Gallo RC (1984). Detection, isolation, and continuous production of cytopathic retroviruses (HTLV-III) from patients with AIDS and pre-AIDS. *Science* 224(4648): 497–500.

Quinn TC, Wawer MJ, Sewankambo N, Serwadda D, Li C, Wabwire-Mangen F, Meehan MO, Lutalo T, and Gray RH (2000). Viral load and heterosexual transmission of human immunodeficiency virus type 1. Rakai Project Study Group. *N Engl J Med* 342(13):921–929.

Ramratnam B, Ribeiro R, He T, Chung C, Simon V, Vanderhoeven J, Hurley A, Zhang L, Perelson AS, Ho DD, and Markowitz M (2004). Intensification of antiretroviral therapy accelerates the decay of the HIV-1 latent reservoir and decreases, but does not eliminate, ongoing virus replication. *J Acquir Immune Defic Syndr* 35(1):33–37.

Reeves JD, and Piefer AJ (2005). Emerging drug targets for antiretroviral therapy. *Drugs* 65(13):1747–1766.

Sackoff JE, Hanna DB, Pfeiffer MR, and Torian LV (2006). Causes of death among persons with AIDS in the era of highly active antiretroviral therapy: New York City. *Ann Intern Med* 145(6):397–406.

Sarngadharan MG, Popovic M, Bruch L, Schupbach J, and Gallo RC (1984). Antibodies reactive with human T-lymphotropic retroviruses (HTLV-III) in the serum of patients with AIDS. *Science* 224(4648): 506–508.

Shattock RJ, and Moore JP (2003). Inhibiting sexual transmission of HIV-1 infection. *Nat Rev Microbiol* 1(1):25–34.

Simon V, and Ho DD (2003). HIV-1 dynamics in vivo: implications for therapy. *Nat Rev Microbiol* 1(3): 181–190.

Simon V, Ho DD, and Abdool Karim Q (2006). HIV/AIDS epidemiology, pathogenesis, prevention, and treatment. *Lancet* 368(9534):489–504.

Spence RA, Kati WM, Anderson KS, and Johnson KA (1995). Mechanism of inhibition of HIV-1 reverse transcriptase by nonnucleoside inhibitors. *Science* 267(5200):988–993.

Staszewski S (1995). Zidovudine and lamivudine: results of phase III studies. *J Acquir Immune Defic Syndr Hum Retrovirol* 10(Suppl. 1):S57.

Stevenson M (2003). HIV-1 pathogenesis. *Nat Med* 9(7): 853–860.

Tashima KT, and Carpenter CC (2003). Fusion inhibition—a major but costly step forward in the treatment of HIV-1. *N Engl J Med* 348(22):2249–2250.

Thomson MM, and Najera R (2005). Molecular epidemiology of HIV-1 variants in the global AIDS pandemic: an update. *AIDS Rev* 7(4):210–224.

UNAIDS (2006). *2006 Report on the Global AIDS Epidemic: A UNAIDS 10th Anniversary Special Edition.* Geneva: UNAIDS.

Weber J, Piontkivska H, and Quinones-Mateu ME (2006). HIV type 1 tropism and inhibitors of viral entry: clinical implications. *AIDS Rev* 8(2):60–77.

[WHO] World Health Organization (2006a). Antiretroviral therapy for HIV infection in adults and adolescents in resource-limited settings: towards universal access. Retrieved September 2006 from http://www.who.int/hiv/pub/guidelines/adult/en/index.html.

[WHO] World Health Organization (2006b). WHO case definitions of HIV for surveillance and revised clinical staging and immunological classification of HIV-related disease in adults and children. Retrieved September 2006 from http://www.who.int/hiv/pub/guidelines/hivstaging/en/index.html.

Zhu T, Korber BT, Nahmias AJ, Hooper E, Sharp PM, and Ho DD (1998). An African HIV-1 sequence from 1959 and implications for the origin of the epidemic. *Nature* 391(6667):594–597.

Chapter 3

Psychoneuroimmunology and HIV

*Adam W. Carrico, Michael H. Antoni,
Lawrence Young, and Jack M. Gorman*

Because of the many the stressors inherent in HIV infection, psychosocial and biomedical issues must be addressed for successful disease management (Schneiderman et al., 1994). The anticipation and impact of HIV antibody test notification; emergence of the first symptoms of disease; changes in vocational plans, lifestyle behaviors, and interpersonal relationships; and the burdens of complex medication regimens are all highly stressful. These multiple challenges can create a state of chronic stress that may overwhelm an individual's coping resources and significantly impair emotional adjustment to ongoing demands of the illness (Leserman et al., 2000). Accordingly, HIV-positive individuals are at increased risk for developing an affective or adjustment disorder across the disease spectrum (Bing et al., 2001). Although reductions in mood disturbance have been observed following the introduction of highly active anti-retroviral therapy (HAART; Rabkin et al., 2000), the risk of developing major depressive disorder is two times higher in HIV-positive samples when compared to HIV-negative peers (Ciesla

and Roberts, 2001; see also Chapters 4 and 9 in this volume).

With substantial reductions in morbidity and mortality following the advent of HAART, clinical care of HIV-positive persons has improved dramatically such that the disease is now commonly conceptualized as a chronic illness (CDC, 1997; Mannheimer et al., 2005). However, not all HIV-positive patients treated with HAART display adequate viral suppression because of the difficulties some patients have adhering to treatment and the emergence of drug-resistant strains of the virus (Bangsberg et al., 2001; Tamalet et al., 2003). Questions also remain regarding the appropriate time to initiate HAART in HIV-positive patients. Variability in the extent of immune reconstitution, an increased incidence of opportunistic infections in the months following initiation, and profound drug-related toxicities have all been reported (Ledergerber et al., 1999; Lederman and Valdez, 2000; Volberding, 2003; Yeni et al., 2004). These issues perpetuate the great uncertainty that surrounds this chronic, albeit unpredictable, disease.

Because HIV-positive persons endure a chronic disease that requires adaptation across a variety of domains, individual differences in the ways they adapt to these challenges may affect not only quality of life but also disease processes. Research in psychoneuroimmunology (PNI) has examined the potential biobehavioral mechanisms whereby psychosocial factors such as stressors, stress responses, coping, and negative affective states influence disease progression (Antoni, 2003a). Psychosocial factors are thought to relate to immune-system function in humans via stress- or distress-induced changes in hormonal regulatory systems (Kiecolt-Glaser et al., 2002). Several adrenal hormones, including cortisol and catecholamines (norepinephrine and epinephrine), are altered as a function of an individual's appraisals of and coping responses to stressors (McEwen, 1998). What is particularly relevant to HIV/AIDS research is the observation that a variety of neuroendocrine abnormalities occur in both clinically depressed (Gillespie and Nemeroff, 2005) and HIV-positive (Kawa and Thompson, 1996) populations. In HIV-positive persons, elevations in these hormones have also been associated with alterations in multiple indices of immune status (Antoni and Schneiderman, 1998). The most definitive PNI work has illuminated such biobehavioral mechanisms through longitudinal and intervention designs where changes in psychosocial factors are mapped onto changes in immunologic indicators and clinical disease progression over time in different HIV-positive populations. In this chapter, we review seminal research findings that support the relevance of PNI pathways in HIV disease progression. Although the majority of PNI investigations with HIV-positive persons were conducted prior to the availability of HAART, more recent findings indicate that enhanced psychological adjustment may facilitate virologic control and bolster immunocompetence, enhancing the effectiveness of HAART.

NEGATIVE LIFE EVENTS

Despite the unprecedented clinical benefits of HAART, HIV-positive persons must continue to cope with a number of chronic, uncontrollable stressors that may hinder optimal management of their illness. This observation is supported by research examining the association between negative life events and HIV disease progression.

Cumulative Life Event Burden

Investigators employing interview-based, contextual methods have observed consistent effects of negative life events on declines in immune system parameters in HIV-positive men who have sex with men (MSM; Leserman, 2003). Specifically, cumulative negative life events were associated with reductions in natural killer (NK) and cytotoxic/suppressor (CD8+) cell counts over a 2-year period in a cohort of HIV-positive MSM recruited in the pre-HAART era (Leserman et al., 1997). The clinical significance of these findings is supported by data indicating that these immune cell subsets may play a key role in suppressing HIV replication (Ironson et al., 2001; Cruess et al., 2003).

Cumulative negative life events have also been associated with increases in HIV viral load in a diverse cohort of HAART-treated, HIV-positive men and women (Ironson et al., 2005). Most notably, individuals classified as experiencing a higher rate (>75th percentile) of cumulative negative life events displayed a twofold increase in HIV viral load over 2 years compared to those with lower rates (<25th percentile), even after controlling for antiretroviral medication adherence. Although no concurrent effects on helper/inducer T-cell (CD4+) counts were observed, results of this investigation demonstrate a continued association between negative life events and immune status in the era of HAART. These data also extend the results of previous investigations to both men and women living with HIV.

Some investigators have also examined relations between life events and clinical-disease outcomes in HIV-positive persons. In a series of studies conducted in the pre-HAART era, Leserman and colleagues demonstrated that cumulative negative life events are associated with faster disease progression in HIV-positive MSM through a 9-year follow-up. Specifically, their findings indicated that higher cumulative negative life events equivalent to one severe stressor doubled the risk of progression to AIDS over 7.5 years (Leserman et al., 1999, Leserman et al., 2000). These results remained unchanged after controlling for demographic variables, baseline CD4+ counts, baseline HIV viral load, number of antiretroviral medications, and serum cortisol. Using similar covariates, a subsequent investigation showed that greater cumulative negative life events (equivalent to one severe stressor) increased the risk of developing an AIDS clinical condition by threefold at 9-year follow-up (Leserman et al., 2002).

Building upon these findings, other investigators have examined the clinical relevance of negative life events in HIV-positive women. Pereira and colleagues (2003a) observed that over a 1-year follow-up in HIV-positive women, greater negative life events during the 6 months prior to follow-up were related to an increased risk for symptomatic genital herpes recurrences, after controlling for indicators of HIV disease status and behavioral factors. These findings remained unchanged after controlling for herpes simplex virus type 2 (HSV-2) immunoglobulin G (IgG) antibody titers at study entry. Greater negative life events were also associated with persistence or progression of cervical squamous intraepithelial lesions (SIL), a preclinical condition to invasive cervical cancer, over the subsequent year (Pereira et al., 2003b). The association between negative life events and the persistence or progression of this preclinical condition in women at risk for AIDS was unchanged after controlling for indicators of HIV disease status (e.g., CD4+ counts), other viral risk factors for SIL (presence or absence of oncogenic human papilloma virus [HPV] infections), and behavioral factors (e.g., tobacco smoking). Taken together, results of these investigations support the relevance of chronic stress in HIV disease progression. Caution is in order, however, when interpreting these findings, as most studies had small samples. Future investigations should examine the prospective association between negative life events and health outcomes in larger, diverse, HAART-treated cohorts of HIV-positive persons. Other investigations have focused on the association between HIV-specific and other salient stressors and immune status.

HIV-Specific Stressful Events

The increase in distress upon learning that one is HIV seropositive has been shown to parallel reductions in CD4+ and NK cell counts (Antoni et al., 1991) and depressed T-lymphocyte responses to mitogenic challenge (Ironson et al., 1990). These findings suggest that stressful experiences early in HIV infection can have negative effects on immune status. One of the most common and recurring stressors for HIV-positive persons is bereavement. Particularly during the pre-HAART era, bereavement and knowledge of HIV serostatus were identified as two important predictors of psychological distress over a 7-year period. Although approximately 50% of HIV-positive men in one sample reported being bereaved each year, the effects of

bereavement on psychological distress diminished over time (Martin and Dean, 1993). However, knowledge of HIV serostatus was a strong predictor of distress over the study period.

Other investigations have focused on bereavement as a predictor of immune status over time in cohorts of HIV-positive MSM. Specifically, bereavement has been related to more rapid declines in CD4+ counts over a 3- to 4-year period (Kemeny and Dean, 1995) and to increases in serum neopterin and impaired lymphoproliferative responses, compared to a matched control group (Kemeny et al., 1995). Other investigations of asymptomatic HIV-positive men have observed that bereavement is associated with decrements in NK cell cytotoxicity over a 1-year period (Goodkin et al., 1996). Although relatively few investigations have examined the relevance of traumatic stressors, one study observed a high rate of exposure to traumatic events in HIV-positive African-American women (Kimmerling et al., 1999). Exposure to a traumatic stressor (especially for participants with posttraumatic stress disorder) was associated with lower CD4+/CD8+ ratios at 1-year follow up. This work suggests that differences in the ways individuals manage newly emerging challenges may affect the status of their immune systems, possibly contributing to health outcomes. The controlled study of individual differences in physiological responsiveness to behavioral and psychosocial challenges enjoys a long history in the use of the "laboratory reactivity" paradigm, mostly as applied to behavioral cardiology research. More recently this paradigm has been used to investigate individual differences in immunocellular reactivity among HIV-positive persons.

STRESS REACTIVITY

What physiologic changes that accompany a person's reaction to stressors could explain the association between life events and HIV disease progression? There is some evidence that distress and other negative mood states may be related to dysregulated hypothalamic-pituitary-adrenal (HPA) activity (e.g., elevated cortisol) in HIV-positive men (Gorman et al., 1991). Alterations in peripheral levels of adrenal hormones could conceivably down-regulate important cellular immune functions. However, there are methodological difficulties inherent in tying physiological stress responses (which may be short-lived) to field stressors or cumulative stressor burden as reported by participants. Consequently, researchers have turned to the laboratory reactivity paradigm to pinpoint endocrine and immune changes that may parallel responses to stressors in HIV-positive persons.

In asymptomatic HIV-positive MSM, investigators have observed blunted adrenocorticotropin hormone (ACTH) responsiveness to a variety of behavioral challenges (Kumar et al., 1993), but no differences in cortisol increases over time compared with HIV-negative men (Starr et al., 1996). The lack of cortisol differences may be an artifact of the timing of blood draws after stressor onset—cortisol responses may lag behind ACTH and catecholamine changes by several minutes. Subsequent investigations have demonstrated that HIV-positive persons show changes in immune cell subsets during an evaluative speech stressor (Hurwitz et al., 2005). Compared to their HIV-negative counterparts, HIV-positive persons showed greater increases in total and activated T-cell counts. Specifically, HIV-positive persons displayed increases in the CD8+ and CD8+38+ T-cell subsets during the speech stressor task. Hurwitz and colleagues (2005) also determined that HIV-positive persons had smaller stressor-induced increases in NK counts and NK cell cytotoxicity as well as impaired lymphoproliferative responsiveness to phytohemagglutinin mitogen. While no group differences in catecholamine reactivity were observed, HIV-positive participants displayed greater increases in CD8+ T-cell count per unit increase in norepinepherine. Most notably, a positive correlation between norepinepherine and CD8+38+ T-cell count was significant only for the HIV-positive group. Taken together, these data highlight that abnormalities in immune cell trafficking observed in HIV-positive persons may be due in part to alterations in sympathoimmune communication.

The relevance of sympathoimmune communication in HIV-positive persons is further supported by results of previous investigations. Because lymphoid organs are a primary site of HIV replication, sympathetic nervous system innervation of these regions may dramatically influence HIV disease progression (Cole and Kemeny, 2001). For example, release of norepinepherine at nerve terminals may down-regulate proliferation of naïve T cells in the lymphoid organs (Felten, 1996). By binding with β_2 receptors on the lymphocyte membrane, norepinepherine induces cellular changes via the G protein–linked adenyl cyclase–cAMP–protein kinase A signaling cascade (Kobilka, 1992). In

vitro data have shown that cellular changes of this nature are associated with decrements in interferon-γ and interleukin-10, which in turn, are associated with elevations in HIV viral load over an 8-day period (Cole et al., 1998).

Other in vivo investigations have specifically examined the role of autonomic nervous system (ANS) activity in HIV-positive persons initiating HAART. Individuals who displayed higher ANS activity at rest prior to beginning HAART subsequently demonstrated poorer suppression of HIV viral load and decreased CD4+ T-cell reconstitution over a 3- to 11-month period (Cole et al., 2001). Furthermore, in a sample of asymptomatic HIV-positive MSM, socially inhibited individuals displayed an eightfold increase in plasma HIV viral load set point and showed poorer responses to HAART (Cole et al., 2003). The effect of social inhibition on higher HIV viral load was mediated by elevated ANS activity, even after controlling for demographic and health status variables. Thus, stress-related alterations in neuroendocrine functioning may continue to influence immune status and health outcomes in the era of HAART. These data also highlight the fact that although negative life events have been shown to substantially influence the course of HIV disease, individuals often have highly variable psychological responses to any given stressor.

COGNITIVE APPRAISALS

Individual differences in cognitive appraisals of stressors may moderate the association between stressful life events and health status in HIV-positive persons. Specifically, one research group has demonstrated that positive illusions and unrealistically optimistic appraisals may confer health-protective benefits (Taylor et al., 2000). Results from an investigation of bereaved HIV-positive men indicated that those who engaged in cognitive processing (deliberate, effortful, and long-lasting thinking) about the death of a close friend or partner were more likely to report a major shift in values, priorities, or perspectives (i.e., finding meaning) following the loss (Bower et al., 1998). For those who were classified as finding meaning, positive health effects appeared to follow. Finding meaning predicted slower CD4+ decline and greater longevity over a 2- to 3-year follow-up period (Bower et al., 1998). Decreased cortisol is one plausible mediator of the effects of finding meaning on health status. In other medical populations (e.g., women being treated for breast cancer) finding benefits in living with a chronic illness predicts concurrent decreases in serum cortisol (Cruess et al., 2000a). In HIV-positive populations, elevated serum cortisol levels have been related to faster progression to AIDS, development of an AIDS-related condition, and mortality over a 9-year period (Leserman et al., 2002). Conversely, lower 15-hour urinary-free cortisol levels are associated with long-term survival with AIDS (Ironson et al., 2002). Importantly, in recent work we have observed that benefit finding uniquely predicted lower 24-hour urinary-free cortisol output in a diverse cohort of HAART-treated HIV-positive persons, even after accounting for the effects of depressive symptoms (Carrico et al., 2006). In other research with HIV-positive MSM conducted in the aftermath of Hurricane Andrew, dispositional optimism was associated with lower Epstein-Barr virus (EBV) and human herpes virus type-6 (HHV-6) IgG antibody titers. These findings suggest better immunologic control over these viruses in participants able to maintain an optimistic attributional style in the wake of a severe environmental stressor (Cruess et al., 2000b).

Other investigators have observed that negative HIV-specific expectancies (i.e., fatalism) are related to elevated risk for symptom onset in bereaved, asymptomatic HIV-positive men (Reed et al., 1999) and to mortality in men with AIDS (Reed et al., 1994). Negative causal attributions about one's self have also been associated with CD4+ count decline over 18 months (Segerstrom et al., 1996). Finally, among HIV-positive women, pessimism has been associated with lower CD8+ percentages and lower NK cell cytotoxicity, after controlling for stressful life events (Byrnes et al., 1998). These findings suggest that across different HIV-positive populations, negative or pessimistic appraisals about stressors or one's efficacy in managing life challenges are associated with poorer immune status and greater risk for disease progression. On the other hand, maintaining optimism and finding benefit in the challenges of HIV/AIDS are associated with lower levels of adrenal stress hormones, better antiviral immunity, and possibly better health outcomes. Importantly, it may be possible to modulate cognitive appraisal processes in HIV-positive persons by way of cognitive-behavioral interventions (Lutgendorf et al., 1998; Carrico et al., 2005b). Before discussing the PNI research on such interventions with HIV-positive persons, it is important to consider the role that negative mood states may play in mediating the associa-tion between cognitive appraisals and health outcomes in HIV/AIDS.

NEGATIVE MOOD

Negative mood states such as depression and anxiety have been associated with additional functional impairment, mortality, and an approximately 50% increase in medical costs for persons managing a variety of chronic medical conditions (Katon, 2003). Because HIV-positive individuals are at increased risk for developing an affective or adjustment disorder across the disease spectrum (Bing et al., 2001), effectively managing negative mood may be an especially relevant task. In fact, elevated negative mood may result in decrements in immune status, HIV disease progression, and mortality (Leserman, 2003). However, the directionality of this relationship has been hotly debated. Because clinically significant reductions in HIV viral load have been observed to predict decreased distress (Kalichman et al., 2002), longitudinal investigations with repeated measurements of psychosocial and immunologic data provide the most reliable findings on the temporal associations between negative mood and HIV disease progression. For example, depressive symptoms were associated with reductions in CD8+ and NK cell counts over a 2-year period, especially among those reporting more stressful life events (Leserman et al., 1997). Although depressive symptoms have been associated with more rapid CD4+ count decline in cohorts of HIV-positive men (Burack et al., 1993; Vedhara et al., 1997) and women (Ickovics et al., 2001), other longitudinal investigations that used *only* baseline measurements of depressive symptoms have not observed similar effects (Lyketsos et al., 1993; Patterson et al., 1996). Another investigation of HIV-positive men and women without AIDS indicated that the relationship between depression and cell-mediated immunity is observed only in participants with low levels of HIV viral burden (Motivala et al., 2003). Specifically, increased distress was associated with lower total CD4+, memory CD4+, and B-cell counts, but only in those with lower viral load (i.e., ≤1 standard deviation below the mean). These findings may partially explain the discrepant results regarding the association between depressive symptoms and CD4+ T-cell counts, suggesting that PNI associations may be more commonly observed at the earliest stages of disease.

Other investigations with HIV-positive women have shown that symptoms of depression and anxiety were associated with more CD8+38+ cells and higher HIV viral load (Evans et al., 2002). In this cross-sectional study, a diagnosis of major depression was also related to lower NK cell cytotoxicity. More importantly, women whose major depression resolved over time showed concurrent increases in NK cell cytotoxicity up to 2 years later (Cruess et al., 2005). The continued relevance of negative mood in the era of HAART is further supported by observations that cumulative depressive symptoms, hopelessness, and avoidant coping scores were associated with decreased CD4+ counts and higher HIV viral load over a 2-year period in a diverse sample of HIV-positive men and women (Ironson et al., 2005). These effects of negative mood and avoidant coping held after controlling for adherence to HAART.

Lending support to the clinical relevance of decrements in immune status are findings highlighting the association between depressive symptoms and disease end points. Specifically, depressive symptoms have been related to faster progression to AIDS (Page-Shafer et al., 1996; Leserman et al., 1999) and development of an AIDS-related clinical condition (Leserman et al., 2002). Other investigations have determined that chronically elevated depressive symptoms are associated with hastened mortality among HIV-positive men (Mayne et al., 1996) and women (Ickovics et al., 2001). Again, the majority of studies reporting no effect of depressive symptoms on hastened mortality used *only* baseline measures (Burack et al., 1993; Lyketsos et al., 1993; Page-Shafer et al., 1996). Interestingly, in a follow-up to one study in which no effects of baseline depressive symptoms were observed on HIV disease progression, participants reported a dramatic increase in depressive symptoms 6 to 18 months before an AIDS diagnosis (Lyketsos et al., 1996). Elevated depressive symptoms in the earlier stages of infection, HIV-related symptoms, unemployment, cigarette smoking, and social isolation were all associated with greater severity of depression as AIDS developed. However, increases in depressive symptomatology during this stage were not associated with mortality. While discrepant findings have been reported, it appears that depressive symptoms may be an important predictor of HIV disease progression. In particular, investigations examining the chronic nature of depressive symptoms over time have yielded the most consistent, replicable findings that demonstrate an effect of depressive symptoms on HIV disease progression.

Although relatively few studies have systematically examined other negative mood states, anger has been associated with faster progression to AIDS (Leserman et al., 2002). Anxiety symptoms have also been related to greater CD8+38+ T-cell counts and higher HIV viral load—both indicators of elevated disease activity (Evans et al., 2002). On the other side of the coin, results of a recent investigation indicate that enhanced positive affect is uniquely associated with longevity in a cohort of HIV-positive MSM (Moskowitz, 2003). Positive and negative affective states have previously been observed to co-occur (Folkman, 1997), and it appears that both states may have implications for HIV disease progression. Thus it is important to measure both positive and negative affect states—as well as positive and negative appraisal processes—when examining the immune and health correlates of individual difference variables in HIV-positive persons.

STRESS MANAGEMENT AND PSYCHIATRIC INTERVENTIONS

Stress management techniques such as relaxation training, cognitive restructuring, and coping skills training may reduce negative mood states in HIV-positive persons by lowering physical tension and increasing self-efficacy (Antoni, 2003a). These affective changes are thought to be accompanied by an improved ability to regulate peripheral catecholamines and cortisol via decreases in ANS activation and improved regulation of the HPA axis, respectively. Neuroendocrine regulation may be associated with a partial "normalization" of immune system functions, providing more efficient surveillance of pathogens such as latent viruses that may increase HIV replication and enhance vulnerability to opportunistic infections or neoplasias. This normalization of stress-associated immune system decrements may ultimately forestall increases in viral load and the manifestation of clinical symptoms over extended periods. A relatively small number of controlled trials have examined the effects of group-based stress management interventions on psychosocial and immune parameters in HIV-positive populations. There is mounting evidence that interventions employing stress management techniques enhance psychological adjustment, improve neuroendocrine regulation, and bolster immune status (Antoni, 2003a).

If stress management can modify negative mood by changing cognitive appraisals, coping responses and social support resources, then neuroendocrine changes and normalization of immune status may follow.

The modal stress management intervention tested in this regard is a 10-week cognitive behavioral stress management (CBSM) intervention for HIV-positive persons. Throughout previous trials, CBSM was tailored to psychosocial sequelae that may follow critical challenges for HIV-positive persons at various disease stages. In the initial trial, a cohort of 65 MSM awaiting HIV serostatus notification were randomly assigned to a 10-week CBSM intervention, a 10-week group-based aerobic exercise intervention, or a no-treatment control group. After 5 weeks of participating in one of these conditions, blood was drawn for antibody testing and the men received news of their HIV serostatus 72 hours later. Among the approximately one-third of men diagnosed as HIV positive (n = 23), those in the control condition reported significant increases in anxiety and depression. In contrast, men in the CBSM and aerobic exercise conditions showed no significant changes in anxiety or depression scores (LaPerriere et al., 1990; Antoni et al., 1991). Whereas HIV-positive men in the control condition showed declines in CD4+ and NK cell counts during this notification period, the HIV-positive men in CBSM displayed significant concurrent increases in CD4+ and NK cell counts as well as small increases in lymphocyte proliferative responses to mitogenic challenge and NK cell cytotoxicity. Thus, CBSM appears to have to "buffered" the notification-associated affective and immunologic changes (Antoni et al., 1991).

There were also changes in indicators of antiviral immunity over the 10-week intervention period. Men assigned to either CBSM or exercise interventions showed significant decreases in IgG antibody titers (reflecting better immunologic control) to EBV and HHV-6, which moved into the normal range for age-matched healthy men. This was in contrast to IgG antibody titer values for assessment-only controls, which remained elevated (Esterling et al., 1992). The reductions in EBV IgG antibody titers in the CBSM group appeared to be mediated by the greater social support levels maintained in this condition (Antoni et al., 1996). Finally, a 2-year follow-up of the HIV-positive men in this trial found that less distress at diagnosis, decreased HIV-specific denial coping after diagnosis, and better participant adherence to CBSM treatment protocol all predicted slower disease progression to symptoms and AIDS (Ironson et al., 1994).

Another 10-week, group-based intervention designed to provide emotional support and coping skills after bereavement was tested in a cohort of 97 HIV-positive asymptomatic MSM dealing with loss. Results of this trial indicated that the bereavement intervention decreased grief and buffered CD4+ decline, and reduced plasma cortisol as well as the number of health care visits over a 6-month period, compared to a no-treatment control condition (Goodkin et al., 1998). In a subset of 36 men, the bereavement intervention also buffered against increases in HIV viral load (Goodkin et al., 2001). Therefore, group-based psychosocial interventions may be adaptable and successful in helping HIV-positive persons deal with different emotional challenges during the early asymptomatic stage of the infection.

In a subsequent trial of CBSM, this intervention was tailored to assist HIV-positive persons in managing the emergence of symptoms. HIV-positive MSM who had mild symptoms (category B of the 1993 CDC definition) were randomly assigned to either a 10-week group-based CBSM intervention or a modified wait-list control group. Men in the wait-list control group completed a 10-week waiting period before they were reassessed and invited to participate in a 1-day CBSM seminar. Results indicated that CBSM decreased depressive symptoms, anxiety, and mood disturbance over the 10-week intervention period (Lutgendorf et al., 1997, 1998). Decreases in depressive symptoms and enhanced social support over the 10-week intervention period partially explained concurrent reductions in HSV-2 IgG antibody titers (Lutgendorf et al., 1997; Cruess et al., 2000c). Subsequently, a buffering effect of CBSM on EBV IgG antibody titers was observed up to 1 year following CBSM (Carrico et al., 2005a). Similar to previous investigations with asymptomatic HIV-positive MSM (Antoni et al., 1996), intervention effects of EBV IgG antibody titers paralleled sustained increases in social support for men randomized to CBSM (Carrico et al., 2005a).

According to a theoretical model (Antoni et al, 1990; Antoni, 2003b) we reasoned that CBSM-related reductions in multiple indices of negative mood should be accompanied by concurrent changes in neuroendocrine regulation that could influence immune system status in this population. CBSM effects on neuroendocrine regulation have been observed in a number of studies, and these effects have been associated with changes in both affective and cellular-immune parameters (Antoni, 2003b). Specifically, CBSM effects on distress have been observed to co-vary with decreases in 24-hour urinary-free cortisol (Antoni et al., 2000b). Lending further support to the PNI model underlying this work, subsequent investigations have determined that reductions in depressed mood and 24-hour urinary-free cortisol during the 10-week intervention period mediate CBSM effects on recovery of transitional naïve T-cell counts over a 6- to 12-month follow-up period (Antoni et al., 2005).

Similarly, reductions in anxiety during the 10-week intervention period have been observed to co-vary with decreases in 24-hour norepinepherine. These intervention-related reductions in norepinepherine mediated the effect of CBSM on maintaining CD8+ T-cell counts through a 6- to 12-month follow-up (Antoni et al., 2000a). This buffering effect was such that men in the control condition had significant declines, while those in the CBSM group maintained CD8+ counts at the same level. CBSM has also been associated with plasma cortisol/DHEA-S decreases (Cruess et al., 1999) and testosterone increases in HIV+ MSM (Cruess et al., 2000d), which paralleled decreases in depressed mood over the 10-week intervention period. Taken together, this series of studies suggests that CBSM may affect hormonal regulation to promote herpesvirus surveillance and immune system reconstitution among HIV-positive MSM. By examining relations among PNI variables changing during the course of these interventions and at follow-up, we have found evidence that meaningful psychological and biological changes may be attributed to the stress management skills learned and the social support increases experienced as a result of participating in these groups (Lutgendorf et al., 1997; Cruess et al., 2000c).

In the HAART era, a variety of behavioral interventions for HIV-positive persons have been developed specifically to support medication adherence. Although psychological adjustment has not been uniformly conceptualized as a mechanism of enhanced adherence, research has supported the efficacy of pharmacist-led, individualized medication adherence training (MAT) interventions and those that employ cognitive-behavioral principles based on self-efficacy theory (Simoni et al., 2003). Consequently, we theorized that a modified form of CBSM may offer benefits in improving mood, health behaviors, and immune status in the era of HAART. In order to test the added value associated with providing stress management training, 130 HIV-positive MSM were recruited for a trial in which the combination of CBSM and MAT (i.e., CBSM+MAT) was compared to MAT alone. In an intent-to-treat analysis, we observed no intervention-related changes in immune status. However, in a secondary analysis with 101 men who had a detectable HIV viral load at baseline, we observed a .56 $\log_{10}$ reduction in HIV viral load over the 15-month investigation period, after controlling for anti-retroviral medication adherence. This clinically interesting effect of CBSM+MAT on HIV viral load was mediated by reductions in depressed mood during the 10-week intervention period. Importantly, these findings held even after controlling for adherence training exposure (each group received MAT) and statistically controlling for individual differences in reported adherence at each time point (Antoni et al., 2006). Thus, there appears to be some added value of reducing depressed mood in persons dealing with the complexities of HAART treatment. It is plausible that reducing depressed mood confers beneficial effects on viral load management by way of *health behavior pathways* (reduced substance use, improved sleep, and less exposure to sexually transmitted infections) and/or PNI *pathways* (better antiviral immunity against coinfections or less neuroendocrine-mediated HIV replication). It remains for future research to incorporate measures of PNI variables as well as indicators of HIV viral load and genetic resistance over extended periods as individuals on multidrug regimens participate in well-controlled psychosocial intervention trials.

It is plausible that an equally efficient strategy for conducting PNI research in HIV-positive individuals is to examine concurrent changes in mood, neuroendocrine, immune, and viral processes in the context of randomized trials of mood-modulating pharmacologic treatments. The work outlined in Chapters 11 and 32 elaborates on some of the contemporary pharmacological strategies available for addressing depressed mood and anxiety symptoms in HIV-positive persons. This seems like a logical starting point for designing future PNI studies that capitalize on the power of a randomized trial. This research approach offers the additional benefit of using a blinded-placebo design, a feature that has been elusive in psychosocial intervention trials.

CONCLUSIONS

If stress and psychiatric symptoms indeed have a negative influence on immune status and medical outcome among people living with HIV/AIDS, this phenomenon may actually be even more relevant since the introduction of HAART. Prior to the availability of these potent antiretroviral regimens, the devastating effects of the HIV may have overshadowed the effects of any other deleterious factors on the immune system. In the HAART era, however, the magnitude of the effects of psychological and behavioral factors on the immune system could be increased, and this may have important implications for health outcomes. The studies reviewed in this chapter suggest that stress and psychiatric symptoms are nontrivial co-factors in HIV disease progression; consequently, getting a definitive answer to these issues is imperative. If this effect is clinically significant, an important remaining question is whether interventions (with psychotherapy and/or medication) decrease HIV-associated morbidity and improve health outcomes.

References

Antoni MH (2003a). Stress management and psychoneuroimmunology in HIV infection. *CNS Spectrums* 8:40–51.

Antoni MH (2003b). Stress management effects on psychological, endocrinological and immune function in men with HIV: empirical support for a psychoneuroimmunological model. *Stress* 6:173–188.

Antoni MH, and Schneiderman N (1998). HIV/AIDS. In A Bellack and M Hersen (eds.), *Comprehensive Clinical Psychology* (pp. 237–275). New York: Elsevier Science.

Antoni M, August S, LaPerriere A, Baggett H.L, Klimas N, Ironson G, et al. (1990). Psychological and neuroendocrine measures related to functional immune changes in anticipation of HIV-1 serostatus notification. *Psychosom Med* 52:496–510.

Antoni MH, Baggett L, Ironson G, August S, LaPerriere A, Klimas N, et al. (1991). Cognitive behavioral stress management intervention buffers distress responses and immunologic changes following notification of HIV-1 seropositivity. *J Consult Clin Psychol* 59:906–915.

Antoni MH, Lutgendorf S, Ironson G, Fletcher M.A, and Schneiderman N (1996). CBSM intervention effects on social support, coping, depression and immune function in symptomatic HIV-infected men. *Psychosom Med* 58:86.

Antoni MH, Cruess DG, Cruess S, Lutgendorf S, Kumar M, et al. (2000a). Cognitive behavioral stress management intervention effects on anxiety, 24-hour urinary catecholamine output, and T-cytotoxic/suppressor cells over time among symptomatic HIV-infected gay men. *J Consult Clin Psychol* 68:31–46.

Antoni MH, Wagner S, Cruess D, Kumar M, Lutgendorf S, Ironson G, et al. (2000b). Cognitive behavioral stress management reduces distress and 24-hour urinary free cortisol among symptomatic HIV-infected gay men. *Ann Behav Med* 22:29–37.

Antoni MH, Cruess D, Klimas N, Carrico AW, Maher K, Cruess S, et al. (2005). Increases in a marker of immune system reconstitution are predated by decreases in 24-hour urinary cortisol output and depressed mood during a 10-week stress management intervention in symptomatic HIV-infected gay men. *J Psychosom Res* 58:3–13.

Antoni MH, Carrico AW, Durán RE, Spitzer S, Penedo F, Ironson G, et al. (2006). Randomized clinical trial of cognitive behavioral stress management on human immunodeficiency virus viral load in gay men treated with highly active antiretroviral therapy. *Psychosom Med* 68:143–151.

Bangsberg DR, Perry S, Charlebois ED, Clark RA, Robertson M, Zolopa AR, et al. (2001). Nonadherence to highly active antiretroviral therapy predicts progression to AIDS. *AIDS* 15:1181–1183.

Bing EG, Burnam MA, Longshore D, Fleishman JA, Sherbourne CD, London, AS, et al. (2001). Psychiatric disorders and drug use among human immunodeficiency virus–infected adults in the United States. *Arch Gen Psychiatry* 58:721–728.

Bower JE, Kemeny ME, Taylor SE, and Fahey JL (1998). Cognitive processing, discovery of meaning, CD4 decline, and AIDS-related mortality among bereaved HIV-seropositive men. *J Consult Clin Psychol* 66:979–986.

Burack JH, Barrett DC, Stall RD, Chesney MA, Ekstrand ML, and Coates TJ (1993). Depressive symptoms and CD4 lymphocyte decline among HIV-infected men. *JAMA* 270:2568–2573.

Byrnes DM, Antoni MH, Goodkin K, Effantis-Potter J, Asthana D, Simon T, et al. (1998). Stressful events, pessimism, natural killer cell cytotoxicity, and cytotoxic/suppressor T cells in HIV+ black women at risk for cervical cancer. *Psychosom Med* 60:714–722.

Carrico AW, Antoni MH, Pereira DB, Fletcher MA, Klimas N, Lechner SC, et al. (2005a). Cognitive behavioral stress management effects on mood, social support, and a marker of anti-viral immunity are maintained up to one year in HIV-infected gay men. *Int J Behav Med* 12:218–226.

Carrico AW, Antoni MH, Weaver KE, Lechner SC, and Schneiderman N (2005b). Cognitive-behavioural stress management with HIV-positive homosexual men: mechanisms of sustained reductions in depressive symptoms. *Chronic Illness* 1:207–215.

Carrico AW, Ironson G, Antoni MH, Lechner SC, Durán RE, Kumar M, et al. (2006). A path model of the effects of spirituality on depressive symptoms and 24-hour urinary-free cortisol in HIV-positive persons. *J Psychosom Res* 61(1):51–58.

Centers for Disease Control and Prevention (1997). Update: trends in AIDS incidence, deaths, and prevalence—United States, 1996. *MMWR Morbid Mortal Wkly Rep* 46(8):165–174.

Cielsa JA, and Roberts JE (2001). Meta-analysis of the relationship between HIV infection and the risk for depressive disorders. *Am J Psychiatry* 158:725–730.

Cole SW, and Kemeny ME (2001). Psychosocial influences on the progression of HIV infection. In R Ader, DL Felten, and S Cohen (eds.), *Psychoneuroimmunology*, third edition. San Diego: Academic Press.

Cole SW, Korin YD, Fahey JL, and Zack JA (1998). Norepinephrine accelerates HIV replication via protein kinase A–dependent effects on cytokine production. *J Immunol* 161:610–616.

Cole SW, Naliboff BD, Kemeny ME, Griswold MP, Fahey JL, and Zack JA (2001). Impaired response to HAART in HIV-infected individuals with high autonomic nervous system activity. *Proc Natl Acad Sci USA* 98:12695–12700.

Cole SW, Kemeny ME, Fahey JL, Zack JA, and Naliboff BD (2003). Psychological risk factors for HIV pathogenesis: mediation by the autonomic nervous system. *Biol Psychiatry*, 54:1444–1456.

Cruess D, Antoni MH, Schneiderman N, Ironson G, Fletcher MA, and Kumar, M (1999). Cognitive behavioral stress management effects on DHEA-S and serum cortisol in HIV seropositive men. *Psychoneuroendocrinology* 24:537–549.

Cruess S, Antoni MH, Cruess D, Fletcher MA, Ironson G, Kumar M, et al. (2000c). Reductions in HSV-2 antibody titers after cognitive behavioral stress management and relationships with neuroendocrine function, relaxation skills, and social support in HIV+ gay men. *Psychosom Med* 62:828–837.

Cruess S, Antoni M, Kilbourn K, Ironson G, Klimas N, Fletcher M.A, et al. (2000b). Optimism, distress, and immunologic status in HIV-infected gay men following Hurricane Andrew. *Int J Behav Med* 7:160–182.

Cruess DG, Antoni MH, McGregor BA, Kilbourn KM, Boyers AE, Alferi SM, et al. (2000a). Cognitive-behavioral stress management reduces serum cortisol by enhancing benefit finding among women being treated for early stage breast cancer. *Psychosom Med* 62:304–308.

Cruess D, Antoni MH, Schneiderman N, Ironson G, McCabe P, Fernandez J, et al. (2000d). Cognitive behavioral stress management increases free testosterone and decreases psychological distress in HIV seropositive men. *Health Psychol* 19:12–20.

Cruess DG, Douglas SD, Petitto JM, Leserman JL, Have TLT, Gettes DL, et al. (2003). Association of depression, CD8 T lymphocytes, and natural killer

cell activity: Implications for morbidity and mortality in human immunodeficiency virus disease. *Curr Psychiatry Rep* 5:445–450.

Cruess DG, Douglas SD, Petitto JM, Have TT, Gettes D, Dube B, et al. (2005). Association of resolution of major depression with increased natural killer cell activity among HIV-seropositive women. *Am J Psychiatry* 162:2125–2130.

Esterling B, Antoni M, Schneiderman N, Ironson G, LaPerriere A, Klimas N, et al. (1992). Psychosocial modulation of antibody to Epstein-Barr viral capsid antigen and herpes virus type-6 in HIV-1 infected and at-risk gay men. *Psychosom Med* 54:354–371.

Evans DL, Ten Have TR, Douglas SD, Gettes D, Morrison CH, Chiappini MS, et al. (2002). Association of depression with viral load, CD8 T lymphocytes, and natural killer cells in women with HIV infection. *Am J Psychiatry* 159:1752–1759.

Felten D (1996). Changes in neural innervation of the lymphoid tissues with age. In N Hall, F Altman, and S Blumenthal (eds.), *Mind–Body Interactions and Disease and Psychoneuroimmunological Aspects of Health and Disease*. Washington, DC: Health Dateline Press.

Folkman S (1997) Positive psychological states and coping with severe stress. *Soc Sci Med* 45(8):1207–1221.

Gillespie CF, and Nemeroff CB (2005). Hypercortisolemia and depression. *Psychosom Med* (Suppl. 1): S26–S27.

Goodkin K, Feaster DJ, Tuttle R, Blaney NT, Kumar M, Baum MK, et al. (1996). Bereavement is associated with time-dependent decrements in cellular immune function in asymptomatic human immunodeficiency virus type 1-seropositive homosexual men. *Clin Diagn Lab Immunol* 3:109–118.

Goodkin K, Feaster D, Asthana D, Blaney NT, Kumar M, Baldewicz T, et al. (1998). A bereavement support group intervention is longitudinally associated with salutary effects on the CD4 cell count and number of physician visits. *Clin Diagn Lab Immunol* 5:382–391.

Goodkin K, Baldewicz T, Asthana D, Khanis I, Blaney N, Kumar M, et al. (2001). A bereavement support group intervention affects plasma burden of HIV-1. *J Hum Virol* 4:44–54.

Gorman JM, Kertzner R, Cooper T, Goetz RR, Lagomasino I, Novacenko H, et al. (1991). Glucocorticoid level and neuropsychiatric symptoms in homosexual men with HIV infection. *Am J Psychiatry* 148:41–45.

Hurwitz BE, Brownley KA, Motivala SJ, Milanovich JR, Kibler JL, Fillion L, et al. (2005). Sympathoimmune anomalies underlying the response to stressful challenge in human immunodeficiency virus spectrum disease. *Psychosom Med* 67:798–806.

Ickovics JR, Hamburger ME, Vlahov D, Schoenbaum EE, Schuman P, Boland RJ, et al. (2001). Mortality, CD4 cell count decline, and depressive symptoms among HIV-seropositive women: Longitudinal analysis from the HIV Epidemiology Research Study. *JAMA* 285:1460–1465.

Ironson G, LaPerriere A, Antoni M, O'Hearn P, Schneiderman N, Klimas N, et al. (1990). Changes in immune and psychological measures as a function of anticipation and reaction to the news of HIV-1 antibody status. *Psychosom Med* 52:247–270.

Ironson G, Friedman A, Klimas N, Antoni M, Fletcher M.A, LaPerriere A, et al. (1994). Distress, denial and low adherence to behavioral interventions predict faster disease progression in gay men infected with human immunodeficiency virus. *Int J Behav Med* 1:90–105.

Ironson G, Balbin G, Solomon G, Fahey J, Klimas N, Schneiderman N, et al. (2001). Relative preservation of natural killer cell cytotoxicity and number in healthy AIDS patients with low CD4 cell counts. *AIDS* 15:2065–2073.

Ironson G, Solomon GF, Balbin EG, O'Cleirigh CO, George A, Kumar M, et al. (2002). The Ironson-Woods Spirituality/Religiousness Index is associated with long survival, health behaviors, less distress, and low cortisol in people with HIV/AIDS. *Ann Behav Med* 24:34–48.

Ironson G, O'Cleirigh C, Fletcher MA, Laurenceau JP, Balbin E, Klimas N, et al. (2005). Psychosocial factors predict CD4 and viral load change in men and women with human immunodeficiency virus in the era of highly active antiretroviral therapy. *Psychosom Med* 67:1013–1021.

Kalichman SC, Difonzo K, Austin J, Luke W, and Rompa D (2002). Prospective study of emotional reactions to changes in HIV viral load. *AIDS Patient Care STDS* 16:113–120.

Katon WJ (2003). Clinical and health services relationships between major depression, depressive symptoms and general medical illness. *Biological Psychiatry* 54:295–306.

Kawa SK, and Thompson EB (1996). Lymphoid cell resistance to glucocorticoids in HIV infection. *J Steroid Biochem Mol Biol* 57:259–263.

Kiecolt-Glaser JK, McGuire L, Robles TF, and Glaser R (2002). Psychoneuroimmunology: Psychological influences on immune function and health. *J Consult Clin Psychol* 70:537–547.

Kemeny ME, and Dean L (1995). Effects of AIDS-related bereavement on HIV progression among New York City gay men. *AIDS Educ Prev* 7(5 Suppl.): 36–47.

Kemeny ME, Weiner H, Durán R, Taylor SE, Visscher B, and Fahey JL (1995). Immune system changes after the death of a partner in HIV-positive gay men. *Psychosom Med* 57:547–554.

Kimmerling R, Calhoun KS, Forehand R, Armistead L, Morse E, Morse P, et al. (1999). Traumatic stress in HIV-infected women. *AIDS Educ Prev* 11:321–330.

Kobilka B (1992). Adrenergic receptors as models for G-protein coupled receptors. *Annu Rev Neurosci* 15:87–114.

Kumar M, Kumar AM, Morgan R, Szapocznik J, and Eisdorfer C (1993). Abnormal pituitary-adrenocortical response in early HIV-1 infection. *J Acquir Immune Defic Syndr Hum Retrovirol* 6:61–65.

LaPerriere A, Antoni MH, Schneiderman N, Ironson G, Klimas N, Caralis P, et al. (1990). Exercise intervention attenuates emotional distress and natural killer cell decrements following notification of positive serologic status for HIV-1. *Biofeedback Self Regul* 15:125–131.

Ledergerber B, Egger M, Erard V, Weber R, Hirschel B, Furrer H, et al. (1999). AIDS-related opportunistic illnesses occurring after the initiation of potent antiretroviral therapy: The Swiss Cohort Study. *JAMA* 282:2220–2226.

Lederman MM, and Valdez H (2000). Immune restoration with antiretroviral therapies: Implications for clinical management. *JAMA* 284:223–228.

Leserman J (2003). HIV disease progression: depression, stress, and possible mechanisms. *Biol Psychiatry* 54:295–306.

Leserman J, Petitto JM, Perkins DO, Folds JD, Golden RN, and Evans DL (1997). Severe stress and depressive symptoms, and changes in lymphocyte subsets in human immunodeficiency virus infected men. *Arch Gen Psychiatry* 54:279–285.

Leserman J, Jackson ED, Petitto JM, Golden RN, Silva SG, Perkins DO, et al. (1999). Progression to AIDS: the effects of stress, depressive symptoms and social support. *Psychosom Med* 61:397–406.

Leserman J, Petitto JM, Golden RN, Gaynes BN, Gu H, Perkins DO, et al. (2000). Impact of stressful life events, depression, social support, coping, and cortisol on progression to AIDS. *Am J Psychiatry* 157:1221–1228.

Leserman J, Petitto JM, Gu H, Gaynes BN, Barroso J, Golden RN, et al. (2002). Progression to AIDS, a clinical AIDS condition and mortality: psychosocial and physiological predictors. *Psychol Med* 32:1059–1073.

Lutgendorf S, Antoni M, Ironson G, Klimas N, Kumar M, Starr K, et al. (1997). Cognitive behavioral stress management decreases dysphoric mood and herpes simplex virus-type 2 antibody titers in symptomatic HIV-seropositive gay men. *J Consult Clin Psychol* 65:31–43.

Lutgendorf SK, Antoni MH, Ironson G, Starr K, Costello N, Zuckerman M, et al. (1998). Changes in cognitive coping skills and social support during cognitive behavioral stress management intervention and distress outcomes in symptomatic human immunodeficiency virus-seropositive gay men. *Psychosom Med* 60:204–214.

Lyketsos CG, Hoover DR, Guccione M, Senterfitt W, Dew MA, Wesch J, et al. (1993). Depressive symptoms as predictors of medical outcomes in HIV infection. *JAMA* 270:2563–2567.

Lyketsos CG, Hoover DR, Guccione M, Dew MA, Wesch JE, Bing EG, et al. (1996). Changes in depressive symptoms as AIDS develops. The Multicenter AIDS Cohort Study. *Am J Psychiatry* 153: 1430–1437.

Mannheimer SB, Matts J, Telzak E, Chesney M, Child C, Wu AW, et al. (2005). Quality of life in HIV-infected individuals receiving antiretroviral therapy is related to adherence. *AIDS Care* 17:10–22.

Martin JL, and Dean L (1993). Effects of AIDS-related bereavement and HIV-related illness on psychological distress among gay men: a 7-year longitudinal study, 1985–1991. *J Consult Clin Psychol* 61:94–103.

Mayne TJ, Vittinghoff E, Chesney MA, Barrett DC, and Coates TJ (1996). Depressive affect and survival among gay and bisexual men infected with HIV. *Arch Intern Med* 156:2233–2238.

McEwen B (1998). Protective and damaging effects of stress mediators. *N Engl J Med* 338:171–179.

Moskowitz JT (2003). Positive affect predicts lower risk of AIDS mortality. *Psychosom Med* 65:620–626.

Motivala SJ, Hurwitz BE, Llabre MM, Klimas N, Fletcher MA, Antoni MH, et al. (2003). Psychological distress is associated with decreased memory helper T-cell and B-cell counts in pre-AIDS HIV seropositive men and women but only in those with low viral load. *Psychosom Med* 65:627–635.

Page-Shafer K, Delorenze GN, Satariano W, and Winkelstein W (1996). Comorbidity and survival in HIV-infected men in the San Francisco Men's Health Survey. *Ann Epidemiol* 6:420–430.

Patterson TL, Williams SS, Semple SJ, Cherner M, McCutchman A, Atkinson JH, et al. (1996). Relationship of psychosocial factors to HIV disease progression. *Ann Behav Med* 18:30–39.

Pereira DB, Antoni MH, Danielson A, Simon T, Efantis-Potter J, Carver CS, et al. (2003a). Stress as a predictor of symptomatic genital herpes virus recurrence in women with human immunodeficiency virus. *J Psychosom Res* 54:237–244.

Pereira DB, Antoni MH, Danielson A, Simon T, Efantis-Potter J, Carver CS, et al. (2003b). Life stress and cervical squamous intraepithelial lesions in women with human papillomavirus and human immunodeficiency virus. *Psychosom Med* 65:427–434.

Rabkin JG, Ferrando SJ, Lin SH, Sewell M, and McElihney M (2000). Psychological effects of HAART: A 2-year study. *Psychosom Med* 62:413–422.

Reed GM, Kemeny ME, Taylor SE, Wang HYJ, and Visscher BR (1994). Realistic acceptance as a predictor of decreased survival time in gay men with AIDS. *Health Psychol* 13:299–307.

Reed GM, Kemeny ME, Taylor SE, and Visscher BR (1999). Negative HIV-specific expectancies and AIDS-related bereavement as predictors of symptoms onset in asymptomatic HIV-positive gay men. *Health Psychol* 18:354–363.

Schneiderman N, Antoni MH, Ironson G, Fletcher MA, Klimas N, and LaPerriere A (1994). HIV-1, immunity and behavior. In R Glaser (ed.), *Handbook of Human Stress and Immunity*. New York: Academic Press.

Segerstrom SC, Taylor SE, Kemeny ME, Reed GM, and Visscher BR (1996). Causal attributions predict rate of immune decline in HIV-seropositive gay men. *Health Psychol* 15:485–493.

Simoni JM, Frick PA, Pantalone DW, and Turner BJ (2003). Antiretroviral adherence interventions: a review of current literature and ongoing studies. *Topics HIV Med* 11:185–197.

Starr KR, Antoni MH, Hurwitz BE, Rodriguez MS, Ironsong G, Fletcher MA, et al. (1996). Patterns of immune, neuroendocrine, and cardiovascular stress responses in asymptomatic HIV serpositive and seronegative men. *Int J Behav Med* 3:135–162.

Tamalet C, Fantini J, Tourres C, and Yashi N (2003). Resistance of HIV-1 to multiple antiretroviral drugs in France: a 6-year survey (1997–2002) based on an analysis of over 7000 genotypes. *AIDS* 17:2383–2388.

Taylor SE, Kemeny ME, Reed GM, Bower JE, and Gruenewald TL (2000). Psychological resources, positive illusions, and health. *Am Psychol* 55: 99–109.

Vedhara K, Nott KH, Bradbeer CS, Davidson EAF, Ong ELC, Snow MH, et al. (1997). Greater emotional distress is associated with accelerated CD4+ cell decline in HIV infection. *J Psychosom Res* 42:379–390.

Volberding PA (2003). HIV therapy in 2003: consensus and controversy. *AIDS* 17(Suppl. 1):S4–S11.

Yeni PG, Hammer SM, Hirsch MS, Saag MS, Schechter M, Carpenter CC, et al. (2004). Treatment for adult HIV infection: 2004 recommendations of the International AIDS Society–USA Panel. *JAMA* 292:251–265.

Chapter 4

Epidemiology of Psychiatric Disorders Associated with HIV and AIDS

Francine Cournos and Karen McKinnon

Mental health problems can occur as risk factors for HIV infection, coincidentally with HIV infection, or as a result of HIV infection and its complications; they are associated with HIV transmission, poor disease prognosis, and poor adherence to antiretroviral regimens (Cournos et al., 2005). The majority of HIV-infected individuals will experience a diagnosable psychiatric disorder (Stoff et al., 2004). Further, the human immunodeficiency virus infects the brain, and a variety of central nervous system complications result. These conditions position psychiatrists and other mental health care providers squarely in charge of treatment decisions that affect the course of patients' illness, the quality of their lives, and, ultimately, containment of the epidemic. HIV-related psychiatric disorders are highly treatable, but they offer a challenge to clinicians in terms of differential diagnosis and management. An understanding of the epidemiology of HIV-related psychiatric disorders can help clinicians gauge the likelihood that symptoms they are presented with are a function of HIV infection and help them intervene in ways that minimize further spread of the virus and its devastating effects on the brain and body.

Epidemiology refers to the incidence, distribution, and control of disease in a population. With respect to HIV, incidence studies of psychiatric disorders are rare, so for our purposes we will focus on the distribution of psychiatric conditions (i.e., their prevalence) across the populations in which they've been studied and on what psychiatrists and other clinicians can do to control the impact of these conditions on people affected by them.

We correctly have moved away from the concept of risk groups, because anyone who engages in risky sexual and drug use behaviors may acquire or transmit HIV. Nonetheless, it remains true that most countries currently have epidemics that are concentrated in vulnerable populations such as injection drug users (IDUs), men who have sex with men (MSM), and sex workers

TABLE 4.1. Substance Use and Other Mental Health Disorders in Concentrated HIV Epidemics

- Injection drug users: high rates of addictive and other psychiatric disorders.
- Men who have sex with men: elevated rates of alcohol/substance use disorders and depression
- Sex workers: high rates of childhood sexual abuse; elevated rates of addictive disorders and post-traumatic stress disorder

(SWs). All three of these vulnerable populations have elevated rates of specific psychiatric disorders (Table 4.1) that may be related to their disenfranchisement from the dominant culture and to the corresponding stigma, legal and other sanctions, and poor access to prevention services. Each of these factors is associated with increased risk behaviors (Cournos et al., 2005).

Underlying the daunting task of preventing the spread of HIV within and beyond vulnerable populations are numerous structural factors, including social discrimination, political indifference or oppression, poverty, and violence. Fundamental changes in behavior within entire populations need to occur, and mental health must become part of the fabric of public health initiatives to accomplish this task. Models of behavior change need to be incorporated into prevention initiatives to understand what motivates people to engage in risky behavior, what incentives are available to change such behavior, and what skills are needed to implement and maintain safer practices. In addition, detecting, understanding, and treating behavioral and psychiatric problems that interfere with safer practices or even promote unsafe practices must be a priority.

This chapter covers rates of psychiatric disorders among people with HIV infection. All prevalences cited in this chapter were derived from U.S. studies unless otherwise stated. We begin with prevalent neuropsychiatric manifestations of HIV's direct effects on the central nervous system. We then discuss the most commonly seen psychiatric disorders among people with HIV in the United States: substance abuse or dependence; depression; anxiety; and psychosis. We also discuss significant psychiatric comorbidities. In addition, we describe what is known about rates of HIV infection among people with substance use disorders and among people with other psychiatric disorders. Where striking or illuminating, we discuss international patterns. We conclude with a delineation of services psy-

chiatrists and other mental health practitioners can provide to help to contain the epidemic and to improve care to their patients.

NEUROPSYCHIATRIC MANIFESTATIONS OF HIV INFECTION

HIV is a neurotropic virus that enters the central nervous system at the time of initial infection and persists there. Subtle neuropsychological impairment may be found in 22% to 30% of otherwise asymptomatic patients with HIV infection (Wilkie et al., 1990; White et al., 1995); these findings may or may not have functional significance. Neuropsychiatric complications of the direct effects of HIV in the brain become more frequent as illness advances (Bartlett and Ferrando, 2004). Common problems include decreased attention and concentration, psychomotor slowing, reduced speed of information processing, executive dysfunction, and, in more advanced cases, verbal memory impairment (Bartlett and Ferrando, 2004). Neuropsychiatric manifestations occur with a range of severity varying from subclinical to specific disorders that include, most commonly, minor cognitive-motor disorder (MCMD) and HIV-associated dementia (HAD). Psychiatric illnesses associated with HAD, where symptoms range from apathy and depression to mania and psychosis, mimic functional psychiatric disorders and require a thorough differential diagnosis. Neuropsychiatric manifestations of HIV are diagnoses of exclusion and the clinician must first eliminate all other possible medical causes, including opportunistic infections, metabolic problems, side effects of antiretrovirals, and substance intoxication or withdrawal. This is an essential task, given that a variety of untreated medical problems can cause irreversible neuronal damage.

Minor Cognitive-Motor Disorder

This disorder has a clinical course and onset that can vary; its diagnosis can be missed, and it does not necessarily progress to dementia. It is characterized by mild impairment in functioning, impaired attention or concentration, memory problems, low energy and/or slowed movements, impaired coordination, and personality change, irritability, or emotional lability. The prevalence of MCMD has been estimated at 20% to 30% for asymptomatic clients and at 60% to 90% for late-stage clients (Goodkin et al., 1997); these rates have remained fairly constant both prior to and after HAART (Neuenberg et al., 2002).

HIV-Associated Dementia

While the prevalence of HAD in the past was estimated to be 15% to 20% of all AIDS patients (Simpson, 1999), the incidence of HAD appears to have been affected by the use of potent combination therapies, and current studies estimate its prevalence at 5% to 10% (Sacktor et al., 1999) since the introduction of combination antiretroviral treatment in 1996. The incidence of HAD reportedly decreased from 21.1/1000 person-years in 1990–1992 to 14.7/1000 person-years in 1995–1997 (Dore et al., 1999; Sacktor et al., 1999). Among patients who received combination antiretroviral treatment, by contrast, the proportion of HAD as a percentage of all AIDS-defining illnesses rose from 4.4% to 6.5% between 1995 and 1997 (Dore et al., 1999). This shift is thought to reflect the decrease in rates of other AIDS-defining conditions, thereby leading to the relative rise in HAD cases.

It is worth noting that the classification of these neuropsychiatric manifestations of HIV infection is undergoing revision after a joint conference of the National Institute of Mental Health and the National Institute of Neurological Disorders and Stroke on June 13, 2005, identified and defined criteria for three levels of HIV-associated neurocognitive disorders or conditions: asymptomatic neurocognitive impairment, mild neurocognitive disorder (previously MCMD), and HIV-associated dementia. Clinicians should update themselves regularly by accessing Web sites such as that of the American Psychiatric Association's Office of HIV Psychiatry (www.psych.org/hiv), which has downloadable curricula on the complete array of HIV-related neuropsychiatric conditions.

One further word about neuropsychiatric manifestations of HIV: hepatitis C virus (HCV) is highly comorbid with HIV, and HCV can create its own neuropsychiatric problems as well as exacerbate those caused by HIV. Screening for HCV is relatively straightforward, but current therapy for HCV infection is poorly tolerated and not effective for a substantial number of patients (Wainberg et al., 2003). Approximately four million people in the United States and probably more than 100 million worldwide are infected with HCV, yet it has been estimated that less than 30% of people with HCV know they are infected (National Institutes of Health Consensus Development Conference Panel, 1997). HCV is an important diagnosis of exclusion when treating neuropsychiatric complications of HIV.

RATES OF PSYCHIATRIC DISORDERS AMONG PEOPLE LIVING WITH HIV INFECTION

Accuracy of available prevalence estimates is unclear because most studies of psychiatric disorders among people with HIV used convenience samples, often of the historic risk groups, had small sample sizes, or were confined to specific geographical areas. Population-based estimates of psychiatric disorders among HIV-positive people are scarce.

The landmark HIV Cost and Services Utilization Study (HCSUS) found that a large, nationally representative probability sample of adults receiving medical care for HIV in the United States in early 1996 (N = 2,864: 2,017 men, 847 women) reported major depression (36%), anxiety disorder (16%), and drug dependence (12%) (Bing et al., 2001; Galvan et al., 2002), as well as heavy drinking at a rate (8%) almost twice that found in the general population and high rates of drug use (50%). The HCSUS study remains the most comprehensive view we have of the prevalence of psychiatric disorders among people living with HIV/AIDS, though the study was not designed as a diagnostic assessment of psychiatric disorders among people with HIV/AIDS and so rates of psychosis, bipolar disorder, alcohol abuse or dependence, and substance abuse, among others, were not obtained. Disorders of alcohol and other drug (AOD) abuse are differentiated from dependence in the *Diagnostic and Statistical Manual of Mental Disorders* (currently in version IV-R) in terms of intensity and duration of use, with dependence indicating a greater severity of addiction. The HCSUS study reported different use thresholds for alcohol than for other substances. Another important aspect of the HCSUS study is that people with HIV who are receiving medical care may be different from those not receiving medical care in terms of underlying comorbidities and their impact on illness progression.

Hospital admissions for AIDS-related illnesses decreased soon after the introduction of highly active antiretroviral therapy (HAART), but a recent study of hospitalizations of 8376 patients in six U.S. HIV care sites showed that among patients hospitalized at least once, the third most common admission diagnosis after AIDS-defining illnesses (21%) and gastrointestinal disorders (9.5%) was a mental illness (9%) (Betz et al., 2005). This study also found that compared with Caucasians, African Americans had higher admission rates for mental illnesses but not for AIDS-defining illnesses. Overall, the majority of these patients were hospitalized for reasons other than AIDS-defining illnesses, and the relatively large number of mental illness admissions highlights the need for comanagement of psychiatric disease, substance abuse, and HIV.

One probability sample study was conducted using South Carolina Hospital Discharge Data from all of the state's 68 hospitals: Among 378,710 adult cases of discharge from all hospitalizations and emergency room visits during 1995, 422 had a diagnosis of HIV/AIDS and mental illness (using ICD 9 criteria), 1353 had a diagnosis of HIV/AIDS alone, and 67,092 had a diagnosis of mental illness alone. People with a mental illness, regardless of race, gender, or age, were 1.44 times as likely to have HIV/AIDS than people without a mental illness (Stoskopf et al., 2001). In this study, two categories of mental illness—alcohol/drug abuse and depressive disorders—were found to have relative risks significantly associated with HIV infection.

Alcohol Use Disorders

The prevalence of current alcohol use disorders among people with HIV infection has been estimated to range from 3% to 12% (Brown et al., 1992; Rabkin, 1996; Dew et al., 1997; Rabkin et al., 1997; Ferrando et al., 1998). In the HCSUS study, participants were screened for heavy drinking in the previous 12 months, and 3% were found to meet criteria for this condition. In the general population, the prevalence of current alcohol use disorders was estimated to be 7% to 10% (Regier et al., 1993; Kessler et al., 1994).

Other Drug Use Disorders

The HCSUS study screened participants for drug dependence in the previous 12 months, and 2.6% were found to meet criteria for this disorder. Specific drugs for which dependence had developed were not reported. Earlier studies had provided estimates of 2% to 19% for current drug use disorders (Brown et al., 1992; Rabkin, 1996; Dew et al., 1997; Rabkin et al., 1997; Ferrando et al., 1998). The general population prevalence for drug use disorders was estimated to be about 3% (Regier et al., 1993; Kessler et al., 1994).

On the basis of these studies, it appears that the prevalence of current AOD use disorders was not different for people living with HIV compared with general-population estimates. However, lifetime prevalence for both alcohol and other drug use disorders does appear to be higher among people with HIV infection than in the general population. Across studies, the lifetime prevalence of alcohol use disorders for people with HIV was 26% to 60% (Rabkin, 1996; Dew et al., 1997; Ferrando et al., 1998) compared with a general population prevalence of 14% (Regier et al., 1990) to 24% (Kessler et al., 1994). Similarly, the lifetime prevalence of drug use disorders for people with HIV was 23% to 56% (Rabkin, 1996; Dew et al., 1997; Ferrando et al., 1998), whereas for the general population it was 6% (Regier et al., 1990) to 12% (Kessler et al., 1994).

Mood and Anxiety Disorders

Although mood disorders encompass the range of unipolar and bipolar conditions, mania secondary to HIV infection is rare, generally occurring in late stages of AIDS. By contrast, depression and anxiety disorders are seen throughout the course of HIV infection, and the conditions commonly coexist (McDaniel and Blalock, 2000). There is an increased likelihood of the emergence of symptoms during pivotal disease points (such as HIV antibody testing, declines in immune status, and occurrence of opportunistic infections).

Depression

Depression is the most common reason for psychiatric referral among people with HIV-infection (Strober et al., 1997). Overall, rates of depression among people with HIV infection are nearly 50% (Bing et al., 2001; Ickovics et al., 2001; Morrison et al., 2002). Among HIV-infected patients referred for psychiatric evaluation, rates of major depression range from 8% to 67% (Acuff et al., 1999), and up to 85% of HIV-seropositive individuals report some depression symptoms (Stolar et al., 2005). In a meta-analysis of published studies, Ciesla and Roberts (2001) found that people with HIV were almost twice as likely as those who were seronegative to be diagnosed with major depression, and that depression was equally prevalent in people with both symptomatic and asymptomatic HIV.

Depression is frequently underdiagnosed and when recognized is often poorly treated, particularly in primary medical settings where HIV/AIDS patients receive care. Clinicians working with HIV/AIDS patients must consider underlying medical causes for depression (for example, medication side effects, brain infections, and endocrine disorders). Rates are generally lower among community-based HIV-positive samples and are highest among IDUs and women engaging in high-risk behaviors. Elevated rates of depression are also seen among patients with more advanced HIV disease, particularly those hospitalized for medical illness. Other risk factors for depression include prior history of depression, substance abuse, unemployment, lack of social support, use of avoidance coping strategies, HIV-related physical symptoms, and multiple losses (Goodkin et al., 1996).

Anxiety

Estimates of the prevalence of anxiety disorders in HIV/AIDS patients range from almost negligible to as high as 40% (Dew et al., 1997; Rabkin et al., 1997; Blalock et al., 2005). The rates vary for numerous reasons, including a host of psychosocial correlates and because anxiety frequently coexists with depression and substance use problems. Higher rates generally are seen as HIV illness progresses. Despite the wide range of prevalence estimates, a pattern emerged in the late 1990s: several studies showed a point prevalence of anxiety disorders in HIV-seropositive patients not significantly different from that of HIV-seronegative clinical comparison groups, even though lifetime rates are higher in the HIV clinical population than in the general population (Dew et al., 1997; Rabkin et al., 1997; Sewell, et al., 2000).

Psychosis

An overview of the literature suggests that the pathophysiology of psychosis in HIV infection is complex, and a multifactorial etiology of psychotic symptoms is likely in many cases. There are many reports of psychotic symptoms in HIV-infected persons in the absence of concurrent substance abuse, iatrogenic causes, evidence of opportunistic infection or neoplasm, or detectable cognitive impairment. A common clinical feature of new-onset psychosis in HIV-infected patients is the acute onset of symptoms. Estimates of the prevalence of new-onset psychosis in HIV-infected patients vary widely, from less than 0.5% to 15%, (Navia et al., 1986; Halstead et al., 1988;

Harris et al., 1991; Prier et al., 1991; Boccellari et al., 1992), with more recent studies from Europe indicating a prevalence closer to 3% for new-onset psychosis (de Ronchi et al., 2000; Alciati et al., 2001). In one study, HIV/AIDS was the leading cause of death among young semirural New York patients experiencing their first hospitalization for a psychotic episode (Susser et al., 1997).

RATES OF HIV INFECTION AMONG PEOPLE WITH SUBSTANCE USE DISORDERS

The extent to which addiction fuels IDU is the most obvious link between psychiatric disorders and HIV transmission. Kral et al. (1998) estimated an overall HIV infection rate among U.S. IDUs of 13%, with wide geographic variability between cities in the East (where rates exceed 40%) and in the Midwest and West (where rates generally are under 5%). Yet many studies of this population did not obtain AOD use disorder diagnoses, so summarizing across studies to generalize rates of HIV infection for specific diagnostic groups is methodologically problematic. People discharged from general hospitals who had documented AOD use disorders were twice as likely to be HIV infected as those without AOD use disorders (Stoskopf et al., 2001). Studies of people admitted to treatment for primary alcohol abuse or dependence reported HIV infection rates of 5% to 10.3% (Avins et al., 1994; Mahler et al., 1994; Woods et al., 2000), and these rates are 10 to 20 times higher than those among the general population (McQuillan et al., 1997).

RATES OF HIV INFECTION AMONG PEOPLE WITH MENTAL ILLNESS

Most studies of rates of HIV infection in psychiatric populations focus on people with severe mental illness (SMI). SMI is a heterogeneous group of psychiatric conditions characterized by acute or persistent duration and functional disability (McKinnon and Rosner, 2000). A significant history of hospitalization and/or maintenance medication typically accompanies these disorders.

Among adults in treatment for such conditions in the United States, infection with HIV has been documented in seroprevalence studies at rates of 3% to

TABLE 4.2. HIV Seroprevalence among Psychiatric Patients in the United States

HIV Seropositive (%)	Patients (N)	Study Region	Sample	Source
5.5		New York City	Inpatients	Cournos et al., 1991
8.9	515	New York City	Inpatients	Volavka et al., 1991
7.1	350	New York City	Inpatients	Sacks et al., 1992
14.4	132	New York City	Inpatients	Lee et al., 1992
6.4	203	New York City	Homeless inpatients	Empfield et al., 1993
19.4	62	New York City	Homeless outpatient men	Susser et al.,1993
4.0	199	New York City	Long-stay inpatients	Meyer et al., 1993
22.4	118	New York City	Dual-diagnosis inpatient	Silberstein, 1994
5.8	533	Baltimore	Inpatients and outpatients	Stewart et al., 1994
19.0	147	New York City	Dual-diagnosis inpatients	Krakow et al., 1998
3.1	931	Connecticut, Maryland, New Hampshire, North Carolina	Inpatients and outpatients	Rosenberg et al., 2001

22% (Table 4.2). Rates found in seroprevalence studies where blood was drawn for HIV antibody testing generally are more reliable than those found in prevalence studies that relied on patient knowledge of their HIV status or on what had been recorded in the medical record; still, generalizability of seroprevalence to other patient populations is limited. All seroprevalence studies were conducted on the East Coast, most in New York City.

Rates established elsewhere in the United States were estimates based on self-report or on archival data. For instance, in the only prevalence study of forensic patients, an infection rate of 5.5% among 223 pretrial detainees in Columbia, South Carolina, was found based on discharge records (Schwartz-Watts et al., 1995). On the West Coast, inpatients at an Oregon state psychiatric hospital showed an infection rate of 2.6% when medical records of 535 chronic patients were reviewed (Meyer, 2003).

Across seroprevalence studies (Cournos and McKinnon, 1997), new admissions to psychiatric units had an overall rate of HIV infection of 8%. A lower rate was found on a long-stay (more than 1 year) psychiatric unit, where 4% of patients were infected. Among patients who were sampled on homeless units, 9% were found to be infected.

Seroprevalence studies support the link between co-occurring psychiatric and AOD use disorders: infection rates were highest in treatment programs for comorbid psychiatric and substance use disorders, where almost 20% of patients were HIV positive (McKinnon

and Cournos, 1998). Among these patients, HIV infection varied by the predominant type of substance use that patients engaged in, with 33.8% among injectors, 15% among non-injectors, 11% among alcohol users, and 3% among those who did not meet criteria for current abuse or dependence diagnoses. The two most recent seroprevalence studies (Krakow et al., 1998; Rosenberg et al., 2001) showed, not surprisingly, that injecting drugs carried a greater than sixfold increase in the likelihood of being HIV seropositive; but even in the absence of injecting, having cocaine as a drug of first choice or using crack ever carried a fourfold increase in the likelihood of being HIV seropositive, and having a co-occurring substance use disorder carried a threefold increase in the likelihood of being HIV seropositive.

These studies provide dramatic evidence that the main driver of the HIV epidemic is substance use, even for sexual transmission, so preventing HIV among people with mental illness, half of whom are likely to develop substance use disorders, can start with the onset of the first disorder (Table 4.3) by ensuring adequate treatment and appropriate prevention of the secondary disorder.

DISENTANGLING COMORBIDITIES AMONG PEOPLE AFFECTED BY HIV/AIDS

More often than not, HIV travels together with other conditions like tuberculosis, particularly in developing

TABLE 4.3. Substance Use and Other Mental Disorder Comorbidity Estimates from the U.S. National Comorbidity Study

- 51% of people with lifetime alcohol or other drug (AOD) use disorders met criteria for at least one other lifetime mental disorder, and vice versa.
- 15% of people with a mental disorder in the past year also met criteria for an AOD disorder in the past year.
- 43% of people with AOD in the past year also met criteria for another mental disorder in the past year.

countries, and hepatitis C worldwide; such conditions are readily identifiable through medical tests routinely offered to people living with HIV. Psychiatric comorbidities also are common but often present considerable difficulty for HIV care providers to recognize and to help their patients manage.

The National Comorbidity Study (Kessler et al., 1996) showed that substance use disorders are highly comorbid with other psychiatric disorders (e.g., bipolar disorder, depression, psychotic disorders, anxiety disorders, and antisocial and borderline personality disorders). Possible explanations for this have been propounded, including that one disorder is a marker for the other disorder; that mental illness leads to self-medication with alcohol and other drugs; and that substance use leads to symptoms of mental illness. It often is impossible to know which disorder came first or is primary, although onset of mental disorders appears to occur at a younger age than that for addictive disorders (Kessler et al., 1996). In clinical settings of any kind it is prudent to screen patients with one type of disorder for the other type of disorder.

Those individuals with dual psychiatric and substance use disorders may be at higher risk for HIV infection than those with either disorder alone (Ferrando and Batki, 2000), and these disorders are likely to be found together across populations of HIV-infected people. The HCSUS study established estimates of the prevalence of co-occurring psychiatric symptoms and either or both drug dependence symptoms or heavy drinking: 13% of their sample had co-occurring psychiatric symptoms and either or both drug dependence symptoms or heavy drinking (Galvan et al., 2003). Sixty-nine percent of those with a substance-related condition also had psychiatric symptoms; 27% of those with psychiatric symptoms also had a substance-related condition.

HOW PSYCHIATRISTS CAN CONTRIBUTE TO CONTAINMENT OF THE MOST CHALLENGING PUBLIC HEALTH PROBLEM THE WORLD HAS FACED ON A GLOBAL SCALE

In the United States, as in most other places in the world, psychiatric disorders are common and undertreated in HIV patients. For instance, less than one-third of the HCSUS sample was taking psychotropic medication, and significant disparities were found between African Americans and others in the prescription of medication for depression (Table 4.4).

The range of mental health issues encountered by HIV/AIDS care providers is broad (e.g., abuse of alcohol, cocaine, crystal methamphetamine; personality disorders; agitation; psychosis) and population-specific (e.g., adolescents, Latinas, people who are homeless or incarcerated). Because service delivery systems (medical care, mental health care, substance abuse treatment) are structured to work separately (historically due to different funding streams), efforts to navigate multiple systems often fail. Integrated HIV mental health care remains rare (Satriano et al., 2007), and comprehensive listings of regional HIV mental health service agencies do not exist. Patients may not themselves recognize the role that mental health problems are playing in their health (Messeri et al., 2002). As a result, HIV/AIDS medical service providers may be unable to integrate adequately HIV/AIDS, mental health, and substance abuse treatment services, even through existing referral networks, let alone to diagnose and treat mental health disorders (Staab and Evans, 2001). Disentangling psychiatric, substance-related, and other comorbidities requires careful differential diagnosis and awareness that the

TABLE 4.4. HIV Cost and Services Utilization Study: Psychotropic Medications among 1489 HIV-Positive Medical Patients

- 27% took psychotropic medication:
  - 21% antidepressants
  - 17% anxiolytics
  - 5% antipsychotics
  - 3% psychostimulants
- About half of patients with depressive disorders did not receive antidepressants; African Americans were overrepresented.

presence of some disorders precludes making other diagnoses.

Yet there are important, basic principles that guide treating mental health problems in HIV illness that all psychiatrists should know (Cournos et al., 2005). These include taking into account multiple comorbidities and knowing how to prioritize their treatment; ruling out a new medical cause for any change in mental status (HIV related or not); starting with lower doses of psychotropic medication and slowly titrating them upward; checking for drug interactions and overlapping toxicities between psychotropics, antiretrovirals, and any other medications being taken (*Psychiatric Medications and HIV Antiretrovirals: A Guide to Interactions for Clinicians*, available at www.nynjaetc .org), including nonprescribed substances; and offering adherence support to patients whose cognitive or psychiatric symptoms interfere with regular medication taking.

We also can foster nonjudgmental prevention (with a wide range of safer-sex and drug use options according to the specific person's needs and lifestyle), educate HIV-infected patients about associated central nervous system problems, monitor psychiatric sequelae, adherence, and quality-of-life issues (e.g., sleep, sexual functioning), and assist in managing the psychosocial impact of the disease on infected people and their relatives.

References

Acuff C, Archambeault J, Greenberg B, Hoeltzel J, McDaniel JS, Meyer Ph, Packer C, Parga FJ, Phillen MB, Ronhovde A, Saldarriaga M, Smith MJW, Stroff D, Wagner D (1999). Mental Health Care for People Living with or Affected by HIV/AIDS: A Practical Guide. Substance Abuse and Mental Health Services Administration monograph (project no. 6031). Rockville, MD: Research Triangle Institute.

Alciati A, Fusi A, D'Arminio Monforte A, Coen M, Ferri A, and Mellado C (2001). New-onset delusions and hallucinations in patients infected with HIV. *J Psychiatr Neurosci* 26:229–324.

Avins AL, Woods WJ, Lindan CP, Hudes ES, Clark W, and Hulley SB (1994). HIV infection and risk behaviors among heterosexuals in alcohol treatment programs. *JAMA* 271:515–518.

Bartleth A and Ferrando SJ (2004). Identification and management of neurologic and psychiatric side effects associated with HIV and HAART. Medscape Retrieved April 25, 2007, from http://www.medscape .com/viewarticle/4700177.

Betz ME, Gebo KA, Barber E, Sklar P, Fleishman JA, Reilly ED, Mathews WC, for the HIV Research Network (2005). Patterns of diagnoses in hospital admissions in a multistate cohort of HIV-positive adults in 2001. *Med Care* 43:3–14.

Bing EG, Burnam A, Longshore D, Fleishman JA, Sherbourne CD, London AS, Turner BJ, Eggan F, Beckman R, Vitiello B, Morton SC, Orlando M, Bozzette SA, Ortiz-Barron L, and Shapiro M (2001). Psychiatric disorders and drug use among human immunodeficiency virus–infected adults in the United States. *Arch Gen Psychiatry* 58:721–728.

Blalock AC, Sharma SM, and McDaniel JS (2005). Anxiety disorders and HIV disease. In K Citron, M-J Brouillette, and A Beckett (eds.), *HIV and Psychiatry: A Training and Resource Manual*, second edition (pp. 120–127). Cambridge, UK: Cambridge University Press.

Boccellari AA, and Dilley JW (1992). Management and residential placement problems of patients with HIV-related cognitive impairment. *Hosp Community Psychiatry* 43:32–37.

Brown GR, Rundell JR, McManis SE, Kendall SN, Zachary R, and Temoshok L (1992). Prevalence of psychiatric disorders in early stages of HIV infection. *Psychosom Med* 54:588–601.

Ciesla JA, and Roberts JS (2001). Meta-analysis of the relationship between HIV-1 infection and risk for depressive disorders. *Am J Psychiatry* 158:725–730.

Cournos F, Empfield M, Horwath E, McKinnon K, Meyer I, Schrage H, Currie C, and Agosin B (1991). HIV seroprevalence among patients admitted to two psychiatric hospitals. *Am J Psychiatry* 148:1225–1230.

Cournos F, and McKinnon K (1997). HIV seroprevalence among people with severe mental illness in the United States: a critical review. *Clin Psychol Rev* 17:259–269.

Cournos F, McKinnon K, and Wainberg M (2005). What can mental health interventions contribute to the global struggle against HIV/AIDS? *World Psychiatry* 4:135–141.

de Ronchi D, Faranca I, Forti P, Ravaglia G, Borderi M, Manfredi R, and Volterra V (2000). Development of acute psychotic disorders and HIV-1 infection. *Int J Psychiatry Med* 30:173–183.

Dew MA, Becker JT, Sanchez J, Caldararo R, Lopez OL, Wess J, Dorst SK, and Banks G (1997). Prevalence and predictors of depressive, anxiety and substance use disorders in HIV-infected and uninfected men: a longitudinal evaluation. *Psychol Med* 27:395–409.

Dore GJ, Correll PK, Li Y, Kaldor JM, Cooper DA, and Brew BJ (1999). Changes to AIDS dementia complex in the era of highly active antiretroviral therapy. *AIDS* 13:1249–1253.

Empfield M, Cournos F, Meyer I, McKinnon K, Horwath E, Silver M, Schrage H, and Herman R (1993). HIV seroprevalence among street homeless patients admitted to a psychiatric inpatient unit. *Am J Psychiatry* 150:47–52.

Ferrando SJ, and Batki SL (2000). Substance abuse and HIV infection. *New Dir Ment Health Serv* 87: 57–67.

Ferrando S, Goggin K, Sewell M, Evans S, Fishman B, and Rabkin J (1998). Substance use disorders in gay/bisexual men with HIV and AIDS. *Am J Addict* 7:51–60.

Galvan FH, Bing EG, Fleishman JA, London AS, Caetano R, Burnam MA, Longshore D, Morton SC, Orlando M, and Shapiro M (2002). The prevalence of alcohol consumption and heavy drinking among people with HIV in the United States: results from the HIV Cost and Services Utilization Study. *J Stud Alcohol* 63:179–186.

Galvan FH, Burnam MA, and Bing EG (2003). Co-occurring psychiatric symptoms and drug dependence or heavy drinking among HIV-positive people. *J Psychoactive Drugs* (SARC Suppl. 1):153–160.

Goodkin K, Forstein M, Beckett A, Bing EG, Cabaj RP, Cournos F, Etemad JG, Fernandez F, Fullilove MJ, Kertzner RM, Kobayashi JS, McDaniel JS, Nicols SE, O'Donnell JH (1996). HIV-related neuropsychiatric complications and treatments. In *AIDS and HIV Disease: A Mental Health Perspective*. Washington DC: AIDS Program Office, American Psychiatric Association.

Goodkin K, Wilkie FL, Concha J, Asthana D, Shapshak P, Douyon R, Fujimura RK, and LoPiccolo C (1997). Subtle neuropsychological impairment and minor cognitive-motor disorder in HIV-1 infection. Neuroradiological, neurophysiological, neuroimmunological, and virological correlates. *Neuroimaging Clin N Am* 3:561–579.

Halstead S, Riccio M, Harlow P, Oretti R, and Thompson C (1988). Psychosis associated with HIV infection. *Br J Psychiatry* 153:618–623.

Harris MJ, Jeste DV, Gleghorn A, and Sewell DD (1991). New-onset psychosis in HIV-infected patients. *J Clin Psychiatry* 52:369–376.

Ickovics JR, Hamburger ME, Vlahov D, Schoenbaum EE, Schuman P, Boland RJ, Moore J, for the HIV Epidemiology Research Study Group (2001). Mortality, CD4 cell count decline, and depressive symptoms among HIV-seropositive women: longitudinal analysis from the HIV Epidemiology Research Study. *JAMA* 285:1466–1474.

Kessler RC, McGonagle KA, Zhao S, Nelson CB, Hughes M, Eshleman S, Wittchen HU, and Kendler KS (1994). Lifetime and 12-month prevalence of DSM III-R psychiatric disorders in the United States: results from the National Comorbidity Study. *Arch Gen Psychiatry* 51:8–19.

Kessler RC, Nelson CB, McGonagle KA, Edlund MJ, Frank RG, and Leaf PJ (1996). The epidemiology of co-occurring addictive and mental disorders: implications for prevention and service utilization. *Am J Orthopsychiatry* 66:17–31.

Krakow DS, Galanter M, Dermatis H, and Westreich LM (1998). HIV risk factors in dually diagnosed patients. *Am J Addict* 7:74–80.

Kral AH, Bluthenthal RN, Booth RE, and Watters JK (1998). HIV seroprevalence among street-recruited injection drug and crack cocaine users in 16 US municipalities. *Am J Public Health* 88:108–113.

Lee HK, Travin S, and Bluestone H (1992). HIV-1 in inpatients. *Hosp Community Psychiatry* 43:181–182.

Mahler J, Yi D, Sacks M, Dermatis H, Stebinger A, Card C, and Perry S (1994). Undetected HIV infection among patients admitted to an alcohol rehabilitation unit. *Am J Psychiatry* 151:439–440.

May M (1990). Organic mental disorders in HIV-1 infection. *AIDS* 4:831–840.

McDaniel JS, and Blalock AC (2000). Mood and anxiety disorders. *New Dir Ment Health Serv* 87:51–56.

McKinnon K, and Cournos F (1998). HIV infection linked to substance use among hospitalized patients with severe mental illness. *Psychiatr Serv* 49:1269.

McKinnon K, and Rosner J (2000). Severe mental illness and HIV-AIDS. *New Dir Ment Health Serv* 87: 69–76.

McQuillan GM, Khare M, Karon JM, Schable CA, and Vlahov D (1997). Update on the seroepidemiology of human immunodeficiency virus in the United States household population: NHANES III, 1988–1994. *J Aquir Immune Defic Syndr Hum Retrovirol* 14:355–360.

Messeri PA, Abramson DM, Aidala AA, Lee F, and Lee G (2002). The impact of ancillary HIV services on engagement in medical care in New York City. *AIDS Care* 14 (Suppl 1):S15–29.

Meyer I, McKinnon K, Cournos F, Empfield M, Bavli S, Engel D, and Weinstock A (1993). HIV seroprevalence among long-stay patients in a state psychiatric hospital. *Hosp Community Psychiatry* 44:282–284.

Meyer JM (2003). Prevalence of hepatitis A, hepatitis B, and HIV among hepatitis C–seropositive state hospital patients: results from Oregon State Hospital. *J Clin Psychiatry* 64:540–545.

Morrison MF, Petitto JM, Ten Have T, Gettes DR, Chiappini MS, Weber AL, Brinker-Spence P, Bauer RM, Douglas SD, and Evans DL (2002). Depressive and anxiety disorders in women with HIV infection. *Am J Psychiatry* 159:789–796.

National Institutes of Health Consensus Development Conference Panel (1997). Management of hepatitis C. *Hepatology* 26:2S–10S.

Navia BA, Jordan BD, and Price RW (1986). The AIDS dementia complex: I. Clinical features. *Ann Neurol* 19:517–524.

Neuenburg JK, Brodt HR, Herndier BG, Bickel M, Bacchetti P, Price RW, Grant RM, and Schlote W (2002). HIV-related neuropathology, 1985 to 1999: rising prevalence of HIV encephalopathy in the era of highly active antiretroviral therapy. *J Acquir Immune Defic Syndr* 31:171–177.

Prier RE, McNeil JG, and Burge JR (1991). Inpatient psychiatric morbidity of HIV-infected soldiers. *Hosp Community Psychiatry* 42:619–623.

Rabkin JG (1996). Prevalence of psychiatric disorders in HIV illness. *Int Rev Psychiatry* 8:157–166.

Rabkin JG, Ferrando SJ, Jacobsberg LB, and Fishman B (1997). Prevalence of axis I disorders in an AIDS cohort: a cross-sectional, controlled study. *Compr Psychiatry* 38:146–154.

Regier DA, Farmer ME, Rae S, Locke BZ, Keith SJ, Judd LL, and Goodwin FK (1990). Comorbidity of mental disorders with alcohol and other drug abuse. *JAMA* 264:2511–2518.

Regier DA, Narrow WE, Rae DS, Manderscheid RW, Locke BZ, and Goodwin FK (1993). The de facto US mental and addictive disorders service system. Epidemiologic Catchment Area prospective 1-year prevalence rates of disorders and services. *Arch Gen Psychiatry* 50:85–94.

Rosenberg SD, Goodman LA, Osher FC, Swartz MS, Essock SM, Butterfield MI, Constantine NT, Wolford GL, and Salyers MP (2001). Prevalence of HIV, hepatitis B, and hepatitis C in people with severe mental illness. *Am J Public Health* 91:31–37.

Sacks MH, Dermatis H, Looser-Ott S, and Perry S (1992). Seroprevalence of HIV and risk factors for AIDS in psychiatric inpatients. *Hosp Community Psychiatry* 43:736–737.

Sacktor NC, Lyles RH, Skolasky RL, Anderson DE, McArthur JC, McFarlane G, Selnes OA, Becker JT, Cohen B, Wesch J, and Miller EN (1999). Combination antiretroviral therapy improves psychomotor speed performance in HIV-seropositive homosexual men: Multicenter AIDS Cohort Study (MACS). *Neurology* 52:1640–1647.

Satriano J, McKinnon K, and Adoff S (2007). HIV service provision for people with severe mental illness in outpatient mental health care settings in New York. *J Prev Interv Community* 33:95–108.

Schwartz-Watts D, Montgomery LD, and Morgan DW (1995). Seroprevalence of human immunodeficiency virus among inpatient pretrial detainees. *Bull Am Acad Psychiatry Law* 23:285–288.

Sewell MC, Goggin KJ, Rabkin JG, Ferrando SJ, McElhiney MC, and Evans S (2000). Anxiety syndromes and symptoms among men with AIDS: a longitudinal controlled study. *Psychosomatics* 41:294–300.

Silberstein C, Galanter M, Marmor M, Lifshutz H, and Krasinski K (1994). HIV-1 among inner city dually diagnosed inpatients. *Am J Drug Alcohol Abuse* 20:101–131.

Simpson DM (1999). Human immunodeficiency virus–associated dementia: review of pathogenesis, prophylaxis, and treatment studies of zidovudine therapy. *Clin Infect Dis* 29:19–34.

Staab JP, and Evans DL (2001). A streamlined method for diagnosing common psychiatric disorders in primary care. *Clin Cornerstone* 3:1–9.

Stewart DL, Zuckerman CJ, and Ingle JM (1994). HIV seroprevalence in a chronic mentally ill population. *J Natl Med Assoc* 86:519–523.

Stoff DM, Mitnick L, and Kalichman S (2004). Research issues in the multiple diagnoses of HIV/AIDS, mental illness and substance abuse. *AIDS Care* 16 (Suppl. 1):S1–S5.

Stolar A, Catalano G, Hakala S, Bright RP, and Fernandez F (2005). Mood disorders and psychosis in HIV. In K Citron, M-J Brouillette, and A Beckett (eds.), *HIV and Psychiatry: A Training and Resource Manual*, second edition (pp. 88–109). Cambridge, UK: Cambridge University Press.

Stoskopf CH, Kim YK, and Glover SH (2001). Dual diagnosis: HIV and mental illness, a population-based study. *Community Ment Health J* 37:469–479.

Strober DR, Schwartz JAJ, McDaniel JS, and Abrams RF (1997). Depression and HIV disease: prevalence, correlates and treatment. *Psychiatr Ann* 27:372–377.

Susser E, Valencia E, and Conover S (1993). Prevalence of HIV infection among psychiatric patients in a New York City men's shelter. *Am J Public Health* 83:568–570.

Susser E, Colson P, Jandorf L, Berkman A, Lavelle J, Fennig S, Waniek C, and Bromet E (1997). HIV infection among young adults with psychotic disorders. *Am J Psychiatry* 154:864–866.

Volavka J, Convit A, Czobor P, Dwyer R, O'Donnell J, and Ventura A (1991). HIV seroprevalence and risk behaviors in psychiatric inpatients. *Psychiatr Res* 39:109–114.

Wainberg M, Cournos F McKinnon K, and Berkman A (2003). HIV and hepatitis C in patients with schizophrenia. In JM Meyer and HA Nasrallah (eds.), *Medical Illness in Schizophrenia* (pp. 115–140). Washington, DC: American Psychiatric Publishing.

White JL, Darko DF, Brown SJ, Miller JC, Hayduk R, Kelly T, and Mitler MM (1995). Early central nervous system response to HIV infection: sleep distortion and cognitive-motor decrements. *AIDS* 9:1043–1050.

Wilkie FL, Eisdorfer C, Morgan R, Loewenstein DA, and Szapocznik J (1990). Cognition in early human immunodeficiency virus infection. *Arch Neurol* 47:433–440.

Woods WJ, Lindan CP, Hudes ES, Boscarino JA, Clark W, and Avins AL (2000). HIV infection and risk behaviors in two cross-sectional surveys of heterosexuals in alcoholism treatment. *J Stud Alcohol* 61:262–266.

Chapter 5

Sociocultural Factors Influencing the Transmission of HIV/AIDS in the United States: AIDS and the Nation's Prisons

Robert E. Fullilove

This chapter examines the sociocultural factors that influence the transmission of HIV, particularly in poor communities in the United States. The primary assertion that guides this examination is that during the first decade of the 21st century, HIV was and continues to be increasingly present in vulnerable, disadvantaged populations.

> From 1990 to 1999, the number of living persons diagnosed with AIDS increased 4-fold, to 312 000 persons. Increasing proportions of persons with AIDS are women, African Americans or Hispanics, IDUs, heterosexuals, and residents of the South, reflecting earlier trends in HIV transmission, differences in testing behaviors, and differential effects of HAART. Our synthesis of surveillance data also shows that the poor are disproportionately affected and that HIV incidence rates are especially high among African Americans with high-risk behavior, and it suggests that HIV incidence has not declined since the early 1990s. (Karon et al., 2001, p. 1068)

At the dawn of the 21st century, the trends observed by Karon and colleagues persisted, as noted in Table 5.1 and Figure 5.1, drawn from Centers for Disease Control and Prevention (CDC) surveillance data examining HIV/AIDS in the period 2001–2004 (CDC, 2005, 2006a). Clearly, communities of color were dramatically overrepresented among new HIV cases during this period. The reasons for the increasing racialization of the HIV/AIDS epidemic, I will argue here, are largely found in the worsening political, social, and economic status of many people of color in the United States. Moreover, I will argue, the "engine" driving these sociocultural trends is the role played by the nation's jails and prisons.

JAILS, PRISONS, AND HEALTH

Social and economic disadvantage is measured in a variety of ways, but at the beginning of the 21st century, social scientists and public health researchers

TABLE 5.1. Racial Disparities and HIV/AIDS: Estimated New Cases of HIV/AIDS among Whites, Blacks, and Hispanics by Sex in 33 States, 2001–2004*

	White		Black		Hispanic		Total[†]	
	N	(%)	N	(%)	N	(%)	N	(%)
Males	38,218	(34)	49,704	(44)	22,062	(20)	112,106	(100)
Female	7,262	(16)	30,483	(68)	6,610	(15)	45,146	(100)
Total	45,479	(29)	80,187	(51)	28,673	(18)	157,252	(100)

*Confidential, name-based reporting was used to determine number of HIV/AIDS cases.

[†]Total includes estimates for Asian/Pacific Islanders and American Indians/Alaska Natives, which are not shown here.

Source: CDC, 2006a.

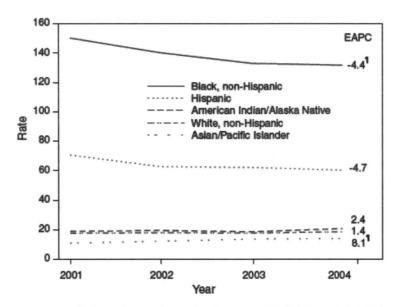

FIGURE 5.1. Estimated annual rates* of cases of HIV/AIDS and EAPC† among males, by race/ethnicity—33 states, § 2001–2004. Reprinted from the Centers for Disease Control, *Morbidity and Mortality Weekly Report*, February 10, 2006; 55(05):121–125.

*Per 100,000 Population

[†]Estimated Annual Percentage Change

[§]Alabama, Alaska, Arizona, Arkansas, Colorado, Florida, Idaho, Indiana, Iowa, Kansas, Louisiana, Michigan, Minnesota, Mississippi, Missouri, Nebraska, Nevada, New Jersey, New Mexico, New York, North Carolina, North Dakota, Ohio, Oklahoma, South Carolina, South Dakota, Tennessee, Texas, Utah, Virginia, West Virginia, and Wyoming.

[¶]Statistically significant (i.e., 95% confidence interval excludes zero) were increasingly focusing their attention on the role of jails and prisons as a "motor" that drives both economic and social inequalities as well as the transmission of HIV in black and brown communities throughout the United States (Fullilove and Fullilove, 1999; Golembeski and Fullilove, 2005; Johnson and Raphael, 2005). As will be demonstrated here, incarceration not only imprisons the population most likely to have been exposed and/or infected with HIV, i.e. drug users, but provides a setting where, as prison inmates, they will quite possibly be exposed to or expose others to a variety of HIV risk behaviors, including risky drug use practices, risky piercing and tattooing practices, and/or consensual and nonconsensual unprotected sexual intercourse (CDC, 2006b).

The poor are disproportionately affected by incarceration in the United States. As noted by Mauer (1999):

> The criminal justice system in general and prison in particular have long served as the principal arena for responding to the crimes of lower-income people. The demographics of the prison population illustrate this well: a 1991 survey of state inmates conducted by the Justice Department found that 65 percent of prisoners had not completed high school, 53 percent earned less than $10,000 in the year prior to their incarceration and nearly one half were either unemployed or working only part-time prior to their arrest. (Mauer, 1999, pp 162–163)

The racial disparities in the system are equally apparent. In 2004, according to the Bureau of Justice Statistics, 41% of prison inmates were black and 19% were Hispanic. Expressed in other terms, within the age group most affected by arrests and incarceration, those aged 25–29, slightly less than 13% of all black males in this age group were in prison or jail as compared with 3.6% of all Hispanic males and 1.7% of white males. Finally, it is estimated that approximately one-third of all black males in the United States will serve time in prison at some time in their lives, in contrast to approximately one-sixth of all Hispanic males and three-fiftieths (3 in 50) of all white males (Sentencing Project, 2006).

One major factor in the growth of the population in state and federal prisons has been the War on Drugs and Get Tough on Crime programs (Mauer, 1999). In 1983, approximately 10% of all jail inmates in the United States had been arrested for drug-related of-

fenses. In 2002, by contrast, approximately 25% of the inmates in the nation's jails were there for drug-related offenses. Among those who have been tried and incarcerated in a state or federal prison, drug offenders constitute a significant portion of the prison population. In 2001, the majority of inmates in federal prison (55%) were drug offenders; one in four (25%) inmates were in state prisons (Sentencing Project, 2006).

Drug use is a particularly important risk factor for HIV infection. HIV infection associated with injection drug use was 2.4 times and 2.6 times more prevalent among blacks and Hispanics, respectively, than among whites living with HIV/AIDS in the United States in 2004. Not surprisingly, injection drug users living with HIV/AIDS pass in and out of the nation's correctional facilities each year. Hammett and colleagues examined data on infectious diseases among correctional inmates for the year 1997 and estimated that "altogether, between 150,000 and 200,000 people living with HIV infection passed through a U.S. correctional facility in 1997, or between 20% and 26% of all people living with HIV in the nation that year" (Hammett et al., 2002, p. 1791). They also estimate that other infectious diseases that are often comorbid with HIV, tuberculosis and hepatitis C, were overrepresented in the population within correctional institutions, with 29% to 43% of all the people in the United States living with hepatitis C and 40% of persons living with tuberculosis passing through correctional facilities in 1997 (Hammett et al., 2002). The authors further note:

> Prevalence statistics for inmates by race and ethnicity are generally lacking, so it was not possible to develop estimates of disease burden by racial and ethnic group. However, the disproportionate incarceration rates experienced by African Americans and Latinos and the already disproportionate burden of diseases under study among the same groups combine to produce a situation in which the vast majority of inmates and releasees with these infectious diseases are African American or Latino. In New York State correctional facilities, 48% of inmates diagnosed with AIDS in 1997 were Black and 45% were Hispanic, compared with the proportions of these groups in the total population of the state of 18% and 14%, respectively. (Hammett et al., 2002, p. 1792–1793)

Correctional facilities are significantly implicated in the disease burden borne by poor communities of color in the United States. The HIV/AIDS epidemic is simply one of many health conditions that are passed from the community to the jails and prisons via a "correctional revolving door" in which inmates pass from jails and prisons, then back to the community, and then, in many cases, back to jails and prisons again as recidivists (Sentencing Project, 2006a).

Prisons impose other burdens on these communities that contribute to the social and economic hardships of their residents. In New York State, for example, state prisons might easily be considered "community institutions" because approximately 7 inmates in 10 are from New York City (Fullilove and Fullilove, 1999). The system to which they are sent has 63 facilities located largely in rural, upstate New York and houses well over 69,000 inmates in any given year (NY State Department of Corrections, 2007). With so many residents of New York City's poorest communities of color in residence in this system or returning to their home communities after completing their terms, prison life is increasingly a part of the life of men, and increasingly women, from poor city neighborhoods, and their loss to their families and friends has costs that extend beyond their being "away upstate."

Prison inmates are counted in the U.S. Census, for example, but they are listed as members of the communities in which the prison facility is located. Thus, important community resources that are based on the census count—representation in legislative bodies, federal grants in aid to name just a few—result in an overall net benefit for the prison community and a net loss for the communities of origin of prison inmates. The biggest loss may be in the revenues lost to poor communities that might have paid for the services that inmates will need to receive upon their release and return home (Golembeski and Fullilove, 2005).

Some of these resources are needed to shore up the medical and public health infrastructures of these poor communities. As Hammett and colleagues note, returning inmates are more likely to need medical care for a variety of conditions, not just HIV/AIDS (Hammett et al., 2002). Poor communities of color are characterized by high rates of morbidity and mortality from diabetes, cardiovascular disease, and certain forms of cancer, a state of affairs that the CDC describes as "health disparities" (Institute of Medicine, 2002; CDC, 2005). Inmates, whose health is generally worse than that of other members of their home communities, represent an increasing burden on already stressed community health care systems when they return home from prison.

Specifically, because approximately 95% of those who are incarcerated in the United States are returned to the streets after serving their time, ex-inmates will find themselves at a dramatic disadvantage in comparison to their neighbors. They will have lost many basic civil rights (in many states, ex-felons permanently lose the right to vote, for example) and will encounter significant difficulty finding employment or housing (Mauer, 1999; Golembeski and Fullilove, 2005). If they are HIV infected or living with AIDS, access to Medicaid services that pay for a significant portion of HIV care for the poor and indigent in this country will be increasingly hard to achieve (Cuellar et al., 2005; Kaiser Family Foundation, 2004).

Many states deny ex-inmates access to housing that is federally financed. These regulations are unevenly applied as states often have a variety of policies for dealing with housing and housing rights. However, homelessness is a major challenge for inmates. Many people who are arrested are homeless at the time of their arrest, and once released, ex-inmates are more likely to be temporarily or semi-permanently homeless while in the community. Kushel and colleagues (2005), for example, studied a sample of homeless and marginally housed adults in San Francisco in 1999 to determine the impact of a history of homelessness on health status and HIV risk behaviors. They concluded that health risks among homeless ex-inmates were higher than among all homeless and marginally housed members of their sample who had not done time. They note the following:

> High rates of imprisonment among homeless populations may be the end result of a system that does not provide access to timely services, including access to housing, health care, mental health care, and substance abuse treatment, and systems that have obstacles preventing receipt of these services by people exiting prison. High rates of HIV infection among homeless ex-prisoners and high rates of continued risky behavior provide motivation for targeting risk reduction efforts at persons exiting prison. The intersection of substance abuse, unemployment, imprisonment, and homelessness is potent and lasting. Efforts to eradicate homelessness also must include the many unmet needs of persons exiting prison. (Kushel et al., 2005, pp. 1751–1752)

IMPRISONMENT AND HIV INFECTION

As noted here repeatedly, prisons are facilities that house many individuals with significant health problems. Additionally, there has been and continues to be speculation that prisons are independent risk factors for HIV infection because inmates engage in sex and engage in unsafe injection practices while "on the inside." In 2005 the Georgia Department of Corrections (GDC) and the Georgia Division of Public Health with assistance from the CDC conducted a study to examine HIV risk behaviors and patterns of HIV transmission within Georgia's correctional system.

In 1988, the Department of Corrections ordered mandatory HIV testing of inmates upon entry to a prison facility "and voluntary testing of inmates on request or if clinically indicated." In the period between July 1988 and February 2005, 88 inmates who were known to have negative HIV tests upon entry into one of the state's correctional facilities were retested and found to be HIV positive.

This study, reported in the *Morbidity and Mortality Weekly Reports* (MMWR) published by the CDC in April of 2006, marked an important set of milestones. It confirmed that HIV risk behaviors do indeed occur in at least one state prison system, and it provided empirical evidence that inmates who engaged in these behaviors did subsequently become infected while incarcerated (CDC, 2006b). However, as shall be shown later, the study leaves many questions unanswered as well.

The study consisted of both an unmatched case-control study as well as a matched case-control study. In the matched study, cases and controls were selected to create two groups whose members had been exposed to HIV risk behaviors for approximately the same period of time (±2 years). In the unmatched study, a larger sample was examined. Control inmates were eligible for inclusion if they had had their HIV-negative status confirmed by repeat HIV testing, including having a negative test upon enrollment in the study. Additionally, in this study, control inmates were randomly selected from seven prisons suspected to house the largest number of seroconverters in the Georgia state system.

The Georgia correctional system has a number of advantages for such a study. The majority of its 44,990 inmates at the time of the study were African American (63%). Although slightly less than 2% of its total inmate population was known to be HIV infected, the system's prevalence of infection rates is significantly higher than the rate of HIV infection for the general U.S. public (approximately 15 per 100,000 during this period). Thus, the primary advantage of the study—from a research standpoint—is that it examines conditions of HIV transmission in an environment that has sufficient numbers of infected persons to ensure that if risk behaviors are present, some HIV transmission is likely to occur. Moreover, the system's policies on HIV testing permit at least some, if not all, inmates to be tested while incarcerated (post-incarceration testing is voluntary). Thus, some, if not all, new infections that occur within prison can be detected and will, in principle, be available for study.

In the unmatched study, in which those who seroconverted were compared with a sample on non-seroconverters from throughout the Georgia Department of Corrections system, HIV seroconversion was associated with "male-male sex in prison, being older, having served five or more years, and a body mass index (BMI) of ≤ 25.4 kg/m on entry." In the matched study, in which an effort was made to match controls and cases with men serving comparable sentences and with comparable lengths of time served, univariate analysis revealed many correlates of HIV infection. However, in multivariate analyses, male-male sex in prison and having a BMI of <25.4 kg (two factors identified in the analysis of unmatched case and control groups) were significantly associated with HIV infection, as were black race and having received a tattoo in prison.

These two studies provide an interesting set of perspectives on the dynamics of HIV transmission behind bars in the Georgia system. In the unmatched case-control study, age and length of time served (≤ 5 years) were significant predictors of HIV infection. Black race was not, however, significantly associated with seroconversion.

The matched case-control study, which involved inmates who were matched for length of sentence and time sentenced, is also revealing. Black race was a significant correlate of HIV seroconversion in this study and, more importantly, sexual behavior was reported by both cases and controls (Table 5.2). Sex with a male inmate was the most frequently reported sexual encounter in both groups. Sex with a prison staff member was reported by both groups, and both groups

TABLE 5.2. Self-Reported HIV Sexual Risk Behaviors of Prison Inmates in a Case-Control Study of the Georgia State Prison System, 2005*

	Case Inmates (N = 68)		Control Inmates (N = 68)	
	n	(%)	n	(%)
Had Sex in Prison	48	(71)	11	(16)
Any male-male sex	48	(71)	11	(16)
New male-male sex[†]	35	(73)	4	(36)
Sex Partner				
Any sex with other male inmate	40	(59)	8	(12)
% within column		[83]		[75]
Any sex with male prison staff	22	(32)	4	(6)
% within column		[67]		[36]
Any sex with female prison staff	15	(22)	6	(9)
% within column		[31]		[54]
Any sex with visitors or prison volunteers	6	(9)	0	(0)
% within column		[13]		[0]
Nature of Encounter				
Consensual sex only	31	(46)	8	(12)
% within column		[65]		[73]
Exchange sex (no rape)	11	(16)	2	(3)
% within column		[23]		[18]
Any rape as victim	6	(9)	1	(1)
% within column		[13]		[9]

*Case inmates (N = 68) were male prison inmates who seroconverted to HIV while in prison; controls (N = 68) were HIV-uninfected male prison inmates with comparable sentence lengths and time served.

[†]Did not engage in male-male sex during the 6 months before incarceration.

Source: CDC, 2006b.

reported having sex with a male staff member as well as with female staff members (although it is impossible to determine if any inmates reported having sex with both male and female staff).

Seven of the HIV-positive case–control sample members reported injection drug use in prison (10% of all case inmates), of which four reported that their first injection use occurred in prison. Although only one control reported injection drug use, he reported that he was also a first-time injector. Finally, 40 cases (59%) and 28 (41%) controls received tattoos in prison. For one-half of the cases and two-thirds of the controls, the prison tattoo was the first tattoo ever received (Table 5.3).

Many caveats must be mentioned. This study is from one prison system. It examines a comparatively small sample, and it does not include HIV-positive inmates who did not volunteer to be tested. Moreover, as the MMWR authors note, it is possible that those inmates, both positive and negative, who volunteered for HIV testing have a different risk profile than those who do not. And, "inmates might have inaccurately reported HIV risk behaviors because sex between inmates, sex with correctional staff, injection drug use, and tattooing are illegal or forbidden by policy in this prison system" (CDC, 2006b, p. 425).

Nonetheless, even using the most conservative interpretation of these data, it is difficult to believe that Georgia is the only state prison system in which there is HIV seroconversion as a result of being incarcerated. It is also difficult to believe that Georgia prisons are the only institutions in which risky sex and injecting drug behavior occur, and where there are sexual relationships between inmates as well as prison staff members of both sexes. Put in other terms, there is ample reason to believe that prisons make an impor-

TABLE 5.3. Characteristics and Risk Behaviors among Prison Inmates Who Became HIV Positive during Incarceration, Compared with Matched Controls, in the Georgia State Prison System, 2005*

Characteristic and Behavior	Case Inmates		Controls		Adjusted Odds Ratio	(95% CI)	p value
	n	(%)	n	(%)			
Any male-male sex in prison	45	(66)	9	(13)	10.1	(3.0–54.9)	<.01
Received tattoo in prison	40	(59)	28	(41)	13.7	(1.5–390.6)	.01
Body mass index $\leq 25.4\,\text{kg/m}^2$ at entry	51	(75)	23	(34)	3.8	(1.2–15.2)	.02
Black race	45	(66)	40	(59)	3.7	(1.1–16.7)	.03

*Case inmates (N = 68) were male prison inmates who seroconverted to HIV while in prison; controls (N = 68) were HIV-uninfected male prison inmates with comparable sentence lengths and time served. This study was done as exact multivariate conditional logistic regression analysis. All values are statistically significant. CI, confidence interval.

Source: CDC, 2006b.

tant, independent contribution to the level of HIV/AIDS in poor communities of color. The fact that HIV-positive inmates had sex with men and women prison staff—people who, in principle, are members of sexual networks outside the prison—also raises the issue of how much this indirect connection to sexual networks in the general community contributes to rates of HIV beyond the prison walls.

MODELING HIV RATES AS A FUNCTION OF INCARCERATION RATES

In a report published by two investigators at the Goldman School of Public Policy at the University of California, Berkeley, a two-stage-least-squares (TSLS) model was used to show the dynamic relationship between male incarceration rates and both male and female HIV infection rates. The results suggested that incarceration rates influence HIV infection rates. Specifically, the authors conclude: "Our results reveal that the higher incarceration rates among black males over this period explain a substantial share of the racial disparity in AIDS infection between black women and women of other racial and ethnic groups" (Johnson and Raphael, 2005, p. 1).

As is the case with research that uses modeling techniques to study casual relationships between two or more factors, Johnson and Raphael acknowledge the degree to which certain assumptions have to be made in the creation of such models. The data supporting model assumptions are extremely important, and in this exercise the authors concede that avail-

able data vary in precision. The major weakness at the time this study was undertaken was the lack of concrete evidence that elevated rates of HIV transmission occurred while individuals were incarcerated.

Such transmission would be affected, they assert, by tattooing, drug use, and high-risk sexual activity. In the Georgia Prison study, all of these behaviors were reported by cases as well as controls, with the self-reported rates of having "received a tattoo in prison" emerging as a particularly significant risk factor for seroconversion in prison. Hence, a significant element of the model receives significant support from these findings.

The Johnson-Raphael model, however, is only partially dependent on the assumption that the disparity between black and white HIV infection rates is a function of in-prison HIV risk behavior. The authors' major focus was to test the degree to which "sexual relationship markets"—that is, the manner in which members of sexually active groups form and break up sexual relationships—are influenced by rates of incarceration.

Of particular importance are the effects of incarceration on the total lifetime number of sex partners and the likelihood of concurrent sexual relationships. The rates at which new relationships form and dissolve impacts the lifetime number of sexual partners at any given age, which affects the risk of sexual contact with an infected person.... The dynamics of prison entry and exit, coupled with a large increase in incarceration rates for men, are likely to impact the rate at which existing sexual relationships dissolve and form. (Johnson and Raphael, 2005, p. 11)

In addition to affecting the rate at which concurrent sexual relationships form and break up, there is evidence that the loss of a significant number of men to jails and prisons affects the degree to which women will insist on condom use and other safe sexual behaviors on the part of their sexual partners (Sampson, 1995). Finally, the impact of missing fathers on families in general, but particularly on their children, is also considerable, given that one of the most important predictors for being imprisoned as a juvenile or as an adult is being a member of a family in which one or more members has done time.

> For example, for children whose parents are imprisoned, feelings of shame, humiliation, and a loss of social status may result (Clear, 1996). Children begin to act out in school or distrust authority figures, who represent the people who removed the parent from the home. Lowered economic circumstances in families experiencing imprisonment also lead to greater housing relocation, resulting in less cohesive neighborhoods. In far too many cases, these children come to represent the next generation of offenders. (Mauer, 1999, p. 185)

CONCLUSIONS

The disparity in HIV infection rates among poor communities of color is increasingly driven by the impact of incarceration on individuals and families in these communities. More importantly, there is evidence that prisons have an even greater impact on the levels of disadvantage in these communities because so many ex-inmates return to neighborhoods that cannot house them, employ them, or care for their illnesses. HIV infection, therefore, is simply one manifestation of this process of prison-mediated community destabilization.

HIV/AIDS research in the United States has often identified poverty, race and racism, and a host of other intractable features of daily life as significant contributors to the transmission of HIV infection. Clearly, these factors do indeed play a significant role. One is often at a loss to determine where, how, and under what circumstances public health and medical professionals and policy specialists can intervene to combat such enormously complicated forces as poverty or racism. Nonetheless, in discussing the role of the prison-industrial complex on HIV/AIDS in particular and on community destabilization in general, I believe it is possible to envision structural interventions that will dramatically affect the dynamics of epidemic transmission described in this chapter.

Blankenship and colleagues (2005) list three areas where interventions can have an impact:

1. Interventions aimed at reducing the likelihood of involvement with the corrections system
2. Interventions aimed at reducing the risks associated with incarceration and supervision
3. Interventions aimed at easing the burden of re-entry

Interventions Aimed at Reducing the Likelihood of Involvement with the Corrections System

As noted earlier, the War on Drugs and the War on Crime have had an enormous impact on increasing rates of incarceration in the United States (Mauer, 1999; Golembeski and Fullilove, 2005). The length of incarceration as a result of violation of drug laws and the likelihood that an offender will go to jail vary significantly by state and municipality. The type of drug, the amount possessed and/or sold, and a host of other factors are often weighed in sentencing and parole decisions. Truth in Sentencing laws also determine how much of a mandatory sentence will be served. All of these factors affect how many people are sent to prison and the number who remain there for a given period of time (Sentencing Project, 2006b). Reducing the length of time served for a first offense, using "drug courts" as a means of dealing with first offenders, and repealing laws, such as syringe possession laws, that add people to the jails and years onto their sentenced are appropriate targets for legislative interventions.

Interventions Aimed at Reducing Risks Associated with Incarceration and Supervision

The editorial note accompanying the CDC study of HIV transmission in Georgia prisons acknowledges the existence of HIV sexual risk behavior in prisons: "Sex among inmates occurs, and laws or policies prohibiting sex among inmates have been difficult to implement or enforce" (CDC, 2006b, p. 423). Because the distribution of condoms is prohibited in all but a few corrections facilities, the study recommends the following: "Departments of corrections with existing condom distribution programs should evaluate these programs to assess their effectiveness; departments of corrections without condom distribution programs should assess relevant state laws, policies, and circumstances to determine the feasibility and benefits and risks of implementing such programs" (CDC, 2006b, p. 425).

The editorial note also recommends that the CDC be on record as recommending that HIV testing, education, prevention, and access to treatment be available to all populations, including inmates. Importantly, the note urges that post-release discharge planning and the provision of links to medical services for those who leave prison HIV infected be made available. Such actions and policies would, quite obviously, reduce much of the HIV risk associated with incarceration.

Interventions Aimed at Easing the Burden of Re-entry

At the outset of this chapter, it was noted that prisons increasingly hold members of poor communities who are both undereducated and unemployed (Mauer, 1999; Golembeski and Fullilove, 2005). The provision of employment training programs, drug treatment programs, and programs designed to increase the educational achievement of many inmates would dramatically improve their ability to function in society upon release. Legislative reforms aimed at restoring the rights of inmates to petition and, ultimately, obtain the right to vote and qualify for student loans and government-sponsored housing would also reverse some of the damage done to inmates and to the families and communities that must house and support ex-inmates upon their release.

One obvious benefit would quite probably be a reduction in the number of ex-inmates who become homeless soon after being released from jail or prison and reductions in the number of recidivists who return to prison because committing crimes is perceived to be the only viable option for survival.

FINAL THOUGHTS

Although jails and prisons are not the causes of the HIV epidemic in poor communities of color, they con-

tribute enormously to making the epidemic and its impact worse.

Structural reforms aimed at changing the role of prisons in the lives of so many poor communities of color are not only within our collective grasp but often involve actions that will prove to be cost-effective in the long run because they may reduce expenditures related to HIV health care. The costs associated with failing to care for HIV-infected, homeless former inmates, many of whom are treated in hospital emergency departments when their HIV disease is significantly advanced, represent just one way in which prisons and the HIV epidemic are slowly but surely ruining the U.S. health care system. The issue is less whether such an impact is reasonable to predict, rather whether as a nation we have the will to do what is so obviously necessary to control the ravages of HIV/AIDS.

References

Blankenship KM, Smoyer AB, Bray SJ, and Mattocks K (2005). Black–white disparities in HIV/AIDS: the role of drug policy in the corrections system. *J Health Care Poor Underserved* 16:140–156

[CDC] Centers for Disease Control and Prevention (2005) Health disparities experienced by Black or African-Americans-United States. *MMWR Morb Mortal Wkly Rep* 54:1–3.

[CDC] Centers for Disease Control and Prevention (2005). *HIV/AIDS Surveillance Report, 2004*. Vol. 16. Atlanta: U.S. Department of Health and Human Services. Retrieved January 25, 2006, at http://www.cdc.gov/hiv/stats/hasrlink.htm.

[CDC] Centers for Disease Control and Prevention (2006a). Racial/ethnic disparities in diagnoses of HIV/AIDS—33 states, 2001–2004. *MMWR Morb Mortal Wkly Rep* 55:121–125.

[CDC] Centers for Disease Control and Prevention (2006b). HIV transmission among male inmates in a state prison system—Georgia, 1992–2005. *MMWR Morb Mortal Wkly Rep* 55:421–426.

Clear TH (1996). *When incarceration increases crime*. Florida State University, Tallahassee, FL. Retrieved April 4, 2007, from www.doc.state.ok.us/offenders/ocjrc/96/Backfire.pdf.

Cuellar AE, Kelleher KJ, Rolls JA, and Pajer K (2005). Medicaid insurance policy for youths involved in the criminal justice system. *Am J Public Health* 95: 1707–1711.

Fullilove RE, and Fullilove MT (1999). HIV prevention and intervention in the African-American community. In PT Cohen, MA Sande, and PA Volberding (eds.), *The AIDS Knowledge Base*, third edition (pp. 911–916). Philadelphia: Lippincott Williams & Wilkens.

Golembeski C, and Fullilove RE (2005). Criminal (in)justice in the city and its associated health consequences. *Am J Public Health* 95:1701–1706.

Hammett TM, Harmon MP, and Rhodes W (2002). The burden of infectious disease among inmates of and releasees from US correctional facilities, 1997. *Am J Public Health* 92:1789–1794.

Institute of Medicine (2002). *Unequal Treatment: Confronting Racial and Ethnic Disparities in Health Care*. Washington, DC: Institute of Medicine.

Johnson RC, and Raphael S (2005). The Effects of Male Incarceration Dynamics on AIDS Infection Rates Among African-American Women and Men. Goldman School of Public Policy, University of California, Berkeley.

Kaiser Family Foundation (2004). *Financing HIV/AIDS Care: A Quilt with Many Holes*. Retrieved April 3, 2007, at http://www.kff.org/hivaids/upload/Financing-HIV-AIDS-Care-A-Quilt-with-Many-Holes.pdf.

Karon JM, Fleming PL, Steketee RW, and DeCock KM (2001). HIV in the United States at the turn of the century: an epidemic in transition. *Am J Public Health* 91:1060–1069.

Kushel MB, Hahn JA, Evans JL, Bangsberg DR, and Moss AR (2005). Revolving doors: imprisonment among the homeless and marginally housed population. *Am J Public Health* 95:1747–1752.

Mauer M (1999). *Race to Incarcerate*. New York: The New Press.

NY State Department of Corrections (2007). Overview. Retrieved March 15, 2007, from http:www.docs.state.ny.us/.

Sampson RJ (1995). Unemployment and imbalanced sex ratios: race-specific consequences for family structure and crime. In MB Tucker and C Mitchell-Kern (eds.), *The Decline in Marriage among African-Americans: Causes, Consequences, and Policy Implications* (pp. 229–260). New York: Russell Sage Foundation.

Sentencing Project (2006a). *Facts about Prisons and Prisoners*. Retrieved April 30, 2006, from http:www.sentencingproject.org/pdfs/1035.pdf.

Sentencing Project (2006b). *Crack Cocaine Sentencing Policy: Unjustified and Unreasonable*. Retrieved April 30, 2006, from http:www.sentencingproject.org/pdfs/1003.pdf

Part II

Comprehensive AIDS
Psychiatric Assessment

———————

Chapter 6

A Biopsychosocial Approach to Psychiatric Consultation in Persons with HIV and AIDS

Mary Ann Cohen and David Chao

All severe and complex medical illnesses have psychosocial and psychological aspects and meanings, and may have associated psychiatric diagnoses. Every patient with a severe and complex medical illness referred for psychiatric evaluation deserves a thorough and comprehensive biopsychosocial assessment. For persons with HIV and AIDS, a thorough and comprehensive assessment has far-reaching implications not only for competent and coordinated care but also for adherence to medical treatment and risk reduction, as well as public health. Psychiatric disorders are associated with inadequate adherence to risk reduction, medical care, and antiretroviral therapy. While adherence to medical care for most medical illnesses has major meaning to patients, loved ones, and families, adherence to medical care for HIV and AIDS has major implications for reduction of HIV transmission and prevention of emergence of drug-resistant HIV viral strains. Most persons with HIV and AIDS have psychiatric disorders (Stoff et al., 2004) and can benefit from psychiatric consultation and care. The rates

of HIV infection are also higher among persons with serious mental illness (Blank et al., 2002).

In 1967 Lipowski provided a classification of commonly encountered problems at the medical–psychiatric interface that is still relevant to AIDS psychiatry today. These problems (with a modification of the fifth item, discussed in Chapter 1 of this book) include psychiatric presentation of medical illness, psychiatric complications of medical illnesses or treatments, psychological response to medical illness or treatments, medical presentation of psychiatric illness or treatments, and comorbid medical and psychiatric illness. These five problems have been illustrated with case vignettes in Chapter 1. Some persons with HIV and AIDS have no psychiatric disorder, while others have a multiplicity of complex psychiatric disorders that are responses to illness or treatments or are associated with HIV/AIDS (such as HIV-associated dementia) or comorbid medical illnesses and treatments (such as hepatitis C, cirrhosis, or HIV nephropathy and end-stage renal disease). Persons with HIV and AIDS may also have comorbid psychiatric disorders that are co-occurring and may be unrelated to HIV (such as schizophrenia or bipolar disorder). The complexity of AIDS psychiatric consultation is illustrated in an article (Freedman et al., 1994) with the title "Depression, HIV Dementia, Delirium, Posttraumatic Stress Disorder (or All of the Above)."

Comprehensive psychiatric evaluations can provide diagnoses, inform treatment, and mitigate anguish, distress, depression, anxiety, and substance use in persons with HIV and AIDS. Furthermore, thorough and comprehensive assessment is crucial because HIV has an affinity for brain and neural tissue and can cause central nervous system (CNS) complications even in healthy seropositive individuals. These complications are described in Chapters 10, 17, and 19 of this book. Because of potential CNS complications as well as the multiplicity of other severe and complex medical illnesses in persons with HIV and AIDS (Huang et al., 2006), every person who is referred for a psychiatric consultation needs a full biopsychosocial evaluation. In this chapter, we provide a basic approach to persons with HIV and AIDS who are referred to an AIDS psychiatrist and a template for a comprehensive psychiatric evaluation. Neuropsychological evaluation can be a valuable adjunct in some persons with HIV and AIDS and is covered in Chapter 7.

SETTINGS FOR AIDS PSYCHIATRIC CONSULTATIONS

Psychiatric consultations are requested in inpatient and ambulatory divisions of acute care facilities and in chronic or long-term care facilities. Consultations may also be requested in other settings including the home care setting, the settings of marginal housing (such as shelters and single room occupancy transitional housing), correctional facilities, and in homeless outreach contexts. The complexities of the many special settings where persons with AIDS may be evaluated are covered in Chapter 31 as well as in Chapter 5, where correctional facility settings are addressed in further detail. Recently published textbooks of psychosomatic medicine (Stern et al., 2004; Levenson, 2005) cover psychiatric assessment of patients in the general-care acute medical setting but do not address specifics of psychiatric evaluation in the ambulatory setting. Since AIDS is now regarded as a chronic severe illness, most persons with HIV and AIDS are seen in outpatient settings, clinics, private offices, and other ambulatory care facilities.

As the medical care of persons with HIV and AIDS has shifted to the ambulatory setting, the psychiatric care for persons with HIV and AIDS has shifted as well, particularly in urban areas where mental health professionals are readily available in academic medical centers. Many models of mental health care delivery are used in the ambulatory setting. There is no clear evidence base to determine the best practice model, but many patients and clinicians are most satisfied with a colocated model of care that is based in the ambulatory HIV setting. Both inpatient and ambulatory evaluations will be presented in these assessments.

COMPREHENSIVE PSYCHOSOCIAL AND PSYCHIATRIC CONSULTATIONS

Outpatient Consultations

A colocated AIDS psychiatry team can provide on-site psychiatric evaluations and consultations as well as follow-up psychiatric care. Since attending a psychiatric clinic and an AIDS clinic may be perceived by some patients as doubly stigmatizing, persons with HIV and AIDS are sometimes relieved to learn that psychiatric care is a routine part of their comprehensive HIV care or HIV prenatal care and may find it more acceptable than having to be seen in a psychiatric outpatient setting. In the setting of the HIV clinic, a consultation may be requested by the primary HIV clinician directly through personal contact, by telephone contact, or by written request. The HIV clinician may indirectly request a consultation through another member of the team, often a social worker or other clinician.

Process of Psychiatric Outpatient Consultation

The consultation begins with a discussion between the HIV clinician and AIDS psychiatrist to determine the reason for the psychiatric referral, the expectations of the consultee, the urgency of the referral (manifest content of the consultation), and some of the feelings that the patient has engendered in consultee (latent content of the consultation). During this discussion, the HIV clinician can provide a summary of the patient's medical history and current condition as well as what medications are being prescribed for the patient. The psychiatrist can review the medical record in further detail. Ideally, if the patient is in the clinic for a scheduled visit with the HIV clinician when the AIDS psychiatrist is available, an introduction by the HIV clinician may prove invaluable and demonstrate the level of coordination of care being offered to the patient. The AIDS psychiatrist can be introduced as an integral member of the multidisciplinary team providing ongoing patient care. The HIV clinician can then discuss his or her concerns about the patient and the reasons for the psychiatric consultation. This open discussion by a sensitive and caring clinician with the psychiatric consultant in the presence of the patient can lead to better acceptance of the referral and set the stage for a continued collaborative relationship. It also serves to diminish anxiety in the patient and perhaps even serves to dispel or at least mitigate frightening myths about psychiatrists and mental health care. It is especially encouraging if the primary provider can discuss the need for the consultation as a means of providing him or her with help in better understanding and caring for the patient. The consultation is scheduled and the consulting AIDS psychiatrist reviews the chart to familiarize himself or herself with the patient's history and medical condition.

Comprehensive Outpatient Psychiatric Consultation

When the patient arrives for the first visit, the AIDS psychiatrist can set the tone for a nonjudgmental evaluation by starting with an introduction that is sensitive to the patient's potential anxiety surrounding the encounter. Suggestions for such an introduction include greeting and shaking hands. Shaking hands is especially important for persons with HIV and AIDS who are exquisitely sensitive to others' fears of contagion and may be reassured by a warm handshake. The introduction includes the AIDS psychiatrist addressing the patient by his or her title and last name (Mr. A), stating his or her title and last name (Dr. P), and accompanying the patient from the waiting area into the psychiatric consulting room. After closing the door to establish privacy and providing for appropriate seating and comfort, the psychiatrist asks the patient "How are you feeling today?" After listening to the response and following leads if applicable, the psychiatrist then describes the reason for the consultation. "Dr. M asked

me to evaluate you for depression. Did she tell you that she was asking me to see you? How do you feel about seeing a psychiatrist?" This may provide an opportunity to ask Mr. A if he has ever seen a psychiatrist or had contact with the mental health system in the past.

During the process of the introduction, the psychiatrist can begin to assess the patient through careful observation. Specific observations are described in detail below under the section on general appearance, manner, and attitude but should begin at the first moment of the encounter.

Chief Complaint and History of Present Illness

The psychiatrist elicits the patient's chief complaint in his or her own words and follows with the history of the present illness, including the onset, course, progression, and medications if any, along with the current medical and psychiatric symptoms and illness chronology. It is important for establishment of rapport to allow the patient to tell the story of the illness in his or her words with minimal interruption or intrusion except for occasional redirection. Although the psychiatrist may wish to have a thorough review of the history in chronological order, it is better to allow the patient to provide the story and for the psychiatrist to reconstruct the chronology by asking questions if the history is unclear. Allowing the patient to tell his or her story enables the psychiatrist to observe for cognitive impairment and to determine whether the patient is an accurate historian. Hearing the history of present illness recounted as a story often provides more information about remote and recent memory than does routine questioning. Following leads is more useful than proceeding on a set course of history-taking that may serve to derail an anxious patient. A comprehensive psychiatric assessment of a person with HIV or AIDS would not be complete without a determination of the patient's understanding of his or her illness and its treatments (Cohen 1986, 1987, 1992; Cohen and Weisman 1988; Cohen and Alfonso 1998, 2004).

Past History

Although there is no special set order, the rest of the history-taking process should follow leads, if possible, and should proceed from less anxiety-provoking to more anxiety-provoking issues. The demographic information and current life situation may be easy for some individuals to start with and may enable the patient to become comfortable and used to the new setting and start to develop a connection while discussing these somewhat less charged issues. It is especially important to learn early on about the patient's occupation or former occupation (if any) and about the patient's family structure and whether or not the patient has a partner, children, or grandchildren. Expression of interest in the patient's occupational and family history can help the patient feel a sense of the psychiatrist's personal interest and perceive that the psychiatrist is thinking about him or her as not just a patient, symptom, or illness, but as a person in the context of family, society, and community.

Medical History

The general health and medical history should include information about medical illnesses and symptoms, hospitalizations, surgery, traumatic injuries as well as medications and other treatments. It is also helpful to determine whether the patient is consulting clinicians other than the primary HIV referring clinician and, if so, whether other medications are being prescribed. Complementary and alternative healing modalities should be explored in a nonjudgmental manner. Additionally, information about nutrition and exercise can be addressed.

Specifics about HIV medical history include how and when the patient first learned about his or her serostatus, current and nadir CD4 counts if known, viral load, course and responses to illness, and treatments and responses to treatments. If the patient is known to have hepatitis C, history of course, treatments, and results are also relevant. Review of laboratory data, X-rays and other imaging studies, and other ancillary data through discussion with the primary physician and/or by a review of the medical record is a necessary part of the psychiatric consultation.

Early Childhood, Developmental, Social, and Family History

Once again, it is helpful to begin with the less affect-laden material, such as age, date of birth, and place of birth. Open-ended questions such as "What was it like for you growing up?" and "Who was in your family when you were growing up?" may be ways to begin. Exploration of relationships with parents, siblings, and other family members as well as discussions about parental drug and alcohol use can follow. Family history also includes information about illness patterns, particularly psychiatric illnesses such as bipolar disorder or schizophrenia. History and chronology of early childhood losses are highly significant and deserve careful interest and documentation. Educational history includes the following questions and is relevant in determination of current level of intellectual and occupational function: (1) "How far did you go in school?" (2) "How did you do in school?" (3) "What was school like for you?" (4) "Were there any problems with learning?"

A thorough housing history includes questions about where the patient lives, whether the patient lives alone or with others, and whether the patient is homeless or marginally housed. Specific information about housing includes whether the patient is in his or her own apartment or home, if the patient is comfortable and has space, privacy, an elevator if mobility is compromised, heat, and hot water, and if the home is free of rodents or other pests. Persons who live in marginal housing, in shelters, or on the street may feel embarrassed to discuss these issues and may not disclose this information as a result.

Family history includes information about family of origin as well as relational history with partners. Since it is hard to suffer an illness in silence, it is important to ask whether the patient has disclosed his or her serostatus to anyone in the family or to any partners. Disclosure may be easier for some patients and difficult to near impossible for other patients. The multidimensional determinants in considerations of disclosure include relational, psychological, social, cultural, spiritual, and political factors. Fear of disclosure to aged parents is often used as a reason for not telling any family member about serostatus.

Ages and health status of parents or dates and causes of death along with number, ages, and health of siblings are relevant. History of medical or mental illnesses and impact on the patient are also significant. Relational history includes information about past and current partners and whether the patient is in a relationship. Allowing the patient to discuss the relationship is important. Such discussions should include questions about disclosure of serostatus to his or her intimate partner. It is important to ask for the number, names, ages, health, and whereabouts of children, if any, along with the status of the parent–child relationship. The complex issues of whether and when to disclose to children are relevant. Dialogue about disclosure can begin during history-taking.

Occupational History

Occupational history is an important determinant of level of function. An individual who never worked may or may not feel distressed by being too ill to work. However, for individuals who have worked and who took pride in their career, the inability to work can be devastating and may be a significant contributor to a sense of loss or distress. It is important to ask questions about occupation in a way that is sensitive to the individual's current condition. If someone is bed-bound and near the end of life, it is helpful to acknowledge clearly that you recognize that the patient is no longer able to work but may have worked in the past. Similarly, in the ambulatory setting it is best not to make assumptions and to elicit information about occupation in a sensitive and compassionate manner. It is also important to be able to use the information in subsequent visits and to record it clearly in the medical record so that the information is available to other members of the team. A former home attendant, professional musician, foreman, teacher, nurse, or superintendent may take considerable pride in his or her hard work. For those individuals who are still able to work this can be a source of validation and meaning for some and a source of stress and fatigue for others.

Trauma History and Response to Trauma History

History of early childhood and other trauma is not easy to obtain. Trauma may be accompanied by amnesia, regardless of whether traumatic brain injury was involved. Trauma may also be followed by intense repression of horrific events. Some patients may refuse to talk about painful experiences whether distant or recent, particularly on a first encounter with the psychiatrist. Furthermore, if there is a history of trauma and such trauma was perpetrated by a parent or other close relative, this absolute violation and betrayal leads to loss of the most significant paradigm and basis for future development of trusting relationships. Hence, the patient may find it difficult to trust physicians and other health professionals who may represent those very figures of parental authority. A brief, supportive statement validating the difficulty of talking about early trauma may serve to mitigate discomfort. Additional reassurance that it is normal for persons who have experienced early-childhood abuse or neglect to have problems with trust can also be comforting.

If the patient is willing to discuss the painful experiences, it is helpful to ask direct and closed-ended questions unless the patient proceeds to tell the story in his or her own words. The patient may, in fact, feel relieved to be able to talk about these secrets after many decades. Questions may include those about physical and emotional abuse as well as neglect. Asking about being a witness to physical or threatened violence on a repeated basis or seeing one parent trying to hurt or kill the other parent may be relieving to the patient who has not been able to tell anyone about it because of threats or fear of reprisals. Specific questions about sexual abuse should elicit information about unwanted touching, molesting, or fondling as well as penetration, intercourse, and rape. It is also important to determine the dates of the traumatic events wherever possible. Later trauma such as rape, life-threatening robbery, kidnapping, or the witnessing of trauma, including combat-related trauma, can be explored in detail as well. Finally, head trauma, often accompanied by amnesia, should be specifically addressed.

A history of trauma is significant in evaluating for trauma sequelae including dissociative phenomena, hyperarousal, depression, eating disorders, substance use disorders, psychiatric disorders (especially posttraumatic stress disorder), domestic violence, and commercial sex work. Specific questions about posttraumatic stress disorder include those about dissociation, intrusive thoughts, flashbacks, nightmares, easy startle, hypervigilance, insomnia, and a sense of a foreshortened future.

Sexual History

Persons with HIV and AIDS have sexual needs as well as needs for companionship, tenderness, love, and romance. Many individuals are extremely uncomfortable discussing sexual feelings and may suffer in silence with problems of arousal, pain, or excitement. Some persons find it difficult to ask a partner to use a condom. Men and women with HIV and AIDS have a high prevalence of alcohol and other drug use and some may continue substance use and associated HIV risk behaviors such as sharing of needles and exchange of sex for drugs or money. The AIDS psychiatrist needs to be comfortable with taking a sexual history and as well as drug and alcohol histories. Suggestions for taking a sexual history are summarized in Table 6.1.

Psychiatric History

Persons with HIV and AIDS have a high prevalence of psychiatric disorders, although some persons with HIV and AIDS have no psychiatric disorders while others

TABLE 6.1. Sexual History-Taking

Setting the Tone

1. Often people with chronic medical illness experience problems with their sexual function. What is your sexual function like since you have been ill?
2. How is your sexual function since you have been physically ill compared with that when you were healthy?
3. Often people with psychiatric illness such as depression experience problems with their sexual function. What is your sexual function like since you have been ill?
4. How is your sexual function since you have been depressed (or had another psychiatric illness) compared with that when you were healthy?
5. Often people who need to take medications experience problems with their sexual function. What is your sexual function like since you have been on (the medication)?
6. How is your sexual function since you have been on (the medication) compared with that before starting on (the medication)?

Sexual Experience

7. When did you have your first period?
8. What was the experience of having your first period like for you?
9. When did you have your first ejaculation?
10. What was the experience of having your first ejaculation like for you?
11. How has your period changed over the years?
12. How have the changes in your hormones affected your sexual function?
13. How enjoyable is sex for you?
14. How enjoyable is masturbation for you?
15. Do you have (a) sexual partner(s)?
16. Are you sexually active?
17. What is the frequency of your sexual activity?
18. Have you noticed a change in the frequency of your sexual activity?
19. How do your religious beliefs affect your sexuality?
20. How do your cultural beliefs affect your sexuality?
21. Which of your sexual practices do you associate with feelings of shame?
22. Which of your sexual practices do you associate with feelings of anxiety?
23. Which of your sexual practices do you associate with feelings of unhappiness?

Safe and Unsafe Sex

24. What methods are you using to prevent yourself from getting sexually transmitted infections (herpes, gonorrhea, syphilis) or HIV infection? How many sexual partners do you have?
25. How many sexual partners have you had?
26. How has your number of sexual partners changed over time?
27. What kind of barrier contraception are you using?
28. What kind of spermicidal preparation are you using?
29. What lubricants do you use during sexual intercourse?
30. Are you aware that petroleum-based lubricants (Vaseline and others) can cause leakage of condoms?
31. How do you put a condom on?
32. At what point during intercourse do you put on a condom?
33. How do you ensure that there is no air bubble trapped inside the condom?
34. While wearing a condom, how do you ensure that there is no leakage during intercourse?
35. How do you ensure that there is no leakage upon condom removal?

may have a multiplicity of serious and often incapacitating psychiatric illnesses. Persons with HIV and AIDS are at especially high risk for cognitive disorders, affective disorders, substance use disorders, and posttraumatic stress disorder. There is also an association between serious mental illness and HIV-related illness, documented in a large study of treated Medicaid recipients. In this study, Blank and colleagues (2002) found a high HIV seroprevalence rate among treated Medicaid recipients with serious mental illness. They found that the HIV seroprevalence rate was four times higher among persons with schizophrenia and five times higher among persons with mood disorder than for persons without serious mental illness. They estimate that the untreated rates may be 10 to 20 times higher for persons with serious mental illness than for persons without serious mental illness.

The prevalence of psychiatric disorders in persons with HIV and AIDS is discussed in depth in Chapter 4 and a comprehensive approach to each of the most prevalent psychiatric disorders is presented in Chapters 8 through 13 of this book.

A comprehensive assessment of prior psychiatric symptoms, a history of psychiatric disorders, and a history of treatment for psychiatric illness include a history of inpatient and outpatient treatment, types of treatment, course of illness, and current involvement in psychiatric care. It is important to ascertain whether the patient is still in the care of other mental health clinicians and to obtain permission to contact the treating mental health clinician if appropriate. A full review of both current psychotropic medications and those previously prescribed is important. Since there is a high prevalence of mood disorders in persons with HIV and AIDS, a history of episodes of depression and mania should be elicited. Because there is a high prevalence of substance use disorders and suicidal ideation among persons with HIV and AIDS, these histories will be delineated separately. Both of these topics are explored in depth in other chapters in this book; suicide is covered in Chapter 18 and substance use disorder is covered in Chapter 8.

Suicide History-Taking

There is no treatment for suicide, only prevention and education. To evaluate for suicide risk in vulnerable persons with HIV and AIDS, AIDS psychiatrists and other clinicians need to be able to take a suicide history, recognize and ensure that depression and other

TABLE 6.2. Risk Factors for Suicide

1. Hopelessness
2. Impulsivity
3. Substance use disorder
4. Previous suicide attempts
5. Recent illness
6. Recent hospitalization
7. Living alone
8. Inexpressible grief
9. Depression

psychiatric disorders are treated, determine risk factors and etiologies, and ultimately help to resolve the suicidal crisis. Psychiatrists need to feel comfortable with taking a suicide history and discussing suicide in depth with a person with HIV and AIDS. This discussion entails the establishment of a trusting relationship, discussion of suicide and death in relation to both the illness and the individual's philosophies and religious beliefs, and awareness of the value of continuity of care and reassurance that the patient will not be abandoned (Cohen, 1992). No suicidal patient ever gets the idea for suicide from talking openly about suicide. Persons who are suicidal are able to admit to suicidal ideation and even to plans for suicide. They are also able to discuss prior attempts as well as precipitants. From these discussions, risk factors for the patient can be determined and crisis intervention initiated. Risk factors for suicide are summarized in Table 6.2 and suicide history-taking is summarized in Table 6.3.

Far from harming the suicidal individual with HIV and AIDS, being able to speak openly about suicidal

TABLE 6.3. Suicide History-Taking

1. Have you ever thought about killing yourself?
2. What specifically made you think of suicide?
3. Have you ever tried to commit suicide?
4. What precipitated your previous attempt or attempts?
5. How did you try to kill yourself?
6. When did you try to kill yourself?
7. Do you know anyone in your family or outside your family who committed suicide?
8. Do you feel like killing yourself now?
9. What would you accomplish?
10. Do you plan to rejoin someone you lost?
11. Who would miss you?
12. What would you miss?
13. Do you have any specific plans?
14. What are they?

thoughts and feelings is highly cathartic. Thoughts of suicide while providing some measure of consolation and control may also be frightening, distressing, and painful. Sharing suicidal feelings with an empathic listener is not only relieving but may also provide the patient with a new perspective. To resolve a suicidal crisis, it is important to reestablish bonds, provide the patient with a supportive network of family, loved ones, friends, and caregivers, and identify and treat psychiatric disorders. Crisis intervention, networking, and ongoing psychiatric care may help prevent suicide.

Drug History-Taking

It is important to be able to take a complete history of substance use for each individual with HIV or AIDS who is referred for psychiatric consultation. Patients are often reluctant to discuss drug addiction and may see their addiction as so much a part of their everyday lives that it is not even given a second thought. This can be as true for a business executive who has a three-martini lunch and continues to drink during and after dinner on a daily basis as it is for a chronic heroin-, cocaine-, or sedative-hypnotic-addicted individual. Furthermore, defensiveness and denial may need to be understood as concomitants of addictive disorders. For each individual, it is important to obtain a history of the chronology of the substance use from the first use to the last. An extremely benevolent and nonjudgmental approach is essential to help diminish defensiveness. An important part of the history-taking is to be able to ask questions that are ego supportive. Addiction history can be obtained after learning about crises, traumas, and losses and later determining if substances may have been used to console or self-medicate at the times of crisis, loss, or trauma. Using "how," "when," and "what" questions generally is useful and can facilitate history-taking and help to avoid the potential blaming aspects of "why" questions. Specific questions for substance use history-taking are summarized in Table 6.4.

The comprehensive and thorough history-taking of substance use can provide information of significance to all members of the treatment team. It is vital to understand what drugs will be induced or inhibited by such substances as heroin or methadone, for example. Drugs that induce isoenzyme cytochrome P4503A4 may lead to lowering opioid levels, resulting in a need for increased heroin use or an increase in the dose of methadone to obtain the same serum levels as before

enzyme induction. If the patient is on an antiretroviral, the patient may stop taking the medication because he or she is feeling uncomfortable symptoms of opioid withdrawal. Other drug–drug interactions, including those with psychotropic medication, are also significant. A patient with comorbid HIV and hepatitis C who stops all alcohol use during interferon treatment and eagerly resumes daily use after successful treatment and eradication of hepatitis C virus puts his or her hepatic function in jeopardy once again. For individuals who have unprotected sexual encounters in the context of alcohol or drug use, history-taking has public health implications. For individuals exposed to drug- or alcohol-related domestic violence, the implications are both tragic and obvious. Hence, for medical, psychological, and social reasons, a comprehensive drug history is essential in persons with HIV and AIDS.

Inpatient General Care Consultations

For patients who are not known to the facility, it is important to obtain as much information as is possible from members of the medical, surgical, obstetric, or other team providing care for the patient. A review of the chart, laboratory data, and a list of current medications should be assessed. Clinicians should ascertain the correct name and room number, and check to be certain that the patient fits the description and that his or her identification bracelet matches the name of the patient referred. This is especially important because of the confidential nature of HIV illness. Specific recommendations for history-taking in the inpatient general care setting are summarized in Table 6.5.

PSYCHIATRIC EXAMINATION

The complete psychiatric assessment of a person with HIV and AIDS includes an evaluation of all the ego functions listed below as part of the examination. Every patient deserves the full baseline cognitive assessment suggested below, since early cognitive changes may be very subtle. A patient may have no evidence of disorientation to person, place, or time, may be able to register and recall, and may not have a subjective awareness of any cognitive difficulty even though executive dysfunction may appear in a clock drawing and preclinical findings may be indicated in constructional apraxia on three-dimensional cube or

TABLE 6.4. Substance Use History-Taking

1. Many people who are ill may use drugs or alcohol to get through difficult times. What have you used to get through these times?

2. Specifically ask about all drugs by name and street name:
   Alcohol
   Heroin—dope, smack, horse
   Cocaine—crack, freebase
   Cannabis—marijuana, weed, dope, pot, joints
   Sedative-hypnotics—primarily benzodiazepines such as alprazolam, Xanax, or sticks
   Hallucinogens
     Lysergic acid dethylamide, LSD, or acid
     Psilocybin or mushrooms
     Methamphetamine or speed, ice, crystal meth, crank
     Dimethoxymethylamphetamine or DOM, STP
     Methylenedioxymethamphetamine or MDMA, Ecstasy, X, XTC
     Ketamine or K, special K, Ket, super K, vitamin K
     Gamma-hydroxybutyric acid or GHB, liquid E, Georgia Home Boy
   Phencylcidine—angel dust

3. Precipitants
   a. What led to your first trying (the specific substance or substances) _____?
   b. What was your reaction to it?
   c. How were you able to get it?
   d. What effect did it have on the problem, crisis, or trauma in your life?

4. Chronology
   a. When did you first use _____?
   b. What happened after that?
   c. What other drugs or alcohol did you use?
   d. How did using _____ effect your school, work, and relationships?
   e. What kind of trouble did you get into?
   f. When did you last use?

5. Amounts, routes, and access
   a. What is the most you can hold or use in a day?
   b. How do you take it?
     Intravenous—with or without sharing of needles or works
     Insufflation or snorting
     Smoking
     Subcutaneous or skin-popping
     Oral
   c. What illegal means did you need to resort to in order to get it?
     Exchange of sex for drugs
     Selling drugs
     Selling belongings
     Selling family belongings
     Robbery, violent crime

6. Course, stage of change, and treatments

Bender-Gestalt drawings. Early-stage dementia may be indicated on formal testing in the comprehensive assessment described. In addition to cognitive disorders, a comprehensive psychiatric examination will provide evidence of any other psychiatric disorders. It will help inform decisions on the patient's ability to adhere to care, as well as lead to psychiatric treatment to alleviate distress and suffering and decrease morbidity and mortality associated with nonadherence to care.

As with history-taking, there is no set order for the psychiatric examination. The least challenging and affect-laden areas should be addressed first and the more complex and difficult ones last. Many of the functions being evaluated will have been observed during the process of meeting the patient and taking the

TABLE 6.5. Recommendations for History-Taking on Inpatient General Care

1. Knock on the door of the room even if it is open, and await a response.
2. Ascertain the patient's identity verbally and also with identification bracelet while beginning introductions.
3. Introduction by name and title: "Good morning Ms. B, I am Dr. P and I am a psychiatrist (while shaking hands).
4. Establish privacy by using the privacy curtains or door of the room.
5. Sit down near the bedside, preferably at the same level as the patient if possible.
6. Attend to distractions with patient's permission.
7. If the television is on at high volume, ask to turn it down.
8. If visitors are present, determine whether to proceed with the interview, request time alone, or reschedule after the visitors leave. Visits by partners, family members, or friends are especially important to persons with HIV and AIDS who, in addition to feeling isolated and alone as with any severe illness, are extremely sensitive to rejection and discrimination and may place a higher value on the presence of visitors.
9. Attend to comfort and address pain or other urgent issues.
10. Obstacles to communication
    a. The sleeping patient
       Since sleep disturbances are prevalent in persons with HIV and AIDS, consider allowing the patient to rest, and come back later.
       One may attempt to arouse the patient and obtain permission to proceed with the introduction and interview with appropriate apology for disturbing his or her sleep.
    b. Pain
       Address pain issues with the primary nurse or physician.
    c. Nausea or vomiting
       Provide an emesis basin and report to primary nurse.
    d. Need for bedpan or assistance to the bedside commode
       Provide bedpan if available or contact nursing assistant.
    e. Sensory deficits
       • Visual impairment
         Describe what you are doing and what is happening and be certain not to touch the patient before fully explaining that you would like to shake hands in greeting and who and where you are.
       • Hearing impairment
         Ascertain that hearing aids are in place or obtain amplifiers.
         Use lip reading if possible.
         Speak slowly, loudly, and clearly and on the side of the ear with the better hearing.
    f. Obtain interpreters if there is a language barrier.
    g. Communication barriers: endotracheal tube, tracheostomy, or ventilator
       Use a clipboard, paper, and pen to enable the patient to write responses to simple questions if possible.
       Make use of a communication board if writing is not feasible because of paralysis or paresis.
       If these measures are not possible, use closed-ended questions with a code such as head-nodding, blinking (1 blink designates "yes" and 2 blinks designates "no"), or finger squeezing (1 squeeze means "yes" and 2 squeezes means "no").

history. However, time has to be set aside to complete a full evaluation of the patient's ego functions and current presentation, including assessment for depression, anxiety, psychosis, suicidality, dangerousness to others, and cognition. The setting of the consultation is meaningful, with a higher prevalence of delirium to be anticipated in acute general-care units and especially intensive care units, and a higher prevalence of HIV-associated dementia can be expected in the nursing home or long-term care facility settings.

General Appearance, Manner, and Attitude

The psychiatrist can observe for signs of medical or psychiatric illnesses: mobility, gait, abnormal movements, general appearance, grooming, appropriateness and neatness of attire, responsiveness, cooperation, and ability to maintain eye contact. Observation for psychomotor retardation (slowing) or agitation can be helpful. The psychiatrist can listen carefully for rate, quality, tone, audibility, modulation, and form of speech, including evidence of prosody, aphasias, or dysphasias. Additionally, observation of skin for icterus, pallor, cyanosis, edema, rashes, or other lesions can be helpful. The psychiatrist should also evaluate whether the patient appears healthy or ill, robust or cachectic, with signs of wasting and protein energy undernutrition. Obvious signs of specific medical illness or organ impairment include seizures, involuntary movements, tremors, paresis, paralysis, facial droop or asymmetry, exophthalmos, neck fullness, spider angiomata, ascites, anascarca, dyspnea, clubbing, and pedal edema. The psychiatrist can look for signs of delirium such as fluctuating levels of consciousness, mood, and behavior and falling asleep during the evaluation. Similarly, delirium related to intoxication or withdrawal can be observed with signs of slurred speech, "nodding out," flattening of the nasal cartilage (due to cocaine insufflation), tremulousness, pinpoint pupils (from use of opioids), dilated pupils (from opioid withdrawal or PCP), tracks and abscesses from injection drug use, and skin lesions indicative of subcutaneous drug use. Finally, the psychiatrist can look for signs of side effects of medications such as lipodystrophy from antiretroviral medications or orobuccolingual movements (tardive dyskinesia) from psychotropic medications.

It is also important to determine whether the patient appears his or her stated age and, if the patient is working, whether he or she is appropriately attired for the occupation. Observing for relational ability, eye contact, handshake, and ability to engage is also significant. The patient's cooperativeness, hostility, depression, anxiety, and fear should be noted.

Affectivity and Mood

Observation of affect includes attention to euthymia, depression, anxiety, elation, irritability, hostility, expansiveness, and constriction or fullness of range. Affectivity is a somewhat objective assessment by the clinician, while mood is more subjective and reflects the patient's assessment of how he or she feels. Moods can be sad, tearful, anxious, angry, or suspicious. Suicidal ideas or intentions as well as plans or thoughts should be explored. Violent or homicidal ideas or plans need to be discussed.

Thought Content and Mental Trend

Delusions, ideas of reference, flight of ideas, tangentiality, preoccupation, paranoid ideation, and expansiveness are important to assess. Specific well-formed and systematic delusions or grandiose ideas as well as general suspiciousness and guarding are indicative of underlying psychotic processes.

Perception

The patient should be asked about perceptions in a supportive manner that does not create defensiveness. Asking whether the patient "ever sees shadows" or feels that his or her "mind may be playing tricks" may be helpful. Specific questions to determine the presence of auditory, visual, olfactory, or tactile (coenesthetic) hallucinations and formication are necessary. Visual hallucinations include those of colorful, frightening, Lilliputian, and specific people either alive or deceased. Observation for signs that the patient is responding to internal stimuli should be documented.

Cognition

This is a crucial part of the evaluation and needs to be done in a systematic and comprehensive and nonthreatening manner. The initial aspects have to do with observation as described above in the section on general appearance, manner, and attitude, observing for level of alertness, consciousness, confusion, fluctuation, somnolence, or stupor. Careful observation may reveal perseveration on words, numbers, or actions. Perseveration may be evident in the absence of hearing impairment when the patient responds to a prior question more than one time as if he or she had not heard the following question. Specific questions as to orientation can be approached in an ego-supportive manner and can be asked as part of the routine. Memory is best tested by observing the patient's ability to provide his or her medical history in an organized manner and asking direct and specific questions about onset, course, and treatments. If a patient spontaneously reveals that memory is a problem, this lead can be followed with a statement such as "Let's see how your memory is working now." This can provide a smooth transition into a formal assessment of cognitive abilities. Memory is tested with evaluation of remote, recent, registration, and recall memory (the four "Rs of memory). Asking the patient to repeat the four words "hat," "car," "tree," and "twenty-six" from a cognitive screening device (Jacobs et al., 1977) and then recall them again 5 minutes later provides a test for registration and 5-minute recall. Drawings can help in the assessment of visuospatial function as well as for perseveration and fine hand tremor. The copying of Bender-Gestalt drawings and a three-dimensional cube assesses for constructional apraxia, as does a clock drawing (Bender, 1938; Lyketsos et al., 2004). Clock drawing is especially helpful in assessing executive function and planning as well as constructional apraxia and hemineglect. Irregular spacing of clock numbers with some too close together or too far apart is indicative of executive dysfunction with difficulty in planning. Left hemineglect may be associated with a lesion in the right parietal lobe.

Repetition of numbers indicates perseveration. The patient should be asked to draw the face of a clock, starting with a circle and placing the numbers on the face. The patient should then be asked to draw the hands to represent a time of 10 after 11 on the clock drawing to assess ability to change mental sets. Further testing for abstract thinking with similarities and proverb interpretation as well as interpretation of current events is helpful. Intellectual function should be assessed in relation to educational and occupational levels and can be tested by observing vocabulary usage, comprehension level, and reasoning. To assess for concentration, calculation, and spelling the patient can be asked to subtract serial 7's or 3's and spell the word "world" both forward and backward. Asking the patient about their understanding of their illness can provide an assessment of insight and judgment as well as abstract thinking.

CONCLUSIONS

A biopsychosocial approach to psychiatric consultation can provide a way to get to know the patient in the context of family, society, and community. This approach is a valuable asset to the comprehensive care of a person with HIV and AIDS.

References

Bender L (1938). A *Visual Motor Gestalt Test and Its Clinical Use*. New York: American Orthopsychiatry Association.

Blank MB, Mandell DS, Aiken L, Hadley TR (2002). Co-occurrence of HIV and serious mental illness among Medicaid recipients. *Psychiatr Serv* 53:868–873.

Cohen MA (1987). Psychiatric aspects of AIDS: A biopsychosocial approach. In GP Wormser, RE Stahl, and EJ Bottone (eds.), *AIDS and Other Manifestations of HIV Infection*. Park Ridge, NJ: Noyes Publishers.

Cohen MA (1992). Biopsychosocial aspects of the HIV epidemic. In GP Wormser (ed.), *AIDS and Other Manifestations of HIV Infection*, second edition (pp. 349–371). New York: Raven Press.

Cohen MA, and Alfonso CA (1998). Psychiatric care and pain management in persons with HIV infection. In GP Wormser (ed.), *AIDS and Other Manifestations of HIV Infection*, third edition. Philadelphia: Lippincott-Raven Publishers.

Cohen MA, and Alfonso CA (2004). AIDS psychiatry: psychiatric and palliative care, and pain management. In GP Wormser (ed.), *AIDS and Other Manifestations of HIV Infection*, fourth edition (pp. 537–576). San Diego: Elsevier Academic Press.

Cohen MA, and Weisman H (1986). A biopsychosocial approach to AIDS. *Psychosomatics* 27:245–249.

Cohen MA, and Weisman HW (1988). A biopsychosocial approach to AIDS. In RP Galea, BF Lewis, and LA Baker (eds.), *AIDS and IV Drug Abusers*. Owings Mills, MD: National Health Publishing.

Freedman JB, O'Dowd MA, Wyszynsk B, Torres JR, and McKegney FP (1994). Depression, HIV dementia, delirium, posttraumatic stress disorder (or all of the above). *Gen Hosp Psychiatry* 16:426–434.

Huang L, Quartin A, Jones D, and Havlir DV (2006). Intensive care of patients with HIV infection. *N Engl J Med* 355:173–181.

Jacobs JN, Bernhard MR, Delgado A, and Strain JJ (1977). Screening for organic mental syndromes in the medically ill. *Ann Intern Med* 86:40–46.

Levenson LL (2005). *American Psychiatric Publishing Textbook of Psychosomatic Medicine* (pp. 3–14). Washington, DC: American Psychiatric Publishing.

Lipowski ZJ (1967). Review of consultation psychiatry and psychosomatic medicine: II. Clinical aspects. *Psychosom Med* 29:201–224.

Lyketsos CG, Rosenblatt A, and Rabins P (2004). Forgotten frontal lobe syndrome or "executive dysfunction syndrome." *Psychosomatics* 43(3):345–355.

Stern TA, Fricchione GL, Cassem NH, Jellinek MS, and Rosenbaum JF (2004). *Massachusetts General Hospital Handbook of General Hospital Psychiatry*, fifth edition (pp. 9–19). Philadelphia: Mosby.

Stoff DM, Mitnick L, and Kalichman S (2004). Research issues in the multiple diagnoses of HIV/AIDS, mental illness and substance abuse. *AIDS Care* 16 (Suppl. 1):S1–S5

Chapter 7

Neuropsychological Evaluation

Elizabeth Ryan and Desiree Byrd

Neuropsychological assessment can be an important part of the care of persons with HIV. The neuropsychological evaluation assesses a patient's cognitive abilities, emotional functioning (i.e., presence of mood disorders, personality functioning), and functional ability complaints (i.e., difficulty performing daily living activities). Patients who may need assistance with daily living or who could benefit from cognitive remediation can be identified through the neuropsychological exam. This chapter provides an overview of issues germane to the neuropsychological assessment of HIV patients, including when to refer a patient for evaluation, the recommended cognitive tests, and current neurocognitive diagnostic algorithms. Given the changing demographics of the HIV/AIDS epidemic, we emphasize the salient issues in the assessment of diverse ethnic populations. We also highlight the neuropsychology of an emerging comorbid condition in HIV—hepatitis C.

NEUROPSYCHOLOGY

Neuropsychology is the subspecialty of psychology that studies the behavioral manifestations of brain dysfunction through the use of tests of cognitive and emotional functioning. Neuropsychology is grounded in psychometric theory, and test selection is based on a test's demonstrated reliability and validity for the population being assessed. Screening instruments (e.g., bedside mental status exams, clock drawing tests) can be useful in the detection of general cognitive impairment but lack the specificity and normative data to be used in isolation. Other than detecting frank impairment, they are not limited in characterizing a patient's cognitive status. Therefore, these types of assessments are generally not endorsed by neuropsychologists, who prefer using well-validated tests. For instance, although the Mental Alternation Test (Jones et al., 1993), a bedside test, has been validated with 62 inpatients in the pre-HAART era, we caution against using this test in isolation, given the changing demographics of seropositive individuals in the HAART era. The Mental Alteration Test requires the patient to say the alphabet and ultimately verbally alternate between numbers and the alphabet in sequence (i.e., 1-A, 2-B, 3-C . . .). Because ethnic minority patients and those from low socioeconomic backgrounds are more likely to have had poor-quality education despite adequate years of education, some members may be less facile with the alphabet. For instance, among a HAART era cohort of predominantly ethnic minority seropositive individuals (17% Caucasian), we found that 44% could not write the alphabet flawlessly, despite having a mean education of 11.9 years (Ryan et al., 2005). Thus, individuals who perform less than 15 alterations in 30 seconds, the required cutoff on the Mental Alteration Test, may not be cognitively impaired but may have low literacy skills.

REFERRING PATIENTS FOR
A NEUROPSYCHOLOGICAL EVALUATION

Although not part of the routine medical care of persons with HIV and AIDS, neuropsychological assessment can provide useful clinical information. The reasons for a neuropsychological evaluation referral may include the following: to obtain prognosis, to diagnose HIV-associated neurocognitive impairment, to screen for cognitive impairment that may affect medication adherence, and to identify the best antiretroviral treatment. Currently it can be less clear which patients require an evaluation, as the relation between cerebrospinal RNA and cognitive impairment observed in the pre-HAART era no longer holds in the HAART era (McArthur, 2004). However, periodic screening of a patient's mental status is good practice, and patients who exhibit a decrement should be referred for a neuropsychological evaluation. Periodic monitoring of mental status is especially important for patients who have been unable to achieve or sustain viral suppression, because in the HAART era, such patients who have cognitive impairment are at increased risk for mortality (Tozzi et al., 2005).

Understandably, practitioners often refer patients when they have complaints. However, a seropositive patient who complains of cognitive difficulty may or may not require a neuropsychological evaluation. Cognitive complaints among persons with HIV are often associated with depression (Moore et al., 1997; Rourke

et al., 1999a). Among seropositive individuals, endorsement of clinical symptoms (i.e., misplacing items like keys, difficulty driving, reading comprehension problems) was associated with depression and anxiety and not neuropsychological impairment; successful treatment of depression alleviated cognitive complaints (Claypoole et al., 1998). Thus, ruling out a mood disorder is particularly important when a patient has cognitive complaints. If a mood disorder exists and cognitive complaints persist despite successful treatment of the disorder, a neuropsychological evaluation is recommended.

In contrast to the overreporting of symptoms among depressed patients, HIV-seropositive patients with bona fide cognitive impairment may be less aware of their cognitive difficulties (Moore et al., 1997, Rourke et al., 1999b). HIV-seropositive patients with frontal-executive disturbance have few subjective memory complaints, but neuropsychological testing has revealed that in addition to conceptual problem-solving deficits, these patients also have memory deficits. Clinicians need to be aware that these patients will be less accurate in their self-appraisals of cognitive functioning, thus complaints from a collateral source (i.e., significant other, social worker, family member) warrant a neuropsychological evaluation referral.

NEUROPSYCHOLOGICAL BATTERY
CONSIDERATIONS

Neuropsychological assessment of the HIV patient targets subcortically mediated cognitive processes (psychomotor speed, attention/working memory, learning and memory, and executive functioning). Below we review the important cognitive domains to assess in the presence of HIV and recommend tests to be used in the assessment. As important as the tests used are, the normative databases used with the tests are even more crucial because they determine impairment. With HIV currently affecting growing numbers of ethnic minorities (CDC, 2004), the cognitive assessment of HIV-seropositive individuals has become more challenging.

Most neuropsychological tests have been normed on primarily Caucasian samples; significant performance differences exist even with neurologically healthy ethnic minorities (compared to Caucasians). Thus it is important to consider culture-related factors in the selection of measures, test performance, and the interpretation of test results. For instance, if the selected battery does not include measures that have been validated with ethnic minority populations or measures that do not have appropriate normative data, the clinician risks an invalid assessment. Evaluations with ethnic minority HIV-seropositive persons may require the clinician to alter the standard battery and substitute or supplement it with measures more appropriate for use with certain ethnic minority groups, especially those with limited English proficiency or poor educational backgrounds.

The administration of neuropsychological tests follows standardized procedures. However, sensitivity to the subtle nuances of cross-cultural interactions with minority clients (e.g., level of formality, comfort and confidence with testing, eye contact, increased importance of rapport) will enhance the evaluation and elicit better test performance. One of the primary challenges encountered with test administration among diverse populations is the assessment of non-native English speakers.

Assessment of patients with limited English proficiency is an especially difficult task, given the language dependence of neuropsychological measures. A practical, though often overlooked, first step to assessment with these patients is the collection of a language history (i.e., proficiency in English and native language, language preference at home, age at first English instruction, and language preference for the assessment). Neuropsychologists who are asked to assess patients who speak an unfamiliar language should first seek and refer patients to colleagues who share the language of the client. When a language-appropriate referral is not available, the use of interpreters may be unavoidable. In such cases, the identification of interpreters with professional training is optimal (e.g., trained psychometrists, court interpreters; Artiola i Fortuny and Mullaney, 1998). Clinicians working with Hispanic seropositive clients can refer to the work of Llorente and colleagues (2001) for a comprehensive list of measures and normative samples useful for neuropsychological assessment in this group.

SUGGESTED NEUROPSYCHOLOGICAL BATTERY

Screening for Cognitive Impairment

The HIV Dementia Scale (HDS) (Power et al., 1995) was designed as a brief screening measure to detect HIV-related cognitive dysfunction. Its four subtests assess *delayed recall* (recall of four words after a 5-minute delay), *psychomotor speed* (timed written alphabet), *constructional praxis* (timed cube copy), and *behavioral inhibition* (antisaccadic errors). Recently the HDS has been shown to be an inadequate screener with ethnically diverse cohorts (Smith et al., 2003; Richardson et al., 2005). The HDS scores have been shown to be related to education and ethnicity (Childers et al., 2002) and do not take into account collateral risk factors for poor neuropsychological performance (i.e., low education) or cognitive impairment (i.e. substance use, psychiatric disorder) that may confound the scores of disenfranchised individuals.

The use of a short battery of tests including the Hopkins Verbal Learning Test-Revised (HVLT-R; the Total Recall index) and the Grooved Pegboard Test (the nondominant hand score) or the HVLT-R Total Recall Index and WAIS-III Digit Symbol (all discussed below) has been found to be more accurate than the HDS in determining impairment (Carey et al., 2004). Alternatively, combining the Modified HDS (M-HDS) (which excludes the antisaccade portion of the test) with the Grooved Pegboard nondominant hand score in a scoring algorithm (Davis et al., 2002) yielded a sensitivity equivalent to the short battery that Carey and colleagues recommend and may be easier for a non-neuropsychologist to administer. The short battery proposed by Carey et al. has the advantage of having ethnically corrected norms for Grooved Pegboard nondominant (Heaton et al., 2004a) and the WAIS-III Digit Symbol test (Tulsky and Price, 2002) and thus may be superior for ethnically diverse clinical populations.

Premorbid Assessment

Estimation of premorbid intellectual functioning is an essential part of interpreting neuropsychological performance following traumatic brain injury and disease-induced brain dysfunction such as HIV illness with brain involvement. Clinical prediction of the presence or degree of HIV illness–induced impairment relies on premorbid estimators, because it is rare that a prior neuropsychological assessment exists. Various premorbid estimation methods have been studied in neuropsychology, including the "best performance" method (which uses the patient's highest test score in the test battery), the use of actuarial or demographic regression formulas, and measurement of cognitive functions assumed to be resistant to disease or injury.

The latter method includes use of tests of reading to predict premorbid functioning. Use of reading level as a premorbid indicator is predicated on the strong correlation of reading with IQ in the general population, its supposed greater resistance to dementia, and its purported reliance on previous knowledge rather than on current cognitive functioning. Reading tests such as the WRAT-4 Reading test (Wilkinson and Robertson, 2006) are commonly used to estimate premorbid functioning in neuropsychology. An important caveat about reading tests is that nationally, ethnic minority populations are overrepresented at the lowest literacy levels (Kirsch et al., 2002) because of disparities in the quality of education they receive. Given that the HIV epidemic has increasing ethnic minority representation, reading tests should be used with caution, as reading levels may underestimate neuropsychological performance in ethnic minorities (Manly et al., 2002; Ryan et al., 2005). Nonverbal tests of intellectual functioning such as the General Ability Measure for Adults (GAMA) (Naglieri and Bardos, 1997) may be better premorbid estimators for HIV patients with low literacy, as HIV is not known to affect visual spatial functioning (Ryan et al., 2006).

In summary, it is essential that a premorbid index not overestimate or underestimate functioning, as this will jeopardize interpretations about the degree or even existence of HIV-related cognitive impairment. If an adequate premorbid estimate cannot be obtained because of a patient's low level of education, poor quality of education, and/or different cultural background, it will be difficult to determine whether the observed performance represents a decline. It may be necessary to follow the patient over time to determine whether the patient is stable or not.

Psychomotor Functioning

HIV has a predilection for the basal ganglia (Berger and Arendt, 2000; von Giessen et al., 2001), which plays a pivotal role in control of movement. Psychomotor slowing (i.e., minor motor deficits) predicts HIV-associated dementia, AIDS, and death (Arendt et al., 1994; Sacktor et al., 1996) but can be ameliorated by HAART (Ferrando et al., 1998; Sacktor et al., 2001). Psychomotor slowing is so central to HIV that it appears to be the underlying cause of the various cognitive deficits in HIV (Becker and Salthouse, 1999).

Psychomotor functioning can be assessed by various tests. The Grooved Pegboard Test (Kløve, 1963),

which assesses psychomotor speed and fine motor control, is sensitive to HIV (Selnes et al., 1995). The score is the total time (in seconds) required to place 25 keyed pegs in a 5 × 5 array of slotted holes. Normative data are available for African Americans (Heaton et al., 2004a). Psychomotor speed can also be assessed with the Symbol Digit Modalities Test (Smith, 1982) and/or the Digit Symbol Test (Wechsler, 1997). These tests require the patient to substitute numbers for symbols (or vice versa) according to a fixed key. The score is the total number of correct items completed in a time limit. The Digit Symbol Test (Wechsler, 1997) also has demographically corrected norms suitable for use with ethnically diverse patient populations (Tulsky and Price, 2002).

Attention and Working Memory

Working memory involves the temporary storage and rehearsal of information; an example of working memory would be memorizing a phone number without writing it down. HIV infection is associated with decrements in working memory (Wood et al., 1998; Hinkin et al., 2002b), which may contribute to other HIV-associated neuropsychological deficits. Working memory can be measured by tests such as Letter Number Sequencing (Wechsler, 1997), in which patients order increasingly longer strings of auditorily presented letters and numbers, and the Paced Auditory Serial Addition Task (PASAT) (Diehr et al., 2003), which involves adding numbers presented auditorily. Both of these tests have demographically adjusted norms.

Learning and Memory

HIV patients exhibit a subcortical pattern of memory deficit with poor leaning and recall of word lists (White et al., 1997) in the absence of rapid forgetting, as seen in cortical dementias. They tend to exhibit a deficit in retrieval, and their memory can be facilitated by presenting them with information in a recognition format rather than asking them to freely recall stimuli. The California Verbal Learning Test-II (CVLT-II) (Delis et al., 2000) is a test of verbal learning and memory that requires the subject to learn a word list over the course of multiple trials and recall it immediately and after a delay. The Hopkins Verbal Learning Test (HVLT-R) is a similar test but has less extensive norms.

Executive Functioning

Executive functioning refers to various interrelated abilities that allow for control over thought and behavior in the service of goal-directed activity, problem solving, and flexible shifting of actions to meet task demands. HIV affects frontostriatal dysfunction and thus, on tests of executive functioning, HIV-positive patients often show impairment (Heaton et al., 1995; Hinkin et al., 1999). Tests of executive functioning include the Wisconsin Card Sorting Test (Kongs et al., 2000), which assesses hypothesis testing, and the Trail Making Test Part B (Reitan and Wolfson, 1985), which requires the patient to consecutively connect numbers and letters, alternating between the two sequences. Norms for African Americans are available for Trail Making Test Part B (Heaton et al., 2004a).

Functional Assessment and Impact

Assessment of a patient's level of everyday functioning is also an important aspect of the neuropsychological evaluation. Typically, functional ability is measured by self- and significant-other reports. Self-reports are used because most objective measures of everyday functioning are laboratory based and are not commercially available like neuropsychological tests are. HIV neuropsychological deficits are associated with complaints about not being able to perform instrumental activities of daily living and vocational functioning (Heaton et al., 1994b; Albert et al., 1995), worse everyday functioning on laboratory-based measures (i.e., shopping, cooking, financial management) (Heaton et al., 2004b), impaired driving ability (Marcotte et al., 2004), increased unemployment (van Gorp et al., 1999; Rabkin et al., 2004), and worse performance on standardized work samples (Heaton et al., 1996). Of particular importance to clinicians is information about a patient's ability to effectively manage his or her medications. Seropositive individuals with impairments in memory, executive function, and psychomotor skills have been found to have significant difficulties on medication management ability and adherence tasks (Hinkin et al., 2002a; Albert et al., 2003). Medication management ability is assessed by means of a laboratory task, the Medication Management Test (Albert et al., 1999), which measures the ability to interpret prescription label information and dispense medication, or by use of the Medication Event Monitoring System (MEMS) (Hinkin et al.,

2002a), in which a computer chip embedded in the top of the pill bottle automatically records the date, time, and duration of pill bottle opening. While these medication management assessment techniques are not part of a traditional neuropsychological battery, patients with neuropsychological deficits and their significant others or caregivers should be asked about their (or the patient's) medication adherence. The Instrumental Activities of Daily Living Scale (Lawton and Brody, 1969) can be used to assess complaints about the inability to accomplish instrumental activities of daily living. This scale assesses the ability to perform tasks such as preparing meals, managing finances, and taking medications properly. For patients with functional impairments, visiting nurse service, a home health aide, or an occupational therapy referral may be appropriate. For patients with cognitive impairments who drive, a driving evaluation is recommended.

INTERPRETATION AND DIAGNOSES

The interpretation of neuropsychological test results is the most decisive stage in the assessment process. It is at this point that clinicians use available evidence to determine whether a patient's pattern of performance is impaired and whether the observed impairment is due to HIV or other contributing factors. In the assessment of ethnic minority persons with HIV and AIDS, the task of test score interpretation is complicated by a number of factors, among them being the disproportionate presence of confounding conditions (e.g., low quality of education, medical illness) and inappropriate normative data. Interpretation difficulties jeopardize the accuracy of the final diagnosis (Manly and Jacobs, 2002a).

Two major diagnostic systems exist to categorize HIV neurocognitive disorders. While a thorough review of the evolution of these diagnostic systems is beyond the scope of this chapter, a brief discussion of the two systems and their interaction with ethnic minority status is presented below.

American Academy of Neurology AIDS Task Force Algorithm and Dana Modification

The most widely accepted rubric for understanding neurocognitive impairment in HIV is the diagnostic criteria established in 1991 by the American Academy of Neurology's (AAN) AIDS task force (AAN, 1991). The AAN criteria functioned to standardize and objectify a rating system for HIV-associated dementia (HAD) and HIV-associated minor cognitive motor disorder (MCMD). Please refer to Chapter 10 of this book for a more extensive discussion of these issues. In general, AAN criteria require impaired cognition in at least two domains (each of which may be represented by a single test), neurological abnormalities or decline in motivation, behavior, or emotional control, and related impairment in functional status. These criteria were further refined and operationalized by the Dana consortium (1996). Importantly, both the Dana modification and the AAN criteria require the use of age- and education-corrected normative data when interpreting neuropsychological data. This recommendation is very important and should not be overlooked. Without the proper matching of demographic characteristics between patients and the normative data used to interpret test results, HIV-seropositive patients, particularly ethnic minorities and those with low levels of education, are at significant risk for misdiagnoses (Ryan et al., 2005). A major critique of the AAN diagnostic system is the low threshold for neuropsychological impairment and lack of adequate consideration of confounding conditions (i.e., lower quality of education, medical illnesses).

Clinical Ratings Method

A clinical ratings approach to evaluating neuropsychological impairment in patients with HIV was developed by the HIV Neurobehavioral Research Center (Heaton et al., 1994a). In this approach, test performances from a large battery of tests are grouped into cognitive domains (i.e., psychomotor functioning, attention and working memory); scores are then transformed into age-, education-, and, where appropriate, ethnicity-corrected standardized scores. Subsequently, clinical ratings are assigned to each cognitive domain by means of a scaled score ranging from 1 (above average) to 9 (severely impaired). A global score is then calculated based on review of domain ratings, with greater weight afforded to impaired domains and considerable leeway granted to premorbid level of functioning. Therefore, significant cognitive dysfunction is necessary before a person is labeled with generalized cognitive impairment. Finally, to meet criteria for an HIV-associated neurocognitive disorder, the patient must demonstrate neuropsychological impairment in

at least two domains and functional impairment in activities of daily living. Though limited in use, this method has proven to have adequate interrater reliability (Woods et al., 2004). Unlike the AAN method or its Dana modification, the clinical ratings method does not require motor, neurological, or emotional impairment for the diagnosis of HAD or MCMD.

Few studies exist that rigorously compare different ratings systems for HIV-associated neurocognitive disorders. Our laboratory recently compared the Dana modification of the AAN and clinical ratings systems for estimating prevalence of neurocognitive disorders in a sample of urban, ethnic minority seropositive adults. Neuropsychological data from 254 seropositive adults (44% African American, 32% Hispanic, and 24% Caucasian) from the Manhattan HIV Brain Bank (http://www.hivbrainbanks.org; Morgello et al., 2001) were reviewed. From a consensus meeting, all patients received a diagnosis of HAD, MCMD, or neuropsychological impairment due to other causes (NPI-O). Though not a formal diagnostic category of the AAN system, labels of NPI-O were assigned to patients with significant confounds (i.e., head trauma, low premorbid functioning) within both systems. Using the Dana modification of the AAN system, ethnic minorities were significantly more likely than Caucasians to be diagnosed with HIV-associated neurocognitive impairment (86% vs. 64%; $\chi_1 = 11.2$, $p = .001$). The clinical ratings method did not generate ethnic disparities and resulted in comparable rates of HAD and MCMD among ethnic minority and Caucasian patients (35% vs. 30%; $p > .05$). Both methods, however, yielded a high rate of NPI-O diagnoses (AAN = 37%, CR = 46%). These results suggest that the AAN method may be overly sensitive and lack specificity in identifying neuropsychological impairment in urban, ethnically diverse seropositive populations, resulting in potentially inflated estimates of HIV-associated neurocognitive disorders. A high prevalence of non-HIV neuropsychological impairment was observed across systems, especially among ethnic minorities. Diagnoses of NPI-O occurred primarily among patients with low levels of education; this group presents a major diagnostic challenge and highlights the need for improved diagnostic tools for seropositive cohorts with multiple confounding characteristics. These data also underscore the importance of consideration of ethnicity in the conceptualization of HIV neurocognitive disorders. Without proper examination of the validity of diagnostic systems in different ethnic groups, estimates of the prevalence and incidence of these disorders risk serious misrepresentation.

The most detrimental consequences of not carefully considering cultural background in the conceptualization of HIV-associated neurocognitive impairment are misdiagnosis and mismanagement of neurocognitive disorders. It is possible that the test performance of neurologically healthy ethnic minority seropositive individuals will be so influenced by their cultural experience that their scores will be classified as impaired when, in fact, no central nervous system (CNS) disease process is present (Manly et al., 1998). When misdiagnoses occur in clinical settings, the potential ramifications for the patient can be daunting and include unnecessary pharmacologic intervention, diagnostic referrals, and psychological distress. The implications of systematic misdiagnoses that occur in the context of research settings are equally harmful, as failure to consider culture in the interpretation of ethnic group performance differences can lead scientists to make erroneous conclusions regarding the prevalence of HIV-associated cognitive disorders by ethnicity, as our data indicate.

Our laboratory's experience with the assessment of culturally diverse seropositive cohorts with poor-quality education has taught us that assessment for this group is best aided by thorough review of possible confounding factors, use of measures to better estimate premorbid cognitive functioning (rather than relying solely on the patient's education level), applying the use of the "best available" demographically corrected normative data and, most importantly, the use of longitudinal assessments (e.g., annual, biannual evaluations) to detect performance decrement. Indeed, longitudinal assessments allow the clinician to compare current performance with past performance, a reliable method for detecting progression. In the absence of better assessment tools and normative data, this technique is likely to yield the most accurate diagnostic data.

HEPATITIS C COMORBIDITY

In developed countries, HAART has largely transformed HIV/AIDS from a fatal to a chronic illness, thus allowing the emergence of significant comorbidities that may affect CNS function. Hepatitis C virus (HCV) infection is a prevalent comorbidity in HIV patients, especially among intravenous drug users, so we will focus primarily on this comorbidity and its cognitive effects. HCV has been shown to cause neuropsychological deficits among HIV- and HCV-positive individuals. Among advanced seropositive participants of the Manhattan HIV Brain Bank, HIV- and HCV-positive coinfected patients were more likely to receive a diagnosis of HIV-associated dementia and have greater impairment in executive functioning (Ryan et al., 2004). These cognitive differences were associated with HCV serology but did not correlate with indices of liver disease severity. Deficits in learning, motor skills (Cherner et al., 2005), attention and concentration, and psychomotor speed (von Geisen et al., 2004; Perry et al., 2005) among coinfected patients have also been reported. Thus, the neuropsychological impairments reported among HCV patients are similar to those of HIV-infected patients, with both diseases affecting cognitive domains subserved by frontal-subcortical circuits.

CONCLUSIONS

While neuropsychological evaluation is not necessary for all seropositive individuals, it can provide information that facilitates treatment planning for individuals who are unable to attain or sustain viral suppression, who have intractable depression or a comorbid medical illness such as hepatitis C, and whose significant other or family member identifies functional decrements. Appropriate selection of neuropsychological tests, normative data, and the interpretive diagnostic system is paramount, given the changing demographics of the HIV epidemic.

References

Albert SM, Marder K, Dooneief G, Bell K, Sano M, Todak G, and Stern Y 1995). Neuropsychologic impairment in early HIV infection: a risk factor for work disability. *Arch Neurol* 52:525–530.

Albert SM, Weber CM, Todak G, Polcano C, Clouse R, McElhiney M, Rabkin J, Stern Y, and Marder K (1999). Neuro-psychological impairment in early HIV infection: a risk factor for work disability. *Arch Neurol* 52:525–530.

Albert SM, Flater SR, Clouse R, Todak G, Stern Y, Marder K, for the NEAD Study Group (2003). Medication management skill in HIV: I. Evidence for adaptation of medication management strategies in people with cognitive impairment. II. Evidence for a pervasive lay model of medication efficacy. *AIDS Behav* 7:329–338.

[AAN] American Academy of Neurology AIDS Task Force (1991). Nomenclature and research case definitions for neurologic manifestations of human immunodeficiency virus-type 1 (HIV-1) infection. *Neurology* 41:778–785.

Arendt G, Hefter H, and Hilperath F (1994). Motor analysis predicts progression in HIV-associated brain disease. *J Neurol Sci* 123:180–185.

Artiola i Fortuny L, and Mullaney, HA (1998). Assessing patients whose language you do not know: can the absurd be ethical? *Clin Neuropsychol* 12:113–126.

Becker JT, and Salthouse TA (1999). Neuropsychological test performance in the acquired immunodeficiency syndrome: independent effects of diagnostic group on functioning. *J Int Neuropsychol Soc* 5(1): 41–47.

Berger JR, and Arendt G (2000). HIV dementia: the role of the basal ganglia and dopaminergic systems. *J Psychopharmacol* 14:214–221.

Carey CL, Woods SP, Rippeth JD, Gonzalez R, Moore DJ, Marcotte TD, Grant I, Heaton RK, for the HIV Neurobehavioral Research Center (HNRC) Group (2004). Initial validation of a screening battery for the detection of HIV-associated cognitive impairment. *Clin Neuropsychol* 18(2):234–248.

[CDC] Centers for Disease Control and Prevention (2004) *HIV/AIDS Surveillance by Race/ Ethnicity*. Retrieved December 12, 2005, from http://www.cdc .gov/hiv/graphics/IMAGES/l238/L238-9.htm.

Cherner M, Letendre S, Heaton RK, Durelle J, Marquie-Beck J, Gragg B, Grant I, and the HIV Neurobehavioral Research Center Group. (2005). Hepatitis C augments cognitive deficits associated with HIV infection and methamphetamine. *Neurology* 64(8): 1343–1347.

Childers M, Ellis R, Deutsch R, Wolfson T, Grant I, and the HNRC Group (2002). The utility and limitations of the HIV Dementia Scale [abstract]. *J Int Neuropsychol Soc* 8:160.

Claypoole KH, Elliott AJ, Uldall KK, Russo J, Dugbartey AT, Bergam K, and Roy-Byrne PP (1998). Cognitive functions and complaints in HIV-1 individuals treated for depression. *Appl Neuropsychol* 5(2): 74–84.

Dana Consortium on Therapy for HIV Dementia and Related Cognitive Disorders (1996). Clinical confirmation of the American Academy of Neurology algorithm for HIV-1 associated cognitive/motor disorder. *Neurology* 47(5):1247–1253.

Davis HF, Skolasky RL Jr, Selnes OA, Burgess DM, and McArthur JC (2002). Assessing HIV-associated dementia: Modified HIV Dementia Scale versus the Grooved Pegboard. *AIDS Reader* 12:29–31, 38.

Delis DC, Kramer JH, Kaplan E, and Ober BA (2000). CVLT-II California Verbal Learning Test, second edition. San Antonio, TX: The Psychological Corporation.

Diehr MC, Cherner M, Wolfson TJ, Miller SW, Grant I, Heaton RK, and the HIV Neurobehavioral Research Center Group (2003). The 50- and 100-item short forms of Paced Auditory Serial Addition Task (PASAT): demographically corrected norms and comparisons with the full PASAT in normal and clinical samples. *J Clin Exp Neuropsychol* 25(4): 571–585.

Ferrando S, van Gorp W, McElhiney M, Goggin K, Sewell M, and Rabkin J (1998). Highly active antiretroviral treatment in HIV infection: benefits for neuropsychological function. *AIDS* 12(8):F65–F70.

Heaton RK, Velin RA, McCutchan JA, Gulevich SJ, Atkinson JH, Wallace MR, Godfrey HP, Kirson DA, and Grant I (1994a) Neuropsychological impairment in human immunodeficiency virus-infection: implications for employment. HIV Neurobehavioral Research Center Group (HNRC). *Psychosom Med* 56(1):8–17.

Heaton RK, Kirson D, Velin R, Grant I, and the HIV Neurobehavioral Research Center Group (1994b). The utility of clinical ratings for detecting cognitive change in HIV infection. In I Grant and A Martin (eds.), *Neuropsychology of HIV Infection* (pp. 188–206). New York: Oxford University Press.

Heaton RK, Grant I, Butters N, White DA, Kirson D, and Atkinson JH (1995). The HNRC 500—neuropsychology of HIV infection at different disease stages. HIV Neurobehavioral Research Center. *J Int Neuropsychol Soc* 1:231–251.

Heaton RK, Marcotte TD, White DA, Ross D, Meredith K, Taylor MJ, Kaplan R, and Grant I (1996). Nature and vocational significance of neuropsychological impairment associated with HIV infection. *Clin Neuropsychol* 10(1):1–14.

Heaton R., Grant I, and Matthews CG (2004a). Revised comprehensive norms for an expanded Halstead-Reitan Battery: demographically adjusted neuropsychological norms for African Americans and Caucasian adults scoring program. Odessa, FL: Psychological Assessment Resources.

Heaton RK, Marcotte TD, Mindt MR, Sadek J, Moore DJ, Bentley H, McCutchan JA, Reicks C, Grant I, and the HIV Neurobehavioral Research Center Group (2004b). The impact of HIV-associated neuropsychological impairment on everyday functioning. *J Int Neuropsychol Soc* 10(3):317–331.

Hinkin CH, Castellon SA, Hardy DJ, Granholm E, Siegle G (1999). Computerized and traditional stroop task dysfunction in HIV-1 infection. *Neuropsychology* 13(2):306–316.

Hinkin CH, Castellon SA, Durvasula RS, Hardy DJ, Lam MN, Mason KI, Thrasher D, Goetz MB, and Stefaniak M (2002a). Medication adherence among HIV+ adults: effects of cognitive dysfunction and regimen complexity. *Neurology* 59(12):1944–1950.

Hinkin CH, Hardy DJ, Mason KI, Castellon SA, Lam MN, Stefaniak M, and Zolnikov B (2002b). Verbal and spatial working memory performance among

HIV-infected adults. *J Int Neuropsychol Soc* 8(4): 532–538.

Jones BN, Teng EL, Folstein MF, and Harrison KS (1993). A new bedside test of cognition for patients with HIV infection. *Ann Intern Med* 119:1001–1004.

Kirsch IS, Jungeblut A, Jenkins L, Kolstad A (2002). Adult literacy in America: a first look at the findings of the National Adult Literacy Survey 2002. Washington, DC: U.S. Department of Education.

Kløve H (1963). *Grooved Pegboard*. Lafayette, IN: Lafayette Instruments.

Kongs SK, Thompson LL, Iverson GL, and Heaton RK (2000). *Wisconsin Card Sorting Test 64 Card Test, Computerized Version*. Lutz, FL: Psychological Assessment Resources.

Lawton MP, and Brody EM (1969). Assessment of older people: Self-maintaining and instrumental activities of daily living. *Gerontologist* 9(3):179–186.

Llorente AM, LoPresti CM, Levy JK, and Fernandez F (2001). Neurobehavioral and neuropsychological manifestations of HIV-1 infection: assessment considerations with Hispanic populations. In M Ponton and J. Leon-Carrion (eds.), *Neuropsychology and the Hispanic Patient: A Clinical Handbook* (pp. 209–241). Mahwah, NJ: Lawrence Erlbaum Associates.

Manly JJ and Jacobs DM (2002). Future directions in neuropsychological assessment with African Americans. In F.R. Ferraro (ed.), *Minority and Cross-Cultural Aspects of Neuropsychological Assessment* (pp. 79–96). Lisse, the Netherlands: Swets & Zeitlinger.

Manly JJ, Miller SW, Heaton RK, Byrd D, Reilly J, Velasquez RJ, Saccuzzo DP, Grant I, and the HIV Neurobehavioral Research Center Group (1998). The effect of African-American acculturation on neuropsychological test performance in normal and HIV positive individuals. *J Int Neuropsychol Soc* 4(3):291–302.

Manly JJ, Jacobs DM, Touradji P, Small SA, and Stern Y (2002). Reading level attenuates differences in neuropsychological test performance between African American and White elders. *J Int Neuropsychol Soc* 8(3):341–348.

Marcotte TD, Wolfson T, Rosenthal TJ, Heaton RK, Gonzalez R, Ellis RJ, Grant I, and the HIV Neurobehavioral Research Center Group (2004). A multimodal assessment of driving performance in HIV infection. *Neurology* 63(8):1417–1422.

McArthur JC (2004). HIV dementia: an evolving disease [review]. *J Neuroimmunol* 157(1-2):3–10.

Moore LH, van Gorp WG, Hinkin CH, Stern MJ, Swales T, and Satz P (1997). Subjective complaints versus actual cognitive deficits in predominantly symptomatic HIV-1 seropositive individuals. J Neuropsychiatry *Clin Neurosci* 9(1):37–44.

Morgello S, Gelman BB, Kozlowski PB, Vinters HV, Masliah E, Cornford M, Cavert W, Marra C, Grant I, and Singer EJ (2001). The National NeuroAIDS Tissue Consortium: a new paradigm in brain banking with an emphasis on infectious disease. *Neuropathol Appl Neurobiol* 27(4):326–335.

Naglieri JA, and Bardos AN (1997). *General Ability Measure for Adults*. Minneapolis: National Computer Systems.

Perry W, Carlson MD, Barakat F, Hilsabeck RC, Schiehser DM, Mathews C, and Hassanein TI (2005). Neuropsychological test performance in patients co-infected with hepatitis C virus and HIV. *AIDS* 19(Suppl. 3):S79–S84.

Power C, Selnes OA, Grim JA, and McArthur JC (1995). HIV Dementia Scale: a rapid screening test. *J Acquir Immune Defic Syndr Hum Retrovirol* 8(3): 273–278.

Rabkin JG, McElhiney M, Ferrando SJ, Van Gorp W, and Lin SH (2004). Predictors of employment of men with HIV/AIDS: a longitudinal study. *Psychosom Med* 66(1):72–78.

Reitan R, and Wolfson D (1985). *The Halstead Reitan Neuropsychological Test Battery*. Tucson, AZ: Neuropsychology Press.

Richardson MA, Morgan EE, Vielhauer MJ, Cuevas CA, Buondonno LM, and Keane TM (2005). Utility of the HIV dementia scale in assessing risk for significant HIV-related cognitive-motor deficits in a high-risk urban adult sample. *AIDS Care* 17(8):1013–1021.

Rourke SB, Halman MH, and Bassel C (1999a). Neurocognitive complaints in HIV infection and their relationship to depressive symptoms and neuropsychological functioning. *J Clin Exp Neuropsychol* 21(6):737–756.

Rourke SB, Halman MH, and Bassel C (1999b). Neuropsychiatric correlates of memory–metamemory dissociations in HIV infection. *J Clin Exp Neuropsychol* 21(6):757–768.

Ryan, E, Morgello, S, Isaacs, K, Naseer, M, Gerits, P, and the Manhattan HIV Brain Bank (2004). Neuropsychiatric impact of hepatitis C on advanced HIV. *Neurology* 62(6):957–962.

Ryan E, Baird L, Rivera R, Mindt M, Byrd D, Monzones, J, and Morgello S (2005). Neuropsychological impairment in racial/ethnic minorities with HIV infection and low literacy levels: effects of education and reading level in participant characterization. *J Int Neuropsychol Soc* 11(6):889–898.

Ryan E, Byrd D, Mindt M, Rivera R, and Morgello S (2006). Assessing premorbid intellectual performance among HIV+ participants with low literacy [abstract]. *J Int Neuropsychol Soc* 12(1):S1, 33.

Sacktor NC, Bacellar H, and Hoover DR (1996). Psychomotor slowing in HIV infection: a predictor of dementia, AIDS and death. *J Neurovirol* 2:404–410.

Sacktor N, Tarwater PM, Skolasky RL, McArthur JC, Selnes OA, Becker J, Cohen B, and Miller EN (2001). Multicenter for AIDS Cohort Study (MACS): CSF antiretroviral drug penetrance and the treatment of HIV-associated psychomotor slowing. *Neurology* 57(3):542–544.

Selnes OA, Galai N, Bacellar H, Miller EN, Becker JT, Wesch J, Van Gorp W, and McArthur JC (1995). Cognitive performance after progression to AIDS: a longitudinal study from the Multicenter AIDS Cohort Study. *Neurology* 45(2):267–275.

Smith A (1982). *Symbol Digit Modalities Test*. Los Angeles: Western Psychological Services.

Smith CA, van Gorp WG, Ryan E, Ferrando SJ, and Rabkin J (2003). Screening subtle HIV-related cognitive dysfunction: the clinical utility of the HIV dementia scale. *J Acquir Immune Defic Syndr* 33(1): 116–118.

Tozzi V, Balestra P, Serraino D, Bellagamba R, Corpolongo A, Piselli P, Lorenzini P, Visco-Comandini U, Vlassi C, Quartuccio ME, Giulianelli M, Noto P, Galgani S, Ippolito G, Antinori A, and Narciso P (2005). Neurocognitive impairment and survival in a cohort of HIV-infected patients treated with HAART. *AIDS Res Hum Retroviruses* 21(8):706–713.

Tulsky D, and Price L (2002). Cross validation of the joint factor structure of the WAIS-III and WMS-III: examination of the structure by ethnic and age groups. In D Tulsky, D Saklofske, RK Heaton, G Chelune, R Ivnik, RA Bornstein, A Prifitera, and M Ledbetter (eds.), *Clinical Interpretation of the WAIS-III and WMS-III*. San Diego: Academic Press.

van Gorp WG, Baerwald JP, Ferrando SJ, McElhiney MC, and Rabkin JG (1999). The relationship between employment and neuropsychological impairment in HIV infection. *J Int Neuropsychol Soc* 5(6):534–539.

von Giesen HJ, Wittsack HJ, Wenserski F, Köller H, Hefter H, and Arendt G (2001). Basal ganglia metabolite abnormalities in minor motor deficits associated with immunodeficiency virus type 1. *Arch Neurol* 58(8):1281–1286.

von Giesen HJ, Heintges T, Abbasi-Boroudjeni N, Kucukkoylu S, Koller H, Haslinger BA, Oette M, and Arendt G (2004). Psychomotor slowing in hepatitis C and HIV infection. *J Acquir Immune Defic Syndr* 35(2):131–137.

Wechsler D (1997). *WAIS-III Administration and Scoring Manual*. Austin, TX: The Psychological Corporation.

White DA, Taylor MJ, Butters N, Mack C, Salmon DP, Peavy G, Ryan L, Heaton RK, Atkinson JH, Chandler JL, and Grant I (1997). Memory for verbal information in individuals with HIV-associated dementia complex. HNRC Group. J Clin Exp Neuropsychol 19(4):357–366.

Wilkinson GS, and Robertson J (2006). *Wide Range Achievement Test (4th edition) Administration Manual*. Lutz, FL: Psychological Assessment Resources.

Wood S, Hinkin CH, Castellon SA, and Yarema K (1998). Working memory deficits in HIV-1 infection. Brain Cogn 37(1):163–166.

Woods SP, Rippeth JD, Frol AB, Levy JK, Ryan E, Soukup VM, Hinkin CH, Lazzaretto D, Cherner M, Marcotte TD, Gelman BB, Morgello S, Singer EJ, Grant I, and Heaton RK (2004). Interrater reliability of clinical ratings and neurocognitive diagnoses in HIV. *J Clin Exp Neuropsychol* 26(6):759–778.

Part III

Psychiatric Disorders
and HIV Infection

Chapter 8

Substance Use Disorders—The Special Role in HIV Transmission

Philip Bialer, Rosalind G. Hoffman, and Jeffrey Ditzell

Injecting drug use (IDU) is a major vector of HIV transmission in many parts of the world. (Needle et al., 2001) While sexual transmission of HIV predominates in endemic areas such as sub-Saharan Africa, IDU and commercial sex are the major transmission modes in South and Southeast Asia, where approximately 7.4 million people are living with HIV (UNAIDS, 2005). IDU is also the main risk behavior in Latin America (HIV prevalence 1.8 million) and Eastern Europe and Central Asia (HIV prevalence 1.6 million; UN-AIDS, 2005). Approximately 27% of the cumulative adult cases of HIV/AIDS in the United States are due to IDU (CDC, 2005). Heterosexual exposure to HIV in the United States most often involves sexual contact with injection drug users (IDUs). When taking this into account along with the category of men who have sex with men and are exposed to IDU, the proportion of HIV/AIDS associated with IDU approaches 50%. In addition, there is a high prevalence of non-injecting drug use among gay and bisexual men (Fer-

rando et al., 1998) that is associated with high-risk sex behavior and seroconversion (Chesney et al., 1998; Woody et al., 1999; Venable et al., 2004). Finally, the potential impact of substance use on HIV progression and neuropsychological functioning gives the subject of substance use disorders (SUDs) very special prominence in HIV/AIDS psychiatry.

Hepatitis C virus (HCV) coinfection has also become a major problem among those with HIV. Of persons injecting drugs for at least 5 years, 60% to 80% are infected with HCV (CDC, 2002). In China, 95% of HIV-positive heroin users were also infected with HCV (Garten et al., 2005). The sharing of contaminated needles can lead to multiple medical problems including skin infections, endocarditis, septicemia, and pulmonary emboli.

One large-scale U.S. study found that 61.4% of adults under care for HIV had used mental health or substance abuse services (Burnham et al., 2001). The drugs most commonly used in the past year

TABLE 8.1. Substance Use Disorders: DSM IV Criteria

Substance Abuse	Substance Dependence
A maladaptive pattern of substance use leading to clinically significant impairment or distress as manifested by one (or more) of the following: • Failure to meet obligations at work, school, or home • Recurrent use in hazardous situations • Use despite legal consequences (e.g., arrests for driving under the influence) • Continued use despite recurrent social or interpersonal problems	A maladaptive pattern of substance use leading to clinically significant impairment or distress as manifested by three (or more) of the following: • Tolerance • Withdrawal • Larger amounts or over greater period than intended • Unsuccessful efforts to cut down • Most time spent in addiction (i.e, activities needed to obtain, use, or recover from the substance) • Important social, occupational, or recreational activities given up • Use despite knowledge of persistent or recurrent medical (e.g., cirrhosis) or psychological (e.g. depression) problems

by this sample were cocaine (62%), analgesics (42%), sedatives (38%), amphetamines (28%), heroin (24%), inhalants (14%), hallucinogens (6%), and marijuana (64%).

TERMINOLOGY AND DEFINITIONS

Clinicians treating patients with HIV/AIDS must have a good working knowledge of SUDs, since most of their patients will have a current or lifetime history of at least one such disorder. Using *Diagnostic and Statistical Manual of Mental Disorders*, fourth edition (DSM IV; American Psychiatric Association, 1994) terminology, SUDs can be divided into three basic categories: substance abuse, substance dependence, and substance-induced disorders. The criteria for abuse and dependence are listed in Table 8.1. *Tolerance* refers to an acquired decrease in the effect of a substance usually manifested by a need for increased amounts of the substance to achieve the desired effect. *Withdrawal* is a substance-specific group of signs and symptoms that follows the abrupt discontinuation, reduction, or antagonistic blockage of a substance. It should be noted that tolerance and physical dependence evidenced by withdrawal symptoms are not sufficient in and of themselves to warrant a diagnosis of substance dependence. Rather, substance dependence should be recognized as a cluster of cognitive, behavioral, and physiological symptoms indicating that a person is continuing to use a substance despite having clinically significant substance-related problems (Cami

and Farre, 2003). The substance-induced disorders are listed in Table 8.2.

INITIAL EVALUATION OF THE PATIENT WITH SUBSTANCE USE DISORDERS

Obtaining a substance use history is essential when evaluating all patients with HIV/AIDS. Some clinicians may have negative feelings about working with patients who exhibit self-destructive behaviors such as substance abuse and dependence. It is important to be aware of these feelings and realize that patients respond better when a working alliance can be established by approaching them in a nonthreatening and nonjudgmental manner. It is also important to reassure the patient that the information they provide will be kept confidential to those outside of the treatment

TABLE 8.2. DSM IV Substance-Induced Disorders

Intoxication
Withdrawal
Mood disorders (depressive or manic)
Psychosis with delusions
Psychosis with hallucinations
Anxiety
Sleep disorders
Sexual dysfunction
Delirium
Dementia
Amnestic disorders

team and be used to develop the safest possible treatment plan. The clinician should ask about specific illicit substances such as heroin, cocaine, marijuana, and the club drugs (see below). For taking a history of alcohol use, some clinicians have suggested the use of the CAGE questionnaire (Ewing, 1984): 1. Can you cut down on your drinking? 2. Are you annoyed when asked to stop? 3. Do you feel guilty about your drinking? 4. Do you need an eye-opener when you wake up in the morning? One should also ask about sedative or stimulant use, whether prescribed or nonprescribed, and any dietary supplements or herbs the patient may be taking. A substance abuse review of systems, focusing on renal, cardiac, gastrointestinal, and, for HIV patients especially, neurological symptoms, is essential. Other points of inquiry are the date the substance was first used; patterns, amount, and frequency of use; and routes of administration and reactions to the use. The time of last use is important to know to determine if the patient is suffering from a substance-induced disorder or is at risk for withdrawal. If the patient has had past substance use treatment it is useful to know the response to this treatment. With the patient's permission, a urine toxicology screen should be obtained, in addition to routine blood tests. Finally, whenever possible, the clinician should try to obtain collateral information about the patient's substance use, since denial is a common defense mechanism in this population.

SUBSTANCES OF ABUSE

Opiates

Injection of heroin may be the most common, though not the only, source of HIV transmission associated with SUD. Opium is one of the oldest medications known, especially for its use in the relief of pain and diarrhea. Morphine and codeine were isolated in the early 1800s and heroin was developed as a semisynthetic opium derivative and introduced into medical practice in 1898. The mu opiate receptor is the main one responsible for analgesia, respiratory depression, decreased gastric motility, miosis, euphoria, and dependence. These receptors appear to stimulate release of dopamine from the ventral tegmental area into the nucleus acumbens, the primary reward pathway of the brain. Heroin reaches peak serum concentration within 1 minute when taken intravenously but actu-

ally begins crossing the blood–brain barrier within 15–20 seconds. Physical signs of acute opiate intoxication include euphoria and tranquility, sedation, slurred speech, problems with memory and attention, and miosis. Signs and symptoms of opioid withdrawal can be both objective (rhinorrhea and lacrimation, nausea and vomiting, diarrhea, piloerection, mydriasis, yawning, and muscle spasms) and subjective (body aches, insomnia, craving, dysphoria, anxiety, hot and cold flashes, and anorexia). Heroin withdrawal usually begins within 4 to 8 hours after last use, whereas with methadone, with its longer elimination half-life, withdrawal may not begin until 24 to 48 hours after last use.

Early in the epidemic, heroin addiction led to a rapid spread of HIV and HCV among IDUs in the United States, since few addicts had access to clean needles and syringes. The increase in the purity and availability of heroin along with a decrease in its street price has led to a resurgence in the use of heroin over the past 15 years. There are 600,000 to 800,000 heroin addicts in the United States; however, less than 20% are currently in treatment for their addiction (Community Epidemiologic Work Group, 2000).

The prevalence of HIV appears to be much higher among long-term heroin users who inject, compared with those who have short-term use or other methods of use. Chitwood and colleagues (2003) found an HIV seroprevalence rate of 25% among long-term IDUs and a rate of 13% among new IDUs or heroin sniffers.

Cocaine and Other Stimulants

Cocaine is an alkaloid extracted from the leaf of the Erythroxylon coca bush. The hydrochloride salt is water soluble and can be administered orally, intravenously, or intranasally. The intravenous route of administration has an onset of action of 10–60 seconds, with a peak effect achieved in minutes and duration of effect that lasts up to 1 hour. Administration of the drug by the intranasal route has an onset of action of up to 5 minutes, with a peak effect achieved in approximately 20 minutes. The total duration of action by the intranasal route is 1 hour. The free-base form, known as crack cocaine, can be heated and smoked. This form has the quickest onset of action of 3–5 seconds, reaching its peak effect in 1 minute. (Lange and Hillis, 2001) The quick and intense effects of crack cocaine may potentially make it the most addictive form of the drug.

The effects of cocaine are mediated by blocking the synaptic reuptake of norepinephrine and dopamine, resulting in an excess of these neurotransmitters at the postsynaptic receptor. It is by this mechanism and the alteration of synaptic transmission that cocaine acts as a powerful sympathomimetic agent. Metabolism of cocaine occurs in the liver and its metabolites are detectable in blood or urine for up to 36 hours after administration. Cardiovascular complications of cocaine use include cerebrovascular accident (CVA), myocardial ischemia and infarct (MI), arrhythmia, and sudden death (McCann and Ricuarte, 2000). Intravenous administration of any substance of abuse increases the risk of the development of bacterial endocarditis. In contrast to the other drugs, endocarditis secondary to intravenous cocaine use more often affects the left-sided valves of the heart (Chambers et al., 1987).

Amphetamines produce many of the same effects as cocaine with similar routes of administration. In contrast to cocaine, amphetamines both stimulate the presynaptic release of dopamine and norepinephrine and then block their reuptake. High doses of amphetamine release 5-hydroxytryptamine (5-HT) and may affect serotonergic receptors. Metabolism occurs in the liver, mediated predominantly by the cytochrome P450 (CYP) 2D6 enzyme. As with cocaine, amphetamines are potent sympathomimetics and can cause MI, seizures, and CVA (Urbina and Jones, 2004).

Methamphetamine use has reached almost epidemic proportions among gay men in urban centers and is often associated with risk behaviors including sharing of needles for those who inject and unprotected sexual activity. Some have suggested that methamphetamines are associated with more intense sexual excitement. When amphetamines are taken along with sildenafil (Viagra), referred to as "sextasy," this combination allows for longer and rougher intercourse, which may promote tears in anal mucosa (Halkitis et al., 2001) and therefore promote HIV transmission. Compared to nonusers, gay men who use methamphetamine have been shown to have more sexual partners and to be more likely to participate in anal receptive intercourse, less likely to use condoms, and more likely to be HIV infected (Molitor et al., 1998; Shoptaw et al., 2002).

There is also a high prevalence of methamphetamine use among predominantly heterosexual men and women in the West and Midwest. One study looking at risk behaviors in this population found that, compared to nonusers, the men who used methamphetamine had more sex partners, had more vaginal and anal insertive intercourse, and were more likely to give or receive money or drugs in exchange for sex (Molitor et al., 1999). The investigators found that the women who used methamphetamine also reported more acts of vaginal intercourse that were not related to prostitution. Both men and women users were less likely to report always using a condom during sex than were nonusers; they were also more likely to use improperly cleaned, used needles and syringes (Molitor et al., 1999). These studies indicate that methamphetamine users may represent a special subpopulation of both injecting and non-injecting drug users that are at particular risk for contracting and spreading HIV.

The mechanisms of action and toxicities for methamphetamine are the same as those for other amphetamines mentioned above. Chronic use leads to reduction of dopamine transporter levels and neuropsychological impairment. Some investigators have suggested that methamphetamine use can enhance neurotoxicity in HIV patients and accelerate the development of HIV-associated dementia (Urbina and Jones, 2004).

Alcohol and Sedatives

The lifetime prevalence of alcohol dependence in the United States is in the range of 14.1% (Kessler et al., 1997), while binge alcohol use and heavy alcohol use within the past month have been reported as 22.8% and 6.9%, respectively (SAMSHA, 2005). Even higher rates are seen among gay men, regardless of their serostatus (Ferrando et al., 1998; Stall et al., 2001).

Alcohol is rapidly absorbed from the duodenum with blood alcohol concentrations of 100–200 mg%, causing impaired motor function and judgment; concentrations of 200–400 mg% lead to stupor and coma. Alcohol activates GABA receptors, inhibits NMDA receptors, and has additional effects on $5-HT_3$, nicotinic, and opioid receptors. It is metabolized by alcohol dehyrogenase at a constant rate of 100 mg/kg/hour. Medical complications of alcohol dependence are listed in Table 8.3. Problems such as anemia, peripheral neuropathy, and dementia are of particular concern in HIV patients, who are already predisposed to these complications. More importantly, alcohol-induced liver disease may be worse in those coinfected

TABLE 8.3. Medical Complications of Alcohol Abuse and Dependence

Gastritis/peptic ulcer	Pancreatitis
Cirrhosis/hepatic failure	Anemia
Pneumonia	Malnutrition
Trauma	Peripheral neuropathy
Subdural hematoma	Dementia
Cardiomyopathy	Wernicke-Korsakoff syndrome

with HCV, as alcoholism doubles the risk of cirrhosis (Maillard and Sorrell, 2005).

Among HIV-positive persons, alcohol abuse leads to additional medical complications because of reduced adherence to treatment. Studies among veterans in care for HIV showed that binge drinkers missed many more doses of medications on drinking days, compared with non-binge drinkers. The study demonstrated that this trend was especially strong for HIV-positive individuals as compared with HIV-negative individuals. The investigators concluded that HIV-positive persons may be particularly sensitive to the negative effects of alcohol consumption (Brathwaite et al., 2005). Additionally, alcohol use is associated with risky sexual behaviors and intravenous drug use, both of which lead to higher rates of HIV transmission (Petry, 1999; Szerlip et al., 2005). Studies abroad have also demonstrated that alcohol intoxication is associated with sexual risk behaviors. A study in China concluded that HIV/AIDS prevention and intervention efforts should include components of alcohol use and abuse prevention for an effective reduction in sexual risk-taking behaviors (Lin et al., 2005).

Club Drugs

In addition to the more commonly thought-of substances of abuse, such as heroin, cocaine, and alcohol, substances used in the context of going to parties or clubs have taken on new significance in the HIV epidemic. These drugs are often used at raves, which are all-night parties in large spaces attended by hundreds to thousands of teenagers and young adults dancing to loud, repetitive electronic music (Weir, 2000). Stimulants and hallucinogens such as LSD and 3, 4-methylenedioxymethamphetamine (MDMA), also known as Ecstasy, are the drugs most commonly used. Circuit parties are another venue where club drugs are used. These are attended mostly by young to middle-aged gay men and may be particularly prob-

lematic in terms of HIV transmission, as the parties often go on for several days, with drug use and sexual activity being the primary objectives. Although some of these parties originally began as fund-raisers for HIV service organizations, most of these organizations have since distanced themselves from such functions and they have taken on independent lives of their own through magazines and Web sites. Drugs commonly used at circuit parties include MDMA, ketamine, gamma-hydroxybutyric acid (GHB), methamphetamine, cocaine, marijuana, and alcohol (Bialer, 2002) The club drugs that are of the most concern in relation to HIV/AIDS are MDMA, GHB, and methamphetamine.

Although MDMA was first synthesized in 1912, its use among youth and gay men has increased greatly only in recent years. One study from Seattle indicated that 41% of gay men aged 20 to 29 years surveyed used Ecstasy at some time in their lives (Community Epidemiologic Work Group, 2000). MDMA seems to achieve its effects by flooding the brain with serotonin. Similar to methamphetamine, it both stimulates the release of serotonin and then inhibits its uptake. It may also be taken along with sildenafil to overcome side effects of sexual dysfunction (to promote "sextasy"), and there has been increasing concern about unsafe sexual activity associated with MDMA and an increase in HIV transmission. Although MDMA is considered a benign drug by many, there are now numerous reports of severe toxic, sometimes fatal, reactions (McCann et al., 1996). Chronic use may lead to mood instability and cognitive impairment, which are particular problems for people with HIV (Bolla et al., 1998; McCann and Ricuarte, 2000; Kalant, 2001).

GHB was initially developed as an anesthetic but was found to have too many side effects to be used regularly. In the club scene, GHB is taken for its sedating and euphoric effects. It has also been used as a date-rape drug, leading to concerns of HIV exposure through unprotected sexual intercourse. Because of its amnestic effects, the victim may not even know that they have been exposed. GHB has a relatively narrow therapeutic range; its toxic effects include seizures, coma, and death. In addition, a severe withdrawal syndrome among chronic users has been reported (Bialer, 2002). Gamma-butyrolactone (GBL) and 1,4-butanediol (1,4- BD) are precursors that can be converted to GHB after ingestion. They are available in a variety of dietary supplements for purported but unproven anabolic effects. Camacho et al. (2004) showed that 52% of their sample of HIV-positive patients reported using GHB or a substance containing GHB, but only 24% of these patients were aware of the toxicities and addictive potential of this drug. GHB has been approved by the U.S. Food and Drug Administration (FDA) for the treatment of cataplexy associated with narcolepsy, although its distribution is highly restricted.

COMORBIDITY

The triple diagnosis of HIV/AIDS, SUD, and psychiatric disorder has long been recognized by those who work with this population. In the general population, approximately 50% of people with psychiatric disorder will meet criteria for SUD in their lifetime (George and Krystal, 2000); 20% of non-alcoholic substance users have a concurrent affective disorder (Kessler et al., 1997). The lifetime prevalence of SUD is even higher, in the range of 70%, among schizophrenics and those with bipolar disease.

Rates of mental disorders and SUD tend to be higher in the HIV population than in the general population. A large national study of HIV-infected patients demonstrated a strong association between SUD and being diagnosed with a mental disorder; screening positive for a psychiatric disorder was also associated with SUD (Bing et al., 2001). Depressive disorders have been found in 33%–40% of HIV-seropositive IDUs (Klinkenberg and Sacks, 2004). In some studies, the rate of depressive disorders was higher among male seropositive IDUs compared to a matching seroncgative sample, but the rates of depression were similar among the female groups studied (Lipsitz et al., 1994; Rabkin et al., 1997). However, in general, women with SUD tend to have a higher rate of comorbidity, particularly posttraumatic stress disorder.

Two major concerns for HIV patients with comorbid SUD and mental disorder are increased risk-taking behavior and the disorders' effects on treatment adherence. Among opiate users, a current and lifetime history of any mental disorder has been associated with a higher frequency of sharing injection equipment and less condom use (Klinkenberg and Sacks, 2004). Compared to other patients with SUD, schizophrenic patients have been found to be more likely to trade sex for money and drugs. Patients with comorbid disorders are also less likely to receive med-

ical treatment or to undergo highly active antiretroviral therapy (HAART; Klinkenberg and Sacks, 2004).

TREATMENT AND MANAGEMENT OF SUBSTANCE USE DISORDERS

To address the unique needs of the HIV patient who is addicted to substances, it is necessary to find the balance between addiction treatment and harm reduction. A greater level of tolerance and flexibility is required than might otherwise be expected in a formalized addiction treatment program that stresses abstinence and the use of 12-step groups. This includes tolerance of ongoing substance use during the course of treatment.

The initial phase of addiction treatment is usually concerned with providing safe and humane detoxification from the substance of abuse. Benzodiazepines are recommended as the treatment of choice in management of alcohol or sedative/hypnotic withdrawal (Mayo-Smith, 1997), although some clinicians have also advocated the use of anticonvulsants (Pages and Ries, 1998; Malcolm et al., 2001). Detoxification can generally be done at the same dosages as those for seronegative patients until the later stages of HIV illness, when lower doses may be necessary.

Methadone detoxification is the preferred method of managing opioid withdrawal. Schedules using buprenorphine and/or clonidine for opioid detoxification are also available (NIH Consensus Development Conference, 1998). Detoxification from cocaine and stimulants is not done pharmacologically.

After medical stabilization and detoxification, the goals of treatment should include maintenance of abstinence when possible and rapid treatment of relapse. Substance abuse treatment is usually provided on an outpatient basis, though treatment communities afford a higher level of care for those with a more severe and refractory SUD. Adjunctive anticraving agents may be used by HIV-positive patients with severe addictive disorders to aid in abstinence. Disulfuram, acamprosate, and naltrexone have all been used to curb alcohol craving. Methadone maintenance therapy has been shown to be effective in managing abstinence from opiates, and recently buprenorphine has been approved for the office management of opiate dependence.

Harm reduction is a strategy that is particularly applicable to the addicted, HIV-positive patient (Ferrando and Batki, 2000). In harm reduction, many individuals in recovery will not maintain abstinence and that treatment strategies should therefore focus on reducing behavior that has potentially harmful consequences, such as the sharing of needles or illicit activities to pay for substance use. Sterile needle–exchange programs have not only been effective in decreasing risk-taking behaviors, but some studies and meta-analyses indicate that they may have contributed to a significant decrease in HIV seroconversion among the IDU population (Cochrane Collaborative Review Group, 2004; Des Jarlais et al., 2005).

Motivational interviewing is a useful method for managing patients with SUD (Miller and Rollnick, 1991). In this process, the practitioner assesses a patient's readiness to change and facilitates movement along a continuum of change (Prochaska and DiClemente, 1986). One goal is to engage the patient in a manner that creates a disparity in wants expressed by the patient and their current reality. In this process the clinician should try to avoid eliciting the patient's defense mechanisms through the expression of empathy, avoid argumentation, create discrepancy, roll with the resistance, and support and reframe the patient's desires, all of which will effectively serve to create an environment that facilitates behavioral change.

Network therapy is an office-based treatment of SUD advocated by Galanter and colleagues (Galanter and Brook, 2001) that employs both psychodynamic and cognitive-behavioral approaches. The treatment includes a therapeutic network of non-abusing family members, significant others, and peers who actively participate with the therapist to provide cohesiveness and support, undermine denial, and promote compliance with treatment. Studies have demonstrated significantly less illicit substance use among patients receiving this treatment for cocaine and opiate abuse. (Galanter et al., 1997, 2004)

Two meta-analyses looking at the outcomes of psychosocial interventions upon risk-taking behavior among IDUs showed that simply undergoing a screening to enroll in the studies seemed to have a beneficial effect of reducing risky behavior in both experimental and comparison groups; there were no significant differences based on the length of time of the interventions (Gibson et al., 1998; Semaan et al., 2002). These studies stress the importance of including information about HIV infection and HIV risk reduction and access to condoms and HIV testing along with other components of any drug intervention program. For those patients with comorbid SUD and mental disorder, successful treatment approaches stress the integration of mental health care and substance abuse treatment along with medical care. Patients receiving ancillary services are more likely to link up with medical care (Klinkenberg and Sacks, 2004).

DRUG–DRUG INTERACTIONS

Potential drug–drug interactions between psychotropics and HIV medications are addressed in Chapter 32 of this volume. Less is known about the specific interactions between HIV medications and substances of abuse.

Nevirapine and efavirenz induce the CYP 3A4 enzyme, which can increase the rate of metabolism of methadone, sometimes causing withdrawal symptoms among patients on maintenance therapy (Altice et al., 1999; Pinzanni et al., 2000). Patients on regimens including these drugs will require higher methadone doses to prevent craving that could lead to risky drug-injecting behaviors. Conversely, if these medications are discontinued, the patient may be at risk for increased sedation if the methadone dose is not adjusted accordingly. Although ritonavir is a potent inhibitor of CYP 3A4, it also induces several P450 enzymes, including 3A4 and 2B6, which could also lead to increased metabolism of methadone and withdrawal (Gerber et al., 2001). Buprenorphine is also metabolized by CYP 3A4 and may have the same interactions as methadone. Finally, methadone has been shown to increase zidovudine levels, potentially causing toxic side effects.

Alcohol consumption has been shown to significantly increase the blood serum level of abacavir by competing for alcohol dehydrogenase (McDowell et al., 2000); however, with chronic use, alcohol can induce CYP 3A4 and may decrease levels of some antiretrovirals (Caballeria, 2003). Ritonavir, and possibly other protease inhibitors, can inhibit the metabolism of alprazolam, which can lead to oversedation and respiratory depression if this drug is being abused. Inhaled marijuana has been shown to decrease the bioavailability of indinavir and nelfinavir, although the precise mechanism is unknown (Kosel et al., 2002).

MDMA and methamphetamine are both metabolized primarily by CYP 2D6. Deaths have been reported among patients who took methamphetamine while being treated with ritonavir, which is an inhibitor of CYP 2D6 (Hales et al., 2000). Similarly, there have been at least two reports of deaths and near-death experiences in patients taking ritonavir and then ingesting MDMA (Henry and Hill, 1998; Harrington et al., 1999). Ketamine (Hijazi and Boulieu, 2002) and phenylcyclidine (Laurenzana and Owens, 1997) appear to be primarily metabolized by CYP 3A4 and patients should be aware of potential interactions with antiretrovirals and other medications that inhibit this enzyme.

PAIN

Pain is highly prevalent among patients with HIV/AIDS, with reports varying from 28% to 97% of patients experiencing pain, depending on the study population and setting. The pain can have many different causes (Cohen and Alfonso, 2004). Studies indicate that there is no difference in the prevalence of pain between HIV patients with a history of IDU and non-drug users; in general, pain is undertreated in all AIDS patients (McCormack et al., 1993; Breitbart et al., 1996; Larue et al., 1997). However, the treatment of pain in HIV patients with a history of SUD, particularly IDU, may be even more problematic. Breitbart et al. (1997) found that among AIDS patients with a history of SUD, only 8% received adequate analgesia compared to 20% of those without SUD. Former drug users are often negatively stereotyped, and clinicians are hesitant to give opioid analgesics to former drug users for fear of being manipulated or fear of promoting substance abuse. The patient may be resistant to taking analgesic medications for fear of causing a relapse. Finally, many practitioners do not feel comfortable treating pain because of their lack of knowledge about pain treatment and inadequate knowledge of the differences between substance dependence, tolerance, and addiction. When pain is undertreated, patients may increase the use of their pain medications or ask for more medication. This behavior has been characterized as "pseudoaddiction" (Weissman and Haddox, 1980) and usually abates once pain is adequately treated.

The assessment and treatment of pain in HIV patients, regardless of history of SUD, should not differ from the treatment of pain in cancer patients and should follow the World Health Organization's analgesic pain ladder (Jacox et al., 1994). Two relatively small open-label studies indicate that opioid analgesics can be used safely and effectively in treating pain in HIV patients with a history of SUD, although higher doses of analgesic may be required (Kaplan et al., 2000; Newshan and Lefkowitz, 2001). When developing a treatment plan for persons with HIV, SUD, and chronic pain, treatment goals should be overtly addressed, limits set with a treatment contract if necessary, and a single provider should write all pain medication prescriptions (Swica and Breitbart, 2002). Some clinicians have suggested the use of methadone for opioid analgesia (Cruciani and Coggins, 2002). Patients in methadone maintenance should be given their usual dose in the morning and then receive additional methadone for analgesia in three or four divided doses. Opioid analgesics should be given around the clock. Maintaining an open line of communication with the patient's maintenance program is essential. We recommend including adjuvant medications and nonpharmacologic modalities in the plan and using a multidisciplinary approach to address the psychosocial problems. The need for high doses of medication to control pain is not in and of itself a sign of misuse. More useful indicators of misuse are noncompliance with the treatment plan, any indications of loss of control with the medications, or indications of alcohol abuse or use of street drugs. Patients on agonist therapy will require higher analgesic doses due to cross-tolerance with the maintenance medication and probable increased pain sensitivity (Alford et al., 2006).

References

Alford DP, Compton P, and Samet JH (2006). Acute pain management for patients receiving maintenance methadone or buprenorphine therapy. *Ann Intern Med* 144:127–134.

Altice FL, Friedland GH, and Cooney EL (1999). Nevirapine induced opiate withdrawal among injection drug users with HIV infection receiving methadone. *AIDS* 13:1957.

American Psychiatric Association (1994). *Diagnostic and Statistical Manual of Mental Disorders*, fourth edition. Washington, DC: American Psychiatric Association.

Bialer PA (2002). Designer drugs in the general hospital. *Psychiatr Clin North Am* 25:231–243.

Bing EG, Burnam AM, Longshore D, et al. (2001). Psychiatric disorders and drug-use among human immunodeficiency virus–infected adults in the United States. *Arch Gen Psychiatry* 58:721–728.

Bolla KI, McCann UD, and Ricuarte GA (1998). Memory impairment in abstinent MDMA ("Ecstasy") users. *Neurology* 51:1532–1537.

Braithwaite RS, McGinnis KA, Conigliaro J, et al. (2005). A temporal and dose–response association between alcohol consumption and medication adherence among veterans in care. *Alcohol Clin Exp Res* 29: 1190–1197.

Breitbart W, Rosenfeld BD, Passik SD, et al. (1996). The undertreatment of pain in ambulatory AIDS patients. *Pain* 65:243–249.

Breitbart W, Rosenfeld B, Passik S, et al. (1997). A comparison of pain report and adequacy of analgesic therapy in ambulatory AIDS patients with and without a history of substance abuse. *Pain* 72:235–243.

Burnham AM, Bing EG, Morton S, et al. (2001). Use of mental health and substance abuse services among adults with HIV in the United States. *Arch Gen Psychiatry* 58:729–736.

Caballeria J (2003). Current concepts in alcohol metabolism. *Ann Hepatol* 2:60–68.

Camacho A, Matthews SC, and Dimsdale JE (2004). Use of GHB compounds by HIV-positive individuals. *Am J Addict* 13:120–127.

Cami J, and Farre M (2003). Mechanisms of disease: drug addiction. *N Engl J Med* 349:975–986.

[CDC] Centers for Disease Control and Prevention (2002). Viral hepatitis and injection drug users (IDU/HIV Prevention fact sheet). Retrieved January 10, 2006, from ww.cdc.gov/idu/hepatitis/viral_hep_drug_use.pdf.

[CDC] Centers for Disease Control and Prevention (2005). *HIV-AIDS Surveillance Report, 2004*. Vol. 16, pp. 1–46. Atlanta: U.S. Department of Health and Human Services, Centers for Disease Control and Prevention.

Chambers HF, Morris DL, Tauber MG, and Modin G (1987). Cocaine use and the risk for endocarditis in intravenous drug users. *Ann Intern Med* 106: 833–836.

Chesney MA, Barrett DC, and Stall R (1998). Histories of substance use and risk behavior: precursors to HIV seroconversion in homosexual men. *Am J Public Health* 88:113–116.

Chitwood DD, Comerford M, and Sanchez J (2003). Prevalence and risk factors for HIV among sniffers, short-term injectors, and long-term injectors of heroin. *J Psychoactive Drugs* 35:445–453.

Cochrane Collaborative Review Group on HIV Infection and AIDS (2004). Evidence assessment strategies for HIV/AIDS prevention treatment and care. University of California, San Francisco, Institute for Global Health. Retrieved January 10, 2006, from www.igh.org/Cochrane/pdfs/Evidence Assessment.pdf.

Cohen MA, and Alfonso CA (2004). AIDS psychiatry: psychiatric and palliative care, and pain management. In GP Wormser (eds.), *AIDS and Other Manifestations of HIV Infection*, fourth edition. San Diego: Elsevier Academic Press.

Community Epidemiologic Work Group (2000). *Epidemiologic Trends in Drug Abuse, Vol. 1: Highlights and Executive Summary* (pp. 81–84). NIH publication No.00-4739A. Bethesda, MD: National Institutes of Health.

Cruciani R, and Coggins C (2002). Current perspectives on pain in AIDS. *Oncology* 16:980–982.

Des Jarlais DC, Perlis T, Arasteh K, et al. (2005). HIV incidence among injection drug users in New York City, 1990 to 2002: use of serologic test algorithm to assess expansion of HIV prevention services. *Am J Public Health* 95:1439–1444.

Ewing J (1984). The CAGE questionnaire. *JAMA* 252: 1903–1907.

Ferrando SJ, and Batki SL (2000). Substance abuse and HIV infection. *New Dir Ment Health Serv* 87:57–67.

Ferrando S, Goggin K, Sewell M, et al. (1998). Substance use disorders in gay/bisexual men with HIV and AIDS. *Am J Addict* 7:51–60.

Galanter M, and Brook D (2001). Network therapy for addiction: bringing family and peer support into office practice. *Int J Group Psychother* 51:101–122.

Galanter M., Keller DS, and Dermatis H (1997). Network therapy for addiction: assessment of the clinical outcome of training. *Am J Drug Alcohol Abuse* 23:355–367.

Galanter M, Dermatis H, Glickman L, et al. (2004). Network therapy: decreased secondary opiate use during buprenorphine maintenance. *J Subst Abuse Treat* 26:313–318.

Garten RJ, Zhang J, Lai S, et al. (2005). Coinfection with HIV and hepatitis C virus among injection drug users in southern China. *Clin Infect Dis* 41(Suppl. 1):S18–S24.

Gerber JG, Gal J, Rosencranz S, et al. (2001). The effect of ritonavir (RTV)/saquinavir (SQV) on stereoselective pharmacokinetics (PK) of methadone (M): results of AIDS Clinical Trial Group (ACTG) 401. *J Acquir Immune Defic Syndr* 27:153–160.

George JP, and Krystal JH (2000). Comorbidity of psychiatric and substance abuse disorders. *Curr Opin Psychiatry* 13:327–331.

Gibson DR, McCusker J, and Chesney M (1998). Effectiveness of psychosocial interventions in preventing HIV risk behavior in injecting drug users. *AIDS* 12:919–929.

Hales G, Roth N, and Smith D (2000). Possible fatal interaction between protease inhibitors and methamphetamine. *Antivir Ther* 5:19.

Halkitis PN, Parsons JT, and Stirratt MJ (2001). A double epidemic: crystal methamphetamine drug use in relation to HIV transmission among gay men. *J Homosex* 41:17–35.

Harrington RD, Woodward JA, Hooton TM, and Horn JR (1999). Life-threatening interactions between HIV-1 protease inhibitors and the illicit drugs MDMA and gamma-hydroxybutyrate. *Arch Intern Med* 159:2221–2224.

Henry JA, and Hill IR (1998). Fatal interaction between ritonavir and MDMA. *Lancet* 352:1751–1752.

Hijazi Y, and Boulieu R (2002). Contribution of CYP3A4, CYP2B6, and CYP2C9 isoforms to N-demethylation of ketamine in human liver microsomes. *Drug Metab Dispos* 30:853–858.

Jacox A, Carr D, Payne R, et al. (1994). *Clinical Practice Guideline Number 9: Management of Cancer Pain.* AHCPR Publ. No. 94-0592. Washington, DC: Agency for Health Care Policy and Research, U.S. Dept of Health and Human Services.

Kalant H (2001): The pharmacology and toxicology of "ecstasy" (MDMA) and related drugs. *CMAJ* 165: 917–928.

Kaplan R, Slywka J, Slagle S, and Ries K (2000). A titrated morphine analgesic regimen comparing substance users and non-users with AIDS-related pain. *J Pain Symptom Manage* 19:265–273.

Kessler RC, Crim RM, Warner LA, et al. (1997). Lifetime co-occurrence of DSM-III-R alcohol abuse and dependence with other psychiatric disorders in the national comorbidity survey. *Arch Gen Psychiatry* 54:313–321.

Klinkenberg WD, and Sacks S (2004). Mental disorders and drug abuse in persons living with HIV/AIDS. *AIDS Care* 16(Suppl. 1):S22–S42.

Kosel BW, Aweeka FT, Benowitz NL, et al. (2002). The effects of cannabinoids on the pharmacokinetics of indinavir and nelfinavir. *AIDS* 16:543–550.

Lange RA, and Hillis DL (2001). Medical progress: cardiovascular complications of cocaine use. *N Engl J Med* 345:351–358.

Larue F, Fountaine A, and Colleau SM (1997). Underestimation and undertreatment of pain in HIV disease. *BMJ* 314:23–28.

Laurenzana EM, and Owens SM (1997). Metabolism of phencyclidine by human liver microsomes. *Drug Metab Dispos* 25:557–263.

Lin D, Li X, Yang H, et al. (2005). Alcohol intoxication and sexual risk behaviors among rural-to-urban migrants in China. *Drug Alcohol Depend* 79:103–112.

Lipsitz JD, Williams JBW, Rabkin JG, et al. (1994). Psychopathology in male and female intravenous drug users with and without HIV infection. *Am J Psychiatry* 151:1662–1668.

Maillard ME, and Sorrell MF (2005): Alcoholic liver disease. In DL Kasper, D Braunwald, AS Fauci AS, et al. (eds.), *Harrison's Textbook of Internal Medicine*, 16th edition. New York: McGraw-Hill.

Malcolm R, Myrick H, Brady KT, and Ballenger JC (2001). Update on anticonvulsants for the treatment of alcohol withdrawal. *Am J Addict* 10(Suppl.):16–23.

Mayo-Smith MT (1997). Pharmacologic management of alcohol withdrawal: a meta-analysis and evidence-based practice guidelines. *JAMA* 278:144–151.

McCann UD, and Ricuarte GA (2000). Drug abuse and dependence: hazards and consequences of heroin, cocaine, amphetamines. *Curr Opin Psychiatry* 13: 321–325.

McCann UD, Slate SO, and Ricuarte GA (1996). Adverse reactions with 3,4-methylenedioxymethamphetamine (MDMA, Ecstasy). *Drug Saf* 15:107–116.

McCormick JP, Li R, Zarowny D, and Singer J (1993). Inadequate treatment of pain in ambulatory HIV patients. *Clin J Pain* 9:279–283.

McDowell JA, Chittick GE, Stevens CP, et al (2000). Pharmacokinetic interaction of abacavir and ethanol in human immunodeficiency virus–infected adults. *Antimicrob Agents Chemother* 44:1686–1690.

Miller WR, and Rollnick S (1991). *Motivational Interviewing: Preparing People to Change Addictive Behavior.* New York: Guilford Press.

Molitor F, Truax SR, Ruiz JD, and Sun RK (1998). Association of methamphetamine use during sex with sexual risk behaviors and HIV infection among non-injection drug user. *West J Med* 168:93–97.

Molitor F, Ruiz JD, Flynn N, et al. (1999). Methamphetamine use and sexual and injection risk behaviors among out-of-treatment injection drug users. *Am J Drug Alcohol Abuse* 25:475–493.

Needle R, Ball A, Des Jarlais D, Whitmore C, and Lambert E (2001). The global research network on HIV prevention in drug-using populations (GRN) 1998–2000: trends in the epidemiology, ethnography, and prevention of HIV/AIDS in injection drug users. In 2000 *Global Research Network Meeting on HIV Prevention in Drug Using Populations: Third Annual Meeting Report*. Washington, DC: NIDA.

Newshan G, and Lefkowitz M (2001). Transdermal fentanyl for chronic pain in persons with AIDS: a pilot study. *J Pain Symptom Manage* 21:69–77.

NIH Consensus Development Conference (1998). Effective medical treatment of opiate addiction. *JAMA* 280:1936–1943.

Pages KP, and Ries RK (1998). Use of anticonvulsants in benzodiazepine withdrawal. *Am J Addict* 7:198–204.

Petry NM (1999). Alcohol use in HIV patients: what we don't know may hurt us. *Int J STD AIDS* 10: 561–570.

PinzanniV, Faucherre V, Peyiere H, et al. (2000). Methadone withdrawal symptoms with nevirapine and efavirenz. *Ann Pharmacother* 34:405–407.

Prochaska JO, and DiClemente CC (1986). Toward a comprehensive model of change. In WR Miller and N Heather (eds.), *Treating Addictive Behaviors: Processes of Change*. New York: Plenum Press.

Rabkin JG, Johnson J, Lin SH, et al. (1997). Psychopathology in male and female HIV-positive and negative injecting drug users: longitudinal course over 3 years. *AIDS* 11:507–515.

[SAMHSA] Substance Abuse and Mental Health Services Administration (2005). *Overview of Findings from the 2004 National Survey of Drug Use and Health*. Office of Applied Studies, NSDUH Series H-27, DHHS Publication No. SMA 05-4061. Rockville, MD: SAMHSA.

Semann S, DesJarlais DC, Sugolow E, et al. (2002). A meta-analysis of the effect of HIV prevention interventions on the sex behaviors of drug users in the United States. *J Acquir Immune Defic Syndr* 30(Suppl.):S73–S93.

Shoptaw S, Reback CJ, and Freese TE (2002). Patient characteristics, HIV serostatus, and risk behaviors among gay and bisexual males seeking treatment for methamphetamine abuse and dependence in Los Angeles. *J Addict Dis* 21:91–105.

Stall R, Paul JP, Greenwood G, et al. (2001). Alcohol use, drug use and alcohol-related problems among men who have sex with men: the Urban Men's Health Study. *Addiction* 96:1589–1601.

Swica Y, and Breitbart W (2002). Treating pain in patients with AIDS and a history of substance use. *West J Med* 176:33–39.

Szerlip MA, DeSalvo KB, and Szerlip HM (2005). Predictors of HIV-infection in older adults. *J Aging Health* 17:293–304.

UNAIDS (2005). *AIDS Epidemic Update: December 2005*. Retrieved February 1, 2006, from http://www.unaids.org/epi/2005/doc/report_pdf.asp.

Urbina A, and Jones K (2004). Crystal methamphetamine, its analogues, and HIV infection: medical and psychiatric aspects. *Clin Infect Dis* 38:890–894.

Venable PA, McKirnan DJ, Buchbinder SP, et al. (2004). Alcohol use and high-risk behavior among men who have sex with men: the effects of consumption level and partner type. *Health Psychol* 23:525–532

Weir E (2000). Raves: a review of the culture, the drugs, and the prevention of harm. *CMAJ* 162:1843–1848.

Weissman DE, and Haddox JD (1980). Opioid pseudoaddiction—an iatrogenic syndrome. *Pain* 36:363–366.

Woody GE, Donnell D, and Seage GR (1999). Non-injection substance use correlates with risky sex among men having sex with men: Data from HIVNET. *Drug Alcohol Depend* 53:197–205.

Chapter 9

Mood Disorders

*Harold W. Goforth, Mary Ann Cohen,
and James Murrough*

Mood disorders have complex synergistic and catalytic interactions with HIV infection. They are significant factors in nonadherence to risk reduction and to medical care. Mood disorders associated with HIV include illness- and treatment-related depression and mania, responses to diagnoses of HIV, and comorbid primary mood disorders such as major depressive disorder and bipolar disorder. While persons with HIV and AIDS may have potentially no or multiple psychiatric disorders, alterations in mood are frequent concomitants of HIV infection. They have a profound impact on quality of life, level of distress and suffering, as well as direct and indirect effects on morbidity, treatment adherence, and mortality. In this chapter we will describe the significance of each of the mood disorders and their impact on the lives of persons with HIV and AIDS and on their families and caregivers. More detailed discussions of the epidemiology and prevalence of mood disorders are found in Chapter 4. Distress is further examined in Chapter 14, insomnia

in Chapter 15, endocrinopathies in Chapter 35, and suicide in Chapter 18.

MOOD DISORDERS AS RESPONSES TO HIV DIAGNOSIS, ILLNESS, AND TREATMENT

Bereavement

Persons with HIV and AIDS may experience not only the losses of loved ones, children, partners, parents, and friends, but also losses related to illness. While such loss is a concomitant of many severe and chronic illnesses such as cancer, diabetes, and neurological illness, persons with AIDS may have all of those illnesses as part of their illness or co-occurring with AIDS. The young woman with AIDS who develops cancer, the older man with AIDS who develops diabetes and end-stage renal disease, and the dancer with

AIDS who is paraplegic due to HIV myelopathy may each be dealing with bereavement in a unique manner. Although far less frequent than before the potent antiretroviral therapies, opportunistic infections such as cytomegalovirus retinitis can lead to loss of vision, HIV-cardiomyopathy to congestive heart failure, and HIV-associated dementia to loss of cognitive function. These occur primarily in persons who lack access to care or are nonadherent to care, and who may also be at increased risk of mood disorders. Loss and grief with mourning and bereavement commonly follow these tragic losses.

Few studies have adequately examined the relationship between bereavement and HIV, although attention to this subject has increased over the last 5 years. Certainly, bereavement is considered a normal reaction to an emotional loss and an expected reaction to the diagnosis of HIV; however, data continue to emerge that suggest a profound role for bereavement in mediating HIV illness and the need to effectively deal with bereavement issues.

A study by Kemeny and Dean (1995) investigated the relationship between early AIDS-related bereavement and subsequent changes in CD4 T-cell levels and overall health over 3 to 4 years of follow-up. The results indicated that those subjects who had experienced an AIDS-related bereavement event showed a more rapid loss of CD4 T cells 2 years post-bereavement, possibly suggesting an ongoing effect from remote bereavement reactions. The authors noted that grief alone did not predict CD4 decline, and T-cell reduction became apparent only in the presence of depressive symptoms reflective of complicated bereavement such as self-reproach. A second study by Kemeny and colleagues (1995) supported this initial finding with data showing that the death of an intimate partner among HIV-positive men was associated with significant immune dysfunction relevant to HIV progression within 1 year.

Subsequent to the results of these studies, multiple intervention-based trials have validated these findings and provided increasing evidence that early intervention at the time of bereavement is an effective and worthwhile strategy to optimize wellness in HIV-infected groups. In a randomized, controlled trial, Goodkin and colleagues (1999) examined the impact of a semistructured bereavement support group on homosexual men who suffered loss of a close friend or intimate partner to AIDS within the prior 6 months, and found that brief group intervention significantly reduced overall distress and accelerated grief reduction. Similar results of improvement in health-related quality of life and grief reduction have been provided by at least two other studies by Sikkema and colleagues (2004, 2005).

One of the most comprehensive studies examining the impact of bereavement intervention on the course of HIV and AIDS (Goodkin et al., 2001) included outcome measures for psychological distress as well as biological markers including viral load and CD4 count. Patients receiving group intervention had a decrease in viral load that was significant even when controlled for the presence of antiviral therapies, prophylactic therapies against secondary infections, CD4 count, viral load, and CDC clinical disease stage (Goodkin et al., 2001). Importantly, this study demonstrated that early psychological intervention for bereavement may not only improve the quality of life in HIV patients but also directly impact the course of HIV disease.

Persons with HIV experience loss in many different ways over the course of their illness, including loss of friends, primary support networks, and physical integrity, and the continuing social stigmata of HIV and AIDS. Unfortunately for many, the loss of family and friends may occur at a time when they are most needed, which may further compound the loss of occupational and recreational capabilities across the course of the disease through both social isolation and physical impairment. Importantly, though, studies have demonstrated that group interventions designed to target maladaptive bereavement processes not only counter psychological distress and improve health-related quality of life but also may have a direct impact on HIV illness progression.

Adjustment Disorder with Depressive Features

Adjustment disorders are defined as brief, maladaptive reactions to significant psychosocial stressors within 3 months of the stressor's onset (DSM-IV-TR; American Psychiatric Association, 2000). The prevalence of these disorders is estimated to be between 2% and 8% of the general population, with women diagnosed twice as often as men. No systematic study has yet adequately addressed the epidemiology of adjustment disorders in an HIV-AIDS population due to a variety of logistical factors including the time-limited duration of the diagnosis, although one study noted that adjustment disorder was the most common Axis I disorder in a group of HIV patients (O'Dowd et al., 1991).

The clinical picture of adjustment disorders can be varied, and subtypes exist for depressed, anxious, conduct disturbance, and mixed subtypes. However, while adjustment disorder is by definition a time-limited diagnosis that gives way to resolution of the psychosocial stressor or a new level of adaptation, it can also be associated with severe reactions, including suicidality. Adjustment disorders may be a frequent concomitant of HIV testing, and present with either negative or positive test results. While the consequences of receiving a positive HIV serology may be more obvious and may provoke both acute anxiety and depressive features, it is equally important to note that a negative serology in some individuals has prompted near euphoria with accompanying disturbances of conduct characterized by paradoxical celebratory actions such as promiscuous sexual encounters and substance abuse (Makulowich, 1997).

Treisman and colleagues (1998) have cautioned against dismissing depressive symptoms in a person with HIV as a variant of a normal reaction to a progressive and fatal illness. While many patients diagnosed with HIV enter a transient period of demoralization and sadness related to normal bereavement and loss, most gradually recover and are able to continue life in a meaningful fashion.

Leserman and colleagues (2002) documented the impact of psychosocial factors such as stressful life events, depressive symptoms, and lack of social support on HIV illness progression, but these studies have not been limited to the diagnosis of adjustment disorder. Therefore, while providing valuable inferential information on the role of adjustment disorder, they are limited to subjects with more profound depressive illness as well as chronic time spans extending beyond the 3-month diagnostic limit (Evans et al., 1997; Leserman et al., 1999, 2000, 2002).

Ideally, adjustment disorders should be treated conservatively with supportive and other appropriate forms of psychotherapy. A psychoeducational approach should be used to dispel misconceptions and increase or sustain healthy behavior as well as bolster existing psychological support. Identification of elements over which the patient has control can help the patient have a sense of empowerment and maintain an internal locus of control. Medications should likely be reserved as augmentation strategies rather than as a primary treatment modality.

MAJOR DEPRESSIVE DISORDER AND MOOD DISORDERS WITH DEPRESSIVE FEATURES DUE TO HIV AND AIDS

Depressive illness is a major cause of distress in patients with HIV and AIDS, and has a severe impact on the quality of life and on medication adherence. Depression is a debilitating condition; its symptoms include sadness, pessimism, anhedonia, guilt, and suicidality in addition to neurovegetative changes such as impaired sleep and appetite. These latter signs can often be confused with the primary illness, as HIV and AIDS often produce fatigue, anorexia, and wasting syndromes, making the diagnosis of depression challenging in this patient group. Additionally, somatic symptoms of depression may be confused with opportunistic infections, further complicating the differential diagnosis and increasing utilization of physicians' time and services.

Major depressive disorder is frequently underdiagnosed and undertreated (Evans et al., 1996–97) in persons with HIV and AIDS. Depression in HIV can be either primary or secondary in nature. When depression develops during the course of HIV infection, it is described typically as a mood disorder due to a medical condition if it is etiologically related to HIV infection, opportunistic disease, antiviral treatments, or comorbid medical conditions. When a person with HIV or AIDS has a longstanding history of depression and/or family history of depression or bipolar disorder, however, it is more likely that the diagnosis of major depressive disorder would be supported.

Secondary Depression

Common aspects of HIV illness that directly impact the emergence of depressive symptoms include endocrine abnormalities, opportunistic disease, nutritional states, comorbid illness, and medication effect. Significant factors and causes of secondary depression are summarized in Table 9.1.

It is unclear what impact HIV progression and stage have on the development of depressive symptoms, and studies have varied in their results. Rabkin identified a cohort of intravenous drug users including 69 seropositive men, 52 seronegative men, 36 seropositive women, and 30 seronegative women who were followed over 3 years. The group that appeared most protected against depressive illness was the seronegative men (15%), whereas seropositive men and seronegative

TABLE 9.1. Significant Factors and Causes of Secondary Depression in HIV and AIDS

Psychiatric Disorders

Substance Use Disorders
Cocaine-induced mood disorder
Sedative-hypnotic-induced mood disorder
Alcohol-induced mood disorder
HIV-associated dementia

Medical Illness

Infections
Hepatitis C
HIV-induced mood disorder
HIV-associated nephropathy and end-stage renal disease
Cirrhosis of the liver

Endorcrine Disorders
Hypothyroidism
Diabetes mellitus
Hypotestosteronism
Adrenal insufficiency

Medications

---

women appeared to be at increased risk (30%). Rabkin and her team were able to correlate the degree of mood decline over time with CD4 T-cell count (Rabkin et al., 1997), suggesting that HIV infection increases the risk of depression among both men and women. Similarly, a more recent study by Creuss and colleagues (2005) encouragingly found that natural killer (NK) cell activity increased in HIV-seropositive individuals with resolution of depressive illness.

Highly active antiretroviral therapy (HAART) has revolutionized the treatment of HIV and has led to increased quality of life and longer lives for those affected. However, HAART-related medications are highly toxic and can produce neurobehavioral disturbances and changes. The most commonly accepted antiviral agent for producing such changes is efavirenz; its effects can include symptoms of depression with suicidal ideation, cognitive changes, headache, dizziness, insomnia, and nightmares. Its neuropsychiatric profile has been shown to be related to blood levels (Gutierrez et al., 2005), but the neurobehavioral symptoms appear to abate gradually as patients continue to receive the agent over time (Clifford et al., 2005).

Hepatitis C virus (HCV) coinfection among HIV-infected populations is problematic and poses a unique set of challenges for the practitioner. Increasing evidence points to a process of neural invasion by HCV with neurocognitive effects similar to those of HIV, but without the associated end-stage dementia (Laskus et al., 2005). Prevalence studies have estimated the 1-month rate of depression in HCV-infected individuals at 28% (Golden et al., 2005), but it is clear that treatment of HCV with interferon-based therapies dramatically increases the risk of depressive symptoms to near 80% (Laguno et al., 2004; Reichenberg et al., 2005; Scalori et al., 2005). These effects on mood, increased fatigue, and worsened quality of life are even greater in patients with concurrent, advanced HIV disease (Ryan et al., 2004), and appear likely to be due to a variety of factors, including biological and sociodemographic ones (Braitstein et al., 2005).

Multiple studies have explored the role of antidepressant treatment to minimize the increased physical and psychological burden associated with interferon therapy, and it appears that selective serotonin reuptake inhibitors show considerable promise in preventing and minimizing interferon-related symptoms (Musselman et al., 2001) in persons with metastatic malignant melanoma. However, a case series describing psychosis in response to interferon in persons with comorbid HIV and HCV indicates that antipsychotic medications and mood stabilizers may be of more benefit with or without antidepressant medication (Hoffman et al., 2003).

Secondary Mania

Secondary manic syndromes due to late-stage disease are not common but can have disastrous consequences for the patient when they do occur. In a chart review, Lyketsos and colleagues (1993) reported that manic syndromes affected approximately 8% of the examined population across a 17-month period. These patients were less likely to have a family history of bipolar disorder but more likely to have concurrent dementia than patients with manic episodes early in the non-AIDS stage of their disease. This link has been substantiated by other retrospective and small case–control studies (Kieburtz et al., 1991; Mijch et al., 1999). Ellen and colleagues (1999) identified mania in 1.2% of HIV-seropositive patients and in 4.3% of those with AIDS-defining illness, findings suggestive of increased rates during the course of disease progression.

Opportunistic infections such as cryptococcal meningitis serve as one of the more common reasons for secondary mania, and any presentation of mania in immunocompromised individuals requires this in the differential diagnosis (Thienhaus and Khosla, 1984; Johannesen and Wilson, 1988). Secondary mania may also be linked to medications such as zidovudine (Maxwell et al., 1988) or didanosine (Brouillette et al., 1994) among the antiretroviral agents, and clarithromycin (Nightingale et al., 1995) or ethambutol (Pickles and Spelman, 1996) in the setting of *Mycobacterium avium* complex (MAC) prophylaxis in individuals with AIDS. In addition, there is a case report of mania with an irritable and expansive presentation due to efavirenz overdose, which resolved within 48 hours after treatment with low-dose risperidone (Blanch et al., 2001).

Treatment is directed toward both symptom control and treatment of the underlying disease, since mania most commonly presents in advanced illness. It is possible that once the viral load is below detectable levels, secondary mania may be less likely to recur, in contrast to idiopathic bipolar affective disorder (Cohen and Alfonso, 2004). Thus, while HIV medications have been sporadically reported as causative agents for mania, they play a pivotal and life-saving role in the treatment of this disease and may actually demonstrate a protective effect against mania in late-stage HIV disease (Mijch et al., 1999).

CONCOMITANT MOOD DISORDERS

Major Depressive Disorder

Major depression is one of the most common mood disorders in HIV-seropositive individuals, and it was the earliest reported mood disturbance of HIV. Rates of depression in HIV have varied widely across studies due to differing sample populations, which are difficult to compare as they share little else in common other than their HIV serostatus. The landmark HIV Cost and Services Utilization Study (HCSUS) identified high rates of drug use (50%), major depression (36%), anxiety disorder (16%), and heavy drinking (12%) among a large representative sample of adults receiving care for HIV in early 1996 (Bing et al., 2001; Galvan et al., 2002). The HCSUS study remains the most well-designed and comprehensive study of the prevalence of psychiatric disorders in an HIV-infected population, although other studies provide snapshots of the high rates of comorbid psychiatric disease in this population (Winiarski et al., 2005). Depression is the most common reason for psychiatric referral among HIV-infected patients (Seth et al., 1991), and

rates of major depression range from 8% to 67% (Acuff et al., 1999); however, up to 85% of HIV-seropositive individuals report the prevalence of some depressive symptoms (Tate et al., 2003) that may not reach diagnostic threshold for a major depressive disorder diagnosis. Examples would include minor depressions and dysthymia. This may especially be true when taking into account the prevalence of depression in other medical illnesses that are comorbid with HIV, including HCV, end-stage renal disease, diabetes mellitus, and other endocrinopathies. Indeed, the impact of HIV disease on mental health was illustrated by a meta-analysis by Ciesla and Roberts (2001), who found that HIV-infected patients were almost twice as likely to be diagnosed with major depressive illness, irregardless of the symptomatic status of their HIV disease. The prevalence and epidemiology of mood disorders are covered more extensively in Chapter 4 of this text.

The early recognition and treatment of serious psychiatric mood disorders such as depression can both alleviate suffering and prevent suicide, covered in more detail in Chapter 18 of this volume. Clinicians need to be aware of particular times during the course of HIV-related illness when individuals may be more vulnerable to suicide as well as psychiatric disorders and other precipitants that may lead to a suicidal crisis.

The pharmacological treatment of depressive illness in persons with HIV and AIDS is guided by both data supporting the direct efficacy of a particular antidepressant and consideration of the adverse-event profile of the agent. Multiple studies of depression have demonstrated that effective treatment not only reduces depressive symptoms but also improves associated quality of life. Importantly, recent evidence has begun to emerge that treatment and resolution of major depression are associated with immune status in HIV patients, which has provided new impetus to the accurate diagnosis and treatment of mood disorders in this population. While multiple studies have supported the efficacy of using antidepressants as a primary therapy for depressive illness in HIV-seropositive patients, little comparison data exist between antidepressants. These topics will be considered in further detail in Chapter 32.

Tricyclic and selective serotonin reuptake inhibitor (SSRI) antidepressants are metabolized through a variety of P450 pathways including 2D6, 1A2, 3A4, and 2C. The oldest SSRI, fluoxetine, is a potent inhibitor of 2D6 and 3A4, and has an extended elimination half-life of approximately 6 weeks when considered with its potent metabolite norfluoxetine. Sertraline, citalopram, and escitalopram have few potential drug–drug interactions, but all can have gastrointestinal side effects including nausea, vomiting, and diarrhea, as well as sleep alterations, weight changes, sexual dysfunction, and extrapyramidal effects such as a high-frequency, low-amplitude tremor. The tricyclics produce significant anticholinergic effects and may induce delirium, cognitive slowing, urinary retention, dry mouth, and orthostasis; these are not recommended for routine use in this vulnerable population. Similarly, monoamine oxidase inhibitors are not recommended for patients with HIV and AIDS. This class of medications poses an extraordinary risk, since persons with HIV and AIDS are often on complex and frequently changing drug regimens and also have the concurrent risk of hypertensive crisis if exposed to certain foods or other medications. These include epinephrine for asthma or meperidine for prevention of rigors from amphotericin B treatment of cryptococcal meningitis or other fungal infections (Cohen and Jacobson, 2000). Psychotherapeutic intervention can have a profound impact on the severity of depressive illness, and multiple studies have supported the efficacy of cognitive-behavioral therapy in treating major depressive illness and reducing the risk of relapse (Hollon et al., 2005), increasing adherence to HAART therapy (Parsons et al., 2005), and having a possible protective effect on the immune system for up to 1 year after completing therapy (Carrico et al., 2005). Importantly, it has been offered in a group therapy model to HIV-infected patients with good success (Blanch et al., 2002).

Similarly, interpersonal therapy (IPT) has demonstrated efficacy in treating major depressive illness in HIV disease (Markowitz et al., 1992, 1995), and IPT may offer advantages to patients who have been recently diagnosed with HIV/AIDS or have recently progressed in their disease severity. IPT is notable for its brevity and can successfully focus on the common problems encountered in HIV disease, including grief, changes of life after disease diagnosis, role identity during times of illness progression, interpersonal disputes related to family strife surrounding diagnosis, issues of homosexuality or drug abuse, and support of existing coping strategies.

Other psychotherapeutic modalities include psychodynamic therapy (brief and extended) as well as supportive therapy, which can work to maximize existing coping strategies in times of heightened stress or turmoil. The role of support groups and other psychosocial interventions within the larger context of psychotherapeutic strategies cannot be underestimated; these will be addressed in more detail in Chapter 27.

Bipolar Disorder

As noted in the chapter segment on depression, HIV-seropositive individuals are at an increased risk of developing mood disorders across the spectrum of their disease as compared to the general population. Mania can occur at any point along the course of HIV illness, but the occurrence generally clusters into two categories: (a) a preexisting bipolar disorder that predated HIV seroconversion or is not directly related to the disease, which can occur at any point during the course of the disease; and (b) the late-stage manic syndrome that occurs most commonly but not exclusively in the context of HIV dementia (Lyketsos et al., 1997; Treisman et al., 1998). Primary bipolar disorder is more likely to appear consistent with the usual course of the illness, including euphoric mood, expansiveness, and signs or symptoms of poor judgment. In addition, the presence of a family history of bipolar disorder is more common in this category, and it is less likely to be associated with a preexisting condition. AIDS mania, though, has been noted to be associated with marked cognitive deficits, a pronounced irritable mood, and greater severity coupled with a rather dismal prognosis (Lyketsos et al., 1993, 1997).

It is has yet to be determined whether there is an increased risk of primary bipolar affective disorder type I in HIV patients, but a few studies have reported an increased prevalence of bipolar type II disease, cyclothymia, and hyperthymic personalities in HIV-positive patients (Perretta et al., 1998). Large-scale epidemiologic studies are required to better define the incidence and prevalence of primary bipolar illness across the spectrum of HIV illness; this topic is further addressed in Chapter 4.

The choice of an effective mood stabilizer in treating patients with bipolar disorder and concurrent HIV disease is complex, and is based both on available supporting evidence of primary efficacy and the potential for pharmacological interactions and potential adverse events. At the time of the writing of this chapter, four mood stabilizers had been approved by the U.S. Food and Drug Administration (FDA) for the treatment of primary bipolar disorder, and of these four agents, three were anticonvulsants—carbamazepine, valproate, lamotrigine, and lithium. There are no data comparing the efficacy of these agents to each other in treating and maintaining bipolar disorder in HIV-infected patients, and there is a dearth of evidence on even the use of any one agent in HIV disease.

The use of carbamazepine is complicated by its induction of the P450-3A4 isozyme, through which protease inhibitors are often metabolized, which may result in subtherapeutic serum concentrations of antiviral agents and the development of viral resistance (Hugen et al., 2000). This is phenomenon particularly troubling, given that resistance to protease inhibitors commonly occurs across the entire class of medications rather than being limited to a single agent (Barry et al., 1997). Carbamazepine also carries significant risk of anticholinergic delirium, which is especially problematic in individuals suffering from an underlying dementing process such as late-stage AIDS. Therefore, at this time, carbamazepine cannot be recommended as a first-line agent for the treatment of bipolar disorder in an HIV population.

The use of valproate derivatives, including divalproex, is a standard first-line therapy in idiopathic bipolar disorder, and may have relative advantages in the management of atypical bipolar disorder over lithium and atypical antipsychotics in patients with HIV illness (Halman et al., 1993) such as a low potential for medication interaction via cytochrome P450 isozymes (Ketter et al., 1999; Ethell et al., 2003). Its use in patients on HAART is complicated, however, by the potential for multiple drug–drug interactions via non-P450 mechanisms as well as the potential for extrapyramidal reactions in this population. Valproate has also been associated with thrombocytopenia, hepatic dysfunction, and pancreatitis, which are adverse events that overlap significantly with those associated with antiretroviral therapies (RachBeisel and Weintraub, 1997). The complexities of these issues will be further explored in Chapter 32.

Valproate in patients with hepatitis C coinfection deserves special caution (Felker et al., 2003), however, as cases of hepatic failure and hyperammonemic encephalopathy have been documented with valproate use even in otherwise healthy adults (Konig et al., 1994). The implications of these findings are especially pertinent for HIV-seropositive intravenous drug users, whose incidence of comorbid HCV is greater than 90%. Persons with HIV/HCV coinfection are especially vulnerable to hepatic complications because of the typically more rapid progression of their disease due to the combined, synergistic effect of HIV and HCV (Brau, 2005).

Lamotrigine is approved by the FDA for maintenance treatment of primary bipolar disorder, but studies examining its use in secondary mania have not been performed, and its relatively long titration period prevents its use to control acute episodes. Lamotrigine is not significantly protein bound, and its metabolism occurs primarily through beta-oxidation with minimal effect on the cytochrome P450 system, making it advantageous when used concurrently with protease inhibitors. It also has significant efficacy in the treatment of painful HIV-associated neuropathy, as demonstrated by Simpson and colleagues (2003) in a randomized, placebo-controlled, double-blind study. However, to date it remains an uncommon agent for treating HIV-associated mania because of concern over potential interaction with the antiretrovirals and the required slow titration schedule.

All atypical antipsychotics have been approved by the FDA for the acute treatment of manic states associated with primary bipolar disorder, and many have secured maintenance indications for primary bipolar as well (Tohen et al., 2000, 2004; Yatham et al., 2003; Bowden et al., 2005; McIntyre et al., 2005; Potkin et al., 2005; Smulevich et al., 2005; Vieta et al., 2005; Sachs et al., 2006). However, no controlled trials of any atypical antipsychotic medication have been performed for either HIV-associated mania or primary bipolar disorder in HIV-seropositive patients.

The use of risperidone in HIV-related psychosis including AIDS-associated (secondary) mania is supported by a case series by Singh and colleagues (1997). However, experience dictates considerable caution when using this agent, as it can provoke severe extrapyramidal reactions, including opisthotonus in our experience. The use of atypical agents is complicated further in HIV patients by the extensive P450 metabolism required of these agents (Meyer et al., 1998), exemplified by a single-dose pharmacokinetic study of olanzapine and ritonavir in healthy volunteers. The study's authors found that concurrent administration effectively reduced the mean half-life of olanzapine from 32 hours to 16 hours (Penzak et al., 2002). This suggests that patients concurrently receiving ritonavir and olanzapine may ultimately require higher doses to achieve similar therapeutic benefit. Little data exist to date regarding other atypical antipsychotic agents in the treatment of HIV patients.

Lithium has been a mainstay of mania treatment, and is the oldest and best characterized mood stabilizer. Its use in HIV and AIDS patients, however, is commonly precluded because of its expansive list of adverse events. The major problem with lithium in treating AIDS patients is the unpredictable fluctuations in serum blood levels due to a variety of mechanisms, making toxicity an ever-present consideration. Shifts in electrolyte balance via sweating, vomiting, diarrhea, or metabolic alkalosis can lead to dangerous elevated lithium levels, as can failure to adequately excrete the drug due to renal impairment from HIV-related nephropathy and heroin nephropathy. Thus, the use of lithium in persons with HIV or AIDS should be exercised with extreme caution (Cohen and Jacobson, 2000).

ADHERENCE DATA

HIV-related hospitalizations and deaths are influenced heavily by nonadherence to prescribed antiviral regimens (Riley et al., 2005; Sabin et al., 2006). Mental illness and drug abuse have been demonstrated in the developed world to be a significant barrier to adherence (Giordano et al., 2005). Depression appears to be an independent risk factor for nonadherence to HAART regimens in particular (Singh et al., 1996; Gordillo et al., 1999; Tuldra et al., 1999; Wagner et al., 2001; Starace et al., 2002; van Servellen et al., 2002; Carrieri et al., 2003; Ammassari et al., 2004; Gonzalez et al., 2004), and may be even more strongly associated with nonadherence than with chronic psychotic mental illness (Walkup et al., 2004). However, treatment for depression is associated with both efficacy and improved quality of life (Cruess et al., 2003; Himelhoch and Medoff, 2005), thus depression may be an easily modified variable to increase adherence to HAART therapy. These issues will be discussed more fully in Chapter 22.

CONCLUSIONS

Mood disorders in the context of HIV disease are varied and encompass almost all of general adult psychiatry, including affective illness, psychosis, substance abuse, psychotherapy, and advanced psychopharmacology. As noted in the introduction, HIV spectrum disease has become today's syphilitic equivalent, and dealing effectively with HIV-associated mood disorders forces the competent practitioner to maintain a high degree of both medical and psychiatric knowledge. Implications for mood disorders in HIV disease include diminished quality of life, heightened risk for suicide, disease progression, and increased rates of nonadherence to HAART therapy. Indirectly, mood disorders may be linked to increased antiviral resistance by virtue of increased rates of nonadherence to HAART therapy and an increased rate of risk-taking behavior including substance abuse.

Treatment of these disorders requires not only a thorough understanding of complicated psychodynamic issues but also a strong basis in advanced psychopharmacology. Medication choice may be dictated by such factors as treatment of comorbid disease, effect on viral activity, and risk of interactions with antiviral agents, as well as guided by data regarding its primary efficacy in HIV disease. Careful choice must be given to all these issues when implementing therapy for this complicated and at-risk group of individuals, and referral to a comprehensive HIV-AIDS center or an HIV-AIDS psychiatrist should remain a viable option for practitioners during these patients' treatment course. Effective treatment offers persons with HIV and AIDS the incalculable advantages of improved quality of life and improved survival in the context of an often devastating illness.

References

American Psychiatric Association (2000). *Diagnostic and Statistical Manual of Mental Disorders*, fourth edition, text revision [DSM IV-TR]. Washington, DC: American Psychiatric Association.

Acuff C, Archambeault J, Greenberg B, Hoeltzel J, McDaniel JS, Meyer P, Packer C, Parga FJ, Pillen MB, Rohhovde A, Saldarriaga M, Smith MJW, Stoff D, Wagner D (1999). *Mental Health Care for People Living with or Affected by HIV/AIDS: A Practical Guide*. Rockville, MD: Research Triangle Institute.

Ammassari A, Antinori A, Aloisi MS, Trotta MP, Murri R, Bartoli L, Monforte AD, Wu AW, and Starace F (2004). Depressive symptoms, neurocognitive impairment, and adherence to highly active antiretroviral therapy among HIV-infected persons. *Psychosomatics* 45(5):394–402.

Barry M, Gibbons S, Back D, and Mulcahy F (1997). Protease inhibitors in patients with HIV disease. Clinically important pharmacokinetic considerations. *Clin Pharmacokinet* 32(3):194–209.

Bing EG, Burnam MA, Longshore D, Fleishman JA, Sherbourne CD, London AS, Turner BJ, Eggan F,

Beckman R, Vitiello B, Morton SC, Orlando M, Bozzette SA, Ortiz-Barron L, Shapiro M (2001). Psychiatric disorders and drug use among human immunodeficiency virus-infected adults in the United States. *Arch Gen Psychiatry* 58(8):721–728.

Blanch J, Corbella B, Garcia F, Parellada E, and Gatell JM (2001). Manic syndrome associated with efavirenz overdose. *Clin Infect Dis* 33(2):270–271.

Blanch J, Rousaud A, Hautzinger M, Martinez E, Peri JM, Andres S, Cirera E, Gatell JM, and Gasto C (2002). Assessment of the efficacy of a cognitive-behavioural group psychotherapy programme for HIV-infected patients referred to a consultation-liaison psychiatry department. *Psychother Psychosom* 71(2):77–84.

Bowden CL, Grunze H, Mullen J, Brecher M, Paulsson B, Jones M, Vagero M, and Svensson K (2005). A randomized, double-blind, placebo-controlled efficacy and safety study of quetiapine or lithium as monotherapy for mania in bipolar disorder. *J Clin Psychiatry* 66(1):111–121.

Braitstein P, Montessori V, Chan K, Montaner JS, Schechter MT, O'Shaughnessy MV, and Hogg RS (2005). Quality of life, depression and fatigue among persons co-infected with HIV and hepatitis C: outcomes from a population-based cohort. *AIDS Care* 17(4):505–515.

Brau N (2005). Chronic hepatitis C in patients with HIV/AIDS: a new challenge in antiviral therapy. *J Antimicrob Chemother* 56(6):991–995.

Brouillette MJ, Chouinard G, and Lalonde R (1994). Didanosine-induced mania in HIV infection. *Am J Psychiatry* 151(12):1839–1840.

Carrico AW, Antoni MH, Pereira DB, Fletcher MA, Klimas N, Lechner SC, and Schneiderman N (2005). Cognitive behavioral stress management effects on mood, social support, and a marker of antiviral immunity are maintained up to 1 year in HIV-infected gay men. *Int J Behav Med* 12(4):218–226.

Carrieri MP, Raffi F, Lewden C, Sobel A, Michelet C, Cailleton V, Chene G, Leport C, Moatti JP, and Spire B for the APROCO Study Group (2003). Impact of early versus late adherence to highly active antiretroviral therapy on immuno-virological response: a 3-year follow-up study. *Antivir Ther* 8(6):585–594.

Ciesla JA, and Roberts JE (2001). Meta-analysis of the relationship between HIV infection and risk for depressive disorders. *Am J Psychiatry* 158(5):725–730.

Clifford DB, Evans S, Yang Y, Acosta EP, Goodkin K, Tashima K, Simpson D, Dorfman D, Ribaudo H, and Gulick RM (2005). Impact of efavirenz on neuropsychological performance and symptoms in HIV-infected individuals. *Ann Intern Med* 143(10):714–721.

Cohen MA, and Alfonso CA (2004). AIDS psychiatry, palliative care and pain management. In G Wormser (ed.), *AIDS and Other Manifestations of HIV Infection*, fourth edition (pp. 537–576). San Diego: Elsevier Academic Press.

Cohen MA, and Jacobson JM (2000). Maximizing life's potentials in AIDS: A psychopharmacologic update. *Gen Hosp Psychiatry* 22:375–388.

Cruess DG, Evans DL, Repetto MJ, Gettes D, Douglas SD, and Petitto JM (2003). Prevalence, diagnosis, and pharmacological treatment of mood disorders in HIV disease. *Biol Psychiatry* 54(3):307–316.

Cruess DG, Douglas SD, Petitto JM, Have TT, Gettes D, Dube B, Cary M, and Evans DL (2005). Association of resolution of major depression with increased natural killer cell activity among HIV-seropositive women. *Am J Psychiatry* 162(11):2125–2130.

Ellen SR, Judd FK, Mijch AM, and Cockram A (1999). Secondary mania in patients with HIV infection. *Aust N Z J Psychiatry* 33(3):353–360.

Ethell BT, Anderson GD, and Burchell B (2003). The effect of valproic acid on drug and steroid glucuronidation by expressed human UDP-glucuronosyl-transferases: *Biochem Pharmacol* 65(9):1441–1449.

Evans DL, Leserman J, Perkins DO, Stern RA, Murphy C, Zheng B, Gettes D, Longmate JA, Silva SG, van der Horst CM, Hall CD, Folds JD, Golden RN, and Petitto JM (1997). Severe life stress as a predictor of early disease progression in HIV infection. *Am J Psychiatry* 154(5):630–634.

Evans DL, Staab J, Ward H, Leserman J, Perkins DO, Golden RN, and Petitto JM (1996–97). Depression in the medically ill: management considerations. *Depress Anxiety* 4(4):199–208.

Felker BL, Sloan KL, Dominitz JA, and Barnes RF (2003). The safety of valproic acid use for patients with hepatitis C infection. *Am J Psychiatry* 160(1):174–178.

Galvan FH, Bing EG, Fleishman JA, London AS, Caetano R, Burnam MA, Longshore D, Morton SC, Orlando M, and Shapiro M (2002). The prevalence of alcohol consumption and heavy drinking among people with HIV in the United States: results from the HIV Cost and Services Utilization Study. *J Stud Alcohol* 63(2):179–186.

Giordano TP, Suarez-Almazor ME, and Grimes RM (2005). The population effectiveness of highly active antiretroviral therapy: are good drugs good enough? *Curr HIV/AIDS Rep* 2(4):177–183.

Golden J, O'Dwyer AM, and Conroy RM (2005). Depression and anxiety in patients with hepatitis C: prevalence, detection rates and risk factors. *Gen Hosp Psychiatry* 27(6):431–438.

Gonzalez JS, Penedo FJ, Antoni MH, Duran RE, McPherson-Baker S, Ironson G, Isabel Fernandez M, Klimas NG, Fletcher MA, and Schneiderman N (2004). Social support, positive states of mind, and HIV treatment adherence in men and women living with HIV/AIDS. *Health Psychol* 23(4):413–418.

Goodkin K, Blaney NT, Feaster DJ, Baldewicz T, Burkhalter JE, and Leeds B (1999). A randomized controlled clinical trial of a bereavement support group intervention in human immunodeficiency virus type 1-seropositive and -seronegative homosexual men. *Arch Gen Psychiatry* 56(1):52–59.

Goodkin K, Baldewicz TT, Asthana D, Khamis I, Blaney NT, Kumar M, Burkhalter JE, Leeds B, and Shapshak P (2001). A bereavement support group intervention affects plasma burden of human immunodeficiency virus type 1. Report of a randomized controlled trial. *J Hum Virol* 4(1):44–54.

Gordillo V, del Amo J, Soriano V, and Gonzalez-Lahoz J (1999). Sociodemographic and psychological variables influencing adherence to antiretroviral therapy. *AIDS* 13(13):1763–1769.

Gutierrez F, Navarro A, Padilla S, Anton R, Masia M, Borras J, and Martin-Hidalgo A (2005). Prediction of neuropsychiatric adverse events associated with long-term efavirenz therapy, using plasma drug level monitoring. *Clin Infect Dis* 41(11):1648–1653.

Halman MH, Worth JL, Sanders KM, Renshaw PF, and Murray GB (1993). Anticonvulsant use in the treatment of manic syndromes in patients with HIV-1 infection. *J Neuropsychiatry Clin Neurosci* 5(4): 430–434.

Himelhoch S, and Medoff DR (2005). Efficacy of antidepressant medication among HIV-positive individuals with depression: a systematic review and meta-analysis. *AIDS Patient Care STDS* 19(12): 813–822.

Hoffman RG, Cohen MA, Alfonso CA, Weiss JJ, Jones S, Keller M, Condemarin JR, Chiu NM, and Jacobson JM (2003). Treatment of interferon-induced psychosis in patients with comorbid hepatitis C and HIV. *Psychosomatics* 44(5):417–420.

Hollon SD, DeRubeis RJ, Shelton RC, Amsterdam JD, Salomon RM, O'Reardon JP, Lovett ML, Young PR, Haman KL, Freeman BB, and Gallop R (2005). Prevention of relapse following cognitive therapy vs. medications in moderate to severe depression. *Arch Gen Psychiatry* 62(4):417–422.

Hugen PW, Burger DM, Brinkman K, ter Hofstede HJ, Schuurman R, Koopmans PP, and Hekster YA (2000). Carbamazepine–indinavir interaction causes antiretroviral therapy failure. *Ann Pharmacother* 34(4):465–470.

Johannesen DJ, and Wilson LG (1988). Mania with cryptococcal meningitis in two AIDS patients. *J Clin Psychiatry* 49:200–201.

Kemeny ME, and Dean L (1995). Effects of AIDS-related bereavement on HIV progression among New York City gay men. *AIDS Educ Prev* 7: 36–47.

Kemeny ME, Weiner H, Duran R, Taylor SE, Visscher B, and Fahey JL (1995). Immune system changes after the death of a partner in HIV-positive gay men. *Psychosom Med* 57(6):547–554.

Ketter TA, Frye MA, Cora-Locatelli G, Kimbrell TA, and Post RM (1999). Metabolism and excretion of mood stabilizers and new anticonvulsants. *Cell Mol Neurobiol* 19(4):511–532.

Kieburtz K, Zettelmaier AE, Ketonen L, Tuite M, and Caine ED (1991). Manic syndrome in AIDS. *Am J Psychiatry* 148(8):1068–1070.

Konig SA, Siemes H, Blaker F, Boenigk E, Gross-Selbeck G, Hanefeld F, Haas N, Kohler B, Koelfen W, and Korinthenberg R (1994). Severe hepatotoxicity during valproate therapy: an update and report of eight new fatalities. *Epilepsia* 35(5):1005–1015.

Laguno M, Blanch J, Murillas J, Blanco JL, Leon A, Lonca M, Larrousse M, Biglia A, Martinez E, Garcia F, Miro JM, de Pablo J, Gatell JM, and Mallolas J (2004). Depressive symptoms after initiation of interferon therapy in human immunodeficiency virus–infected patients with chronic hepatitis C. *Antivir Ther* 9(6):905–909.

Laskus T, Radkowski M, Adair DM, Wilkinson J, Scheck AC, and Rakela J (2005). Emerging evidence of hepatitis C virus neuroinvasion. *AIDS* 19:S140–S144.

Leserman J, Petitto JM, Gu H, Gaynes BN, Barroso J, Golden RN, Perkins DO, Folds JD, and Evans DL (1999). Progression to AIDS: the effects of stress, depressive symptoms, and social support. *Psychosom Med* 61(3):397–406.

Leserman J, Petitto JM, Golden RN, Gaynes BN, Gu H, Perkins DO, Silva SG, Folds JD, and Evans DL (2000). Impact of stressful life events, depression, social support, coping, and cortisol on progression to AIDS. *Am J Psychiatry* 157(8):1221–1228.

Leserman J, Petitto JM, Gu H, Gaynes BN, Barroso J, Golden RN, Perkins DO, Folds JD, and Evans DL (2002). Progression to AIDS, a clinical AIDS condition and mortality: psychosocial and physiological predictors. *Psychol Med* 32(6):1059–1073.

Lyketsos CG, Hoover DR, Guccione M, Senterfitt W, Dew MA, Wesch J, VanRaden MJ, Treisman GJ, and Morgenstern H (1993). Depressive symptoms as predictors of medical outcomes in HIV infection. Multicenter AIDS Cohort Study. *JAMA* 270(21): 2563–2567.

Lyketsos CG, Schwartz J, Fishman M, and Treisman G (1997). AIDS mania. *J Neuropsychiatry Clin Neurosci* 9(2):277–279.

Makulowich GS (1997). Bereavement increases sexual risk-taking behaviors among gay men. *AIDS Patient Care STDS* 11(5):379–380.

Markowitz JC, Klerman GL, and Perry SW (1992). Interpersonal psychotherapy of depressed HIV-positive outpatients. *Hosp Community Psychiatry* 43(9):885–890.

Markowitz JC, Klerman GL, Clougherty KF, Spielman LA, Jacobsberg LB, Fishman B, Frances AJ, Kocsis JH, and Perry SW 3rd (1995). Individual psychotherapies for depressed HIV-positive patients. *Am J Psychiatry* 152(10):1504–1509.

Maxwell S, Scheftner WA, Kessler HA, and Busch K (1988). Manic syndrome associated with zidovudine treatment. *JAMA* 259(23):3406–3407.

McIntyre RS, Brecher M, Paulsson B, Huizar K, and Mullen J (2005). Quetiapine or haloperidol as monotherapy for bipolar mania—a 12-week, double-blind, randomised, parallel-group, placebo-controlled trial. *Eur Neuropsychopharmacol* 15(5):573–585.

Meyer JM, Marsh J, and Simpson G (1998). Differential sensitivities to risperidone and olanzapine in a human immunodeficiency virus patient. *Biol Psychiatry* 44(8):791–794.

Mijch AM, Judd FK, Lyketsos CG, Ellen S, and Cockram A (1999). Secondary mania in patients with HIV infection: are antiretrovirals protective? *J Neuropsychiatry Clin Neurosci* 11(4):475–480.

Musselman DL, Lawson DH, Gumnick JF, Manatunga AK, Penna S, Goodkin RS, Greiner K, Nemeroff CB, and Miller AH (2001). Paroxetine for the prevention of depression induced by high-dose interferon alpha. *N Engl J Med* 344(13):961–966.

Nightingale SD, Koster FT, Mertz GJ, and Loss SD (1995). Clarithromycin-induced mania in two patients with AIDS. *Clin Infect Dis* 20(6):1563–1564.

O'Dowd MA, Natali C, Orr D, and McKegney FP (1991). Characteristics of patients attending an HIV-related psychiatric clinic. *Hosp Community Psychiatry* 42(6): 615–619.

Parsons JT, Rosof E, Punzalan JC, and Di Maria L (2005). Integration of motivational interviewing and cognitive behavioral therapy to improve HIV medication adherence and reduce substance use among HIV-positive men and women: results of a pilot project. *AIDS Patient Care STDS* 19(1):31–39.

Penzak SR, Hon YY, Lawhorn WD, Shirley KL, Spratlin V, and Jann MW (2002). Influence of ritonavir on olanzapine pharmacokinetics in healthy volunteers. *J Clin Psychopharmacol* 22(4):366–370.

Perretta P, Akiskal HS, Nisita C, Lorenzetti C, Zaccagnini E, Della Santa M, and Cassano GB (1998). The high prevalence of bipolar II and associated cyclothymic and hyperthymic temperaments in HIV-patients. *J Affect Disord* 50(2-3):215–224.

Pickles RW, and Spelman DW (1996). Suspected ethambutol-induced mania. *Med J Aust* 164(7):445–446.

Potkin SG, Keck PE Jr, Segal S, Ice K, and English P (2005). Ziprasidone in acute bipolar mania: a 21-day randomized, double-blind, placebo-controlled replication trial. *J Clin Psychopharmacol* 25(4): 301–310.

Rabkin JG, Johnson J, Lin SH, Lipsitz JD, Remien RH, Williams JB, and Gorman JM (1997). Psychopathology in male and female HIV-positive and negative injecting drug users: longitudinal course over 3 years. *AIDS* 11(4):507–515.

RachBeisel JA, and Weintraub E (1997). Valproic acid treatment of AIDS-related mania. *J Clin Psychiatry* 58(9):406–407.

Reichenberg A, Gorman JM, and Dieterich DT (2005). Interferon-induced depression and cognitive impairment in hepatitis C virus patients: a 72-week prospective study. *AIDS* 19:S174–S178.

Riley ED, Bangsberg DR, Guzman D, Perry S, and Moss AR (2005). Antiretroviral therapy, hepatitis C virus, and AIDS mortality among San Francisco's homeless and marginally housed. *J Acquir Immune Defic Syndr* 38(2):191–195.

Ryan EL, Morgello S, Isaacs K, Naseer M, Gerits P, for the The Manhattan HIV Brain Bank (2004). Neuropsychiatric impact of hepatitis C on advanced HIV. *Neurology* 62(6):957–962.

Sabin CA, Smith CJ, Youle M, Lampe FC, Bell DR, Puradiredja D, Lipman MC, Bhagani S, Phillips AN, and Johnson MA (2006). Deaths in the era of HAART: contribution of late presentation, treatment exposure, resistance and abnormal laboratory markers. *AIDS* 20(1):67–71.

Sachs G, Sanchez R, Marcus R, Stock E, McQuade R, Carson W, Abou-Gharbia N, Impellizzeri C, Kaplita S, Rollin L, and Iwamoto T (2006). Aripiprazole in the treatment of acute manic or mixed episodes in patients with bipolar I disorder: a 3-week placebo-controlled study. *J Psychopharmacol* 20(4):536–546.

Scalori A, Pozzi M, Bellia V, Apale P, Santamaria G, Bordoni T, Redaelli A, Avolio A, Parravicini P, Pioltelli P, and Roffi L (2005). Interferon-induced depression: prevalence and management. *Dig Liver Dis* 37(2):102–107.

Seth R, Granville-Grossman K, Goldmeier D, Lynch S (1991). Psychiatric illnesses in patients with HIV infection and AIDS referred to the liaison psychiatrist. *Br J Psychiatry* 159:347–350.

Sikkema KJ, Hansen NB, Kochman A, Tate DC, and Difranceisco W (2004). Outcomes from a randomized controlled trial of a group intervention for HIV positive men and women coping with AIDS-related loss and bereavement. *Death Stud* 28(3):187–209.

Sikkema KJ, Hansen NB, Meade CS, Kochman A, and Lee RS (2005). Improvements in health-related quality of life following a group intervention for coping with AIDS-bereavement among HIV-infected men and women. *Qual Life Res* 14(4):991–1005.

Simpson DM, McArthur JC, Olney R, Clifford D, So Y, Ross D, Baird BJ, Barrett P, Hammer AE, for the Lamotrigine HIV Neuropathy Study Team (2003). Lamotrigine for HIV-associated painful sensory neuropathies: a placebo-controlled trial. *Neurology* 60(9):1508–1514.

Singh N, Squier C, Sivek C, Wagener M, Nguyen MH, and Yu VL (1996). Determinants of compliance with antiretroviral therapy in patients with human immunodeficiency virus: prospective assessment with implications for enhancing compliance. *AIDS Care* 8(3):261–269.

Singh AN, Golledge H, and Catalan J (1997). Treatment of HIV-related psychotic disorders with risperidone: a series of 21 cases. *J Psychosom Res* 42(5):489–493.

Smulevich AB, Khanna S, Eerdekens M, Karcher K, Kramer M, and Grossman F (2005). Acute and continuation risperidone monotherapy in bipolar mania: a 3-week placebo-controlled trial followed by a 9-week double-blind trial of risperidone and haloperidol. *Eur Neuropsychopharmacol* 15(1):75–84.

Starace F, Ammassari A, Trotta MP, Murri R, De Longis P, Izzo C, Scalzini A, d'Arminio Monforte A, Wu AW, Antinori A, for the AdICoNA Study Group (2002). NeuroICoNA Study Group: depression is a risk factor for suboptimal adherence to highly active antiretroviral therapy. *J Acquir Immune Defic Syndr* 31: S136–S139.

Tate D, Paul RH, Flanigan TP, Tashima K, Nash J, Adair C, Boland R, and Cogen RA (2003). The impact of apathy and depression on quality of life in patients infected with HIV. *AIDS Patient Care and STDs* 17(3):115–120.

Thienhaus OJ, and Khosla N (1984). Meningeal cryptococcosis misdiagnosed as a manic episode. *Am J Psychiatry* 141:1459–1460.

Tohen M, Jacobs TG, Grundy SL, McElroy SL, Banov MC, Janicak PG, Sanger T, Risser R, Zhang F, Toma V, Francis J, Tollefson GD, and Breier A (2000). Efficacy of olanzapine in acute bipolar mania: a double-blind, placebo-controlled study. The Olanzipine HGGW Study Group. *Arch Gen Psychiatry* 57(9):841–849.

Tohen M, Chengappa KN, Suppes T, Baker RW, Zarate CA, Bowden CL, Sachs GS, Kupfer DJ, Ghaemi SN, Feldman PD, Risser RC, Evans AR, and Calabrese JR (2004). Relapse prevention in bipolar I disorder: 18-month comparison of olanzapine plus mood stabiliser v. mood stabiliser alone. *Br J Psychiatry* 184:337–345.

Treisman G, Fishman M, Schwartz J, Hutton H, and Lyketsos C (1998). Mood disorders in HIV infection. *Depress Anxiety* 7(4):178–187.

Tuldra A, Ferrer MJ, Fumaz CR, Bayes R, Paredes R, Burger DM, and Clotet B (1999). Monitoring adherence to HIV therapy. *Arch Intern Med* 159(12): 1376–1377.

van Servellen G, Chang B, Garcia L, and Lombardi E (2002). Individual and system level factors associated with treatment nonadherence in human immunodeficiency virus–infected men and women. *AIDS Patient Care STDS* 16(6):269–281.

Vieta E, Bourin M, Sanchez R, Marcus R, Stock E, McQuade R, Carson W, Abou-Gharbia N, Swanink R, Iwamoto T, on behalf of the Aripoprazole Study Group (2005). Effectiveness of aripiprazole v. haloperidol in acute bipolar mania: double-blind, randomised, comparative 12-week trial. *Br J Psychiatry* 187:235–242.

Wagner JH, Justice AC, Chesney M, Sinclair G, Weissman S, Rodriguez-Barradas M, for the VACS 3 Project Team (2001). Patient- and provider-reported adherence: toward a clinically useful approach to measuring antiretroviral adherence. *J Clin Epidemiol* 54:S91–S98.

Walkup JT, Sambamoorthi U, and Crystal S (2004). Use of newer antiretroviral treatments among HIV-infected Medicaid beneficiaries with serious mental illness. *J Clin Psychiatry* 65(9):1180–1189.

Winiarski MG, Greene LI, Miller AL, Palmer NB, Salcedo J, and Villanueva M (2005). Psychiatric diagnoses in a sample of HIV-infected people of color in methadone treatment. *Community Ment Health J* 41(4):379–391.

Yatham LN, Grossman F, Augustyns I, Vieta E, and Ravindran A (2003). Mood stabilisers plus risperidone or placebo in the treatment of acute mania. International, double-blind, randomised controlled trial. *Br J Psychiatry* 182:141–147.

Chapter 10

HIV-Associated Neurocognitive Disorders

Stephen J. Ferrando and Constantine G. Lyketsos

Since the beginning of the HIV epidemic, the neuro-cognitive manifestations of the infection have been widely recognized. HIV infection is associated with a range of cognitive and behavioral symptoms that become more frequent and severe as the immune system declines and symptomatic illness and AIDS ensue. In order to approach the neuropsychiatric evaluation and treatment of the HIV patient, it is critical that the clinician develop a working understanding of central nervous system (CNS) manifestations of HIV disease, including HIV-associated neurocognitive disorders.

The clinical and neuropathological manifestations of the AIDS dementia complex (ADC) were described in two classical papers by Navia and colleagues in 1986 (Navia et al., 1986a, 1986b). These authors described what came to be known as the ADC triad of *cognitive, motor,* and *behavioral* symptoms that occurred in nearly one-fourth of AIDS patients and was often progressive to severe dementia. In autopsy specimens of patients with the disorder, the authors described characteristic changes in the white matter and subcortical structures, including diffuse white matter pallor and rarefaction, and lymphocyte and macrophage infiltration (signs of inflammation). In most cases, these changes correlated well with the clinical manifestations of the disorder. See Chapter 19 for a thorough review of the neuropathology of HIV.

In response to work in this area during the first 10 years of the epidemic, the American Academy of Neurology (AAN) published in 1991 diagnostic criteria for two HIV-associated CNS disorders: HIV-associated minor cognitive motor disorder (MCMD) and HIV-associated dementia (HAD, known previously as ADC) (American Academy of Neurology AIDS Task Force, 1991). These criteria contained the classical triad of clinical symptoms and stipulated that the symptoms must cause everyday functional impairment in order to make a diagnosis. In the years prior to the advent of highly active combination antiretroviral therapy (HAART), the criteria were modified and validated in longitudinal studies (Dana Consortium on Therapy for HIV Dementia and Related Cognitive

Disorders, 1996). These disorders were found to predict shorter survival, even after statistically controlling for other HIV illness markers (Sacktor et al., 1996; Wilkie et al., 1998).

The landscape changed with the advent and widespread use of HAART in the mid-1990s. The *incidence* of HAD has declined (Sacktor et al., 2001a), but, since patients live longer, these disorders may have a stable or increasing *prevalence*. Further, milder forms of impairment persist in a substantial proportion of patients (Ferrando et al., 1998; Starace et al., 2002), with higher levels of immune functioning (Dore et al., 1999), and the course is highly variable, including fluctuation over time, progression, or even regression of the symptoms. Motor manifestations, while continuing to occur in some cases, are less frequent. Finally, comorbid and differential diagnostic considerations for the cause of these disturbances have shifted away from opportunistic infections toward entities such as substance abuse, hepatitis C coinfection, and the neuropsychiatric and metabolic side effects of antiretroviral medications. To account for these shifts, the diagnostic criteria for HIV-associated neurocognitive disorders are undergoing revision.

This chapter provides an overview of the diagnostic criteria, differential diagnosis, assessment, and treatment of the HIV-associated neurocognitive disorders. See Chapters 7 and 19 for review of neuropsychological assessment and HIV neuropathology.

CLINICAL MANIFESTATIONS AND DIAGNOSTIC CRITERIA

Neuropsychological deficits in HIV-associated neurocognitive disorders reflect underlying subcortical-frontal pathology (see Chapter 19 for a full discussion of neuropsychological deficits in HIV infection). Briefly, impairments are seen in the areas of attention, concentration, psychomotor processing speed, speed of information processing, executive function (abstraction, divided attention, shifting cognitive sets, response inhibition), and verbal memory (particularly retrieval of stored information) (Heaton et al., 1995). Disorders of language, visuospatial abilities, and praxis generally occur in later-stage dementia. Associated neuropsychiatric symptoms include apathy, depression, mania, and psychosis.

In considering the diagnosis of an HIV-associated neurocognitive disorder, it is important to remember that there is a range in the number and severity of neuropsychological deficits and that some patients may have abnormal neuropsychological test scores but no functional impairment. This "asymptomatic neuropsychological impairment" cannot be applied to make a diagnosis of a neurocognitive disorder. Further, it is important to remember that in the context of HIV infection, there is a broad differential diagnosis for neuropsychological test abnormalities, and other etiologies must be ruled out to make a diagnosis of an HIV-associated neurocognitive disorder (see below).

Table 10.1 contains the 1991 AAN diagnostic criteria for HIV-associated minor cognitive motor disorder (MCMD) and HIV-associated dementia (HAD). Note that diagnostic criteria for both disorders are based primarily on severity of neuropsychological test impairment and on degree of functional impairment, with the disorders differing according to levels of severity in these domains. In addition, neuropsychiatric and motor symptoms are emphasized in making the diagnosis of HAD.

As mentioned previously, the diagnostic criteria for HIV-associated neurocognitive disorders are being modified (Forstein et al., 2006), for several reasons. First is the recognition that asymptomatic cognitive impairment, even when not associated with functional impairment, is a risk factor for subsequent functional decline. Second is the recognition of the primacy of cognitive symptoms relative to the motor and neuropsychiatric symptoms. Third is the need to precisely specify the neurocognitive domains to be tested and the degree of impairment needed to qualify for a diagnosis of neurocognitive disorder. Finally, the course of the neurocognitive disorder varies, thus allowing for course specifiers. Figure 10.1 depicts suggested modified diagnostic criteria for the HIV-associated neurocognitive disorders. Publication of these modified criteria is forthcoming.

EPIDEMIOLOGY

The incidence of MCMD and HAD in the HAART era has not been precisely estimated. Prior to 1991, the incidence of HAD within 2 years of AIDS diagnosis was 7% per year (McArthur, 1994). Since the advent of HAART, the overall incidence of HIV-associated dementia has declined. A study of the incidence of CNS complications of HIV in the Multicenter AIDS Cohort (MACS) from 1990 through 1997 documented

TABLE 10.1. American Academy of Neurology Criteria for HIV-Associated Neurocognitive Disorders

HIV-1-Associated Dementia (HAD)*

Criteria for 1 and 2 must be met:
1. Scores 1 standard deviation (SD) below age- and education-adjusted norms on two of eight neuropsychological tests or 2 SD below the norms on one of eight tests
2. Requires assistance or has difficulty (due to either physical or cognitive deficit) in at least one of the following instrumental activities of daily living:
   Using the telephone
   Handling money
   Taking medication
   Performing light housekeeping
   Doing laundry
   Preparing meals
   Shopping for groceries
   Getting to places out of walking distance
and must meet either 1 or 2 of the following:

1. Any impairment in the following: lower extremity strength, coordination, finger tapping, alternating hand movements, leg agility, or performance on grooved pegboard 2 SDs below mean (dominant hand)
2. Self-reported frequent depression that interferes with function, loss of interest in usual activities or emotional lability, or irritability

Staging of HAD: mild, moderate or severe, based on degree of functional deficit

HIV-Associated Minor Cognitive/Motor Disorder (MCMD)*

Does not meet criteria for HAD and meets 1 and 2 of the following:

1. Deficit in at least two of the following:
   Mental slowing: digit symbol at least 1 SD below age- and education-adjusted norms
   Memory: Rey Auditory Verbal Learning Test (total) at least 1 SD below norms
   Motor dysfunction: any impairment in finger tapping, or pronation or supination
   Incoordination: mild impairment in gait or clumsiness
   Emotional lability, or apathy or withdrawal
and
2. Deficit in at least one of the role function measures attributed in part to cognitive function:
   Need for frequent rests
   Cut down on amount of time in activities
   Accomplish less than desired
   Cannot perform activities as carefully as one would like
   Limited in work or activities
   Difficulty performing activities
   Require special assistance to perform activities

*Symptoms should not be exclusively caused by other etiologies, i.e., CNS opportunistic infections, systemic disease, substance abuse.

Source: Adapted from American Academy of Neurology AIDS Task Force, 1991.

a decline in probable or possible HAD from 30 cases per 1000 person-years to 17 per 1000 person-years (Sacktor et al., 2001a). CNS opportunistic infections including toxoplasmosis, cryptococcal meningitis, and lymphoma declined similarly during this time period. Researchers from Australia found a similar decline in CNS AIDS-defining illnesses (ADIs) between 1992 and 1997 (Dore et al., 1999). However, over this time period, they found that HAD comprised a greater proportion of new-onset ADIs, rising from 4.4% in 1992 to 6.5% in 1997. Further, the average CD4 count of patients with HAD increased from 70 cells/µl to 170 cells/µl during this time period. This relative rise in the proportion of ADIs that are HAD may be due to variable CNS penetration of antiretroviral medications. Thus, while HIV patients taking HAART may have enhanced immune function and survive longer without HIV-associated cognitive decline, the prevalence of all-cause dementia in HIV-infected patients likely has remained stable or increased.

DIFFERENTIAL DIAGNOSIS

Differential diagnosis is paramount in evaluating neurocognitive symptoms in HIV/AIDS medical inpatients, especially when investigating for medical and neuropsychiatric etiological factors related to HIV illness and its treatment. Table 10.2 lists the major differential diagnostic considerations.

Multiple studies have indicated that 60%–70% of patients with HIV infection have one or more psychiatric disorders prior to contracting HIV illness (Perry et al., 1990; Williams et al., 1991; Lyketsos et al., 1995). Patients with Axis I disorders, including depression, bipolar disorder, schizophrenia, and substance abuse, may present with cognitive complaints or impairment. Substance intoxication and/or withdrawal are also common causes of cognitive impairment, particularly delirium. CNS opportunistic illnesses (OIs) and cancers can also present with a wide range of cognitive and neuropsychiatric symptoms, most often in the context of delirium, as a result of both focal and generalized neuropathological processes. Table 10.3 lists the major CNS OIs, their major symptom presentation, and diagnostic workup.

Hepatitis C infection, independent of HIV coinfection and interferon/ribavirin therapy, is characterized by multiple neuropsychiatric complaints, most frequently fatigue (up to 97% of patients), depression

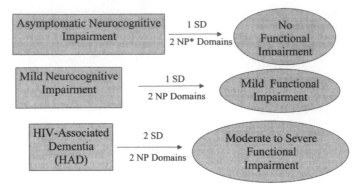

FIGURE 10.1. Schematic depiction of proposed modified criteria for HIV-associated neurocognitive disorders. NP, neuropsychological; SD, standard deviation. Forstein M et al., 2006.

(up to 25% of patients meet criteria for a current depressive disorder and up to 70% have elevated scores on depression rating scales), and cognitive dysfunction (up to 82% impairment on some measures) (Crone and Gabriel, 2003). Compared to patients with HIV alone, patients with comorbid HIV and hepatitis C are more likely to have disturbances in executive function and dementia (Ryan et al., 2004). The pattern of cognitive impairment associated with hepatitis C is similar to that of HIV. Patients with mild liver disease tend to have impairment in attention and concentration, and patients with more severe liver fibrosis have problems with learning, psychomotor speed, and cognitive flexibility. Patients with end-stage liver disease and cirrhosis experience superimposed delirium ("hepatic encephalopathy"). Combination pegylated interferon alpha 2a and ribavirin treatment for hepatitis C is well known to be a cause of dysphoria, suicidal ideation, anxiety, sleep disturbance, fatigue, mania, psychosis, confusion, and cognitive dysfunction (Crone and Gabriel, 2003).

Several antiretroviral and other medications used in the context of HIV have been associated with neuropsychiatric side effects. These include zidovudine (Maxwell et al., 1998), didanosine (Brouillett et al., 1994), abacavir (Foster et al., 2004), nevirapine (Morlese et al. 2002), efavirenz (Bartlett and Ferrando, 2004), interferon alpha 2a (Crone and Gabriel, 2003), and clarithromycin (Colebunders and Florence, 2002). Most of these effects are infrequent and causal relationships linking them to the medications have been difficult to discern (Johnson et al., 2003). The most widespread clinical concern has been generated by reports of sudden-onset depression and suicidal ideation after treatment with interferon alpha 2a (discussed above) and/or efavirenz. Early reports suggested that efavirenz may be associated with at least transient neuropsychiatric side effects in excess of 50% of patients (Staszewski et al., 1999). Reported effects are protean and include depression, suicidal ideation, vivid nightmares, anxiety, insomnia, psychosis, cognitive dysfunction, and antisocial behavior (Bartlett and Ferrando, 2004). Some, but not all, reports suggest that patients with a prior history of substance use or other psychiatric disorders are at greater risk for the neuropsychiatric side effects of efavirenz (Bartlett and Ferrando,

TABLE 10.2. Differential Diagnosis of HIV-Associated Neurocognitive Disorders

- Delirium (from multiple possible etiologies, often superimposed on underlying neurocognitive disorder)
- Primary or comorbid psychiatric disorder (e.g., depression)
- Primary or comorbid neurodegenerative disorder (e.g., Alzheimer disease, vascular dementia)
- CNS opportunistic illnesses and cancers (e.g., cytomegalovirus or herpes simplex encephalitis, progressive multifocal leukoencephalopathy)
- Substance intoxication and/or withdrawal
- Neuropsychiatric complications of hepatitis C and its treatments
- Neuropsychiatric side effects of HIV medications
- Metabolic complications of HIV medications (e.g., diabetes, cerebrovascular and cardiovascular disease)
- Drug interactions
- Endocrinological abnormalities (e.g., hypogonadism, adrenal insufficiency)

TABLE 10.3. Opportunistic Illnesses of the Central Nervous System in AIDS

Opportunistic Illness	CD4	Signs	Focal	CT/MRI	Lumbar Puncture
Toxoplasmosis	<100	Fever Delirium Headache Seizures	Y	Ring-enhancing lesions Basal ganglia Gray–white junction	*T. gondii* antibody or PCR High specificity or low sensitivity
Cytomegalovirus	<50	Delirium Infections found at diagnosis: Retina Blood Adrenal gland GI tract	N (Y)	Ventricular enlargement Increased periventricular signal (T2 image)	CMV PCR Variable specificity or sensitivity Elevated protein level, pleocytosis, hypoglycorrhachia
Cryptococcal meningitis	<100	Fever Delirium Not universally seen Increase in ICP (50%) Seizures	N [Y] [10%]	Nonspecific	*C. neoformans,* India ink, latex agglutination or PCR High specificity or sensitivity
Progressive multifocal leukoencephalopathy	<100	Mono or Hemiparesis Dysarthria Gait disturbance Sensory deficit Progressive dementia Occasional Visual loss Seizures	Y	Attenuated signal/non-enhancing (T2 images) Periventricular white matter Other areas: Gray matter Brain stem Cerebellum Spinal cord	JCV PCR High specificity or sensitivity Other routine CSF studies not generally diagnostic
Central nervous system neoplasms/lymphoma	<100	Afebrile Delirium Seizures 10% Increased ICP	Y	Lesions: Hypodense or patchy Nodular enhancing SPECT thallium: Differentiates from toxoplasmosis	EBV PCR High specificity or sensitivity Other routine CSF evaluation not useful

CMV, cytomegalovirus; CSF, cerebrospinal fluid; EBV, Epstein-Barr virus; ICP, intracranial pressure; JCV, Jakob Creutzfelt virus; PCR, polymerase chain reaction; SPECT, single photon emission computed tomography.

2004). In contrast to early and uncontrolled reports, the only prospective study (Bartlett and Ferrando, 2004) found that vivid dreams and vestibular dysfunction symptoms were significantly more frequent among patients treated with an efavirenz-based regimen than those treated with a triple nucleoside regimen. These symptoms were primarily seen in week 1 and resolved thereafter (Clifford et al., 2005). Efavirenz treatment was in fact associated with overall improvement in neuropsychological performance.

Drug interactions between antiretroviral and psychotropic medications, covered extensively in Chapter 32, are an important aspect of differential diagnosis and treatment in evaluating and treating cognitive dysfunction. Clinically significant drug interactions are more often seen in acute care settings because of medical illness severity, prior substance abuse, the likelihood of multiple medications being initiated simultaneously, changes in volume of distribution or protein binding, and hepatic or renal impairment.

Patients with HIV or AIDS often experience endocrinological derangements that may produce cognitive and behavioral symptoms. These include clinical and subclinical hypothyroidism (Beltran et al., 2003), hypogonadism (Mylonakis et al., 2001), adrenal insufficiency (Mayo et al., 2002), and Grave's disease (autoimmune thyroiditis) (Chen et al., 2005). Multiple etiological mechanisms have been hypothesized, including viral and other opportunistic infections, neoplastic infiltration of endocrine glands, antiretroviral therapy, and autoimmune phenomena, including immune reconstitution inflammatory syndrome (IRIS) (Beltran et al., 2003; Chen et al., 2005). Thyroid deficiency, including subclinical forms, is present in approximately 16% of HIV-infected patients (Chen et al., 2005). Testosterone deficiency, with clinical symptoms of hypogonadism, is present in up to 50% of men with symptomatic HIV or AIDS and is likely to be present with concurrent acute illness (Rabkin et al., 1999; Mylonakis et al., 2001). Deficiency of adrenal glucocorticoid production is present in up to 50% of severely ill HIV patients (Marik et al., 2002; Mayo et al., 2002). Similarly, deficiency in adrenal androgens, particularly dehydroepiandrosterone (DHEA), is also common in both HIV-infected men and women and is associated with advanced HIV disease and loss of lean body mass (Rabkin et al., 2000). These endocrine deficiencies have been associated with fatigue, low mood, low libido, and loss of lean body mass, symptoms that may be ameliorated by correction of the deficiency state. Graves disease in the acute stages presents with activation symptoms including anxiety, irritability, insomnia, weight loss, mania, and agitation. Endocrine disorders are covered in detail in Chapter 35 of this text.

COGNITIVE AND FUNCTIONAL ASSESSMENT

The assessment for neurocognitive disorders presents challenges in the HIV clinical setting. The neuropsychological literature suggests that patient self-reports of cognitive problems ("metacognitive" complaints) are more likely to be secondary to depression or other forms of distress than to cognitive impairment assessed by neuropsychological tests (Hinkin et al., 1996). Thus, when patients present with cognitive complaints, it is first important to assess for depression, anxiety, and other Axis I psychiatric disorders.

Formal neuropsychological assessment, administered by a licensed clinical neuropsychologist, is the gold standard for assessing for HIV-associated neurocognitive disorders (see Chapter 7 for a full review of this topic). Several batteries sensitive to HIV-associated deficits have been proposed (Butters et al., 1990). Unfortunately, such testing is time intensive, expensive, and not readily available in HIV clinics. Regardless of the availability of neuropsychological testing, a thorough psychiatric and cognitive assessment, such as that suggested in Chapter 6, is an important aide in making a diagnosis of neurocognitive disorder. In this context, commonly used bedside cognitive assessments, such as the Mini Mental Status Exam (Folstein et al., 1975), are typically insensitive to HIV-associated deficits, since they were designed to assess the global deficits found in cortical dementias. The HIV Dementia Scale (HDS) was developed as a rapid screening test to assess for HIV-associated dementia (Power et al., 1995). The HDS assesses psychomotor processing speed, verbal memory, constructional ability, and executive function (response inhibition, set shifting) (Fig. 10.2). While it is a useful dementia screen, its utility for assessing mild HIV-associated cognitive deficits in the clinical setting is limited (Smith et al., 2003). This test also exists in a modified form (eliminating the antisaccadic subtest, which is often difficult to administer), which has been validated for use in both determining the presence

MAXIMUM SCORE	PATIENT SCORE	TEST
		MEMORY - REGISTRATION Give 4 words to recall (dog, hat, green, peach) and 1 second to say each. Then ask the patient to repeat all 4 after you have said them.
4		ATTENTION Antisaccadic eye movements (20 commands): ____ errors out of 20 ≤ 3 errors = 4; 4 errors = 3; 5 errors = 2; 6 errors = 1; > 6 errors = 0
6		PSYCHOMOTOR SPEED Ask patient to write the alphabet in uppercase letters horizontally across the page (use back of form) and record time: ____ seconds ≤ 21 sec = 6; 21.1-24 sec = 5; 24.1-27 sec = 4; 27.1-30 sec = 3; 30.1-33 sec = 2; 33.1-36 sec = 1; >36 sec = 0
4		MEMORY - RECALL Ask for the 4 words from MEMORY – REGISTRATION TEST above. Give 1 point for each correct. For words not recalled, prompt with a semantic clue as follows: animal (dog); piece of clothing (hat); color (green); fruit (peach). Give 1/2 point for each correct word after prompting.
2		CONSTRUCTION Copy the cube below. Record time ____ seconds < 25 sec = 2; 25-35 sec = 1; >35 sec = 0 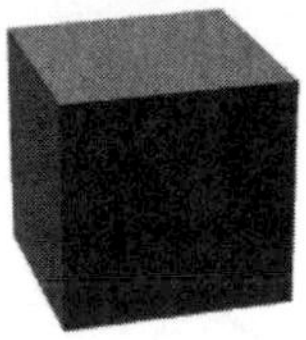

FIGURE 10.2. HIV Dementia Scale. Adapted from Power et al., HIV Dementia Scale: a rapid screening test. *Journal of Acquired Immune Deficiency Syndrome and Human Retrovirology* 1995; 8:273–278. Used with permission.

and severity of HAD, and may be more usable clinically (Davis et al., 2002).

The presence of everyday functional impairment is necessary to diagnose HIV-associated neurocognitive disorders. In patients with HIV, cognitive dysfunction has been associated with impairments in both basic and instrumental activities of daily living (Schiffitto et al., 2001), poor adherence to HAART (Hinkin et al., 2002), and reduced ability to work (Rabkin et al., 2004a). There is no uniformly accepted or validated measure of functional impairment in HIV infection. Assessment should focus on instrumental activities of daily living (IADL), functions that allow individuals to live independently. These include shopping, cooking, cleaning and laundry, using the telephone, managing money, and adherence to medication (Lawton and Brody, 1969; Albert et al., 2003). As with cognitive complaints, self-reported functional impairment correlates poorly with neuropsychological test performance. Therefore, observations of family members, caregivers, and clinical assessment over time are key components of documenting functional decline.

LABORATORY TESTING

The laboratory evaluation of patients with HIV or AIDS who have neurocognitive impairment is consistent with the broad differential diagnosis and is focused on identifying potentially reversible underlying etiologies. A thorough psychiatric evaluation, including presenting symptoms and personal and family history of psychiatric illness and substance abuse, and a cognitive functioning examination are essential. While a complete medical evaluation is implicit, the psychiatric consultant may suggest additional diagnostic testing based on the clinical situation. Table 10.4 contains a listing of possible diagnostic tests.

In general, the diagnostic workup should include complete blood count with differential, CD4 lymphocyte count, HIV-1 viral load, serum chemistries (including liver and renal function tests, fasting glucose and creatine phosphokinase), chest X-ray, electrocardiogram, blood and urine cultures (if indicated), toxicology screen, and psychotropic medication serum levels (when available). Based on the clinical presentation,

TABLE 10.4. Clinical and Laboratory Evaluation of Patients with HIV and Neurocognitive Symptoms

- Medical evaluation with screening laboratories: complete blood count, chemistry screen (including liver and renal function tests), urinalysis, chest X-ray, electrocardiogram, blood and urine cultures (when applicable)
- CD4 lymphocyte count, HIV-1 plasma viral load
- Psychiatric diagnostic interview including personal and family history
- Cognitive screen (HIV Dementia Scale)
- Additional laboratories when applicable: illicit drug toxicology screen, serum psychotropic drug levels, thyroid function tests, antithyroid antibodies, vitamin B12 and B6 levels, total or bioavailable testosterone, dehydroepiandrosterone sulfate, adrenocorticotropic stimulation test, 24-hour urine cortisol
- Evaluation for hepatitis C (including viral load)
- Review of antiretroviral regimen for neuropsychiatric side effects
- Review of psychotropic mediations for efficacy, neuropsychiatric side effects, drug interactions
- Neuroimaging (MRI, MR spectroscopy, diffusion tensor imaging)
- Lumbar puncture (including CSF HIV-1 viral load if available)
- Review of antiretroviral medication for CNS penetrance

assays of thyroid function, vitamins B6 and B12, *Treponema pallidum* IgG and IgM, serum total and/or bioavailable testosterone, adrenocorticotropic hormone (ACTH) stimulation, and 24-hour urinary cortisol may be obtained.

A lumbar puncture may also be obtained, if necessary, under sedation with fluoroscopic guidance. Results are often nonspecific, but important tests include opening pressure, culture (viral, fungal, mycobacterial), cell count, protein, neopterin, beta-2 microglobulin, and, if available, polymerase chain reaction (PCR) testing for cytomegalovirus, Epstein Barr virus, Jakob Creutzfelt virus, herpes simplex virus, and HIV-1. While measurement of cerebral spinal fluid (CSF) HIV-1 viral load is probably the best way to monitor virologic susceptibility to and effectiveness of HAART for neurocognitive symptoms (Ellis et al., 1997; McArthur et al., 1997; Price et al., 1997; DiStefano et al., 1998), some studies suggest that plasma viral load measurements correlate with neurocognitive symptoms (Staprans et al., 1999; Sacktor et al., 2003).

In terms of static neuroimaging approaches, contrast magnetic resonance imaging (MRI) of the brain with gadolinium is preferred over computed tomography as it provides better visualization of subcortical and posterior fossa structures and focal lesions; however, MRI is less feasible in agitated patients. Functional brain imaging, including magnetic resonance spectroscopy (Sacktor et al., 2005) and diffusion tensor imaging (Filippi et al., 2001), may be helpful in detecting submacroscopic functional changes associated with HIV-associated neurocognitive disorders.

TREATMENT

The availability of HAART renewed hope that there would be effective prevention and treatment for HIV-associated neurocognitive disturbances. However, a problem with HAART is that different antiretrovirals are not equivalent in their ability to penetrate the blood–brain barrier (BBB) (Enting et al., 1998). This fact produced concern early in the advent of HAART that otherwise healthy individuals might develop progressive cognitive decline and dementia and, further, that viral resistance to these poorly penetrating drugs might develop in the CNS and "seed" the peripheral circulation, rendering treatment ineffective. Further, sufficient BBB penetration may be necessary to achieve adequate HIV-1 inhibitory concentrations in the CNS for durable antiretroviral efficacy against neurocognitive disorders.

The nucleoside/nucleotide reverse-transcriptase inhibitors (NRTIs) zidovudine, stavudine, lamivudine, and abacavir, and the non-nucleoside reverse transcriptase inhibitor (NNRTI) nevirapine penetrate the BBB effectively (Enting et al., 1998; Ravitch and Moseley, 2001). While efavirenz is highly protein bound and only a minimal percentage of plasma concentration reaches the CSF, it has been found to achieve sufficient concentration to inhibit HIV replication

(Tashima et al., 1999). Zidovudine monotherapy at standard and higher doses has been shown to improve neuropsychological performance and dementia (Schmitt et al., 1988; Martin et al., 1999) and was associated with the decline in the incidence of dementia from the late 1980s to the early 1990s. However, these benefits of zidovudine monotherapy are temporary, due to the emergence of viral resistance (Gulevitch et al., 1993). Didanosine monotherapy has also been shown effective in improving psychomotor function. Furthermore, the addition of stavudine to zidovudine after a period of zidovudine monotherapy effectively improves motor performance (Arendt et al., 2001).

The protein inhibitors (PIs), with the exception of indinavir (Brinkman et al., 1998), have poor BBB penetration, generating concern that PI-based HAART might not benefit CNS disease. However, HAART regimens containing various PIs have been associated with reductions in CSF viral load to undetectable levels (Gisslen et al., 1997), with reversal of white matter lesions on MRI (Filippi et al., 1998) and reversal of brain metabolic abnormalities on magnetic resonance spectroscopy (Chang et al., 1999).

As previously discussed, the HAART era has seen a dramatic decline in the incidence of HAD. Numerous cross-sectional and longitudinal studies have documented the benefits of heterogeneous HAART regimens for the full range of HIV-associated neurocognitive symptoms (Ferrando et al., 1998, 2003; Tozzi et al., 1999; Sacktor et al., 1999), with the most consistent improvements seen in psychomotor processing speed. Some authors report that regimens containing multiple CNS penetrating drugs are no better in improving psychomotor processing speed than regimens containing only one CNS-penetrating drug (Sacktor et al., 2001b). Others have found that HAART regimens containing three or more CSF-penetrating antiretroviral drugs correlate with the ability to suppress HIV RNA in CSF (DeLuca et al., 2002; Letendre et al., 2004). Marra and colleagues (2003) reported that HAART regimens containing zidovudine and indinavir were superior to other regimens in improving neurocognitive performance.

In addition to using antiretroviral therapy for HIV-associated neurocognitive disorders, other neuroprotective and adjunctive agents are in various stages of investigation for their potential to block aspects of the neurotoxic immune cascade or, more modestly, to augment important neurotransmitters, such as dopamine. Neuroprotective agents studied to date include pentoxifylline, a tumor necrosis factor-alpha inhibitor (Melton et al., 1997); nimodipine, a calcium channel blocker (Navia et al., 1998); memantine, an N-methyl-D-aspartate receptor antagonist (Anderson et al., 2004); selegiline, a monoamine oxidase type B inhibitor, antioxidant, and antiapoptotic (Dana Consortium on the Therapy of HIV Dementia and Related Cognitive Disorders, 1998); and platelet-activating factor antagonists (Persitsky et al., 2001). The psychostimulants, particularly methylphenidate and dextroamphetamine, which augment dopamine neurotransmission, have shown some promise in improving cognitive and psychomotor impairment in advanced HIV illness (Holmes et al., 1989).

Modafinil, a wakefulness agent, was shown to increase cognitive performance in HIV-infected patients whose primary complaint was fatigue (Rabkin et al., 2004b). Finally, in a recent open-label study of lithium 600–1200 mg/day on a background of HAART, cognitively impaired patients experienced significant cognitive improvement (Letendre et al., 2006). While some of these neuroprotective and neuromodulatory agents have shown promise in preliminary study, none has shown the magnitude of benefit of HAART.

CONCLUSION

In the past several years, much has been learned about the neuropathogenesis, clinical presentation, and treatment of HIV-associated neurocognitive disorders. Despite these advancements, patients with HIV continue to suffer from functionally significant neurocognitive disorders. Thus, effective and well-tolerated antiretroviral, neuroprotective, and adjunctive treatments need to be developed.

References

Albert SM, Flater SR, Claus R, et al. (2003). Medication management skill in HIV: I. Evidence for adaptation of medication management strategies in people with cognitive impairment. II. Evidence for a pervasive lay model of medication efficacy. *AIDS Behav* 7:329–338.
American Academy of Neurology AIDS Task Force (1991). Nomenclature and research case definitions for neurologic manifestations of human immunodeficiency virus-type 1 (HIV-1) infection. Report of a Working Group of the American Academy of Neurology AIDS Task Force. *Neurology* 41:778–785.
Anderson ER, Gendelman HE, and Xiong H (2004). Memantine protects hippocampal neuronal function

in murine human immunodeficiency virus type 1 encephalitis. *J Neurosci* 24:7194–7198.

Arendt G, von Giesen HJ, Hefter H, and Theisen A (2001). Therapeutic effects of nucleoside analogues on psychomotor slowing in HIV infection. 15:493–500.

Bartlett JA, and Ferrando S (2004). Identification and management of neurologic and psychiatric side effects associated with HIV and HAART. *Medscape* Retrieved April 25, 2007, from http://www.medscape.com/viewarticle/470017.

Beltran S, Lescure F-X, Desailloud R, Douadi Y, Smail A, El Esper I, Arlot S, Schmit J-L, for the Thyroid and VIH (THYVI) Group (2003). Increased prevalence of hypothyroidism among human immunodeficiency virus–infected patients: a need for screening. *Clin Infect Dis* 37:579–583.

Brinkman K, Kroon F, Hugen PW, and Burger DM (1998). Therapeutic concentrations of indinavir in cerebrospinal fluid of HIV-1-infected patients. *AIDS* 12:537.

Brouillette MJ, Chouinard G, and Laloonde R (1994). Didanosine-induced mania in HIV infection. *Am J Psychiatry* 151:1839–1840.

Butters N, Grant I, Haxby J, et al. (1990). Assessment of AIDS-related cognitive changes: recommendations of the NIMH Workshop on Neuropsychological Assessment Approaches. *J Clin Exp Neuropsychol* 12:963–978.

Chang L, Ernst T, Leonido-Yee M, et al. (1999). Highly active antiretroviral therapy reverses brain metabolite abnormalities in mild HIV dementia. *Neurology* 53:782–789.

Chen F, Day SL, Metcalfe RA, Sethi G, Kapembwa MS, Brook MG, Churchill D, De Ruiter A, Robinson S, Lacey CJ, and Weetman AP (2005). Characteristics of autoimmune thyroid disease occurring as a late complication of immune reconstitution in patients with advanced human immunodeficiency virus (HIV) disease. *Medicine (Baltimore)* 84(2): 98–106.

Clifford DB, Evans S, Yang Y, et al. (2005). Impact of efavirenz on neuropsychological performance and symptoms in HIV-infected individuals. *Ann Intern Med* 143:714–721.

Colebunders R, and Florence E (2002). Neuropsychiatric reaction induced by clarithromycin. *Sex Transm Infect* 78:75–76.

Crone C, and Gabriel GM (2003). Comprehensive review of hepatitis C for psychiatrists: risks, screening, diagnosis, treatment and interferon-based therapy complications. *J Psychiatr Pract* 9:93–110.

Dana Consortium on Therapy for HIV Dementia and Related Cognitive Disorders (1996). Clinical confirmation of the American Academy of Neurology algorithm for HIV-1-associated cognitive/motor disorder. *Neurology* 47:1247–1253.

Dana Consortium on the Therapy of HIV Dementia and Related Cognitive Disorders (1998). A randomized, double-blind, placebo-controlled trial of deprenyl and thioctic acid in human immunodeficiency virus-associated cognitive impairment. *Neurology* 50:645–651.

Davis HF, Skolasky RL Jr, Selnes OA, et al. (2002). Assessing HIV-associated dementia: modified HIV Dementia Scale versus the grooved pegboard. *AIDS Read* 12:29–31, 38.

De Luca A, Ciancio BC, Larussa D, et al. (2002). Correlates of independent HIV-1 replication in the CNS and of its control by antiretrovirals. *Neurology* 59: 342–347.

Di Stefano M, Monno L, Fiore JR, et al. (1998). Neurological disorders during HIV-1 infection correlate with viral load in cerebrospinal fluid but not with virus phenotype. *AIDS* 12:737–743.

Dore G, Correll PK, Li Y, et al. (1999). Changes to AIDS dementia complex in the era of highly active antiretroviral therapy. *AIDS* 13:1249–1253.

Ellis RJ, Hsia K, Spector SA, et al. (1997). Cerebrospinal fluid human immunodeficiency virus type 1 RNA levels are elevated in neurocognitively impaired individuals with acquired immunodeficiency syndrome. HIV Neurobehavioral Research Center Group. *Ann Neurol* 42:679–688.

Enting RH, Hoetelmans RM, Lange JM, Burger DM, Beijnen JH, and Portegies P (1998). Antiretroviral drugs and the central nervous system. *AIDS* 12: 1941–1955.

Ferrando S, van Gorp W, McElhiney M, Goggin K, Sewell M, and Rabkin J (1998). Highly active antiretroviral treatment in HIV infection: benefits for neuropsychological function. *AIDS* 12:F65–F70.

Ferrando SJ, Rabkin JG, van Gorp W, Lin SH, and McElhiney M (2003). Longitudinal improvement in psychomotor processing speed is associated with potent combination antiretroviral therapy in HIV-1 infection. *J Neuropsychiatry Clin Neurosci* 15:208–214.

Filippi CG, Sze G, Farber SJ, Shahmanesh M, and Selwyn PA (1998). Regression of HIV encephalopathy and basal ganglia signal intensity abnormality at MR imaging in patients with AIDS after the initiation of protease inhibitor therapy. *Radiology* 206: 491–498.

Filippi CG, Ulug AM, Ryan E, Ferrando SJ, and van Gorp W (2001). Diffusion tensor imaging in HIV patients with normal-appearing white matter on brain MR scans. *AJNR Am J Neuroradiol* 22:277–283.

Folstein MF, Folstein SE, and McHugh PR (1975). "Mini-Mental State." A practical method for grading the cognitive state of patients for the clinician. *J Psychiatr Res* 12:189–198.

Forstein M, Cournos F, Douaihy A, Goodkin K, Wainberg ML, and Wapenyi KH (2006). *Guideline Watch: Practice Guideline fort the Treatment of Patients with HIV/AIDS*. Arlington, VA: American Psychiatric Association.

Foster R, Taylor C, and Everall IP (2004). More on abacavir-induced neuropsychiatric reactions. *AIDS* 18:2449.

Gisslen M, Hagberg L, Svennerholm B, and Norkrans G (1997). HIV-1 RNA is not detectable in the cerebrospinal fluid during antiretroviral combination therapy. *AIDS* 11:1194.

Gulevich SJ, McCutchan JA, Thal LJ, et al. (1993). Effect of antiretroviral therapy on the cerebrospinal fluid of patients seropositive for the human immunodeficiency virus. *J Acquir Immune Defic Syndr* 6:1002–1007.

Heaton RK, Grant I, Butters N, et al. (1995). The HNRC 500—neuropsychology of HIV infection at different disease stages. HIV Neurobehavioral Research Center. *J Int Neuropsychol Soc* 1:231–251.

Hinkin CH, van Gorp W, Satz P, et al. (1996). Actual versus self-reported cognitive dysfunction in HIV-1 infection: memory—metamemory dissociations. *JClin Exp Neuropsychol* 18:431–443.

Hinkin CH, Castellon SA, Durvasula RS, et al. (2002). Medication adherence among HIV+ adults: effects of cognitive dysfunction and regimen complexity. *Neurology* 59:1944–1950.

Holmes VF, Fernandez F, and Levy JK (1989). Psychostimulant response in AIDS-related complex patients. *J Clin Psychiatry* 50:5–8.

Johnson MO, Stallworth T, and Neilands TB (2003). The drugs or the disease? Causal attributions of symptoms held by HIV-positive adults on HAART. *AIDS Behav* 7:109–117.

Lawton MP, and Brody EM (1969). Assessment of older people: self-maintaining and instrumental activities of daily living. *Gerontologist* 9(3):179–186.

Letendre SL, McCutchan JA, Childers ME, et al. (2004). Enhancing antiretroviral therapy for human immunodeficiency virus cognitive disorders. *Ann Neurol* 2004 56(3):416–423.

Letendre SL, Woods SP, Ellis RJ, et al. (2006). Lithium improves HIV-associated neurocognitive impairment. *AIDS* 20(14):1885–1888.

Lyketsos CG, and Federman EB (1995). Psychatric disorders and HIV infection: impact on one another. *Epidemol Rev* 17:152–164.

Marik PE, Kiminyo K, and Zaloga GP (2002). Adrenal insufficiency in critically ill patients with human immunodeficiency virus. *Crit Care Med* 30(6):1267–1273.

Marra CM, Lockhart D, Zunt JR, Perrin M, Coombs RW, and Collier AC (2003). Changes in CSF and plasma HIV-1 RNA and cognition after starting potent antiretroviral therapy. *Neurology* 60:1388–1390.

Martin EM, Pitrak DL, Novak RM, Pursell KJ, and Mullane KM (1999). Reaction times are faster in HIV-seropositive patients on antiretroviral therapy: a preliminary report. *J Clin Exp Neuropsychol* 21:730–735.

Maxwell S, Scheftner WA, Kessler HA, and Busch K (1988). Manic syndrome associated with zidovudine treatment. *JAMA* 259:3406–3407.

Mayo J, Callazos J, Martinez E, and Ibarra S (2002). Adrenal function in the human immunodeficiency virus–infected patient. *Arch Intern Med* 162:1095–1098.

McArthur J (1994). Neurological and neuropathological manifestations of HIV infection. In I Grant and J Martin (eds.), *The Neuropsychology of HIV Infection* (pp. 56–107). New York: Oxford University Press.

McArthur JC, McClernon DR, Cronin MF, et al. (1997). Relationship between human immunodeficiency virus–associated dementia and viral load in cerebrospinal fluid and brain. *Ann Neurol* 42:689–698.

Melton ST, Kirkwood CK, and Ghaemi SN (1997). Pharmacotherapy of HIV dementia. *Ann Pharmacother* 31:457–473.

Morlese JF, Qazi NA, Gazzard BG, and Nelson MR (2002). Nevirapine-induced neuropsychiatric complications, a class effect of non-nucleoside reverse transcriptase inhibitors? *AIDS* 16:1840–1841.

Mylonakis E, Koutkia P, and Grinspoon S (2001). Diagnosis and treatment of androgen deficiency in human immunodeficiency virus–infected men and women. *Clin Infect Dis* 33:857–864.

Navia BA, Jordan BD, and Price RW (1986a). The AIDS dementia complex: I. Clinical features. *Ann Neurol* 19:517–524.

Navia BA, Cho ES, Petito CK, and Price RW (1986b). The AIDS dementia complex: II. Neuropathology. *Ann Neurol* 19:525–535.

Navia BA, Davni U, Simpson D, et al. (1998). A phase I/II trial of nimodipine for HIV-related neurologic complications. *Neurology* 51:221–228.

Perry S, Jacobsberg LB, Fishman B, Frances A, Bobo J, and Jacobsberg BK (1990). Psychiatric diagnosis before serological testing for the human immunodeficiency virus. *Am J Psychiatry* 147:89–93.

Persitsky Y, Limoges J, Rasmussen J, et al. (2001). Reduction in glial immunity and neuropathology by a PAF antagonist and an MMP and TNF-alpha inhibitor in SCID mice with HIV-1 encephalitis. *J Neuroimmunol* 114:57–68.

Power C, Selnes OA, Grim JA, and McArthur JC (1995). HIV Dementia Scale: a rapid screening test. *J Acquir Immune Defic Syndr Hum Retrovirol* 8:273–278.

Price RW, and Staprans S (1997). Measuring the "viral load" in cerebrospinal fluid in human immunodeficiency virus infection: window into brain infection? *Ann Neurol* 42:675–678.

Rabkin JG, Wagner GJ, and Rabkin R (1999). Testosterone therapy for human immunodeficiency virus–positive men with and without hypogonadism. *J Clin Psychopharmacol* 19:19–27.

Rabkin JG, Ferrando SJ, Wagner GJ, and Rabkin R (2000). DHEA treatment for HIV+ patients: effects on mood, androgenic and anabolic parameters. *Psychoneuroendocrinology* 25:53–68.

Rabkin JG, McElhiney, Ferrando SJ, and van Gorp WG (2004a). Predictors of employment of men with HIV/AIDS: a longitudinal study. *Psychosom Med* 66:72–78.

Rabkin JG, McElhiney M, Rabkin R, and Ferrando SJ (2004b). Modafinil treatment for fatigue in HIV+ patients: a pilot study. *J Clin Psychiatry* 65(12):1688–1695.

Ravitch IR, and Moseley CG (2001). High-performance liquid chromatographic assay for abacavir and its two major metabolites in human urine and cerebrospinal fluid. *J Chromatogr B Biomed Sci Appl* 762:165–173.

Ryan EL, Morgello S, Isaacs K, et al. (2004). Neuropsychiatric impact of hepatitis C on advanced HIV. *Neurology* 62(6):957–962.

Sacktor NC, Bacellar H, Hoover DR, et al. (1996). Psychomotor slowing in HIV infection: a predictor of dementia, AIDS and death. *J Neurovirol* 2:404–410.

Sacktor NC, Lyles RH, Skolasky RL, et al. (1999). Combination antiretroviral therapy improves psychomotor speed performance in HIV-seropositive homosexual men. Multicenter AIDS Cohort Study (MACS). *Neurology* 52:1640–1647.

Sacktor N, Lyles RH, Skolasky R, et al. (2001a). HIV-associated neurologic disease incidence changes: Multicenter AIDS Cohort Study, 1990–1998. *Neurology* 56:257–260.

Sacktor N, Tarwater PM, Skolasky RL, et al. (2001b). CSF antiretroviral drug penetrance and the treatment of HIV-associated psychomotor slowing. *Neurology* 57:542–544.

Sacktor N, Skolasky RL, Tarwater PM, et al. (2003). Response to systemic HIV viral load suppression correlates with psychomotor speed performance. *Neurology* 61:567–569.

Sacktor N, Skolasky RL, Ernst T, et al. (2005). A multicenter study of two magnetic resonance spectroscopy techniques in individuals with HIV dementia. *J Magn Reson Imaging* 21:325–333.

Schifitto P, Kieburz K, McDermott MP, et al. (2001). Clinical trials in HIV-associated cognitive impairment: cognitive and functional outcomes. *Neurology* 56:415–418.

Schmitt FA, Bigley JW, McKinnis R, Logue PE, Evans RW, and Drucker JL. (1988). Neuropsychological outcome of zidovudine (AZT) treatment of patients with AIDS and AIDS-related complex. *N Engl J Med* 319:1573–1578.

Smith CA, van Gorp WG, Ryan ER, Ferrando J, and Rabkin J (2003). Screening subtle HIV-related cognitive dysfunction: the clinical utility of the HIV dementia scale. *J Acquir Immune Defic Syndr* 33:116–118.

Staprans S, Marlowe N, Glidden D, et al. (1999). Time course of cerebrospinal fluid responses to antiretroviral therapy: evidence for variable compartmentalization of infection. *AIDS* 13:1051–1061.

Starace F, Bartoli L, Aloisi MS, et al. (2002). Cognitive and affective disorders associated to HIV infection in the HAART era: findings from the NeuroICONA study. *Acta Psychiatr Scand* 106:20–26.

Staszewski S, Morales-Ramirez J, Tashima KT, et al. (1999). Efavirenz plus zidovudine and lamivudine, efavirenz plus indinavir, and indinavir plus zidovudine and lamivudine in treatment of HIV-1 infection in adults. Study 006 team. *N Engl J Med* 341:1865–1873.

Tashima KT, Caliendo AM, Ahmad M, et al. (1999). Cerebrospinal fluid human immunodeficiency virus type 1 (HIV-1) suppression and efavirenz drug concentrations in HIV-1-infected patients receiving combination therapy. *J Infect Dis* 180:862–864.

Tozzi V, Balestra P, Galgani S, et al. (1999). Positive and sustained effects of highly active antiretroviral therapy on HIV-1-associated neurocognitive impairment. *AIDS* 13:1889–1897.

Wilkie FL, Goodkin K, Eisdorfer C, et al. (1998). Mild cognitive impairment and risk of mortality in HIV-1 infection. *J Neuropsychiatry Clin Neurosci* 10:125–132.

Williams JBW, Rabkin JG, Remien RH, Gorman JM, and Ehrhardt AA (1991). Multidisciplinary baseline assessment of homosexual men with and without human immunodeficiency virus infection II. Standardized clinical assessment of current and lifetime psychopathology. *Arch Gen Psychiatry* 48:124–130

Chapter 11

Anxiety Disorders

Mary Ann Cohen, Sharon M. Batista,
and Jack M. Gorman

Anxiety is a painful and ubiquitous concomitant of most severe medical illness, and AIDS is no exception. Anxiety may be experienced as a symptom, as one of the anxiety disorders, as a consequence of AIDS-associated illness, or as a result of one of its treatments. It can occur at any stage, from the realization of being at risk, to the anxiety about a possible symptom, to the time of HIV testing, diagnosis, disclosure, disease progression, and severe illness and dying. This chapter will explore the complexities of anxiety as it relates to HIV and AIDS as well as to risk reduction and medical care.

ANXIETY THROUGH THE COURSE OF HIV AND AIDS

Persons with HIV and AIDS may experience anxiety from the first realization of being at risk to the existential anxiety that may accompany inexorable progression of illness near the end of life. Pathologic anxiety is differentiated from normal fear response in that it is out of proportion with respect to the environmental stimulus in question, has significant intensity and duration, and results in either impairment of coping, disruption of normal function, or abnormal behaviors (Pollack et al., 2004). The determinants of severity of anxiety are multifactorial and are related to social support and experience with prior stressors and illnesses, as well as coping capacity, defensive structure, adaptive capacity, resilience, and the presence or absence of other psychiatric disorders. In addition to the psychological and social factors, severity and presence of comorbid medical conditions play a significant role in the level of anxiety experienced.

ANXIETY DISORDERS AND RISK FOR HIV INFECTION

While there have been reports of posttraumatic stress disorder (PTSD) in response to receipt of an HIV diagnosis (Kelly et al., 1998; Olley et al., 2005), Hutton and colleagues (2001) have proposed that PTSD may also have an association with risky behaviors that lead to HIV exposure, such as commercial sex and receptive anal sex. A study of 357 people infected with HIV showed that an overwhelming percentage had been victims of sexual assault since age 15 (68% of women and 35% of men) and that these assault survivors reported greater anxiety, depression, and symptoms of borderline personality disorder, and were more likely to report unprotected sexual intercourse (Kalichman et al., 2002). Studies to date do not agree on the impact of knowledge of serostatus on risk behaviors (Iniciardi et al., 2005). A high level of anxiety may lead to denial of awareness of risk and self-medication with alcohol or other drugs, leading to further risk due to disinhibition. Similarly, among persons who are dependent on alcohol or other drugs, such anxiety may lead to increased use of substances leading to diminished awareness of the possible consequences of risky behaviors. Blumberg and Dickey (2003) surveyed American adults with and without mental illness and found that adults with a mental disorder were more likely to report risk of becoming infected with HIV, to have been tested in the past year, and to expect to be tested in the upcoming year.

Intense anxiety may develop when a person first recognizes that he or she is at risk for infection. A healthy coping mechanism would be to assess the situation, explore options for testing, and consider a change in their risky behavior. Examples of more severe consequences of awareness of risk include PTSD in response to a needle-stick with HIV-contaminated blood (Howsepian, 1998), "AIDS-panic" as a result of exaggerated fear of contracting HIV (O'Brien and Hassanyeh, 1985; Brotman and Forstein, 1988), or even obsessive-compulsive disorder (OCD) (Schechter et al., 1991; Bruce and Stevens, 1992; Kraus and Nicholson, 1996). Some level of anxiety about risky sexual behavior may be necessary to modify highly risky sexual practices and ensure that condoms are available (or clean needles for injection drug use) and appropriate use or monogamy occurs.

Anxiety may ensue when a person develops both an awareness of being at risk and symptoms associated with HIV infection, such as night sweats or lymphadenopathy (Rundell et al., 1986). Braunstein's (2004) study of 40 HIV-negative and 101 HIV-positive (34 asymptomatic and 30 symptomatic patients, and 37 symptomatic patients with an AIDS diagnosis) demonstrated that while the patients did not vary overall in possession of irrational beliefs or death anxiety, the presence of irrational beliefs and HIV-positive serostatus strongly predicted the presence of death anxiety. Again, if anxiety leads to adaptive behavior, the individual will obtain counseling and testing for sexually transmitted infections. Anxiety about testing may lead to procrastination or avoidance of medical visits, being tested but not returning to receive results, or learning of HIV seropositivity without obtaining needed health care. If knowledge of serostatus alone carried more immediate psychological consequences, we would expect such behavior to be protective, but this is not known to be the case (Perry et al., 1993). Similarly, anxiety over disease progression can be so severe that it can prevent a person from being tested for CD4 count or viral load or from obtaining test results for fear of having to confront feelings about mortality. A low CD4 count or high viral load can mean that the patient's HIV illness is not responsive to treatment, is progressing, or is undertreated. Cohen and colleagues (2002) found that patients with low CD4 counts or high viral loads as well as those who were younger were more likely to be distressed when assessed with the Distress Thermometer (described by Roth et al., 1998) and were particularly more likely to have higher anxiety or depression scores on the Hospital Anxiety and Depression Scale (HADS), developed by Zigmond and Snaith (1983).

Anxiety about seropositivity may lead to both adaptive and maladaptive behaviors and responses. Adaptive responses include discussions with a partner, former partners, and trusted family members and friends. Just as learning about any serious threat to health can result in a need to talk, to ventilate fears, and mobilize a system of support, so too can learning of seropositivity lead to similar needs. Persons with HIV are understandably anxious about health and mortality. Many feel anxious and angry over the uncertainty surrounding their illness and treatment (Dilley et al., 1985). There is a fine line between vigilance in monitoring symptoms and incapacitating anxiety that interferes with function or results in relentless pursuit of minor medical complaints. As with any severe illness, symptoms such as unexplained weakness, dizziness, glandular swelling, fever, diarrhea, fatigue, headache, or night sweats may result in anxiety until they resolve or can be explained. Since these are symptoms that may be ubiquitous in persons with or without HIV infection or AIDS and are more common in persons with HIV infection, they are frequently a source of anxiety. Fear of death is omnipresent, especially in late-stage AIDS, described by one of our patients as being "like a fish always nibbling away at my toes—and always there if I want to notice." While some anxiety may help encourage patients to seek care for complications of HIV or for symptoms associated with antiretroviral medications, excessive anxiety may influence patients to stop taking antiretrovirals if such symptoms are perceived as side effects. Anxiety over fear of progression of illness can have painful implications, including devastating feelings about missing important milestones such as seeing a small child grow up, seeing a teenager graduate from high school, or enjoying the birth of a first grandchild.

For some patients, the very first symptom of HIV infection or HIV-related illness can be overwhelming and can shatter well-developed defenses of denial or suppression. Similarly, disease progression and the beginning of treatment with antiretroviral medication can also result in anxiety. With antiretroviral therapy, most HIV-positive patients are forced to confront their infection as a chronic, slowly debilitating illness (Tiamson, 2002). Consequences of such an illness are end-of-life issues, such as debilitating physical illness and subsequent loss of function (Zegans et al., 1994; Selwyn and Forstein, 2003), loss of ability to care for oneself, and alteration in roles within the patient's relationships (Farber and McDaniel, 1999). As AIDS or AIDS-related illness progresses, anxiety about loss of function intensifies. Inability to work can be overwhelming to individuals whose sense of self is related to independence and financial stability. Loss of ability to work may also be unrelated to AIDS progression, but rather entirely coincidental, as illustrated in the following vignette.

Case Vignette

Ms. B is a 50-year-old woman with HIV who worked as a home attendant until she sustained a comminuted fracture of her elbow as well as a shoulder injury when she fell during a job-related accident. The resultant disability prevented her from resuming her job as a home attendant. Until that time, she had been fully independent, hardworking, and able to support herself. She experienced intense anxiety and distress when she was faced with having to apply for entitlements for the first time in her life, in addition to being dependent financially for food and shelter.

HIV infection leads to physical deterioration through a wide range of infectious processes, such as opportunistic infections, in addition to noninfectious processes. Severe illness with opportunistic infections during late-stage AIDS is a cause of intense anxiety. Anxiety due to HIV-related illnesses other than opportunistic infections can also be severe and incapacitating. These illnesses include pulmonary hypertension, community acquired pneumonia, and cardiac disease, such as HIV-cardiomyopathy or coronary artery disease (Prendergast, 2003; Eaton, 2005), and can result in severe and overwhelming dyspnea, functional limitation, and existential anxiety. Anxiety can also be secondary to pain (Cabaj, 1996) or to side effects of antiretroviral therapy (Moreno et al., 2003; Damsa et al., 2005; Hawkins et al., 2005) and other medications used as prophylaxis of opportunistic infections.

Finally, in addition to the anxiety that results from the stress of HIV-related illness, comorbid anxiety disorders and anxieties related to other medical illnesses further complicate the course of HIV and AIDS. The psychological concomitants of comorbid medical illnesses are addressed in Chapters 33 through 37.

PSYCHOIMMUNOLOGY OF ANXIETY IN HIV INFECTION

The role of neuroendocrine pathways, namely the hypothalamic-pituitary-adrenal axis and the sympathetic adrenomedullary system, in anxiety disorders is only partially understood. To date, studies do not agree on the relationship between immune function and psychological distress in persons with HIV and AIDS (Antoni et al., 1991; Sahs et al., 1994; Kimmerling et al., 1999; Sewell et al., 2000; Antoni, 2003; Delahanty et al., 2004). One challenge of such studies is that the physiologic effects of HIV must be distinguished from those attributed to anxiety. For further details regarding the interaction between HIV, psychiatric illness, and the immune system, please refer to Chapter 3.

ANXIETY DISORDERS

As a result of improved care, persons with HIV are living longer and rather than developing solely HIV-related complications, also develop non-HIV-related illnesses such as cardiac disease, hypertension, diabetes mellitus, osteoarthritis, cancer, pulmonary hypertension, and chronic obstructive pulmonary disease. Symptoms of fatigue, insomnia, and pruritus may occur in the absence of specific medical or psychiatric pathology. Fatigue is a particularly disabling symptom that is not associated with advanced HIV disease or the use of highly active antiretroviral therapy (HAART) but rather with psychological distress (Henderson et al., 2005). Anxiety related to these symptoms as well as to life stresses can be devastating. Added to these commonly encountered sources of anxiety is the diagnosis of AIDS itself as well as some of its symptoms such as memory impairment, diarrhea, incontinence, and even cachexia.

In reviewing the specific anxiety disorders commonly seen in persons with HIV and AIDS, it is important to recognize that these are often superimposed on the anxiety that is experienced in the general population and commonly in the population with chronic symptomatic medical illness (Wells et al., 1988, 1989). Earlier in the epidemic, it was unclear whether the prevalence of anxiety disorders in HIV-positive patients exceeded that of persons without HIV infection (Fell et al., 1993; Dew et al., 1997), but recently it has been shown that HIV-positive persons do suffer from anxiety symptoms (Sewell et al., 2000) and anxiety disorders at increased rates (Morrison et al., 2002). The lifetime prevalence of anxiety disorders in the general population is about 25% (Kessler et al., 1994, 2005) and is an especially common complaint in the ambulatory medical setting (Schurman et al., 1985; Spitzer et al., 1999). The prevalence of anxiety in the waiting room population of an urban HIV clinic was 70% (Cohen et al., 2001). Given that anxiety disorders in HIV patients can masquerade as physical illness (Pollack et al., 2004), when evaluating a patient for diagnosis and treatment of an anxiety disorder it is important to be cognizant of the potential for organic etiology of such pathologic behavior. Upon initial evaluation, a thorough medical history, physical exam, and appropriate basic screening tests (EKG, CBC, thyroid function test, blood chemistry, urinalysis, RPR/VDRL, urine toxicology) should be performed to aid in diagnosis and to rule out contributing medical illness (Basu et al., 2005). Rarely, endocrine dysfunction, cardiovascular illness, or drug intoxication or withdrawal may be mistaken for an anxiety disorder (Pollack et al., 2004). In addition to neuropsychiatric disease secondary to HIV infection, those with anxiety due to an organic etiology often suffer from alcohol,

benzodiazepine, and stimulant dependence, which may result in confusion regarding symptomatology and affect treatment efficacy (Batki, 1990). The possibility of this scenario makes it especially important to investigate substance use and medication history, including both prescribed and over-the-counter or herbal medications.

Generalized Anxiety Disorder

Persons suffering from chronic illness and comorbid anxiety disorders have been shown to exhibit lower levels of function than those without anxiety disorders or those with comorbid depressive disorders, especially with respect to physical function, emotional health problems, social function, pain, fatigue or energy, emotional well-being, and health perception (Sherbourne et al., 1996). Anxiety and depression are prevalent in HIV-infected populations regardless of symptom status or HAART (Sewell et al., 2000; Lambert et al., 2005). HIV-positive women have been shown to have significantly higher anxiety symptom scores than HIV-negative women (Morrison et al., 2002). In contrast, there were no significant differences in the prevalence of anxiety in gay men with HIV and AIDS and HIV-negative gay men (Sewell et al., 2000). However, gay men who were HIV-negative or HIV-positive (with or without progression to AIDS) reported more anxiety symptoms and stress in comparison to the general population (Sewell et al., 2000).

While anxiety is a common ailment, it is still necessary to screen patients for symptoms of distress. In doing so, a full psychiatric evaluation is not always necessary to identify a pathologic anxious behavior or feelings, although there is no agreement on which screening tools to employ (Savard et al., 1998; Krefetz et al., 2004).

Posttraumatic Stress Disorder

The relationship between PTSD and HIV infection is complex; many researchers agree that there is a high rate of comorbidity between these two illnesses. The prevalence of PTSD in persons with HIV and AIDS ranges from 30% (Kelly et al., 1998) to 42% (Cohen et al., 2002) and is significantly correlated with the number of traumatic life events that the individual has experienced (Martinez et al., 2002). The severity of HIV-related PTSD symptoms is associated with a greater number of HIV-related physical symptoms, extensive history of pre-HIV trauma, decreased social support, increased perception of stigma, and negative life events (Katz and Nevid, 2005). In a study of 64 HIV-positive people, it was found that acute stress reactions (as defined by the DSM-IV definition of acute stress disorder) to recent events were significantly positively correlated with PTSD symptoms related to prior trauma but did not differ based on gender, AIDS status, or whether the patient had received group therapy (Koopman et al., 2002).

Posttraumatic stress disorder is often a concomitant of other psychiatric disorders as well as medical disorders, and HIV/AIDS is no exception. Olley and colleagues (2005) performed a study of 149 recently diagnosed South African persons with HIV/AIDS in which they found that other psychiatric conditions were likely to be associated with PTSD, such as major depressive disorder, suicidality, and social anxiety disorder. In this study, it was found that persons with PTSD and HIV did not differ demographically from those without PTSD. Olley and colleagues reported significant work impairment, as well as higher rates of alcohol use among persons with PTSD. Posttraumatic stress disorder has also been noted to have an association with pain (Smith et al., 2002; Tsao et al., 2004) and depressive symptoms (Sledjeski et al., 2005). Treatment of patients with multiple comorbidities is challenging, especially if the patient is nonadherent to either psychiatric or medical therapies, although it has been shown that therapies can be successfully tailored to the individual provided that the patient's barriers to care are identified and addressed in a compassionate manner (Batki et al., 1988, Treisman et al., 2001; Ricart et al., 2002). Case reports (Cohen et al., 2001; Ricart et al., 2002) and studies (Hutton et al., 2001; Sledjeski et al., 2005) have indicated a correlation between early childhood–induced PTSD and nonadherence to risk reduction and medical care in persons with HIV and AIDS. In comparison to depressed persons with lower CD4 counts, persons with greater PTSD symptoms are more likely to adhere to HAART regimens.

Antiretroviral medications, namely efavirenz and zidovudine, have been postulated to be responsible for recurrence or exacerbation of PTSD symptoms in a small number of patients (Moreno et al., 2003; Damsa et al., 2005). While unusual, such case reports are significant because they show that even medications used to treat HIV infection can have psychiatric consequences.

Posttraumatic stress disorder is prevalent among persons with HIV and AIDS, results in considerable distress, and may contribute significantly to nonadherence to risk reduction and medical care. The recognition and treatment of PTSD may improve not only quality of life but also overall health and well-being of persons with HIV/AIDS.

Panic Disorder

There are few reports or studies regarding panic disorder in HIV patients. Earlier in the HIV epidemic the mortality of HIV infection was extremely high because of a lack of treatment options and lack of support systems for victims. Summers and colleagues (1995) conducted a study between 1989 and 1993, when HAART was just being developed, and found that there was an increased incidence of major depression and panic disorder among those with unresolved grief. Panic disorder also has a strong association with pain in HIV patients (Tsao et al., 2004).

Obsessive-Compulsive Disorder

Obsessive-compulsive disorder is known to occur in conjunction with HIV infection (Schechter et al., 1991; Bruce and Stevens, 1992; Kraus and Nicholson, 1996; Cohen, 1998), but no studies exist to date.

Specific Phobias

There are several reports of AIDS-specific phobias (Freed, 1983; Jacob et al., 1987; Brotman and Forstein, 1988). Rapaport and Braff (1985) described a paranoid schizophrenic patient who experienced delusions about AIDS as a component of his "homosexual panic," which consisted of persecutory delusions that others believed he was gay.

There are also several case reports describing patients with an irrational fear or belief that they have AIDS despite medical evidence that they are HIV negative (Miller et al., 1986; Jacob et al., 1987; Brotman and Forstein, 1988; Kausch, 2004). On the basis of this limited quantity of case reports, it appears that illness-related phobias have some qualities in common with OCD (Logsdail et al., 1991), such as pervasive preoccupations, ritualistic behaviors, and an unfounded fear that is resistant to reassurance. The morbidity of this disorder is tremendous: many of these patients attempt or complete suicide at a rate higher than would be predicted by their lifestyle alone (Vuorio et al., 1990). In the early 1980s, it was particularly difficult to reassure such patients, given that a test to detect HIV was not available until several years into the epidemic. Miller and colleagues (1985) describe one such patient, later diagnosed with chronic anxiety, who presented with various ailments that he attributed to AIDS but that were differentiated from symptomatic HIV disease by a knowledgeable clinician.

TREATMENT

Treatment of anxiety disorders in HIV-positive patients follows guidelines similar to those for treating persons with other chronic medical illnesses, with particular attention to medication dosing, metabolism, potential for drug interactions, and potential for side effects (Farber and McDaniel, 2002). This will be discussed further in Chapter 32. While the DSM-IV guidelines prove helpful in diagnosing specific disorders, it is generally more appropriate to treat the anxiety on the basis of a patient's symptoms and symptom severity. To minimize adverse effects, medications should be started at low doses and titrated up slowly to the desired effect. Side effect profiles should also be taken into account.

Generalized Anxiety Disorder

Psychotherapy is an excellent first-line therapy for patients suffering from mild anxiety symptoms or can be used in combination with medication for those in need of more immediate relief or those suffering from more severe symptoms. Psychotherapeutic treatments have been shown to be effective in alleviating the distress of patients suffering from anxiety disorders. A therapeutic modality should be chosen that takes into account a patient's physical and psychological symptomatology, social supports, stressors, prior therapy or medication experience, ability to cope, cultural or religious background, and goals (Zegans et al., 1994). Numerous studies have demonstrated the overall benefits of group therapy as an intervention that ameliorates symptoms of depression, anxiety, and distress, and enhances coping in patients suffering from chronic illnesses, including HIV (Mulder et al., 1994; Sherman et al., 2004). Cognitive-behavioral stress management has been shown to result in significant stress reduction (Antoni et al., 2000; Cruess et al., 2000b) as

well as decreased mood disturbance and anxious mood (Cruess et al., 2000a) in HIV-positive patients. A similar study demonstrated that behavioral stress management techniques such as self-induced relaxation using progressive muscle relaxation, electromyographic (EMG) biofeedback, self-hypnosis, and meditation resulted in improvement in anxiety, mood, and self-esteem (Taylor, 1995). Lutgendorf and colleagues (1998) also observed improvement in cognitive coping strategies, namely positive reframing and acceptance in addition to improvements in social supports.

Selective serotonin reuptake inhibitors (SSRIs) are useful as first-line therapy for treating chronic anxiety disorders (Ferrando and Wapenyi, 2002, Pollack et al., 2004), although benzodiazepines are most frequently used (Cabaj, 1996). Benzodiazepines are especially useful as an adjunct to SSRIs for those who cannot wait for several weeks while an SSRI is titrated to an effective dose, or for those patients who require acute relief of distressing symptoms such as panic. Many clinicians are wary of using benzodiazepines because they have potential for abuse and dependence in patients with substance abuse history (Fernandez and Levy, 1994; Ferrando and Wapenyi, 2002; Douaihy et al., 2003) and if used chronically put the patient at risk for withdrawal symptoms when the medication is stopped. An alternative is buspirone, which is a nonbenzodiazepine agent shown to be useful in the treatment of generalized anxiety. Compared to benzodiazepines, buspirone has a relatively low risk of excessive sedation (Ferrando and Wapenyi, 2002), low risk of drug interactions (McDaniel et al., 2000), low potential for abuse (Ferrando and Wapenyi, 2002), but has been reported to induce psychosis in an HIV-positive man (Trachman, 1992). It is primarily used as a second-line agent, for long-term relief, or prophylaxis of anxiety symptoms. For rapid anxiolysis, Ferrando and Wapenyi (2002) comment that alternatives to buspirone include antihistamines such as diphenhydramine, hydroxyzine, sedating tricyclic antidepressants, and trazodone.

AIDS Phobia and OCD

One challenge in treating patients with phobias as well as OCD is that such patients are highly hesitant to refrain from engaging in rituals. In light of infection control practices, it can be difficult to avoid compulsive washing and cleaning behaviors (Bruce and Stevens, 1992). Case reports are the only current evidence of treatment of AIDS phobia or OCD. Jenike and Pato (1986) reported on a patient with irrational and persistent fear of HIV infection, successfully treated with imipramine. Five of the seven patients discussed by Logsdail and colleagues (1991) achieved both reduction of fears and improved social functioning with 7 to 10 sessions of exposure-based treatment that included response prevention following a model similar to that for treatment of individuals suffering from OCD. There is a dearth of clinical trials on treatment of HIV/AIDS-related OCD. McDaniel and Johnson (1995) successfully treated two patients with fluoxetine.

Panic Disorder

Standard therapy for panic disorders consists of medication to relieve and prevent symptoms (tricyclic antidepressants [TCAs], SSRIs, monoamine oxidase inhibitors [MAOIs], serotonin-norepinephrine reuptake inhibitors [SNRIs], benzodiazepines, with or without the addition of beta-adrenergic antagonists to modify some of the physiologic symptoms of panic disorder) as well as possible augmentation of therapy with psychotherapeutic modalities such as cognitive-behavioral therapy. Fernandez and Levy (1991, 1994) prefer to treat HIV patients suffering from either panic disorder or delusions with anxious features with neuroleptics instead of benzodiazepines because the latter drug class is behaviorally disinhibiting. It should be noted that beta-adrenergic antagonists are not effective when used alone, are contraindicated in patients who abuse cocaine, and may also cause depression, fatigue, and sexual dysfunction.

Posttraumatic Stress Disorder

The literature regarding treatment of PTSD in HIV-infected persons is limited. In the general population, it has been demonstrated that antidepressant medications, particularly SSRIs, are excellent first-line pharmacotherapy for PTSD (Cooper et al., 2005). Cohen and colleagues (2001) have reported three cases in which patients responded well to weekly psychodynamic psychotherapy in addition to outreach via telephone. In agreement with this, Ricart and colleagues (2002) demonstrated that one of the more important aspects of care for a patient with PTSD is establishment of a therapeutic alliance with the patient in an ego-supportive manner: the patient feels cared for, is able to trust his or her caretakers, and so is able to form attachments to both the individual caretakers as well as to the clinic or hospital itself. Forming such an attachment is instrumental in working toward adherence to psychiatric and medical therapies, especially given that persons suffering from PTSD often experience difficulty in forming trusting relationships because of past violations of their trust and the symptoms of their illness. Medications are also useful for treating HIV-infected persons with PTSD; two of the patients in the Cohen et al. (2001) study noted improved symptoms with combinations of medications such as citalopram, gabapentin, and/or hydroxyzine. It is promising that recent studies of non-HIV-infected individuals have demonstrated the utility of cognitive-behavioral therapy in the treatment of patients suffering from PTSD complicated by substance use disorder (Cohen and Hien, 2006) as well as that of psychosocial interventions such as eye movement desensitization and reprocessing (Rothbaum et al., 2005). Further information on the psychopharmacology of PTSD can be found in Chapters 27 and 32 of this text.

SUMMARY

Anxiety is a concomitant to all severe illness and is significant among persons with HIV and AIDS. The recognition and treatment of anxiety throughout the course of HIV, from time of awareness of risk to end-stage illness, can help reduce suffering and improve adherence to risk reduction and medical care.

References

Antoni MH (2003). Stress management effects on psychological, endocrinological, and immune functioning in men with HIV infection: empirical support for a psychoneuroimmunological model. *Stress* 6(3): 173–188.

Antoni MH, Schneiderman N, Klimas N, LaPerriere A, Ironson G, and Fletcher MA (1991). Disparities in psychological, neuroendocrine, and immunologic patterns in asymptomatic HIV-1 seropositive and seronegative gay men. *Biol Psychiatry* 29(10):1023–1041.

Antoni MH, Cruess DG, Cruess S, Lutgendorf S, Kumar M, Ironson G, Klimas N, Fletcher MA, and Schneiderman N (2000). Cognitive-behavioral stress management intervention effects on anxiety, 24-hr urinary norepinephrine output, and T-cytotoxic/suppressor cells over time among symptomatic HIV-infected gay men. *J Consult Clin Psychol* 68(1):31–45.

Basu S, Chwastiak LA, and Bruce RD (2005). Clinical management of depression and anxiety in HIV-infected adults. *AIDS* 19(18):2057–2067.

Batki SL (1990). Buspirone in drug users with AIDS or AIDS-related complex. *J Clin Psychopharmacol* 10(3 Suppl.):111S–115S.

Batki SL, Sorensen JL, Faltz B, and Madover S (1988). Psychiatric aspects of treatment of I.V. drug abusers with AIDS. *Hosp Community Psychiatry* 39(4): 439–441.

Blumberg SJ, and Dickey WC (2003). Prevalence of HIV risk behaviors, risk perceptions, and testing among US adults with mental disorders. *J Acquir Immune Defic Syndr* 32(1):77–79.

Braunstein JW (2004). An investigation of irrational beliefs and death anxiety as a function of HIV status. *Journal of Rational-Emotive and Cognitive-Behavioral Therapy* 22(1):21–38.

Brotman AW, and Forstein M (1988). AIDS obsessions in depressed heterosexuals (case report). *Psychosomatics* 29:428–431.

Bruce BK, and Stevens VM (1992). AIDS-related obsessive compulsive disorder: a treatment dilemma. *J Anxiety Disord* 6:79–88.

Cabaj RP (1996). Management of anxiety and depression in HIV-infected patients. *J Int Assoc Physicians AIDS Care* 2(6):11–16.

Cohen LR, and Hien DA (2006). Treatment outcomes for women with substance abuse and PTSD who have experienced complex trauma. *Psychiatr Serv* 57(1):100–106.

Cohen MAA (1998): Psychiatric care in an AIDS nursing home. *Psychosomatics* 39:154–161.

Cohen MA, Alfonso CA, Hoffman RG, Milau V, and Carrera G (2001). The impact of PTSD on treatment adherence in persons with HIV infection. *Gen Hosp Psychiatry* 23(5):294–296.

Cohen MA, Hoffman RG, Cromwell C, Schmeidler J, Ebrahim F, Carrera G, Endorf F, Alfonso CA, and Jacobson JM (2002). The prevalence of distress in persons with human immunodeficiency virus infection. *Psychosomatics* 43(1):10–15.

Cooper J, Carty J, and Creamer M (2005). Pharmacotherapy for posttraumatic stress disorder: empirical review and clinical recommendations. *Aust N Z J Psychiatry* 39(8):674–682.

Cruess DG, Antoni MH, Kumar M, and Schneiderman N (2000a). Reductions in salivary cortisol are associated with mood improvement during relaxation training among HIV-seropositive men. *J Behav Med* 23(2):107–122.

Cruess DG, Antoni MH, Schneiderman N, Ironson G, McCabe P, Fernandez JB, Cruess SE, Klimas N, and Kumar M (2000b). Cognitive-behavioral stress management increases free testosterone and decreases psychological distress in HIV-seropositive men. *Health Psychol* 19(1):12–20.

Damsa C, Bandelier C, Maris S, Lazignac C, Vidailhet P, Andreoli A, and Bianchi-Demicheli F (2005).

Recurrence of post-traumatic stress disorder and antiretrovirals. *Scand J Infect Dis* 37(4):313–316.

Delahanty DL, Bogart LM, and Figler JL (2004). Posttraumatic stress disorder symptoms, salivary cortisol, medication adherence, and CD4 levels in HIV-positive individuals. *AIDS Care* 16(2): 247–260.

Dew MA, Becker JT, Sanchez J, Caldararo R, Lopez OL, Wess J, Dorst SK, and Banks G (1997). Prevalence and predictors of depressive, anxiety and substance use disorders in HIV-infected and uninfected men: a longitudinal evaluation. *Psychol Med* 27(2):395–409.

Dilley JW, Ochitill HN, Perl M, and Volberding PA (1985). Findings in psychiatric consultations with patients with acquired immune deficiency syndrome. *Am J Psychiatry* 142(1):82–86.

Douaihy AB, Jou RJ, Gorske T, and Salloum IM (2003). Triple diagnosis: dual diagnosis and HIV disease, part 2. *AIDS Read* 13(8):375–382.

Eaton ME (2005). Selected rare, noninfectious syndromes associated with HIV infection. *Top HIV Med* 13(2):75–78.

Farber EW, and McDaniel JS (1999). Assessment and psychotherapy practice implications of new combination antiretroviral therapies for HIV disease. *Prof Psychol Res Pr* 30:173–179.

Farber EW, and McDaniel JS (2002). Clinical management of psychiatric disorders in patients with HIV disease. *Psychiatr Q* 73(1):5–16.

Fell M, Newman S, Herns M, Durrance P, Manji H, Connolly S, McAllister R, Weller I, and Harrison M (1993). Mood and psychiatric disturbance in HIV and AIDS: changes over time. *Br J Psychiatry* 162:604–610.

Fernandez F, and Levy JK (1991). Psychopharmacotherapy of psychiatric syndromes in asymptomatic and symptomatic HIV infection. *Psychiatr Med* 9(3): 377–394.

Fernandez F, and Levy JK (1994). Psychopharmacology in HIV spectrum disorders. *Psychiatr Clin North Am* 17(1):135–148.

Ferrando SJ, and Wapenyi K (2002). Psychopharmacological treatment of patients with HIV and AIDS. *Psychiatr Q* 73(1):33–49.

Freed E (1983). AIDophobia (letter). *Med J Aust* 2:479.

Hawkins T, Geist C, Young B, Giblin A, Mercier RC, Thornton K, and Haubrich R (2005). Comparison of neuropsychiatric side effects in an observational cohort of efavirenz- and protease inhibitor-treated patients. *HIV Clin Trials* 6(4):187–196.

Henderson M, Safa F, Easterbrook P, and Hotopf M (2005). Fatigue among HIV-infected patients in the era of highly active antiretroviral therapy. *HIV Med* 6(5):347–352.

Howsepian AA (1998). Post-traumatic stress disorder following needle-stick contaminated with suspected HIV-positive blood. *Gen Hosp Psychiatry* 20: 123–127.

Hutton HE, Treisman GJ, Hunt WR, Fishman M, Kendig N, Swetz A, and Lyketsos CG (2001). HIV risk behaviors and their relationship to posttraumatic stress disorder among women prisoners. *Psychiatr Serv* 52(4):508–513.

Inciardi JA, Surratt HL, Kurtz SP, and Waever JC (2005). The effect of serostatus on HIV risk behaviour change among women sex workers in Miami, Florida. *AIDS Care* 17(Suppl. 1):S88–S101.

Jacob KS, John JK, Verghese A, and John TJ (1987). AIDS-phobia. *Br J Psychiatry* 150:412–413.

Jenike MA, and Pato C (1986). Disabling fear of AIDS responsive to imipramine. *Psychosomatics* 27:143–144.

Kalichman SC, Sikkema KJ, DiFonzo K, Luke W, and Austin J (2002). Emotional adjustment in survivors of sexual assault living with HIV-AIDS. *J Trauma Stress* 15(4):289–296.

Katz S, and Nevid JS (2005). Risk factors associated with posttraumatic stress disorder symptomatology in HIV-infected women. *AIDS Patient Care STDS* 19(2):110–120.

Kausch O (2004). Irrational fear of AIDS associated with suicidal behavior. *J Psychiatr Pract* 10(4):266–271.

Kelly B, Raphael B, Judd F, Perdices M, Kernutt G, Burnett P, Dunne M, and Burrows G (1998). Posttraumatic stress disorder in response to HIV infection. *Gen Hosp Psychiatry* 20(6):345–352.

Kessler RC, McGonagle KA, Zhao S, Nelson CB, Hughes M, Eshleman S, Wittchen HU, and Kendler KS (1994). Lifetime and 12-month prevalence of DSM-III-R psychiatric disorders in the United States. Results from the National Comorbidity Survey. *Arch Gen Psychiatry* 51(1):8–19.

Kessler RC, Demler O, Frank RG, Olfson M, Pincus HA, Walters EE, Wang P, Wells KB, and Zaslavsky AM (2005). Prevalence and treatment of mental disorders, 1990 to 2003. *N Engl J Med* 352(24):2515–2523.

Kimerling R, Calhoun KS, Forehand R, Armistead L, Morse E, Morse P, Clark R, and Clark L (1999). Traumatic stress in HIV-infected women. *AIDS Educ Prev* 11(4):321–330.

Koopman C, Gore-Felton C, Azimi N, O'Shea K, Ashton E, Power R, De Maria S, Israelski D, and Spiegel D (2002). Acute stress reactions to recent life events among women and men living with HIV/AIDS. *Int J Psychiatry Med* 32(4):361–378.

Kraus RP, and Nicholson IR (1996). AIDS-related obsessive compulsive disorder: deconditioning based on fluoxetine-induced inhibition of anxiety. *J Behav Ther Exp Psychiatry* 27(1):51–56.

Krefetz DG, Steer RA, Jermyn RT, and Condoluci DV (2004). Screening HIV-infected patients with chronic pain for anxiety and mood disorders with the Beck anxiety and depression inventory—fast screens for medical settings. *J Clin Psychol Med Settings* 11(4):283–289.

Lambert S, Keegan A, and Petrak J (2005). Sex and relationships for HIV positive women since HAART: a quantitative study. *Sex Transm Infect* 81(4):333–337.

Logsdail S, Lovell K, Warwick H, and Marks I (1991). Behavioural treatment of AIDS-focused illness phobia. *Br J Psychiatry* 159:422–425.

Lutgendorf SK, Antoni MH, Ironson G, Starr K, Costello N, Zuckerman M, Klimas N, Fletcher MA, and Schneiderman N (1998). Changes in cognitive coping skills and social support during cognitive behavioral stress management intervention and distress outcomes in symptomatic human immunodeficiency virus (HIV)-seropositive gay men. *Psychosom Med* 60(2):204–214.

Martinez A, Israelski D, Walker C, and Koopman C (2002). Posttraumatic stress disorder in women attending human immunodeficiency virus outpatient clinics. *AIDS Patient Care STDS* 16(6):283–291.

McDaniel JS, and Johnson KM (1995). Obsessive-compulsive disorder in HIV disease. Response to fluoxetine. *Psychosomatics* 36(2):147–150.

McDaniel JS, Chung JY, Brown L, Cournos F, Forstein M, Goodkin K, and Lyketsos C (2000). Work Group on HIV/AIDS. Practice guidelines for the treatment of patients with HIV/AIDS. *Am J Psychiatry* 157:11.

Miller D, Green J, Farmer R, and Carroll G (1985). A "pseudo-AIDS" syndrome following from fear of AIDS. *Br J Psychiatry* 146:550–551.

Miller F, Weiden P, Sacks M, and Wizniak J (1986). Two cases of factitious acquired immune deficiency syndrome (letter to the editor). *Am J Psychiatry* 147:91.

Moreno A, Labelle C, and Samet JH (2003). Recurrence of post-traumatic stress disorder symptoms after initiation of antiretrovirals including efavirenz: a report of two cases. *HIV Med* 4(3):302–304.

Morrison MF, Petitto JM, Ten Have T, Gettes DR, Chiappini MS, Weber AL, Brinker-Spence P, Bauer RM, Douglas SD, and Evans DL (2002). Depressive and anxiety disorders in women with HIV infection. *Am J Psychiatry* 159(5):789–796.

Mulder CL, Emmelkamp PM, Antoni MH, Mulder JW, Sandfort TG, and de Vries MJ (1994). Cognitive-behavioral and experiential group psychotherapy for HIV-infected homosexual men: a comparative study. *Psychosom Med* 56(5):423–431.

O'Brien G, and Hassanyeh F (1985). AIDS-panic: AIDS-induced psychogenic states (letter). *Br J Psychiatry* 147:91.

Olley BO, Zeier MD, Seedat S, and Stein DJ (2005). Post-traumatic stress disorder among recently diagnosed patients with HIV/AIDS in South Africa. *AIDS Care* 17(5):550–557.

Perry S, Jacobsberg L, Card CA, Ashman T, Frances A, and Fishman B (1993). Severity of psychiatric symptoms after HIV testing. *Am J Psychiatry* 150(5):775–779.

Pollack MH, Otto MW, Bernstein JG, and Rosenbaum JF (2004). Anxious patients. In TA Stern, GL Fricchione, NH Cassem, MS Jellinek, and JF Rosenbaum (eds.), *Massachusetts General Hospital Handbook of General Hospital Psychiatry*, fifth edition. Philadelphia: Mosby.

Prendergast BD (2003). HIV and cardiovascular medicine. *Heart* 89(7):793–800.

Rapaport M, and Braff DL (1985). AIDS and homosexual panic. *Am J Psychiatry* 142(12):1516.

Ricart F, Cohen MA, Alfonso CA, Hoffman RG, Quinones N, Cohen A, and Indyk D (2002). Understanding the psychodynamics of non-adherence to medical treatment in persons with HIV infection. *Gen Hosp Psychiatry* 24(3):176–180.

Roth AJ, Kornblith AB, Batel-Copel L, Peabody E, Scher HI, and Holland JC (1998). Rapid screening for psychologic distress in men with prostate carcinoma: a pilot study. *Cancer* 82(10):1904–1908.

Rothbaum BO, Astin MC, and Marsteller F (2005). Prolonged exposure versus eye movement desensitization and reprocessing (EMDR) for PTSD rape victims. *J Trauma Stress* 18(6):607–616.

Rundell JR, Wise MG, and Ursano RJ (1986). Three cases of AIDS-related psychiatric disorders. *Am J Psychiatry* 143:777–778.

Sahs JA, Goetz R, Reddy M, Rabkin JG, Williams JB, Kertzner R, and Gorman JM (1994). Psychological distress and natural killer cells in gay men with and without HIV infection. *Am J Psychiatry* 151(10):1479–1484.

Savard J, Laberge B, Gauthier JG, Ivers H, and Bergeron MG (1998). Evaluating anxiety and depression in HIV-infected patients. *J Pers Assess* 71(3):349–367.

Schechter JB, Myers MF, and Solyom L (1991). A case of obsessive-compulsive disorder related to AIDS: psychopharmacologic treatment. *Can J Psychiatry* 36:118–120.

Schurman RA, Kramer PD, and Mitchell JB (1985). The hidden mental health network. Treatment of mental illness by nonpsychiatrist physicians. *Arch Gen Psychiatry* 42(1):89–94.

Selwyn PA, and Forstein M (2003). Overcoming the false dichotomy of curative vs. palliative care for late-stage HIV/AIDS. *JAMA* 290(6):806–814.

Sewell MC, Goggin KJ, Rabkin JG, Ferrando J, McElhiney MC, and Evans S (2000). Anxiety syndromes and symptoms among men with AIDS: a longitudinal controlled study. *Psychosomatics* 41(4):294–300.

Sherbourne CD, Wells KB, Meredith LS, Jackson CA, and Camp P (1996). Comorbid anxiety disorder and the functioning and well-being of chronically ill patients of general medical providers. *Arch Gen Psychiatry* 53(10):889–895.

Sherman AC, Mosier J, Leszcz M, Burlingame GM, Ulman KH, Cleary T, Simonton S, Latif U,

Hazelton L, and Strauss B (2004). Group interventions for patients with cancer and HIV disease: Part I: Effects on psychosocial and functional outcomes at different phases of illness. *Int J Group Psychother* 54(1):29–82.

Sledjeski EM, Delahanty DL, and Bogart LM (2005). Incidence and impact of posttraumatic stress disorder and comorbid depression on adherence to HAART and CD4+ counts in people living with HIV. *AIDS Patient Care STDS* 19(11):728–736.

Smith MY, Egert J, Winkel G, and Jacobson J (2002). The impact of PTSD on pain experience in persons with HIV/AIDS. *Pain* 98(1-2):9–17.

Spitzer RL, Kroenke K, and Williams JB (1999). Validation and utility of a self-report version of PRIME-MD: the PHQ primary care study. Primary Care Evaluation of Mental Disorders. Patient Health Questionnaire. *JAMA* 282:1737–1744.

Summers J, Zisook S, Atkinson JH, Sciolla A, Whitehall W, Brown S, Patterson T, and Grant I (1995). Morbidity associated with acquired immune deficiency syndrome-related grief resolution. *J Nerv Ment Dis* 183(6):384–389.

Taylor DN (1995). Effects of a behavioral stress-management program on anxiety, mood, self-esteem, and T-cell count in HIV positive men. *Psychol Rep* 76(2):451–457.

Tiamson ML (2002). Challenges in the management of the HIV patient in the third decade of AIDS. *Psychiatr Q* 73(1):51–58.

Trachman SB (1992). Buspirone-induced psychosis in a human immunodeficiency virus–infected man. *Psychosomatics* 33:332–335.

Treisman GJ, Angelino AF, and Hutton HE (2001). Psychiatric issues in the management of patients with HIV infection. *JAMA* 286(22):2857–2864.

Tsao JCI, Dobalian A, and Naliboff BD (2004). Panic disorder and pain in a national sample of persons living with HIV. *Pain* 109:172–180.

Vuorio KA, Aarela E, and Lehtinen V (1990). Eight cases of patients with unfounded fear of AIDS. *Int J Psychiatry Med* 20(4):405–411.

Wells KB, Golding JM, and Burnam MA (1988). Psychiatric disorder in a sample of the general population with and without chronic medical conditions. *Am J Psychiatry* 145(8):976–981.

Wells KB, Golding JM, and Burnam MA (1989). Chronic medical conditions in a sample of the general population with anxiety, affective, and substance use disorders. *Am J Psychiatry* 146(11):1440–1446.

Zegans LS, Gerhard AL, and Coates TJ (1994). Psychotherapies for the person with HIV disease. *Psychiatr Clin North Am* 17(1):149–162.

Zigmond AS, and Snaith RP (1983). The hospital anxiety and depression scale. *Acta Pscyhiatr Scand* 67:361–370.

Chapter 12

Psychotic Disorders and Severe Mental Illness

Julia Skapik, Alexander Thompson, Andrew Angelino, and Glenn Treisman

Since HIV/AIDS became a chronic illness in the United States, its prevalence has remained high, affecting an estimated 0.6% of the adult population (UNAIDS, 2006). In the population of individuals with known mental illnesses the prevalence is far higher, with a review of studies finding a mean HIV prevalence of 7.8% among people with mental illness, while the prevalence in the general population at that time was 0.4% (Cournos and McKinnon, 1997). Given the increased rates of HIV among people with mental illness, it is justified to recognize that HIV/AIDS is an epidemic in this population. Persons with mental illness and HIV/AIDS are at high risk to have poor outcomes because of lack of access to health care, poor social and financial support, cognitive limitations, difficult environmental factors, and vulnerability to high risk behaviors. Compared with HIV positive individuals without mental illness, persons with mental illness receive their HIV diagnoses later, are less likely to receive treatment, less likely to benefit from treatment, and more likely to experience morbidity and mortality.

Delays in HIV treatment for persons with HIV and mental illness may be due to concerns about inadequate adherence and emergence of viral resistance, a sense of futility about outcomes, and patients' lack of cooperation and adherence to treatment recommendations. Although persons with HIV and chronic mental illness are less likely to be treated with antiretroviral therapy, (Fairfield et al., 1999), they may be the patients most immediately in need of treatment. Invariably, substance abuse, which is present in at least half of most samples with severe mental illness, is seen as complicating and worsening treatment outcomes and disease progression.

The treatment of mental illness with HIV coinfection requires greater attention, more resources, and a multidisciplinary setting. This approach results in better outcomes and reduced cost. Medical comorbidities are common among people with mental illness, including HIV/AIDS (McDaniel et al., 1997; McKinnon et al., 2002; Green et al., 2003). Persons with mental illness and HIV/AIDS often frustrate their HIV clinicians who may not have adequate training to treat the comorbid mental conditions. Primary HIV providers may find it difficult to provide adequate medical treatment for persons with HIV and severe mental illness. Psychiatric treatment provided collaboratively in the medical setting results in better medical outcomes and improved patient–provider relationships (Murphy et al., 2004).

The cost of untreated psychiatric illness includes disability, increased medical expenditure, and societal costs such as crime and increased transmission of communicable diseases such as HIV and hepatitis B and C. The potential benefits of preventing crime and HIV transmission, and reducing disability far outweigh the added costs of treatment. The addition of psychiatric services to existing HIV/AIDS clinics can cost as little as a few hundred dollars per week and can prevent emergence of multidrug-resistant viral strains through improved adherence, decrease HIV transmission by reduction in risk behaviors, and decrease disability in patients.

The most compelling reason to provide adequate and comprehensive treatment for HIV/AIDS and mental illness is that it is the right thing to do. Patients in successful treatment have a better quality of life, can better care for themselves, and participate in family and community life. As such, the goals for HIV/AIDS clinics and clinicians should be to improve quality of life by providing support, changing damaging beliefs, and reducing harmful behavior; improve medical therapy by enabling patients to participate and tolerate treatment; and decrease risk of transmission of HIV to others through behavior modification and decreased viral loads.

TREATMENT OF PSYCHIATRIC DISORDERS IN THE CONTEXT OF HIV

Specific considerations should be given to patients with HIV and severe, chronic mental illness. Approximately 2.6% of persons in the United States meet the criteria (based on duration, disability, and diagnosis) for severe mental illness (SMI) in a given year (Kessler et al., 1996). Most individuals with SMI have schizophrenia, bipolar disorder, and major depressive disorder

(MDD), requiring extended or frequent hospitalizations (Regier et al., 1990). Schizophrenia and bipolar disorder impair a person's ability to perceive HIV risk, modify behavior, and participate in treatment. Adequate consideration and treatment of the specific symptoms in individual patients will maximize their adherence to a comprehensive treatment plan.

SEVERE MENTAL ILLNESS AND HIV RISK

Chronically mental ill patients have an increased risk of acquiring HIV through practicing risky sexual behaviors, abusing substances, and taking part in social networks that have a higher prevalence of HIV. Individuals with mental illness have variable knowledge of HIV risks and safer sex practices, with a diagnosis of schizophrenia being a specific predictor of having poor knowledge of such risks and practices. More importantly, increased knowledge of HIV risk behaviors does not translate to less risk behaviors on the part of individuals with mental illness. In fact, some studies have found that mentally ill individuals who practice risky behaviors had greater knowledge of HIV risks than those who did not (Chuang and Atkinson, 1996, McKinnon et al., 1996). Risk behaviors more common among psychiatric patients include multiple partners, partners with known HIV-positive status, substance use during sex, trading sex for money, drugs, or housing, and lack of condom use (Treisman and Angelino, 2004). Interestingly, compared to individuals with substance abuse alone, patients with severe mental illness and substance abuse have similar numbers of sexual partners and rates of unprotected oral, anal, and vaginal sex, but significantly increased rates of very high–risk behaviors, such as trading sex for money or gifts, being forced to have sex, having sex with intravenous drug users and persons with known HIV-positive status, and sharing needles (Dausey and Desai, 2003). Coercive sexual behavior and physical violence in particular have been shown to be frequent among chronically mental ill patients (Carey et al., 1997; Lamb, 1982). Many individuals with mental illness have unstable housing and finances, making access to condoms and clean works more difficult (McKinnon et al., 2002; Drake and Wallach, 1989).

Many providers use counseling about risk as the primary means of HIV prevention. Data on psychiatric patients indicate that, at baseline, persons with mental illness have more difficulty with behavior self-modification and furthermore, better knowledge of HIV prevention does not translate to behavior change (Carey et al., 1997). Thus, the HIV clinician and clinic need to provide knowledge as well as active interventions to facilitate behavior change. It is important to cover beliefs related to HIV risk, means of improving sexual or drug paraphernalia hygiene, negotiation of condom use, recognition of vulnerable emotional states, ways of avoiding risky behaviors, and sexual empowerment. Thorough screening must be done to identify individual risk factors. Patients with mental illness consistently underestimate the risk of their own behaviors (Carey et al., 1997). Helping patients to find other financial support or substance abuse treatment is critical to reduce the exchange of sex for money or drugs. Screening and treatment for victims of sexual abuse and assault should be addressed, since in one group of psychiatric outpatients, 13% reported being pressured for sex and 14% reported being coerced or forced into sex in the past year (Carey et al., 1997). Same-sex partnerships should be discussed in all settings, as some subgroups of mentally ill individuals have been shown to have increased rates of same-sex activity, particularly men (McKinnon et al., 2002).

Psychiatric treatment is especially important for individuals with psychosis, as there is a strong correlation between positive symptoms and high-risk behaviors. Successful reduction of positive symptoms of schizophrenia leads to a reduction in risk behaviors. Antidepressant therapy can be helpful, as individuals with depression may also engage in risky behavior because of a sense of hopelessness. It is critical that patients set goals toward healthy partnerships, and discuss what a healthy relationship entails, as many patients may never have experienced a stable romantic relationship. Having positive goals toward loving relationships also helps patients maintain a positive focus and appeals to reward-seeking extroverts; HIV risk counseling often focuses solely on risks and thus appeals less to extroverts who are less risk avoidant. Although HIV risk counseling can produce significant reductions in risk behavior after fewer than 10 treatment sessions (McKinnon et al., 2002), the practice of risk reduction fades over time, thus sessions that help maintain risk reduction may help to sustain subsequent benefits.

The importance of substance abuse treatment in the care of mentally ill patients with HIV/AIDS can-

not be emphasized enough. To maximize risk reduction, substance abuse should be addressed in all settings, including behavioral interventions, support for maintaining risk reduction, and medical and psychiatric appointments with health care professionals. Numerous studies have shown that patients with schizophrenia and other chronic mental illnesses have high rates of substance abuse, generally ranging from 40%–75% depending on the substances considered and method of ascertainment (Regier et al., 1990; Test et al., 1989; Miller and Tannenbaum, 1989; Toner et al., 1992; Caton et al., 1989; Horwath et al., 1996).

Various explanations have been given for the use of substances by psychiatric patients, one being that mentally ill patients self-medicate with substances in an attempt to alleviate symptoms or ameliorate side effects of medicines (Dixon et al., 1991; Test et al., 1989; Lamb, 1982; Mueser et al., 1990). Another theory is that chronically ill patients have disruptions of social functioning and use substances as a means of connecting with others (Alterman et al., 1982), which has been supported by interviews with SMI patients that showed 44.4% of substance abusers cited "something to do with friends" as a reason for their substance abuse (Test et al., 1989). Although these explanations help clinicians treat dually diagnosed patients, the fact remains that patients with severe mental illnesses use substances frequently and should be considered at greater risk for HIV.

Substance abuse affects every aspect of HIV/AIDS treatment. It worsens prognosis and compliance, interferes with the creation and maintenance of healthy social relationships, increases risk behaviors, and decreases judgment and insight (Drake and Wallach, 1989; McKinnon et al., 2002). Studies have shown that substance abuse or dependence concurrent with HIV/AIDS is associated with a more severe course of illness and poor medication compliance (RachBeisel et al., 1999). Thus substance abuse, by worsening psychiatric disorders, may cause more symptoms or worsen one's coping ability and lead to increased high-risk behavior. Intravenous drug use (IVDU) must be addressed, as any lifetime IVDU increases the risk of HIV infection from two- to ten-fold (Horwath et al., 1996). Five to 26 percent of psychiatric patients report prior injection and 1%–8% report IVDU in the past 3–12 months (Susser et al., 1996; Carey et al., 1997; Rosenberg et al., 2001). It is critical to inquire about IVDU at all visits, as IVDU among people with severe mental illness is often intermittent (McKinnon et al., 2002; Horwath et al., 1996). People with mental illness are more likely to be part of social networks that include intravenous drug users, increasing the risk of sexual transmission as well as IVDU-related infection.

Although abstinence from mood- or cognitive-altering substances is often considered the ideal, agonist-based therapies may provide a particularly effective form of treatment for opiate users. Methadone maintenance therapy is highly useful in the management of opiate addiction among the chronically mentally ill. Adherence to a methadone program has been shown to decrease HIV risk behavior (Wong et al., 2003); it removes individuals from high-risk behaviors and environments while reducing motivation to seek IVDU in the community. It also keeps the individual actively participating in a treatment community. Individuals on methadone maintenance therapy demonstrate better adherence to highly active antiretroviral therapy (HAART), which decreases the overall cost of health care (Sambamoorthi et al., 2000). Methadone can be used by providers to give positive reinforcement for desired behaviors, such as rewarding a patient with take-home methadone after several months of negative toxicology screens. Methadone maintenance decreases drug-related morbidity and mortality and crime and improves patient function, leading to improved ability to participate in care. For patients who have failed abstinence-based treatment or are unwilling to attempt opiate cessation, methadone is a useful adjunct to HIV treatment.

Although IVDU often receives more attention in addressing HIV risk and care from providers, all forms of substance abuse contribute to risk and patient level of function. Alcohol, cocaine, and methamphetamine abuse are particularly important to address in HIV treatment, as their use is associated with high-risk sexual behaviors (McKinnon et al., 2002). Most importantly, substance abuse stands between the goals of HIV treatment and helping the patient with chronic mental illness as it demoralizes patients, prevents them from achieving stable living situations, work, and healthy relationships, and increases the severity of underlying psychiatric illness. Without the ability to achieve consistency and stability in life, patients have little opportunity to achieve consistent treatment adherence and improved functional outcome. Substance abuse among individuals with chronic mental illness is widespread, leads to practice of HIV risk behaviors, and is a poor prognostic factor for psychiatric treatment as well as HIV treatment.

Schizophrenia

Schizophrenia has a worldwide prevalence of about 1%. It is a lifelong disorder that usually has an onset in the teens and 20s for men and in the 20s and 30s for women, occurring with roughly equal prevalence in both sexes. Schizophrenia is a chronic condition that may be described as a disease of executive function, the ability to plan and carry out complex tasks using adaptability to internal and environmental cues. The essential deficit is the inability to plan and carry out complex tasks that require the ability to respond appropriately to certain variables, such as understanding and using social cues and organizing goal-directed behavior. As such, this disorganization interferes with treatment of medical conditions like HIV and the ability to manage risks and modify behaviors. Patients are thus predisposed to chaotic, unstable life situations and are vulnerable to sexual abuse, substance use, and dysfunctional relationships.

Schizophrenia is characterized by both positive and negative features. The more chronic and disabling negative features are often the least well understood by medical providers, and yet may most profoundly influence the relationship with the provider. These features were originally described by Bleuler in 1911, and are often referred to as the four "A's" of schizophrenia: flattened *a*ffect (a decrease in both expressed and experienced emotions), *a*mbivalence, *a*utism (an inability to make meaningful emotional connections with others), and loose *a*ssociations. These features impede the ability of patients to "connect" with providers. They make patients ambivalent about all elements of treatment and make it hard for patients to engage with their providers.

The "positive" features include episodes of psychosis in which patients develop hallucinations (usually auditory), delusions (often paranoid and bizarre), and disordered thinking. These intrusive experiences are often disturbing and can lead to unpredictable and bizarre behavior that alienates patients from others and may be dangerous to the patient or others. These experiences and behaviors are considered positive symptoms because they add to the patient's otherwise normal experience. Over time, most patients develop apathy, withdraw from social functioning, and become increasingly disconnected in social interactions.

At an extreme, patients can be catatonic, living entirely in a separate mental world that others cannot access. This loss of connection leaves patients without emotional and social support and removes any motivation to achieve a better quality of life. Patients are often described as having been odd and withdrawn before the development of psychotic symptoms. The condition is a lifelong illness and is progressively disabling in most patients. It is associated with early mortality and increased morbidity.

Currently there is no significant difference between the pharmacologic treatment of schizophrenia in an HIV-infected individual and the treatment of an uninfected person. It is important to take into consideration interactions between HAART medications and antipsychotics; psychiatrists and HIV practitioners must work together closely during initiation of or changes in antiretroviral or antipsychotic treatment, as concomitant alterations in dosing may be needed. Many antipsychotics are associated with severe side effects, such as tardive dyskinesia and Parkinsonian syndromes known as extrapyramidal symptoms (EPS). They also have effects on metabolism, including weight gain, increased insulin resistance, and increased lipids that may complicate similar effects produced by antiviral medications. There may be drug interactions with antiviral treatment as well, although these remain unpredictable for the most part (Treisman and Angelino, 2004). Antipsychotic medications have been shown to be poorly adhered to by patients and may contribute to poor adherence to medications in general. It is unclear how much of this nonadherence is related to their mental health and how much is related to the medication side effects.

Treatment principles for patients with schizophrenia apply universally. They include medications for the control of hallucinations, delusions, thought disorders, and negative symptoms, as well as psychosocial rehabilitation for reintegration into the community. Studies have shown that adequate treatment of positive symptoms leads to significant reductions in HIV risk behaviors (McKinnon et al., 1996). The treatment of negative symptoms may help to motivate and engage the patient in treatment. Reality testing should be supported at all times, and the confrontation of delusional thoughts should be gentle and appropriately timed.

Patients should be given support for medication compliance. Substance abuse in particular leads to poor compliance in patients with schizophrenia

(Drake and Wallach, 1989). The incorporation of friends and family into the treatment plan can improve adherence to treatment and reinforce consistency of the treatment message, as well as provide support to these caregivers. Occasionally, issues arise because of delusions the schizophrenic patient has concerning the HIV infection itself. The most common of these is the belief that the patient does not have an HIV infection and that the situation is a hoax, created to monitor the patient's activity or somehow control the patient (Treisman and Angelino, 2004). Again, adequate antipsychotic treatment combined with a consistent but supportive message from the family, psychiatric team, and HIV team can address delusions and hallucinations that interfere with HIV treatment.

Bipolar Disorder

Bipolar disorder (previously called manic-depressive illness) is an illness that impacts the affective domain of one's mental health and accounts for many patients with severe mental illness. Often presenting with psychosis, this condition may be misdiagnosed as schizophrenia when severe. In the classic descriptions of manic-depressive illness, patients spend extended periods of time depressed, usually weeks to months at a time, followed by shorter periods when they are in an elevated, euphoric, and energized state, referred to as mania. Most often, patients cycle from one type of mood to the other, these cycles often interspersed with periods of normal moods but occasionally with intermediate mixed states that have features of both depressive and elevated mood states simultaneously or in rapid succession. The emotions and emotional changes in patients with bipolar disorder run their lives and can have a strong effect on their attitude toward treatment from minute to minute (Treisman and Angelino, 2004). Bipolar disorder is covered in more detail in Chapter 9 of this book.

In contrast to the bipolar disorder found in the general population, another type of mania appears to be specifically associated with late-stage HIV infection (CD4 count <200 per mm^3), and it occurs in cognitive impairment or dementia (Kiburtz et al., 1991). This syndrome has been called "AIDS mania" and probably represents a related but different condition, as the patients show a lack of previous episodes or family history (Lyketsos et al., 1997). Clinically, patients with AIDS mania may be difficult to distinguish from those with delirium, because the sleep–wake cycle is often disturbed and patients show a good deal of confusion and cognitive impairment. For this reason, the workup begins with a careful evaluation of the causes of delirium. Patients with AIDS mania may differ clinically from those with familial bipolar disorder, as the predominant mood tends to be irritability rather than elation or euphoria. A review at a hospital AIDS clinic found that 8% of patients with AIDS experienced a manic syndrome at some point during the course of the illness (Lyketsos et al., 1993). Of these patients experiencing manic syndromes, half had no personal or family history of bipolar disorder and were more likely to have later stage AIDS. Personal or family history, imaging findings, and other clinical indicators may help to distinguish between AIDS mania and bipolar mania associated with AIDS (Lyketsos et al., 1993).

Major Depressive Disorder

Depression is the most common psychiatric disorder and as such is common among individuals with HIV/AIDS. A meta-analysis of studies reported active depression in 9.4% of individuals with HIV/AIDS compared with 5.2% in HIV-negative individuals (Ciesla and Roberts, 2001). Individuals with depression are predisposed to greater HIV/AIDS risk for several reasons. Higher HIV risk may result from a sense of hopelessness about the future. Additionally, persons with depression may seek to alleviate their symptoms with alcohol and other drugs. Alcohol abuse and dependence are prevalent among persons with depression. For patients with depression, alcohol use is a major source of HIV risk, as patients under the influence of alcohol are more likely to engage in risky sexual behaviors and IVDU because of decreased inhibition (McKinnon et al., 2002). Lack of memory and attention may distract depressed individuals from self-care and risk reduction behaviors. It can also keep patients from being diagnosed or entering treatment. Chronic depression, particularly when complicated by psychotic features, also adds to the population of patients with chronic and severe mental illness. This is particularly true when combined with chronic stimulant or alcohol use, leading to complex and difficult to understand symptoms at presentation.

Patients with major depression can be strongly resistant to HIV therapy. They may have difficulty engaging in treatment and maintaining treatment adherence. Because depressed patients feel hopeless, they are less likely to seek care or testing and counseling. It is difficult to engage depressed patients in treatment because they are preoccupied with negative ideas and low mood. Once involved in treatment, extra effort must be employed to maintain their engagement, because depression leads to low motivation and energy. This can be partially overcome through the use of incremental goals and rewards (Treisman and Angelino, 2004). Because depression causes decreased memory and concentration, patients have a more difficult time with medication adherence. Visual cues and memory aids may help improve adherence, and social support can improve morale and adherence. It is therefore necessary to treat depression concomitantly with HIV/AIDS if providers wish to succeed in viral suppression. Major depressive disorder is covered in further detail in Chapter 9 of this book.

MEDICAL MANAGEMENT
OF INDIVIDUALS WITH SEVERE
MENTAL ILLNESS

Patients with severe mental illness have worse medical outcomes than their unaffected counterparts. Psychiatric patients generally have a poor appreciation of their medical conditions and are both less aware of their physical condition and less likely to have or seek adequate medical care. The treatment of mentally ill patients is often more difficult and time consuming for providers than for those without mental illness. Because they are a more difficult population to treat, providers are hesitant to accept them as patients, and they are at higher risk for being discharged from care. Psychiatric patients also have decreased ability to participate in their care because of cognitive and emotional limitations. They often fail to appreciate benefits of treatment that are not immediately apparent and are focused concretely on the here and now. Patients with apathy and low mood may feel that treatment is pointless or feel that they just don't have the energy to participate. Decreased concentration and memory in many conditions may cause patients to forget medications and appointments.

HIV and medical screening of psychiatric patients is inadequate in psychiatric and medical settings. Patients with severe, chronic mental illness may receive limited medical attention in general and therefore are at risk for sequelae of undiagnosed disorders, such as neurosyphilis and chronic pelvic inflammatory disease. Women with chronic psychiatric illnesses are less likely to receive prenatal care during pregnancy (Turner et al., 1996) and thus are more likely to spread infection to their offspring. Individuals with chronic mental illness are less likely to have access to medical care and are more likely to be without insurance, homeless, and unemployed (Folsom et al., 2005; Meade and Sikkema, 2005). Unsurprisingly, outcomes are worse for individuals with severe mental illness (Goldman, 2000; Cournos et al., 2005).

It is therefore necessary to aggressively screen individuals with mental illness for both HIV and other medical illnesses, such as diabetes, hepatitis, hypertension, and heart disease. It is helpful for both patients and providers to centralize care as much as possible, making all providers aware of all medical problems as well as the current treatment plan to provide a consistent message (Treisman and Angelino, 2004). Frequent pregnancy testing and on-site prenatal care may improve outcomes for pregnant women with HIV. It is important to incorporate preventative medicine whenever possible, including smoking cessation, weight management, and risk reduction; this counseling has been often overlooked in patients with multiple medical problems and with HIV, but is even more crucial now that HIV/AIDS has become a chronic illness. We emphasize that psychiatric providers should be vigilant about screening for medical illnesses, even using a standard medical review questionnaire for the periodic assessment of a patient's medical status. Patients with altered mental status in particular need special attention and careful physical examinations because they may be less likely or able to report symptoms. In addition, we urge medical providers in clinics to take extra care in examining the chronically mentally ill, because often their illnesses, or the stigma attached to them, prevent open lines of communication.

In medicine, physicians often seek to educate patients about risks to their health and benefits of treatment and health maintenance in an effort to influence patients' behavior toward compliance and improved quality of life. Providers treating people with chronic mental illness, however, have to take a different approach to therapy. In this population increasing knowledge does not usually affect behavior; thus patients with severe psychiatric illnesses require assistance with behavior modification. As discussed above, chronically mentally ill individuals with HIV who engage in

risky behaviors are often better educated about risks than their HIV-positive counterparts who are not mentally ill (Chuang and Atkinson, 1996, McKinnon et al., 1996), perhaps because of their providers' efforts to motivate them to change through increased education about HIV risk. This suggests that education alone may be successful in increasing knowledge in this population, but not in changing behavior. Cognitive behavioral therapy can be useful in this regard; identifying harmful attitudes, ideas, and behaviors and creating a framework of new, healthy attitudes and behaviors is helpful for patients who struggle to modify their behavior. Interventions in which patients actively practice health hygiene, behavior modification, safe-sex negotiation, and positive interactions with others help patients to realize their own ability to retrain patterns of harmful behaviors.

Many individuals with mental illness are unstable extroverts who are reward focused and somewhat indifferent to risk. Furthermore, physician education often focuses on risks and negative outcomes that result from failing to be compliant with treatment. We suggest that providers focus strongly on the benefits of treatment, such as improved energy, a more stable living situation due to substance abstinence, better relationships with others, improvement in lab values as a result of good treatment adherence, and decreased time spent in the hospital (Treisman and Angelino, 2004). Although education is essential, and negative outcomes must be discussed with patients, an optimistic, behavior-focused plan for patients is more helpful than general discussion of health risks. We encourage providers to take small steps in behavior modification, setting one or two concrete goals at each visit and following their progress, praising success and exploring the cause of failures. These steps also help patients to build rapport with providers and build confidence in patients as well as providers, who tend to get discouraged with negative outcomes of mentally ill patients.

ADHERENCE TO THERAPY IN PERSONS WITH SEVERE MENTAL ILLNESS

Nonadherence to treatment is one of the major problems in treating individuals with HIV/AIDS. It has been demonstrated that greater than 90% adherence to a HAART regimen is needed to achieve effective suppression in most patients (Moreno et al., 2000; Paterson et al., 2000). One study that examined individuals with directly observed therapy (DOT) found that 93% adherence led to 85% of patients achieving an undetectable viral load (Kirkland et al., 2002). Good adherence to HAART is related to HIV-related mortality, morbidity, and hospitalization (Press et al., 2002). Difficulty with adherence is compounded among patients with chronic mental illness because they have characteristics predisposing them to poor adherence, including trouble with memory and concentration, medication cost, lack of transportation, lack of stable housing, homelessness, unemployment, and lack of social support (Chander et al., 2006). Thus each patient with HIV/AIDS should be given a thorough assessment for access to medications, transportation, housing, social support, work and ability to work, finances, including ability to afford necessities, and cognitive abilities. A strong patient–provider relationship not only improves adherence but also enables the physician to anticipate barriers to adherence and intervene early. Because many patients with chronic mental illness are concretely focused and may be asymptomatic, they may focus on immediate side effects without appreciating the benefits of treatment. It is important to treat side effects and symptoms whenever possible to improve patients' ability to realize the benefits of treatment.

The patient's belief system about treatment and their diagnoses can strongly affect their willingness to take medications. The belief that treatment will be successful improves adherence. Factors adversely affecting adherence the most for HIV-positive individuals with severe mental illness are problems with planning, lack of interaction with others, failure to use cues, and HIV/AIDS treatment issues related to lack of motivation, side effects, and hopelessness (Kemp-painen et al., 2004). The burden of regular appointments and daily medication is greater on this population, and demoralized patients may easily give up on treatment, sometimes citing futility of treatment due to lack of a cure for HIV. Patients experiencing depression have less ability to perform self-care and subjectively experience more pain than when they are well; treating pain adequately may improve adherence. Patients with decreased memory, concentration, or other cognitive limitations should have reminders or alarms placed in their home and, ideally, a friend or family member to help remind them or even observe the patient taking medications and provide encouragement of treatment. Psychiatric consults and referrals can also help address these issues, as remis-sion of illness maximizes the ability to tolerate medical therapy. Adherence is addressed in detail in Chapter 22 of this book.

COMPREHENSIVE HIV SERVICES LEAD TO IMPROVED OUTCOMES FOR PATIENTS AND PROVIDERS

We envision the ideal HIV treatment for individuals with chronic mental illness as a comprehensive care center that provides treatment for HIV, other medical conditions, psychiatric disorders, substance abuse, and psychosocial problems in one location. Initially, our clinic performed psychiatric evaluations on site and referred patients to outside psychiatric care. In the first year of referrals, we referred 94 patients, of whom 89 agreed to be referred. Upon follow-up we learned that none of these 89 patients ever attended follow-up care (Treisman and Angelino, 2004). This convinced us that on-site psychiatric care was necessary in the HIV clinic. The care team should work together to present a unified front to patients and prevent splitting of providers. Collaboration by providers has the potential to actually improve the quality of care, with physicians educating each other in their respective specialties, prevent unnecessary care, and help physicians diagnose new problems earlier.

Patients who are able to make one visit to take care of all their needs will have greater ability to attend necessary appointments, as additional transportation and multiple appointments are then avoided. On-site counseling, risk reduction, social work, and substance abuse treatment could be incorporated into each visit as needed. Ideally, on-site housing could be incorporated for patients who require living assistance or are homeless. For sites that lack funding for a comprehensive treatment center, addition of psychiatric services is cost-effective, requires little equipment or facilities, and can still retain many of the benefits of collaboration between medical and psychiatric providers. In an ideal HIV treatment program, the treatment team would use role induction to outline the conditions of care and give the patient an opportunity to see that providers are working together. The program would ideally incorporate cognitive behavioral therapy to aid with behavior modification and risk reduction, substance abuse treatment, social services, job training and assistance, and medical and psychiatric treatment. The program should also have an on-site pharmacy that offers adherence programs to support patients' compliance with medications, make it easier to track medications dispensed, and increase the ability of patients with limited mobility or transportation to obtain medications. A program that incorporates family members or significant others can improve social support for patients and for family members as well as improve treatment adherence.

The more integrated services are, the better patients can be incorporated into a treatment regimen with a team of health care professionals to provide support. In our multidisciplinary clinic, HIV-positive patients with psychiatric disorders were more likely to receive HAART and had reduced mortality compared to the general HIV-positive population and our own clinic population before the integration of services, presumably because of increased support and more advocacy by mental health professionals. These improved results in turn led to better viral suppression and reduced risk (Himelhoch et al., 2004). Our experience shows that we can have success treating this population and that the appropriate management of psychiatric disorders can facilitate improved quality of life and survival in patients with HIV/AIDS.

References

Alterman AI, Erdlen FR, and LaPorte DJ (1982). Effects of illicit drug use in an inpatient psychiatric population. Addict Behav 7:231–242.

Bleuler, E (1911). Dementia praecox oder Gruppe der Schizophrenien', In: G. Aschaffenburg (ed.), Handbuch der Psychiatrie. Spezieller Teil. 4. Abteilung, 1. Hälfte. Leipzig und Wien: Franz Deuticke.

Carey MP, Carey KB, Weinhardt LS, and Gordon CM (1997). Behavioral risk for HIV infection among adults with a severe and persistent mental illness: patterns and psychological antecedents. Community Ment Health J 33(2):133–142.

Caton CLM, Gralnick A, Bender S, and Robert S (1989). Young chronic patients and substance abuse. Hosp Community Psychiatry 40:1037–1040.

Chander G, Himelhoch S, and Moore RD (2006). Substance abuse and psychiatric disorders in AIDS patients: epidemiology and impact on antiretroviral therapy. Drugs 66(6):769–789.

Chuang HT, and Atkinson M (1996). AIDS knowledge and high-risk behavior in the chronic mentally ill. Can J Psychiatry 41(5):269–272.

Ciesla JA, and Roberts JE (2001). Meta-analysis of the relationship between HIV infection and risk for depressive disorder. Am J Psychiatry 158(5):725–730.

Cournos F, and McKinnon K (1997). HIV seroprevalence among people with severe mental illness in the United States: A critical review. Clin Psychol Rev 17(3):259–269.

Cournos F, McKinnon K, and Sullivan G (2005). Schizophrenia and comorbid human immunodeficiency virus and hepatitis C. J Clin Psychiatry 66(S6):27–33.

Dausey DJ, and Desai RA (2003). Psychiatric comorbidity and the prevalence of HIV infection in a sample of patients in treatment for substance abuse. J Nerv Ment Dis 191(1):10–17.

Dixon L, Hass G, Weiden PJ, Sweeny J, and Frances AJ (1991). Drug abuse in schizophrenic patients: clinical correlates and reasons for use. Am J Psychiatry 148:224–230.

Drake RE, and Wallach MA (1989). Substance abuse among the chronic mentally ill. Hosp Community Psychiatry 40:1041–1046.

Drake RE, Osher FC, and Wallach MA (1989). Alcohol use and abuse in schizophrenia. J Nerv Ment Dis 177:40.

Drake RE, Mueser KT, Clark RE, and Wallach MA (1996). The course, treatment, and outcome of substance disorder in persons with severe mental illness. Am Orthopsychiatr Assoc 66:42–51.

Fairfield KM, Libman H, Davis RB, Eisenberg DM, and Philips RS (1999). Delays in protease inhibitor use in clinical practice. J Gen Intern Med 14:395–401.

Folsom DP, Hawthorne W, Lindamer L, Gilmer T, Bailey A, Golshan S, Garcia P, Unutzer J, Hough R, and Jeste DV (2005). Prevalence and risk factors for homelessness and utilization of mental health services among 10,340 patients with serious mental illness in a large public mental health system. Am J Psychiatry 162(2):370–376.

Goldman LS (2000). Comorbid medical illness in psychiatric patients. Curr Psychiatry Rep 2(3):256–263.

Green AI, Canuso CM, Brenner MJ, and Wojcik JD (2003). Detection and management of comorbidity in schizophrenia. Psychiatr Clin North Am 26:115–139.

Himelhoch S, Moore RD, Treisman G, and Gebo KA (2004). Does the presence of a current psychiatric disorder in AIDS patients affect the initiation of antiretroviral treatment and duration of therapy? J Acquir Immune Defic Syndr 37(4):1457–1463.

Horwath E, Cournos F, McKinnon K, Guido JR, and Herman R (1996). Illicit-drug injection among psychiatric patients without a primary substance abuse disorder. Psychiatr Serv 47:181–185.

Kemppainen JK, Levine R, Buffum M, Holzemer W, Finley P, and Jensen P (2004). Antiretroviral adherence in persons with HIV/AIDS and severe mental illness. J Nerv Ment Dis 192(6):395–404.

Kessler RC, Nelson CB, McGonagle KA, Liu J, Swartz M, and Blazer DG (1996). Comorbidity of DSM-III-R major depressive disorder in the general population: results from the US National Comorbidity Survey. Br J Psychiatry Suppl (30):17–30.

Kiburtz K, Zettelmaier AE, Ketonen L, Tuite M, and Caine EC (1991). Manic syndrome in AIDS. *Am J Psychiatry* 98:1068–1070.

Kirkland LR, Fischl MA, Tashima KT, Paar D, Gensler T, Graham NM, Gao H, Rosenzweig KR, McClernon DR, Pittman G, Hessenthaler SM, Hernandez JE, for the NZTA4007 Study Team (2002). Response to lamivudine-zidovudine plus abacavir twice daily in antiretroviral-naive, incarcerated patients with HIV taking directly observed treatment. *Clin Infect Dis* 34(4):511–518.

Lamb HR (1982). Young adult chronic patients: the new drifters. *Hosp Community Psychiatry* 7:197–203.

Lyketsos CG, Hanson AL, Fishman M, Rosenblatt A, McHugh PR, and Treisman GJ (1993). Manic syndrome early and late in the course of HIV. *Am J Psychiatry* 150:326–327.

Lyketsos CG, Schwartz J, Fishman M, and Treisman G (1997). AIDS mania. *J Neuropsychiatry Clin Neurosci* 9:277–279.

McDaniel JS, Purcell DW, and Farber EW (1997). Severe mental illness and HIV-related medical and neuropsychiatric sequelae. *Clin Psychol Rev* 17(3): 311–325.

McKinnon K, Cournos F, Sudgen R, Guido JR, and Herman R (1996). The relative contributions of psychiatric symptoms and AIDS knowledge to HIV risk behaviors among people with severe mental illness. *J Clin Psychiatry* 57:506–513.

McKinnon K, Cournos F, and Herman R (2002). HIV among people with chronic mental illness. *Psychiatry Q* 73(1):17–31.

Meade CS, and Sikkema KJ (2005). HIV risk behavior among adults with severe mental illness: a systematic review. *Clin Psychol Rev* 25(4):433–457.

Miller FT, and Tanenbaum JH (1989). Drug abuse in schizophrenia. *Hosp Community Psychiatry* 40: 847–849.

Moreno A, Perez-Elias MJ, Casado JL, Munoz V, Antela A, Dronda F, Navas E, Foran J, Quereda C, and Moreno S (2000). Effectiveness and pitfalls of initial highly active retroviral therapy in HIV-infected patients in routine clinical practice. *Antivir Ther* 5(4):243–248.

Mueser KT, Yarnold PR, Levinson DF, Singh H, Bellack AS, Kee K, Morrison RI, and Yadalam KG (1990). Revalence of substance abuse in schizophrenia: demographic and clinical correlates. *Schizophr Bull* 16:31–49.

Mueser KT, Bellack AS, and Blanchard JJ (1992). Comorbidity of schizophrenia and substance abuse: implications for treatment. *J Consult Clin Psychiatry* 60:845–856.

Murphy DA, Marelich WD, Hoffman D, and Steers WN (2004). Predictors of antiretroviral adherence. *AIDS Care* 16(4):471–484.

Paterson DL, Swindells S, Mohr J, Brester M, Vergis EN, Squier C, Wagener NM, and Singh N (2000). Adherence to protease inhibitor therapy and outcomes in patients with HIV infection. *Ann Intern Med* 133:21–30.

Press N, Tyndall MW, Wood E, Hogg RS, and Montaner JSG (2002). Virologic and immunologic response, clinical progression, and highly active antiretroviral therapy adherence. *J Acquir Immune Defic Syndr* 31:S112–S117.

RachBeisel J, Scott J, and Dixon L (1999). Co-occurring severe mental illness and substance use disorders: a review of recent research. *Psychiatr Serv* 50(11): 1427–1434.

Regier DA, Farmer ME, Rae DS, Locke BJ, Keith SJ, Judd LL, and Goodwin FK (1990). Comorbidity of mental disorders with alcohol and other drug abuse. Results from the Epidemiologic Catchment Area (ECA) Study. *JAMA* 264(19):2511–2518.

Rosenberg SD, Trumbetta SL, Mueser KT, Goodman LA, Osher FC, Vidaver RM, and Metzger DS (2001). Determinants of risk behavior for human immunodeficiency virus/acquired immunodeficiency syndrome in people with severe mental illness. *Comp Psychiatry* 42(4):263–271.

Sambamoorthi U, Warner LA, Crystal S, and Walkup J (2000). Drug abuse, methadone treatment, and health services use among injection drug users with AIDS. *Drug Alcohol Depend* 60(1):77–89.

Susser E, Miller M, Valencia E, Colson P, Roche B, and Conover S (1996). Injection drug use and risk of HIV transmission among homeless men with mental illness. *Am J Psychiatry* 153(6):794–798.

Test MA, Wallisch LS, Allness DJ, and Ripp K (1989). Substance use in young adults with schizophrenic disorders. *Schizophr Bull* 15:465–476.

Toner BB, Gillies LA, Prendergasst P, Cote FH, and Browne C (1992). Substance use disorders in a sample of Canadian patients with chronic mental illness. *Hosp Community Psychiatry* 43:251–254.

Treisman GJ, and Angelino AF (2004). *The Psychiatry of AIDS: A Guide to Diagnosis and Treatment*. Baltimore, MD: Johns Hopkins University Press.

Turner BJ, McKee LJ, Silverman NS, Hauck WW, Fanning TR, and Markson LE. Prenatal care and birth outcomes of a cohort of HIV-infected women. *J Acquir Immune Defic Syndr Hum Retrovirol* 12(3):259–267.

UNAIDS (2002). *Report on the Global AIDS Epidemic*. Geneva: UNAIDS.

Wong KH, Lee SS, Lim WL, and Low HK (2003). Adherence to methadone is associated with a lower level of HIV-related risk behaviors in drug users. *J Subst Abuse Treat* 24(3):233–239.

Chapter 13

The Role of Personality in HIV Risk Behaviors: Implications for Treatment

Heidi E. Hutton and Glenn J. Treisman

The risk behaviors that transmit HIV and complicate HIV treatment are often influenced by psychiatric disorders. Major depression, substance abuse, and chronic mental illness are problems that commonly complicate HIV treatment, but none can generate more distress and dissention among medical providers than personality problems. Caregiver burnout, failure to establish stable medical care relationships, and "excessive resource utilization" have been associated with certain personality traits and disorders. There has been relatively little research on the role of personality traits in HIV despite their stable, durable, and heritable influence on thoughts, feelings, and behavior. Certain traits, however, appear to increase the likelihood of: engaging in HIV risk behaviors, having poorer quality of life and management of HIV, and adhering to treatment regimens. Effective HIV prevention and treatment programs should consider specific personality traits that render some individuals more vulnerable to engaging in behavior that further endangers their health as well as the health of others.

Recognizing these personality traits or disorders will be useful in developing more specific, effective risk reduction strategies and improving overall health outcomes.

DEFINING PERSONALITY

Personality is defined by the emotional and behavioral characteristics or traits that constitute stable and predictable ways that an individual relates to, perceives, and thinks about the environment and the self (Rutter, 1987; Rothbart and Ahadi, 1994; Livesley, 2001). Early observations of the nature of personality begin with classical scholars such as Hippocrates, Plato, Aristotle, and Galen and later with philosophers such as Aquinas, Machiavelli, Hobbes, Locke, and Nietzsche. Current personality theory, exemplified by the work of Hans Eysenck (1990), Paul T. Costa, Jr. (Costa and Widiger, 2002) and C. Robert Cloninger (1999), has extended these early observations by refining personality descriptions, developing measurement tools, and documenting their influence on functioning. Despite differences in details, the work in the field of personality agrees on these fundamental ideas: (1) individuals vary in the degree to which they possess a given trait and in the way it influences behavior; (2) traits are not positive or negative, but rather are adaptive in one setting and maladaptive in another; and (3) personality is a combination of temperament (or constellation of heritable traits) and character (environmental experience).

Extroversion–Introversion

Most personality taxonomies identify dimensions of extroversion–introversion and stability–instability or neuroticism. The dimension of extroversion–introversion refers to the individual's basic tendency to respond to stimuli with either excitation or inhibition. Individuals who are *extroverted* are (1) present oriented, (2) feeling directed, and (3) reward seeking (Eysenck, 1990; Lucas et al., 2000). Their chief focus is their immediate and emotional experience. Feelings dominate thoughts, and the predominant motivation is immediate gratification or relief from discomfort. Extroverts are charismatic, sociable, venturesome, optimistic, and impulsive. By contrast, *introverted* individuals are (1) future and past oriented, (2) cognition directed, and (3) consequence avoidant. Logic and function predominate over feelings. Introverts are motivated by appraisal of past experience and avoidance of future adverse consequences. They are unlikely to engage in a pleasurable activity if it might pose a threat in the future. Introverted individuals are quiet, dislike excitement, and distrust the impulse of the moment. They tend to be orderly, reliable, and rather pessimistic.

The second dimension, stability–instability, defines the degree of emotionality or lability. The emotions of *stable* individuals are aroused slowly and predictably and have low amplitude. By contrast, *unstable* individuals have intense, mercurial emotions that are easily and unpredictably aroused. What will cause an extreme reaction at one time will not necessarily provoke an emotional response at another time.

IMPLICATIONS FOR HIV RISK BEHAVIOR

If these two trait dimensions are juxtaposed (Fig. 13.1), four personality types emerge (Jung, 1923; Eysenck, 1990; Costa and Widger, 2002). At the extremes of these dimensions are the types of personality-disordered patients likely to be seen at the psychiatry service of an HIV clinic. Of the four types, unstable extroverts are the most prone to engage in HIV risk behavior, and therefore will be the primary focus of this chapter. These patients are preoccupied by, and act upon, their feelings, which are evanescent and changeable (Eysenck and Eysenck, 1975; Eysenck, 1990; Lucas et al., 2000). Thus, their actions tend to be unpredictable and inconsistent. Most striking is the inconsistency found between thought and action. In spite of intellectual ability or knowledge of HIV, unstable extroverts can engage in behavior associated with high risk of HIV infection. Past experience and future consequences have little salience in decision making for the individual who is ruled by feeling; the present is paramount. Goals are dictated by emotions—either to achieve pleasure or remove pain—with little regard for circumstances. Furthermore, as part of their emotional instability, they experience intense fluctuations in their feelings and moods. It is difficult for them to tolerate uncomfortable or painful affect, such as boredom, sadness, or unresolved drive; they want to escape or avoid such feelings as quickly and easily as possible. Thus, they are motivated to pursue pleasurable, dramatic, and emotionally intense experiences, however risky, and avoid low moods or boredom. They are attracted to emotionally intense interactions and stimuli.

Psychiatric patients characterized by unstable extroversion are more likely to engage in behaviors that place them at risk for HIV infection. Their spontaneity and impulsivity make them less likely to plan ahead and carry condoms and therefore more likely to have unprotected sex. They are more fixed upon the rewards of sex, particularly sex that is emotionally provocative, and less attentive to the sexually transmitted disease (STD) they may acquire without a condom. Unstable extroverts are also less likely to accept the diminution of intensity or spontaneity associated with the use of condoms or, once aroused, to interrupt the "heat of the moment" to use condoms. Similarly, unstable extroverts are more vulnerable to alcohol and drug abuse. They are drawn to alcohol and drugs as a quick route to pleasure or relief from discomfort or boredom. They are more likely to experiment with different kinds of drugs and to use greater quantities. Unstable extroverts are also more likely to inject drugs because the experience is more intense. They are also less likely to defer this intensity in the interest of safety.

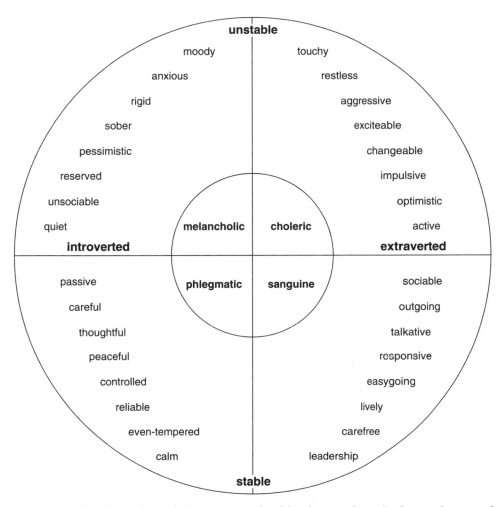

FIGURE 13.1. Hans Eysenck's circle. The inner circle of this diagram shows the famous doctrine of the four temperaments; the outer circle shows the results of numerous modern experiments involving ratings and self-ratings of behavior patterns of large groups of people. There is considerable agreement between the inner and outer circles, and a considerable part of personality can be described in terms of two major dimensions, here labeled introversion–extroversion and unstable–stable. Reprinted from Eysenck HJ: (1970). Principles and methods of personality description, classification, and diagnosis. In *Readings in Extraversion-Introversion, I. Theoretical and Methodological Issues*. Eysenck HJ (ed.) Wiley Interscience, p. 36, with permission from Edits Publishers.

Disorders of personality characterized by stable extroversion also engage in HIV risk behaviors, but the motivations are somewhat different from those associated with unstable extroversion. These patients, too, are present oriented and pleasure seeking; however, their emotions are not as intense, as easily provoked, or mercurial. Hence, they are not as strongly driven to achieve pleasure. Their emotional "flatness" may generate a kind of indifference to HIV risk more than a drive to seek pleasure at any cost. Stable ex-

troverts may be at risk because they are too optimistic or sanguine to believe that they will become HIV infected.

Introverted personalities are less likely to engage in HIV risk behaviors. Their focus on the future, avoidance of negative consequences, and preference for cognition over feeling render them more likely to engage in protective and preventive behaviors. The dimension of emotional instability–stability has a significant role in determining HIV risk for introverts.

Patients who are unstable introverts are anxious, moody, and pessimistic. Typically these patients seek drugs and/or sex not for pleasure but for relief or distraction from pain. They are concerned about the future and adverse outcomes, but believe that they have little control over their fates. Stable introverts are risk adverse and controlled, and are the least likely to engage in spontaneous or hedonistic behaviors. If these individuals present to the HIV clinic, it is usually because of an environmental exposure. This exposure could be a blood transfusion or an occupational needle stick. Alternatively, the environmental exposure could be a severely traumatic event that alters their characteristic functioning.

Clinical observations of the influence of extroversion and emotional instability on HIV risk behavior are supported by empirical investigation, although the research in this area has been limited. The Eysenck Personality Questionnaire (EPQ; Eysenck and Eysenck, 1975) and the NEO Personality Inventory (NEO-PI-R) of the Five Factor Model of personality (Costa and McCrae, 1992) have high reliability and validity in measuring these traits. High Extroversion is associated with sexual promiscuity, desire for sexual novelty, multiple sex partners (Eysenck, 1976; McCown 1991, 1993; Trobst et al., 2000) and heroin and other drug addictions (Francis and Bennett 1992; Lodhi and Thakur, 1993). Among HIV-positive substance abusers in treatment, those who had attempted suicide scored significantly higher on the EPQ's Neuroticism scale (Kosten and Rounsaville, 1988).

Sensation Seeking

The third construct elaborated by most personality models identifies a trait that Eysenck entitled "psychoticism–socialization" but has been defined in other theories as "flight versus aggression" or sensation seeking (Zuckerman et al., 1978; Zuckerman, 1994). Zuckerman (1994) described sensation seeking as "the seeking of varied, novel, complex, and intense sensations and experiences, and the willingness to take physical, social, legal, and financial risks for the sake of such experience" (p. 27). A reliable and well-validated measurement called the Sensation Seeking Scale measures this trait (Zuckerman et al., 1978). An adaptation of Zuckerman's scale measures the tendency to seek out novel or risky sexual stimulation (Sexual Sensation Seeking Scale, SSSS; (Kalichman et al.,

1994, Kalichman and Rompa, 1995) Among HIV-positive and HIV at-risk women and men, high scorers on the SSSS were more likely to engage in unprotected anal sex, unprotected anal sex with multiple partners, or unprotected vaginal sex. High scorers were also more likely to have unprotected intercourse 6 months later. Sexual sensation seeking was also related to expectancies about alcohol enhancing sexual pleasure or prowess that in turn was related to alcohol use during sex and, ultimately, to unprotected sex (Kalichman et al., 1996, 2005; Kalichman and Cain, 2004).

PERSONALITY DISORDER IN HIV AT-RISK AND HIV-POSITIVE INDIVIDUALS

When traits found in certain individuals exceed the levels found in most of society and are sufficiently rigid and maladaptive to cause subjective distress or functional impairment, a personality disorder is usually diagnosed (Rutter, 1987; Paris, 1996). Personality disorders represent extremes of normal personality characteristics and are disabling conditions in environments where the trait is maladaptive. Defining personality extremes into categories and specific entities (rather than traits that are dimensionally distributed) facilitates diagnosis and research that has contributed to our understanding of the relationship between HIV and personality.

Personality disorder is a risk factor for HIV infection (Brooner et al., 1993). Prevalence rates of personality disorders among HIV-positive (19%–36%) and HIV at-risk (15%–20%) individuals (Perkins et al., 1993; Jacobsberg et al., 1995; Johnson et al., 1995) are high and significantly exceed rates found in the general population (10%) (Weissman, 1993). Antisocial (ASPD) and borderline (BPD) personality disorders are the most common (Golding and Perkins, 1996). Individuals with personality disorder, particularly ASPD, have high rates of substance abuse and are more likely to inject drugs and share needles compared to those without an Axis II diagnosis (Kleinman et al., 1994; Hudgins et al., 1995; Dinwiddie et al., 1996). Approximately, half of drug abusers meet criteria for a diagnosis of ASPD (Hudgins et al. 1995; Dinwiddie et al., 1996). Individuals with ASPD are also more likely to have higher numbers of lifetime sexual partners, engage in unprotected anal sex, and contract STDs, compared to individuals without ASPD (Brooner et al., 1990; Ellis et al., 1995; Ladd and Petry, 2003). The highest rates of substance use disorders and HIV risk appear to be among individuals with an Axis I disorder and a comorbid diagnosis of ASPD (Disney et al., 2006). On the other hand, the highest rates of HIV testing among psychiatric patients appear to be among nonpsychotic patients with co-occurring BPD, which was attributed to their tendency to engage in impulsive sexual and substance abuse behaviors (Meade and Sikkema, 2005).

The diagnosis of personality disorders in the clinic setting must be undertaken cautiously. Making a DSM-IV diagnosis according to Axis II of the *Diagnostic and Statistical Manual of Mental Disorders*, fourth edition, text revision (DSM-IV-TR; American Psychiatric Association, 2000) requires considerable time and experience, but does little to explain behavior or suggest intervention strategies. Classifying individuals along a continuum of personality traits rather than in DSM-IV Axis II discrete categories has been shown to be a better predictor of HIV risk behavior (Tourian et al., 1997). Furthermore, a diagnosis of antisocial or borderline personality disorder can be stigmatizing, particularly in a general medical clinic where care providers may have less experience managing such patients.

PERSONALITY AND DISEASE PROGRESSION

A relatively new area of personality research in HIV is examining the relationship between temperament and disease progression. Specifically, social inhibition (introversion, reduced emotional expression, and social avoidance) is associated with elevated levels of autonomic nervous system activity. This specific characteristic appears to place individuals with this temperament at heightened risk for elevated HIV-1 viral load and impaired response to antiretroviral therapy (Cole et al., 2003).

IMPLICATIONS FOR MEDICATION ADHERENCE

Medication adherence across a variety of diseases and patients has been consistently estimated at 50% (Sackett and Snow, 1979). In HIV, however, greater than 95% adherence to highly active antiretroviral therapy (HAART) is necessary to achieve viral load suppression, improve immune function, and prevent viral mutations. Such adherence is especially challenging in HIV because it is associated with all of the components of low treatment adherence: long duration of treatment, preventative rather than curative treatment, asymptomatic periods, and frequent and complex medication dosing (Kruse et al., 1991; Blackwell, 1996; Icovics and Meade, 2002).

Our clinical experience suggests that unstable extroversion is the personality trait mostly likely to influence adherence. The same personality characteristic that increases risk of HIV also reduces ability to adhere to demanding drug regimens. Specifically, present-time orientation, combined with reward seeking, makes it more difficult for these patients to tolerate uncomfortable side effects from HAART, whose treatment effects may not be immediately apparent. It is also difficult for feeling-driven individuals to maintain consistent, well-ordered routines. Hence, following frequent, rigid dosing schedules can also be problematic. Unstable, extroverted patients may be intent on following the schedule, but their mercurial and sometimes chaotic emotions are more likely to interfere with and disrupt daily routines. For example, a patient may report that he became very angry with a partner and miss several doses of his antiretroviral medicines, despite knowing the risks of missing medication doses. These same patients also appear to differ in their appraisals of side effects of medicines. The principal reason for discontinuing HAART across studies is the side effects of medicines or anticipated side effects of medicines. Some patients are less able or willing to tolerate side effects in the present to prevent poor health in the future.

There is a relative paucity of research examining the association between personality and adherence to HAART. Personality traits were indirectly related to adherence in one study. On the NEO-PI-R (Costa and McCrae, 1992), HIV-positive patients high in neuroticism reported lower overall and HIV-specific quality of life that was associated with HAART nonadherence. By contrast, patients higher in extroversion, as well as other personality traits, reported better overall and HIV-specific quality of life that was associated with HAART adherence (Penedo et al., 2003). Neuroticism (instability) was also found to moderate the effect of perceived stress on adherence although not viral load.

Specifically, individuals high in neuroticism on the EPQ were less likely to be adherent to HAART as their level of perceived stress increased (Bottonari et al., 2005). Neuroticism is the trait that best distinguishes borderline patients from patients without this personality disorder (Morey and Zanarini, 2000). It is not surprising, therefore, that preliminary research on personality disorders and adherence suggests that BPD is associated with nonadherence to HAART. In a convenience sample of 107 triply diagnosed methadone patients (HIV positive with at least one psychiatric diagnosis and at least one substance use diagnosis), only BPD of all the Axis I and II psychiatric disorders was associated with less than 95% adherence in a 3-day recall of medications taken (Palmer et al., 2003).

TREATMENT

Traditional approaches in risk reduction counseling emphasize the avoidance of negative consequences in the future, such as using a condom during sexual intercourse to prevent STDs. But such educational approaches have been ineffective with individuals with marked personality problems, such as unstable extroverts, who engage in risky behaviors (Kalichman et al., 1996; Trobst et al., 2000). Psychiatric and medical treatment of patients with this personality type is challenging. Such patients are often baffling or frustrating for physicians and other medical providers because they engage in high-risk sex and drug behaviors in spite of knowing the risks, or fail to adhere to treatment regimens for HIV infection in spite of knowing the consequences. Because of their focus on feelings and interests of the moment, they can constantly change what they want from treatment and change their goals for their care. Patients may complain that a selective serotonin reuptake inhibitor gives them a mild headache while seeming to be untroubled by shooting heroin in a carotid artery. After 6 months of missed medical appointments, such individuals may impulsively leave the clinic if the primary care provider is 15 minutes late for the appointment. Such personality traits reflect relatively stable, lifelong modes of responding; thus, direct efforts to change these traits are unlikely to be successful. It is possible, however, to modify the behavior that is an expression of the trait. By recognizing individual differences in risk-related personality characteristics, interventions can be better targeted and their impact maximized.

We have found that a cognitive-behavioral approach is most effective in treating patients who present with extroverted and/or emotionally unstable personalities. Four principles guide our standard care:

1. Focus on thoughts, not feelings. Unstable, extroverted personalities benefit from learning how they are predisposed to act in certain ways. Often, they recognize that they are highly emotional and are driven by their feelings. They may be equally baffled by their own actions. These patients fail to understand why they intend to stay clean but later find themselves "shooting dope." The mental health professional can identify the role that strong feelings play, so that these patients can begin the process of understanding their own chaotic, often irrational, behavior. Simultaneously, the mental health professional can encourage their cognitive, logical side. Patients can focus on doing what is right or healthy rather than what is immediately pleasurable. The task is to build consistency into behavior. For some patients whose severe emotionality is severe enough to warrant a diagnosis of borderline personality disorder, there is a high likelihood of occult mood disorder such as major depression or bipolar disorder type II, and the addition of psychotropic medication such as an antidepressant or mood stabilizer may be beneficial in stabilizing emotional fluctuations.

2. Use a behavioral contract. A behavioral contract is developed with all patients. The contract outlines goals for treatment, often only a day or a week at a time. While patients and mental health professionals may develop the contract, the focus of treatment is *not* on what patients want or are willing to do to get off of drugs, but rather on established methods, such as drug treatment and Narcotics Anonymous or Alcoholics Anonymous. The importance of the behavioral contract lies in the creation of a *stable* plan that supersedes the emotional meanderings of these patients. Unstable extroverts present an ever-changing array of concerns and priorities. The task of the mental health professional is to order the priorities with patients and help them follow through on these, regardless of changing emotions.

3. Emphasize rewards. In developing the behavioral contract and in treatment, the purpose is cast in terms of the rewards that will follow from their behavioral change. Positive outcomes, not

adverse consequences, are salient to extroverts. Exhortations to use condoms to avoid STDs are unpersuasive. More success has been achieved with extroverts by eroticizing the use of condoms (Tanner and Pollack, 1988) or by the addition of novel sexual techniques (erotic massage, use of sex toys) into sexual repertoires (Abramson and Pinkerston, 1995). Similarly, the rewards of abstaining from drugs or alcohol are emphasized, such as having money to buy clothing, having a stable home, or maintaining positive relationships with children.

In building adherence to antiretroviral therapies, the focus is on the rewards of an increased CD4 count and reduced viral load, rather than avoiding illness. Using the viral load as a strategy to build adherence can increase acceptance in all patients, but is especially effective in reward-driven extroverts.

4. Coordinate treatment with medical care providers. Medical care providers are often frustrated or discouraged when treating unstable, extroverted patients. It is useful to provide education about a patient's personality and how it influences behavior. Particularly effective is the development of a coordinated treatment plan, where medical care provider and mental health professional work in tandem to develop behavioral contracts to reduce HIV risk behaviors and build medication adherence. This is particularly useful when patients' lives are too chaotic to begin HAART. A step-wise plan that begins with stabilization on psychiatric medication and enrollment in psychotherapy can be rewarded by initiating HAART.

CONCLUSION

Personality characteristics and personality disorders reflect relatively stable, lifelong propensities that are difficult to change. This does not mean, however, that HIV risk reduction efforts are necessarily futile. Rather, by understanding certain personality characteristics and their role in HIV risk behaviors and medication adherence, the mental health professional can develop more effective, specific treatment strategies for psychiatric patients with personality vulnerabilities. Patients who can identify aspects of their personality that might influence intentions to practice safer behavior, and then develop strategies for dealing with these situations, may be less susceptible to high-risk situations. Finally, the mental health professional can provide

valuable assistance to medical care providers to improve health outcomes for these patients.

References

Abramson PR, and Pinkerton SD (1995). *With Pleasure: Thought on the Nature of Human Sexuality*. New York: Oxford University Press.

American Psychiatric Association (2000). *Diagnostic and Statistical Manual of Mental Disorders*, fourth edition, text revision (DSM-IV-TR) Washington, DC: American Psychiatric Press.

Blackwell B (1996). From compliance to alliance: a quarter century of research. *Netherlands J Med* 48: 140–149.

Bottonari KA, Roberts JE, Ciesla JA, and Hewitt RG (2005). Life stress and adherence to antiretroviral therapy among HIV-positive individuals: a preliminary investigation. *AIDS Patient Care STDS* 19: 719–727.

Brooner RK, Bigelow GE, Strain E, and Schmidt CW (1990). Intravenous drug users with antisocial personality disorder: increased HIV risk behavior. *Drug Alcohol Depend* 26:39–44.

Brooner RK, Greenfield L, Schmidt, CW, and Bigelow GE (1993). Antisocial personality disorder and HIV infection among intravenous drug users. *Am J Psychiatry* 150:53–58.

Cloninger CR (1999). *Personality and Psychopathology*. Washington, DC: American Psychiatric Press.

Cole SW, Kemeny ME, Fahey JL, Zack JA, Naliboff BD (2003). Psychological risk factors for HIV pathogenesis: mediation by the autonomic nervous system. *Biol Psychiatry* 54:1444–1456.

Costa PT Jr, and McCrae RR (1992). *Revised NEO Personality Inventory (NEO PI-R) and NEO Five-Factor Inventory (NEO-FFI) Professional Manual*. Odessa, FL: Psychological Assessment Resources.

Costa PT Jr, and Widiger TA (2002). *Personality Disorders and the Five-Factor Model of Personality*, second edition. Washington, DC: American Psychological Association.

Dinwiddie SH, Cottler L, Compton W, and Ben Aabdallah A (1996). Psychopathology and HIV risk behaviors among injection drug users in and out of treatment. *Drug Alcohol Depend* 43:1–11.

Disney E, Kidorf M, Kolodner K, King V, Peirce J, Beilenson P, and Brooner RK (2006). Psychiatric comorbidity is associated with drug use and HIV risk syringe exchanges participants. *J Nerv Ment Dis* 194:577–583.

Ellis D, Collins I, and King M (1995). Personality disorder and sexual risk taking among homosexually active and heterosexually active men attending a genitorurinary medicine clinic. *Psychosom Res* 39:901–910.

Eysenck HJ (1976). *Sex and Personality*. London: Open Books.

Eysenck HJ (1990). Genetic and environmental contributions to individual differences: the three major dimension of personality. *J Pers* 58:245–261.

Eysenck HJ, and Eysenck SBG (1975). *Eysenck Personality Questionnaire*. San Diego: EditTS/Educational and Industrial Testing Service.

Francis LJ, and Bennett GA (1992). Personality and religion among female drug misusers. *Drug Alcohol Depend* 30(1):27–31.

Golding M, and Perkins DO (1996). Personality disorder in HIV infection. *Int Rev Psychiatry* 8:253–258.

Hudgins R, McCusker J, and Stoddard A (1995). Cocaine use and risky injection and sexual behaviors. *Drug Alcohol Depend* 37:7–14.

Ickovics JR, and Meade CS (2002). Adherence to HAART among patients with HIV: breakthroughs and barriers. *AIDS Care* 14:309–318.

Jacobsberg L, Frances A, and Perry S (1995). Axis II diagnoses among volunteers for HIV testing and counseling. *Am J Psychiatry* 152:1222–1224.

Johnson JG, Williams JB, Rabkin JG, Goetz PR, and Remien RH (1995). Axis I psychiatric symptomatology associated with HIV infection and personality disorder. *Am J Psychiatry* 152:551–554.

Jung C (1923). *Psychological Types*. New York: Harcourt Brace.

Kalichman SC, and Cain D (2004). A prospective study of sensation seeking and alcohol use as predictors of sexual risk behaviors among men and women receiving sexually transmitted infection clinic services. *Psychol Addict Behav* 18:367–373.

Kalichman SC, and Rompa D (1995). Sexual sensation seeking and Sexual Compulsivity Scales: reliability, validity, and predicting HIV risk behavior. *J Pers Assess* 65:586–601.

Kalichman SC, Johnson JR, Adair V, Rompa D, Multhauf K, and Kelly JA (1994). Sexual sensation seeking: scale development and predicting AIDS-risk behavior among homosexually active men. *J Pers Assess* 62:385–397.

Kalichman SC, Heckman T, and Kelly JA (1996). Sensation-seeking as an explanation for the association between substance use and HIV-related risky sexual behavior. *Arch Sex Behav* 25:141–154.

Kalichman SC, Cain D, Knetch J, and Hill J (2005). Patterns of sexual risk behavior change among sexually transmitted infection clinic patients. *Arch Sex Behav* 34:307–319.

Kleinman PH, Millman RB, Robinson H, Lesser M, Hsu C, Engelhart P, and Finkelstein I (1994). Lifetime needle sharing: a predictive analysis. *J Subst Abuse Treat* 11:449–455.

Kosten T, and Rounsaville B (1988). Suicidality among opioid addicts: 2.5 year follow-up. *Am J Drug Alcohol Abuse* 14:357–369.

Kruse W, Eggert-Kruse W, Rampmaier J, Runnebaum B, and Weber E (1991). Dosage frequency and drug-compliance behavior—a comparative study on compliance with a medication to be take twice or four times daily. *Eur J Clin Pharmacol* 41:589–592.

Ladd GT, and Petry NM (2003). Antisocial personality in treatment-seeking cocaine abusers: psychosocial functioning and HIV risk. *J Subst Abuse Treat* 24:323–330.

Livesley WJ (2001). Conceptual and taxonomic issues. In: WH Livesley (ed.), *Handbook of Personality Disorders* (pp. 3–38). New York: Guilford Press.

Lodhi PH, and Thakur S (1993). Personality of drug addicts: Eysenckian analysis. *Pers Individ Diff* 15:121–128.

Lucas RE, Diener E, Grob A, Suh EM, and Shao L (2000). Cross-cultural evidence for the fundamental features of extraversion. *J Pers Soc Psychol* 79:452–468.

McCown W (1991). Contributions of the EPN paradigm to HIV prevention: a preliminary study. *Pers Individ Diff* 12:1301–1303.

McCown W (1993). Personality factors predicting failure to practice safer sex by HIV-positive males. *Pers Individ Diff* 14:613–615.

Meade CS, and Sikkema KJ (2005). Correlates of HIV testing among psychiatric outpatients. *AIDS Behav* 9:465–473.

Morey LC, and Zanarini MC (2000). Borderline personality: traits and disorder. *J Abnorm Psychol* 109:733–737.

Palmer NB, Salcedo J, Miller AL, Winiarski M, and Arno P (2003). Psychiatric and social barriers to HIV medication adherence in a triply diagnosed methadone population. *AIDS Patient Care STD* 17:635–644.

Paris J (1996). *Social Factors in the Personality Disorders: A Biopsychosocial Approach to Etiology and Treatment*. Cambridge, UK: Cambridge University Press.

Penedo FJ, Gonzalez JS, DAhn JR, Antoni M, Malow R, Costa PT Jr, and Schneiderman N (2003). Personality, quality of life and HAART adherence among men and women living HIV/AIDS. *J Psychosom Res* 59:271–278.

Perkins DO, Davidson EJ, Leserman J, Liao D, and Evans DL (1993). Personality disorder in patients infected with HIV: a controlled study with implications for clinical care. *Am J Psychiatry* 150:309–315.

Rothbart MK, and Ahadi SA (1994). Temperament and the development of personality. *J Abnorm Psychol* 103:55–66.

Rutter M (1987). Temperament, personality and personality disorder. *Br J Psychiatry* 150:443–458.

Sackett DL, and Snow JS (1988). The magnitude of compliance and noncompliance. In RB Haynes, DW Taylor, and D.L. Sackett (eds.), *Compliance in Health Care* (pp. 11–45). Baltimore: Johns Hopkins University Press.

Tanner WM, and Pollack RH (1988). The effect of condom use and erotic instructions on attitudes towards condoms. *J Sex Res* 25:537–541.

Tourian K, Alterman A, Metzger D, Rutherford M, Cacciola JS, and McKay JR (1997). Validity of three measures of antisociality in predicting HIV risk behaviors in methadone-maintenance patients. *Drug Alcohol Depend* 47:99–107.

Trobst KK, Wiggins JS, Costa PT, Jr, Herbst JH, McCrae RR, and Masters HL III (2000). Personality psychology and problem behaviors: HIV risk and the five-factor model. *J Pers* 68:1232–1252.

Weissman MM (1993). The epidemiology of personality disorders: a 1990 update. *J Pers Dis* 7(Suppl.):44–62.

Zuckerman M (1994). *Behavioral Expressions and Biosocial Bases of Sensation Seeking* (p. 27). New York: Cambridge University Press.

Zuckerman M, Eysenck S, and Eysenck HJ (1978). Sensation seeking in England and America: cross-cultural, age, and sex comparisons. *J Consult Clin Psychol* 46:139–149.

Part IV

Unique Psychiatric Manifestations of HIV Infection

Chapter 14

Distress in Persons with HIV and AIDS

*Harold W. Goforth, Mary Ann Cohen,
Sami Khalife, and Alicia Hurtado*

Distress is defined as "pain or suffering affecting the body, a bodily part, or the mind" (Webster's Online Dictionary, 2006). Thus, psychological distress can be seen as an unsettling psychological state that interferes with a person's overall well-being. In this chapter, we will attempt to understand these sources from a bio-psychosocial approach, exploring some of the physical and social factors that affect psychological distress, including cultural and political components. We will also present ways to screen for, recognize, and cope with psychological distress.

Persons with HIV infection and AIDS have high levels of distress from multiple sources including symptoms (such as fatigue, pruritus, and insomnia), medical and psychiatric illness, discrimination and stigma, as well as social, occupational, and financial stresses. AIDS can affect nearly every organ and system with severe and multiple illnesses. Individuals with HIV and AIDS may have severe psychiatric illnesses as well. Psychiatric sources of distress were present in 52% of patients presenting to an HIV clinic

for evaluation and treatment in a study by Lyketsos and colleagues (1996). Actual distress rates of homeless persons with AIDS who do not self-present for treatment are likely higher. Persons with AIDS are also subject to the same losses, stresses, and life changes as the rest of the population and, because they are living longer, and are subject to other non-HIV-related illnesses such as heart disease, hypertension, diabetes mellitus, osteoarthritis, cancer, and chronic obstructive pulmonary disease. The symptoms of fatigue, insomnia, and pruritus may occur even in the absence of specific medical or psychiatric pathology. Persons with AIDS may also have symptoms related to highly active antiretroviral therapy (HAART) or interferon treatment for concomitant hepatitis C. An overview of the biopsychosocial determinants of distress is presented in Table 14.1.

This chapter will explore the myriad of biopsychosocial sources of distress in persons with HIV and AIDS in order to provide a brief but comprehensive summary. The specific issues that may cause distress are

TABLE 14.1. Biopsychosocial Determinants of Distress in Persons Living with HIV Infection

Biological	Psychological	Social
Pain	Depression	Alienation
Confusion	Anxiety	Social isolation
Cognitive decline	Psychosis	Stigma
Disfigurement	Mania	Discrimination
Dyspnea	Withdrawal	Spiritual isolation
Insomnia	Intoxication	Financial loss
Fatigue	Substance misuse	Unemployment
Nausea	Existential anxiety	Loss of housing
Vomiting	Bereavement	Loss of key roles
Diarrhea	Suicidality	Loss of meaning
Blindness		Loss of independence
Paralysis		
Weakness		
Cachexia		
Incontinence		
Pruritus		
Hiccups		

covered in more depth throughout this text. Chapter 1 addresses stigma, Chapter 4, the prevalence of psychiatric disorders, Chapter 5, sociocultural vulnerabilities, Chapters 3 through 13, the psychiatric disorders, Chapters 14 through 18, special symptoms and psychiatric manifestations of HIV, Chapters 19, 20, and 33 through 37, the medical illnesses, and Chapter 39, end-of-life issues.

MEASURING DISTRESS

Distress, depression, and anxiety can be measured rapidly and easily by means of the Distress Thermometer (DT) and the Hospital Anxiety and Depression Scale (HADS). Roth and colleagues (1998) and Cohen and colleagues (2002) have demonstrated the feasibility of using these scales in waiting-room convenience samples of persons with cancer and AIDS, respectively. Cohen et al. found a 72.3% prevalence of distress on the DT, 70.3% prevalence of anxiety on the HADS, 45.5% prevalence of depression on the HADS, and 53.5% prevalence of both anxiety and depression on the HADS in a waiting-room sample of persons registered at an HIV clinic. The DT and HADS are also valuable for screening persons with HIV and hepatitis C virus (HCV) prior to interferon-ribavirin treatment to provide a baseline score and to follow patients during the course of treatment to determine the need for

antidepressant or antipsychotic medications. The rapidity (5 minutes in total for both the DT and HADS) and feasibility of the DT and HADS make them excellent tools for screening for distress in a busy HIV clinic.

DISTRESS ON THREE CONTINENTS

Distress and suffering are ubiquitous phenomena and occur across all cultures, although the specific expressions of distress and suffering may differ across cultural systems. Studies of distress in persons with HIV and AIDS have been done in many different parts of the world, including North America, Africa, the Caribbean, and South America. The results of these studies illustrate the need for effective interventions designed to improve the quality of life for affected individuals.

It is well known that HIV infection is not equally distributed in the general population, and in the United States, African Americans and Latinos (who constitute 25% of the general U.S. population) are, respectively, 11 and 4 times more likely than non-Latino whites to be diagnosed with AIDS (CDC, 2002). Approximately 70% of new HIV infections are among African American and Latino individuals, and this pattern extends to at-risk adolescent and young men, whose incident rates are much higher than those among white groups, even when controlling for socioeconomic status (Valleroy et al., 2000). This disparity creates significant distress in multiple ways— minorities are at higher risk of racial and ethnic discrimination than non-minority groups because of limited opportunities for employment, housing, education, and health care, and are more likely to experience unfair treatment (Cain and Kington, 2003). These perceptions produce a wide array of negative emotional and stress responses that predict a range of negative physical and mental health outcomes (Williams et al., 2003).

HIV infection among Asians and Pacific Islanders (API) in the United States continues to increase given the escalating prevalence of HIV in Asia and the increasing number of immigrants from these regions (Operario et al., 2005). Asians and Pacific Islanders often face unnecessary delays in accessing medical and supportive services (Eckholdt and Chin, 1997; Eckholdt et al., 1997; Pounds et al., 2002) for treatment of their HIV. Distress related to disclosure of HIV status due to fears of discrimination by peers, employers, and family members (Chin et al., 1999; Yoshioka et al., 2001) is further compounded by discrimination based on race, immigration status, culturally disapproved lifestyle, and sexual orientation (Herek, 1999; Kang and Rapkin, 2003; Kang et al., 2003).

Studies have also shown the interconnection between distress and engaging in risky sexual behavior, as exemplified by a study of Latino gay men recruited from social venues (bars, clubs, and weeknight events) in the cities of New York, Miami, and Los Angeles (Diaz et al., 2004). Diaz found that a substantial number of reported experiences of social discrimination on the basis of sexual orientation were combined with racial and ethnic discrimination within the context of the gay community. Symptoms of psychological distress reported for 6 months were highly prevalent in this group: 61% reported sleep problems; 44% reported symptoms of anxiety and panic on at least one occasion; 80% reported a sad or depressed mood at least once; and 17% reported suicidal ideation at least once.

Africa has one of the world's highest prevalence rates of HIV and AIDS, and has limited access to effective therapy. The effect of HIV on Africa has been devastating; 11 million children in sub-Saharan Africa alone have witnessed the death of at least one parent to complications of AIDS (Atwine et al., 2005). Shawn and colleagues (2005) noted that palliative care for

HIV is currently the standard treatment in Africa because of limited access to antiviral treatment. They noted that pain, skin complaints, respiratory infections, fatigue, anger, and social isolation figured prominently in patients' lives (Shawn et al., 2005). Poor quality of life and high levels of distress have been noted in other South African studies as well (O'Keefe and Wood, 1996). Likewise, Atwine and colleagues (2005) investigated the psychosocial consequences of AIDS for 123 orphans with AIDS in rural Uganda and found that orphan status was a significant predictor of increased distress associated with higher rates of anxiety, depression, and anger.

The impact of increased distress is not limited to those who have been orphaned as a result of AIDS, but includes those who are forced to care for family members living with HIV and other chronic and severe illness. In systematic interviews of caregivers of HIV patients in Botswana, older women reported feeling overwhelmed with the complexity and magnitude of the tasks facing them, often neglecting their own health and experiencing high levels of exhaustion, malnourishment, and depression. Among younger girls there were high rates of physical and sexual abuse, depression, and truancy from school, and all ages experienced poverty and had high rates of social isolation (Lindsey et al., 2003).

The experience of gays, lesbians, and bisexuals in Botswana and, by extrapolation, sub-Saharan Africa is equally poor, as same-sex activities are illegal in many sub-Saharan countries, punishable by imprisonment or death. Varying levels of distress in up to two-thirds of this population have been documented, and distress appears to stem predominantly from health concerns, discrimination, and sexual violence (Ehlers et al., 2001). Botswana has been noted to have one of Africa's leading health care systems (Ehlers et al., 2001); therefore, the distress level in many regions may actually be higher than the 64% rate encountered in Ehlers's study.

HIV is a growing problem in most South American and Caribbean countries, and it is endemic in Haiti in proportions equal to those of many sub-Saharan African regions. Distress levels associated with HIV in these countries reflects those of the African experience, with rates exceeding 50%. A survey of HIV-associated distress in an ambulatory HIV clinic in the Dominican Republic indicated prevalence rates of distress of 49% on the DT; anxiety, 58% on the HADS; depression, 44% on the HADS; and an overall HADS rate of 49%

(A. Hurtado, 2005, unpublished data). Fewer resources dedicated to HIV care are available in these countries, and increasing infection rates drain existing medical resources and tax populations as a whole.

MEDICAL COMPLICATIONS AS SOURCES OF DISTRESS

Other factors causing distress are the multiple complications resulting from immunological suppression, including visual loss, neurological illness, and fears of progressive health decline and changes in one's ability to care for one's self independently. Cytomegalovirus (CMV) retinopathy is one of the most distressing complications of HIV disease, as it results in vision loss with accompanying social isolation, loss of independence, and loss of function.

Visual Loss as a Source of Distress

The advent of HAART therapy has altered the natural progression of HIV and has changed the incidence, natural history, management, and sequelae of HIV-associated retinopathy, especially CMV-associated retinopathy. Before use of HAART, CMV retinitis was common, occurring in 20%–40% of seropositive patients. Patients were relegated to indefinite intravenous therapy, and between 25% and 50% suffered retinal detachment. Survival after development of CMV retinitis was 6–10 months. The incidence of CMV retinitis declined by approximately 80% after the advent of HAART therapy, and mean survival has increased to over 1 year from time of diagnosis (Holbrook et al., 2003; Goldberg et al., 2005). However, visual loss and blindness from multiple etiologies are still significant causes for concern and sources of distress for patients with HIV (Ng et al., 2000; Kestelyn and Cunningham 2001; Hill and Dubey 2002; Oette et al., 2005).

Specific studies examining the quality of life and distress experienced by persons with visual loss have not been performed among persons with HIV disease. However, data on distress among patients with macular degeneration and other acquired forms of visual loss may be used to better understand the sense of isolation, psychological distress, and limitations these patients experience on a routine basis. Data from patients with acquired macular degeneration indicated a strong association between decline in vision and

functional impairment, along with high rates of depression, anxiety, and emotional distress (Berman and Brodaty, 2006). In a study focusing on patients' attitudes toward visual loss from subfoveal choroidal neovascularization, patients reported that they would rather suffer medical illnesses such as dialysis-dependent renal failure and AIDS than visual impairment (Bass et al., 2004). Similar findings have been noted in studies of diabetes mellitus–associated visual loss (Cox et al., 1998). Clearly, across multiple medical conditions, acquired visual loss has a profound impact on self-perception of overall health-related quality of life, distress, and suffering.

Neurological Decline and HIV Disease

Cognitive disorders, vacuolar myelopathy, and sensory neuropathies are the most common neurological disorders in patients with HIV disease and are a great source of fear and distress in this population. One of the most disturbing aspects of advancing HIV disease is the prospect of progressive physical and cognitive impairment leading to eventual complete incapacity. Since the advent of HAART therapy, however, there has been an approximate 50% reduction in HIV-related neurological complications (Maschke et al., 2000; Sacktor, 2002). Distress and fear of loss of independence and functionality continue among patients nonetheless.

Mapou and colleagues (1993) studied neuropsychological performance of 79 military medical beneficiaries infected with HIV and that of 27 HIV-seronegative control subjects. Seropositive subjects who complained of subjective difficulties had more deficits in attention, response speed, motor function, and memory than those not reporting difficulties. Seropositive individuals also had increased rates of anxiety and depression, illustrating the need for screening for both disturbances in seropositive individuals, as each may become a significant source of distress. The pathophysiology and potential treatment of dementia are discussed further in Chapters 3, 10, and 19.

Pain and Distress in HIV Disease

Pain is an incapacitating symptom in many people with HIV and AIDS, and untreated pain leads to an increase in psychological distress and a reduction in quality of life. Sources of pain are varied and range from neuropathic pain to chronic pain of malignancy, and all types of pain are associated with increased suicidal risk. Pain is undertreated particularly in patients with HIV and AIDS, in part because of the common prevalence of substance abuse disorder. Pain is especially common in this setting and ranges from 28% to 97% across various studies (Schoefferman, 1988; Lebovits et al., 1989; McCormack et al., 1993; Reiter and Kudler, 1996).

Abdominal pain and neuropathic pain were the most common pain complaints in one study at a pain consultation service; other causes included odynophagia, dysphagia, headache, cutaneous pain, musculoskeletal pain, and postherpetic neuralgia (Newshan and Wainapel, 1993). Inadequate pain assessment is a major factor in the undertreatment of pain, and use of standardized pain assessment measures may assist in both assessment and treatment. Practitioners need to be educated to address myths such as (a) people overestimate their pain; (b) minority groups exaggerate their pain complaints; (c) people with a past history of addiction routinely lie about pain to secure drugs; (d) pain is often psychogenic in etiology; and (e) the etiology of pain remains obscure in most cases. In fact, patients have been shown to be reluctant to volunteer pain complaints. Thus routine assessment is needed (Von Roenn et al., 1993), with instruments such as the Wisconsin Brief Pain Inventory (BPI), which measures adequacy of analgesia and impact of pain on related psychosocial factors. Further discussion of pain assessment and management can be found in Chapters 20 and 30, which deal with neurological complications in HIV and palliative care for persons with HIV, respectively.

Cardiopulmonary Disease in HIV

HIV-associated cardiomyopathy can be a direct result of HIV disease, HIV treatment, comorbid conditions, and other etiologies. Cardiomyopathy has been identified in up to 20% of HIV-seropositive patients (Fisher and Lipschultz, 2001). It appears to have a more pernicious course in HIV-positive patients, with symptoms including dyspnea, peripheral and pulmonary edema, hepatosplenomegaly, and arrhythmias (Currie et al., 1994). Dilated cardiomyopathy is the most frequently identified cardiac disease associated with HIV and is an independent predictor of mortality, but other manifestations include myocarditis, bacterial and fungal endocarditis, pulmonary hypertension, malignancy, accelerated atherosclerosis, and autonomic dysfunction (Dakin et al., 2006).

Similarly, respiratory events and illnesses such as opportunistic infections, tuberculosis, malignancies, adult respiratory distress syndrome, and pulmonary fibrosis (Rosen et al., 1997) remain common in HIV-seropositive populations, especially among those with CD4 counts $<200/mm^3$ and injection drug abusers. Importantly, the risk of these disorders appears to increase with advancing HIV disease despite the widespread use of antibiotic prophylaxis (Wallace et al., 1993; Hirschtick et al., 1995).

Distress in these populations is created by both the psychological implications of advancing HIV disease and the imposition of severe physical limitations related to cardiopulmonary disease. Such limitations further isolate this population and limit individuals' ability to perform previously enjoyable coping activities such as exercise. In advanced cases, they impinge directly on patients' ability to maintain independence and perform activities of daily living, serving as a constant reminder of impending mortality.

Diarrhea in HIV Disease

Another common potential source of distress among HIV-seropositive patients is bacterial diarrhea, which has been noted to predict increased use of hospital resources, longer hospital admissions, and an increased prevalence of opportunistic infections such as *Pneumocystis carinii* pneumonia. *Clostridium difficile* colitis and associated diarrhea were the etiology in approximately 32% of study patients in a large, Chicago-based, public hospital study. It appears that this disorder is more likely to present among advanced-HIV patients (Pulvirenti et al., 2002). Other notable causes include *Shigella*, *Campylobacter*, and *Salmonella* species, which may reflect progressive deficits in mucosal immune function in advanced HIV disease (Sanchez et al., 2005).

From a mental health standpoint, bacterial diarrhea can cause significant distress in that it both limits environmental freedom and self-sufficiency and serves as a marker and reminder of advancing disease. Fears of loss of bowel control and fecal incontinence further isolate a high-risk population from available social support. These conditions can also be a source of HIV-associated wasting and general decline. While no specific studies have addressed the issue of distress in this population, in our experience the associated distress and impairment from chronic diarrhea can be profoundly embarrassing, with significant limitation in life satisfaction.

Itching in HIV Disease

Medical sources of distress are not limited to major organ systems such as cardiorespiratory and gastrointestinal systems but include a variety of scenarios and organ systems. Pruritus is a common manifestation of advancing liver disease, which is discussed further in the context of HIV in Chapter 33. Likewise, renal disease with associated uremia can produce significant symptoms of itching; renal complications associated with HIV disease are covered more extensively in Chapter 34. Studies of distress in relation to HIV disease and itching have not been performed, but quality-of-life studies of chronic urticarial illness have demonstrated marked reductions in quality of life in terms of both social functioning and emotional capacity (Staubach et al., 2006).

Insomnia

One area that has been linked to distress and a reduction in quality of life in HIV is insomnia. Complaints of lack of sleep from persons with HIV disease are ubiquitous, but etiologies are varied and often include a combination of comorbid Axis I conditions, medical conditions affecting sleep quality, and potentially a direct role of HIV on the brain. In a review of insomnia in the setting of HIV, Reid and Dwyer (2005) noted that up to 60% of HIV-positive individuals experienced sleep disturbances, and greater psychological distress appeared to be related to greater sleep difficulties and lower numbers of CD3 and CD8 cells. This review highlights the importance of effective interventions designed to improve sleep quality and in turn potentially reduce distress and improve life quality. Further details of HIV-associated sleep abnormalities are addressed in Chapter 15.

Fatigue

Fatigue is one of the most limiting of the HIV syndromes in terms of quality of life and its incremental impact on dealing effectively with advancing HIV disease, comorbid depression, and hepatitis C coinfection. HIV-related fatigue decreases functional status, which in turn can lead to symptoms of isolation,

inability to perform required self-care, and nonadherence to medications. In fact, fatigue, along with neurological symptoms, is one of two domains that independently predicts functional decline in instrumental activities of daily living, even when controlling for sociodemographic variables (Wilson and Cleary, 1997).

In a cross-sectional survey of ambulatory AIDS patients, Breitbart and colleagues (1998) found that over 50% of respondents had fatigue according to self-report with the Memorial Symptom Assessment Scale. Women appeared significantly more likely to experience fatigue than men, and fatigue was associated with several other variables, including the number of AIDS-related physical symptoms, the current treatment of HIV disease, anemia, and pain. Those subjects reporting significant fatigue suffered increased rates of both psychological distress and lower quality of life across several standardized rating scales (Breitbart et al., 1998).

Fatigue also plays an important role in HCV infection, as fatigue is a common complaint among sufferers of HCV both prior to and during treatment with biological agents such as interferon-based therapies. Four hundred and eighty-four HIV-seropositive subjects participated in a self-report trial which confirmed that HCV-coinfected patients demonstrated significantly more elements of distress compared to the HIV-only group in social, psychological, and biological arenas. The patients were also more likely to be in unstable social situations and to experience depression, fatigue, and reduced quality of life (Braitstein et al., 2005).

The treatment of fatigue is an important area for psychiatrists treating patients with HIV, as it can directly improve quality of life, alleviate distress, and improve functioning. Breitbart and colleagues (2001) and others have described effective and safe treatments with either methylphenidate or pemoline. The role of antidepressants, androgenic steroids, and modafinil in treating fatigue has also been examined (Rabkin et al., 2004a, 2004b). Further discussion of HIV-associated fatigue can be found in Chapter 16.

AIDS PALLIATIVE CARE AND DEATH AND DYING

End-of-life issues involve complex decision making, and issues such as wills and estates take on overtones of the finality of life. They can also provide an impetus for overall life review, which can prove quite distressing to a patient who is unprepared for this process. These decisions are increasingly complicated and distressing, as recent political actions have been taken to limit the ability of same-sex couples to enter contracts approximating marriage with survival benefits. Dying patients must struggle with the impact of their dying on loved ones and caregivers, and caregiver distress can frequently lead to burnout and suboptimal care for the patient.

AIDS palliative care has been defined as comprehensive, multidisciplinary care that focuses on alleviating suffering and maximizing life potentials across all stages of disease severity, independent of stage or prognosis (personal communication, Daniel Fischberg). Most clinicians associate palliative care with end-stage illness only, but the true nature of palliative care makes it appropriate at every stage by focusing on comfort. Comfort gradually assumes a more important role as the disease progresses and cures of specific complications become less likely. This gradual transition to a comfort-care model minimizes sources of distress associated with an abrupt change from a curative model to a comfort-care-only model that can occur in the terminal phases of HIV.

Different methods of comfort care such as pastoral care, hypnosis, music, relaxation, meditation, writing, and art can be incorporated with much success, and these methods need to be integrated and offered to persons during the entire course of their illness on a routine basis (Cohen, 1999). Depression, anxiety, pain, and other mental health disorders need to be addressed with both psychotherapy and pharmacotherapy using multiple models, including crisis, individual, group, and family therapy, over the entire spectrum of illness. Integration of spiritual care has been shown to provide comfort and solace to persons suffering with cancer (Saunders, 1988; Jacox et al., 1994). Attempts to provide these interventions across the spectrum of HIV illness will improve the seamless attention given to the associated suffering and distress.

We have noted that untreated pain and pruritus are associated with severe psychological reactions, including depression, anxiety, and suicidality. Dyspnea inspires feeling of anxiety, panic, and fear of death by asphyxiation. Periods of prolonged hiccups can lead to exhaustion and feelings of helplessness, and untreated psychological symptoms can exacerbate somatic complaints. Prompt attention to psychological distress complements palliative symptom management strategies.

Being physically present with the patient is important at the end of life and can alleviate the fear of abandonment often experienced by dying individuals. Simple acts such as talking, holding hands, and surrounding the patient with loved ones provide muchneeded healing and comfort at this stage. Clinicians who can cope with and tolerate the intimacy and evoked feelings of such moments can also experience significant healing and personal rewards.

TREATMENT OF DISTRESS OCCURRING IN THE CONTEXT OF HIV INFECTION

Use of HAART has dramatically improved the lives of millions of patients living with HIV/AIDS and has transformed HIV into a chronic illness. Few studies have investigated adequately the impact of HAART on the psychological well-being of infected individuals, but currently available evidence does suggest the beneficial role of HAART on psychological well-being (Rabkin et al., 2000). The effect of HAART on reducing distress has been shown in other studies as well (BeLow-Beer et al., 2000). Other interventions can begin by identifying distress through routine use of screening instruments. Prompt identification and treatment of comorbid psychiatric disease can allow initiation of effective interventions and minimize suffering. Attention to psychological coping mechanisms and bolstering of social and spiritual supports can limit the impact of loneliness and social isolation, thus enabling a higher quality of life in this vulnerable population.

CONCLUSIONS

Persons living with HIV and AIDS have witnessed radical shifts in the prognosis and treatment associated with this devastating illness over the last 25 years. The advent of potent antiretroviral medications has transformed AIDS from a fatal illness with serial health crises into a chronic illness with a focus on long-term considerations and health maintenance. However, HIV and AIDS continue to cause distress through multiple mechanisms involving biologic processes, psychological states, and social situations. Persons with AIDS can live more comfortable lives through the establishment of nurturing and supportive health-care paradigms. Education about medical and psychiatric care, pain management, and decision-making capacity can help persons with HIV and their caregivers meet the challenges of this illness with optimism and dignity.

References

Atwine B, Cantor-Graae E, and Bajunirwe F (2005). Psychological distress among AIDS orphans in rural Uganda. *Soc Sci Med* 61:555–564.

Bass EB, Marsh MJ, Mangione CM, Bressler NM, Childs AL, Dong LM, Hawkins BS, Jaffee HA, and Miskala P (2004). Submacular Surgery Trials Research Group. Patients' perceptions of the value of current vision: assessment of preference values among patients with subfoveal choroidal neovascularization. The Submacular Surgery Trials Vision Preference Value Scale: SST Report No. 6. *Arch Ophthalmol* 122:1856–1867.

BeLow-Beer S, Chan K, Yip B, et al. (2000). Depressive symptoms decline among persons on HIV protease inhibitors. *J Acquir Immune Defic Syndr* 23:295–301.

Berman K, and Brodaty H (2006). Psychosocial effects of age-related macular degeneration. *Int Psychogeriatr* 1:1–14.

Braitstein P, Montessori V, Chan K, Montaner JS, Schecter MT, O'Shaughnessy MV, and Hogg RS (2005). Quality of life, depression and fatigue among persons co-infected with HIV and hepatitis C: outcomes from a population-based cohort. *AIDS Care* 17:105–115.

Breitbart W, McDonald MV, Rosenfeld B, Monkman ND, and Passik S (1998). Fatigue in ambulatory AIDS patients. *J Pain Symptom Manage* 15:159–167.

Breitbart W, Rosenfeld B, Kaim M, and Funesti-Esch J (2001). A randomized, double-blind, placebo-controlled trial of psychostimulants for the treatment of fatigue in ambulatory patients with human immunodeficiency virus disease. *Arch Intern Med* 161:411–120.

Cain VS, and Kington RS (2003). Investigating the role of racial/ethnic bias in health outcomes. *Am J Public Health* 93:191–192.

[CDC] Centers for Disease Control and Prevention (2002). *HIV/AIDS Surveillance Report 2002*, Vol. 14. Retreived March 26, 2007, from www.cdc.gov/hiv/topics/surveillance/resources/reports/2002report/default.htm.

Chin D, and Kroesen KW (1999). Disclosure of HIV infection among API American women: cultural stigma and support. *Cultur Divers Ethnic Minor Psychol* 5:222–235.

Cohen MA (1999). Psychodynamic psychotherapy in an AIDS nursing home. *J Am Acad Psychoanal* 27:121–133.

Cohen MA, Hoffman RG, Cromwell C, Schmeidler J, Ebrahim F, Carrera G, Endorf F, Alfonso CA, and Jacobson JM (2002). The prevalence of distress in persons with human immunodeficiency virus infection. *Psychosomatics* 43:10–15.

Cox DJ, Kiernan BD, Schroeder DB, and Cowley M (1998). Psychosocial sequelae of visual loss in diabetes. *Diabetes Educ* 24:481–484.

Currie PF, Jacob AJ, Foreman AR, Elton RA, Brettle RP, and Boon NA (1994). Heart muscle disease related to HIV infection: prognostic implications. *BMJ* 309:1605–1607.

Dakin CL, O'Connor CA, and Patsdaughter CA (2006). HAART to heart: HIV-related cardiomyopathy and other cardiovascular complications. *AACN Clin Issues* 17:18–29.

Diaz RM, Ayala G, and Bein E (2004). Sexual risk as an outcome of social oppression: data from probability sample of Latino gay men in three US cities. *Cultur Divers Ethnic Minor Psychol* 10:255–267.

Eckholdt H, and Chin J (1997). *Pneumocystis carini* pneumonia in Asians and Pacific Islanders. *Clin Infect Dis* 24:1265–1267.

Eckholdt HM, Chin JJ, Manzon-Santos JA, and Kim DD (1997). The needs of Asians and Pacific Islanders living with HIV in New York City. *AIDS Educ Prev* 9:493–504.

Ehlers VJ, Zuverduin A, and Oosthuizen MJ (2001). The well-being of gays, lesbians and bisexuals in Botswana. *J Adv Nurs* 35:848–856.

Fisher SD, and Lipshultz SE (2001). Epidemiology of cardiovascular involvement in HIV disease and AIDS. *Ann NY Acad Sci* 946:13–22.

Goldberg DE, Smithen LM, Angelilli A, Freean WR. HIV-associated retinopathy in the HAART era. *Retina* 25:633–649.

Herek GM (1999). AIDS and stigma. *Am Behav Sci* 42:1106–1116.

Hill D, and Dubey JP (2002). *Toxoplasma gondii*: transmission, diagnosis and prevention. *Clin Microbiol Infect* 8:634–640.

Hirschtick RE, Glassroth J, Jordan MC, Wilcosky TC, Wallace JM, Kvale PA, Markowitz N, Rosen MJ, Mangura BT, and Hopewell PC (1995). Bacterial pneumonia in persons infected with the human immunodeficiency virus. Pulmonary Complications of HIV Infection Study Group. *N Engl J Med* 333:845–851.

Holbrook JT, Jabs DA, Weinberg DV, Lewis RA, Davis MD, and Friedberg D (2003). Studies of Ocular Complications of AIDS (SOCA) Research Group. Visual loss in patients with cytomegalovirus retinitis and acquired immunodeficiency syndrome before widespread availability of highly active antiretroviral therapy. *Arch Ophthalmol* 121:99–107.

Jacox AJ, Carr DB, and Payne R (1994). New clinical practice guidelines for the management of pain in patients with cancer. *N Engl J Med* 330:651.

Kang E, and Rapkin B (2003). Adherence to antiretroviral medication among undocumented Asians living with HIV disease in New York City. *Community Psycholog* 36:35–38.

Kang E, Rapkin B, Springer C, and Kim JH (2003). The "demon plague" and access to care among Asian undocumented immigrants living with HIV disease in New York City. *J Immigr Health* 5:49–58.

Kestelyn PG, and Cunningham ET Jr (2001). HIV/AIDS and blindness. *Bull World Health Organ* 79:208–213.

Lebovits AH, Lefkowitz M, McCarthy D, Simon R, Wilpon H, Jung R, and Fried E (1989). The prevalence and management of pain in patients with AIDS: a review of 134 cases. *Clin J Pain* 5(3):245–248.

Lindsey E, Hirschfeld M, and Tlou S (2003). Home-based care in Botswana: experiences of older women and young girls. *Health Care Women Int* 24:486–501.

Lyketsos CG, Hutton H, Fishman M, Schwartz J, and Treisman GJ (1996). Psychiatric morbidity on entry to an HIV primary care clinic. *AIDS* 10:1033–1039.

Mapou RL, Law WA, Martin A, Kampen D, Salazar AM, and Rundell JR (1993). Neuropsychological performance, mood, and complaints of cognitive and motor difficulties in individuals infected with the human immunodeficiency virus. *J Neuropsychiatry Clin Neurosci* 5:86–93.

Maschke M, Kastrup O, Esser S, Ross B, Hengge U, and Hufnagel A (2000). Incidence and prevalence of neurological disorders associated with HIV since the introduction of highly active antiretroviral therapy (HAART). *J Neurol Neurosurg Psychiatry* 69:376–380.

McCormack JP, Li R, Zarowny D, and Singer J (1993). Inadequate treatment of pain in ambulatory HIV patients. *Clin J Pain* 9:279–283.

Newshan GT, and Wainapel SF (1993). Pain characteristics and their management in persons with AIDS. *J Assoc Nurses AIDS Care* 4:53–59.

Ng CW, Lam MS, and Paton NI (2000). Cryptococcal meningitis resulting in irreversible visual impairment in AIDS patients: a report of two cases. *Singapore Med J* 41:80–82.

Oette M, Hemker J, Feldt T, Sagir A, Best J, and Haussinger D (2005). Acute syphilitic blindness in an HIV-positive patient. *AIDS Patient Care STDS* 19:209–211.

O'Keefe EA, and Wood R (1996). The impact of human immunodeficiency virus (HIV) infection on quality of life in a multiracial South African population. *Qual Life Res* 5:275–280.

Operario D, Nemoto T, Ng T, Syed J, and Mazarei M (2005). Conducting HIV interventions for Asian Pacific Islander men who have sex with men: challenges and compromises in community collaborative research. *AIDS Educ Prev* 17:334–346.

Pounds MB, Conviser R, Ashman JJ, and Bourassa V (2002). Ryan White CARE Act service use by Asian/Pacific Islanders and other clients in three California metropolitan areas (1997–1998). *J Community Health* 27:403–417.

Pulvirenti JJ, Mehra T, Hafiz I, DeMarais P, Marsh D, Kocka F, Meyer PM, Fischer SA, Goodman L, Gerding DN, and Weinstein RA (2002). Epidemiology and outcome of *Clostridium difficile* infection and diarrhea in HIV infected inpatients. *Diagn Microbiol Infect Dis* 44:325–330.

Rabkin JG, Ferrando SJ, Lin Sh, Sewell M, McElhiney M (2000). Psychological effects of HAART: a 2-year study. *Psychosom Med* 62:413–422.

Rabkin JG, McElhiney MC, Rabkin R, and Ferrando SJ (2004a). Modafinil treatment for fatigue in HIV+ patients: a pilot study. *J Clin Psychiatry* 65:1688–1695.

Rabkin JG, Wagner GJ, EcElhiney MC, Rabkin R, and Lin SH (2004b). Testosterone versus fluoxetine for depression and fatigue in HIV/AIDS: a placebo-controlled trial. *J Clin Psychopharmacol* 24:379–385.

Reid S, and Dwyer J (2005). Insomnia in HIV infection: a systematic review of prevalence, correlates, and management. *Psychosom Med* 67:260–269.

Reiter GS, and Kudler NR (1996). Palliative care and HIV, part II: systemic manifestations and late-stage issues. *AIDS Clin Care* 8:27–36.

Roth AJ, Kornblith AB, Batel-Copel L, Peabody E, Scher HI, and Holland JC (1998). Rapid screening for psychological distress in men with prostate carcinoma: a pilot study. *Cancer* 82:1904–1908.

Sacktor N (2002). The epidemiology of human immunodeficiency virus–associated neurological disease in the era of highly active antiretroviral therapy. *J Neurovirol* 8(Suppl. 2):115–121.

Sanchez TH, Brooks JT, Sullivan PS, Juhasz M, Mintz E, Dworkin MS, and Jones JL (2005). Adult/Adolescent Spectrum of HIV Disease Study Group. Bacterial diarrhea in persons with HIV infection, United States, 1992–2002. *Clin Infect Dis* 41:1621–1627.

Saunders C (1988). Spiritual pain. *J Palliat Care* 4:29–32.

Schofferman J (1988). Pain: diagnosis and management in the palliative care of AIDS. *J Palliat Care* 4:46–49.

Shawn ER, Campbell L, Mnguni MB, Defilippi KM, and Williams AB (2005). The spectrum of symptoms among rural South Africans with HIV infection. *J Assoc Nurses AIDS Care* 16:12–23.

Staubach P, Eckhardt-Henn A, Dechene M, Vonend A, Metz M, Magerl M, Breuer P, and Maurer M (2006). Quality of life in patients with chronic urticaria is differentially impaired and determined by psychiatric comorbidity. *Br J Dermatol* 154:294–298.

Valleroy LA, MacKellar DA, Karon JM, Rosen DH, McFarland W, Shehan DA, Stoyanoff SR, LaLota M, Celentano DD, Koblin BA, Thiede H, Katz MH, Torian LV, and Janssen RS (2000). HIV prevalence and associated risks in young men who have sex with men. Young Men's Survey Study Group. *JAMA* 284:198–204.

Von Roenn JH, Cleeland CS, Gonin R, Hatfield AK, and Pandya KJ (1993). Physician attitudes and practice in cancer pain management. A survey from the Eastern Cooperative Oncology Group. *Ann Intern Med* 119:121–126.

Wallace JM, Rao AV, Glassroth J, Hansen NI, Rosen MJ, Arakaki C, Kvale PA, Reichman LB, and Hopewell PC (1993). Respiratory illness in persons with human immunodeficiency virus infection. The Pulmonary Complications of HIV Infection Study Group. *Am Rev Respir Dis* 148:1523–1529.

Webster's Online Dictionary. Accessed May 22, 2006.

William DR, Neighbors HW, and Jackson JS (2003). Racial/ethnic discrimination and health: findings from community studies. *Am J Public Health* 93:200–208.

Wilson IB, and Cleary PD (1997). Clinical predictors of declines in physical functioning in persons with AIDS: results of a longitudinal study. *J Acquir Immune Defic Syndr Hum Retrovirol* 16:343–349.

Yoshioka MR, and Schustack A (2001). Disclosure of HIV status: cultural issues of Asian patients. *AIDS Patient Care STDs* 15:77–82.

Chapter 15

Insomnia and HIV:
A Biopsychosocial Approach

Mary Alice O'Dowd
and Maria Fernanda Gomez

Sleep that knits up the ravel'd sleave of care,
The death of each day's life, sore labor's bath,
Balm of hurt minds, great nature's second course
Chief nourisher in life's feast
—Macbeth, II, ii, 36

Shakespeare's Macbeth recognized the vital role of sleep in the renewal and nourishment of mind and body, but until recently, medical science has tended to give sleep disorders scant attention. Insomnia, the most common sleep disorder, can be a symptom of many disorders and has been described as a major public health problem that impacts the lives of millions of individuals, their families, and communities (NIH, 2005). However, random studies of adults have found that the majority of those with sleep complaints are unlikely to broach the topic with a health care provider (Martin and Ancoli-Israel, 2003). When a patient does complain of insomnia, the complaint may be either given short shrift by the clinician or a sleep medication may be prescribed for short-term use without much attention to the etiology of the complaint or to follow-up. Insomnia is not just an annoyance. It has been shown to affect cognitive functioning, quality of life, and even longevity (Martin and Ancoli-Israel, 2003). Before discussing the specific issue of insomnia in individuals living with HIV infec-

tion, it may be helpful to review the physiology of healthy sleep.

PHYSIOLOGY OF HEALTHY SLEEP

Normal sleep is made up of rapid eye movement (REM) sleep and non-REM sleep. In non-REM sleep, the sleeper passes from wakefulness into stage I, a light sleep that is easily disrupted by environmental stimuli. Stage II is deeper and most stimuli will pass unnoticed by the sleeper. Stages III and IV are deeper still and the sleeper's electroencephalogram (EEG) shows higher-voltage slow waves, leading to these stages of sleep being described as deep, slow-wave, or delta-wave sleep. Here environmental stimuli go unnoticed unless extreme and prolonged. The normal sleep cycle consists of passage from wakefulness to stage I, then through the stages to the deeper levels of sleep. The sleeper then returns to stage II, which occupies the greater part of the night, and from that level into a period of REM sleep. During

REM sleep, the sleeper is dreaming and exhibits high levels of cortical activation but with muscle atonia that prevents the movements usually associated with such activation.

This cycle repeats itself several times over the course of the average night's sleep. Deep sleep tends to occur earlier in the night's rest while REM periods occur later and become longer (Krahn and Richardson, 2005). These cycles of sleep and wakefulness are thought to be the result of intricate interactions between circadian rhythms and sleep homeostasis that promote the ideal of 8 uninterrupted hours of sleep and 16 hours of wakefulness, with periods in the daily cycle that are more or less conducive to falling asleep (Pack and Mackiewicz, 2003). Such patterns are the basis for recommendation of a regular schedule that takes advantage of these natural rhythms as part of "sleep hygiene." Insomnia can affect sleep onset, maintenance, or duration. Causes are often multifactorial and an individual may have several physiological and psychological factors contributing to one or more sleep disorders.

SLEEP DISTURBANCE IN HIV

Clinicians have long been aware of the frequency with which insomnia and fatigue figure in the complaints of individuals living with HIV. Fatigue and sleep disturbance can affect a wide range of activities and even health itself in this population, as the healing benefits of sleep are lost at the time when patients have the greatest need of rest and renewal. A study that compared HIV-positive and HIV-negative homosexual men found that the HIV-infected patients were significantly more likely to report a problem with fatigue, although they slept more and napped more than the HIV-negative subjects. This fatigue interfered with important activities such as employment and driving and was also correlated with measures of immunosuppression and inflammation (Darko et al., 1992). Why do HIV-positive individuals feel fatigued and sleep poorly? Although these two complaints are obviously interrelated, they are not synonymous. Some patients with HIV infection may sleep relatively well, wake up rested, but develop fatigue as the day progresses, while those with insomnia sleep poorly, wake up unrefreshed, feel tired all day, and yet are still unable to fall asleep or remain asleep when night falls.

Fatigue is discussed in Chapter 16; this chapter will focus more specifically on the sleep disorders seen among individuals living with HIV infection.

Formal sleep studies and self-reports (Norman et al., 1990, Moeller et al., 1991) have shown that sleep in individuals living with HIV is impaired in both quantity and quality, although studies have been inconsistent as to whether these impairments are significantly related to stage of illness. A study by Wiegand and colleagues (1991) found a number of changes suggestive of disrupted sleep in individuals living with HIV, including increased sleep latency and nocturnal awakening and a decrease in the percentage of stage II sleep. The International Classification of Sleep Disorders divides sleep disorders into the primary disorders, which include dysomnias and parasomnias, and the more common secondary sleep disorders related to another mental, neurological, or medical disorder or induced by the use of substances (Silber, 2005). The recently released NIH Draft Statement on Insomnia (2005), by contrast, recommends the use of the term "comorbid insomnia," both to avoid undertreatment of the insomnia and because of the still limited understanding of causality. The forms of insomnia found in an HIV-positive population most often fall into this category of the secondary or comorbid insomnias, with all of the comorbid causes of insomnia mentioned above having a high prevalence in this population. Thus, treatment should focus first on identification and treatment of the comorbid causes of the insomnia, taking a broad biopsychosocial approach in this complex population, then on addressing the primary insomnia if the complaint persists.

Medical Disorders

HIV infection itself has been linked to insomnia. Studies in sleep laboratories have identified changes in sleep architecture among even asymptomatic HIV-infected patients (Terstegge et al., 1993). In asymptomatic HIV infection, slow-wave sleep is increased, particularly toward the later portion of the sleep period (Norman et al., 1992; Ferini-Strambi et al., 1995). This finding is unique to HIV infection and may be due to immune peptides, including tumor necrosis factor and interleukin. These peptides are elevated in the blood of HIV-infected individuals and have been found to be somnogenic in both clinical studies and animal models (Darko et al., 1995, Pollmacher et al., 1995). The human immunodeficiency virus and other lenti viruses may affect sleep more directly by resetting circadian rhythms, leading to altered sleep patterns and fatigue (Clark et al., 2005). Dysregulation of the growth hormone axis has also been implicated as a possible cause of sleep disturbance, with studies showing differences in the coupling between delta-frequency sleep EEG amplitude and growth hormone secretion in HIV-positive versus HIV-negative subjects, a change that occurs early in the course of the infection (Darko et al., 1998).

Looking at the problem from another direction, in non-HIV-infected populations, chronic insomnia has been found to affect immune function, with good sleepers having higher levels of CD3+, CD4+, and CD8+ cells than those with sleep difficulties (Savard et al., 2003). Studies with animal models have found that prolonged sleep deprivation can lead to compromised immune function and even death from sepsis (Bergman et al., 1996). Thus, insomnia may be both a cause of and a result of immune dysfunction.

Sleep Disorders Related to Another Mental Disorder

Mood disorders, anxiety disorders, and cognitive disorders, all of which have a high prevalence in populations living with HIV, have been linked with both acute and chronic insomnia. A study of 115 HIV-positive individuals, including women and injection drug users, found that overall, 73% met criteria for having a sleep disturbance, while 100% of the patients diagnosed with a cognitive disorder also had comorbid insomnia. Both cognitive impairment and depression were the best predictors of insomnia, although there was also a trend toward a higher prevalence among drug-using patients. Despite the high prevalence of disturbed sleep in all groups in this study, only 33% of the patients with insomnia had any mention of sleep disturbance in their medical records (Rubenstein and Selwyn, 1998). Reid and Dwyer (2005) undertook a systematic review of 29 articles dealing with insomnia in HIV infection and found that while an AIDS-defining illness, cognitive impairment, and treatment with efavirenz were all significant risk factors for insomnia, the most notable association was with psychological morbidity. Another recent study found both depression and anxiety among the variables related to sleep quality in an HIV-infected population (Robbins et al., 2004).

Depression

Studies in other populations have found an extensive comorbidity between psychiatric disorders and insomnia, with depression being the psychiatric diagnosis most commonly associated with insomnia (Martin and Ancoli-Israel, 2003). Patients with depression often report difficulties falling asleep and staying asleep, as well as early morning awakening. REM sleep has been found to occur earlier in sleep in depressed subjects and to decrease as the night progresses, reversing the normal cycle (Kloss and Szuba, 2003). Major depression is common in an HIV-infected population, with a prevalence estimated at 15%–40% (American Psychiatric Association, 2000), leaving this cohort vulnerable to the range of sleep disorders seen in conjunction with depression. Insomnia has been found to be more closely correlated with worsening depression in an HIV-infected population than CD4 count and disease progression (Perkins et al., 1995).

If insomnia develops during an episode of major depression, treatment of the depressive symptoms should take priority, as the insomnia will often resolve as the depression remits. An antidepressant with sedation as a side effect, such as mirtazapine, may relieve symptoms of insomnia while treating the depression. Another option is to combine antidepressant treatment with the short-term use of a sedative-hypnotic agent. The addition of cognitive-behavioral therapy may help remedy both depression and insomnia (Kloss and Szuba, 2003).

Mania

Less need for sleep and difficulty falling asleep are common symptoms of mania. In individuals living with HIV, mania may represent exacerbation of a preexisting bipolar disorder, may be part of the organic manic syndrome that can be seen in the context of advanced HIV infection, or may be associated with treatment with steroids or zidovudine (Della Penna and Triesman, 2005). Identification and treatment of the underlying cause of the organic mania and treatment of the mania itself with mood stabilizers or antipsychotics may resolve the insomnia, although hypnotics can be added if necessary.

Anxiety Disorders

Anxiety can occur at any stage of HIV infection, as patients must adapt to ever-changing circumstances. From the initial diagnosis, the patient may experience a number of anxiety-producing events, including changes in health or medication regimens, anticipation of results of tests and procedures, and changing family and financial circumstances, to mention just a few. Anxiety disorders may antedate seroconversion, and symptoms of anxiety may also occur in the context of substance abuse or withdrawal. In patients with more advanced illness or those who have lost loved ones to HIV infection, anxiety may take the form of resistance to falling asleep for fear of never awakening. Studies of patients with anxiety in other settings have found that 50%–70% report sleep difficulties affecting all stages of sleep (Kloss and Szuba, 2003).

Anxiolytics and/or antidepressants are usually effective in decreasing anxiety, although the use of anxiolytics in patients with a history of substance abuse may raise another set of issues. The possibility of drug–drug interactions with highly active antiretroviral therapy (HAART) may also limit the choice of agent.

Posttraumatic Stress Disorder

It has been suggested that individuals living with HIV may experience a higher prevalence of posttraumatic stress disorder (PTSD) than that among the general population (Della Penna and Triesman, 2005) and that the diagnosis of HIV itself may lead to PTSD (Kelly et al., 1998). Painful medical treatments or intensive-care unit stays can also lead to PTSD. Disturbing nightmares are part of the symptom cluster of PTSD and may reflect changes in REM sleep, such as increased REM density and, in most studies, an increased REM percent (Kloss and Szuba, 2003). Treatment with a selective serotonin reuptake inhibitor (SSRI) is recommended for the primary symptom, and use of a sedative-hypnotic may be helpful while waiting for the full SSRI effect.

Grief and Bereavement

Because HIV infection can affect multiple members of a family, a social network, or even a community, loss and bereavement are not uncommon. Acute grief can lead to insomnia, which may be relieved by short-term use of hypnotics. Lack of social support or pre-existing poor coping skills may interfere with adaptation to loss and lead to persistence of insomnia and other markers of bereavement. Individual or group psychotherapy may provide emotional support and teach adaptational skills.

Cognitive Impairment and Dementia

As previously mentioned, studies have found an association between the presence of dementia and insomnia in advanced HIV infection. In non-HIV-infected populations, the level of dementia has been found to contribute to poor sleep quality. Those individuals with cognitive impairment who reside in nursing homes have been found to have more disturbed circadian rhythm, more fragmented sleep, and even reversal of the sleep–wake cycle (Martin and Ancoli-Israel, 2003). Both these findings could be relevant to sleep disorders in the later stages of HIV infection.

Pain

Pain clearly can interfere with all stages of sleep. Chronic pain in HIV-positive patients may still be underestimated and undertreated despite data demonstrating that pain is a common symptom in this population (Breitbart et al., 1996; Larue et al., 1997) Disrupted sleep may result when doctors are hesitant to prescribe sufficient analgesic medications to treat complaints of pain from patients with a history of substance abuse, or they may undertreat pain when the cause of pain in an HIV-infected patient remains uncertain even after a thorough workup.

Other Physical Causes

Diarrhea is a common complaint of patients living with opportunistic infections and can lead to fragmented and non-restful sleep, as can urinary frequency, hot flashes, muscle cramping, pruritus, dyspnea, and other physical complaints. Obstructive sleep apnea due to adenotonsillar hypertrophy has been estimated to have a prevalence of 7% among individuals living with HIV, even in the absence of obesity (Epstein et al., 1995). It has also been associated with increased neck fat hypertrophy, which is due to the deposit of adipose tissue around the neck as part of HIV-associated lipodystrophy (Schulz et al., 2003). Decreased levels of testosterone can also lead to insomnia.

Medication Side Effects

Methylphenidate and other psychostimulants used to treat apathy and fatigue in HIV-infected patients can cause insomnia, although restriction of dosing schedules to the earlier part of the day should avoid this side effect. Insomnia and non-restful sleep have been reported early in treatment with efavirenz and may also cause more chronic sleep difficulty. Studies have found longer sleep latency and shorter duration of deep sleep in patients treated with efavirenz compared with controls as well as higher efavirenz plasma levels in patients with insomnia and/or reduced sleep efficiency than in those being treated with efavirenz who did not have sleep complaints (Gallego et al., 2004). In addition, efavirenz has been associated with vivid dreams and nightmares (American Psychiatric Association, 2000) that may result in disturbed and less restful sleep. Abacavir, stavudine, didanosine, and zidovudine (AZT) have also been linked to insomnia, with placebo-controlled studies showing more insomnia in patients treated with AZT than in those given placebo treatment (Worth and Volberding, 1994; Fellay et al., 2001). Other medications, including steroids, caffeine, theophylline, calcium channel agonists, L-dopa, amantadine, certain antineoplastic agents, and even buspirone, have also been implicated in sleep disturbance (Sateia and Nowell, 2004; Krahn and Richardson, 2005). Both use and abrupt discontinuation of substances of abuse, including alcohol and nicotine, can lead to sleep disturbance, as can abrupt discontinuation of many prescribed medications.

DIAGNOSIS

As with many diagnoses, a high index of suspicion is the best diagnostic tool. The HIV-infected population is best served by a broad biopsychosocial approach to diagnosis. A good sleep assessment should certainly be done whenever a patient complains of fatigue or insomnia, but the clinician should also take the initiative and ask all patients about symptoms of initial, middle, or late insomnia. History from partners or other family members may be helpful, as some patients actually adapt to their insomnia and may lose insight into the degree of nighttime insomnia and daytime sleepiness. The Epworth Sleepiness Scale (Johns, 1991) is a brief self-rating instrument that may be helpful in identifying daytime sleepiness; insomnia

can best be diagnosed by careful interview augmented by a sleep log, in which the patient details over a week or more pre-sleep events and amount of time spent in bed asleep or trying to sleep. Referral to a sleep lab for assessment is usually not indicated unless evidence of disordered breathing, periodic limb movements, or lack of response to treatment suggests need for a more thorough evaluation (Sateia and Nowell, 2004; Silber, 2005).

For the diagnosis to be made, the patient should report taking more than 30 minutes to fall asleep and/ or difficulty maintaining sleep, have wakeful periods of more than 30 minutes, and have an overall sleep efficiency (the ratio of sleep time to time spent in bed) of less than 85%. In addition, sleep disturbance should occur at least 3 nights/week, total sleep duration should be less than 6 hours/night and be nonrestorative, and the sleep disturbance must cause distress or significant impairment in daytime functioning (Savard and Morin, 2001). A careful history should include a review of the sleep schedule and daytime napping; information on the sleep environment, including adequacy of housing or homelessness, and presence of a partner, children, or pets in the bed; use of prescription medication, over-the-counter remedies, or herbal preparations; use of alcohol, tobacco, street drugs, or caffeine; involvement in shift work or pre-bedtime exercise; the presence of pain, periodic leg movements, or loud snoring; details and frequency of daytime sleepiness; and the frequency of vivid nightmares. The history of the complaint should include questions regarding prior assessments, treatments, and their results; childhood and family sleep history; and, if the symptom had a sudden onset, possible precipitants such as trauma, change of sleep partners, location, or routine; and new diagnoses or treatments (Stepanski et al., 2003; Krahn and Richardson, 2005). Both clinicians and researchers have found the Pittsburgh Sleep Quality Index, a sleep problem questionnaire, useful in documenting the presence and severity of insomnia (Buysse et al., 1989).

If the patient has a regular sleep partner, this individual should also be interviewed about the patient's pre-sleep behaviors, sleep patterns, snoring, and respiratory pauses. As previously noted, a good psychiatric history can be an important part of the evaluation of insomnia; symptoms of depression, anxiety, posttraumatic stress disorder, and other psychiatric disorders that might contribute to insomnia should be reviewed. Insomnia can precipitate the psychiatric disorder or can be secondary to it, thus correlation of onset of psychiatric symptoms with the onset of insomnia can be essential in determining treatment.

TREATMENT

Not every individual with insomnia requires treatment. In one epidemiological survey only one in four patients who met criteria for a diagnosis of insomnia reported actual sleep dissatisfaction (Morin, 1993). Thus, treatment is reserved for those with clinically significant insomnia and resultant daytime dysfunction. Because insomnia often has a multifactorial etiology, with both onset and course affected by predisposing, precipitating, and perpetuating factors (Morin, 2003), treatment should take a biopsychosocial approach to address all aspects of the problem. As noted previously, the impact of HIV on the brain may underlie much of the insomnia seen in this population and, insofar as this impact is not related to disease stage or progression, may not be directly treatable. What is treatable is the symptom of poor sleep as well as other factors that may contribute to it.

Underlying physical and psychiatric conditions should be diagnosed and treated, and behaviors that work against a good night's sleep should be identified and, if possible, changed. Many people with insomnia have developed poor sleep habits that make restful sleep less likely. The longer insomnia lasts, the more dysfunctional and ingrained the patient's maladaptive sleep patterns may become; behaviors that were initially adopted to relieve the problem, such as napping or spending more time in bed, eventually become part of the problem (Hauri, 2003).

The first step toward successful treatment is to make sure that every patient is aware of good sleep hygiene—the pattern of behaviors that take advantage of circadian rhythms and predispose to sleep. Some easy steps that the patient can take include avoiding naps, limiting time in bed to 8 hours, getting daily exercise, but completing this at least 4 hours before bedtime, keeping the same schedule 7 days/week rather than attempting to make up lost sleep, and using bright lights in the morning and avoiding them at night (Krahn and Richardson, 2005).

The next set of behaviors that need be targeted are those that may promote or disrupt sleep. Promotion of sleep can include developing a consistent and soothing bedtime ritual and making sure the bedroom is comfortable in terms of light, noise, and temperature. This may be challenging for patients in congregate or overcrowded housing or who are homeless. In such situations, working toward a safe environment where good sleep is possible needs to be part of the treatment. Patients may need help getting adequate bedding, earplugs when the environment is noisy, or even a fan, which can provide white noise and offer relief in conjunction with medications when dyspnea is limiting sleep. Alcohol, caffeine, nicotine, large meals, and excessive liquids should be avoided in the pre-sleep hours. Chronic insomnia may lead to increased anxiety, as bedtime and the bed itself become associated with frustration and arousal rather than sleep. Treatment for this includes stimulus control therapy to restructure such attitudes and reestablish circadian rhythms. Patients are advised not to use the bed for anything but sleep or sex, moving outside the bed for other activities such as reading, snacking, or watching TV. Bedtime should be postponed until the patient is tired, and if sleep is not quickly achieved, the patient should get out of bed and pursue non-stimulating activity, returning to bed only when drowsy. This pattern is repeated until sleep is achieved to reassociate the bedroom, bed, and bedtime with sleep (Silber, 2005).

Although it may seem counterintuitive, sleep restriction may also be helpful. Using the sleep log, the patient's sleep efficiency is calculated (total sleep/time in bed). If efficiency is over 90%, time in bed is increased by 15 minutes daily; for sleep efficiency under 80%, time in bed is decreased by the same amount, using the sleep log as a guide for further readjustment every 5–7 days until an efficiency of 85% is achieved (Sateia and Nowell, 2004). If worry or stress is a consistent factor in poor sleep, the patient may need to work on strategies to avoid taking worries to bed. This may involve learning muscle relaxation techniques or attention-focusing procedures such as imagery training, hypnosis, meditation, or even biofeedback (Morin, 2003). Another helpful technique is paradoxical intention, in which patients are advised to focus on remaining awake, thereby reducing performance anxiety (Sateia and Nowell, 2004).

Cognitive therapy can be used to identify maladaptive, erroneous, and distorted cognitions about sleep and replace these with more helpful attitudes. A combination of some or all of the nonpharmacological treatments outlined above can lead to clinically significant and durable improvement (Sateia and Nowell,

2004). Such cognitive-behavioral therapies have been found to be as effective as prescriptions medication for short-term treatment of insomnia, with individual therapy being more helpful than group therapy (Silber, 2005), Unlike medications, these therapies can have effects that last well beyond the termination of treatment (NIH, 2005). Self-help books and tapes for the insomniac are also available.

If pain, nausea, pruritus, dyspnea, other physical complaints, or medication side effects are limiting sleep, the patient's primary care doctor may need to be brought into the treatment process to help identify and treat these comorbidities. Working with patients on harm reduction to decrease use and ultimately abstain from drugs, nicotine, and alcohol can be an important step toward improving sleep.

Another avenue of approach to the treatment of insomnia is through the resetting of circadian rhythms. Sleep and rhythms can become dissociated by shift work, travel to other time zones, seasonal changes, and irregular sleep habits. Melatonin is produced by the pineal gland in response to the daily cycle of light and dark and plays a role in the maintenance of circadian rhythm. Bright light in the morning and/or melatonin taken at night can shift the circadian rhythm to facilitate sleep and reduce sleep latency (Sack et al., 2003). Melatonin can be bought over the counter and in health food stores. Because of varying bioavailability and the presence of contaminants long-term use in medically compromised populations should not be encouraged, nor has such use been studied. Ramelteon, a melatonin agonist, has been reported to help the initiation of sleep. Other herbal preparations such as valerian, kava-kava, broom, and passionflower are also reported to promote sleep but raise similar concerns regarding bioavailability, efficacy, and drug interactions (Krahn and Richardson, 2005). L-tryptophan, an endogenous amino acid, has been suggested as a possible sleep aid, but studies have been limited and drug interactions may lead to toxicity (NIH, 2005).

For many decades, the mainstay of insomnia treatment has been the sedative-hypnotic class of medications. Conventional wisdom has held that these medications lose efficacy if used on a daily basis for more than a few weeks (Sateia and Nowell, 2004), and most are approved by the U.S. Food and Drug Administration (FDA) for short-term use only. However, some authors see this as an unproven and mistaken belief that leads to undertreatment and that de-

veloped only because of the short length of most drug trials (Mendelson, 2003). What is clear is that many patients take these medications for months and even years and feel benefit from them despite concerns about side effects and the accumulation of metabolites. A few longer-terms studies (Ancoli-Israel et al, 2005; Winkelman and Pies, 2005) have been done with the newer non-benzodiazipine agents that suggest that total sleep time may be preserved despite an increase in sleep latency with long-term use. A study of subjects who were taking benzodiazepines for sleep found that 100% of the subjects felt that the medications were still helping almost 5 years after beginning treatment (Mendelson, 2003). Without sleep studies it is difficult to confirm the veracity of such findings, as patients' anxieties and misperceptions about the nature of sleep lend themselves to the possibility of a placebo response. It is preferable that patients use such medications only as needed, a common recommendation being that after a night of use, the patient should try to sleep the following night without medication. If sleep is unsatisfactory, a second night without medication should be attempted on the grounds that the patient will now be tired and thus more likely to sleep. However, if the second night's sleep is also unsatisfactory, medication should be used on the third night and then the cycle repeated. In practice, however, many patients prefer the security of nightly long-term medication, despite the recommendation of the NIH Draft Statement (2005) of further study of long-term effectiveness of these agents.

Medications from a number of different classes, each with its own advantages and drawbacks, have been used for the relief of insomnia. The benzodiazepines have a long record of use and relative safety, but regular use can lead to dependence. Agents with a more rapid onset and shorter half-life may be most useful for early and middle insomnia, while those with a longer half-life may be more appropriate for treatment of later insomnia. However, even brief use of shorter-acting medications, such as triazolam, can lead to rebound insomnia not seen with longer-acting agents (Silber, 2005). Other drawbacks include misuse, diversion to the street market, accumulation of metabolites with impairment of daytime function, and slower metabolism for some members of this class in the context of liver dysfunction.

For individuals living with HIV, the risk of drug–drug interactions with HAART further limits treatment options. Metabolism of alprazolam, triazolam, and midazolam is significantly inhibited by ritonavir, amprenavir, efavirenz, and delaviradine through the cytochrome 3A4 enzyme system, potentially causing respiratory depression, fatigue, and depression or worsening cognitive impairment (Wyszynski et al., 2003). Lorazepam, oxazepam, and temazepam, which bypass oxidative metabolism, avoid these interactions and may be better options. The non-benzodiazepine hypnotics, zaleplon and zolpidem, act at the benzodiazepine receptors, have rapid onset, and have little or no residual effect on next-day wakefulness, although the effect on the CYP3A4 system remains unclear (Silber, 2005). Zolpidem is reported to have less effect on sleep stages than the benzodiazepines, as it maintains time spent in stages III and IV. Because of their rapid onset, these agents are most useful for those individuals with early insomnia, although a slow-release form of zolpidem is now available and may be helpful in treating middle and late insomnia. Because of very rapid onset, only minimal physical tolerance to zaleplon develops and rapid discontinuance is possible (NIH, 2005). Eszopiclone is the newest member of this class, has a longer duration of action, and has been found to have sustained effectiveness in a 6-month study, although side effects are disturbing to a substantial number of patients; this agent also uses the CYP3A4 system for metabolism (Silber, 2005).

The use of both over-the-counter and prescribed medications approved for other conditions to help sleep has become increasingly common; however, no long-term studies have been done on the effectiveness of these agents, and the risk/benefit ratio may not be favorable to their use (NIH, 2005). Antihistamines, particularly H1 receptor antagonists such as diphenhydramine, can have sedation as a desired side effect and are often considered safe alternatives to sleep medications. In addition, they are inexpensive and can be bought without a prescription. However, these agents can have anticholinergic side effects and cause daytime sleepiness as well as interact with other medications.

The tricyclic antidepressants have been used to promote sleep, again making use of their well-known side effect of sedation, and may be a good choice if depressive symptoms are present. Doxepin, which has strong antihistaminic and sedating properties, can be helpful if pruritus is contributing to poor sleep. However, these agents are far from benign, can be lethal in overdose, and have a broad profile of potentially harmful side effects in addition to sedation. Trazodone has found a niche as a sleep medication, is nonaddictive,

and may treat concomitant depression, although it has been reported to cause priapism and postural hypotension as well as lower seizure threshold. The sedating antipsychotics have also been used and clearly have a role when psychosis is also present. These are not drugs to be prescribed lightly, however, as the risks of using these agents are well known and include anticholinergic side effects, weight gain, development of metabolic syndrome, neuroleptic malignant syndrome, or tardive dyskinesia, and even increased risk of stroke and death. Gabapentin is a relatively benign agent that may help sleep and is safe in the context of liver disease because of renal excretion. In a medically fragile population receiving multiple medications, starting doses of all these agents should be reduced.

CONCLUSION

Insomnia can be a draining and debilitating result of HIV infection and may even worsen outcome. Physician awareness of insomnia may facilitate its diagnosis and a biopsychosocial approach is necessary for effective treatment. Because of the burden imposed by insomnia, the benefits of the supervised use of appropriate hypnotic agents may outweigh the risks. Further study needs to be done to determine the efficacy of medication for long-term use, although caution must be used in this medically fragile population. Treatment that includes a cognitive-behavioral approach may lessen dependence on medication and reduce the frequency of use. Awareness of a patient's specific medical needs and social milieu may help target treatment most effectively.

References

American Psychiatric Association, Work Group on HIV/ AIDS (2000). Practice guideline for the treatment of patients with HIV/AIDS. *Am J Psychiatry* 157(11 Suppl.):1–62.

Ancoli-Israel S, Richardson GS, Mangano RM, Jenkins L, Hall P, Jones WS (2005). Long term use of sedative hypnotics in older patients with insomnia. *Sleep Med* 6(2):107–113.

Bergman BM, Gilliland MA, Feng PF, Russell DR, Shaw P, Wright M, Rechtschaffen A, and Alverdy JC (1996). Are physiological effects of sleep deprivation in the rat mediated by bacterial invasion? *Sleep* 19:554–562.

Breitbart W, Rosenfeld BD, Passik SD, McDonald MV, Thaler H, and Portenoy RK (1996). The undertreatment of pain in ambulatory AIDS patients. *Pain* 65(2-3):243–249.

Buysse DJ, Reynolds CF, Monk TH, Berman SR, and Kupfer DJ (1989). The Pittsburgh Sleep Quality Index: a new instrument for psychiatric practice and research. *Psychol Res* 28:193–213.

Clark JP, Sampair CS, Kofuji P, Nath A, and Ding JM (2005). HIV protein, transactivator of transcription, alters circadian rhythms though the light entrainment pathway. *Am J Physiol Regul Integr Comp Physiol* 289:R656–R662.

Darko DF, McCutchan JA, Kripke DF, Gillin, JC, and Golshan S (1992). Fatigue, sleep disturbance, disability and indices of progression of HIV infection. *Am J Psychiatry* 149:514–520.

Darko DF, Mitler MM, and Henriksen SJ (1995). Lentiviral infection, immune response peptides and sleep. *Adv Neuroimmunol* 5:57–77.

Darko DF, Mitler MM, and Miller JC (1998). Growth hormone, fatigue, poor sleep and disability in HIV infection. *Neuroendocrinology* 67:317–324.

Della Penna ND, and Treisman GJ (2005). HIV/AIDS. In J Levenson (ed.), *American Psychiatric Publishing Textbook of Psychosomatic Medicine* (pp. 599–627). Washington, DC: American Psychiatric Publishing.

Epstein LJ, Strollo PJ, Donegan RB, Delman J, Hendrix C, and Westbrook PR (1995). Obstructive sleep apnea in patients with human immunodeficiency virus (HIV) disease. *Sleep* 18:368–376.

Fellay J, Boubaker K, Ledergerber B, Bernasconi E, Furrer H, Battegay M, Hirschel B, Vernazza P, Francioli P, Greub G, Flepp M, and Talenti A (2001). Prevalence of adverse events associated with potent antiretroviral treatment: Swiss HIV Cohort Study. *Lancet* 358:1322–1327.

Ferini-Strambi L, Oldani A, Tirloni G, Zuconi M, Castagna A, Lazzarin A, and Smirne S (1995). Slow wave sleep and cyclic alternative pattern (CAP) in HIV-infected asymptomatic men. *Sleep* 18:446–450.

Gallego L, Barreiro P, del Rio R, Gonzalez de Requena D, Rodriguez-Albarino A, Gonzalez-Lahoz J, and Soriano V (2004). Analyzing sleep abnormalities in HIV-infected patients treated with efavirenz. *Clin Infect Dis* 38:430–432.

Hauri PJ (2003). Clinical work with insomnia: state of the art (circa 2004). In MP Szuba, JD Kloss, and DF Dinges (eds.), *Insomnia, Principles and Management* (pp. 75–82). Cambridge, UK: Cambridge University Press.

Johns M (1991). A new method for measuring daytime sleepiness: the Epworth Sleepiness Scale. *Sleep* 14:540–545.

Kelly B, Raphael B, Judd F, Perdices M, Kernutt G, Burnett P, Dunne M, and Burrows G (1998). Posttraumatic stress disorder in response to HIV infection. *Gen Hosp Psychiatry* 20:345–352.

Krahn LE, and Richardson JW (2005). Sleep disorders. In J Levenson (ed.), *American Psychiatric Publishing Textbook of Psychosomatic Medicine* (pp. 335–358). Washington, DC: American Psychiatric Publishing.

Kloss JD, and Szuba MP (2003). Insomnia in psychiatric disorders. In MP Szuba, JD Kloss, and DF Dinges (eds.), *Insomnia, Principles and Management* (pp. 43–72). Cambridge, UK: Cambridge University Press.

Larue F, Fontaine A, and Colleau SM (1997). Underestimation and undertreatment of pain in HIV disease: multicentre study. *BMJ* 314(7073):23–28.

Martin JL, and Ancoli-Israel S (2003). Insomnia in older adults. In MP Szuba, JD Kloss, and DF Dinges (eds.), *Insomnia, Principles and Management* (pp. 136–154). Cambridge, UK: Cambridge University Press.

Mendelson W (2003). Long-term use of hypnotic medications. In MP Szuba, JD Kloss, and DF Dinges (eds.), *Insomnia, Principles and Management* (pp. 115–124). Cambridge, UK: Cambridge University Press.

Moeller AA, Oechsner M, Backmund HC, Popescu M, Emminger C, and Holsboer F (1991). Self-reported sleep quality in HIV infection: correlation to the stage of infection and zidovudine therapy. *J Acquir Immune Defic Syndr* 4:1000–1003.

Morin C (1993). *Insomnia: Psychological Assessment and Management.* New York: Guilford Press.

Morin CM (2003). Treating insomnia with behavioral approaches: evidence for efficacy, effectiveness, and practicality. In MP Szuba, JD Kloss, and DF Dinges (eds.), *Insomnia, Principles and Management* (pp. 83–95). Cambridge, UK: Cambridge University Press.

[NIH] National Institutes of Health State-of-the-Science Conference Statement. Manifestations and management of chronic insomnia in adults, June 13–15, 2005.

Norman SE, Chediak AD, Kiel M, and Cohn MA (1990). Sleep disturbance in HIV-infected homosexual men. *AIDS* 4:775–778.

Norman SE, Chediak AD, Freeman C, Kiel M, Mendez A, Duncan R, Simoneau J, and Nolan B. (1992). Sleep disturbances in men with asymptomatic human immunodeficiency (HIV) infection. *Sleep* 15:150–155.

Pack AI, and Mackiewicz M (2003). Molecular approaches to understanding insomnia. In MP Szuba, JD Kloss, and DF Dinges (eds.), *Insomnia, Principles and Management* (pp. 150–155). Cambridge, UK: Cambridge University Press.

Perkins DO, Lesserman J, Stern RA, Baum SF, Liao D, Golden RN, and Evans DL (1995). Somatic symptoms and HIV infection: relation to depressive symptoms and indicators of HIV infection. *Am J Psychiatry* 155:1776–1781.

Pollmacher T, Mullington J, Korth C, and Hinze-Selch D (1995). The influence of host defense activation on sleep in humans. *Adv Neuroimmunol* 5(2):155–169.

Reid S, and Dwyer J (2005). Insomnia in HIV infection: a systematic review of prevalence, correlates and management. *Psychosom Med* 67(2):260–269.

Robbins JL, Phillips KD, Dudgeon WD, and Hand GA (2004). Physiological and psychological correlates of sleep in HIV infection. *Clin Nurs Res* 13:33–52.

Rubinstein ML, and Selwyn PA (1998). High prevalence of insomnia in an outpatient population with HIV infection. *J Acquir Immune Defic Syndr Hum Retrovirol* 19:260–265.

Sack, RL, Hughes RJ, Pires ML, and Lewy AJ (2003). The sleep-promoting effects of melatonin. In ML Szuba, JD Kloss, and DF Dinges (eds.), *Insomnia, Principles and Management* (pp. 96–114). Cambridge, UK: Cambridge University Press.

Sateia MJ, and Nowell PD (2004). Insomnia. *Lancet* 364:1959–1973.

Savard J, and Morin CM (2001). Insomnia in the context of cancer: a review of a neglected problem. *Clin Oncol* 19:895–908.

Savard J, Laroche L, Simard S, Ivers H, and Morin CM (2003). Chronic insomnia and immune functioning. *Psychosom Med* 65:211–221.

Schulz R, Lohmeyer J, and Seeger W (2003). Obstructive sleep apnea due to HIV associated lipodystrophy. *Clin Infect Dis* 37:1398–1399.

Silber MH (2005). Clinical insomnia. *N Engl J Med* 353:803–810.

Stepanski E, Rybarczyk G, Lopez M, and Stevens S (2003). Assessment and treatment of sleep disorders in older adults: a review for rehabilitation psychologists. *Rehabil Psychol* 48:23–36.

Terstegge K, Henkes H, Scheuler W, Hansen ML, Ruf B, and Kubicki S (1993). Spectral power and coherence analysis of sleep EEG in AIDS patients: decrease in interhemispheric coherence. *Sleep* 16:137–145.

Wiegand M, Moller AA, Schreiber W, Kreig JC, Fuchs D, Wachter H, and Holsboer F (1991). Nocturnal sleep EEG in patients with HIV infection. *Eur Arch Psychiatry Clin Neurosci* 240:153–180.

Winkelman J, and Pies R (2005). Current patterns and future directions in the treatment of insomnia. *Ann Clin Psychiatry* 17(1):31–40.

Worth LA, and Volberding PA (1994). Clinical applications of antiretroviral therapy. In PT Cohen, M Sande, and P Volberding (eds.), *The AIDS Knowledge Base* (pp. 1–33). Boston: Little, Brown and Company.

Wyszynski AA, Bruno B, Ying P, Chuan L, Friedlander M, and Rubenstein B (2003). The HIV infected patient. In AA Wyszynski and B Wyszynski (eds.), *Manual of Psychiatric Care for the Medically Ill* (pp. 171–201). Washington, DC: American Psychiatric Publishing.

Chapter 16

Fatigue and HIV

William Breitbart and Anna L. Dickerman

Fatigue is a common symptom reported by patients with HIV and AIDS and is associated with reduced quality of life and impaired physical functioning (Breitbart et al., 1998; Ferrando et al., 1998; Vogl et al. 1999). Patients regard fatigue as an important condition to be addressed because it is disabling (Sharpe and Wilks, 2002), yet typically it has been overlooked and undertreated by physicians (Dittner et al., 2004). Increasingly, clinicians caring for persons with HIV and AIDS have been giving more attention to symptom management and quality of life and thus should be familiar with major issues in fatigue assessment and treatment. This is especially true for psychiatrists treating psychosomatic disorders, given their ability to distinguish between medical and psychiatric contributors to fatigue and their proficiency in both psychotherapeutic and psychopharmacologic interventions for reducing fatigue or helping the patient better cope with fatigue. This chapter reviews the definition and assessment of fatigue, the prevalence of fatigue in HIV/AIDS and its impact on patients, medical and psychological causes of fatigue, and evidence-based strategies for intervention.

DEFINING FATIGUE

Fatigue is a poorly defined symptom that may involve physical, mental, emotional, and motivational components (Smets et al., 1993; Ream and Richardson, 1996; Sharpe and Wilks, 2002). It is typically defined as extreme and persistent tiredness, weakness, or exhaustion that may be mental, physical, or both (Dittner et al., 2004). Thus, fatigue can refer to a subjective sensation or to objectively impaired performance (Sharpe and Wilks, 2002). Furthermore, patients use various words to describe fatigue (Smets et al., 1993), each of which may point to a different underlying etiology. For example, fatigue described as "anhedonia" (loss of interest and enjoyment) suggests depression, whereas prominent "sleepiness" indicates potential sleep disruption, which may in turn be due to a variety of possible factors (Greenberg, 1998; Sharpe and Wilks, 2002). It is important, therefore, to obtain a descriptive account of the nature of the patient's fatigue to investigate all possible causes and facilitate accurate diagnosis (Greenberg, 1998).

Recognizing the need for a standardized definition of fatigue, Cella and colleagues (1998) have proposed a set of diagnostic criteria, currently undergoing validation for inclusion in the International Classification of Diseases, tenth revision (ICD-10). The criteria listed in Table 16.1 were originally developed in the context of cancer, but can also be applied to patients with HIV/AIDS. A study evaluating this clinical syndrome approach reported preliminary evidence of its reliability and validity (Sadler et al., 2002). Fifty-one patients received a standardized interview designed

to identify the presence of a clinical syndrome of cancer-related fatigue; these patients also completed self-report measures of fatigue, depression, and health-related quality of life. Comparisons among independent raters demonstrated high rates of reliability for the presence or absence of a cancer-related fatigue syndrome and its symptoms. Twenty-one percent of the patients met diagnostic criteria for a cancer-related fatigue syndrome. These patients reported more severe, frequent, and pervasive fatigue than did patients who did not meet diagnostic criteria; they also demonstrated poorer role function, less vitality, and more depressive symptomatology. Thus, this newly developed clinical syndrome approach appears to have great utility in identifying patients who experience clinically significant, illness-related fatigue.

ASSESSMENT OF FATIGUE

Fatigue is a concept that is not only difficult to define but also challenging to quantify. Nonetheless, reliable and valid tools for assessment are crucial for improved management and research progress (Dittner et al., 2004). There are a variety of standardized self-report scales, most of which have been developed in the context of cancer and chronic illnesses other than HIV, that can also be used to measure fatigue in patients with HIV and AIDS. These are summarized in Table 16.2. Not surprisingly, the information provided by these scales depends on the questions asked and, therefore, reflects the scale writer's own understanding of fatigue. The patient, in turn, may have his or her own interpretation of the questions. Thus, different scales may measure fundamentally different aspects, or even potentially distinct conceptions, of fatigue. The challenge facing the clinician or researcher, then, is to choose a reliable and valid tool for the measurement of fatigue that is most adequately suited to his or her purposes (Dittner et al., 2004).

The oldest scales assessing fatigue are dichotomous, meaning that fatigue is measured as either present or absent. These include the Pearson-Byars Fatigue Checklist (Pearson and Byars, 1956), Profile of Mood States (POMS) Fatigue and Vigor Subscale (Cella et al., 1987), the Fatigue Severity Scale (Krupp et al., 1989b), and the European Organization for Research and Treatment of Cancer Quality of Life Questionnaire (EORTC-QLQ-C30) Fatigue Subscale (Aaronson et al., 1993).

TABLE 16.1. Proposed (1998 draft) ICD-10 Criteria for Cancer-Related Fatigue

Six (or more) of the following symptoms have been present every day or nearly every day during the same 2-week period in the past month, and at least one of the symptoms is (A1) significant fatigue:

A1. Significant fatigue, diminished energy, or increased need to rest, disproportionate to any recent change in activity level
A2. Complaints of generalized weakness or limb heaviness
A3. Diminished concentration or attention
A4. Decreased motivation or interest to engage in usual activities
A5. Insomnia or hypersomnia
A6. Experience of sleep as unrefreshing or nonrestorative
A7. Perceived need to struggle to overcome inactivity
A8. Marked emotional reactivity (e.g., sadness, frustration, or irritability) to feeling fatigued
A9. Difficulty completing daily tasks attributed to feeling fatigued
A10. Perceived problems with short-term memory
A11. Postexertional malaise lasting several hours
B. The symptoms cause clinically significant distress or impairment in social, occupational, or other important areas of functioning.
C. There is evidence from the history, physical examination, or laboratory findings that the symptoms are a consequence of cancer or cancer therapy.
D. The symptoms are not primarily a consequence of comorbid psychiatric disorders such as major depression, somatization disorder, somatoform disorder, or delirium.

Source: Cella D, Peterman A, Passik S, et al. Progress toward guidelines for the management of fatigue. Oncology 1998;12:369–377, with permission from Karga AG, Basel.

TABLE 16.2. Fatigue Measures and Assessment Tools

Scales Using a Dichotomous Approach

1. Pearson-Byars Fatigue Checklist (Pearson and Byars, 1956)
2. Profile of Mood States Fatigue and Vigor Subscale (Cella et al., 1987)
3. Fatigue Severity Scale (Krupp et al., 1986)
4. European Organization for Research and Treatment of Cancer Quality of Life Questionnaire Fatigue Subscale (Aaronson et al., 1993)

Scales Using a Unidimensional Approach

1. Visual Analogue Scale for Fatigue (Lee et al., 1991)
2. Karnofsky Performance Status (Schag et al., 1984)
3. Global Fatigue Index (Bormann et al., 2001)

Scales Using a Multidimensional Approach

1. Piper Fatigue Scale (Piper et al., 1989)
2. Fatigue Symptom Inventory (Hann et al., 1998)
3. Brief Fatigue Inventory (Mendoza et al., 1999)
4. Multidimensional Assessment of Fatigue (Belza, 1995)

Specific Scales for the HIV Population

1. Sleep and Infection Questionnaire (Darko et al., 1992)
2. HIV-Related Fatigue Scale (Barroso and Lynn, 2002)

Source: Dufour N, Dubé B, Breitbart W (2005). HIV-related fatigue. In J DeLuca (ed.), *Fatigue as a Window to the Brain* (pp. 188–207). Cambridge, MA: The MIT Press, with permission.

Newer scales have taken a unidimensional approach. The Visual Analogue Scale for Fatigue (VAS-F), for example, chiefly probes intensity (Lee et al., 1991). The VAS-F is organized into energy and fatigue dimensions and has good psychometric properties (Dittner et al., 2004). The Karnofsky Performance Status, by contrast, probes mainly consequences of fatigue (Schag et al., 1984). The limitations of such unidimensional scales include the presence of confounding factors such as pain.

Multidimensional scales include the Fatigue Symptom Inventory (Hann et al., 1998) and the Brief Fatigue Inventory (Mendoza et al., 1999), both originally developed to assess the severity and impact of fatigue in cancer and palliative care populations. The Piper Fatigue Scale (PFS) was originally developed for use in cancer patients (Piper et al., 1989). It consists of affective, cognitive, sensory, and severity subscales and has been used to measure fatigue in individuals with HIV. Its major shortcomings include the lengthy amount of time it takes to complete it and the difficulty some patients have in understanding it (Dittner et al.,

2004). The Multidimensional Assessment of Fatigue (MAF) scale is a revision of the Piper Fatigue Scale developed for use among patients with rheumatoid arthritis (Belza, 1995). The Global Fatigue Index (GFI) stems from the MAF and has been validated for use in HIV patients (Bormann et al., 2001). The scale is easily administered and takes only about 5 minutes to complete. The ultimate GFI score is unidimensional.

Although there is no widely recognized gold-standard assessment scale for HIV-related fatigue, there are several recently developed fatigue scales that are specific to HIV and AIDS. The Sleep and Infection Questionnaire developed by Darko et al. (1992), for example, is an 11-item scale that examines the affect of fatigue on mental agility, but does not encompass the full fatigue experience in HIV. The HIV-Related Fatigue Scale (HRFS) developed by Barroso and Lynn (2002) consists of 56 items, incorporating elements from five preexisting scales (MAF, General Fatigue Scale, Fatigue Impact Scale, Fatigue Assessment Index, and the Sleep and Infection Questionnaire) plus four additional items. The HRFS probes three domains: intensity, consequences, and circumstances of fatigue. It shows much promise for assessing fatigue in HIV/AIDS, as it encompasses most elements of fatigue specific to persons with HIV and AIDS.

Given the multifactorial nature of fatigue, accessory scales (e.g., depression scales) and measurements of certain biological parameters (e.g., disease progression indicators such as viral load and CD4 count) should be used in addition to fatigue assessment tools to obtain the most complete evaluation of a patient's fatigue. In particular, the complex interrelationships between fatigue and psychiatric disturbances such as depression and anxiety merit special attention and will be further explored later on in this chapter.

PREVALENCE AND IMPACT OF FATIGUE IN HIV/AIDS

The high frequency and distressing nature of fatigue in both "asymptomatic" individuals with HIV and patients with advanced AIDS has been well documented. These findings are summarized in Table 16.3. Estimates of the prevalence of HIV-related fatigue range from 2%–27% among individuals with early, "asymptomatic" HIV seropositivity to 30%–54% among patients with AIDS (Longo et al., 1990; Miller et al., 1991; Hoover et al., 1993; Anderson and Grady, 1994;

TABLE 16.3. Prevalence of Fatigue in HIV/AIDS

Study	Population	Prevalence
Longo et al., 1990	Gay men with AIDS	41%
Darko et al., 1992	HIV+ gay men	57% CDC stage IV 11% CDC stage III 10% HIV-negative controls
Hoover et al., 1993	HIV+ "asymptomatic" gay men	9% HIV+ 6% HIV-negative controls
Vlahov et al., 1994	HIV+ male and female intravenous drug users	19.4%–30%, depending on CD4 counts
Breitbart et al., 1998	Ambulatory HIV/AIDS patients	54%
Ferrando et al., 1998	HIV+ gay or bisexual men	6%–17%, depending on CD4 counts
Vogl et al., 1999	AIDS outpatients	85.1%

Source: Dufour N, Dubé B, Breitbart W (2005). HIV-related fatigue. In J DeLuca (ed.), *Fatigue as a Window to the Brain* (pp. 188–207). Cambridge, MA: The MIT Press, with permission.

Revicki et al., 1994; Vlahov et al., 1994). Darko and colleagues (1992), for example, found that more than 50% of a sample of 14 AIDS patients suffered from fatigue, in comparison to 10% of 50 HIV-seronegative controls. This study found that AIDS patients with fatigue sleep more than AIDS patients without fatigue. Fatigued patients also experienced greater interference with work, self-care, social interactions, and daily activities. In a study conducted by Longo and colleagues (1990), fatigue was identified as a "major physical concern" in 41% of a sample of 34 AIDS patients. Vlahov and colleagues (1994) examined a sample of 562 HIV-seropositive intravenous drug abusers who did not satisfy criteria for AIDS, and found that 19%–30% of the sample experienced fatigue. Other studies have demonstrated similar findings (Richman et al., 1987; Crocker, 1989; Miller et al., 1991, Anderson and Grady, 1994, Revicki et al., 1994).

In a comprehensive study of fatigue in a heterogeneous population of 429 ambulatory AIDS patients, Breitbart and colleagues (1998) assessed the frequency of fatigue and its medical and psychological correlates. They administered the Memorial Symptom Assessment Scale (MSAS) and the AIDS Physical Symptom Checklist (PSC) to divide patients into fatigue and no-fatigue groups. Those patients that endorsed both of the fatigue items from the MSAS and the AIDS physical symptom checklists were classified as having fatigue. Self-report inventories were also used to assess psychological stress, depression, and quality of life in the subjects. More than 85% of the AIDS patients endorsed "lack of energy" on the MSAS, while greater than 55% endorsed "persistent or frequent fatigue lasting 2 weeks or longer" on the PSC. Of the patients studied, 46.9 % were distressed by their lack of energy, while 39.9% were "somewhat" distressed. Both MSAS and PSC fatigue items were endorsed by 52.7% of the patients. There were no associations found between fatigue and education, age, or race. However, women were found to be significantly more susceptible to fatigue than men. This is not a surprising finding, given that fatigue has been reported as more common among women in both the general population and cancer patients (Curt et al., 2000; Sharpe and Wilks, 2002), and female gender is considered a predisposing factor for fatigue (Sharpe and Wilks, 2002). Men whose primary risk behavior was having sex with men were less likely to experience fatigue than persons whose primary risk behavior was injection drug use or heterosexual contact. The study also found a correlation between the number of AIDS-related symptoms present on the PSC, particularly pain, and fatigue. Finally, Breitbart et al. (1998) also indicated that fatigue was associated with (1) treatment for AIDS-related medical conditions, (2) decreased serum hemoglobin, and (3) higher psychological distress, more depressive symptoms, and greater hopelessness (as measured by the Brief Symptom Inventory, Beck Depression Inventory, Beck Hopelessness Scale, and the Functional Living Inventory for Cancer [modified for AIDS]).

In a later study also using the MSAS, Vogl and colleagues (1999) replicated some of the above findings in a population of AIDS outpatients. For example, this particular study found that fatigue was highly prevalent (present in 85% of the sample) and that both the number of symptoms and symptom distress were highly associated with psychological distress and poor quality of life. However, Vogl et al. found no association between fatigue and gender. There has also been some discrepancy in findings regarding the correlation between fatigue and immunologic compromise in patients with HIV disease. Several studies reported a higher prevalence of fatigue in patients with immunologic compromise (Lee et al., 1991; Hoover et al., 1993; Walker et al., 1997), while others found no association between viral load and fatigue (Vlahov et al., 1994; Breitbart et al., 1998; Ferrando et al., 1998; Vogl et al., 1999). These differences probably result from methodological inconsistencies that are beyond the scope of this chapter.

Voss (2005) studied variation in the intensity of fatigue according to selected demographic, cultural, and health/illness variables in 372 patients with HIV/AIDS. The UCSF Symptom Management Model was used to assess fatigue severity in a sample including 73% African Americans and 63% males; 58% of patients experienced moderate to severe fatigue intensity. Women, Hispanics, disabled persons, and those with inadequate income or insurance reported higher fatigue intensity scores. Braitstein and colleagues (2005) reported similar findings in a study comparing HIV-monoinfected individuals to patients coinfected with HIV and hepatitis C (HCV). Coinfected patients reported more symptoms consistent with depression, increased fatigue, and poorer quality of life. However, upon multivariate modeling, it was determined that this negative impact of HCV was better explained by the sociodemographic factors related to poverty and injection drug use than by HCV itself. The authors concluded that patients coinfected with HIV and HCV represent a patient population with significant physical and mental health challenges primarily related to socioeconomic issues rather than HCV infection. The results of these two studies suggest the need for further gender and ethnic-specific fatigue research, as well as symptom cluster research, in patients with HIV and AIDS.

ETIOLOGIES OF FATIGUE IN HIV/AIDS

Fatigue among patients with HIV is multifaceted and should be viewed as the final common pathway for a variety of causal factors (Sharpe and Wilks, 2002). Fatigue may be due to preexisting conditions in HIV-infected individuals (e.g., congestive heart failure), opportunistic infections, or other medical complications encountered throughout the illness. Finally, there are complex connections between psychiatric disturbances and fatigue in HIV illness. The underlying mechanisms of fatigue remain unclear, as certain hypotheses have not been tested adequately. These include fatigue as a potential result of the build-up of waste products such as pyruvic and lactic acid (Simonson, 1971). It has also been suggested that cytokine activation may lead to abnormalities in the hypothalamic-pituitary-adrenal axis or to neurophysiological changes in the brain that ultimately cause fatigue (Ur et al., 1992). Finally, hepatocyte toxicity may cause fatigue in HIV patients. Bartlett and colleagues demonstrated that 75% of HIV-seropositive patients had abnormal liver function (Bartlett, 1996). HIV messenger RNA was present in hepatocytes and HIV p24 in Kupffer cells and endothelial cells, findings suggesting that HIV can involve the liver directly. It is unclear, however, whether liver damage results from primary damage by the virus itself or occurs through a secondary mechanism such as hepatitis. Aside from these theoretical issues, there are several commonly recognized mechanisms of HIV-related fatigue; these are reviewed below and summarized in Table 16.4.

Anemia

Anemia is one of numerous hematologic complications that may occur in patients with HIV disease, including thrombocytopenia, lymphopenia, and neutropenia. It is considered a prognostic marker of disease progression and death in HIV patients, independent of viral load and CD4 count (Moyle, 2002). Studies have reported that anemia occurs in 10%–20% of asymptomatic HIV-seropositive individuals and in 66%–85% of patients with advanced AIDS (Doweiko and Groopman, 1998). There are multiple potential etiologies of anemia in HIV disease, including opportunistic infections; neoplasia (mostly lymphoma); chronic inflammation (which can lead to erythropoietin deficiency); dietary deficiency due to poor appetite, oral lesions, or difficulty with digestion or absorption; diarrhea; blood loss; histiocytosis; or bone marrow abnormalities such as myelodysplasia, myelofibrosis, or bone marrow suppression (Volberding, 2000). Up-regulation of cytokines (interferons, interleukin-1, tumor necrosis factor, and transforming growth factor) may also impair erythropoietin response and result in ineffective red blood cell production (Means, 1997). Finally, anemia may be iatrogenic, as pharmacologic interventions for

TABLE 16.4. Etiologies of Fatigue in HIV/AIDS

Physiological Factors

Direct Effects of HIV/AIDS
Peripheral and central nervous system
Hepatocyte toxicity
Cytokines

Comorbid Medical Conditions
Anemia
Hypogonadism
Hypo- or hyperthyroidism
Adrenal insufficiency
Opportunistic infections
Nutritional deficincies

Treatment Effects
Medication side effects

Exacerbating Factors
Sleep disturbances
Lack of exercise
Inactivity
Pain syndromes

Psychological Factors

Depression
Anxiety
Coping with a chronic illness

Source: Dufour N, Dubé B, Breitbart W (2005). HIV-related fatigue. In J DeLuca (ed.), *Fatigue as a Window to the Brain* (pp. 188–207). Cambridge, MA: The MIT Press, with permission.

HIV may lead to myelosuppression. Specifically, dideoxynucleoside analogues as well as antimicrobials (e.g., pentamidine, trimethoprim, sulfonamides, ganciclovir, pyrimethamine) are among the more common pharmacologic causes of myelosuppression in HIV treatment (Pluda et al., 1991).

Endocrinopathies

Hormonal imbalances are another potential contributing factor to fatigue in individuals with HIV. The HIV virus affects immunologic cytokines, which may in turn influence various endocrine processes. The clinical correlates of these effects, however, remain unclear (Briggs and Beazlie, 1996). The HIV-related endocrinopathies are covered in depth in Chapter 35 of this book.

Hypogonadism and Low Testosterone

The most prevalent endocrinopathy present in HIV disease is hypogonadism. This encompasses impair-

ment in testicular or ovarian function that may ultimately lead to low testosterone levels (Klauke et al., 1990). Decreased testosterone is associated with fatigue, low libido, impotency, anorexia, weight loss, and depression. Approximately 25% of asymptomatic, untreated HIV-infected men and approximately 45% of untreated men diagnosed with AIDS are estimated to have low testosterone levels (Dobs et al., 1988). Possible mechanisms of hypogonadism include insufficient production of testosterone due to low stimulation by brain hormones, testicular damage, and side effects of medication.

Other Endocrine Abnormalities

Adrenal insufficiency is yet another possible physiological cause of fatigue in HIV patients (Norbiato et al., 1994; Abbott et al., 1995; Piedrola et al., 1996). Possible mechanisms include infection (with HIV, cytomegalovirus, or tuberculosis), drugs, or psychological stress, which may increase the activity of the hypothalamic-pituitary-adrenal axis. While it has been consistently demonstrated that cortisol levels are higher in individuals with HIV than in those without HIV (Enwonwu et al., 1996; Clerici et al., 1997; Rondanelli et al., 1997), these patients also have a reduced cortisol response to adrenocorticotropin hormone (ACTH) stimulation (Stolarczyk et al., 1998).

Hyperthyroidism and hypothyroidism can also both induce fatigue, and should be considered when diagnosing a patient presenting with fatigue.

Malnutrition

In the era of highly active antiretroviral therapy (HAART), severe malnutrition states are no longer seen frequently in AIDS patients with access to care. Less severe malnutrition, however, is still seen, and can contribute significantly to fatigue. Thus, it is important to identify and treat potential malnutrition. Persons with HIV and AIDS may have decreased appetite for a variety of possible reasons. These include nausea induced by medication, difficulty swallowing due to painful candida esophagitis, or malabsorption due to gastrointestinal parasitic infection (*Cryptosporidium*, *Microsporidium*), viral infection (cytomegalovirus), or neoplasia (Kaposi sarcoma). A frequent cause of nutritional deficits in HIV is medication-induced nausea. Patients often experience reduced appetite and take in less food because of nausea and/or vomiting caused by pharmacologic interventions. This is particularly true for patients receiving multidrug antiretroviral (ARV) therapy. Often this ARV-induced nausea occurs only upon initiation of therapy (Janoff and Smith, 2001).

Treatment-Related Causes of Fatigue

As described above, there are a variety of iatrogenic mechanisms of fatigue in HIV. Highly active antiretroviral therapy is especially likely to cause such processes. Interferon (IFN)-alpha 2b used in combination with HAART for HCV coinfection can also induce fatigue, as well as neutropenia and malaise. Krown and colleagues (2006) conducted a phase I study in 14 patients with AIDS-associated Kaposi sarcoma and found that these toxicities occurred at IFN doses 5 million IU/day. To summarize, the major treatment-induced causes of fatigue in HIV patients are myelosuppression and subsequent anemia, endocrinopathies such as hypogonadism, and malnutrition resulting from nausea and/or vomiting (Table 16.5).

Psychiatric Disturbances and Fatigue

Mood Disorders

Anxiety and depression are the most commonly reported psychiatric disturbances in HIV-infected individuals. Mood disorders and anxiety disorders are covered extensively in Chapters 9 and 11, respectively,

of this book. Up to 83% of HIV patients are diagnosed with depressive spectrum disturbances and 10%–20% of HIV patients suffer from major depression (Perdices et al., 1992). It can be very challenging to sort out fatigue, depression, and anxiety in patients with HIV (Walker et al., 1997), particularly because fatigue can be a symptom of both HIV-related disease and mood disorders. There are also symptoms common to both fatigue and depression in particular, such as decreased energy and motivation, sleep disruptions, diminished concentration and attention, and problems with short-term memory. Finally, anxiety and depression are highly prevalent in HIV patients. Thus, it is necessary to clarify the relationship between mood disturbances (particularly anxiety and depression) and fatigue for both clinicians and researchers to effectively evaluate and treat individuals with HIV disease.

Jacobsen and Weitzner (2003) proposed four important questions as a theoretical framework for this task. Although these questions were originally developed in the context of cancer, they are also applicable to HIV-related fatigue. They address (1) the conceptual similarities and differences between depression or anxiety and fatigue, (2) the extent to which anxiety and depression coexist with fatigue, and how they can be distinguished, (3) the causal link between fatigue and depression and anxiety, and (4) treatment implications of the relationship of fatigue to depression and anxiety. Jacobsen and Weitzner found that fatigue, anxiety, and depression have been assessed through three separate approaches in HIV/AIDS: the clinical-syndrome

TABLE 16.5. Antiretroviral Side Effects Leading or Contributing to Fatigue

Drug Class	Side Effect		
	Fatigue	Nausea, vomiting	Anemia
Nucleoside reverse transcriptase inhibitors	Lamivudine, abacavir	Lamivudine, zalcitabine, zidovudine	Zidovudine
Nucleotide reverse transcriptase inhibitors		Tenofovir	
Nonnucleoside reverse transcriptase inhibitors		Efavirenz	
Protease inhibitors	Amprenavir, saquinavir, lopinavir/ritonavir, ritonavir	Amprenavir, saquinavir, lopinavir/ritonavir, ritonavir, melfinavir	Indinavir

Source: Dufour N, Dubé B, Breitbart W (2005). HIV-related fatigue. In J DeLuca (ed.), Fatigue as a Window to the Brain (pp. 188–207). Cambridge, MA: The MIT Press, with permission.

approach, which determines whether or not a mood disorder is present; the symptom-cluster approach, in which multiple symptoms of anxiety and depression are measured; and the single-symptom approach, which specifically measures symptoms of anxious and depressed mood. Fatigue has also been evaluated using these same methods.

There is an overlap among these three approaches in studies that have measured the relationship between fatigue, anxiety, and depression. Some of this research has suggested that fatigue in HIV patients is secondary to depression. For example, Lyketsos and colleagues (1996) conducted a longitudinal study of AIDS patients to examine the temporal relationship between fatigue and anxiety. They reported that depressive symptoms and fatigue are associated in close chronological proximity across various stages of HIV disease. Because they found no correlation between fatigue and immune or HIV illness measures, these researchers ultimately concluded that fatigue is a symptom of depression. In a study conducted with 20 HIV-seropositive men without AIDS, O'Dell and colleagues (1996) reported similar findings; they found no significant association between fatigue and physiological parameters (total protein, albumin, hematocrit, hemoglobin, and physical dimension score on the Sickness Impact Profile). Thus, they concluded that fatigue is more strongly correlated with psychological rather than physical parameters. Henderson and colleagues (2005) also found that the presence of fatigue in HIV-infected individuals was more strongly associated with psychological factors than with advanced disease or the use of HAART. Thus, these researchers also concluded that fatigue may suggest underlying depression and anxiety in these patients. In a study of asymptomatic men with HIV, Perkins et al. (1995) found that depressive symptoms and major depression significantly predict the severity of fatigue at baseline and at 6-month follow-up. These results suggest that fatigue may be a manifestation of depression in the early stages of HIV disease.

Other research, however, has indicated that the relationship between depression and fatigue in HIV disease may be more complex. For example, Ferrando and colleagues (1998) reported that depressed men with HIV are more likely to experience clinical fatigue. However, after a 1-year follow-up, these researchers found an increase in depressive symptoms without a similar variance in fatigue. They concluded that although fatigue is associated with major depression and depressive symptoms, fatigue in advanced HIV illness may not merely be a symptom of depression. Breitbart and colleagues (1998) reported similar findings in the previously mentioned study of ambulatory AIDS patients. While they found that greater than 70% of patients likely to have a depressive order suffered from fatigue, the majority (58%) of the sample with fatigue did not demonstrate any increase in depressive symptoms. Moreover, fatigue and depression provided unique contributions to the prediction of psychological distress and quality of life. Thus, the authors suggested that fatigue may be a symptom of depression in some, but certainly not all, fatigued patients with AIDS, and that the impact of fatigue on psychological function and quality of life is not merely a reflection of underlying depression. They also reported that patients with fatigue had significantly higher scores on measures assessing cognitive symptoms of depression and psychological distress, indicating the possibility that depression may in fact be the result of fatigue. Finally, Barroso and colleagues (2002) conducted a longitudinal study of 36 HIV-seropositive gay men for 7.5 years and found that fatigue was predicted by both physiological (CDC clinical status) and psychological (anxiety, hopelessness, social conflict, lack of satisfaction with support) risk factors. They reported, however, that depression was predicted only by psychological risk factors. Depression was strongly correlated with premorbid depression and fatigue correlated with premorbid fatigue. Depression present at the previous visit was correlated with fatigue, and fatigue at the previous visit correlated with depression scores. Thus, these results suggest that fatigue and depression play roles in mutually predicting one another in gay men with HIV disease.

In light of these findings, future research is necessary to aid in the clarification between depression and fatigue in persons with HIV and AIDS. In the meantime, we know that depressive symptoms due to fatigue are typically less severe, and that patients tend to attribute such symptoms to the consequences of fatigue. Depression, on the other hand, is more likely in the presence of hopelessness, feelings of worthlessness and/or guilt, suicidal ideation, and a family history of depression (see Table 16.6).

Fatigue and Neuropsychological Function

Preliminary research has suggested a potential relationship between fatigue and central nervous system

TABLE 16.6. Differentiating Fatigue and Depression in HIV

Symptoms Common to Both Syndromes

Fatigue
Decreased energy
Increased need to rest
Anhedonia
Decreased motivation
Sadness, frustration, irritability
Insomnia or hypersomnia
Diminished concentration/attention
Perceived short-term memory problems

Symptoms and Factors Suggestive of Depression

Feelings of hopelessness, worthlessness, or guilt
Suicidal ideation, desire for death
History or family history of depression

(CNS) involvement in HIV. Perkins et al. (1995) examined the relationship between insomnia and fatigue to indicators of mood disturbance and HIV severity. To assess disease severity, they measured CD4 counts and performed neuropsychological testing that encompassed both global and motor performance. They found that severity of depressive symptoms and self-reported dysphoric mood were related to the level of fatigue and insomnia, but that global and motor neuropsychological function were not significantly related to either fatigue or insomnia. However, at 6-month follow-up, there was a reduction in motor neuropsychological function that was associated with more complaints of fatigue. This finding was consistent even after controlling for depression. The researchers suggested that there might be a relationship between fatigue and HIV effects on the brain, proposing that fatigue may be a possible earlier indicator of CNS involvement.

TREATMENT STRATEGIES

Early, active management of fatigue is preferable before the symptom becomes chronic. Education is an important initial step in this respect, particularly because patients tend not to report fatigue unless directly asked. Patients and members of their support networks should be taught how to recognize signs and symptoms of fatigue to aid in its detection and treatment. Precipitating factors, such as acute physical stresses and

psychological stresses, should be identified, as should perpetuating factors such as physical inactivity and ongoing psychological or social stresses (Sharpe and Wilks, 2002). Finally, clinicians should engage in discussion with the patient, giving ample information so that the patient knows what to expect from the treatment of their fatigue.

Given the multidimensional nature of HIV-related fatigue, a broad biopsychosocial approach is recommended for treatment of fatigue in this population (Sharpe and Wilks, 2002). Cella and colleagues (1998) have proposed a three-stage hierarchy for the management of fatigue: (1) identify and treat any underlying causes of fatigue; (2) treat the symptoms of fatigue directly while the etiology of fatigue is determined; and (3) address and manage the consequences of fatigue. Outlined below are fatigue intervention strategies in HIV/AIDS; these are summarized in Table 16.7.

Treatment of Physiological Causes of Fatigue

In accordance with the paradigm proposed by Cella et al. (1998), potential physiological causes of fatigue should be identified and treated, and nonessential centrally acting drugs should be eliminated. If anemia is the main cause of fatigue, for example, the physician should determine the necessity of a transfusion in severely symptomatic patients. Recombinant human erythropoietin (rHuEPO) is recommended for patients with hemoglobin levels below 11g/dl, regardless of whether they are being treated with zidovudine (Fischl et al., 1990; Henry et al., 1992; Phair et al., 1993). Clinical trials have shown that anemic patients have improved energy and less fatigue after rHuEPO treatment. Therapy with rHuEPO can be administered either intravenously or subcutaneously, three times weekly. It is generally well tolerated.

If hypogonadism is identified as the underlying cause of fatigue, exogenous testosterone or synthetic anabolic steroids may be administered (Dufour et al., 2005). However, patients receiving this treatment are susceptible to anabolic and androgenic effects such as increased heart rate, increased blood pressure, and hirsutism. Testosterone therapy may take the form of injections, pills, patches, gels, or creams. This treatment has been shown to have a beneficial effect on not only fatigue but also sexual interest, appetite, wasting, energy levels, and even concomitant depression. It

TABLE 16.7. Fatigue Intervention Strategies in HIV/AIDS

Cause-Specific Interventions

Anemia	Transfusions, rHuEPO
Hypogonadism	Testosterone
Adrenal insufficiency	Corticosteroids
Hypothyroidism	Levothyroxine
Infections	Antibiotic, antiviral, or antifungal therapy
Malnutrition	Nutritional supplement, megestrol acetate
Depression	Antidepressants, psychotherapy
Inactivity	Exercise, training
Sleep disturbances	Sleep aids

Nonspecific Pharmacological Interventions

Selective serotonin-reuptake inhibitors
Tricyclic antidepressants
Psychostimulants
   Methylphenidate
   Dextroamphetamine
   Pemoline
Modafinil
Anti-cytokine agents
   Thalidomide
   Pentoxifylline

Nonpharmacological Interventions

Good sleep hygiene
Education
Meditation, relaxation
Energy conservation and restoration
Cognitive-behavioral therapy

Source: Dufour N, Dubé B, Breitbart W (2005). HIV-related fatigue. In J DeLuca (ed.), *Fatigue as a Window to the Brain* (pp. 188–207). Cambridge, MA: The MIT Press, with permission.

can be used in women, although patients must be carefully monitored for any potential virilizing effects, which may be irreversible.

Primary adrenal insufficiency can be treated with oral hydrocortisone or dexamethasone replacement therapy (Dufour et al., 2005). Hypothyroidism improves with levothyroxine administration, which has also been found to improve quality of life and energy levels in HIV patients with no evidence of hypothyroidism (Derry, 1995).

Treatment of Psychological Causes of Fatigue

Once potential underlying organic causes of fatigue have been ruled out and treated, psychotherapeutic and pharmacologic treatments may be explored for the management of any mood disturbances.

Pharmacologic Interventions

Underlying depression should be treated with selective serotonin reuptake inhibitors (SSRIs), which are generally better tolerated than tricyclic antidepressants by patients with HIV and AIDS (Elliot et al., 1998; Schwarz and McDaniel, 1999). The notable exception is fluvoxamine, which is less well tolerated despite its efficacy in treating depression (Grassi, 1995). Since fatigued patients with HIV and AIDS are especially sensitive to antidepressant side effects compared to patients without fatigue (Sharpe and Wilks, 2002), treatment should be initiated at very low doses. Because concomitant antiretroviral therapy is frequently used, drug–drug interactions should also be carefully monitored by prescribing physicians. Excellent reviews of such psychopharmacologic considerations have been carried out by Robinson and Qagish (2002) and

Thompson et al. (2006). Psychopharmacologic treatment issues in AIDS psychiatry are also addressed in depth in Chapter 32 of this book.

Psychotherapeutic Interventions

Much less research, however, has been conducted about psychotherapeutic interventions for depressed HIV patients. Most of this literature supports group cognitive-behavioral therapy approaches as a means of improving mental health–related quality of life indices (Lechner et al., 2003) and relieving depression (Blanch et al., 2002). Although individual psychotherapy has not been as well investigated, it is an integral part of the American Psychiatric Association's practice guidelines for the treatment of patients with HIV/AIDS (American Psychiatric Association, 2000).

Direct Treatment of Fatigue

Once the potential physiological and psychological causes of fatigue have been addressed, residual effects of fatigue can be treated directly. There are several pharmacologic agents that may be used to directly treat fatigue in persons with HIV and AIDS who may or may not be depressed.

Psychostimulants such as methylphenidate, pemoline, and dextroamphetamine have shown great promise in the treatment of fatigued patients with cancer and multiple sclerosis (Krupp et al., 1989a; Weinshenker et al., 1992). These drugs have also been used safely and successfully in HIV patients with fatigue (Holmes et al., 1989; Wagner and Rabkin, 2000; Breitbart et al., 2001). Breitbart and colleagues (2001) conducted the first randomized, double-blind, placebo-controlled trial of two psychostimulants for the treatment of fatigue in ambulatory patients with HIV disease. They found that both methylphenidate hydrochloride (Ritalin) and pemoline (Cylert) were equally effective and significantly superior to placebo in decreasing fatigue severity with minimal side effects. Fifteen patients (41%) of 144 ambulatory HIV patients taking methylphenidate and 12 patients (36%) taking pemoline experienced clinically significant improvement, as compared to 6 patients (15%) taking placebo. The significantly improved fatigue was also associated with improved quality of life, decreased depression, and decreased psychological distress. Although subjects experienced minimal side

effects, "jitteriness" was reported by some patients (31.8% of subjects taking methylphenidate; 25.6% of subjects taking pemoline). Thus, the use of psychostimulants may be appropriate as part of a comprehensive approach to the treatment of fatigue in HIV patients (Breitbart et al., 2001).

Modafinil, a norepinephrine agonist in the human hypothalamus (McClellan and Spencer, 1998), is a wakefulness-promoting agent that has been used off-label to augment antidepressants in small studies (Menza et al., 2000; Schwartz et al., 2002). It is currently used as a first-line agent for the treatment of severe fatigue in multiple sclerosis (MacAllister and Krupp, 2005). One pilot study has shown promising results for modafinil in the alleviation of HIV-related fatigue (Rabkin et al., 2004a). Further research will be necessary to validate these results.

Finally, one study has shown that testosterone administration may be effective for the treatment of fatigue in depressed men with HIV and AIDS. Rabkin et al. (2004b) conducted a double-blind, randomized, placebo-controlled trial comparing the outcomes of fluoxetine, testosterone, and placebo administration in 123 HIV-seropositive men with a depressive disorder. The Clinical Global Impressions Scale for mood and fatigue, the Hamilton Rating Scale for Depression, and the Chalder Fatigue Scale were used to assess patient symptoms. The conclusions did not support prescription of testosterone as a first-line treatment for depression in men with HIV disease. However, testosterone was significantly superior to both fluoxetine and placebo in terms of reducing fatigue.

Managing the Consequences of Fatigue

The negative impact of HIV-related fatigue on quality of life has been emphasized throughout this chapter. Addressing the consequences of fatigue is also crucial to improve the patient's quality of life. Treatment of fatigue should not merely involve the restoration or amelioration of energy, but also the preservation of energy to improve the patient's level of functioning. This may entail appropriate rest, pacing of energy-consuming activities, stress reduction, meditation or relaxation techniques, aerobic exercise (if it is not contraindicated), and participation in pleasurable activities. Counseling and communication can help patients re-prioritize their activities, adjust to their limitations, and restructure their goals and expectations accordingly. Throughout this process sustaining a sense of purpose and meaningfulness is vital (Winningham et al., 1994).

CONCLUSIONS

Fatigue is a serious clinical problem that is highly prevalent among patients with HIV/AIDS and is associated with decreased quality of life. The complaint of fatigue needs to be explored specifically to explore different etiologies. Several simple, reliable, and valid measurement scales are available for the assessment of fatigue. Discrete medical causes of fatigue should be treated directly. Certain psychiatric syndromes, particularly mood disorders, can cause acute fatigue in the absence of HIV disease; thus diagnosis and treatment of these disturbances are also necessary. There are a number of therapeutic strategies that can benefit fatigued patients with HIV, though further research is warranted. Patients need to be educated and informed about their diagnosis and treatment so they can prepare and adjust accordingly. Finally, the psychiatrist has a unique ability to provide both medical treatment and psychosocial support to HIV patients with fatigue. Ameliorating treatable causes of fatigue can add to the stores of physical and emotional energy needed to cope with HIV/AIDS and even thrive in the face of this illness.

References

Aaronson NK, Ahmedzai S, Bergman B, Bullinger M, Cull A, Duez NJ, Filibert A, Flechtner H, Fleishman SB, de Haes JC, et al. (1993). The European Organization for Research and Treatment of Cancer QLQ-C30: a quality-of-life instrument for use in international clinical trials in oncology. *J Natl Cancer Inst* 85:365–763.

Abbott M, Khoo SH, Hammer MR, and Wilkins EGL (1995). Prevalence of cortisol deficiency in late HIV disease. *J Infect* 31:1–4.

American Psychiatric Association (2000). Practice guidelines for the treatment of patients with HIV/AIDS. *Am J Psychiatry* 157:1–62.

Anderson R, and Grady C (1994). Symptoms reported by "asymptomatic" HIV-infected subjects [abstract]. Proceedings of the 7th Annual Association of Nurses in AIDS Care in Nashville, TN, November 10–12, 1994.

Barroso J, and Lynn ML (2002). Psychometric properties of the HIV-Related Fatigue Scale. *J Assoc Nurses AIDS Care* 13:66–75.

Barroso J, Preisser JS, Leserman JL, Gaynes BN, Golden RN, and Evans DN (2002). Predicting fatigue and depression in HIV-positive gay men. *Psychosomatics* 43:317–325.

Bartlett JG (1996). *Medical Management of HIV Infection*. Glenview, IL: Physicians and Scientists Publishing.

Belza BL (1995). Comparison of self-reported fatigue in rheumatoid arthritis and controls. *J Rheumatol* 22: 639–643.

Blanch J, Rousaud A, Hautzinger M, Martinez E, Peri JM, Andres S, Cirera E, Gatell JM, and Gasto C (2002). Assessment of the efficacy of cognitive-behavioral group psychotherapy program for HIV-infected patients referred to a consultation-liaison psychiatry department. *Psychother Psychosom* 71: 77–84.

Bormann J, Shively M, Smith TL, and Gifford AL (2001). Measurement of fatigue in HIV-positive adults: reliability and validity of the Global Fatigue Index. *J Assoc Nurses AIDS Care* 12:75–83.

Braitstein P, Montessori V, Chan K, Montaner JS, Schechter MT, O'Shaughnessy MV, and Hogg RS (2005). Quality of life, depression and fatigue among persons co-infected with HIV and hepatitis C: outcomes from a population-based cohort. *AIDS Care* 17(4):505–515.

Breitbart W, McDonald MV, Rosenfeld B, Monkman ND, and Passik S (1998). Fatigue in ambulatory AIDS patients. *J Pain Symptom Manage* 15:159–167.

Breitbart W, Rosenfeld B, Kaim M, and Funesti-Esch J (2001). A randomized, double-blind, placebo-controlled trial of psychostimulants for the treatment of fatigue in ambulatory patients with human immunodeficiency virus disease. *Arch Intern Med* 161:411–420.

Briggs JM, and Beazlie LH (1996). Nursing management of symptoms influenced by HIV infection of the endocrine system. *Nurs Clin North Am* 31:845–865.

Cella DF, Jacobsen PB, Orav EJ, Holland JC, Silberfarb PM, and Rafla S (1987). A brief POMS measure of distress for cancer patients. *J Chronic Dis* 40:939–942.

Cella D, Peterman A, Passik S, Jacobsen P, and Breitbart W (1998). Progress toward guidelines for the management of fatigue. *Oncology* 12:369–377.

Clerici M, Trabattoni D, Piconi S, Fusi ML, Ruzzante S, Clerici C, and Villa ML (1997). A possible role for the cortisol/anticortisols imbalance in the progression of human immunodeficiency virus. *Psychoneuroendocrinology* 22(Suppl. 1):S27–S31.

Crocker KS (1989). Gastrointestinal manifestations of the aquired immunodeficiency syndrome. *Nurs Clin North Am* 24:395–406.

Curt GA, Breitbart W, Cella D, Groopman JE, Horning SJ, Itri LM, Johnson DH, Miaskowski C, Scherr SL, Portenoy RK, and Vogelzang NJ (2000).

Impact of cancer-related fatigue on the lives of patients: new findings from the Fatigue Coalition. *Oncologist* 5:353–360.

Darko DF, McCutchan JA, Kripke DF, Gillin JC, and Golshan S (1992). Fatigue, sleep disturbance, disability, and indices of progression of HIV infection. *Am J Psychiatry* 149:514–520.

Derry DM (1995). Thyroid therapy in HIV-infected patients. *Med Hypotheses* 45:121–124.

Dittner AJ, Wessely SC, and Brown RG (2004). The assessment of fatigue: a practical guide for clinicians and researchers. *J Psychosom Res* 56:157–170.

Dobs AS, Dempsey MA, Ladenson PW, and Polk BF (1988). Endocrine disorders in men infected with HIV. *Am J Med* 84:611–616.

Doweiko J, and Groopman J (1998). Hematologic manifestations of HIV infection. In G Wormser (ed.), *AIDS and Other Manifestations of HIV Infection* (pp. 542–557). Philadelphia: Lippincott-Raven.

Dufour N, Dubé B, and Breitbart W (2005). HIV-related fatigue. In J DeLuca (ed.), *Fatigue as a Window to the Brain* (pp. 188–207) Cambridge, MA: MIT Press.

Elliot AJ, Uldall KK, Bergam K, Russo J, Claypoole K, and Roy-Byrne PP (1998). Randomized, placebo-controlled trial of paroxetine versus imipramine in depressed HIV-positive outpatients. *Am J Psychiatry* 155:367–372.

Enwonwu CO, Meeks VI, and Sawiris PG (1996). Elevated cortisol levels in whole saliva in HIV infected individuals. *Eur J Oral Sci* 104:322–324.

Ferrando S, Evans S, Goggin K, Sewell M, Fishman B, and Rabkin J (1998). Fatigue in HIV illness: relationship to depression, physical limitations, and disability. *Psychosom Med* 60:759–764.

Fischl M, Galpin JE, Levine JD, Groopman JE, Henry DH, Kennedy P, Miles S, Robbins W, Starret B, Zalusky R, et al. (1990). Recombinant human erythropoietin for patients with AIDS treated with zidovudine. *N Engl J Med* 322:1488–1492.

Grassi B (1995). Notes on the use of fluvoxamine as a treatment of depression in HIV-1 infected subjects. *Pharmacopsychiatry* 28:93–94.

Greenberg DB (1998). Fatigue. In JC Holland, et al. (eds.), *Psycho-oncology* (pp. 485–493) New York: Oxford University Press.

Hann DM, Jacobsen PB, Azzarello LM, Martin SC, Curran SL, Fields KK, Greenberg H, and Lyman G (1998). Measurement of fatigue in cancer patients: development and validation of the Fatigue Symptom Inventory. *Qual Life Res* 7:301–310.

Henderson M, Safa F, Easterbrook P, and Hotopf M (2005). Fatigue among HIV-infected patients in the era of highly active antiretroviral therapy. *HIV Med* 6(5):347–352.

Henry DH, Beall GN, Benson CA, Carey J, Cone LA, Eron LJ, Fiala M, Fischl MA, Gabin SJ, Gottlieb MS, et al. (1992). Recombinant human erythropoietin in the treatment of anemia associated with HIV infection and zidovudine therapy: overview of four clinical trials. *Ann Intern Med* 117:739–748.

Holmes VF, Fernandez F, and Levy JK (1989). Psychostimulant response in AIDS-related complex patients. *J Clin Psychiatry* 50:5–8.

Hoover DR, Saah AJ, Bacellar H, Murphy R, Visscher B, Anderson R, and Kaslow R (1993). Signs and symptoms of "asymptomatic" HIV-1 infection in homosexual men. *J Acquir Immune Defic Syndr* 6:66–71.

Jacobsen PB, and Weitzner MA (2003). Evaluating the relationship of fatigue to depression and anxiety in cancer patients. In RK Portenoy and E Bruera E (eds.), *Issues in Palliative Care Research* (pp. 127–149). New York: Oxford University Press.

Janoff EN, and Smith PD (2001). Emerging concepts in gastrointestinal aspects of HIV-1 pathogenesis and management. *Gastroenterology* 120:607–621.

Klauke S, Falkenbach A, Schmidt K, et al. (1990). Hypogonadism in males with AIDS. [abstract FB]. *Int Conf AIDS* 6:209.

Krown SE, Lee JY, Lin L, Fischl MA, Ambinder R, and Von Roenn JH (2006). Interferon-alpha2b with protease inhibitor–based antiretroviral therapy in patients with AIDS-associated Kaposi sarcoma: an AIDS malignancy consortium phase I trial. *J Acquir Immune Defic Syndr* 41(2):149–153.

Krupp LB, Coyle PK, Cross AH, et al. (1989a). Amelioration of fatigue with pemoline in patients with multiple sclerosis. *Ann Neurol* 26:155–156.

Krupp LB, LaRocca NG, Mur-Nash J, and Steinberg AD (1989b). The Fatigue Severity Scale. *Arch Neurol* 46:1121–1123.

Lechner SC, Antoni MH, Lydston D, LaPerriere A, Ishii M, Devieux J, Stanley H, Ironson G, Schneiderman N, Brondolo E, Tobin JN, and Weiss S (2003). Cognitive-behavioral interventions improve quality of life in women with AIDS. *J Psychosom Res* 54: 253–261.

Lee KA, Hicks G, and Nino-Murcia G (1991). Validity and reliability of a scale to assess fatigue. *Psychiatry Res* 36:291–298.

Longo MB, Spross JA, and Locke AM (1990). Identifying major concerns of persons with acquired immunodeficiency syndrome: a replication. *Clin Nurse Spec* 4:21–26.

Lyketsos CG, Hoover DR, Cuccione M, Dew MA, Wesch JE, Bing EG, and Treisman GJ (1996). Changes in depressive symptoms as AIDS develops. *Am J Psychiatry* 153:1430–1437.

MacAllister WS, and Krupp LB (2005). Multiple sclerosis–related fatigue. *Phys Med Rehabil Clin N Am* 16(2):483–502.

McClellan KJ, and Spencer CM (1998). Modafinil: a review of its pharmacology and clinical efficacy in the management of narcolepsy. *CNS Drugs* 9:311–324.

Means R Jr (1997). Cytokines and anemia in HIV infection. *Cytokines Cell Mol Ther* 3:179–186.

Mendoza TR, Wang XS, Cleeland CS, Morrissey M, Johnson BA, Wendt JK, and Huber SL (1999). The rapid assessment of fatigue severity in cancer patients: use of the Brief Fatigue Inventory. *Cancer* 85:1186–1196.

Menza MA, Kaufman KR, and Castellanos A (2000). Modafinil augmentation of antidepressant in depression. *J Clin Psychiatry* 61:378–381.

Meynell J, and Barroso J (2005). Bioimpedance analysis and HIV-related fatigue. *J Assoc Nurses AIDS Care* 16(2):13–22.

Miller RG, Carson PJ, Moussavi RS, Green AT, Baker AJ, and Weiner MW (1991). Fatigue and myalgia in AIDS patients. *Neurology* 41:1603–1607.

Moyle G (2002). Anemia in persons with HIV infection: prognostic marker and contributor to morbidity. *AIDS Rev* 4:13–20.

Norbiato G, Galli M, Righini V, and Moroni M (1994). The syndrome of acquired glucocorticoid resistance in HIV infection. *Ballieres Clin Endocrinol Metab* 8:77–787.

O'Dell MW, Meighen M, and Riggs RV (1996). Correlates of fatigue in HIV prior to AIDS: a pilot study. *Disabil Rehabil* 18:249–254.

Pearson PG, and Byars GE (1956). The Development and Validation of a Checklist Measuring Subjective Fatigue (report no. 56–115). Randolph AFB, Texas: School of Aviation, U.S. Air Force.

Perdices M, Dundar N, Grunseit A, Hall W, and Cooper DA (1992). Anxiety, depression, and HIV-related symptomatology across the spectrum of HIV disease. *Aust N Z J Psychiatry* 26:560–566.

Perkins DO, Leserman J, Stern RA, Baum SF, Liao D, Golden RN, and Evans DL (1995). Somatic symptoms of HIV infection: relationship to depressive symptoms and indicators of HIV disease. *Am J Psychiatry* 152:1776–1781.

Phair JP, Abels RI, McNeill MV, and Sullivan DJ (1993). Recombinant human erythropoietin treatment: investigational new drug protocol for the anemia of the acquired immunodeficiency syndrome: overall results. *Arch Intern Med* 153:2669–2675.

Piedrola G, Casado JL, Lopez E, Moreno A, Perez-Elias MJ, and Garcia-Robles R (1996). Clinical features of adrenal insufficiency in patients with acquired immunodeficiency syndrome. *Clin Endocrinol* 45:97–101.

Piper B, Lindsey A, Dodd M, et al. (1989). Development of an instrument to measure the subjective dimension of fatigue. In S Funk, et al. (eds.), *Key Aspects of Comfort: Management of Pain, Fatigue and Nausea* (pp. 199–208). New York: Springer-Verlag.

Pluda JM, Mitsuya H, and Yarchoan R (1991). Hematologic effects of AIDS therapies. *Hematol Oncol Clin N Am* 5:229–248.

Rabkin JG, McElhiney MC, Rabkin R, and Ferrando SJ (2004). Modafinil treatment for fatigue in HIV+ patients: a pilot study. *J Clin Psychiatry* 65(12):1688–1695.

Rabkin JG, Wagner GJ, McElhiney MC, Rabkin R, and Lin SH (2004). Testosterone versus fluoxetine for

depression and fatigue in HIV/AIDS: a placebo-controlled trial. *J Clin Psychopharmacol* 24(4):379–385.

Ream E, and Richardson A (1996). Fatigue: a concept analysis. *Int J Nurs Stud* 33:519–529.

Revicki DA, Brown RE, Henry DH, McNeill MV, Rios A, and Watson T (1994). Recombinant human erythropoietin and health-related quality of life of AIDS patients with anemia. *J Acquir Immune Defic Syndr* 7:474–484.

Richman DD, Fischl MA, Grieco MH, Gottlieb MS, Volberding PA, Laskin OL, Leedom JM, Groopman JE, Mildvan D, Hirsch MS, et al. (1987). The toxicity of azidothymidine (AZT) in the treatment of patients with AIDS and AIDS-related complex. *N Engl J Med* 317:192–197.

Robinson MJ, and Qaqish RB (2002). Practical psychopharmacology in HIV-1 and acquired immunodeficiency syndrome. *Psychiatr Clin North Am* 25:149–175.

Rondanelli M, Solerte SB, Fioravanti M, Scevola D, Locatelli M, Minoli L, and Ferrari E (1997). Circadian secretory pattern of growth hormone, insulin-like growth factor type 1, cortisol, adrenocorticotropic hormone, thyroid-stimulating hormone, and prolactin during HIV infection. *AIDS Res Hum Retroviruses* 13:1243–1249.

Sadler IJ, Jacobsen PB, Booth-Jones M, Belanger H, Weitzner MA, and Fields KK (2002). Preliminary evaluation of a clinical syndrome approach to assessing cancer-related fatigue. *J Pain Symptom Manage* 23(5):406–416.

Schag CC, Heinrich RL, and Ganz PA (1984). Karnofsky Performance Status revisited: reliability, validity, and guidelines. *J Clin Oncol* 2:187–193.

Schwartz TL, Leso L, Beale M, Ahmed R, and Naprawa S (2002). Modafinil in the treatment of depression with severe comorbid medical illness. *Psychosomatics* 43:336–337.

Schwarz JA, and McDaniel JS (1999). Double-blind comparison of fluoxetine and desipramine in the treatment of depressed women in advanced HIV disease: a pilot study. *Depress Anxiety* 9:70–74.

Sharpe M, and Wilks D (2002). Fatigue. *BMJ* 325:480–483.

Simonson E (1971). *Physiology of Work Capacity and Fatigue.* Springfield, IL: Thomas.

Smets EM, Garssen B, Schuster-Uitterhoeve AL, and deHaesm JC (1993). Fatigue in cancer patients. *Br J Cancer* 68:220–224.

Stolarczyk R, Rubio SI, Smolyar D, Young IS, and Poretsky L (1998). Twenty-four-hour urinary free cortisol in patients with acquired immunodeficiency syndrome. *Metabolism* 47:690–694.

Thompson A, Silverman B, Dzeng L, and Treisman G (2006). Psychotropic medications and HIV. *Clin Infect Dis* 42(9):1305.

Ur E, White PD, and Grossman A (1992). Hypothesis: cytokines may be activated to cause depressive illness and chronic fatigue syndrome. *Eur Arch Psychiatry Clin Neurosci* 241:317–322.

Vlahov D, Munoz A, Solomon L, Astemborski J, Lindsay A, Anderson J, Galai N, and Nelson KE (1994). Comparison of clinical manifestations of HIV infection between male and female injecting drug users. *AIDS* 8:819–823.

Vogl D, Rosenfeld B, Breitbart W, Thaler H, Passik S, McDonald M, and Portenoy RK (1999). Symptom prevalence, characteristics, and distress in AIDS outpatients. *J Pain Symptom Manage* 18: 253–262.

Volberding P (2000). Consensus statement: anemia in HIV infection current trends, treatment options, and practice strategies. Anemia in HIV Working Group. *Clin Ther* 22:1004–1020.

Voss JG (2005). Predictors and correlates of fatigue in HIV/AIDS. *J Pain Symptom Manage* 29(2):173–184.

Wagner GJ, and Rabkin R (2000). Effects of dextroamphetamine on depression and fatigue in men with HIV: a double-blind, placebo-controlled trial. *J Clin Psychiatry* 61:436–440.

Walker K, McGown A, Jantos M, and Anson J (1997). Fatigue, depression, and quality of life in HIV-positive men. *J Psychosoc Nurs Ment Health Serv* 35:32–40.

Weinshenker BG, Penman M, Bass B, Ebers GC, and Rice GP (1992). A double-blind, randomized crossover trial of pemoline in fatigue associated with multiple sclerosis. *Neurology* 42:1468–1471.

Winningham ML, Nail LM, Burke MB, Brophy L, Cimprich B, Jones LS, Pickard-Holley S, Rhodes V, St. Pierre B, Beck S, et al. (1999). Fatigue and the cancer experience: the state of the knowledge. *Oncol Nurs Forum* 21:23–36.

Wolfe G (1999). Fatigue in patients with HIV/AIDS. *Care Manage* 3:8–11.

Chapter 17

Unique Manifestations
of HIV-Associated Dementia

James Murrough and Mary Ann Cohen

Currently persons with HIV are living longer and healthier lives than earlier in the epidemic. As the average length of survival increases, new challenges emerge in the diagnosis, management, and treatment of behavioral and cognitive manifestations of HIV infection. In a cohort study reported by Cohen (1998), 83% of patients admitted to an AIDS-dedicated nursing home had a diagnosis of dementia. Although the overall prevalence rate for HIV-associated dementia (HAD) is decreasing with the use of potent antiretroviral therapies, its rate in AIDS nursing homes may not reflect the benefits of antiretroviral therapy on central nervous system (CNS) infection. Persons with AIDS may be admitted to nursing homes because of both late-stage AIDS and dementia resulting from nonadherence to care. Dementia is a cognitive disorder involving loss of function in multiple cognitive domains (e.g., memory, attention, judgment, abstract thinking) severe enough to interfere with an individual's social or occupational functioning. Patients with advanced HIV infection are vulnerable to multiple causes of dementia, the most common of which is HAD. HIV-associated dementia is a metabolic encephalopathy caused by viral replication in brain macrophages and microglia and associated inflammatory and neurotoxic host responses (Gendelman et al., 1998; Zink et al., 1999; Anderson et al., 2002; Kaul et al., 2005). HAD is characteristic of a subcortical dementia in which cognitive decline, motor slowing, and behavior changes are predominant (Clifford, 2002). For a more detailed and thorough description of HAD we refer the reader to Chapters 3 and 19 of this volume. In this chapter we describe some of the behavioral consequences of HAD and their impact on persons with HAD, on their families, and on their caregivers. Caregivers of persons with HAD face multiple challenges that require special education and training. Some of the unique manifestations of HAD include accidental firesetting, violent behavior, and the repetitive taking of other persons' property.

ACCIDENTAL FIRESETTING

Firesetting is a unique manifestation of HAD. Cohen and Alfonso (1998) have described several cases of firesetting behavior among persons with cognitive impairment and HIV infection and suggest a multifactorial etiology for the behavior. Accidental firesetting often occurs in the context of cigarette smoking by persons both with and without cognitive impairment. The cognitive impairment concomitant with HAD exaggerates the lapses in attention, memory, or judgment that may lead to accidental firesetting from lit cigarettes. HAD is characterized by motor abnormalities such as tremor and bradykinesia, which may contribute to fine motor dyscontrol, thereby increasing the risk of, for example, dropping a lit cigarette. In addition to encephalopathy, persons with HIV may have HIV-associated neuropathy, which may further increase the likelihood of an accident by decreasing the perception of heat. A person with visual acuity limited by cytomegalovirus (CMV) retinitis would have further difficulty in not being able to perceive a dangerous situation until it is too late.

It is important that caregivers be aware of this potentially dangerous behavior among persons with HIV. We strongly recommend programs of smoking cessation. Ideally, all health care environments should be smoke free for fire prevention and for the health of both patients and staff. Smoking should be prohibited except with direct staff supervision and preferably out of doors with supervision. Staff education and frequent fire drills are important. Warning signs of unsafe smoking include severe dementia, delirium, visual impairment, and neuropathy. Specific measures that can be taken to decrease the risk of firesetting include limiting unsupervised cigarette smoking, providing flame-retardant clothing, and encouraging smoking cessation.

VIOLENT BEHAVIOR

There are multiple pathways to violent behavior of persons with advanced HIV infection, including biological, psychological, and social factors. HAD, like other forms of dementia, may lead to violence through a process of behavioral disinhibition related to cortical and subcortical dysfunction and the resultant neurocognitive impairment. Delirium is a frequent precursor to violence. Patients with advanced HIV are vulnerable to many causes of delirium, such as toxic-metabolic insults, hepatic encephalopathy, drug or alcohol intoxication or withdrawal, CNS opportunistic infections and neoplasms, or traumatic brain injury. Lesions involving the temporal lobes or partial complex seizures are associated with violent outbursts.

In terms of the psychosocial factors associated with violent behavior, patients with HIV often suffer considerable loss in the context of their illness—for example, the loss of significant relationships and occupational functioning. The potential for significant physical disability due to a general systemic illness or HIV-related neurological deficit further compounds the potential for personal loss and the attendant emotional or behavioral disturbance. Finally, the risk of violence may be increased in HIV patients with comorbid Axis I disorders, such as schizophrenia or bipolar disorder, or Axis II disorders, such as borderline personality disorder or antisocial traits.

Prevention is the most important aspect of managing violent behavior of persons with HIV. Caregivers of persons with HIV must be alert for early warning signs of violent behavior. These include verbal aggression, physical aggression against objects (e.g., slamming doors, throwing things), physical aggression against self, and threats of physical aggression against others. Risk factors for violence in general include a history of violence, early childhood abuse, exposure to serious trauma, substance abuse, dementia, and schizophrenia.

Violent behavior may be prevented by working with the patient who has a history or potential for violence to encourage self-recognition and self-awareness of violent tendencies. Patients should be counseled about reaching out to staff when they sense the potential within themselves for imminent violence. Patients may learn to request soothing foods in an effort to prevent escalating emotional or behavioral dyscontrol. Potentially violent patients may also benefit from the use of relaxation techniques and biofeedback. Cohen and Alfonso (1998) assert that hope is the most important deterrent to violence, which is often lacking in patients with HIV and AIDS. Caregivers should be cognizant of this fact and work to cultivate hope in their patients.

Cohen and Alfonso (1998) advocate a multidimensional approach to the management and treatment of violent behavior among persons with HIV. The approach includes early recognition, crisis intervention, alternative outlets, and psychotherapy. The elements to early recognition and the prediction of violent behavior have been discussed above. Crisis intervention should be carried out by trained personnel, with an objective to preserve the dignity of the patient and allow the patient to regain self-control. The patient should not be cornered and the caregiver should speak in a gentle, reassuring voice. In addition to offering medicine, foods such as cookies or ice cream may be helpful in the de-escalation of violence.

After the need for crisis intervention has passed, caregivers may work with patients to develop extracurricular activities to minimize aggressive behavior. Alternative outlets for aggressive impulses include painting, creative writing, dance, exercise, and arts and crafts. Patients may be encouraged to keep a personal diary. Specific activities or therapies based on an individual patient's deficits may be helpful, such as movement therapy for patients with motor deficits or the use of talking books for the visually impaired.

Psychotherapy should be used for the development of coping skills and stress management. Patients with advanced HIV will invariably have multiple serious life stressors to process and work through. It is important for caregivers to provide ongoing supportive and interpersonal therapy during this time. Specific issues that patients with HIV may have include a distorted need for physical contact and closeness and the need for negative attention (Cohen and Alfonso, 1998).

Sutor and colleagues have addressed the problem of managing agitation in dementia and recommend a behavioral approach whenever possible (Sutor, 2002; Sutor et al., 2006). These authors point out that behavior, even in dementia, is a form of communication, and behaviors that may appear random may in fact be adaptive or goal directed from the patient's point of view. Agitation may thus result from the frustration of perceived goals on the part of the patient. Successful redirection of the patient is more likely to be achieved if the caregiver attends to the emotional content of the patient's behavior. For example, a patient's agitation may be provoked by anxiety related to missing her family. Furnishing the patient's room with photos and messages from his or her family may go some way toward relieving the patient's anxiety. The authors also point out that since behaviors compete with each other in real time, difficult behaviors can be decreased by increasing desired behaviors. Desired behaviors can be encouraged by tailoring activities to fit the patient's level of function and premorbid interests and talents. For example, a former school

teacher may be soothed by being made the "lunch room monitor."

The successful management of agitated behavior in dementia begins with a thorough assessment of the patient's living environment. Sutor and colleagues emphasize that managing the antecedents of behavior is key to reducing the frequency of difficult behavior in dementia. The authors recommend that staff or family keep a log of the patient's behavior, noting exacerbating and ameliorating factors. As dementia progresses, the patient becomes less adaptive to his or her environment. This may be compensated for to a certain extent by making the environment more adaptive to the patient. Caregivers should thus be aware that modifying a patient's environment and customizing the manner in which care is delivered may be key to reducing difficult behavior and increasing desired behavior.

Sutor and colleagues (2006) describe a three-step approach to redirection of an agitated patient. Step 1 is to validate. The caregiver should seek to understand and acknowledge where the patient is coming from and what the behavior means to the patient, as discussed above. Step 2 is to join with the patient. Here the caregiver is encouraged to be an ally of the patient; for example, the caregiver might say, "You're looking for your children? Let's look together." Step 3 is to distract. Once the caregiver has gained an emotional understanding of the patient's position and established a common goal with the patient it may be easier to distract the patient by pointing out another activity or goal.

It should be emphasized that maximizing treatment of medical, neurological, and psychiatric disorders in potentially violent persons with HIV is a key to prevention of violent behavior. This includes stabilization of complex partial seizures, treatment of CNS infection, treatment of psychosis, and correction of metabolic or electrolyte disturbances. When there is a new onset of agitated behavior, a full medical history and physical exam are indicated. New medications, pain, changes in oxygenation, and poor sleep are all common contributors to agitation in patients with dementia.

Medication for violent behavior is indicated when behavioral and psychosocial interventions fail. Recommended medications include both atypical and older antipsychotics (quetiapine, olanzapine, aripiprazole, haloperidol, and perphenazine), anticonvulsants (gabapentin and valproic acid), benzodiazepines (lorazepam, oxazepam), and beta-adrenergic blockers (propanolol). Specific doses are covered below in the section on repetitive taking of other people's property. Medications should be selected with special consideration of the vulnerabilities that patients with HIV face, such as bone marrow suppression, seizures, liver disease, wasting, and anticholinergic and extrapyramidal side effects. Oral medication, rather than parenteral administration, should be used whenever possible to maintain the patient's dignity and avoid further exacerbating a violent situation.

In weighing the risks and benefits of antipsychotic treatment for patients with dementia, Sutor and colleagues point out that atypical antipsychotics have been the treatment of choice for some practitioners (Alexopoulos et al., 2005; Sink et al., 2005; Sutor et al., 2006). Although the U.S. Food and Drug Administration (FDA) has issued a black-box warning on the use of atypical antipsychotics in elderly patients with dementia, estimating an increased risk of death at 1.6 to 1.7 times the baseline rates (FDA, 2005; Schneider et al., 2005), there are currently no data addressing the safety of these medications in patients with HAD.

Sutor and colleagues recommend a targeted approach to the pharmacologic treatment of behavioral problems in patients with dementia (Sutor et al., 2006). If depression is a predominant symptom, an SSRI in the low therapeutic range is recommended. If agitation predominates, atypical antipsychotic medications and anticonvulsant mood stabilizers can be helpful.

REPETITIVE TAKING OF OTHER PERSON'S PROPERTY

Patients with HAD may exhibit the repetitive taking of other persons' property (Cohen and Alfonso, 1998). This behavior can be dangerous to the patient because of potential violent retaliation from the victims of the theft. Dementia can predispose persons with HAD to repetitive theft through several mechanisms, including cortical disinhibition, behavioral dyscontrol, and impaired memory function. Persons with advanced dementia are known to exhibit regression such that their thought patterns and behaviors appear childlike. Patients with HAD may have difficulty distinguishing right from wrong or ownership from desire, as in the toddler who points to an object of desire and shouts "mine." The development of HAD may also exacer-

bate an underlying tendency toward theft, as in kleptomania or antisocial personality disorder.

Often the objects of theft are associated with cravings, such as food or cigarettes. The cortical disinhibition evidenced in dementia may result in patients' difficulty controlling their cravings. This may be compounded by short-term memory impairment and perseveration, so that persons addicted to nicotine may seek a cigarette immediately following the smoking of a cigarette, having forgotten that they had just satisfied their craving.

Approaches to the management of theft behavior of patients with HAD include psychological, behavioral, social, and pharmacologic modalities. Supportive psychotherapy should focus on ego lending and the encouragement of mature defenses. Simple cognitive approaches include establishing a plan to follow when, for example, the patient experiences a cigarette craving: "When you need a cigarette, ask for one at the nurse's station." Or a more general statement regarding theft can be used: "If you see something that you want, ask a staff or family member if it would be possible to obtain your own." Group therapy may be helpful as a forum for some patients in a structured setting to reinforce the fact that taking other persons' property is unacceptable.

In terms of behavior, creative outlets such as creative writing, artwork, or music may help to sublimate destructive tendencies. A reward system with positive reinforcement for not taking others' property may prove useful. The staff and the patient may cooperate to keep a written record of the patient's behavior and devise rewards such as food or privileges for consecutive days without theft.

As part of a social intervention to prevent the taking of other persons' property, it is important to identify and develop a network of family and friends or volunteers to supply the patients with items of desire such as cigarettes, food, or money. Education of family, friends, and staff is important so that the theft behavior is understood as part of the illness. The repetitive taking of other persons' property is regressive, childlike behavior resulting from the dementia, thus retaliation is not appropriate.

Pharmacologic intervention should be used when other approaches are ineffective and especially if the patient is in danger of violent retaliation from victims of the theft behavior. Since behavioral manifestations of dementia are often worse in the evening ("sundowning"), medication can be administered in the evening or throughout the day if necessary. Adjunctive treatment for the repetitive taking of other persons' property include antipsychotics (quetiapine 50–400 mg, olanzapine 2.5–20 mg, aripiprazole 10 mg, perphenazine 2–10 mg, haloperidol 0.5–5 mg), anticonvulsants (gabapentin 100–3600 mg, valproate 250–750 mg, carbamazepine 200–1000 mg), and anxiolytics (lorazepam 1–2 mg, oxazepam 15–30 mg). It is recommended that treatment start with an antipsychotic. If an antipsychotic alone is inadequate to control the behavior, an anticonvulsant should be added. If a combination of an antipsychotic and anticonvulsant is inadequate, an anxiolytic should be added. Both valproate and carbamazepine should be used with caution. Valproate can cause drug–drug interactions and carbamazepine can cause leukopenia and anticholinergic side effects. Anxiolytic benzodiazepines can worsen dementia and regressive behavior and should also be used with caution.

CONCLUSION

HIV-associated dementia is a metabolic encephalopathy uniquely associated with several cognitive and behavioral disturbances that caregivers of persons with advanced HIV must be aware of to minimize dangers to both patients and staff. These unique manifestations include accidental firesetting, violent behavior, and the repetitive taking of other persons' property. A combination of staff education, psychosocial support, treatment of underlying medical illness, and appropriate pharmacotherapy may significantly reduce suffering and improve the quality of life for persons with HAD.

References

Alexopoulos GS, Jeste DV, Chung H, et al. (2005). The Expert Consensus Guideline Series: Treatment of Dementia and Its Behavioral Disturbances. Minneapolis, MN: McGraw-Hill.

Anderson E, Zink W, Xiong H, and Gendelman HE (2002). HIV-1-associated dementia: a metabolic encephalopathy perpetrated by virus-infected and immune-competent mononuclear phagocytes. J Acquir Immune Defic Syndr 31:43–54.

Clifford DB (2002). AIDS dementia [review]. Med Clin North Am 86(3):537–550.

Cohen MA (1998). Psychiatric care in an AIDS nursing home. Psychosomatics 39:154–161.

Cohen MA, and Alfonso CA (1998). Psychiatric care and pain management of persons with HIV infection. In GP Wormser (ed.), AIDS and Other Manifestations of HIV Infection, third edition (pp. 475–503). Philadelphia: Lippincott-Raven.

[FDA] U.S. Food and Drug Administration (2005).FDA Talk Paper. The FDA issues public health advisory for antipsychotic drugs used to for treatment of behavioral disorders in elderly patients. Retrieved March 26, 2007, from http://www.fda.gov/bbs/topics/ANSWERS/2005/ANS01350.html.

Gendelman HE, Zheng J, Coulter CL, Ghorpade A, Che M, Thylin M, Rubocki R, Persidsky Y, Hahn F, Reinhard J Jr, and Swindells S (1998). Suppression of inflammatory neurotoxins by highly active antiretroviral therapy in human immunodeficiency virus-associated dementia. J Infect Dis 178:1000–1007.

Kaul M, Zheng J, Okamoto S, Gendelman HE, and Lipton SA (2005). HIV-1 infection and AIDS: consequences for the central nervous system. Cell Death Differ 12:878–892.

Schneider LS, Dagerman LS, and Insel P (2005). Risk of death with atypical antipsychotic drug treatment for dementia: meta-analysis of randomized controlled trials. JAMA 294:1934–1943.

Sink KM, Holden KF, and Yaffe K (2005). Pharmacological treatment of neuropsychiatric symptoms of dementia: a review of the evidence. JAMA 293:596–608.

Sutor B (2002). Behavioral problems in demented nursing home residents: a multifaceted approach to assessment and management. Compr Ther 28:183–188.

Sutor B, Nykamp LJ, and Smith GE (2006). Get creative to manage dementia-related behaviors. Curr Psychiatry 5:81–96.

Zink WE, Zheng J, Persidsky Y, Poluektova L, and Gendelman HE (1999). The neuropathogenesis of HIV-1 infection. FEMS Immunol Med Microbiol 26:233–241.

Chapter 18

Suicide

César A. Alfonso and Mary Ann Cohen

Living with HIV infection and AIDS is arduous and can become intolerable. Even after more effective antiretroviral treatments were developed and the mortality of HIV infection has been significantly reduced in countries with access to these treatments, psychological and medical comorbidities continue to create great distress, and psychosocial issues such as stigma and discrimination compound the distress experienced by persons with AIDS. Suicide is always multifactorial and requires a multidimensional approach for its prevention. Suicide is preventable even when hopelessness is tangible, overwhelming, and contagious. By identifying the treatable predisposing psychosocial factors and reducing distress, clinicians will be able to anchor the ambivalent suicidal patient and prevent deliberate self-harm.

HIV seropositivity and AIDS continue to be independent risk factors for suicide. HIV-positive persons with comorbid psychiatric and medical illnesses are at an even higher risk of dying by suicide. Although completed suicides in the general population are statistically relatively rare events, the majority of persons with HIV infection frequently experience thoughts of suicide and commonly engage in suicidal behavior, and a substantial number end their lives by suicide. Caring for suicidal persons poses a great challenge to significant others, family members, and clinicians. Suicidal behavior among the medically ill, a psychiatric emergency, is one of the most common reasons for psychiatric consultation in inpatient and outpatient settings and demands great clinical expertise for its management.

In this chapter we will discuss the epidemiology of suicide of HIV-infected persons and describe the known predisposing factors of suicidal behavior. We will also focus on the protective factors against suicide by discussing the psychosocial profile of nonsuicidal HIV-positive persons, and elaborate on the psychodynamics of suicide. Finally, assessment and prevention strategies essential to the treatment of suicidal persons are described.

EPIDEMIOLOGY

The epidemiology of suicide and HIV infection is complex. Prevalence estimates of suicidal behavior and completed suicides vary depending on the population studied. In addition, suicides of persons with AIDS may be underreported in certain parts of the world and acts of deliberate self-harm are often recorded as accidental overdoses or accidental deaths (Carvajal et al., 1995; Semela et al., 2000). Inadequate reporting is particularly relevant when completed suicides among intravenous drug users, who may choose to end their lives by drug overdose, escape our awareness. Since drug overdose is the most common method of completed suicide among HIV-infected persons (Cote et al., 1992; Rajs and Fugelstad, 1992), the suicide rate may actually be higher than what has been reported because of incorrect reporting of suicides as accidental deaths or overdoses. This section summarizes the epidemiology of suicide in the general population, in the medically ill, and in persons with HIV infection with or without associated comorbidities.

The suicide rate in the general population varies from country to country and among immigrant groups with different levels of acculturation. Approximately one million lives are lost worldwide each year to suicide. Reported suicide statistics range from the highest in Eastern European countries, with rates up to 27 per 100,000, to the United States at mid-range, with a rate 11 per 100,000, to some Latin American countries, with rates as low as 6.5 per 100,000 persons/year (Mann et al., 2005). In general, suicide rates among recent immigrants approximate that of the country of origin (Malenfant, 2004); as acculturation occurs it increases or decreases to match that of the new host country (Pavlovic and Marusic, 2001).

It is estimated that 98% of persons who die by suicide have psychiatric or medical conditions (Pokornoy, 1966; Mann et al., 2005). While psychiatric disorders are widely known to increase suicide risk (Guze and Robins, 1970; Barraclough et al., 1974; Blumenthal, 1988; Leibenluft and Goldberg, 1988; Mann, 2005), certain chronic medical illnesses have also been independently associated with higher suicide rates (Harris and Barraclough, 1994; McHugh, 1994).

The psychiatric disorders with the highest suicide rate are mood disorders, which are present in 60% of all suicides (Guze and Robins, 1970), and alcohol abuse and dependence, present in up to 35% of completed suicides (Pirkola et al., 2000). Up to 13%

of persons with schizophrenia die by suicide (Roy, 1986; Pompili et al., 2004). Diagnoses of intravenous drug use disorders (Vaillant, 1966; James, 1967; Marzuk et al., 1992), borderline personality disorder (Frances, 1986; Blumenthal, 1988), dementia (Alfonso and Cohen, 1994), and delirium (Glickman, 1980) also carry a suicide risk significantly higher than that of the general population.

Medical disorders that carry an increased risk for suicide independent of their psychiatric comorbidities include Huntington disease (Huntington, 1872; Schoenfeld et al., 1984), end-stage renal disease (Abram et al., 1971; Kurella et al., 2005), cardiorespiratory illnesses (Farberow et al., 1966; Quan et al., 2002), systemic lupus erythematosus (Harris and Barraclough, 1994), multiple sclerosis (Kahana et al., 1971), and certain cancers such as head and neck, melanoma, and pancreatic tumors (Louhivuori and Hakama, 1979; Breitbart, 1987).

Reports suggesting an association between HIV seropositivity and suicidal behavior in the United States can be found in the medical literature during the first decade of the epidemic (Rundell et al., 1986; Pierce, 1987; Frierson and Lippmann, 1988). A more definitive association of HIV infection as an independent risk factor for suicide was established by autopsy studies (Glass, 1988; Kizer et al., 1988; Marzuk et al., 1988; Plott et al., 1989; Cote et al., 1992). These autopsy studies from cohorts in the United States showed decreasing suicide rates from 66 to 7.4 times greater in persons with HIV infection than in the general population, as we moved from the first to the second decade of the epidemic. But even after the introduction of highly active antiretroviral therapy (HAART), which has substantially reduced morbidity and mortality in areas with access to these treatments, recent studies in the United States (Marzuk et al., 1997), Australia (Ruzicka et al., 2005), and France (Lewden et al., 2005) continue to show an increased risk of suicide among persons with HIV infection.

Clinical studies, likewise, demonstrate high rates of suicidal behavior in persons with HIV infection. In a primary care setting that serves patients with a wide range of demographic characteristics in New York City, 63% of HIV-seropositive subjects acknowledged current or past suicidal ideation (Gil et al., 1998). In a cohort from Missouri, 17% of HIV-positive gay men reported serious thoughts or plans to end their lives at the time of routine clinical interview (Goggin et al., 2000). In a rural cohort of small communities in eight

U.S. states, 38% of persons with HIV infection admitted that they had suicidal thoughts 1 week prior to responding to self-administered surveys (Heckman et al., 2002). Similarly, 27% of middle-aged and older persons living with HIV admitted to suicidal ideation within 1 week prior to a clinical survey (Kalichman et al., 2000). In a municipal general hospital in New York City, suicidal behavior was present in one out of every five persons with HIV infection (Alfonso et al., 1994).

PREDISPOSING FACTORS

Predisposing factors that have cumulative or synergistic effects on increasing suicide risk are multidimensional, with biological, psychological, social, and cultural determinants. In this section we will discuss the predisposing factors associated with completed suicides among persons with HIV infection and AIDS.

The demographic characteristics of persons with HIV infection who die by suicide show different patterns from those of persons with unknown HIV status who completed suicide. General-population suicide statistics show that death by suicide among men is three times higher than among women (McIntosh, 2003). Among persons with HIV infection, women are at a significantly higher risk for attempting and dying by suicide (Brown and Rundell, 1989; Rundell et al., 1992; Roy, 2003; Cohen and Alfonso, 2004). Also, whereas general-population completed suicides occur primarily during late life for men and peak in mid-life and then decrease for women (Kaplan and Klein, 1989), persons with HIV infection can be suicidal at any time from diagnosis to end-stage illness (Cohen and Alfonso, 2004). In fact, clinicians in Europe, Asia, America, and Africa have observed that suicidality has a bimodal distribution, with peaks at the time of diagnosis with HIV seropositivity or infection and at end-stage illness with AIDS (Gala et al., 1982; Perry et al., 1990; Sindiga and Lukhando, 1993; Gotoh et al., 1994; Sherr, 1995; Kelly et al., 1998, Cooperman and Simoni, 2005). While in the United States most completed general-population suicides are older Caucasian men, a New York City autopsy study showed that among those with HIV infection, younger and middle-aged Latino and African-American men had the highest suicide rate (Marzuk et al., 1997).

A family history of suicide attempts or death by suicide is a strong predictor of suicide in individuals with HIV infection (Roy, 2003). Persons with a history of early childhood trauma with or without a diagnosis of posttraumatic stress disorder are also at increased risk for suicide (Miles, 1977; Roy, 2003; Cooperman and Simoni, 2005). Suicide risk increases in states of bereavement (Sherr, 1995), in particular during holidays or anniversary dates relevant to the deceased. Suicidal behavior increases when persons have poor social support, decreased social integration, poor family relations, and a restricted social environment (Kalichman et al., 2000; Haller and Miles, 2003). One study showed that suicidal behavior increases when persons disclose their positive serostatus (Kalichman et al., 2000), and several studies have shown that being burdened by caregiving and having an HIV-positive spouse or children can increase suicide risk (Rosengard and Folkman, 1997; Chandra et al., 1998).

The medical comorbidities of HIV infection can trigger thoughts of suicide and suicidal behavior. Incapacitating nociceptive and neuropathic pain, pruritus, hiccups, insomnia, dyspnea, nausea, emesis, intractable diarrhea, severe wasting, blindness, motor deficits, and paresis may compound hopelessness and lead to suicide (Alfonso et al., 1994; Chandra et al., 1998; Cohen and Alfonso, 2004). It is important to recognize that when persons with AIDS have access to HAART and to effective treatments for their opportunistic infections they can live longer and healthier lives. As persons with HIV infection age, they may develop other chronic illnesses with a high prevalence of suicide that can complicate prognosis and increase suicide risk.

Psychiatric comorbidities associated with increased suicide risk among persons with HIV infection include psychiatric disorders, subthreshold conditions and symptoms, medication side effects, and negative affective states. Elevated suicide rates are found among persons with HIV infection and comorbid depressive disorders, bereavement, posttraumatic stress disorder (Kelly et al., 1998; Haller and Miles, 2003), schizophrenia and other psychotic states (Wood et al., 1997; Haller and Miles, 2003), personality disorders, psychoactive substance use disorders (Haller and Miles, 2003), dementia, and delirium (Alfonso and Cohen, 1994). Clinical researchers have recently identified a particularly high suicide rate with comorbid major depression and posttraumatic stress disorder (Oquendo et al., 2005a; Sher et al., 2005), which are common coexisting conditions in persons with HIV infection (Cohen et al., 2001). Even though affective states of depression, guilt, anger, fear, and shame are commonly present and increase suicide risk in HIV-positive patients, the affective state with the strongest association with suicide is hopelessness (Beck et al., 1985; Cohen and Alfonso, 2004).

Studies of the neurobiology of suicide have consistently shown serotonergic dysfunction. HIV-infected individuals have decreased levels of cerebrospinal fluid (CSF) 5-HT and 5-HIAA, suggesting that the virus may interfere with serotonin production in the brain (Larsson et al., 1989; Kumar et al., 2001).

Impulsivity and behavioral disinhibition that can precipitate suicidal behavior can occur in patients undergoing alcohol and opioid withdrawal and are also common in advanced stages of HIV dementia. Medication side effects, such as akathisia secondary to aripripazole, fluphenazine, or risperidal (Shear et al., 1983; Drake and Ehrlich, 1985; Scholten and Selten, 2005), and dysphoria secondary to alpha-interferon have been associated with suicidal behavior in persons with HIV infection as well as comorbid medical and psychiatric disorders.

Stressful life events in the context of poor social support can heighten suicide risk (Kalichman et al., 2000; Haller and Miles, 2003). Persons with HIV infection can have distorted perceptions of illness. Just as an asymptomatic HIV-positive individual can become suicidal upon learning of his or her HIV serostatus, changes in immune parameters can also trigger a suicidal crisis. Learning that one has an increased viral load or decreased CD4 cell count can precipitate a suicidal crisis, even with reassurance that a change in medical treatment can easily reverse the situation (Alfonso et al., 1994; Haas et al., 1997).

Having access to lethal means can make a predisposed individual who is ambivalently contemplating suicide more likely to end his or her life. HIV-seropositive persons have a higher rate of self-inflicted burns and of death by self-immolation (Cohen et al., 1990; Castellani et al., 1995). By providing flame-retardant hospital clothing and restricting access to firearms and prescription drugs, caregivers can protect a suicidal person from deliberate self-harm. Other suicide prevention strategies will be discussed later in this chapter.

PROTECTIVE FACTORS

HIV-seropositive persons who use escape and avoidance coping skills tend to have a poorer prognosis and attempt suicide more often, whereas persons who use positive-reappraisal coping are protected from suicide thoughts and actions (Kalichman et al., 2000).

Experience gathered from individual and group psychotherapy of suicidal persons with HIV infection indicates that several factors can protect an individual from a premature self-inflicted death and from self-destructive behaviors. Protective factors include a "taking-charge" attitude rather than passivity, an adequate understanding of illness, denial that does not interfere with adherence with medical treatment, increasing social support via networking, and optimism (Alfonso and Cohen, 1997; Rosengard and Folkman, 1997; Cohen, 1998, 1999).

There is very little research that systematically addresses the protective factors that prevent development of suicidal behavior in persons with HIV infection. Studies of nonsuicidal persons with psychiatric disorders and unknown HIV serostatus and clinical interviews of HIV-positive, long-term survivors can be used, however, to highlight possible psychosocial variables that may ultimately prevent the development of suicidal and self-destructive behavior.

Clinical researchers have examined the protective factors against suicidal acts for persons with diverse psychopathology and high suicide risk. While prior attempted suicide and hopelessness are the strongest predictors of completed suicides, protective factors include more feelings of responsibility toward family, more fear of social disapproval, greater survival and coping skills, and a greater fear of suicide (Malone et al., 2001). These same factors proved protective in a cohort of Latino patients diagnosed with major depression whose depressive symptomatology did not result in suicidal behavior (Oquendo et al., 2005b).

Studies of long-term survivors with AIDS in the New York City area have demonstrated that high levels of hope and low levels of distress and depressive symptoms result in psychological resiliency and an extended life span (Rabkin et al., 1990, 1993). Another study in Miami showed that higher emotional expression and depth processing, including positive cognitive appraisal change, experiential involvement, self-esteem enhancement, and adaptive coping strategies, were significantly related to long-term survival status of men and women with AIDS, as well as to lower viral load and higher CD4 cell count in women with AIDS (O'Cleirigh et al., 2003). The clinical implications of these studies underscore the importance of psychotherapy in the treatment of suicidal persons with HIV infection. The psychotherapeutic component of treatment will be elaborated on further in the section on prevention strategies below.

PSYCHODYNAMICS

Although common psychodynamic formulations may be relevant to suicidal patients with HIV infection, individual life experiences will influence and determine behavior and clinicians should not adopt any universal set of dynamics as absolute or paradigmatic. Commonality of certain life experiences, nevertheless, can propel a predisposed individual to engage in acts of deliberate self-harm.

Freud and Abraham's original contributions on the dynamics of grief and depression shed some light on the meaningfulness of suicide. They observed that depression often follows either real or imagined loss. Ambivalent anger toward the lost loved one can be turned against the self in an act of aggression. Suicide can be understood as a cathartic expression of rage and sadness that symbolically attempts to recapture what has been lost (Abraham, 1911, 1924; Freud, 1917).

Suicidal behavior is never random. Unbearable situations create intolerable distress, and suicide serves as an escape from intense suffering. Suicidal persons with HIV infection are often plagued by unendurable negative affects. These may include shame, sadness, rage, guilt, anxiety, and hopelessness. Suicidal persons are truly blinded by their suffering and see no options to alleviate their distress. This constriction of cognition (Litman, 1989) results in the distorted view that suicide serves as the only way out, and when psychic pain is unbearable, cessation of life — "ending it all" — serves the purpose of and becomes synonymous with remediation of pain and suffering.

Other dynamic factors that may be enacted as self-destruction include conflicts over relinquishing autonomy and intolerable dependency. Persons with chronic or incapacitating medical illnesses fear that losing control over their bodily functions will be dehumanizing and make life not worth living. Interpersonal conflicts and inability to trust or accept help from significant others magnify the distress created by pain, disfigurement, blindness, weakness, and depression associated with some of the infections that affect persons with AIDS. Those who value autonomy over life itself experience suicidal behavior as a better alternative than relying on others.

Social dynamics that drive people to end their lives include the forces of stigma and discrimination. HIV seropositivity and a diagnosis of AIDS often bring to surface feelings of shame and guilt. Negative social attitudes result in social oppression, which can further precipitate these affective states, alienating individuals into hopelessness and despair that can culminate in suicide (Cohen and Alfonso, 2004).

Suicidal individuals with a history of harmful use of alcohol or illicit drugs have experienced social isolation, loneliness, and alienation from their families and communities. A diagnosis of HIV and deteriorating health can exacerbate their sense of expendability (Sabbath, 1969; Cohen and Merlino, 1983), leading to suicidal behavior as a way to control one's destiny and escape overwhelming hopelessness, extreme isolation, and despair.

HIV-seropositive individuals with a history of early childhood trauma with or without a current diagnosis of posttraumatic stress disorder can experience a sense of foreshortened future that may further increase their suicide risk (Cohen et al., 2001; Ricart et al., 2002). The dynamics of posttraumatic stress disorder are complex and an understanding of them is essential for effective psychotherapeutic work to occur with persons with AIDS. These dynamics are discussed further in Chapter 11 of this volume.

To recapitulate, the psychodynamics of suicide need to be understood in the context of the individual's unique life experiences. Suicide is often a reaction to loss, either loss of loved ones, present and past, or loss of function and vitality. In addition to anger and sadness, the predominant affects of depression, and other emotional states such as shame, guilt, and hopelessness precede suicidal behavior. Interpersonal conflicts resulting in inability to trust and accept others into one's life need to be worked through to prevent the intolerable loneliness and distress that could result in suicide. The suicidal person with AIDS is often in the midst of a crisis of expendability. Stigma and discrimination further compound the hopelessness and psychic distress, heightening the possibility of death by suicide.

PREVENTION STRATEGIES

Suicide prevention starts with taking a suicide history of every patient with HIV. Clinicians need to feel comfortable discussing suicide in depth.

Countertransference reactions play a major role in being able to have a productive dialogue with the suicidal patient and establishing a therapeutic alliance. Feelings are contagious, and the overwhelming hopelessness of a suicidal individual may interfere with the clinician's ability to infuse hope and help the patient find alternatives to premature death. Far from harming the patient, being able to put feelings into words to express suicidal impulses is highly relieving and can prevent acting out aggressively. When a suicidal person verbalizes his or her suicidal ideas and plans, a different perspective can be attained as unendurable affects are expressed. Listening with empathy at a moment of crisis can begin to dissipate hopelessness and mobilize the will to live.

An adequate suicide history includes an assessment of present suicidal ideas and plans by asking direct and open-ended questions. Since past suicide attempts are, along with hopelessness, the strongest predictors of future completed suicide, the clinician must always ask about previous attempts and elicit a family history of suicide. Timely treatment of the psychiatric disorders associated with heightened suicide risk could prevent suicide in individuals at risk. Antidepressants should be prescribed to depressed and anxious suicidal patients, but it is important to remember that anhedonia and psychomotor retardation lift first when these are prescribed, and hopelessness, dysphoria, and suicidal behavior take longer to improve (Mann, 2005). Psychotherapy can reduce a sense of alienation, provide symptomatic relief, increase networking, and promote conflict resolution. Psychotherapy modalities that can help suicidal patients include interpersonal, cognitive-behavioral, psychodynamic, and supportive, in both individual and group therapy settings.

Physical symptoms compound psychological distress and can precipitate death by suicide. Providing symptomatic relief and palliation of nociceptive and neuropathic pain, pruritus, diarrhea, nausea, emesis, and anorexia can avert a suicidal crisis in persons with HIV infection.

There is no treatment for suicide, only prevention. Thus there may be times when a person with HIV or AIDS is overwhelmed with suicidal feelings, and the person may or may not have a prior relationship with a psychiatrist or other mental health clinician. If there is a suicide attempt or an expression of suicidal ideation, primary physicians, psychiatrists, and other mental health professionals in an emergency setting, or psychosomatic medicine psychiatrists in general care

may need to assess for suicidality. In such situations, an emergency psychiatric hospitalization may be indicated if the person is found to be actively suicidal and in the midst of a suicidal crisis. Close observation by staff is essential to ensure that the suicidal individual is safe during the process of the transfer. If the medical condition does not permit transfer, then one-on-one observation should be maintained until the suicidal crisis resolves or the transfer can be accomplished.

Since suicidal persons are ambivalent by definition and will oscillate from wanting to live and opting to die, it is important to identify family members or friends who can be called on to accompany and protect patients during a time of crisis. Family members or friends can also be of assistance in minimizing access to lethal means.

In order for the suicidal person with HIV infection to resolve a suicide crisis, it is important to establish trusting relationships, reconnect with family members and significant others, restore hope, find meaning in life, and develop goals to attain a sense of fulfillment and connectedness. With support, companionship, networking, conflict resolution, palliative care, adequate medical treatment, and alleviation of psychological distress, persons with HIV infection may realize that suicide is not the only option.

References

Abram HS, Moore GL, and Westervelt FB (1971). Suicidal behavior in chronic dialysis patients. *Am J Psychiatry* 127:119–124.

Abraham K (1911). Notes on the psychoanalytical investigation and treatment of manic-depressive insanity and allied conditions. In *Selected Papers on Psychoanalysis* (pp. 137–156). Translated by D Byran D and A Strachey. New York: Basic Books, 1960.

Abraham K (1924). A short study of the development of the libido, viewed in the light of mental disorders. In *Selected Papers on Psychoanalysis* (pp. 418–501). Translated by D Byran and A Strachey. New York: Basic Books, 1960.

Alfonso CA, and Cohen MA (1994). HIV dementia and suicide. *Gen Hosp Psychiatry* 16:45–46.

Alfonso CA, and Cohen MA (1997). The role of group psychotherapy in the care of persons with AIDS. *J Am Acad Psychoanal* 25:623–638.

Alfonso CA, Cohen MA, Aladjem AD, Morrison F, Powell DR, Winters RA, and Orlowski BK (1994). HIV seropositivity as a major risk factor for suicide in the general hospital. *Psychosomatics* 35:368–373.

Barraclough B, Bunch J, Nelson B, and Sainsbury P (1974). A hundred cases of suicide: clinical aspects. *Br J Psychiatry* 25:355–372.

Beck AT, Steer RA, Kovacs M, and Garrison B (1985). Hopelessness and eventual suicide: a 10-year prospective study of patients hospitalized with suicidal ideation. *Am J Psychiatry* 142:559–563.

Blumenthal SJ (1988). Suicide: a guide to risk factors, assessment, and treatment of suicidal patients. *Med Clin North Am* 72:937–971.

Breitbart W (1987). Suicide in cancer patients. *Oncology* 4:49–54.

Brown GR, and Rundell JR (1989). Suicidal tendencies in women with human immunodeficiency virus infection. *Am J Psychiatry* 146:556–557.

Carvajal MJ, Vicioso C, Santamaria JM, and Bosco A (1995). AIDS and suicide issues in Spain. *AIDS Care* 7:135–138.

Castellani G, Beghini D, Barisoni D, and Marigo M (1995). Suicide attempted by burning: a 10-year study of self-immolation deaths. *Burns* 21(8):607–609.

Chandra PS, Ravi V, Desai A, and Subbakrishna DK (1998). Anxiety and depression among HIV-infected heterosexuals—a report from India. *J Psychosom Res* 45:401–409.

Cohen MA (1998). Psychiatric care in an AIDS nursing home. *Psychosomatics* 39:154–161.

Cohen MA (1999). Psychodynamic psychotherapy in an AIDS nursing home. *J Am Acad Psychoanal* 27:121–133.

Cohen MA, and Alfonso CA (2004). AIDS psychiatry, palliative care and pain management. In GP Wormser (ed.), *AIDS and Other Manifestations of HIV Infection*, fourth edition (p. 566). San Diego: Elsevier Academic Press.

Cohen MA, and Merlino JP (1983). The suicidal patient on the surgical ward: multidisciplinary case conference. *Gen Hosp Psychiatry* 5:65–71.

Cohen MA, Aladjem AD, Brenin D, and Ghazi M (1990). Firesetting by patients with the acquired immunodeficiency syndrome (AIDS). *Ann Intern Med* 112:386–387.

Cohen MA, Alfonso CA, Hoffman R, Milau V, and Carrera G (2001). The impact of PTSD on treatment adherence in persons with HIV infection. *Gen Hosp Psychiatry* 23(5):294–296.

Cooperman NA, and Simoni JM (2005). Suicidal ideation and attempted suicide among women living with HIV/AIDS. *J Behav Med* 28(2):149–156.

Cote TR, Biggar RJ, and Dannenberg AL (1992). Risk of suicide among persons with AIDS. *JAMA* 268:2066–2068.

Drake RE, and Ehrlich J (1985). Suicide attempts associated with akathisia. *Am J Psychiatry* 142(4):499–501.

Farberow L, McKelligott JW, Cohen S, and Darbonne A (1966). Suicide among patients with cardiorespiratory illnesses. *JAMA* 195:422–428.

Frances A (1986). Personality and suicide. *Ann N Y Acad Sci* 487:281–293.

Freud S (1917). *Mourning and Melancholia*. In *Standard Edition of the Complete Psychological Works of Sigmund Freud*, Vol. 14 (pp. 237–260). Translated and edited by J Strachey. London: Hogarth Press, 1957.

Frierson RL, and Lippmann SB (1988). Suicide and AIDS. *Psychosomatics* 29:226–231.

Gala C, Pergami A, Catalan J, Riccio M, Durbano F, Musicco M, Baldeweg T, and Invernizzi G (1982). Risk of deliberate self-harm and factors associated with suicidal behaviors among asymptomatic individuals with human immunodeficiency virus infection. *Acta Psychiatr Scand* 86:70–75.

Gil F, Passik S, Rosenfeld B, and Breitbart W (1998). Psychological adjustment and suicidal ideation in patients with AIDS. *AIDS Patient Care STDs* 12(12):927–930.

Glass RM (1988). AIDS and suicide. *JAMA* 259:1369–1370.

Glickman LS (1980). The suicidal patient. In LS Glickman (ed.), *Psychiatric Consultation in the General Hospital* (pp. 181–202). New York: Marcel Dekker.

Goggin K, Sewell M, Ferrando S, Evans S, Fishman B, and Rabkin J (2000). Plans to hasten death among gay men with HIV/AIDS: relationship to psychological adjustment. *AIDS Care* 12(2):125–136.

Gotoh T, Ajisawa A, Negishi M, and Yamaguchi T (1994). A study of suicide and attempted suicide in HIV carriers and patients with AIDS. Xth International Conference on AIDS, Yokohama, Japan. 10:400 [abstract].

Guze SB, and Robins E (1970). Suicide and primary affective disorder. *Br J Psychiatry* 117:437–438.

Haas DW, Morgan ME, and Harris VL (1997). Increased viral load and suicidal ideation in an HIV-infected patient. *Ann Intern Med* 126(1):86–87.

Haller DL, and Miles DR (2003). Suicidal ideation among psychiatric patients with HIV: psychiatric morbidity and quality of life. *AIDS Behav* 7(2):101–108.

Harris EC, and Barraclough BM (1994). Suicide as an outcome for medical disorders. *Medicine* 73:281–296.

Heckman TG, Miller J, Kochman A, Kalichman SC, Carlson B, and Silverthorn M (2002). Thoughts of suicide among HIV-infected rural persons enrolled in a telephone-delivered mental health intervention. *Ann Behav Med* 24(2):141–148.

Huntington G (1872). On chorea. *Med Surg Reporter* 26:317–321.

James IP (1967). Suicide and mortality among heroin addicts in Britain. *Br J Addict* 62:391–398.

Kahana E, Lebowitz W, and Alter M (1971). Cerebral multiple sclerosis. *Neurology (Minn)* 21:1179–1185.

Kalichman SC, Heckman T, Kochman A, Sikkema K, and Bergholte J (2000). Depression and thoughts of suicide among middle-aged and older persons living with HIV-AIDS. *Psychiatr Serv* 51:903–907.

Kaplan A, and Klein R (1989). Women and suicide. In D Jacobs and H Madison (eds.), *Suicide: Understanding and Responding* (pp. 257–282). Madison, CT: International Universities Press.

Kelly B, Raphael B, Judd F, Perdices M, Kernutt G, Burnett P, Dunne M, and Burrows G (1998). Suicidal ideation, suicide attempts, and HIV infection. *Psychosomatics* 39:405–415.

Kizer KW, Green M, Perkins CI, Doebbert G, and Hughes MJ (1988). AIDS and suicide in California. *JAMA* 260:1881.

Kumar AM, Berger JR, Eisdorfer C, Fernandez JB, Goodkin K, and Kumar M (2001). Cerebrospinal fluid 5-hydroxytryptamine and 5-hydroxyindoleacetic acid in HIV-1 infection. *Neuropsychobiology* 44(1):13–18.

Kurella M, Kimmel PL, Young BS, and Chertow GM (2005). Suicide in the United States end-stage renal disease program. *J Am Soc Nephrol* 16(3):774–781.

Larsson M, Hagberg L, Norkrans G, and Forsman A (1989). Indole amine deficiency in blood and cerebrospinal fluid from patients with human immunodeficiency virus infection. *J Neurosci Res* 23(4): 441–446.

Leibenluft E, and Goldberg RL (1998). The suicidal terminally ill patient with depression. *Psychosomatics* 29:379–386.

Lewden C, Salmon D, Morlat P, Bevilacqua S, Jougla E, Bonnet F, Heripret L, Costagliola D, May T, and Chene G (2005). Causes of death among human immunodeficiency virus (HIV)-infected adults in the era of potent antiretroviral therapy: emerging role of hepatitis and cancers, persistent role of AIDS. *Int J Epidemiol* 34(1):130–131.

Litman R (1989). Suicides: what do they have in mind? In D Jacobs and H Brown (eds.), *Suicide: Understanding and Responding* (pp. 143–154). Madison, CT: International Universities Press.

Louhivuori KA, and Hakama M (1979). Risk of suicide among cancer patients. *Am J Epidemiol* 109:59–65.

Malenfant EC (2004). Suicide in Canada's immigrant population. *Health Reports* 5:9–17.

Malone KM, Oquendo MA, Haas GL, Ellis SP, Li S, and Mann JJ (2000). Protective factors against suicidal acts in major depression: reasons for living. *Am J Psychiatry* 157(7):1331–1332.

Mann JJ (2005). The medical management of depression. *N Engl J Med* 353:1819–1834.

Mann JJ, Apter A, Bertolote J, Beautrais A, Currier D, Haas A, Hegerl U, Lonnqvist J, Malone K, Marusic A, Mehlum L, Patton G, Phillips M, Rutz W, Rihmer Z, Schmidtke A, Shaffer D, Silverman M, Takahashi Y, Varnik A, Wasserman D, Yip P, and Hendin H (2005). Suicide prevention strategies—a systematic review. *JAMA* 294(16):2064–2074.

Marzuk PM, Tierney H, Tardiff K, Gross EM, Morgan EB, Hsu MA, and Mann JJ (1988). Increased risk of suicide in persons with AIDS. *JAMA* 259:1333–1337.

Marzuk PM, Tardiff K, Leon AC, Stajic M, Morgan EB, and Mann JJ (1992). Prevalence of cocaine use among residents of New York City who committed suicide during a one-year period. *Am J Psychiatry* 149:371–375.

Marzuk PM, Tardiff K, Leon AC, Hirsch CS, Hartwell N, Portera L, and Iqbal MI (1997). HIV seroprevalence among suicide victims in New York City, 1991–1993. *Am J Psychiatry* 154:1720–1725.

McHugh PR (1994). Suicide and medical afflictions. *Medicine* 73:297–298.

McIntosh J (2003). *U.S.A. Suicide: Suicide Data* (p. 2001). Washington, DC: American Association of Suicidology.

Miles CP (1977). Conditions predisposing to suicide: a review. *J Nev Ment Dis* 164:231–246.

O'Cleirigh C, Ironson G, Antoni M, Fletcher MA, McGuffey L, Balbin E, Schneiderman N, and Solomon G (2003). Emotional expression and depth processing of trauma and their relation to long-term survival in patients with HIV/AIDS. *J Psychosom Res* 54(3):225–235.

Oquendo M, Brent DA, Birmaher B, Greenhill L, Kolko D, Stanley B, Zelazny J, Burke AK, Firinciogullari S, Ellis SP, and Mann JJ (2005a). Posttraumatic stress disorder comorbid with major depression: factors mediating the association with suicidal behavior. *Am J Psychiatry* 162(3):560–566.

Oquendo MA, Dragatsi D, Harkavy-Friedman J, Dervic K, Currier D, Burke AK, Grunebaum MF, and Mann JJ (2005b). Protective factors against suicidal behavior in Latinos. *J Nerv Ment Dis* 193(7):438–443.

Pavlovic E, and Marusic A (2001). Suicide in Croatia and in Croatian immigrant groups in Australia and Slovenia. *Croat Med J* 42(6):669–672.

Perry S, Jacobsberg L, and Fishman B (1990). Suicidal ideation and HIV testing. *JAMA* 263:679–682.

Pierce C (1987). Underscore urgency of HIV counseling: several suicides follow positive tests. *Clin Psychiatry News* October 1.

Pirkola SP, Isometsa ET, Heikkinen ME, and Lonnqvist JK (2000). Suicides of alcohol misusers and nonmisusers in a nationwide population. *Alcohol Alcohol* 35(1):70–75.

Plott RT, Benton SD, and Winslade WJ (1989) Suicide of AIDS patients in Texas: a preliminary report. *Tex Med* 85:40–43.

Pokorny AD (1966). A follow-up study of 618 suicidal patients. *Am J Psychiatry* 122:1109–1116.

Pompili M, Ruberto A, Girardi P, and Tatarelli R (2004). Suicide in schizophrenia. What are we going to do about it? *Ann Ist Super Sanita* 40(4):463–467.

Quan H, Arboleda-Florez J, and Flick G (2002). Association between physical illness and suicide among the elderly. *Soc Psychiatry Psychiatr Epidemiol* 37:190–197.

Rabkin JG, Williams JB, Neugebauer R, Remien RH, and Goetz R (1990). Maintenance of hope in

HIV-spectrum homosexual men. *Am J Psychiatry* 147(10):1322–1326.

Rabkin JG, Remien R, Katoff L, and Williams JB (1993). Resilience in adversity among long-term survivors of AIDS. *Hosp Community Psychiatry* 44(2):162–167.

Rajs J, and Fugelstad A (1992). Suicide related to human immunodeficiency virus infection in Stockholm. *Acta Psychiatr Scand* 85:234–239.

Ricart F, Cohen MA, Alfonso CA, Hoffman RG, Quinones N, Cohen A, and Indyk D (2002). Understanding the psychodynamics of non-adherence in persons with PTSD and HIV infection. *Gen Hosp Psychiatry* 24(3):176–180.

Rosengard C, and Folkman S (1997). Suicidal ideation, bereavement, HIV serostatus and psychosocial variables in partners of men with AIDS. *AIDS Care* 9(4):373–384.

Roy A (1986). Suicide in schizophrenia. In A Roy (ed.), *Suicide* (pp. 97–112). Baltimore: Williams & Wilkins.

Roy A (2003). Characteristics of HIV patients who attempt suicide. *Acta Psychiatr Scand* 107(1):41–44.

Rundell JR, Wise ME, and Ursano RJ (1986). Three cases of AIDS-related psychiatric disorders. *Am J Psychiatry* 143:777–778.

Rundell JR, Kyle KM, Brown GR, and Thomason JL (1992). Risk factors for suicide attempts in a human immunodeficiency virus screening program. *Psychosomatics* 33:24–27.

Ruzicka LT, Choi CY, and Sadkowsky K (2005). Medical disorders of suicides in Australia: analysis using a multiple-cause-of-death approach. *Soc Sci Med* 61(2):333–341.

Sabbath J (1969). The suicidal adolescent: the expendable child. *J Am Acad Child Psychiatry* 8:272–289.

Schoenfeld M, Myers RH, Cupples LA, Berkman B, Sax DS, and Clark E (1984). Increased rate of suicide among patients with Huntington's disease. *J Neurol Neurosurg Psychiatry* 47:1283–1287.

Scholten MR and Selten JP (2005). Suicidal ideations and suicide attempts after starting on aripiprazole, a new antipsychotic drug. *Ned Tijdschr Geneeskd* 149(41):2296–2298.

Semela D, Glatz M, Hunziker D, Scmid U, and Vernazza PL (2000). Cause of death and autopsy findings in patients of the Swiss HIV Cohort Study (SHCS). *J Suisse Med* 130:1726–1733.

Shear MK, Frances A, and Weiden P (1983). Suicide associated with akathisia and depot fluphenazine treatment. *J Clin Psychopharmacol* 3(4):235–236.

Sher L, Oquendo MA, Burke AK, Grunebaum MF, Zalsman G, Huang YY, and Mann JJ (2005). Higher cerebrospinal fluid homovanillic acid levels in depressed patients with comorbid posttraumatic stress disorder. *Eur Neuropsychopharmacol* 15(2):203–209.

Sherr L (1995) Suicide and AIDS: lessons from a case note audit in London *AIDS Care* 7 (Suppl 2):109–116.

Sindiga I, and Lukhando M (1993). Kenyan university students' views on AIDS. *East Afr Med J* 70:713–716.

Vaillant GE (1966). A twelve-year follow-up of New York narcotic addicts. *Am J Psychiatry* 122:727–737.

Wood KA, Nairn R, Kraft H, Siegel (1997). Suicidality among HIV-positive psychiatric in-patients. *AIDS Care* 9(4):385–389.

Part V

Neuropathologic Manifestations of HIV Infection

Chapter 19

HIV and the Central Nervous System

Ashley Reynolds, Georgette Kanmogne, Irena Kadiu, and Howard E. Gendelman

Significant progress has been achieved as a result of global research efforts into the pathogenesis, epidemiology, and developmental therapeutics for human immunodeficiency virus (HIV) infection and disease (Giulian et al., 1990; Genis et al., 1992; McArthur et al., 1993; Kaul et al., 2001; Sacktor et al., 2001; McArthur, 2004). Simply put, since the discovery more than 23 years ago of HIV as the virus that causes the acquired immune deficiency syndrome (AIDS) (Barre-Sinoussi et al., 1983; Gallo et al., 1983), the molecular structure, function, regulation, tropism, and methods for viral persistence have been well elucidated (Gray et al., 2005; Burton, 2006; Ribeiro et al., 2006). Perhaps most important is that potent antiretroviral therapies (ART) and treatments for a myriad of opportunistic infections are widely available in the developed world (Egger et al., 2002; Manzardo et al., 2005; Walensky et al., 2006). A significant global political, social, and basic research effort is now emerging to make the same drug formulations available to developing countries (Mukherjee et al., 2003; Tassie

et al., 2003; Chulamokha et al., 2005; Dou et al., 2006). All together, HIV is now a treatable and chronic disorder in which the immune system can be protected through ART reductions of viral load. However, complexities and toxicities of antiretroviral medicines abound. Indeed, drugs are not always effective, especially when administered over prolonged time periods and after a protracted and often complicated clinical course (Chen et al., 2002; Badley et al., 2003; Fellay et al., 2005; Green et al., 2005; Azzam et al., 2006). The emergence of viral drug resistance, consequent immune deterioration, treatment interruptions, and short- and long-term toxicities commonly make the outcome of HIV disease at best uncertain.

Of all the complications of HIV disease, the most foreboding, long-term one is the disease's effects on the nervous system. Indeed, early after the description of AIDS, neurological impairments were described and associated with advanced disease and profound immune suppression (Navia et al., 1986a, 1986b). These can often become severe with a triad of cognitive, motor, and behavioral disturbances (Wilkie et al., 2003; Griffin et al., 2004; Weed and Steward, 2005; Worlein et al., 2005). Although ART has reduced disease severity, the prevalence of disease is on the rise. Newer medicines, improved delivery platforms, and effective adjunctive therapies are needed along with better insights into the disease diagnosis, course, and progression.

This review serves to highlight both the research advances made in understanding the effects of HIV on the nervous system and what remains undone. Particular attention is given to the effects of the virus on the nervous system at the molecular and cellular levels as well as within the infected human host. A parallel focus is on prospects for increasing ART effectiveness and availability. An emerging and interesting aspect of disease pathogenesis remains in the many similarities now known between the pathogenesis of HIV-associated cognitive impairments and that of other neurodegenerative disorders (for example, Parkinson's and Alzheimer's disease). Similarities abound at the level of glial inflammation and dysregulation of innate immune responses. Whether caused by virus or misfolded and aggregated proteins, all of these processes underlie the tempo and progression of disease (Hirsch et al., 2003; Butovsky et al., 2005; Minghetti, 2005; Zhang et al., 2005; Craft et al., 2006; Ghafouri et al., 2006; Wu et al., 2006). A significant body of data has emerged in the past quarter century on how HIV affects the brain and causes progressive clinical impairment (Navia et al., 1986a, 1986b; McArthur et al., 1993; Masliah et al., 1997; Everall et al., 1999). The key to future research strategies remains in discovering ways to protect the brain, reverse the process of impairment, or attenuate it.

CLINICAL DISEASE MANIFESTATIONS OF HIV-ASSOCIATED COGNITIVE IMPAIRMENTS

Virus invades the brain early after exposure to HIV and likely before the development of humoral and cellular immune responses (Koenig et al., 1986; Michaels et al., 1988; Gartner, 2000; Aquaro et al., 2005). An aseptic meningitis is known to occur and is characterized by nuchal rigidity, fever, and altered mentation (Brown et al., 1992; Huang et al., 2005). In most patients, the HIV-seroconversion reaction is commonly subclinical and often passes unnoticed; others

may present with a mild influenza-like illness and rarely a mononucleosis-like syndrome (Martin et al., 1992; Beckett and Forstein, 1993; Huang et al., 2005). A portion of these individuals will develop headaches, fever, myalgia, anorexia, rash, and/or diarrhea within the first 2 weeks (Schacker et al., 1996; Lindback et al., 2000; Tyrer et al., 2003; Pilcher et al., 2004). Prior to seroconversion, the acute phase of viral infection is characterized by a rapid HIV-mediated loss of memory CD4+CCR5+ T cells within the mucosal tissues that results in potentially irreversible immune suppression (Veazey et al., 1998; Brenchley et al., 2004; Mehandru et al., 2004; Derdeyn and Silvestri, 2005). During this acute HIV infection, high levels of viremia and viral shedding at mucosal sites occur. Genital and oral ulcers, cancers, and coinfections with a number of sexually transmitted microbial pathogens, including herpes simplex and hepatitis viruses, syphilis, and gonorrhea, can also manifest during the HIV seroconversion reaction (Stamm et al., 1988; Bagdades et al., 1992; Kinloch-de Loes et al., 1993; Bollinger et al., 1997).

The transition from the acute to chronic phase of infection is accompanied by generation of HIV-1-specific adaptive immune responses (Cao et al., 1995; Poluektova et al., 2004; Draenert et al., 2006). Initially, HIV-specific cytotoxic CD8+ T-cell responses and humoral responses (for example, neutralizing antibodies) function to reduce viral replication to a set-point level that is characteristic of chronic HIV infection (Borrow et al., 1997; Schmitz et al., 1999; Letvin and Walker, 2003; Montefiori et al., 2003; Goulder and Watkins, 2004; Koup, 2004). Although this is a robust initial immune response, it is not enough to eradicate virus infection (Musey et al., 1997; Oxenius et al., 2004; Draenert et al., 2006). Continuous low-level or restricted infection of naïve CD4+ T cells and mononuclear phagocytes (monocytes, tissue macrophages, and dendritic cells) during acute infection effectively evades immune surveillance (Zhang et al., 1999; Blankson et al., 2000). The persistence of these quiescent but infected cellular reservoirs makes it difficult to eradicate HIV infection.

Despite early HIV nervous system infection, most infected individuals remain neurologically intact until late stages of AIDS. After years of viral infection and associated profound losses in CD4+ T lymphocytes and viral loads, infected patients commonly succumb to behavioral, motor, and cognitive impairment. During the early days of the AIDS epidemic, cases of unexplained diffuse and often profound neurological impairment were reported in patients who were in the advanced stages of disease (Snider et al., 1983; Nielsen et al., 1984; Navia et al., 1986a, 1998). Neurological manifestations were ascribed to HIV-1 infection itself following the identification of virus in brains at autopsy from neurologically impaired individuals (Koenig et al., 1986; Navia et al., 1986a; Price and Brew, 1988; Price et al., 1988; Cherner et al., 2002).

Dementia is perhaps the most common manifestation of HIV disease, the resultant neuropsychiatric consequences termed by a variety of names: HIV-1 dementia, HIV-1 encephalopathy (the name used commonly for infected children), HIV-associated cognitive/motor complex, AIDS dementia complex, and now, most commonly, HIV-1 associated dementia (HAD) (Swindells et al., 1999; Wilkie et al., 2003; Griffin et al., 2004; Weed and Steward, 2005; Worlein et al., 2005). A clinical diagnosis is based on findings of developmental delays, psychomotor slowing, forgetfulness, personality changes, and decreased knowledge acquisition (Beckett and Forstein, 1993; Sidtis et al., 1993; Sacktor and McArthur, 1997; Schifitto et al., 2001; Cysique et al., 2006). Before use of antiretroviral therapy (ART), HAD developed in 20%–50% of AIDS patients, indicating that HIV-associated central nervous system (CNS) disease does not manifest in all infected individuals. Currently with ART, the rates of disease are around 7%–10%. The more serious neurological manifestations typically occur in patients with high peripheral viral loads, generally when an individual has advanced immune suppression and systemic HIV disease or AIDS (Beckett and Forstein, 1993; Martin-Garcia and Rodriguez-Scarano, 2005). Dementia related to direct HIV infection of the brain is only one of the protean manifestations of AIDS that may be associated with decline in mental status in an infected person. Among the complications of AIDS that must be considered in the differential diagnosis of dementia are the direct effect of HIV on the CNS, opportunistic fungal, viral, and or parasitic infections, neoplasm (lymphoma), ischemic or hemorrhagic lesions, and metabolic abnormalities. These include, for example, toxoplasmosis, cryptococcal meningitis, progressive multifocal leukoencephalopathy (PML), and tuberculosis, among others (Kure et al., 1991; Manzardo et al., 2005). Although there are no definitive tests for HAD, diagnosis is most commonly made following exclusion of common opportunistic and cancerous brain diseases, with screening tests such as neuropsychological test batteries for psychomotor speed and the HIV Dementia Scale (Power et al., 1995; Davis et al., 2002; Cysique et al., 2006). A variety of biomarkers have been discovered in recent years, but none are used in clinical practice (Genis et al., 1992; Gelbard et al., 1994; Mellors et al., 1997; Sporer et al., 2004; McArthur et al., 2005; Schifitto et al., 2005).

BIOMARKERS FOR HIV-1 ASSOCIATED COGNITIVE IMPAIRMENTS

The search for biomarkers including viral and immune factors in diagnosing and monitoring HIV-associated neurological impairments has increased significantly in recent years (Ammassari et al., 2000; Carlson et al., 2004a, 2004b; Ciborowski et al., 2004; Wojna et al., 2004; Helke et al., 2005; Zink et al., 2005; Ciborowski and Gendelman, 2006). In the past, routine cerebrospinal fluid (CSF) evaluation of patients with HAD reflected nonspecific abnormalities with only mild elevations of protein and cellular pleocytosis in about a third of patients (Heyes et al., 1991). Biomarkers include elevated levels of proinflammatory and antiviral cytokines (tumor necrosis factor-alpha [TNF-α], interleukin-1 [IL-1], interleukin-6 [IL-6], and interferon alpha [IFN-α]) (Martin et al., 1992; Brew et al., 1996; Brew, 2001; Roberts et al., 2003), redox-related factors and HIV cellular proteins (Heyes et al., 1991; Sacktor et al., 2001, 2004), as well as soluble receptors and cell adhesion molecules intercellular adhesion molecule-1 (ICAM-1), vascular cell adhesion molecule-1 (VCAM-1), and E-selectin (Gattegno et al., 1995; Vasilescu et al., 2004; Nasi et al., 2005) and monocyte chemotactic protein-1 (MCP-1). Increased levels of these agents are strongly correlated with the development of HIV and simian immunodeficiency virus (SIV) CNS disease (Kelder et al., 1998; Zink et al., 2001; Gonzalez et al., 2002; Sui et al., 2003). CSF viral loads can also correlate with the development of cognitive impairments in a susceptible person (Brew et al., 1997; McArthur et al., 1997; Robertson et al., 1998). In addition, HIV-1-specific cytotoxic T lymphocytes are commonly found in the CSF of patients with HAD (Jassoy et al., 1992; Borrow et al., 1997; Schmitz et al., 1999; Letvin and Walker, 2003; Montefiori et al., 2003; Goulder and Watkins, 2004; Koup, 2004).

With the advent of polymerase chain reaction (PCR) technology, virus load in CSF and plasma can be quantified and its relationship to dementia explored. HIV-1 RNA levels in CSF appear to correlate with cognitive impairment more than do levels seen in plasma (Brew et al., 1997; McArthur et al., 1997; Robertson et al., 1998; Stankoff et al., 1999). However, CSF HIV-1 RNA levels may not be the best predictor of viral burden in the brain, as viral load in the CSF may also be increased by other CNS infections. Because the amount of HIV in the CNS is small even in patients with neurological disease, CSF RNA levels are often relatively low (usually <1 log of plasma levels). This reflects the false-negative rate of CSF RNA as a marker for HIV-1 brain dysfunction. The relationship between CSF HIV-1 RNA and HAD remains thus unresolved. Indeed, minor neurological dysfunction is not always associated with high CSF HIV RNA levels (Brew et al., 1997; Ellis et al., 1997; Cysique et al., 2005).

Evaluation of CSF of HIV-positive individuals has also led to the detection of various neurotoxins that are secreted excessively during HIV-1 infection. Many of these toxins induce excitotoxicity in neurons and are variously associated with cognitive dysfunction. These include HIV-1 viral proteins Tat (Bonavia et al., 2001) and glycoprotein (gp)120 (Lipton, 1998), proinflammatory cytokines (Conant et al., 1996; Shi et al., 1998), arachidonic acid metabolites, and platelet activating factor (PAF), which appear to act on neurons via pathways that converge on elevated PAF signaling (Perry et al., 1998) and subsequent N-methyl-D-aspartate (NMDA) receptor–mediated excitotoxicity (Giulian et al., 1990). PAF is increased in HAD (Gelbard et al., 1994) and has been shown to mediate NMDA excitotoxicity (Ogden et al., 1998) through the up-regulation of glutamate (Clark et al., 1992) and quinolinate (Smith et al., 2001) release from presynaptic terminals. PAF has also been shown to promote dendrite injury following elevated synaptic activity in hippocampal slices, paralleling HIV-1-associated dendrite pathology (Bellizzi et al., 2005). Subsequent genomic analysis has shown the up-regulation of STAT transcripts, resulting in the increased production of IFN-αβ and IFN-γ (Roberts et al., 2004). The implication for HIV is underscored by the discovery that IFN-α may induce expression of the TNF-α receptor (Lau et al., 1991). The role of TNF-α in neurotoxicity and neuronal apoptosis is well established. In fact, new research is being done to val-

idate the utility of extracellular TNF receptors to prevent TNF-α-induced neurotoxicity (Williams et al., 2005). In particular, TNF-α and FasL can induce neuronal death or potentiate the effects of viral proteins gp120 and tat (Jeohn et al., 1998; Sacktor et al., 2004). Other biomarkers have been used as predictors for clinical outcome, including major histocompatibility complex (MHC) class II, the macrophage-specific marker CD68, T-cell intracytoplasmic antigen 1, CSF MCP-1, p38 mitogen-activated protein kinase, and beta-amyloid precursor protein (Zink et al., 2005). It has also been proposed that the level of 14-3-3 protein in CSF is an early marker for neuronal damage, viral replication, and CNS disease (Helke et al., 2005).

Increased prostaglandin production has also been correlated with infection. Prostaglandin E2 is abundantly secreted from several types of cancer cells, and secretion is increased following HIV infection (Foley et al., 1992; Nokta et al., 1995; Rahmouni et al., 2004). Increased prostaglandin E2 has been shown by various laboratories to induce anergy of cytotoxic T cells, thereby suppressing T-cell function (Foley et al., 1992; Rahmouni et al., 2004). Recent findings suggest that prostaglandin E2 induces expression of the functional inhibitory receptors, CD94/NKG2A in human CD8+ T lymphocytes, which inhibit cell-mediated cytotoxicity upon interaction with MHC class I gene products (Zeddou et al., 2005). The abnormal up-regulation of the inhibitory receptor on cytotoxic T cells could be responsible for the failure of the host immune system to attenuate HIV infection (Jeohn et al., 1998; Sacktor et al., 2004).

Ongoing investigations using methods for protein profiling have revealed additional potential biomarkers for HAD (Carlson et al., 2004a; Ciborowski et al., 2004; Wojna et al., 2004; Berger et al., 2005; Pocernich et al., 2005; Ciborowski and Gendelman, 2006), including disordered matrix metalloproteinase (MMP-2, 7, and 9) secretion (Chong et al., 1998; Marshall et al., 1998; Kumar et al., 1999; Ciborowski et al., 2004), and elevated levels of beta 2-microglobulin (Brew et al., 1989, 1992; McArthur et al., 1992), neopterin (Fuchs et al., 1989; Brew et al., 1990), and quinolinate (Brouwers et al., 1993). MMP-9, for example, is known to affect neuronal function. The down-regulation of MMP-9 in infected macrophages, normally up-regulated during macrophage maturation, parallels a more undifferentiated cell phenotype, which suggests that components of monocyte-macrophage differentiation can be regulated during viral infection. Infection of monocytes with HIV-1 is an abortive infection, whereas infection of matured macrophages is more permissive (Zheng et al., 2001). Matrix metalloproteinases are proteolytic enzymes believed to mediate the pathogenesis of disease (Ghorpade et al., 2001). Indeed, expression of MMP-2 and MMP-9 is induced following stimulation of astrocytes and microglia with lipopolysaccharide (LPS), and this expression is markedly attenuated following treatment with antiretroviral drugs (indinavir [IDV] and zidovudine [ZDV]) (Liuzzi et al., 1994). An epidemiological study measuring levels of proinflammatory mediators in children revealed that MMP-9 expression parallels decline in CSF HIV RNA levels (McCoig et al., 2004). The elucidation of new biomarkers for early diagnosis of HAD is essential to establish a more definitive diagnosis of disease. With the aid of new, developing technologies, the efficacy of various treatments can also be examined for therapeutic benefit and monitoring as treatment expands from the use of antiretroviral medications to combination therapy with adjunct medications.

NEUROIMAGING

Diagnostic decisions can often be clouded by concomitant depression, motor impairments, and lethargy that follow debilitating immune suppression and weight loss. In reality, cognitive, motor, and behavior abnormalities underlie a variety of neurological dysfunctions associated with advanced HIV-1 infection. Thus, combinations of clinical, laboratory, and neuroimaging tests, while not irrefutably conclusive, are essential to provide diagnostic support (Syndulko et al., 1994; Boska et al., 2004; Tucker, 2004).

Neuroimaging techniques have the potential to identify underlying neurological processes involved in disease progression (Tucker et al., 2004). Brain imaging with magnetic resonance imaging (MRI), computed tomography (CT), or diffusion tensor imaging (DTI) is often used to supplement clinical and neurological examinations for the diagnosis of HIV-1-associated cognitive impairments (Lawrence and Major, 2002; Thompson et al., 2005; Thurnher et al., 2005). These radiographic and functional imaging tests can delineate the structural and metabolic effects of HIV on the brain and differentiate them from those caused by other types of infectious diseases or cancerous lesions. CT, MRI, and DTI easily depict brain

atrophy. Computerized tomography of the brain characteristically shows cerebral atrophy in most patients with moderate to severe dementia, but atrophic changes may also be present in asymptomatic individuals (Gonzalez et al., 2002). MRI and DTI studies of patients with HAD show increased ventricular size, sulcal widening, diffuse white matter abnormalities, and atrophy (Heyes et al., 1991; Hall et al., 1996; Pomara et al., 2001; Anderson et al., 2002; Thompson et al., 2005; Thurnher et al., 2005). On MRI these lesions appear as a fluffy, nonfocal signal hyperintensity on T2-weighted images, involving bilaterally the periventricular and centrum semiovale white matter (Diesing et al., 2002; Nelson et al., 2005). The distribution and existence of such lesions do not necessarily correlate with the clinical picture, and a certain degree of parenchymal involvement, often missed by CT scan, may be visible in asymptomatic patients. Extensive white matter involvement is more likely to be symptomatic. These changes usually appear in the later stages of disease and thus are not useful for diagnosis (Chong et al., 1993; Post et al., 1993; Anderson et al., 2002).

More advanced techniques assess functional changes in brain metabolism. These include single-photon emission computed tomography (SPECT), positron-emission tomography (PET), functional MRI (fMRI), and magnetic resonance spectroscopy (^{1}H MRS). These techniques have the potential advantage of detecting early functional abnormalities before morphological changes occur.

^{1}H MRS has emerged as an effective way to detect early brain dysfunction in HAD through measurements of brain metabolites (McConnell et al., 1994; Jarvik et al., 1996; Tracey et al., 1998). ^{1}H MRS is a noninvasive method of quantifying neuronal loss indicated by conventional resonance imagers. Assessment of in vivo metabolism gives biochemical information that complements the structural information from the MRI examination, in a quantitative fashion (Diesing et al., 2002). ^{1}H MRS has shown that in early stages of HAD, frontal white matter exhibits changes suggestive of glial proliferation and cell membrane injury, evaluated through measurement of N-acetyl compounds. Individuals with minor cognitive disorder have abnormalities confined to the frontal white matter, whereas those with HAD have metabolite abnormalities throughout the frontal cortex white matter and basal ganglia (Chang et al., 1999a; Vinters, 2004; Nelson et al., 2005). Several groups have reported a reduction in N-acetylaspartate (NAA), a marker for neuronal loss, using in vivo proton ^{1}H MRS in patients with advanced HIV disease (Chang et al., 1999a, 1999b). The ratio of NAA to creatine (CR) reflects neuronal density and correlates with cognitive impairment in HIV-1-associated cognitive dysfunction (Becker et al., 1997). ^{1}H MRS has also demonstrated progressive neuronal loss over time in HIV-infected individuals, and the degree of neuronal loss observed correlates with neurological impairment (Swindells et al., 1995, 1999). Similarly, the ratio of both choline (CHO) and myoinositol (MI) to CR reflects glial density, and both are elevated in HAD (McConnell et al., 1994; Jarvik et al., 1996; Tracey et al., 1998). Increased CHO levels reflect glial membrane turnover indicative of the astrocytosis that follows HIV encephalitis (HIVE).

^{1}H MRS may also be helpful in the differential diagnosis of HAD and other neurological disorders associated with HIV disease, for example, other metabolic encephalopathies (Swindells et al., 1995). Although ^{1}H MRS imaging is not often applied in clinical settings, studies in which brain metabolite concentrations predict response to treatment and correlate with cognitive dysfunction (Chang et al., 1999a, 1999b) are prospective applications for these tests. Moreover, such technologies may be helpful in monitoring therapeutic responses to antiretroviral therapies (Chang et al., 1999b). The advent of new technologies, including the development of quantitative MRS imaging (Boska et al., 2004), has led to improved diagnostic possibilities for HAD. As these technologies improve, metabolic alterations and neuronal loss can be determined much earlier and with broader clinical applicability.

NEUROPATHOLOGY AND ITS ASSOCIATIONS WITH COGNITIVE IMPAIRMENTS

HIV-associated dementia is commonly associated with the neuropathological correlates of HIVE. HIV-1 can be localized to the CNS by immunohistochemistry, in situ hybridization, or PCR methods. Neuropathological abnormalities seen in brain tissues of patients with HAD are usually diffuse and predominantly localized to the white and deep gray matter regions (Navia et al., 1986a). These include myelin pallor and inflammatory infiltrates composed of macrophages and multinucleated giant cells (MGC), widespread reactive astrogliosis and neuronal dropout (in areas responsible for cognition and motor function), and dendritic and synaptic damage, all considered to be hallmarks of the disease process (Sharer et al., 1985; Navia et al., 1986a; Price and Brew, 1988; Price et al., 1991; Gray et al., 1993). Neuropathological evidence of HIVE and the severity of HAD suggest that HIV-1 infection appears to be confined to microglia and perivascular macrophages and that both the presence and frequency of infected cells are highly correlated with histopathological findings of HIVE (Fischer-Smith et al., 2004; Vinters, 2004). Focal necrosis and demyelination associated with only mild neuronal loss, and minor inflammatory changes consisting of perivascular macrophage infiltrates and microglial nodules are less common. In situ PCR studies of brain tissues from patients who are HIV-1 seropositive but asymptomatic suggest that there is early infection of brain microglia, astrocytes and microvascular endothelial cells (Schmid et al., 1994).

Although HIV invades the brain early after viral exposure, functional changes in the CNS occur many years later (Swindells et al., 1999; Gartner and Liu, 2002). These are usually associated with the breakdown of innate and acquired immune mechanisms that serve to control ongoing viral replication, both in the periphery and the brain. Unlike many other viral infections of the brain, which directly infect neurons, HIV-1 mediates neural damage through brain mononuclear phagocytes (MP) by inducing autocrine and paracrine immune amplification of neurotoxic secretions and affecting subsequent neuropathology (Gelbard et al., 1994; Gendelman et al., 1994; Xiong et al., 2000; Jiang et al., 2001; Zheng et al., 2001). These cells exert their neurotoxic effects primarily through secretory factors (Lipton, 1992, 1993; Dreyer and Lipton, 1995; Kaul et al., 2001; Anderson et al., 2002; Garden, 2002; Gendelman and Persidsky, 2005; Ghorpade et al., 2005; Kaul and Lipton, 2006). Mononuclear phagocytes serve as a reservoir for persistent viral infection, a vehicle for dissemination of virus throughout the brain and a major source of neurotoxic products that affect neuronal function and lead to deficits in cognition. The predominant mechanism for disease is through soluble MP neurotoxins. Viral replication appears to be necessary but not sufficient for disease (Gartner and Liu, 2002; Harrold et al., 2002; Persidsky and Gendelman, 2003). Moreover, clinical disease correlates more with the number of activated macrophages than with viral load in the brain (Glass et al., 1995).

The indirect effects of virus on neural function by glial inflammatory products have led to the term *metabolic encephalopathy* for HAD. By definition, HIV-1 is essential for the development of HAD and viral load within the brain. Increasing viral load is associated with worsening neuronal damage, and this damage has been correlated with the onset of early cognitive impairment (Ellis et al., 1997, 2002; Langford et al., 2005). However, many patients never develop HAD, despite persistent high levels of HIV-1 RNA and a rapidly progressive disease course (Ellis et al., 2002, 2003). Likewise, not all patients with HAD have high virus loads. Thus, the association between virus load and neurological disease is complex, and the onset and progression of HAD presumably reflect its complex pathogenic mechanisms.

CNS TARGETS FOR HIV INFECTION

Mononuclear Phagocytes

The pathogenesis of HIV-associated CNS disease centers around the macrophage. Macrophages are the principal cell infected in the brain and become activated and recruited into tissue during inflammation and emigrate into the CNS during disease (Koenig et al., 1986; Schrier et al., 1993; Gabuzda and Wang, 1999; Gartner and Liu, 2002). This influx is transient, however, and will revert to a quiescent state after the inflammatory process has subsided. For HIVE and HAD, the process never subsides, as brain inflammation is continuous and induced by ongoing viral replication. One population of MP, meningeal macrophages, is characteristically infected early after the initial seroconversion reaction, paralleling the development of aseptic meningitis. Later in the course of the disease perivascular macrophages and microglia are infected preferentially (Kure et al., 1990; Devadas et al., 2004).

The perivascular macrophage is an actively studied MP cell type involved in HAD pathogenesis. In natural conditions, these cells exist between the glia limitans and basement membrane of the choroid plexus and CNS capillaries. Perivascular macrophages are derived from circulating monocytes but will not become fully active macrophages. They are in close association with the bone microvascular endothelial cells

(BMVEC), and this position allows them to serve as sentinels for the CNS. They are, in fact, intermediates between the circulation and the microglia. Since microglia are in contact with these macrophages, signals may be rapidly communicated deep into the CNS from interactions at the perivascular space. Transmission of virus and/or inflammatory responses in the brain may occur between these perivascular macrophages and glial cells (Pulliam et al., 1991; Gendelman et al., 1994; Kaul et al., 2001; Williams and Hickey, 2002; Persidsky and Gendelman, 2003; Devadas et al., 2004; Gonzalez-Scarano and Martin-Garcia, 2005).

Current data strongly suggest that perivascular macrophages are likely responsible for most of the transmission of virus into the CNS (Pulliam et al., 1991; Gartner and Liu, 2002; Williams and Hickey, 2002; Devadas et al., 2004). Several observations support this hypothesis, including findings of perivascular macrophages infected with virus, often at high levels (Rappaport et al., 1999; Williams and Hickey, 2002). Through such cells, virus can be readily transferred to microglia upon microglial activation, since there is close contact between the two. The perivascular macrophages are the critical CNS-resident MP acting as an antigen-presenting cell to T cells (Tyor et al., 1992). Thus, they are at high risk for exposure and contact with infected T cells and/or inducing T-cell protective immunity. Moreover, there is relatively frequent turnover of perivascular macrophages, compared with that of microglia (Kennedy and Abkowitz, 1997; Ghorpade et al., 1998). They may bring virus into the CNS after being infected in the periphery, and release or transmit virus after cell death or through interactions with T cells or microglia.

Parenchymal microglia occur in significant numbers in the CNS and may constitute up to 10% of CNS cells. They enter the CNS during gestation and have a very low turnover rate (Kaur and Ling, 1991; Alliot et al., 1999). There are two morphological subtypes of microglia (Ling, 1982a). Ramified microglia are resting cells with reduced secretory and phagocytic activity (Ling, 1982a; Glenn et al., 1992). They make up the web of microglia that spans the CNS. In contrast to perivascular macrophages, they have weak antigen-presenting capability. The second morphological subtype, amoeboid in form, is a morphological intermediate and transitional cell between the ramified microglia and the brain macrophages. This subtype is not found in the normal adult CNS but rather in inflammatory and demyelinating conditions (Ling, 1982b; Kaur et al., 1985; Ling and Wong, 1993).

Infection of brain MPs leads to formation of multinucleated giant cells (MGC). These cells result from the fusion of HIV-1-infected brain MP with uninfected monocyte-derived macrophages (MDM) or microglia (Budka, 1986, 1991; Pontow et al., 2004). This fusion is mediated by HIV-envelope glycoproteins present at the surface of infected cells with CD4 and chemokine receptors at the surface of uninfected cells (Dalgleish et al., 1984; Lifson et al., 1986a, 1986b; Matthews et al., 1987). The MGC are large, irregularly round, elongated or polyhedral, with dense eosinophilic cytoplasm in the center and vacuolated at the periphery (Budka et al., 1988; Pontow et al., 2004). Giant cell formation is found throughout the brain in HIV disease, but is characteristically seen primarily in the deep brain structures and most commonly in subcortical white matter. Although pathognomonic of HAD, giant cells are only found in 50% of patients (Sharer et al., 1985, 1988; Dickson, 1986).

Moreover, CNS macrophages are protected from most antiviral medication in part because of the blood–brain barrier (BBB). The nature of this viral reservoir and its abilities to harbor and support virus growth remain a key obstacle to eradication of HIV-1 infection in the CNS.

Astrocytes

Astrocyte function, critical for the survival of neurons, may be impaired in the context of HIV-1 infection. Astrocytes are responsible for maintaining homeostasis in the CNS and are important in the detoxification of excess excitatory amino acids such as extracellular glutamate levels (Wesselingh and Thompson, 2001; Deshpande et al., 2005). However, infected astrocytes can produce cellular factors that may adversely affect neuronal survival (Lawrence and Major, 2002). Astrocytes play a dual role in the pathogenesis of HIV-related encephalopathy. In HIV-1 infection, astrocyte glutamate reuptake is impaired, possibly due to interactions with infected macrophages (Fine et al., 1996; Jiang et al., 2001). In addition, glutamate release from the astrocyte is induced by activated macrophages (Vesce et al., 1997; Bezzi et al., 2001). Activation of the CXCR4 receptor by stromal cell-derived factor 1 (SDF-1) results in the release of extracellular TNF-α and downstream release of glu-

tamate (Bezzi et al., 2001). During HIV-1 infection there is an amplification or regulation of neurotoxic signals among astrocytes and microglia (Genis et al., 1992; Nottet et al., 1995). The HIV protein Tat induces expression in astrocytes of MCP-1, a chemoattractant for macrophages, and IL-8 and inducible protein-10 (IP-10), which attract multiple leukocyte types (Conant et al., 1998; Kutsch et al., 2000).

Astrocytes both proliferate and undergo apoptosis in HIV-1 CNS infection (Wesselingh and Thompson, 2001). The level of astrocyte apoptosis correlates strongly with both the severity and rate of progression of HIV dementia. Astrocytes can be infected (Wiley, 1986) in the absence of classical CD4 receptor through other chemokine receptors (Lawrence and Major, 2002), such as CXCR4 (Bezzi et al., 2001). Astrocytes may also serve as a reservoir for virus. In contrast to primary infection in MP, HIV-1 infection of astrocytes is not considered productive. The molecular events that limit HIV infection in primary astrocytes have been attributed to the inefficient translation of HIV structural proteins (Wesselingh and Thompson, 2001). The actual percentage of restrictively infected astrocytes in brains of patients with HIVE is unknown but thought to be relatively small.

T Cells

Impaired immune response is characteristic of late stages of HIV-1 neurodegeneration and HAD pathogenesis. This could be as a result of infection of CD4+ T cells, which occurs frequently and in the early stage of disease. T-cell abnormalities such as CD4+ T-cell lymphopenia, characterized by decreased lymphoproliferation and a decreased number of cells having a naïve phenotype, are seen in HIV-1-infected individuals (Devadas et al., 2004). An uninfected individual normally has 800 to 1200 CD4+ T cells per cubic millimeter of blood, but during HIV infection these cell numbers progressively decline. In addition, infiltrating CD8+ cells lose their protective role in later stages of infection, ultimately exhibiting impaired cytokine production and cytolysis, possibly as a result of anergy and the inability to eliminate HIV-1-infected cells in the setting of functionally impaired helper CD4+ T lymphocytes (Lewis et al., 1994; Liegler and Stites, 1994; Oxenius et al., 2004).

CD4+ T cells also serve as important reservoirs of HIV; a small proportion of these cells harbor HIV in a stable, inactive form. Normal immune processes may activate these cells, resulting in the production of new HIV virions. Once past the BBB, T cells are able to instigate cell-to-cell spread of HIV through CD4-mediated fusion of an infected cell with an uninfected cell. In addition, phagocytosis of CD4+ T cells by MP can result in the spread of virus (Budka, 1991; Lima et al., 2002). Activated T cells penetrate the BBB after insult to the CNS and can initiate both protective and toxic inflammatory responses (Petito et al., 1986). Protective responses are elicited through elimination of the ongoing infectious agent by innate, humoral, and cytotoxic immune activities. Nonetheless, widespread inflammation in the setting of HIV often leads to damage of the BBB and further transendothelial migration of leukocytes entering the nervous system (Persidsky et al., 2000). Inflammation of the brain and spinal cord actively attracts T cells to the CNS. Macrophage inflammatory protein-1 alpha (MIP-1α) and MIP-1β are relevant to the cellular recruitment and immune activation during HIV infection (Canque et al., 1996; Jennes et al., 2004), as both use CCR5 as their receptor (Farzan et al., 1997; Navenot et al., 2001; Miyakawa et al., 2002). MIP-1α selectively attracts CD8+ and MIP-1β recruits CD4+ lymphocytes. Both MIP-1α and MIP-1β are produced by HIV-1-infected monocytes and are closely linked to viral replication (Schmidtmayerova et al., 1996).

During HIV-1 infection, more T cells are activated to a blast phase (Marcondes et al., 2001; Chen et al., 2005; Holm and Gabuzda, 2005). Once within the CNS, the lymphoblasts search for antigen as they migrate through the parenchyma. Such cells can easily encounter and engage perivascular macrophages through direct cell-to-cell contact or through soluble factors released. CD4+ T lymphocytes are responsible for most of the HIV replication in the periphery. HIV-1 may enter the CNS in infected lymphocytes during the late stage of the disease. As the T cells migrate through the parenchyma, they secrete the cytokines that lead to activation of MP and an amplification of inflammatory cell responses throughout the CNS region involved (Weidenheim et al., 1993). If these activated T cells are infected, they will shed virus as they migrate. At the same time, they induce CD4 expression on cells susceptible to HIV infection, rendering them even more susceptible. T cells expressing the CD40 ligand (soluble and bound forms) can activate both infected and noninfected monocytes that express TNF-α and CD40 receptors (Kornbluth et al., 1998; Zhang et al., 2004; Chen et al., 2006). Macrophages become activated by

way of scavenger receptors as they clear the debris of dead virus-infected cells (Lima et al., 2002, 2006). Since viral replication occurs mostly within CD4+ T cells, direct cytopathic effects of HIV-1 may be attributed to cell death (Zhang et al., 1999). The decline in CD4+ T lymphocytes allows macrophages, without control, to express a metabolically active, tissue-destructive phenotype.

MOLECULAR PATHOGENESIS OF HIV-ASSOCIATED DEMENTIA

HIV Replication and Innate Immunity: A First Failed Response to Combat Viral Growth

The disease pathogenesis revolves around a number of genetic and environmental factors: host genetics, advanced immune suppression, high viral loads, and late-stage disease. There are several innate immune responses that serve to curtail viral growth but the in end fail. One is the formation of giant cells. The pathological hallmark of HIVE and a correlate to cognitive dysfunction is the multinucleated giant cell, which results from fusion of infected and uninfected macrophage and microglia in an active but ultimately vein host attempt to limit ongoing viral growth (Dalgleish et al., 1984; Sharer et al., 1985; Budka, 1986, 1991; Dickson, 1986; Lifson et al., 1986a, 1986c; Sodroski et al., 1986; Wiley et al., 1986; Matthews et al., 1987; Michaels et al., 1988; Epstein and Gendelman, 1993; Pontow et al., 2004). Similar mechanisms are used by the macrophage for mycobacterial, fungal, and parasitic infections, with similar pathological and functional outcomes (Handa et al., 1996; Suparak et al., 2005; Tambuyzer and Nouwen, 2005).

The second immune response is the production of interferons. Monocytes, macrophages, and most commonly dendritic cells secrete interferons, predominantly IFN-α and IFN-β, after engagements with virus. This response is limited and not self-sustaining. Indeed, later in the course of disease the appearance of interferons is correlated negatively with viral growth and ongoing replication (Woelk et al., 2004; Bower et al., 2006; Chen et al., 2006).

The third response is a combination of phagocytosis and intracellular killing mechanisms that evolve through phagolysosomal fusion (Pittis et al., 1993; Newman et al., 2005). The virus quickly adapts to such responses, however, so the mechanism is essentially inoperative to control ongoing infections (Pittis et al., 1993, 1996; Moorjani et al., 1996).

Finally, virus can use Fc gamma receptors for entry into MP with the emergence of enhancing antibodies. This process has been shown in Dengue hemorrhagic fever as well as in the setting of HIV infections (Payeras et al., 2002; Pham et al., 2005; Holl et al., 2006). All together, the innate immune responses that often characterize macrophage control of microbial infection are either inoperative or have a paradoxical effect on viral growth. In the setting of adaptive immune compromise, these responses ultimately yield to accelerated HIV replication and the host of metabolic and immune events that lead to advancing disease (da Silva, 2003; Poluektova et al., 2004; Peut and Kent, 2006).

Entry into Brain Cells: Receptors for Mononuclear Phagocytes and Transmigration into the Central Nervous System

HIV is thought to gain entry to the protected environment of the CNS either when HIV-infected lymphocytes and monocytes cross the BBB or as it enters through the choroids plexus, with subsequent seeding of the brain (Nottet et al., 1996; Persidsky et al., 2000; Berger and Avison, 2004). Several mechanisms have been proposed by which HIV-1 gains entry into the brain (Toborek et al., 2005). In one such model, HIV-1 enters the brain inside infected macrophages that migrate into the brain parenchyma through BBB disruption and establishment of a chemokine gradient. This model is commonly referred to as the "Trojan horse hypothesis," since virus buds into intracytoplasmic vesicles in macrophages with limited expression of viral proteins on the cell surface and escapes from immune surveillance (Zink et al., 1999; Persidsky and Gendelman, 2003). A second theory is that cell-free HIV-1 virus directly infects the endothelial cells and astrocytes of the BBB. The major problem with this theory is the low or nonproductive infection of cells of the BBB (Kanmogne et al., 2000). In another model, the transcytosis model, HIV-1 invades the CNS through internalization of the virion by endothelial cells or by astrocyte foot processes by macropinocytosis or endosomes, with subsequent transfer of the virus to CNS cells (Eugenin et al., 2005).

Infected monocytes, macrophages, and perhaps CD4+ T lymphocytes act as vehicles through which virus enters the brain. Activated microglia and, to a lesser extent, astrocytes express MHC class I and II antigens and adhesion molecules and secrete cytokines and reactive oxygen intermediates. All are shown to be important factors contributing to HAD (Tyor et al., 1992; Lipton et al., 1994). Microglia and astrocytes produce chemokines and control monocyte migration across the BBB (Nottet et al., 1995, 1996; Persidsky et al., 2000; Aquaro et al., 2005; Nottet, 2005). The event(s) triggering monocyte invasion into the nervous system likely involves the secretion of macrophage attractant chemokines and the up-regulation of adhesion molecules on activated endothelial and immune cells (Fig. 19.1). Proinflammatory factors induce cytokines and chemokines (such as IL-8, IFN-γ, IP-10, growth-related oncogene α [GRO-α], MIP-1a, MIP-1b, RANTES, and MCP-1) found in infected brain tissue and may also participate directly in the disease process (Nottet, 2005). Both cytokines and HIV-1 Tat induce expression of E-selectin on BMVEC. The likelihood of this event is increased by the release of nitric oxide (NO). TNF-α and Il-1β also induce expression of VCAM-1 on the BMVEC (Brabers and Nottet, 2006). This induction of adhesion molecules allows binding of HIV-infected cells to the brain endothelium (Nottet, 2005). Virus and activated macrophage entry into the brain is likely precipitated by BBB damage heralded by activation of brain MP. Neuronal damage and alterations in the integrity of tight junction and/or regulation of its immune function occur as consequences of viral and cellular secretory products and are crucial to HIV-1 brain transport (Persidsky et al., 2000).

Hickey and colleagues (2005) have proposed that the principle culprits in carrying HIV into the nervous system are the perivascular cells. They claim that these cells' kinetics of replacement is sufficiently frequent that it would permit a significant number of viral-laden cells to enter the brain or spinal cord over a few years. In addition, immunohistological examination of brain tissue from patients with HIVE most frequently demonstrates virus in the perivascular macrophages. Furthermore, these cells are in prolonged, intimate contact with parenchymal microglia cells, and thus have the potential to pass virus to them when the microglia have entered a susceptible, activated state. Finally, in patients with HIV-associated CNS syndromes

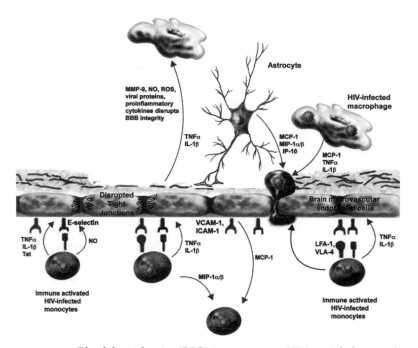

FIGURE 19.1. Blood–brain barrier (BBB) impairment in HIV encephalities and HIV-associated dementia. Alterations in capillary endothelial cells and basement membrane and disruption of tight junctions by HIV-1-infected monocytes and macrophages lead to a compromise of the structural integrity of the BBB following HIV-1 infection of the nervous system. Disruption of the BBB is affected by a number of inflammatory factors, including proinflammatory cytokines (TNF-α and IL-1β) secreted by perivascular HIV-1-infected monocytes and macrophages. TNF-α, IL-1β, and HIV-1 Tat induce expression of E-selectin on brain microvascular endothelial cells (BMVEC), which mediates rolling of HIV-infected monocytes on the vessel wall. TNF-α and IL-1β also induce the expression of the adhesion molecules VCAM-1 and ICAM-1 on BMVEC to allow for the binding of HIV-infected monocytes to the brain endothelium. These neurotoxic factors may contribute to breakdown of the BBB and affect the generation of a chemokine gradient through interactions between HIV-infected monocytes and BMVEC and lead to enhanced transendothelial migration of cells from blood to brain. This interaction results in the production of monocyte-derived chemokines MIP-1α, MIP-1β, and the endothelial-derived chemokine MCP-1. These chemokines will attract more mononuclear phagocytic cells into the brain parenchyma, resulting in expansion of the viral load within the central nervous system. NO, nitric oxide; ROS, reactive oxygen species.

attributable to neural dysfunction, there is BBB breakdown (Hickey et al., 2005).

The blood–brain barrier consists of a monolayer of specialized, nonfenestrated, microvascular endothelial cells. Associated with the BBB is a capillary basement membrane on the abluminal side of the monolayer. Tight junctions connect the BMVEC, and there

are no transcellular pores. These together serve to restrict movement of cells and macromolecules, including virus throughout much of HIV-1 infection. Nonetheless, a number of biological situations enable the trafficking of cells across the BBB as a result of HIV-1 infection. Virus enters the brain early after the acute seroconversion reaction, carried into the CNS inside infected cells, macrophages and/or CD4+ T lymphocytes, or alternatively as cell-free viral particles. The movement of virus from the periphery into the brain is facilitated through its immune and structural BBB compromise. This process occurs, in large measure, late in the course of disease and serves to speed the overall pathogenic process. HIV-1 infection alters the BBB itself (Banks et al. 1998, 2001; Andras et al., 2003); numerous functional and structural abnormalities are operative, including damage to the basement membrane, damage to tight junction proteins, morphological and functional alterations of the BMVEC (Kanmogne et al., 2005, 2007), and subsequent protein leakage (Nottet et al., 1996). In this pathologic setting, HIV-1-infected monocytes and/or CD4+ T lymphocytes as well as cell-free virus are able to cross the BBB (Wu et al., 2000; Banks et al., 2001).

Inflammation serves to enhance trafficking of cells across the BBB. ICAM-1, VCAM-1, and E-selectin are up-regulated on the surface of BMVEC and astrocytes after exposure to proinflammatory cytokines (for example, TNF-α and IL-1β) secreted from microglia and astrocytes and/or activated leukocytes from the periphery. These serve to augment the process of adhesion molecule expression on not only BMVEC but also astrocytes (Conant et al., 1994; Nottet et al., 1996). Late in the disease process, inflammatory cytokines are produced at high levels and allow the BBB to be more easily breached. These proinflammatory cytokines induce a transient increase in endothelial permeability by increasing secretion of endothelial vasoactive factors, such as NO (Diesing et al., 2002). TNF-α and IL-1β increase the production of other inflammatory mediators, including arachidonic acid–derived PAF (Nottet and Gendelman, 1995; Nottet et al., 1996; Lawrence and Major, 2002). These serve to promote monocyte migration across the BBB and ultimately into the brain parenchyma (Nottet et al., 1996). The adhesion molecules ICAM-1 and VCAM-1 on the luminal surface of the BMVEC bind LFA-1 and Vl-4 on the monocyte, resulting in migration of the monocyte between the endothelial cells during the early stages of viral infection.

Other inflammatory factors and changes in cellular biophysiology that are induced as a consequence of inflammation also influence transmigration of inflammatory cells into the CNS. For example, chemokines are secreted at sites of inflammation, in all tissues including the CNS, and guide leukocytes in a concentration-dependent manner. Importantly, specific chemokines will attract specific populations of leukocytes. MIP-1α and MCP-1 levels are increased during HIV encephalitis and are potent chemoattractants for macrophages as well as CD4+ T lymphocytes (Schmidtmayerova et al., 1996; Lawrence and Major, 2002). Increasing damage to the BBB impairs its ability to protect the CNS from the periphery. Cells and toxins are then able to reach the CNS unchecked. Levels of inflammatory factors greatly increase and lead to a cascade of events culminating in further BBB dysfunction. These processes, taken together, affect MP-induced neuronal destruction during HAD.

The first event during the course of HIV-1 infection is attachment of the virus particle to the cell surface, followed by fusion of the viral and cellular membranes delivering the viral core into the cytoplasm of the cell. This process of attachment and fusion is mediated by the interaction of viral glycoproteins with the CD4 receptor and a seven-transmembrane coreceptor (Lifson et al., 1986a, 1986b; Devadas et al., 2004), either CCR5 or CXCR4. In the brain, monocyte-derived macrophages and microglia are the main cell types infected by HIV-1 (Kure et al., 1990; Devadas et al., 2004; Vinters, 2004). The virus replicates in the infected macrophages and can infect other cells such as microglia. In addition to macrophages and microglia, other cell types such as astrocytes and capillary endothelial cells have been found to contain HIV-1 protein and DNA in infected individuals (Devadas et al., 2004). It is likely that, depending on the infected brain macrophage population, the extent of CNS inflammation and the numbers of recruited MDM into the brain predict the course and extent of neurological impairment.

More important, there is a positive correlation between the profundity of the acute syndrome and both a more rapid rate of progression to AIDS (Vanhems et al., 2000) and an earlier development of HIV-associated cognitive impairment (Wallace et al., 2001). The tempo of disease may also rely on the emergence of neurotropic and neurovirulent viral strains. In truth, the neuroinvasiveness of HIV-1 is a consequence of viral tropism for macrophages and microglia, inducing neuronal injury involving a set of cellular interactions that ultimately lead to neuronal loss, gliosis, and diffuse and perivascular infiltration of macrophages and emergence of multinucleated giant cells (Gendelman et al., 1994).

HIV-1 infection of the brain begins soon after initial viral infection. It has been suggested that the early CNS infection most probably induces immune activation of the brain parenchyma with a subsequent increase in the number of microglial cells, up-regulation of MHC class II expression, and local production of cytokines (Martin-Garcia and Gonzalez-Scarano, 2005). In the normal CNS, neurons, oligodendrocytes, astrocytes, and microlgia are intimately associated with each other, and they communicate through specialized synapses and cell junctions. There is a need for direct cell contact for the mature or inhibited phenotype of glia. For glia to undergo transformation to an activated amoeboid phenotype, they need to be freed from inhibitory neural and astrocytic responses (Lee and Dickson, 2005) (Fig. 19.2A). In neurodegenerative disorders associated with synaptic degeneration and disruption of normal intracellular junctions, microglial and astrocytic activation is imminent.

Macrophage activation during HIV-1 infection may occur by several mechanisms. Proinflammatory cytokines such as IFN-γ and TNF-α are potent macrophage activators. TNF-α allows astrocytes and macrophages to amplify the immune activation, resulting in co-activation of other macrophages. Other mechanisms of macrophage activation involve injury of the axon. Axonal injury results in activation of microglia in the CNS. For example, injury to peripheral processes such as the axon of a motor neuron causes activation of the microglia within the anterior horn. Another theory is that there is exhaustion of the T cells late in the disease state, with compensation by the granulocytes and phagocytes that are excessively stimulated. Chemokines are yet another method of macrophage activation. MIP-1α and RANTES act through CCR5 (Cocchi et al., 1995) on the cell surface, and SDF-1α through CXCR4 (Oberlin et al., 1996). Fractalkine, a brain chemokine expressed by neurons, astrocytes, and endothelial cells, binds CX3CR1 to mediate macrophage recruitment and activation (Tong et al., 2000). T cells will also activate macrophages by cytokines as well as by direct contact. Activated T cells will enter the blast phase and enter the CNS. As they migrate through the parenchyma, they secrete the cytokines that serve as a source for macrophage activation (Diesing et al., 2002; Lawrence and Major, 2002). As these T cells die in the brain, the debris is removed by the brain macrophages, also contributing to macrophage activation.

Activated macrophage and microglia are the primary perpetrator of neuronal injury in HIV-1-associated CNS disease. It is widely accepted that these mononuclear phagocytes act to bring about neuronal injury primarily through indirect mechanisms. These indirect mechanisms are alterations in secretory function of chemokines, cytokines, arachidonic acid derivatives and PAF, as well as NO, free radicals, and excitatory amino acids (Kadiu et al., 2005). Direct mechanisms also bring about neurotoxicity, but probably play a lesser role. These mechanisms consist of soluble viral proteins and glycoproteins that work through neuronal receptors (D'Aversa et al., 2005).

Changes in secretory profiles of glia play an important role in the pathogenesis of neurodegenerative disorders due to changes in proinflammatory cytokine production and to a degree the regulation of adaptive immune responses. Indeed, MP products including cytokines, chemokines, and excitotoxins, together with proteins of the classical complement cascade and pentraxins, play a critical role in the pathogenesis of neurodegenerative diseases. Such mechanisms are operative in a wide variety of diseases regardless of the insult. HIV infection of the brain involves activation of innate immune responses resulting in subacute and chronic disease mediated by the same glial factors including proinflammatory cytokines, free radicals, excitotoxins, and arachidonic acid and its metabolites (Fig. 19.2B). Indeed, increased expression of both proinflammatory and noninflammatory cytokines including TGF-β, IL-1α, IL-1β, IL-6, and TNF-α, have been documented in the brain and/or CSF of patients with AIDS, particularly those with HAD (Martin et al., 1992; Brew et al., 1996; Brew, 2001; Roberts et al., 2003; Gonzalez-Scarano and Martin-Garcia, 2005).

Chemokines and their receptors also play a central role in HIV-1-associated encephalopathy. A chemokine gradient established through inflammatory responses resulting from viral infection can initiate monocyte transendothelial migration increases in the viral reservoir and provide additional cell sources for neurotoxic products. Chemokines engage their receptors on neurons, and glia then activate intracellular signaling pathways that alter synaptic transmission and neural functions. For example, gp120 and SDF-1 both interact with CXCR4, initiating intracellular signaling pathways that can either directly lead to neuronal apoptosis (Oberlin et al., 1996) or stimulate microlgia and astrocytes to excrete TNF-α. The presence of

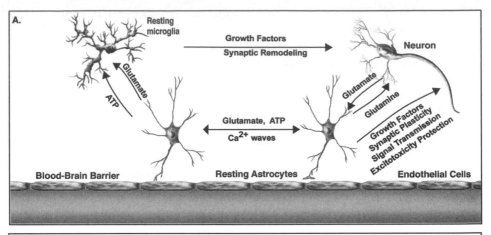

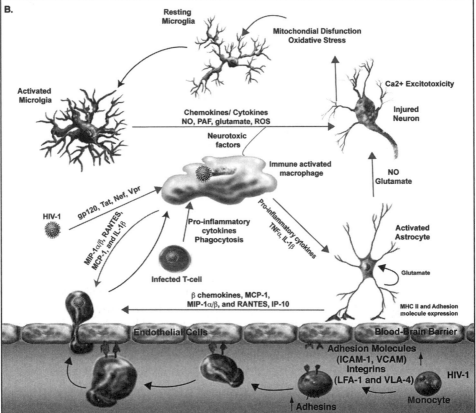

FIGURE 19.2. Pathobiology of the central nervous system (CNS) under normal conditions and in disease. (A) In the normal adult brain, there is constant crosstalk among resident neuroglia and neurons that serves to maintain homeostasis through secretion of trophic factors, immune surveillance, and regulation of metabolic factors. (B) During the disease state, mononuclear phagocytes (MP) may be primed by virus or viral proteins and secondarily activated by factors such as proinflammatory cytokines and chemokines, or by T cells trafficking in and out of the nervous system. The primed and immune-activated MP secrete a variety of neurotoxic factors (cytokines, chemokines, platelet-activating factor [PAF], quinolinic acid, glutamate, and nitric oxide [NO]) that affect neural function and CNS inflammation. These factors may contribute to the breakdown of the blood–brain barrier and affect transendothelial migration of leukocytes into the brain, perpetuating the inflammatory cascade. Depending on their functional status, astrocytes may suppress or increase MP secretory functions and toxicity. ROS, reactive oxygen species.

chemokine receptors on neural cells also supports the notion that chemokines can regulate neuronal physiology.

The primary role of the macrophage in HIV neuropathogenesis is neurotoxin secretion. Among these toxins are the excitatory amino acids (EAA). Neurotoxicity activity as mediated through NMDA receptors has been demonstrated in many studies. Investigators have characterized likely EAA toxins as candidates, such as Ntox (Giulian et al., 1990) and quinolate (Heyes et al., 1991). Excitotoxicity is brought about by repeated and excessive stimulation of NMDA neuronal receptors. Glutamate is a well-known neurotoxin able to increase cell calcium conductance, eventually leading to further release of glutamate (Tremolizzo et al., 2002). Quinolinate is another such EAA that acts via the neuronal NMDA glutamate receptor to induce excitotoxicity. There is a strong correlation between quinolinate levels in the CNS and dementia (Potula et al., 2005). Macrophages have been shown to be the primary source of quinolinate in the CNS. Indoleamine 2,3 dioxygenase (IDO), the rate-limiting enzyme in the generation of quinolinic acid-enzymatic activity, is up-regulated in the brain of a subset of HIV-1 infected individuals with severe immune suppression and high peripheral viral loads (Potula et al., 2005). An increase of functional IDO enzymatic activity in the brain could lead to the enhanced production of neurotoxins.

Oxidative stress plays a significant role in the neuropathogenesis of HIV-1. Free radical formation combined with impaired antioxidant capabilities brings about this stress (Bal-Price and Brown, 2001). The free radical species in this situation are superoxide anions, NO, and peroxynitrite. Nitric oxide is produced by neurons in response to excitation and changes in intracellular calcium. Neurons can be exposed to additional NO released from astrocytes, macrophages, and microglia that have been stimulated with proinflammatory cytokines such as TNF-α and IL-1β, and the viral proteins HIV-1 gp120 and HIV-1 gp41 (Bal-Price and Brown, 2001; Devadas et al., 2003, 2004). HIV-1 gp120 and Tat protein treatment of primary neurons results in a release of superoxide (Jana and Pahan, 2004; Price et al., 2005). It was confirmed that p22phox is responsible for gp120-induced superoxide production (Jana and Pahan, 2004). These observations led to the elucidation of NADPH oxidase involvement in gp120-induced neuronal cell death; gp120 leads to neuronal apo-

ptosis and cell death via NADPH oxidase–mediated activation of neutral sphingomyelinase (NSMase) (Jana and Pahan, 2004). In HIV-1 infection, astrocyte re-uptake of extracellular glutamate is impaired by gp120 and infection of the astrocyte itself (Patton et al., 2000). In addition, glutamate release from the astrocyte is induced by activated macrophages.

The HIV-1 Tat protein also induces toxicity that correlates with an increase in intracellular calcium, stimulating the production of reactive oxygen intermediates and activation of the apoptosis pathways by caspase (Devadas et al., 2004). In addition, the levels of inducible nitric oxide synthase (iNOS) in HIV-infected patients are elevated (Liu et al., 2002; Bagetta et al., 2004; Saha and Pahan, 2006). Further complicating the pathogenesis, HIV-1-infected patients lack the antioxidant glutathione (Ogunro et al., 2006) and have reduced levels of the hydrogen peroxide scavenger catalase in CD8+ T cells (Yano et al., 1998). This illustrates HIV-1-infected patients' impaired ability to clear free radicals. These factors contribute to a chronic state of oxidative stress in HIV-1-infected patients.

Establishing a Central Nervous System Viral Reservoir

In the past 25 years since AIDS was first described, a significant amount of work has been done to discover how the virus penetrates and evolves in the brain and how it targets cells, and to investigate modes of viral brain persistence and mechanisms of neurotoxicity (Gray et al., 2005; Burton, 2006; Ribeiro et al., 2006). HIV-1 seeds the brain early after systemic infection (Davis et al., 1992; An and Scaravelli, 1997), but neurological disease occurs years later in association with BBB compromise and significant immune dysfunction. What ensues is a second wave of viral entry into the brain years after the initial seroconversion reaction and coincident with a robust peripheral immune activation (Gray et al., 1996). Along with the emergence of CD14/CD16 and CD/CD69 monocyte subsets there is a profound immune activation with concomitant up-regulation of cell adhesion molecules (VCAM-1 and E-selectin) on brain microvascular endothelial cells and macrophage, microglial, and astrocyte secretion of the chemoattractant molecules, most notably MCP-1, and establishment of a chemokine gradient and robust monocyte penetration through the BBB (Pulliam et al., 1997; Maslin et al.,

2005). Such disease-specific events contribute to viral entry into the brain as cell-associated free progeny virions (Sato et al., 1992). The more monocytes and macrophages that gain entry into brain, the broader the viral reservoir, serving as a cell nidus for productive viral replication (Porcheray et al., 2006).

Ultimately, this process accelerates disease by enhancing the levels of virus present in the CNS and by serving as a source of cells for secretion of neurotoxins (Anderson et al., 2002). Thus, immune activation serves as a trigger for virus growth, and viral growth in turn serves as a trigger for immune activation, leading to a cascade of innate neuroinflammatory responses amplified by interactions among MP, astrocytes, endothelial cells, and neurons in a paracrine and autocrine manner (Tyor et al., 1992; Minagar et al., 2002; Kaul et al., 2005) (Fig.19.3). Over the past decade and

a half, MP secretory neurotoxins have been identified and include arachidonic acid and its metabolites (Nottet and Gendelman, 1995), PAF (Gelbard et al., 1994), proinflammatory cytokines (such as TNF-α or IL-1β) (Genis et al., 1992), quinolinic acid (Heyes et al., 1991a, 1991b; Kerr et al., 1998), Ntox (Giulian et al., 1990), NO (Bukrinsky et al., 1995; Adamson et al., 1996), reactive oxygen species, and TNF-related apoptosis-inducing ligand (TRAIL) and matrix metalloproteinases (MMP) (Conant et al., 1999; Ghorpade et al., 2001; Williams and Hickey, 2002).

There are several HIV-1 proteins that are potentially neurotoxic. The structural viral proteins such as gp120 (Brenneman et al., 1988), gp41 (Adamson et al., 1996), and the nonstructural proteins Tat (New et al., 1997; Price et al., 2005), Nef, Vpr, and Rev secreted by infected MP can all negatively affect neuronal

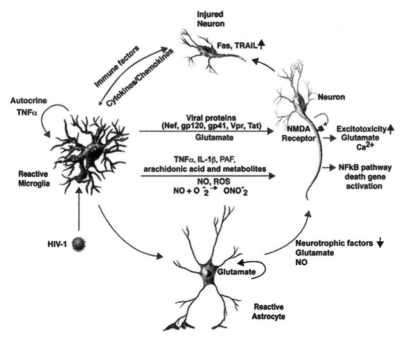

FIGURE 19.3. HIV-related neuronal damage. Immune-activated and HIV-infected mononuclear phagocytes (MP) release potentially neurotoxic substances. These substances induce neuronal injury, dendritic and synaptic damage, and apoptosis. The enhanced production of cytokines TNF-α and IL-1β, reactive oxygen species (ROS), and viral proteins from macrophages stimulates astrocytosis and the subsequent production of nitric oxide (NO). In addition, neurotoxins released from macrophages impair astrocyte clearing of the neurotransmitter glutamate and thus contribute to excitotoxicity. The neurotoxic product also directly affects neuronal function. Taken together, the secretion of neurotoxic products and the decreased neurotropic capacity of astrocytes contribute to the destruction of proximal neurons.

function (Price et al., 2006). The HIV-1 coat protein gp120 can directly disrupt glial and neuronal function through alteration of calcium homeostasis (Lannuzel et al., 1995) and induction of reactive oxygen and nitrogen species (Mollace et al., 1993), induce apoptosis, or promote MP to secrete proinflammatory cytokines such as TNF-α and IL-1β as well as arachidonic acid metabolites implicated in HIV-1 neuropathogenesis (Jana and Pahan, 2004). Secretion of Tat can also cause direct or indirect injury to neurons through similar mechanisms (Nath, 2002; Song et al., 2003). In addition, Tat may contribute to the disruption of the BBB (Andras et al., 2003). Tat has been shown to contribute to the inflammatory cascade through promotion of TNF-α and IL-1 production by MP and stimulate the production of several chemokines including RANTES and MCP-1 in astrocytes, which may propagate neuronal toxicity (Nath, 2002; El-Hage et al., 2005). The regulatory protein Vpr might also be neurotoxic. Intracellular and extracellular Vpr have been demonstrated to induce apoptosis by increasing caspase-8 activation (Pomerantz, 2004) and through cell cycle arrest (Jowett et al., 1995; Stewart et al., 1997).

Altogether, secretory products and immune-competent and virus-infected MP along with cell–cell immune cross-talk adversely affect neuronal function (Tyor et al., 1992; McArthur et al., 1993; Gelbard et al., 1994) and lead to a metabolic encephalopathy (Zheng et al., 2001; Anderson et al., 2002). This is characterized clinically by behavioral, motor, and cognitive impairments (Wilkie et al., 2003; Griffin et al., 2004; Weed and Steward, 2005; Worlein et al., 2005). Moreover, ongoing inflammatory responses in the brain change microglial function and inevitable unresponsiveness to environmental cues, leading to lack of control for innate immunity (Ghorpade et al., 2005). The end result is the continuous entry of macrophages from blood to brain, with ensuing enhanced neurotoxic secretions (Nottet et al., 1995; Zheng and Gendelman, 1997; Poluektova et al., 2005; Kanmogne et al., 2007).

HIV REPLICATION AND PERSISTENCE IN THE BRAIN

HIV-1 is neuroinvasive and enters the CNS early in infection (Budka, 1986; Lewin, 1986; Brew et al., 1988; Diesing et al., 2002). Once inside, the CNS

brain macrophages and microglia and, to lesser extent, astrocytes serve as a reservoir for virus. Neuroinvasive viral strains infect predominantly MP (M-tropic), the more prevalent viral subtype, early in the course of infection. In contrast, T-lymphocyte-tropic (T-tropic) strains predominate later in the course of disease, when levels of proinflammatory cytokines rise and serve to amplify the entry and replication of the virus through activated brain MP. Infection typically begins when an HIV particle, which contains two copies of the HIV RNA, encounters a cell with a surface molecule called cluster designation 4 (CD4). Cell-to-cell spread of HIV can also occur through the CD4-mediated fusion of an infected cell with an uninfected cell (Lifson et al., 1986a, 1986b). Recent research has shown that most infecting strains of HIV use a coreceptor molecule called CCR5, in addition to the CD4 molecule, to enter certain of its target cells. One or more of the virus's gp120 molecules binds tightly to CD4 molecule(s) on the cell's surface (Lyerly et al., 1987). The membranes of the virus and the cell fuse, a process that probably involves the envelope of HIV and a second coreceptor molecule on the cell surface. Following fusion, the virus's RNA, proteins, and enzymes are released into the cell. Although CD4+ T cells appear to be HIV's main target, other immune system cells with CD4 molecules on their surfaces are infected as well. Among these are long-lived monocytes and macrophages, which apparently can harbor large quantities of the virus without being killed, thus acting as reservoirs of HIV.

Infection and activation of macrophages contribute to the release of toxins, cytokines, arachidonic acid, PAF, and NO, which, in turn, lead to dysfunction of neurons and astrocytes. In vivo, infected astrocytes preferentially express HIV-1 regulatory proteins Nef, Rev, and Tat, whereas late structural proteins such as Gag and Env are rarely detected in these cells (Ranki et al., 1995; Kohleisen et al., 2001; Olivetta et al., 2003; Zhou et al., 2004; Di Stefano and Chiodi, 2005). Infection has been shown to lead to transient viral production and recovery of replicating virus only upon coculture with susceptible CD4+ cells. The restricted virus production can be overcome by the addition of TNF-α and IL-1β, resulting in increased expression of early HIV genes (Di Stefano and Chiodi, 2005).

Viral genetic diversity is an important determinant of neuropathogenesis and evasion of the host immune response. In the brain, monocyte-derived macrophages and microlgia are the main cell types infected by HIV-1. The virus replicates in the infected macrophages and can infect other cells such as microglia. In addition to macrophages and microglia, other cell types such as astrocytes and capillary endothelial cells have been found to contain HIV-1 protein and DNA in infected individuals (Devadas et al., 2004). The V3 hypervariable region of HIV-1 gp120 viral protein (Cann et al., 1992; Shioda et al., 1992; Diesing et al., 2002) largely determines tropism of HIV-1 in macrophages. HIV-1 gp120 binds CD4 to the surface of mononuclear phagocytes and T cells among other CD4+ cell types. CD4 is mandatory for infection of these cells but not sufficient for effective infection by all strains of virus. The V3 function is distinct from the HIV-1 gp120 CD4 requirement and is more associated with post-CD4-binding interactions such as proteolytic cleavage and fusion, all of which is critical for productive infection of brain MP (Ebenbichler et al., 1993; Diesing et al., 2002). Nonetheless, the V3 region is crucial to the tropism of HIV-1, although it is not the only factor. The V1/V2 region may also contribute independently or in concert with V3. Chemokine receptors are associated with viral tropism as well (Morikita et al., 1997; Diesing et al., 2002). The chemokine receptor CCR5 expressed on macrophages is a determinant on M-tropic strains, while T-tropic strains are associated with the chemokine receptor CXCR4. T cells may be infected by either strain of virus.

HIV IN THE BRAIN

Immunoregulation

Persistent viral infection of the CNS involves a number of innate and acquired immune factors that contribute in a significant manner to neural cell damage. Commonly, HIV infection of the brain results in activation of innate immune responses leading to subacute and chronic disease mediated by the same glial factors, including proinflammatory cytokines, free radicals, excitotoxins, and arachidonic acid and its metabolites, among others operative in most neurodegenerative disorders (Gendelman and Folks, 1999; Wesselingh and Thompson, 2001; Persidsky and Gendelman, 2003).

Profound immunodeficiency is characteristic of AIDS, although it is clear that inflammatory responses from activated monocytes and lymphocytes occur during HIV-1 infection as well. Antibody synthesis occurs systemically and in the brain early after HIV-1 infection, during the asymptomatic phase (Chiodi et al., 1988). Increased levels of proinflammatory cytokines such as IL-1, IFN-γ, and especially TNF-α and soluble cytokine receptors are found in the CSF of AIDS patients (Martin et al., 1992; Gattegno et al., 1995; Brew et al., 1996; Lawrence and Major, 2002; Roberts et al., 2003; Vasilescu et al., 2004; Nasi et al., 2005). Moreover, the levels of cytokine production in the CNS correlate with the severity of neurological symptoms. Although activated macrophages are the source of these proinflammatory cytokines in the CNS during initial infection, astrocytes, neurons, and endothelial cells, when stimulated by activated macrophages or HIV-1 membrane proteins, have the capacity for cytokine production as well (Genis et al., 1992; Lawrence and Major, 2002; Roberts et al., 2003).

One of the pivotal cytokines induced by HIV-1 infection of brain MP is TNF-α. In diseased and inflammatory brain tissue, TNF-α has toxic effects on neurons when produced in abundance. TNF-α exerts such effects by interfering with signaling of growth factors or by affecting the regulation of other cytokines either at the receptor levels, at downstream signaling pathways, or by intraneuronal receptor crosstalk (Bezzi et al., 2001; Perry et al., 2002). For example, activation of CXCR4 by SDF-1 and subsequent glutamate release by astrocytes is dependent on the release of TNF-α (Bezzi et al., 2001). In addition, it has been shown that TNF-α and IL-1β enhance HIV-1 replication through increased production and viral DNA binding of the NFκB transcription factor in macrophages (Lawrence and Major, 2002; Olivetta et al., 2003).

Another aspect of the immune response important in the process of HIVE is chemokine production in the brain. Chemokines comprise a small family of cytokines produced by infected cells that work in a gradient fashion to activate and attract specific subsets of cells from the immune system to the site of damage. Chemokines can also increase adhesion molecules on various cell types, including responding cells and the endothelial cells of the BBB, facilitating the entry of the responding cells from the blood into the damaged areas of the brain (Weiss et al., 1998; Wu et al., 2000; Biernacki et al., 2001; Lawrence and Major, 2002). In HIV encephalopathy, chemokines contribute to the pathogenesis by trafficking into the brain increasing numbers of infected and/or activated monocytes and CD4+ T lymphocytes, another source for both viral and cellular toxins that affect neuronal function and survival.

Morphological Changes

Neuropathological nomenclature of HIV-1 infection–induced pathology in the CNS includes HIV encephalitis, HIV leukoencephalopathy, vacuolar myelopathy and vacuolar leukoencephalopathy, lymphocytic meningitis, diffuse poliodystrophy, and cerebral vasculitis (Budka, 2005). As is evident, there is not one but several sets of morphological correlates of HIV-1 infection and associated dementia. Damage to the cerebral white matter is nonetheless traditionally described as the most conspicuous neuropathology in AIDS. Indeed, advanced HAD correlates with significant white matter lesions (Broderick et al., 1993; Budka, 2005; Langford et al., 2005).

HIV encephalitis is a multifocal process with foci widely scattered throughout the white matter, including corpus collosum and anterior commissure, basal ganglia (preferentially), and brainstem. Inflammatory changes of HIVE may also spread to ventricle walls and meninges (Post et al., 1988; Budka, 2005). Another common histopathological feature of HAD is leukoencephalopathy. Unlike HIVE, leukoencephalopathy is a diffuse neurodegenerative process, often observed without prominent signs of inflammation. Here considerable damage to white matter or myelin attenuation is seen in association with astrogliosis, macrophage accumulation, and multinucleated giant cells. Damage to the white matter frequently includes characteristic microvascular changes with BBB leakage and postdyshoric agiocentric foci, morphological evidence for vascular disturbance in the brain damage of AIDS (Krupp et al., 1985; Gray et al., 1987; Budka, 2005; Langford et al., 2005). Other HIV-associated CNS pathology includes lymphocytic meningitis and cerebral vasculitis, as well as diffuse poliodystrophy. Diffuse poliodystrophy consists of reactive astrogliosis and microglia inflammation in gray matter often with associated neuron loss or dendritic damage (Budka, 2005).

Although in AIDS the preponderance of conditions usually manifest in the brain, the spinal cord may also be affected. This most prominent spinal cord disease in AIDS is vacuolar myelopathy, characterized as a subacute combined degeneration of the spinal cord

(Budka, 2005). This condition affects multiple areas of the spinal cord but is predominant in the dorsolateral tracts, consistent with numerous vacuolar swellings and macrophages residing in vacuoles.

NEUROPSYCHOLOGICAL ABNORMALITIES ASSOCIATED WITH HIV

Manifestations of HIV-Associated Dementia

The likelihood of a particular neurological syndrome correlates with the clinical stage of HIV infection as reflected by viral load, immune response, and CD4+ lymphocyte count. This in turn is related to the severity of immunodeficiency and autoimmunity and to serum and tissue cytokine levels. Approximately one-third to one-half of all persons infected with HIV exhibit neuropsychological impairment, with greater proportions of incipient cognitive dysfunction emerging in later stages of disease (Woods et al., 2006).

The occurrence of neurological manifestations in some patients followed soon after the onset of the HIV-1 pandemic and could not be ascribed to an opportunistic infection but to the HIV infection itself. Shortly thereafter, HIV was identified in CNS tissues obtained at autopsy from neurologically impaired, HIV-1-positive individuals (Koenig et al., 1986; Navia et al., 1986a, 1986b; Price and Brew, 1988; Price et al., 1988; Cherner et al., 2002; Martin-Garcia and Gonzalez-Scarano, 2005). The resultant neuropsychiatric entity has been termed HIV-1 dementia, HIV-1 encephalopathy, HIV-associated cognitive/motor complex, AIDS dementia complex, and HIV-associated dementia.

Early manifestations of HAD include cognitive impairment (slowing, impaired attention and concentration, forgetfulness), motor abnormalities, and behavioral changes (reduced spontaneity, apathy, and social withdrawal). Late in the disease, an affected patient shows profound mental status changes (psychomotor slowing, impaired word reversal and serial subtraction, blunted affect) and further motor deterioration. Onset of dementia is insidious, with steady progression occurring thereafter over months or years. Often in the presence of systemic illness, deterioration may occur more abruptly (Vinters, 2004; McMurtray et al., 2006). Neuropsychological findings will vary according to HIV disease stage, disease markers, presence of opportunistic infections, and the effectiveness of treatment with antiviral medications.

Studies have shown that neurological and neuropsychological abnormalities are associated with symptomatic but not asymptomatic HIV-1 infection (Stern et al., 2001; Vinters, 2004). Indeed, most patients with cognitive impairment have neurodegeneration, and those with a normal neuropsychological profile show preservation of their synaptodendritic organization (Langford et al., 2005). In addition, neuropsychological dysfunction has been associated with lower CD4 counts and higher viral load in the CSF (Woods et al., 2006).

The introduction of antiretroviral therapy has increased the life expectancy of people infected with HIV-1 and resulted in an immediate decrease in the incidence of severe dementia. Indeed, in a case study, participants have demonstrated remarkable improvement in cognitive function with almost a complete reversal of associated symptoms of HAD over the course of 7 years (Gendelman et al., 1998). In the last decade, however, there has actually been an increase in the prevalence of HAD, perhaps because of the poor penetration of antiretrovirals into the CNS. As a result, antiretroviral therapy has failed to prevent the development of HAD or to reverse the disease in most cases (Major et al., 2000).

Experimental Behavioral and Long-Term Potentiation Studies

Impaired cognition is a distinguishing feature of HAD. In 2002, Zink and colleagues reported on the relevancy of a mouse model of HIV-1 encephalitis in studying spatial cognition and synaptic potentiation during the course of disease. Using this mouse model, they examined spatial cognition through Morris water maze testing. A frank inability to learn is manifested by final mean escape latency being statistically indistinguishable from initial latency. These mice demonstrated impaired spatial cognition and synaptic potentiation, both of which are observed in patients diagnosed with HAD.

Alterations in neuronal physiology also occur as a consequence of viral replication and inflammatory responses in these HIVE mouse models. Later studies by the same group provided evidence of hippocampal synaptic dysfunction in the same mouse model, implicating this feature with cognitive impairment seen in humans (Anderson et al., 2003). Impairment in hippocampal function can be shown by input–output function tests and deficits in long-term potentiation (LTP), which parallel deficiencies in cognitive function. In the hippocampus, LTP is an NMDA receptor–dependent function and relies on protein kinases as well. To produce LTP, the membrane must be sufficiently depolarized to expel Mg^{2+} from NMDA channels (Anderson et al., 2003). Thus, LTP is effectively reliant on membrane potential and secondary messenger systems. The LTP test results in the HIVE mouse model study indicated that differences between HIVE and sham groups were observed at days 7 and 15 after inoculation with HIV-1 virus, but not at day 3 (Anderson et al., 2003). By separating the phases of LTP over time, evoked responses were interpreted according to the cellular mechanisms involved. The impairment in the ability to induce and maintain LTP in HIVE groups may be due to exceedingly impaired membrane quality and to disruption of secondary messenger systems.

PEDIATRIC NEUROAIDS: HIV-1 ENCEPHALOPATHY

Children infected with HIV-1 are at risk for developing CNS disease characterized by impairments in cognitive, language, motor, and behavioral functions. Children with HIV infection exhibit three main patterns of CNS dysfunction: (1) encephalopathy, (2) CNS compromise, and (3) apparently normal functioning (Wolters and Brouwers, 2005). Neurological dysfunction in HIV-infected children is associated with poor mental and psychomotor development, which suggests that the CNS is the primary pathway through which HIV affects mental and psychomotor development (Knight et al., 2000).

The predominant clinical neurological findings seen in the pediatric population with HIV-1 infection represent a well-defined triad: impaired brain growth, progressive motor dysfunction, and loss or an inadequate rate of acquisition of neurodevelopmental milestones (Tudor-Williams et al., 1992; Epstein and Gendelman, 1993; Brouwers et al., 1994). In children with frank HIVE, the effects of HIV disease on the CNS tend to be generalized and affect brain function and structure severely and globally, leading to a general decline in cognitive function. Language abnormalities are common in pediatric HIV disease, with expressive language being more impaired than receptive language. This differential deficit has been attributed to a more general HIV-related impairment of expressive behavior, including motor function and emotional language (Brouwers et al., 1994). Motor impairments are a frequent manifestation of HIV CNS disease in children. Abnormalities in muscle tone and loss of acquired motor milestones have been reported in infants and young children. Oral motor functioning such as swallowing might also be impaired, resulting in difficulty eating and swallowing and in articulation (Brouwers et al., 1994). Children with HIVE may exhibit maladaptive psychological reactions, such as anxiety and depression, as well as impairments in adaptive functioning (Tudor-Williams et al., 1992; Brouwers et al., 1994; Knight et al., 2000; Wolters and Brouwers, 2005). Behavioral manifestations usually develop as a result of HIV-1 effects on the CNS and psychological stresses of living with HIV.

NEUROINFLAMMATION: LINKS BETWEEN HIV-ASSOCIATED DEMENTIA AND OTHER NEURODEGENERATIVE DISORDERS

The etiology of neurodegenerative disorders is multifactorial, consisting of progressive neuronal loss and chronic inflammation that is incited by interactions between the aging brain, environmental exposure, genetic predisposition, and altered oxidative metabolism. The key component that propagates the inflammatory process in the brain is the MP. Underlying MP cellular functions is inflammation, the same type that often proves detrimental in localized and systemic diseases, including those of the brain and in neurodegenerative disease. Not intrinsically bad, inflammation enables the host to fend off various disease-causing microbes including bacteria, viruses, and parasites. The moment virulent microorganisms enter the body inflammation enables a defense that serves to eliminate the invader along with damaged tissue. All together, this process, orchestrated primarily by macrophages, is a vital sensor against invasion by microbial pathogens and is a vital component of wound healing following acute tissue infection or injury. However, inflammatory responses can also prove deadly to tissue and to the host. Inflammatory responses are closely linked to a number of degenerative states including, but not limited to, cancer, arthritis, cardiovascular disease, and autoimmune diseases. With regard to the

nervous system, recent data suggest that neuroinflammation perpetrated through activation of MP, other glial elements including astrocytes, and, to a lesser degree, endothelial cells may act in concert as a central pathway in a diverse set of neurodegenerative diseases, including HAD, Alzheimer disease (AD), Parkinson disease (PD), and amyotrophic lateral sclerosis (ALS), among others.

Although several cell types have been implicated as contributors to inflammation-mediated neurodegeneration, microglia are critical components of the immunological insult to neurons. Indeed, microglial activation is a feature of virtually every CNS disorder. In most cases this is considered a secondary process, but in certain autoimmune and infectious disorders, such as HIVE, it can rightly be considered a primary process. Inflammatory mediators produced by microglia in turn control the fate of neurons and other glia. Glia-derived cytokines and chemokines such as, IL-6, granulocyte-macrophage colony stimulating factor (GM-CSF), and TNF-α (Campbell, 2004) have been shown to modulate neuronal toxicity in several CNS disorders. Thus, disorders with widely differing etiologies—viral infections, autoimmune disorders, stroke, and neurodegenerative diseases—may have shared pathogenic mechanisms, including common neurotoxins such as TNF-α, NO, superoxide, or excitotoxic amino acids or downstream effectors (Nottet and Gendelman, 1995; Price et al., 1997; Tu et al., 1997; Wie et al., 1997; Campbell, 2004; Lee and Dickson, 2005). Furthermore, as the brain ages, inflammatory events are up-regulated (David et al., 1997; Streit et al., 1999). It is possible that this is due to compromise of the BBB, leading to activation and proliferation of both microglial and astrocytic cells. As a consequence of BBB breakdown and local immune activation, the brain's resident macrophages or microglia can release a plethora of neurotoxins such as proteases, glutamate, and arachidonic acid and its metabolites, including PAF and reactive oxygen species, that affect synaptic transmission and lead to neuronal damage. Along with microglial activation, reactive astrogliosis is frequently observed in the lesioned regions in the brains of patients with HAD, AD, and PD. Astrogliosis induces the production of proinflammatory and neurotoxic factors such as NO and IL-1β (Brosnan et al., 1997; Liu and Hong, 2003). Interestingly, reactive astrogliosis usually lags behind the occurrence of microgliosis. Breakdown of the BBB also enables leukocytes to enter into the brain, propagating the CNS inflammatory cascade.

Alzheimer's Disease

Alzheimer's disease was one the first neurodegenerative diseases associated with neurotoxic microglial activation. It is the leading cause of dementia; neuronal damage results in the loss of language skills, followed by memory decline and finally delusion (Braak and Braak, 1994). Pioneering work by McGeer and colleagues (1987) proposed that neuronal death in AD could be caused by activated microglia found around the amyloid-beta (AB)-containing plaques in postmortem AD tissue. Amyloid beta has since been shown to both recruit and activate microglia (Davis et al., 1992; Meda et al., 1995), where AB enables the release of neurotoxic factors from microglia, such as NO (Ii et al., 1996), TNF-α (Dheen et al., 2005), and superoxide (Qin et al., 2002). Therapeutic inhibition of AB-induced inflammation is neuroprotective in animal AD models (Craft et al., 2004), and inhibition of microglial activation in vitro results in a reduction of AB-induced neurotoxicity (Liu et al., 2003). An increase in neuroinflammation is also seen in patients with AD. Levels of TNF-α in the CSF of patients with mild cognitive impairment who after 9 months progressed to AD are significantly higher than those in controls (Tarkowski et al., 2003). Taken together, these studies indicate that inflammation and microglia are critical for the ongoing process of neurodegeneration in AD.

Parkinson's Disease

Parkinson's disease (PD) is characterized by the progressive degeneration of dopaminergic neurons in the substantia nigra and the nerve terminals in the striatum, resulting in resting tremor, rigidity, bradykinesia, and gait disturbance in the patient (Jellinger, 2001). Dopaminergic neurons are particularly susceptible to the deleterious effects of microglial activation. The selective mechanism of microglia-mediated dopaminergic neurotoxicity is thought to be due to the generation of oxidative insult from microglia. Dopaminergic neurons in particular posses reduced antioxidant capacity as a result of low intracellular glutathione, which renders dopaminergic neurons more vulnerable to oxidative stress and microglial activation than other cell types (Loeffler et al., 1994).

Early work by McGeer and colleagues (1988) first documented the microglial response to the selective loss of dopaminergic neurons. The persistent activation of microglia in response to dopaminergic neuron injury and the active neurotoxic consequences of this microglial activation have since been investigated using the MPTP neurotoxin. Work from several laboratories has documented that microglia play an active role in the process of neuronal death, as MPTP-induced neurotoxicity is clearly linked with microglial activation (Wu et al., 2003; McGeer and McGeer, 2004). Further studies have shown that MPTP neurotoxicity may be attenuated in mice deficient in proinflammatory function, demonstrating that microglial-derived proinflammatory factors play a significant role in overall neurotoxicity (Feng et al., 2002; Sriram et al., 2002; Teismann et al., 2003; Wu et al., 2003).

Activated microglia contribute to the degeneration of dopamine (DA)-containing neurons by releasing neurotoxic factors such as NADPH oxidase–derived superoxide and cytokines (Gao et al., 2003). Cytokines released from the activated microglia bind their cognate receptors located on DA-containing neurons to activate transduction pathways resulting in apoptosis or the expression of iNOS and cyclooxygenase 2 (COX-2) within glial cells or neuronal cells (Du et al., 2001). Reactive oxygen species products can cause toxic events in dopaminergic neurons by either intensifying other cytotoxic factors or elevating the generation of neurotoxic factors in microglia. Oxidation and nitration of α-synuclein leads to formation of aggregates and the stabilization of assembled filaments found to be a major component of Lewy bodies, the hallmark lesions of PD. Microglial activation and neurotoxicity are associated with degenerating dopaminergic neurons and deposition of α-synuclein in the SNpc in PD (Croisier et al., 2005). Laboratory studies from our lab and others have shown that native and oxidized α-synuclein can activate microglia with release of reactive oxygen species and neurotoxicity (Zhang et al., 2005). The combination of reactive oxygen species from activated microglia and subsequent production of oxidative agents may be one of the most influential contributors to the pathogenesis of PD.

Amyotrophic Lateral Sclerosis

Amyotrophic lateral sclerosis (ALS) is a progressive, fatal neurodegenerative disease in which motor neurons in the brain and spinal cord are selectively destroyed

(Campbell, 2004). The pathology of ALS is characterized by neuronal degeneration and atrophy confined almost entirely to the upper and lower motor neurons (Weydt et al., 2005). The hypothesized mechanisms that support this pathology, such as glutamate toxicity, exogenous factors, neurofilament accumulation, neuroinflammation, and oxidative stress (Strong and Rosenfeld, 2003; Bruijn et al., 2004), could be independent factors or could cooperate to cause motor neuron loss.

A key discovery in ALS research took place when missense mutations were found in the gene on chromosome 21 encoding for a Cu/Zn binding protein called superoxide dismutase (SOD1) (Weydt et al., 2005). Indeed, approximately 20% of familial ALS cases have been linked to a mutation in the copper-zinc superoxide dismutase (*SOD1*) gene. SOD1 is an enzyme involved in the conversion of superoxide to hydrogen peroxide and dioxygen, thus decreasing the levels of superoxide in its surroundings (Weydt et al., 2005). The ALS phenotype is caused by gain of a novel, unknown toxic property of the SOD1 mutant enzyme, rather than by diminished SOD1 activity (Valentine and Hart, 2003), resulting in apoptotic degeneration of motor neurons. This can be potentiated by reduced glutamate transport and depressed through supplementation of antioxidant N-acetylcysteine, which suggests the involvement of reactive oxygen species in this pathology. Mutations of the *SOD* gene may have two adverse effects on the cell: (1) reduced ability to scavenge the superoxide radical, and (2) enhanced affinity to peroxynitrite, which could have the consequence of inactivating, through nitration, several critical components of motor neurons, such as the neurofilaments and tyrosine kinase receptors (Cui et al., 2004). Oxidative stress appears to be a major culprit in the pathogenesis of ALS. Mutant forms of SOD have altered enzyme activity and can result in increased superoxide radicals such that the formation of peroxynitrite from superoxide and nitric oxide would be favored. In transgenic mice overexpressing *SOD1*, levels of genes associated with inflammation and apoptosis are increased before symptoms of the disease and neuronal death are apparent (Yoshihara et al., 2002). It is believed that cell death as a result of the *SOD* mutation is in part mediated by chronic glial activation. Indeed, an inhibitor of microglial activation, minocycline, has been shown to not only delay the onset of ALS but also dose-dependently increase the survival of *SOD1* transgenic mice (Van den Bosch et al., 2002)

ADJUNCTIVE THERAPIES FOR NEURODEGENERATIVE DISORDERS

Many diverse mechanisms, factors, and pathways are involved in neurodegenerative disorders, thus several different therapeutic methods have been developed to target a specific factor or a whole intricate pathway with the intent of ameliorating, preventing, or reversing neuronal cell damage. Inflammation and oxidative stress form a commonality between many neurodegenerative diseases; therefore most therapeutic modalities currently under investigation target MP activation to decrease the magnitude of the inflammatory responses (Fig. 19.4). The targets of these therapies include, but are not restricted to, enhancement of neurotrophic factors (brain-derived neurotrophic factor [BDNF], glia cell-line derived neurotrophic factor [GDNF], and nerve growth factor [NGF]), up-regulation of anti-inflammatory cytokines (IL-4, IL-10, and TGF-β1), inhibition of enzymatic activities that encourage neurotoxicity (GSK-3β, γ-secretase), Ca^{2+} and glutamate excitotoxicity blockers that inhibit NMDA receptor function, suppression of neuronal cytotoxicity (memantine, lithium, sodium valproate), and attenuation of inflammation by anti-inflammatory drugs (NSAID, minocycline) (Fig. 19.4A). Novel approaches are currently being developed to attenuate aggregation of misfolded proteins with antibodies and the use of T-cell-mediated immune responses to attenuate neuroinflammation. Anti-inflammatory and/or anti-oxidative therapies could be used in conjunction to form combinational therapies targeting multiple sites of oxidative stress that contribute to inflammation responses and progressive disease.

Presently there is a push for interdisciplinary research designed to find specific biomarkers for earlier diagnosis of disease. This research has been made possible by the development of novel proteomic, genomic, and metabolomic assays and cellular systems designed to replicate human disease. The development of sensitive clinical tests and advancement of imaging capabilities with SPECT and MRI will also lead to earlier diagnosis. Currently, treatment for neurodegenerative diseases begins long after neurodegeneration has started, after its detrimental effects become symptomatic. The failure in late- or end-stage clinical trials of promising therapeutic modalities emphasizes the need for presymptomatic treatment.

Neurodegeneration in HAD, PD, AD, ALS, and other neurodegenerative diseases seems to be

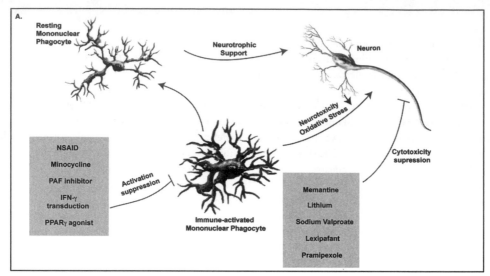

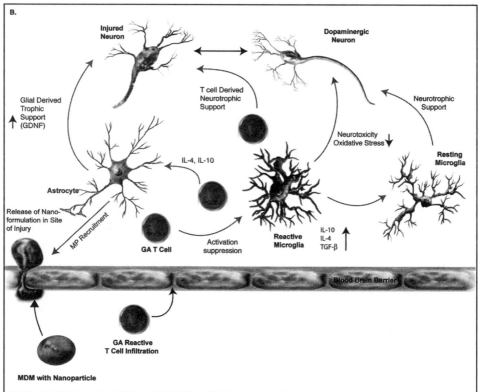

FIGURE 19.4. Adjunctive treatments of HIV-1 and other neurodegenerative disorders. A number of adjunctive therapies are being developed for treatment of HIV-1-associated cognitive impairments. These are directed at pathogenic mechanisms for disease, including those that affect viral replication, modulate neuroinflammation, interdict cell signaling events that lead to neuronal demise, or affect cell migration into the brain or the viral replication cycle (A). Novel approaches are now under development to harness the host's own immune system to combat disease. These methodologies currently involve direct immunization strategies and novel nanoparticle delivery systems (B). GA, glatiramer acetate; MDM, monocyte derived macrophages; MP, mononuclear phagocyte; PAF, platelet-activating factor; PPARγ, peroxisome proliferator-activated receptor gamma.

multifactorial, in that a complex set of toxic reactions including inflammation, glutamatergic neurotoxicity, increases in iron and nitric oxide, depletion of endogenous antioxidants, reduced expression of trophic factors, dysfunction of the ubiquitin-proteasome, and expression of pro-apoptotic proteins leads to the demise of neurons. As a result, the gradual accumulation of neuronal death and the increase in disease severity across time is a unifying theme across the diverse classifications of neurodegenerative disease. Thus, while the triggers of various neurodegenerative diseases are diverse, inflammation may be a basic mechanism driving the progressive nature of multiple neurodegenerative diseases. With complete comprehension of the cellular and molecular mechanisms and of the specificities of inflammation in these neurological disorders, therapeutic strategies to prevent or slow the progression of these destructive diseases can be delineated. The combinatorial use of therapeutic modalities that target inflammatory processes might aid in providing supportive treatment of HAD, AD, PD, and ALS.

The dementia produced by CNS infection with HIV elicits a cascade of events involving both resident and invading cell types and ultimately the devastating loss of neuronal function and increase in cognitive deterioration. Treatment failures, viral mutation drug-associated disease, and evolving neurological syndromes support the importance of neurological impairments as a significant part of the overall disease complex. In the past decade we have seen a milder phenotype and decreased incidence of HAD, largely due to the widespread use of combination chemotherapy to reduce viral burden. However, the prevalence of neurological disease in people living with HIV-1 has actually increased, raising significant concerns that new therapeutic strategies, directed at restoring neuronal and glial homeostasis and signaling in the CNS, as opposed to directly interfering with the life cycle of HIV-1, must be developed. Researchers developing new agents and strategies for the management of HIV-1 disease are focusing on regimens that include novel targets and are simpler and better tolerated, with decreased potential for development of viral resistance. Because the disease process occurs in a stepwise fashion, it provides the opportunity for development of therapeutics directed at discrete pathogenic mechanisms. Although antiretroviral agents are currently the only therapy in general use for treatment of AIDS dementia, a clearer understanding of the neuropathogenesis of HIVE and HAD has al-

lowed the selection of rational adjunctive therapies for HAD that are now in development. Phase 1 clinical trials for adjunctive (i.e., chemotherapeutic agents that do not have a primary antiretroviral mechanism of action) therapy in patients with HAD have been conducted.

There are several reasons for the demand for such therapies. First, antiretroviral therapy, while successful in decreasing viral burden and delaying the onset of HAD, does not prevent it. Second, combination antiretroviral therapies are not always well tolerated. Third, only a very limited fraction of the global population of HIV-infected persons has access to antiretrovirals. Fourth, HIV-1 is able to adapt to most of the antiretroviral agents. Also, most antiretroviral agents do not freely cross the BBB. Finally, overlapping pathogenic mechanisms are operative for other neurodegenerative disorders containing an inflammatory component, making it likely that agents will have crossover potential for treatment of a wide range of neurodestructive processes.

Antiretrovirals

Prior to the advent of potent antiretroviral therapy, HIV infection was characterized as an acute, systemic infection that rapidly led to immune suppression and cognitive decline. With the development of antiretroviral therapies, extended life expectancies and a better quality of life never before anticipated for patients with AIDS have been achieved. The decision to start antiretroviral therapy is largely based on CD4+ T-cell count thresholds, although higher viral load has been shown to increase risk of disease progression. Current guidelines recommend treatment for all patients with symptomatic HIV disease or AIDS and for asymptomatic patients with CD4+ T-cell counts <200 cells/mm^3 (Swindells et al., 1999). Since HIV-1-infected brain MP initiate the inflammatory neuro-immune cascade in the brain, leading to neuronal dysfunction, it is vital that any therapeutic strategy includes the use of antiretroviral agents to decrease the CNS viral load. Indeed, sufficient doses of 3'-azido-3'-deoxythymidine (AZT) can produce clinical improvement in the mental function of HIV-1-infected individuals (Schmitt et al., 1988; Llorente et al., 2001). Many antiretroviral agents are currently in use; these can be classified into specific categories based on function, including nucleoside reverse transcriptase inhibitors (e.g., zidovudine [AZT], didanosine

[DDI]), nonnucleoside reverse transcriptase inhibitors (e.g., nevirapine, delavirdine), protease inhibitors (e.g., indinavir, ritonavir), and combination antiretroviral therapy (Chang et al., 1999b; Ammassari et al., 2000; Gray and Keohane, 2003; Dou et al., 2004). While antiretroviral agents are beneficial in attenuating viral load, complications associated with infection are still prevalent, as the virus is never wholly eliminated. Antiretroviral medicines fail to completely eradicate the virus, in part because of a latent form of the virus that persists in resting memory CD4+ T cells (Finzi et al., 1997; Ho et al., 1998; Silician et al., 2003) and select viral mutations that result in viral resistance to antiretroviral drugs (Johnson et al., 2005). Viral reservoirs represent a potentially lifelong persistence of replication-competent forms of HIV-1, recovered from resting CD4 T cells (Finzi et al., 1997) and peripheral blood monocytes (Crowe and Sonza, 2000), that cannot be suppressed by current antiretroviral treatments. Primary and acquired antiretroviral resistance rates reflect the relative usage of different antiretroviral drugs in the population, as well as the inherent genetic barrier to the development of resistance associated with individual drugs. Data on antiretroviral resistance rates, gleaned from the growing HIV-1-infected population treated with a continuously increasing number of antiretroviral drugs and drug combinations, provide insight to the relative ease by which HIV-1 escapes the selective pressure of chronic drug exposure. Strains of HIV-1 that are resistant to reverse transcriptase and protease inhibitors arise in the majority of treated patients who have either poor adherence to the treatment regime or low plasma drug levels for other reasons (Kedzierska et al., 2003). Most important, virus resistance to drugs heralds increased viral loads, immune suppression, and the onset of neurological impairments associated with advanced viral infection. The development of novel adjunctive immunotherapies to use in combination with antiretroviral drugs provide new therapeutic strategies to combat infection that will be better tolerated and have a decreased potential for the emergence of viral resistance. New research will continue to provide more options for such patients, with new treatments and eventually vaccines on the horizon.

Glutamate Receptor Antagonists

The use of NMDA-receptor antagonists is a good example of this approach. Neuronal dysfunction and death that occur in HIVE and are associated with HAD might ultimately be mediated by pathologic activation of excitatory subtypes of glutamate receptors, in particular the NMDA receptor (Lipton, 1992, 1994; Lipton et al., 1994). Numerous examples in the literature demonstrate the involvement of NMDA and non-NMDA receptor activation in vulnerable neurons after exposure to HIV-1-associated neurotoxins. One problem in designing a practical therapeutic approach to ameliorating excitotoxic neuronal damage is that most of the available small-molecule agents that block ionotropic receptors function as uncompetitive or noncompetitive channel antagonists. Thus, administration of such an agent at concentrations that might be neuroprotective in the CNS might also significantly interfere with fast excitatory neurotransmission. Thus far, the most promising NMDA antagonist currently in clinical trials for HIV-1-related neurological disease is memantine. This NMDA-receptor antagonist is an open channel blocker and has been shown to attenuate the neuronal damage induced by HIV-infected macrophages and gp120 (Jain, 2000).

GSK-3 Inhibitors

The GSK-3 inhibitor sodium valproate (VPA) has been proposed to possess neuroprotective properties as a result of its effects on GSK-3β activity (Tong et al., 2000) and because of its cytoprotective effect on neurons exposed to candidate HIV neurotoxins. VPA has already been used in HIV-1-infected individuals to manage psychiatric disorders and was generally well tolerated. VPA is preferable to the other presently available inhibitor of GSK-3β, lithium, in light of its greater tolerability in HIV-positive individuals and lack of toxic side effects.

Dopaminergic Agents

In HIV-1-infected individuals, neurological disease has been linked to changes in DA metabolism, and DA levels within the CSF are reduced. Furthermore, experiments conducted with cell culture have shown that HIV-1 gp120 is toxic for dopaminergic neurons (Bennett et al., 1995). On the basis of these findings, it has been proposed that alterations in DA metabolism may contribute to motor deficits in persons with HAD and possibly to other aspects of this disease. Therefore, DA agonists such as pramipexole, shown to be neuroprotective in a mouse model in the context of MPTP-induced injury, have been proposed for treatment of HIV infection (Hall et al., 1996; Cassarino et al., 1998; Kitamura et al., 1998a, 1998b). Pramipexole had been shown to up-regulate the expression of anti-apoptotic proteins such as Bcl-2, and to protect cultured neurons from pro-apoptotic insults (Takata et al., 2000). Furthermore, Bcl-2 can mediate neuroprotection against candidate HIV-1 neurotoxins, including HIV-1 Tat and TNF-α.

PAF Receptor Antagonist

PAF is a phospholipid mediator that may play a key role in NMDA receptor activation in HAD (Bito et al., 1982). Intriguingly, in vivo experiments using the SCID mouse model of HIVE demonstrate that PAF receptor antagonists are neuroprotective (Persidsky et al., 2001). A phase I trial of tolerability of the PAF receptor antagonist lexipafant in a cohort of patients with varying stages of HAD demonstrated trends in improvement of neuropsychological parameters, including verbal memory (Schifitto et al., 1999, 2001). These trends were promising enough to extend the cohort size and dosing schedule into an ongoing trial of efficacy.

PPARγ Agonists

Peroxisome proliferator-activated receptor gamma (PPARγ) is a nuclear receptor involved in monocyte-derived macrophage differentiation. Agonists for this receptor, such as cyPG, PgJ, and troglitazone, have been shown to inhibit HIV-1 replication in vitro in T-cell lines (Hughes-Fulford et al., 1992) in chronically infected macrophages (Rozera et al., 1996) and, more recently, in acutely infected monocytes (Hayes et al., 2002; Skolnik et al., 2002).

Immunotherapy

There is renewed interest in the use of immunotherapy as an adjunct to antiretrovirals in the treatment of HIV disease. A number of cytokines have been proposed as modulators of HIV-specific effector functions, the most studied being IL-2. Subcutaneous IL-2 administered to patients with HIV-1 infection has been shown to facilitate CD4+ T-cell expansion, facilitated by the selective induction of the alpha chain (CD25) of the high-affinity IL-2 receptor complex on CD4+ T cells (Kovacs et al., 1996a, 1996b; Pett and Emery, 2001). Clinical trials have demonstrated that intermittent administration of IL-2 to HIV-1-infected patients in combination with antiretrovirals results in substantial and significantly higher CD4+ T-cell increases than those achieved with antiretroviral therapy alone (Kovacs et al., 1996a, 1996b; Davey et al., 1997; Pett and Emery, 2001). Other cytokines that contribute to enhancing macrophage function, including GM-CSF and IFN-γ, have also been proposed as immunomodulators for use in immunotherapy. The main caveat however, is that without effective antiretroviral therapy, these cytokines can promote HIV-1 replication (Kaplan et al., 1991; Krown et al., 1992a, 1992b). Indeed, GM-CSF is known to stimulate the proliferation and differentiation of cells of the macrophage lineage; it has also been shown to increase the phagocytic activity of these cells (Krown et al., 1992b; Eischen et al., 2001). Even so, GM-CSF has been shown to augment the effects of antiretroviral therapy. Data show that patients receiving GM-CSF in combination with antiretroviral therapy experienced a decrease in viral load and an increase in CD4+ T-cell count (Brites et al., 2000).

Glatiramer Acetate Immunization

Glatiramer acetate (GA, Copaxone, copolymer-1) is an FDA-approved immunomodulatory drug for the treatment of multiple sclerosis (MS). GA immunization induces Th2 regulatory T lymphocytes secreting anti-inflammatory cytokines in mice and humans. These T cells migrate to the brain and provide bystander suppression against neuroinflammation. GA was shown to be an effective immunomodulatory treatment for neuroprotection in animal models of experimental autoimmune encephalomyelitis, optic nerve crush, PD, and AD (Kipnis et al., 2000; Benner et al., 2004; Weber et al., 2004; Frenkel et al., 2005; Wolinsky, 2006). In addition, clinical trials are ongoing in the use of GA in the treatment of ALS (Gordon et al., 2006). A newly completed study in our own lab tested the effects of GA immunization on neuropathological outcomes in rodent models of HIVE. GA administration resulted in significant neuroprotection accompanied by increased levels of IL-10 and BDNF (Gorantla et al., submitted). Immunization with GA is probable, as it is already approved for treatment of MS, it is able to boost immune responses of both the Th1 and Th2 phenotype, and it has been used without side effects in a phase 1 study of ALS (Weber et al., 2004; Gordon et al., 2006).

Nanoparticle Drug Delivery

The limitations of antiretroviral therapy in the long-term treatment of HIV-1, which include cost, treatment failures, dosing complexities, and drug toxicity, are beginning to be realized (Chen et al., 2002; Chulamokha et al., 2005). As a result, a global effort has been undertaken to develop novel therapeutic strategies to address these limitations. Recently, we described a nanoparticle (NP) system that was developed in our lab, in conjunction with Baxter Pharmaceuticals. The nanoformulation is designed to improve therapeutic efficacy of antiretroviral drugs through a delivery system capable of distributing drug to areas of active viral replication, as well as to extend dosing intervals (Dou et al., 2006). Because of the small and highly stable NP formulation, we were able to package the particles within macrophages to be delivered through systemic trafficking within the host. In a single dose, the NP containing the drug trafficked to the site of inflammation in the CNS (visualized by MRSI), had sustained drug release over a period of 2 weeks, and presented with antiretroviral activity. Toxicity was not evident during the administration period (Fig. 19.4B). The treatment of HIV-1, which requires lifelong therapy, with a similar nanoformulation could affect therapeutic outcome and drug usage in the developing world.

SUMMARY

Progressive HIV infection is associated with a broad range of neurological and neuropsychiatric disorders that are either caused by opportunistic viral, bacterial, fungal, and protozoan infections, malignancies, or directly linked to progressive HIV infection. These disorders follow profound CD4+ T-lymphocyte depletion and high viral loads. Cognitive impairments are linked to HIV-1 infection of the nervous system and are characterized by a triad of memory, motor, and behavioral disturbances. These neurological deficits result from a metabolic encephalopathy in which brain mononuclear phagocytes (brain macrophages and microglia) affect neuronal function through the secretion of inflammatory and viral toxins, known in its most severe form as HIV-associated dementia (HAD). Ultimately, if left untreated, the process rapidly leads to substantive neurodegeneration, characterized pathologically by multinucleated giant cell encephalitis with profound neuroinflammation and neuronal, dendritic, and synaptic cleft losses. Further investigation of the mechanisms by which the virus invades the nervous system and induces neurological deficits and the signaling pathways responsible for the neuroinflammatory cascade is key to a better understanding of disease mechanisms and to improved therapies.

With the advent of potent antiretroviral therapy and longer survival of HIV-infected individuals, HAD has been transformed from a subacute and often lethal disorder to a chronic and protracted medical condition, more commonly known as HIV-1-associated cognitive impairment. During progressive HIV-1 infection, the brain is affected by a spectrum of inflammatory changes, dendritic and synaptic damage, and neuronal loss. Further complicating the situation, patients with AIDS show varying degrees of damage to the white matter and cerebral microvasculature. Increasing viral load is associated with worsening neuronal damage, and this damage correlates with the onset of early cognitive impairment. Recent advances in antiretroviral regimens have slowed the progression of HIV disease in affected individuals and decreased the incidence of dementia. Moreover, because infection and activation of MP are necessary for macrophage-mediated neuronal damage, adjunctive anti-inflammatory and/or neuroprotective therapeutic strategies have received intense attention.

The complex relationship between disease pathobiology, cognitive impairment, and neurodegeneration is now being widely investigated by many laboratories throughout the world. Perhaps most interesting is the fact that disease mechanisms uncovered for HIV/AIDS within the CNS parallel those of other neurodegenerative disorders. Indeed, treatments aimed at disabling macrophage activation and/or its neurotoxic secretions within the brain may lead to not only therapeutic benefit but also neural tissue repair and improvements in mental function for a variety of disorders of the nervous system.

ACKNOWLEDGMENTS   This work was supported in part by National Institute of Health grants 2 R37 NS36126, 1 P01 NS043985-01, 5 P01 MH64570-03, P20 RR15635 (to H.E.G.), and KO1 MH068214 (to G.K.) and by a University of Nebraska Medical Center Graduate Fellowship (to A.R.). We thank Robin Taylor for excellent editorial assistance.

References

Adamson D, Wildemann B, Sasaki M, Glass JD, McArthur JC, Christov VI, Dawson TM, and Dawson VL (1996). Immunologic NO synthase: elevation in severe AIDS and induction by HIV-1 gp41. *Science* 274:1917–1921.

Alliot F, Godin I, and Pessac B (1999). Microglia derive from progenitors, originating from the yolk sac, and which proliferate in the brain. *Brain Res Dev Brain Res* 117(2):145–152.

Ammassari A, Cingolani A, Pezzotti P, et al. (2000). AIDS-related focal brain lesions in the era of highly active antiretroviral therapy. *Neurology* 55(8):1194–1200.

An SF, and Scaravilli F (1997). Early HIV infection of the central nervous system. *Arch Anat Cytol Pathol* 45:94–105.

Anderson E, Zink W, Xiong H, and Gendelman HE (2002). HIV-1-associated dementia: a metabolic encephalopathy perpetrated by virus-infected and immune-competent mononuclear phagocytes. *J Acquir Immune Defic Syndr* 31(Suppl. 2):S43–S54.

Anderson ER, Boyle J, Zink WE, et al. (2003). Hippocampal synaptic dysfunction in a murine model of human immunodeficiency virus type 1 encephalitis. *Neuroscience* 118(2):359–369.

Andras IE, Pu H, Deli MA, et al. (2003). HIV-1 Tat protein alters tight junction protein expression and distribution in cultured brain endothelial cells. *J Neurosci Res* 74(2):255–265.

Aquaro S, Ronga L, Pollicita M, et al. (2005). Human immunodeficiency virus infection and acquired immunodeficiency syndrome dementia complex: role of cells of monocyte-macrophage lineage. *J Neurovirol* 11(Suppl. 3):58–66.

Azzam R, Lal L, Goh SL, et al. (2006). Adverse effects of antiretroviral drugs on HIV-1-infected and -uninfected human monocyte-derived macrophages. *J Acquir Immune Defic Syndr* 42(1):19–28.

Badley AD, Roumier T, Lum JJ, and Kroemer G. (2003). Mitochondrion-mediated apoptosis in HIV-1 infection. *Trends Pharmacol Sci* 24(6):298–305.

Bagdades EK, Pillay D, Squire SB, et al. (1992). Relationship between herpes simplex virus ulceration and CD4+ cell counts in patients with HIV infection. *AIDS* 6(11):1317–1320.

Bagetta G, Piccirilli S, Del Duca C, et al. (2004). Inducible nitric oxide synthase is involved in the mechanisms of cocaine enhanced neuronal apoptosis induced by HIV-1 gp120 in the neocortex of rat. *Neurosci Lett* 356(3):183–186.

Bal-Price A, and Brown GC (2001). Inflammatory neurodegeneration mediated by nitric oxide from activated glia-inhibiting neuronal respiration, causing glutamate release and excitotoxicity. *J Neurosci* 21(17):6480–6491.

Banks WA, Akerstrom V, and Kastin AJ (1998). Adsorptive endocytosis mediates the passage of HIV-1 across the blood-brain barrier: evidence for a post-internalization coreceptor. *J Cell Sci* 111(Pt. 4):533–540.

Banks WA, Freed EO, Wolf KM, et al. (2001). Transport of human immunodeficiency virus type 1 pseudoviruses across the blood–brain barrier: role of envelope proteins and adsorptive endocytosis. *J Virol* 75(10):4681–4691.

Barre-Sinoussi F, Chermann JC, Rey F, Nugeyre MT, Chamaret S, Gruest J, Daughet C, Axler-Blin C, Vezinet-Brun F, Rouzioux C, Rozenbaum W, and Montagnier L (1983). Isolation of T-lymphotropic retrovirus from a pateint at risk for acquired immune deficiency syndrome. *Science* 220:868–871.

Becker JT, Sanchez J, Dew MA, et al. (1997). Neuropsychological abnormalities among HIV-infected individuals in a community-based sample. *Neuropsychology* 11(4):592–601.

Beckett A, and Forstein M (1993). Psychological manifestations. In H Libman and RA Witzburg (eds.), *HIV Infection: A Clinical Manual* (pp. 219–229). Boston: Little, Brown and Company.

Bellizzi M, Lu S-M, Masliah E, and Gelbard HA (2005). Synaptic activity becomes excitoxic in neurons exposed to elevated levels of platelet activating factor. *J Clin Invest* 115(11):3185–3192.

Benner EJ, Mosley RL, Destache CJ, et al. (2004). Therapeutic immunization protects dopaminergic neurons in a mouse model of Parkinson's disease. *Proc Natl Acad Sci U S A* 101(25):9435–9440.

Bennett BA, Rusyniak DE, and Hollingsworth CK (1995). HIV-1 gp120-induced neurotoxicity to midbrain dopamine cultures. *Brain Res* 705(1-2):168–176.

Berger JR and Avison M (2004). The blood brain barrier in HIV infection. *Front Biosci* 9:2680–2685.

Berger JR, Avison M, Mootoor Y, and Beach C (2005). Cerebrospinal fluid proteomics and human immunodeficiency virus dementia: preliminary observations. *J Neurovirol* 11(6):557–562.

Bezzi P, Domercq M, Brambilla L, et al. (2001). CXCR4-activated astrocyte glutamate release via TNFalpha: amplification by microglia triggers neurotoxicity. *Nat Neurosci* 4(7):702–710.

Biernacki K, Prat A, Blain M, and Antel JP (2001). Regulation of Th1 and Th2 lymphocyte migration by human adult brain endothelial cells. *J Neuropathol Exp Neurol* 60(12):1127–1136.

Bito LZ, Nichols RR, and Baroody RA (1982). A comparison of the miotic and inflammatory effects of biologically active polypeptides and prostaglandin E2 on the rabbit eye. *Exp Eye Res* 34(3):325–337.

Blankson J, Finzi D, Pierson TC, et al. (2000). Biphasic decay of latently infected CD4+ T cells in acute human immunodeficiency type 1 infection. *J Infect Dis* 182:1636–1642.

Bollinger RC, Brookmeyer RS, Mehendale SM, et al. (1997). Risk factors and clinical presentation of acute primary HIV infection in India. *JAMA* 278:2085–2089.

Bonavia R, Bajetto A, Barbero S, et al. (2001). HIV-1 Tat causes apoptotic death and calcium homeostasis alterations in rat neurons. *Biochem Biophys Res Commun* 288(2):301–308.

Borrow P, Lewicki H, Wei X, et al. (1997). Antiviral pressure exerted by HIV-1-specific cytotoxic T lymphocytes (CTLs) during primary infection demonstrated by rapid selection of CTL escape virus. *Nat Med* 3(2):205–211.

Boska MD, Mosley RL, Nawab M, et al. (2004). Advances in neuroimaging for HIV-1 associated neurological dysfunction: clues to the diagnosis, pathogenesis and therapeutic monitoring. *Curr HIV Res* 2(1):61–78.

Bower WA, Culver DH, Castor D, et al. (2006). Changes in hepatitis C virus (HCV) viral load and interferon-alpha levels in HIV/HCV-coinfected patients treated with highly active antiretroviral therapy. *J Acquir Immune Defic Syndr* 42(3):293–297.

Braak H, and Braak E (1994). Morphological criteria for the recognition of Alzheimer's disease and the distribution pattern of cortical changes related to this disorder. *Neurobiol Aging* 15(3):355–356; discussion 379–380.

Brabers NA, and Nottet HS (2006). Role of the pro-inflammatory cytokines TNF-alpha and IL-1beta in HIV-associated dementia. *Eur J Clin Invest* 36(7): 447–458.

Brenchley JM, Schacker TW, Ruff LE, et al. (2004). CD4+ T cell depletion during all stages of HIV disease occurs predominantly in the gastrointestinal tract. *J Exp Med* 200(6):749–759.

Brenneman D, Westbrook GL, Fitzgerald SP, Ennist DL, Elkins KL, Ruff MR, and Pert CB (1988). Neuronal cell killing by the envelope protein of HIV and its prevention by vasoactive intestinal peptide. *Nature* 335:639–642.

Brew BJ (2001). Markers of AIDS dementia complex: the role of cerebrospinal fluid assays. *AIDS* 15(14): 1883–1884.

Brew BJ, Rosenblum M, and Price RW (1988). AIDS dementia complex and primary HIV brain infection. *J Neuroimmunol* 20(2–3):133–140.

Brew BJ, Bhalla RB, Fleisher M, et al. (1989). Cerebrospinal fluid beta 2 microglobulin in patients infected with human immunodeficiency virus. *Neurology* 39(6):830–834.

Brew BJ, Bhalla RB, Paul M, et al. (1990). Cerebrospinal fluid neopterin in human immunodeficiency virus type 1 infection. *Ann Neurol* 28(4):556–560.

Brew BJ, Bhalla RB, Paul M, et al. (1992). Cerebrospinal fluid beta 2-microglobulin in patients with AIDS dementia complex: an expanded series including response to zidovudine treatment. *AIDS* 6(5):461–465.

Brew BJ, Dunbar N, Pemberton L, and Kaldor J (1996). Predictive markers of AIDS dementia complex: CD4 cell count and cerebrospinal fluid concentrations of beta 2-microglobulin and neopterin. *J Infect Dis* 174(2):294–298.

Brew BJ, Pemberton L, Cunningham P, and Law MG (1997). Levels of human immunodeficiency virus type 1 RNA in cerebrospinal fluid correlate with AIDS dementia stage. *J Infect Dis* 175(4):963–966.

Brites C, Gilbert JM, Pedral-Sampaio D, et al. (2000). A randomized, placebo-controlled trial of granulocyte-macrophage colony-stimulating factor and nucleoside analogue therapy in AIDS. *J Infect Dis* 182(5):1531–1535.

Broderick DF, Wippold FJ 2nd, Clifford DB, et al. (1993). White matter lesions and cerebral atrophy on MR images in patients with and without AIDS dementia complex. *AJR Am J Roentgenol* 161(1): 177–181.

Brosnan CF, Lee SC, and Liu J (1997). Regulation of inducible nitric oxide synthase expression in human glia: implications for inflammatory central nervous system diseases. *Biochem Soc Trans* 25(2): 679–683.

Brouwers P, DeCarli C, Tudor-Williams G, et al. (1994). Interrelations among patterns of change in neurocognitive, CT brain imaging and CD4 measures associated with anti-retroviral therapy in children with symptomatic HIV infection. *Adv Neuroimmunol* 4(3):223–231.

Brouwers P, Heyes MP, Moss HA, et al. (1993). Quinolinic acid in the cerebrospinal fluid of children with symptomatic human immunodeficiency virus type 1 disease: relationships to clinical status and therapeutic response. *J Infect Dis* 168(6):1380–6138.

Brown GR, Rundell JR, McManis SE, et al. (1992). Prevalence of psychiatric disorders in early stages of HIV infection. *Psychosom Med* 54(5):588–601.

Bruijn LI, Miller TM, and Cleveland DW (2004). Unraveling the mechanisms involved in motor neuron degeneration in ALS. *Annu Rev Neurosci* 27: 723–749.

Budka H (1986). Multinucleated giant cells in brain: a hallmark of the acquired immune deficiency syndrome (AIDS). *Acta Neuropathol (Berl)* 69(3-4): 253–258.

Budka H (1991). Neuropathology of human immunodeficiency virus infection. *Brain Pathol* 1(3):163–175.

Budka H (2005). The neuropathology of HIV-associated brain disease. In HE Gendelman, I Grant, IP Everall, SA Lipton, and S Swindells (eds.), *The Neurology of AIDS* (pp. 375–391). New York: Oxford University Press.

Budka H, Maier H, and Pohl P (1988). Human immunodeficiency virus in vacuolar myelopathy of the acquired immunodeficiency syndrome. *N Engl J Med* 319(25):1667–1668.

Bukrinsky MI, Nottet HS, Schmidtmayerova H, et al. (1995). Regulation of nitric oxide synthase activity in human immunodeficiency virus type 1 (HIV-1)-infected monocytes: implications for HIV-associated neurological disease. *J Exp Med* 181(2):735–745.

Burton DR (2006). Structural biology: images from the surface of HIV. *Nature* 441(7095):817–818.

Butovsky O, Talpalar AE, Ben-Yaakov K, and Schwartz M (2005). Activation of microglia by aggregated beta-amyloid or lipopolysaccharide impairs MHC-II expression and renders them cytotoxic whereas IFN-gamma and IL-4 render them protective. *Mol Cell Neurosci* 29(3)381–393.

Campbell IL (2004). Chemokines as plurifunctional mediators in the CNS: implications for the pathogenesis of stroke. *Ernst Schering Res Found Workshop* 45:31–51.

Cann AJ, Churcher MJ, Boyd M, et al. (1992). The region of the envelope gene of human immunodeficiency virus type 1 responsible for determination of cell tropism. *J Virol* 66(1):305–309.

Canque B, Rosenzwajg M, Gey A, et al. (1996). Macrophage inflammatory protein-1alpha is induced by human immunodeficiency virus infection of monocyte-derived macrophages. *Blood* 87(5):2011–2019.

Cao Y, Qin L, Zhang L, Safrit J, and Ho DD (1995). Virologic and immunologic characterization of long-term survivors of human immunodeficiency virus type 1 infection. *N Engl J Med* 332(4):201–208.

Carlson KA, Ciborowski P, Schellpeper CN, et al. (2004a). Proteomic fingerprinting of HIV-1-infected human monocyte-derived macrophages: a preliminary report. *J Neuroimmunol* 147(1-2):35–42.

Carlson KA, Limoges J, Pohlman GD, et al. (2004b). OTK18 expression in brain mononuclear phagocytes parallels the severity of HIV-1 encephalitis. *J Neuroimmunol* 150(1-2):186–198.

Cassarino DS, Fall CP, Smith TS, and Bennett JP Jr (1998). Pramipexole reduces reactive oxygen species production in vivo and in vitro and inhibits the mitochondrial permeability transition produced by the parkinsonian neurotoxin methylpyridinium ion. *J Neurochem* 71(1):295–301.

Chang L, Ernst T, Leonido-Yee M, Walot I, and Singer E (1999a). Cerebral metabolite abnormalities correlate with clinical severity of HIV-1 cognitive motor complex. *Neurology* 52(1):100–108.

Chang L, Ernst T, Leonido-Yee M, Witt M, et al. (1999b). Highly active antiretroviral therapy reverses brain metabolite abnormalities in mild HIV dementia. *Neurology* 53(4):782–789.

Chen AM, Khanna N, Stohlman SA, and Bermann CC (2005). Virus-specific and bystander CD8 T cells recruited during virus-induced encephalomyelitis. *J Virol* 79(8):4700–4708.

Chen K, Huang J, Gong W, et al. (2006). CD40/CD40L dyad in the inflammatory and immune responses in the central nervous system. *Cell Mol Immunol* 3(3):163–169.

Chen RY, Westfall AO, Raper JL, et al. (2002). Immunologic and virologic consequences of temporary antiretroviral treatment interruption in clinical practice. *AIDS Res Hum Retroviruses* 18(13):909–916.

Cherner M, Masliah E, Ellis RJ, et al. (2002). Neurocognitive dysfunction predicts postmortem findings of HIV encephalitis. *Neurology* 59(10):1563–1567.

Chiodi F, Sonnerborg A, Albert J, et al. (1988). Human immunodeficiency virus infection of the brain. I. Virus isolation and detection of HIV specific antibodies in the cerebrospinal fluid of patients with varying clinical conditions. *J Neurol Sci* 85(3):245–257.

Chong WK, Sweeney B, Wilkinson ID, et al. (1993). Proton spectroscopy of the brain in HIV infection: correlation with clinical, immunologic, and MR imaging findings. *Radiology* 188(1):119–124.

Chong YH, Seoh JY, and Park HK (1998). Increased activity of matrix metalloproteinase-2 in human glial and neuronal cell lines treated with HIV-1 gp41 peptides. *J Mol Neurosci* 10(2):129–141.

Chulamokha L, DeSimone JA, and Pomerantz RJ (2005). Antiretroviral therapy in the developing world. *J Neurovirol* 11(Suppl. 1):76–80.

Ciborowski P, and Gendelman HE (2006). Human immunodeficiency virus–mononuclear phagocyte interactions: emerging avenues of biomarker discovery, modes of viral persistence and disease pathogenesis. *Curr HIV Res* 4(3):279–291.

Ciborowski P, Enose Y, Mack A, et al. (2004). Diminished matrix metalloproteinase 9 secretion in human immunodeficiency virus–infected mononuclear phagocytes: modulation of innate immunity and implications for neurological disease. *J Neuroimmunol* 157(1-2):11–6.

Clark G, Happel LT, Zorumski CF, and Bazan NG (1992). Enhancement of hippocampal excitatory synaptic transmission by platelet activating factor. *Neuron* 9(6):1211–1216.

Cocchi F, DeVico AL, Garzino-Demo A, et al. (1995). Identification of RANTES, MIP-1 alpha, and MIP-1 beta as the major HIV-suppressive factors produced by CD8+ T cells. *Science* 270(5243):1811–1815.

Conant K, Tornatore C, Atwood W, et al. (1994). In vivo and in vitro infection of the astrocyte by HIV-1. *Adv Neuroimmunol* 4(3):287–289.

Conant K, Ma M, Nath A, and Major EO (1996). Extracellular human immunodeficiency virus type 1 Tat protein is associated with an increase in both NF-kappa B binding and protein kinase C activity in primary human astrocytes. *J Virol* 70(3):1384–1389.

Conant K, Garzino-Demo A, Nath A, et al. (1998). Induction of monocyte chemoattractant protein-1 in HIV-1 Tat-stimulated astrocytes and elevation in AIDS dementia. *Proc Natl Acad Sci U S A* 95(6):3117–3121.

Conant K, McArthur JC, Griffin DE, et al. (1999). Cerebrospinal fluid levels of MMP-2, 7, and 9 are elevated in association with human immunodeficiency virus dementia. *Ann Neurol* 46(3):391–398.

Craft JM, Watterson DM, Frautschy SA, and Van Eldik LJ (2004). Aminopyridazines inhibit beta-amyloid-induced glial activation and neuronal damage in vivo. *Neurobiol Aging* 25(10):1283–1292.

Craft JM, Watterson DM, and Van Eldik LJ (2006). Human amyloid beta–induced neuroinflammation is an early event in neurodegeneration. *Glia* 53(5): 484–490.

Croisier E, Moran LB, Dexter DT, et al. (2005). Microglial inflammation in the parkinsonian substantia nigra: relationship to alpha-synuclein deposition. *J Neuroinflammation* 2:14.

Crowe SM, and Sonza S (2000). HIV-1 can be recovered from a variety of cells including peripheral blood monocytes of patients receiving highly active antiretroviral therapy: a further obstacle to eradication. *J Leukoc Biol* 68(3):345–350.

Cui LY, Liu MS, and Tang SF (2004). Single fiber electromyography in 78 patients with amyotrophic lateral sclerosis. *Chin Med J (Engl)* 117(12):1830–1833.

Cysique LA, Brew BJ, Halman M, et al. (2005). Undetectable cerebrospinal fluid HIV RNA and beta-2 microglobulin do not indicate inactive AIDS dementia complex in highly active antiretroviral therapy–treated patients. *J Acquir Immune Defic Syndr* 39(4):426–429.

Cysique LA, Maruff P, Darby D, and Brew BJ (2006). The assessment of cognitive function in advanced HIV-1 infection and AIDS dementia complex using a new computerised cognitive test battery. *Arch Clin Neuropsychol* 21(2):185–194.

Dalgleish AG, Beverley PC, Clapham PR, et al. (1984). The CD4 (T4) antigen is an essential component of the receptor for the AIDS retrovirus. *Nature* 312(5996):763–767.

da Silva J (2003). The evolutionary adaptation of HIV-1 to specific immunity. *Curr HIV Res* 1(3):363–371.

D'Aversa TG, Eugenin EA, and Berman JW (2005). NeuroAIDS: contributions of the human immunodeficiency virus-1 proteins Tat and gp120 as well as CD40 to microglial activation. *J Neurosci Res* 81(3): 436–446.

Davey RT Jr, Chaitt DG, Piscitelli SC, et al. (1997). Subcutaneous administration of interleukin-2 in human immunodeficiency virus type 1–infected persons. *J Infect Dis* 175(4):781–789.

David JP, Ghozali F, Fallot-Bianco C, et al. (1997). Glial reaction in the hippocampal formation is highly correlated with aging in human brain. *Neurosci Lett* 235(1-2):53–56.

Davis HF, Skolasky RL Jr, Selnes OA, et al. (2002). Assessing HIV-associated dementia: modified HIV dementia scale versus the Grooved Pegboard. *AIDS Read* 12(1):29–31, 38.

Davis JB, McMurray HF, and Schubert D (1992). The amyloid beta-protein of Alzheimer's disease is chemotactic for mononuclear phagocytes. *Biochem Biophys Res Commun* 189(2):1096–1100.

Derdeyn CA, and Silvestri G (2005). Viral and host factors in the pathogenesis of HIV infection. *Curr Opin Immunol* 17(4):366–373.

Deshpande M, Zheng J, Borgmann K, et al. (2005). Role of activated astrocytes in neuronal damage: potential links to HIV-1-associated dementia. *Neurotox Res* 7(3):183–192.

Devadas K, Zhou P, Tewari D, and Notkins AL (2003). Inhibition of HIV-1 replication by the combined action of anti-gp41 single chain antibody and IL-16. *Antiviral Res* 59(1):67–70.

Devadas K, Hardegen NJ, Wahl LM, et al. (2004). Mechanisms for macrophage-mediated HIV-1 induction. *J Immunol* 173(11):6735–6744.

Dheen ST, Jun Y, Yan Z, Tay SS, and Ling EA (2005). Retinoic acid inhibits expression of TNF-alpha and iNOS in activated rat microglia. *Glia* 50(1): 21–31.

Dickson DW (1986). Multinucleated giant cells in acquired immunodeficiency syndrome encephalopathy. Origin from endogenous microglia? *Arch Pathol Lab Med* 110(10):967–968.

Diesing TS, Swindells S, Gelbard H, and Gendelman HE (2002). HIV-1-associated dementia: a basic science and clinical perspective. *AIDS Read* 12(8): 358–368.

Di Stefano M, Sabri F, and Chiodi F (2005). HIV-1 structural and regulatory proteins and neurotoxicity. In HE Gendelman, I Grant, IP Everall, SA Lipton, and S Swindells (eds.), *The Neurology of AIDS* (pp. 49–56). New York: Oxford University Press.

Dou H, Kingsley JD, Mosley RL, et al. (2004). Neuroprotective strategies for HIV-1 associated dementia. *Neurotox Res* 6(7-8):503–521.

Dou H, Destache CJ, Morehead JR, et al. (2006). Development of a macrophage-based nanoparticle system for anti-retroviral drug delivery. *Blood* 108(8): 2827–2835.

Draenert R, Allen TM, Liu Y, et al. (2006). Constraints on HIV-1 evolution and immunodominance revealed in monozygotic adult twins infected with the same virus. *J Exp Med* 203(3):529–539.

Dreyer EB, and Lipton SA (1995). The coat protein gp120 of HIV-1 inhibits astrocyte uptake of excitatory amino acids via macrophage arachidonic acid. *Eur J Neurosci* 7(12):2502–2507.

Du Y, Ma Z, Lin S, et al. (2001). Minocycline prevents nigrostriatal dopaminergic neurodegeneration in the MPTP model of Parkinson's disease. *Proc Natl Acad Sci U S A* 98(25):14669–14674.

Ebenbichler C, Westervelt P, Carrillo A, et al. (1993). Structure–function relationships of the HIV-1 envelope V3 loop tropism determinant: evidence for two distinct conformations. *AIDS* 7(5):639–646.

Egger M, May M, Chene G, et al. (2002). Prognosis of HIV-1-infected patients starting highly active antiretroviral therapy: a collaborative analysis of prospective studies. *Lancet* 360(9327):119–129.

Eischen CM, Packham G, Nip J, et al. (2001). Bcl-2 is an apoptotic target suppressed by both c-Myc and E2F-1. *Oncogene* 20(48):6983–6993.

El-Hage N, Gurwell JA, Singh IN, et al. (2005). Synergistic increases in intracellular Ca2+, and the release of MCP-1, RANTES, and IL-6 by astrocytes treated with opiates and HIV-1 Tat. *Glia* 50(2):91–106.

Ellis RJ, Hsia K, Spector SA, et al. (1997). Cerebrospinal fluid human immunodeficiency virus type 1 RNA levels are elevated in neurocognitively impaired individuals with acquired immunodeficiency syndrome. HIV Neurobehavioral Research Center Group. *Ann Neurol* 42(5):679–688.

Ellis RJ, Moore DJ, Childers ME, et al. (2002). Progression to neuropsychological impairment in human immunodeficiency virus infection predicted by elevated cerebrospinal fluid levels of human immunodeficiency virus RNA. *Arch Neurol* 59(6):923–928.

Ellis RJ, Childers ME, Zimmerman JD, et al. (2003). Human immunodeficiency virus-1 RNA levels in cerebrospinal fluid exhibit a set point in clinically stable patients not receiving antiretroviral therapy. *J Infect Dis* 187(11):1818–1821.

Epstein LG, and Gendelman HE (1993). Human immunodeficiency virus type 1 infection of the nervous system: pathogenetic mechanisms. *Ann Neurol* 33(5):429–436.

Eugenin EA, Dyer G, Calderon TM, and Berman JW (2005). HIV-1 tat protein induces a migratory phenotype in human fetal microglia by a CCL2 (MCP-1)-dependent mechanism: possible role in Neuro-AIDS. *Glia* 49(4):501–510.

Everall IP, Heaton RK, Marcotte TD, et al. (1999). Cortical synaptic density is reduced in mild to moderate human immunodeficiency virus neurocognitive disorder. HNRC Group. HIV Neurobehavioral Research Center. *Brain Pathol* 9(2):209–217.

Farzan M, Choe H, Martin KA, et al. (1997). HIV-1 entry and macrophage inflammatory protein-1beta-mediated signaling are independent functions of the chemokine receptor CCR5. *J Biol Chem* 272(11):6854–6857.

Fellay J, Marzolini C, Decosterd L, et al. (2005). Variations of CYP3A activity induced by antiretroviral treatment in HIV-1 infected patients. *Eur J Clin Pharmacol* 60(12):865–873.

Feng ZH, Wang TG, Li DD, et al. (2002). Cyclooxygenase-2-deficient mice are resistant to 1-methyl-4-phenyl1, 2, 3, 6-tetrahydropyridine-induced damage of dopaminergic neurons in the substantia nigra. *Neurosci Lett* 329(3):354–358.

Fine SM, Angel RA, Perry SW, et al. (1996). Tumor necrosis factor alpha inhibits glutamate uptake by primary human astrocytes. Implications for pathogenesis of HIV-1 dementia. *J Biol Chem* 271(26):15303–15306.

Finzi D, Hermankova M, Pierson T, et al. (1997). Identification of a reservoir for HIV-1 in patients on highly active antiretroviral therapy. *Science* 278(5341):1295–1300.

Fischer-Smith T, Croul S, Adeniyi A, et al. (2004). Macrophage/microglial accumulation and proliferating cell nuclear antigen expression in the central nervous system in human immunodeficiency virus encephalopathy. *Am J Pathol* 164(6):2089–2099.

Foley P, Kazazi F, Biti R, Sorrell TC, and Cunningham AL (1992). HIV infection of monocytes inhibits the T-lymphocyte proliferative response to recall antigens, via production of eicosanoids. *Immunology* 75:392–397.

Frenkel D, Maron R, Burt DS, and Weiner HL (2005). Nasal vaccination with a proteosome-based adjuvant and glatiramer acetate clears beta-amyloid in a mouse model of Alzheimer disease. *J Clin Invest* 115(9):2423–2433.

Fuchs D, Chiodi F, Albert J, et al. (1989). Neopterin concentrations in cerebrospinal fluid and serum of individuals infected with HIV-1. *AIDS* 3(5):285–288.

Gabuzda D, and Wang J (1999). Chemokine receptors and virus entry in the central nervous system. *J Neurovirol* 5(6):643–658.

Gallo RC, Sarin PS, Gelmann EP, et al. (1983). Isolation of human T-cell leukemia virus in acquired immune deficiency syndrome (AIDS). *Science* 220(4599):865–867.

Gao HM, Liu B, and Hong JS (2003). Critical role for microglial NADPH oxidase in rotenone-induced degeneration of dopaminergic neurons. *J Neurosci* 23(15):6181–6187.

Garden GA (2002). Microglia in human immunodeficiency virus–associated neurodegeneration. *Glia* 40(2):240–251.

Gartner S (2000). HIV infection and dementia. *Science* 287(5453):602–604.

Gartner S, and Liu Y (2002). Insights into the role of immune activation in HIV neuropathogenesis. *J Neurovirol* 8(2):69–75.

Gattegno L, Bentata-Peyssare M, Gronowski S, et al. (1995). Elevated concentrations of circulating intercellular adhesion molecule 1 (ICAM-1) and of vascular cell adhesion molecule 1 (VCAM-1) in HIV-1 infection. *Cell Adhes Commun* 3(3):179–185.

Gelbard H, Nottet HS, Swindells S, Jett M, Dzenko KA, Genis P, White R, Wang L, Choi YB, Zhang D, Lipton SA, Tourtellotte WW, Epstein LG, and Gendelman HE (1994). Platelet activating factor: a candidate human immunodeficiency virus type 1–induced neurotoxin. *J Virol* 68:4628–4635.

Gendelman HE, and Folks DG (1999). Innate and acquired immunity in neurodegenerative disorders. *J Leukoc Biol* 65(4):407–408.

Gendelman HE, and Persidsky Y (2005). Infections of the nervous system. *Lancet Neurol* 4(1):12–13.

Gendelman HE, Genis P, Jett M, Zhai QH, and Nottet HS (1994). An experimental model system for HIV-1-induced brain injury. *Adv Neuroimmunol* 4(3): 189–193.

Gendelman HE, Zheng J, Coulter CL, et al. (1998). Suppression of inflammatory neurotoxins by highly active antiretroviral therapy in human immunodeficiency virus–associated dementia. *J Infect Dis* 178(4):1000–1007.

Genis P, Jett M, Bernton EW, et al. (1992). Cytokines and arachidonic metabolites produced during human immunodeficiency virus (HIV)–infected macrophage–astroglia interactions: implications for the neuropathogenesis of HIV disease. *J Exp Med* 176(6):1703–1718.

Ghafouri M, Amini S, Khalili K, and Sawaya BE (2006). HIV-1 associated dementia: symptoms and causes. *Retrovirology* 3:28.

Ghorpade A, Nukuna A, Che M, et al. (1998). Human immunodeficiency virus neurotropism: an analysis of viral replication and cytopathicity for divergent strains in monocytes and microglia. *J Virol* 72(4): 3340–50.

Ghorpade A, Persidskaia R, Suryadevara R, et al. (2001). Mononuclear phagocyte differentiation, activation, and viral infection regulate matrix metalloproteinase expression: implications for human immunodeficiency virus type 1–associated dementia. *J Virol* 75(14):6572–6583.

Ghorpade A, Persidsky Y, Swindells S, et al. (2005). Neuroinflammatory responses from microglia recovered from HIV-1-infected and seronegative subjects. *J Neuroimmunol* 163(1-2):145–156.

Giulian D, Vaca K, and Noonan CA (1990). Secretion of neurotoxins by mononuclear phagocytes infected with HIV-1. *Science* 250:1593–1596.

Glass JD, Fedor H, Wesselingh SL, and McArthur JC (1995). Immunocytochemical quantitation of human immunodeficiency virus in the brain: correlations with dementia. *Ann Neurol* 38(5):755–762.

Glenn JA, Ward SA, Stone CR, Booth PL, and Thomas WE (1992). Characterisation of ramified microglial cells: detailed morphology, morphological plasticity and proliferative capability. *J Anat* 180(Pt. 1):109–118.

Gonzalez E, Rovin BH, Sen L, et al. (2002). HIV-1 infection and AIDS dementia are influenced by a mutant MCP-1 allele linked to increased monocyte infiltration of tissues and MCP-1 levels. *Proc Natl Acad Sci U S A* 99(21):13795–13800.

Gonzalez-Scarano F, and Martin-Garcia J (2005). The neuropathogenesis of AIDS. *Nat Rev Immunol* 5(1):69–81.

Gorantla S, Lui J, Sneller H, et al. (submitted for publication). Glatiramer acetate induces adaptive immune anti-inflammatory glial and neuroprotective responses in a murine model of HIV-1 encephalitis.

Gordon PH, Doorish C, Montes J, et al. (2006). Randomized controlled phase II trial of glatiramer acetate in ALS. *Neurology* 66(7):1117–1119.

Goulder PJ, and Watkins DI (2004). HIV and SIV CTL escape: implications for vaccine design. *Nat Rev Immunol* 4(8):630–640.

Gray F, and Keohane C (2003). The neuropathology of HIV infection in the era of highly active antiretroviral therapy (HAART). *Brain Pathol* 13(1):79–83.

Gray F, Gherardi R, Baudrimont M, et al. (1987). Leukoencephalopathy with multinucleated giant cells containing human immune deficiency virus–like particles and multiple opportunistic cerebral infections in one patient with AIDS. *Acta Neuropathol (Berl)* 73(1):99–104.

Gray F, Hurtrel M, and Hurtrel B (1993). Early central nervous system changes in human immunodeficiency virus (HIV)-infection. *Neuropathol Appl Neurobiol* 19(1):3–9.

Gray F, Scaravilli F, Everall I, et al. (1996). Neuropathology of early HIV-1 infection. *Brain Pathol* 6(1):1–15.

Gray L, Sterjovski J, Churchill M, et al. (2005). Uncoupling coreceptor usage of human immunodeficiency virus type 1 (HIV-1) from macrophage tropism reveals biological properties of CCR5-restricted HIV-1 isolates from patients with acquired immunodeficiency syndrome. *Virology* 337(2):384–398.

Green DA, Masliah E, Vinters HV, et al. (2005). Brain deposition of beta-amyloid is a common pathologic feature in HIV positive patients. *AIDS* 19(4):407–411.

Griffin WC 3rd, Middaugh LD, Cook JE, and Tyor WR (2004). The severe combined immunodeficient (SCID) mouse model of human immunodeficiency virus encephalitis: deficits in cognitive function. *J Neurovirol* 10(2):109–115.

Hall M, Whaley R, Robertson K, et al. (1996). The correlation between neuropsychological and neuroanatomic changes over time in asymptomatic and symptomatic HIV-1-infected individuals. *Neurology* 46(6):1697–1702.

Handa R, Wali JP, Kaushick P, et al. (1996). Toxoplasma encephalitis in AIDS. *J Assoc Physicians India* 44(11):838.

Harrold SM, Wang G, McMahon DK, et al. (2002). Recovery of replication-competent HIV type 1-infected circulating monocytes from individuals receiving antiretroviral therapy. *AIDS Res Hum Retroviruses* 18(6):427–434.

Hayes MM, Lane BR, King SR, et al. (2002). Peroxisome proliferator-activated receptor gamma agonists inhibit HIV-1 replication in macrophages by transcriptional and post-transcriptional effects. *J Biol Chem* 277(19):16913–16919.

Helke KL, Queen SE, Tarwater PM, et al. (2005). 14-3-3 protein in CSF: an early predictor of SIV CNS disease. *J Neuropathol Exp Neurol* 64(3):202–208.

Heyes MP, Brew BJ, Martin A, Markey SP, et al. (1991a). Quinolinic acid in cerebrospinal fluid and serum in HIV-1 infection: relationship to clinical and neurological status. *Ann Neurol* 29(2):202–209.

Heyes MP, Brew B, Martin A, Price RW, et al. (1991b). Cerebrospinal fluid quinolinic acid concentrations are increased in acquired immune deficiency syndrome. *Adv Exp Med Biol* 294:687–690.

Hickey WF, Williams KC, Corey S, and Kim WK (2005). Mononuclear phagocyte heterogeneity and the blood brain barrier: a model for HIV-1 neuropathogenesis. In HE Gendelman, I Grant, IP Everall, SA Lipton, and S Swindells (eds.), *The Neurology of AIDS* (pp. 71–83). New York: Oxford University Press.

Hirsch EC, Breidert T, Rousselt E, et al. (2003). The role of glial reaction and inflammation in Parkinson's disease. *Ann N Y Acad Sci* 991:214–228.

Ho WZ, Lai JP, Bouhamdan M, et al. (1998). Inhibition of HIV type 1 replication in chronically infected monocytes and lymphocytes by retrovirus-mediated gene transfer of anti-Rev single-chain variable fragments. *AIDS Res Hum Retroviruses* 14(17):1573–1580.

Holl V, Peressin M, Decoville T, et al. (2006). Nonneutralizing antibodies are able to inhibit human immunodeficiency virus type 1 replication in macrophages and immature dendritic cells. *J Virol* 80(12):6177–6181.

Holm GH, and Gabuzda D (2005). Distinct mechanisms of CD4+ and CD8+ T-cell activation and bystander apoptosis induced by human immunodeficiency virus type 1 virions. *J Virol* 79(10):6299–6311.

Huang ST, Lee HC, Liu KH, Lee NY, and Ko WC (2005). Acute human immunodeficiency virus infection. *J Microbiol Immunol Infect* 38(1):65–68.

Hughes-Fulford M, McGrath MS, Hanks D, Erickson S, and Pulliam L (1992). Effects of dimethyl prostaglandin A1 on herpes simplex virus and human immunodeficiency virus replication. *Antimicrob Agents Chemother* 36(10):2253–2258.

Ii M, Sunamoto M, Ohnishi K, and Ichimori Y (1996). Beta-amyloid protein-dependent nitric oxide production from microglial cells and neurotoxicity. *Brain Res* 720(1-2):93–100.

Jain KK (2000). Evaluation of memantine for neuroprotection in dementia. *Expert Opin Investig Drugs* 9(6):1397–1406.

Jana A, and Pahan K (2004). Human immunodeficiency virus type 1 gp120 induces apoptosis in human primary neurons through redox-regulated activation of neutral sphingomyelinase. *J Neurosci* 24(43): 9531–9540.

Jarvik JG, Lenkinski RE, Saykin AJ, et al. (1996). Proton spectroscopy in asymptomatic HIV-infected adults: initial results in a prospective cohort study. *J Acquir Immune Defic Syndr Hum Retrovirol* 13(3):247–253.

Jassoy C, Johnson RP, Navia BA, Worth J, and Walker BD (1992). Detection of a vigorous HIV-1-specific cytotoxic T lymphocyte response in cerebrospinal fluid from infected persons with AIDS dementia complex. *J Immunol* 149(9):3113–3119.

Jellinger KA (2001). The pathology of Parkinson's disease. *Adv Neurol* 86:55–72.

Jennes W, Vereecken C, Fransen K, de Roo A, and Kestens L (2004). Disturbed secretory capacity for macrophage inflammatory protein (MIP)-1 alpha and MIP-1 beta in progressive HIV infection. *AIDS Res Hum Retroviruses* 20(10):1087–1091.

Jeohn GH, Kong LY, Wilson B, Hudson P, and Hong JS (1998). Synergistic neurotoxic effects of combined treatments with cytokines in murine primary mixed neuron/glia cultures. *J Neuroimmunol* 85(1):1–10.

Jiang ZG, Piggee C, Heyes MP, et al. (2001). Glutamate is a mediator of neurotoxicity in secretions of activated HIV-1-infected macrophages. *J Neuroimmunol* 117(1-2):97–107.

Johnson V, Brun-Vezinat F, Clotet B, Conway B, Kuritzkes DR, Pillay D, Schapiro J, Telenti A, and Richman D (2005). Update of the drug resistance mutations in HIV-1: 2005. *Top HIV Med* 13(1):51–57.

Jowett JB, Planelles V, Poon B, Shah NP, Chen ML, and Chen IS (1995). The human immunodeficiency virus type 1 vpr gene arrests infected T cells in the G2 + M phase of the cell cycle. *J Virol* 69(10):6304–6313.

Kadiu I, Glanzer JG, Kipnis J, Gendelman HE, and Thomas MP (2005). Mononuclear phagocytes in the pathogenesis of neurodegenerative diseases. *Neurotox Res* 8(1-2):25–50.

Kanmogne GD, Grammas P, and Kennedy RC (2000). Analysis of human endothelial cells and cortical neurons for susceptibility to HIV-1 infection and co-receptor expression. *J Neurovirol* 6(6):519–528.

Kanmogne GD, Primeaux C, and Grammas P (2005). HIV-1 gp120 proteins alter tight junction protein expression and brain endothelial cell permeability: implications for the pathogenesis of HIV-associated dementia. *J Neuropathol Exp Neurol* 64(6):498–505.

Kanmogne GD, Schall K, Leibhart J, et al. (2007). HIV-1 gp120 compromises blood–brain barrier integrity and enhances monocyte migration across blood–brain barrier: implication for viral neuropathogenesis. *J Cereb Blood Flow Metab.* 27(1):123–124.

Kaplan MH, Sadick NS, and Talmor M (1991). Acquired trichomegaly of the eyelashes: a cutaneous marker of acquired immunodeficiency syndrome. *J Am Acad Dermatol* 25(5 Pt. 1):801–804.

Kaul M, and Lipton SA (2006). Mechanisms of neuronal injury and death in HIV-1 associated dementia. *Curr HIV Res* 4(3):307–318.

Kaul M, Garden GA, and Lipton SA (2001). Pathways to neuronal injury and apoptosis in HIV-associated dementia. *Nature* 410(6831):988–994.

Kaul M, Zheng J, Okamoto S, Gendelman HE, and Lipton SA (2005). HIV-1 infection and AIDS:

consequences for the central nervous system. *Cell Death Differ* 12(Suppl. 1):878–892.

Kaur C, and Ling EA (1991). Study of the transformation of amoeboid microglial cells into microglia labelled with the isolectin *Griffonia simplicifolia* in postnatal rats. *Acta Anat (Basel)* 142(2):118–125.

Kaur C, Ling EA, and Wong WC (1985). Transformation of amoeboid microglial cells into microglia in the corpus callosum of the postnatal rat brain. An electron microscopical study. *Arch Histol Jpn* 48(1): 17–25.

Kedzierska K, Azzam R, Ellery P, Mak J, Jaworowski A, and Crowe SM (2003). Defective phagocytosis by human monocyte/macrophages following HIV-1 infection: underlying mechanisms and modulation by adjunctive cytokine therapy. *J Clin Virol* 26:247–263.

Kelder W, McArthur JC, Nance-Sproson T, McClernon D, and Griffin DE (1998). B Chemokines MCP-1 and RANTES are selectively increased in cerebrospinal fluid of patients with human immunodeficiency virus–associated dementia. *Ann Neurol* 44: 831–835.

Kennedy DW, and Abkowitz JL (1997). Kinetics of central nervous system microglial and macrophage engraftment: analysis using a transgenic bone marrow transplantation model. *Blood* 90(3):986–993.

Kerr SJ, Armati PJ, Guillemin GJ, and Brew BJ (1998). Chronic exposure of human neurons to quinolinic acid results in neuronal changes consistent with AIDS dementia complex. *AIDS* 12(4):355–363.

Kinloch-de Loes S, de Saussure S, Sauret JH, et al. (1993). Symptomatic primary infection due to human immunodeficiency virus type 1: review of 31 cases. *Clin Infect Dis* 17:59–65.

Kipnis J, Yoles E, Porat Z, et al. (2000). T cell immunity to copolymer 1 confers neuroprotection on the damaged optic nerve: possible therapy for optic neuropathies. *Proc Natl Acad Sci U S A* 97(13):7446–7451.

Kitamura Y, Furukawa M, Matsuoka Y, et al. (1998a). In vitro and in vivo induction of heme oxygenase-1 in rat glial cells: possible involvement of nitric oxide production from inducible nitric oxide synthase. *Glia* 22(2):138–148.

Kitamura Y, Matsuoka Y, Nomura Y, and Taniguchi T (1998b). Induction of inducible nitric oxide synthase and heme oxygenase-1 in rat glial cells. *Life Sci* 62(17-18):1717–1721.

Knight WG, Mellins CA, Levenson RL Jr, Arpadi SM, and Kairam R (2000). Brief report: effects of pediatric HIV infection on mental and psychomotor development. *J Pediatr Psychol* 25(8):583–587.

Koenig S, Gendelman HE, Orenstein JM, et al. (1986). Detection of AIDS virus in macrophages in brain tissue from AIDS patients with encephalopathy. *Science* 233(4768):1089–1093.

Kohleisen B, Hutzler P, Shumay V, Ovod V, and Erfle V (2001). HIV-1 Nef co-localizes with the astrocyte-specific cytoskeleton protein GFAP in persis-tently nef-expressing human astrocytes. *J Neurovirol* 7(1):52–55.

Kornbluth R, Kee SK, and Richman DD (1998). CD40 ligand (CD154) stimulation of macrophages to produce HIV-1-suppressive beta-chemokines. *Proc Natl Acad Sci U S A* 95(9):5205–5210.

Koup RA (2004). Reconsidering early HIV treatment and supervised treatment interruptions. *PLoS Med* 1(2):e41.

Kovacs A, Hinton DR, Wright D, et al. (1996a). Human immunodeficiency virus type 1 infection of the heart in three infants with acquired immunodeficiency syndrome and sudden death. *Pediatr Infect Dis J* 15(9):819–824.

Kovacs JA, Vogel S, Albert JM, et al. (1996b). Controlled trial of interleukin-2 infusions in patients infected with the human immunodeficiency virus. *N Engl J Med* 335(18):1350–1356.

Krown SE, Paredes J, Bundow A, et al. (1992a). Interferon-alpha, zidovudine, and granulocyte-macrophage colony-stimulating factor: a phase I AIDS Clinical Trials Group study in patients with Kaposi's sarcoma associated with AIDS. *J Clin Oncol* 10(8):1344–13451.

Krown SE, Paredes J, Gold JW, et al. (1992b). Clinical potential of GM-CSF in HIV-infected patients: Studies at the Memorial Sloan Kettering Cancer Center. *Pathol Biol (Paris)* 39(9):963.

Krupp LB, Lipton RB, Swerdlow ML, Leeds NE, and Llena J (1985). Progressive multifocal leukoencephalopathy: clinical and radiographic features. *Ann Neurol* 17(4):344–349.

Kumar A, Dhawan S, Mukhopadhyay A, and Aggarwal BB (1999). Human immunodeficiency virus-1-tat induces matrix metalloproteinase-9 in monocytes through protein tyrosine phosphatase-mediated activation of nuclear transcription factor NF-kappaB. *FEBS Lett* 462(1-2):140–144.

Kure K, Lyman WD, Weidenheim KM, and Dickson DW (1990). Cellular localization of an HIV-1 antigen in subacute AIDS encephalitis using an improved double-labeling immunohistochemical method. *Am J Pathol* 136(5):1085–1092.

Kure K, Llena JF, Lyman WD, et al. (1991). Human immunodeficiency virus-1 infection of the nervous system: an autopsy study of 268 adult, pediatric, and fetal brains. *Hum Pathol* 22(7):700–710.

Kutsch O, Oh J, Nath A, and Benveniste EN (2000). Induction of the chemokines interleukin-8 and IP-10 by human immunodeficiency virus type 1 tat in astrocytes. *J Virol* 74(19):9214–9221.

Langford TD, Everall IP, and Masliah E (2005). Current concepts in HIV-neuropathogenesis, neuronal injury, white matter disease, and neurotrophic factors. In HE Gendelman, I Grant, IP Everall, SA Lipton, and S Swindells (eds.), *The Neurology of AIDS* (pp. 405–414). New York: Oxford University Press.

Lannuzel A, Lledo PM, Lamghitnia HO, et al. (1995). HIV-1 envelope proteins gp120 and gp160 potentiate NMDA-induced [Ca2+]i increase, alter [Ca2+]i homeostasis and induce neurotoxicity in human embryonic neurons. *Eur J Neurosci* 7(11): 2285–2293.

Lau AS, Der SD, Read SE, and Williams BR (1991). Regulation of tumor necrosis factor receptor expression by acid-labile interferon-alpha from AIDS sera. *AIDS Res Hum Retroviruses* 7(6):545–552.

Lawrence DM, and Major EO (2002). HIV-1 and the brain: connections between HIV-1-associated dementia, neuropathology and neuroimmunology. *Microbes Infect* 4(3):301–308.

Lee SC, and Dickson D (2005). Common immune pathways of neural injury in neurodegenerative disorders. In HE Gendelman, I Grant, IP Everall, SA Lipton, and S Swindells (eds.), *The Neurology of AIDS* (pp. 85–93). New York: Oxford University Press.

Letvin NL, and Walker BD (2003). Immunopathogenesis and immunotherapy in AIDS virus infections. *Nat Med* 9:861–866.

Lewin R. (1986). AIDS virus entry pinpointed in brain. *Science* 233(4760):160.

Lewis DE, Tang DS, Adu-Oppong A, et al. (1994). Anergy and apoptosis in CD8+ T cells from HIV-infected persons. *J Immunol* 153(1):412–420.

Liegler TJ, and Stites DP (1994). HIV-1 gp120 and anti-gp120 induce reversible unresponsiveness in peripheral CD4 T lymphocytes. *J Acquir Immune Defic Syndr* 7(4):340–348.

Lifson J, Coutre S, Huang E, and Engelman E (1986a). Role of envelope glycoprotein carbohydrate in human immunodeficiency virus (HIV) infectivity and virus-induced cell fusion. *J Exp Med* 164(6):2101–2106.

Lifson JD, Feinberg MB, Reyes GR, et al. (1986b). Induction of CD4-dependent cell fusion by the HTLV-III/LAV envelope glycoprotein. *Nature* 323(6090):725–728.

Lifson JD, Reyes GR, McGrath MS, Stein BS, and Engelman EG (1986c). AIDS retrovirus induced cytopathology: giant cell formation and involvement of CD4 antigen. *Science* 232(4754):1123–1127.

Lima RG, Van Weyenbergh J, Saraiva EM, et al. (2002). The replication of human immunodeficiency virus type 1 in macrophages is enhanced after phagocytosis of apoptotic cells. *J Infect Dis* 185(11):1561–1566.

Lima RG, Moreira L, Paes-Leme J, et al. (2006). Interaction of macrophages with apoptotic cells enhances HIV type-1 replication through PGE(2), PAF, and vitronectin receptor. *AIDS Res Hum Retroviruses* 22(8):763–769.

Lindback S, Thorsstenson R, Karlsson AC, et al. (2000). Diagnosis of primary HIV-1 infection and duration of follow-up after HIV exposure. *AIDS* 14:2333–2339.

Ling EA (1982a). A light microscopic demonstration of amoeboid microglia and microglial cells in the retina of rats of various ages. *Arch Histol Jpn* 45(1): 37–44.

Ling EA (1982b). Influence of cortisone on amoeboid microglia and microglial cells in the corpus callosum in postnatal rats. *J Anat* 134(Pt. 4):705–717.

Ling EA, and Wong WC (1993) The origin and nature of ramified and amoeboid microglia: a historical review and current concepts. *Glia* 7(1):9–18.

Lipton SA (1992). Requirement for macrophages in neuronal injury induced by HIV envelope protein gp120. *Neuroreport* 3(10):913–915.

Lipton SA (1993). Human immunodeficiency virus–infected macrophages, gp120, and N-methyl-D-aspartate receptor-mediated neurotoxicity. *Ann Neurol* 33(2):227–228.

Lipton SA (1994). Laboratory basis of novel therapeutic strategies to prevent HIV-related neuronal injury. *Res Publ Assoc Res Nerv Ment Dis* 72:183–202.

Lipton SA (1998). Neuronal injury associated with HIV-1: approaches to treatment. *Annu Rev Pharmacol Toxicol* 38:159–177.

Lipton SA, Yeh M, and Dreyer EB (1994). Update on current models of HIV-related neuronal injury: platelet-activating factor, arachidonic acid and nitric oxide. *Adv Neuroimmunol* 4(3):181–188.

Liu B, and Hong JS (2003). Role of microglia in inflammation-mediated neurodegenerative diseases: mechanisms and strategies for therapeutic intervention. *J Pharmacol Exp Ther* 304(1):1–7.

Liu X, Jana M, Dasgupta S, et al. (2002). Human immunodeficiency virus type 1 (HIV-1) tat induces nitric-oxide synthase in human astroglia. *J Biol Chem* 277(42):39312–39319.

Liu Y, Qin L, Li G, et al. (2003). Dextromethorphan protects dopaminergic neurons against inflammation-mediated degeneration through inhibition of microglial activation. *J Pharmacol Exp Ther* 305(1): 212–218.

Liuzzi G, Mastroianni CM, Latronico T, Mengoni F, and Fasano A (1994). Anti-HIV drugs decrease the expression of matrix metalloproteinases in astrocytes and microglia. *Brain Pathol* 127(2):398–407.

Llorente AM, van Gorp WG, Stern MJ, et al. (2001). Long-term effects of high-dose zidovudine treatment on neuropsychological performance in mildly symptomatic HIV-positive patients: results of a randomized, double-blind, placebo-controlled investigation. *J Int Neuropsychol Soc* 7(1):27–32.

Loeffler DA, DeMaggio AJ, Juneau PL, Havaich MK, and LeWitt PA (1994). Effects of enhanced striatal dopamine turnover in vivo on glutathione oxidation. *Clin Neuropharmacol* 17(4):370–379.

Lyerly HK, Matthews TJ, Langlois AJ, et al. (1987). Human T-cell lymphotropic virus IIIB glycoprotein (gp120) bound to CD4 determinants on normal lymphocytes and expressed by infected cells serves as target for immune attack. *Proc Natl Acad Sci U S A* 84(13):4601–4605.

Major EO, Rausch D, Marra C, and Clifford D (2000). HIV-associated dementia. *Science* 288(5465):440–442.

Manzardo C, Del Mar Ortega M, Sued O, et al. (2005). Central nervous system opportunistic infections in developed countries in the highly active antiretroviral therapy era. *J Neurovirol* 11(Suppl.3):72–82.

Marcondes MC, Burudi EM, Huitron-Resendiz S, et al. (2001). Highly activated CD8(+) T cells in the brain correlate with early central nervous system dysfunction in simian immunodeficiency virus infection. *J Immunol* 167(9):5429–5438.

Marshall DC, Wyss-Coray T, and Abraham CR (1998). Induction of matrix metalloproteinase-2 in human immunodeficiency virus-1 glycoprotein 120 transgenic mouse brains. *Neurosci Lett* 254(2):97–100.

Martin A, Heyes MP, Salazar AM, et al. (1992). Progressive slowing of reaction time and increasing cerebrospinal fluid concentrations of quinolinic acid in HIV-infected individuals. *J Neuropsychiatry Clin Neurosci* 4(3):270–279.

Martin-Garcia J, and Gonzalez-Scarano F (2005). Viral receptors and the mechanisms of HIV-1 entry into cells and the central nervous system. In HE Gendelman, I Grant, IP Everall, SA Lipton, and S Swindells (eds.), *The Neurology of AIDS* (pp. 125–146). New York: Oxford University Press.

Masliah E, Heaton RK, Marcotte TD, et al. (1997). Dendritic injury is a pathological substrate for human immunodeficiency virus–related cognitive disorders. HNRC Group. The HIV Neurobehavioral Research Center. *Ann Neurol* 42(6):963–972.

Maslin CL, Kedzierska K, Webster NL, et al. (2005). Transendothelial migration of monocytes: the underlying molecular mechanisms and consequences of HIV-1 infection. *Curr HIV Res* 3(4):303–317.

Matthews TJ, Weinhold KJ, Lyerly HK, et al. (1987). Interaction between the human T-cell lymphotropic virus type IIIB envelope glycoprotein gp120 and the surface antigen CD4: role of carbohydrate in binding and cell fusion. *Proc Natl Acad Sci U S A* 84(15):5424–5428.

McArthur JC (2004). HIV dementia: an evolving disease. *J Neuroimmunol* 157(1-2):3–10.

McArthur JC, Nance-Sproson TE, Griffin DE, et al. (1992). The diagnostic utility of elevation in cerebrospinal fluid beta 2-microglobulin in HIV-1 dementia. Multicenter AIDS Cohort Study. *Neurology* 42(9):1707–1712.

McArthur J, Hoover DR, Bacellar H, Miller EN, Cohen BA, and Becker JT (1993). Dementia in AIDS patients: incidence and risk factors. *Neurology* 43:2245–2252.

McArthur JC, McClernon DR, Cronin MF, et al. (1997). Relationship between human immunodeficiency virus–associated dementia and viral load in cerebrospinal fluid and brain. *Ann Neurol* 42(5):689–698.

McArthur JC, Brew BR, and Nath A. (2005). Neurological complications of HIV infection. *Lancet Neurol* 4(9):543–555.

McCoig C, Castrejon MM, Saavedra-Lozano A, et al. (2004). Cerebrospinal fluid and plasma concentrations of proinflammatory mediators in human immunodeficiency virus–infected children. *Pediatr Infect Dis J* 23(2):114–118.

McConnell JR, Swindells S, Ong CS, et al. (1994). Prospective utility of cerebral proton magnetic resonance spectroscopy in monitoring HIV infection and its associated neurological impairment. *AIDS Res Hum Retroviruses* 10(8):977–982.

McGeer PL, and McGeer EG (2004). Inflammation and neurodegeneration in Parkinson's disease. *Parkinsonism Relat Disord* 10(Suppl. 1):S3–S7.

McGeer PL, Itagaki S, Tago H, and McGeer EG (1987). Reactive microglia in patients with senile dementia of the Alzheimer type are positive for the histocompatibility glycoprotein HLA-DR. *Neurosci Lett* 79(1-2):195–200.

McGeer PL, Itagaki S, Boyes BE, and McGeer EG (1988). Reactive microglia are positive for HLA-DR in the substantia nigra of Parkinson's and Alzheimer's disease brains. *Neurology* 38(8):1285–1291.

McMurtray A, Clark DG, Christine D, and Mendez MF (2006). Early-onset dementia: frequency and causes compared to late-onset dementia. *Dement Geriatr Cogn Disord* 21(2):59–64.

Meda L, Cassatella MA, Szendrei GI, et al. (1995). Activation of microglial cells by beta-amyloid protein and interferon-gamma. *Nature* 374(6523):647–650.

Mehandru S, Poles MA, Tenner-Racz K, et al. (2004). Primary HIV-1 infection is associated with preferential depletion of CD4+ T lymphocytes from effector sites in the gastrointestinal tract. *J Exp Med* 200(6):761–770.

Mellors JW, Munoz A, Giorgi JV, et al. (1997). Plasma viral load and CD4+ lymphocytes as prognostic markers of HIV-1 infection. *Ann Intern Med* 126(12):946–954.

Michaels J, Sharer LR, and Epstein LG (1988). Human immunodeficiency virus type 1 (HIV-1) infection of the nervous system: a review. *Immunodefic Rev* 1(1):71–104.

Minagar A, Shapshak P, Fujimura R, Ownby R, Heyes M, and Eisdorfer C (2002). The role of macrophage/micrglia and astrocytes in the pathogenesis of three neurological disorders: HIV-associated dementia, Alzheimer's disease and multiple sclerosis. *J Neurol Sci* 202:13–23.

Minghetti L (2005). Role of inflammation in neurodegenerative diseases. *Curr Opin Neurol* 18(3):315–321.

Miyakawa T, Obaru K, Maeda K, Harada S, and Mitsuya H (2002). Identification of amino acid residues critical for LD78beta, a variant of human macrophage inflammatory protein-1alpha, binding to CCR5 and inhibition of R5 human immunodeficiency virus type 1 replication. *J Biol Chem* 277(7):4649–4655.

Mollace V, Colasanti M, Persichini T, et al. (1993). HIV gp120 glycoprotein stimulates the inducible isoform of no synthase in human cultured astrocytoma cells. *Biochem Biophys Res Commun* 194(1):439–445.

Montefiori DC, Altfeld M, Lee PK, et al. (2003). Viremia control despite escape from a rapid and potent autologous neutralizing antibody response after therapy cessation in an HIV-1-infected individual. *J Immunol* 170(7):3906–3914.

Moorjani H, Craddock BP, Morrison SA, and Steigbigel RT (1996). Impairment of phagosome–lysosome fusion in HIV-1-infected macrophages. *J Acquir Immune Defic Syndr Hum Retrovirol* 13(1):18–22.

Morikita T, Maeda Y, Fujii S, et al. (1997). The V1/V2 region of human immunodeficiency virus type 1 modulates the sensitivity to neutralization by soluble CD4 and cellular tropism. *AIDS Res Hum Retroviruses* 13(15):1291–1299.

Mukherjee JS, Farmer PE, Niyizonkiza D, et al. (2003). Tackling HIV in resource-poor countries. *BMJ* 327(7423):1104–1106.

Musey L, Hughes J, Schacker T, et al. (1997). Cytotoxic-T-cell responses, viral load, and disease progression in early human immunodeficiency virus type 1 infection. *N Engl J Med* 337(18):1267–1274.

Nasi M, Pinti M, Bugarini R, et al. (2005). Genetic polymorphisms of Fas (CD95) and Fas ligand (CD178) influence the rise in CD4+ T cell count after antiretroviral therapy in drug-naive HIV-positive patients. *Immunogenetics* 57(9):628–635.

Nath A (2002). Human immunodeficiency virus (HIV) proteins in neuropathogenesis of HIV dementia. *J Infect Dis* 186(Suppl. 2):S193–S198.

Navenot JM, Wang ZX, Trent JO, et al. (2001). Molecular anatomy of CCR5 engagement by physiologic and viral chemokines and HIV-1 envelope glycoproteins: differences in primary structural requirements for RANTES, MIP-1 alpha, and vMIP-II binding. *J Mol Biol* 313(5):1181–1193.

Navia B, Cho ES, Petito CK, and Price RW (1986a). The AIDS dementia complex: II Neuropathology. *Ann Neurol* 19:525–535.

Navia BA, Jordan BD, et al. (1986b). The AIDS dementia complex: I. Clinical features. *Ann Neurol* 19(6):517–524.

Navia BA, and Price RW (1998). Clinical and biological features of the AIDS dementia complex. In HE Gendelman, SA Lipton, and L Epstein (eds.), *The Neurology of AIDS* (pp. 229–240). New York: Chapman Hall.

Nelson JA, Dou H, Ellison B, et al. (2005). Coregistration of quantitative proton magnetic resonance spectroscopic imaging with neuropathological and neurophysiological analyses defines the extent of neuronal impairments in murine human immuno-

deficiency virus type-1 encephalitis. *J Neurosci Res* 80(4):562–575.

New D, Ma M, Epstein LG, Nath A, and Gelbard HA (1997). Human immunodeficiency virus type-1 tat protein induces death by apoptosis in primary human neuron cultures. *J Neurovirol* 3:168–173.

Newman SL, Bhugra B, Holly A, and Morris RE (2005). Enhanced killing of *Candida albicans* by human macrophages adherent to type 1 collagen matrices via induction of phagolysosomal fusion. *Infect Immun* 73(2):770–777.

Nielsen SL, Petito CK, Urmacher CD, and Posner JB (1984). Subacute encephalitis in acquired immune deficiency syndrome: a postmortem study. *Am J Clin Pathol* 82(6):678–682.

Nokta M, Hassan M, Loesch KA, and Pollard RB (1995). HIV-induced TNF alpha regulates arachidonic acid and PGE2 release form HIV-infected mononuclear phagocytes. *Virology* 208:590–600.

Nottet HS (2005). The blood–brain barrier: monocyte viral entry into the brain. In HE Gendelman, I Grant, IP Everall, SA Lipton, and S Swindells (eds.), *The Neurology of AIDS* (pp. 155–161). New York: Oxford University Press.

Nottet HS, and Gendelman HE (1995). Unraveling the neuroimmune mechanisms for the HIV-1-associated cognitive/motor complex. *Immunol Today* 16(9):441–448.

Nottet HS, Jett M, Flanagan CR, et al. (1995). A regulatory role for astrocytes in HIV-1 encephalitis. An overexpression of eicosanoids, platelet-activating factor, and tumor necrosis factor-alpha by activated HIV-1-infected monocytes is attenuated by primary human astrocytes. *J Immunol* 154(7):3567–3581.

Nottet HS, Persidsky Y, Sasseville VG, et al. (1996). Mechanisms for the transendothelial migration of HIV-1-infected monocytes into brain. *J Immunol* 156(3):1284–1295.

Oberlin E, Amara A, Bachelerie F, et al. (1996). The CXC chemokine SDF-1 is the ligand for LESTR/fusin and prevents infection by T-cell-line-adapted HIV-1. *Nature* 382(6594):833–835.

Ogden F, DeCoster MA, and Bazan NG (1998). Recombinant plasma type platelet activating factor acetylhydrolase attenuates NMDA-induced hippocampal neuronal apoptosis. *J Neurosci Res* 53:677–684.

Ogunro PS, Ogungbamigbe TO, Elemie TO, et al. (2006). Plasma selenium concentration and glutathione peroxidase activity in HIV-1/AIDS infected patients: a correlation with the disease progression. *Niger Postgrad Med J* 13(1):1–5.

Olivetta E, Percario Z, Fiorucci G, et al. (2003). HIV-1 Nef induces the release of inflammatory factors from human monocyte/macrophages: involvement of Nef endocytotic signals and NF-kappa B activation. *J Immunol* 170(4):1716–1727.

Oxenius A, Price DA, Trkola A, et al. (2004). Loss of viral control in early HIV-1 infection is temporally associated with sequential escape from CD8+ T cell responses and decrease in HIV-1-specific CD4+ and CD8+ T cell frequencies. *J Infect Dis* 190(4):713–721.

Patton HK, Zhou ZH, Bubien JK, Benveniste EN, and Benos DJ (2000). gp120-induced alterations of human astrocyte function: Na(+)/H(+) exchange, K(+) conductance, and glutamate flux. *Am J Physiol Cell Physiol* 279(3):C700–C708.

Payeras A, Martinez P, Mila J, et al. (2002). Risk factors in HIV-1-infected patients developing repetitive bacterial infections: toxicological, clinical, specific antibody class responses, opsonophagocytosis and Fc(gamma) RIIa polymorphism characteristics. *Clin Exp Immunol* 130(2):271–278.

Perry S, Hamilton JA, Tjoelker LW, et al. (1998). Platelet activating factor receptor activation. An initiator step in HIV-1 neuropathogensis. *J Biol Chem* 273:17660–17664.

Perry SW, Dewhurst S, Bellizzi MJ, and Gelbard HA (2002). Tumor necrosis factor-alpha in normal and diseased brain: conflicting effects via intraneuronal receptor crosstalk? *J Neurovirol* 8(6):611–624.

Persidsky Y, and Gendelman HE (2003). Mononuclear phagocyte immunity and the neuropathogenesis of HIV-1 infection. *J Leukoc Biol* 74(5):691–701.

Persidsky Y, Zheng J, Miller D, and Gendelman HE (2000). Mononuclear phagocytes mediate blood–brain barrier compromise and neuronal injury during HIV-1-associated dementia. *J Leukoc Biol* 68(3):413–422.

Persidsky Y, Limoges J, Ramssen J, Zheng J, Gearing A, and Gendelman HE (2001). Reduction in glial immunity and neuropathology by a PAF antagonist and an MMP and TNFalpha inhibitor in SCID mice with HIV-1 encephalitis. *J Neuroimmunol* 114:57–68.

Petito CK, Cho ES, Lemann W, Navia BA, and Price RW (1986). Neuropathology of acquired immunodeficiency syndrome (AIDS): an autopsy review. *J Neuropathol Exp Neurol* 45(6):635–646.

Pett SL, and Emery S (2001). Immunomodulators as adjunctive therapy for HIV-1 infection. *J Clin Virol* 22(3):289–295.

Peut V, and Kent SJ (2006). Fitness constraints on immune escape from HIV: implications of envelope as a target for both HIV-specific T cells and antibody. *Curr HIV Res* 4(2):191–197.

Pham VT, Wen L, McCluskey P, et al. (2005). Human retinal microglia express candidate receptors for HIV-1 infection. *Br J Ophthalmol* 89(6):753–757.

Pilcher C, Eron JJ Jr, Galvin S, Gay C, and Cohen MS (2004). Acute HIV revisited: new opportunities for treatment and prevention. *J Clin Invest* 113(7):937–945.

Pittis MG, Sternik G, Sen L, et al. (1993). Impaired phagolysosomal fusion of peripheral blood monocytes from HIV-infected subjects. *Scand J Immunol* 38(5):423–427.

Pittis MG, Prada F, Sternik G, and Sen L (1996). Recombinant human immunodeficiency virus type 1 (HIV-1) Tat protein inhibits phagolysosomal fusion in human peripheral blood monocytes. *Viral Immunol* 9(3):169–174.

Pocernich CB, Boyd-Kimball D, Poon HF, et al. (2005). Proteomics analysis of human astrocytes expressing the HIV protein Tat. *Brain Res Mol Brain Res* 133(2):307–316.

Poluektova L, Gorantla S, Faraci J, et al. (2004). Neuroregulatory events follow adaptive immune-mediated elimination of HIV-1-infected macrophages: studies in a murine model of viral encephalitis. *J Immunol* 172(12):7610–7617.

Poluektova L, Meyer V, Walters L, Paez X, and Gendelman HE (2005). Macrophage-induced inflammation affects hippocampal plasticity and neuronal development in a murine model of HIV-1 encephalitis. *Glia* 52(4):344–353.

Pomara N, Crandall DT, Choi SJ, Johnson G, and Lim KO (2001). White matter abnormalities in HIV-1 infection: a diffusion tensor imaging study. *Psychiatry Res* 106(1):15–24.

Pomerantz RJ (2004). Effects of HIV-1 Vpr on neuroinvasion and neuropathogenesis. *DNA Cell Biol* 23(4):227–238.

Pontow SE, Heyden NV, Wei S, and Ratner L (2004). Actin cytoskeletal reorganizations and coreceptor-mediated activation of rac during human immunodeficiency virus–induced cell fusion. *J Virol* 78(13): 7138–7147.

Porcheray F, Samah B, Leone C, Dereuddre-Bosquet N, and Gras G (2006). Macrophage activation and human immunodeficiency virus infection: HIV replication directs macrophages towards a pro-inflammatory phenotype while previous activation modulates macrophage susceptibility to infection and viral production. *Virology* 349(1):112–120.

Post MJ, Tate LG, Quencer RM, et al. (1988). CT, MR, and pathology in HIV encephalitis and meningitis. *AJR Am J Roentgenol* 151(2):373–380.

Post MJ, Berger JR, Duncan R, et al. (1993). Asymptomatic and neurologically symptomatic HIV-seropositive subjects: results of long-term MR imaging and clinical follow-up. *Radiology* 188(3):727–733.

Potula R, Poluektova L, Knipe B, et al. (2005). Inhibition of indoleamine 2,3-dioxygenase (IDO) enhances elimination of virus-infected macrophages in an animal model of HIV-1 encephalitis. *Blood* 106(7): 2382–2390.

Power C, Selnes OA, Grim JA, and McCarthur JC (1995). HIV Dementia Scale: a rapid screening test. *J Acquir Immune Defic Syndr Hum Retrovirol* 8(3):273–278.

Price DB, Inglese CM, Jacobs J, et al. (1988). Pediatric AIDS. Neuroradiologic and neurodevelopmental findings. *Pediatr Radiol* 18(6):445–448.

Price DL, Wong PC, Borchelt DR, et al. (1997). Amyotrophic lateral sclerosis and Alzheimer disease. Lessons from model systems. *Rev Neurol (Paris)* 153(8-9):484–495.

Price RW, and Brew B (1988). Infection of the central nervous system by human immunodeficiency virus. Role of the immune system in pathogenesis. *Ann N Y Acad Sci* 540:162–175.

Price RW, Sidtis JJ, and Brew BJ (1991). AIDS dementia complex and HIV-1 infection: a view from the clinic. *Brain Pathol* 1(3):155–162.

Price TO, Ercal N, Nakaoke R, and Banks WA (2005). HIV-1 viral proteins gp120 and Tat induce oxidative stress in brain endothelial cells. *Brain Res* 1045(1-2):57–63.

Price TO, Uras F, Banks WA, and Ercal N (2006). A novel antioxidant N-acetylcysteine amide prevents gp120- and Tat-induced oxidative stress in brain endothelial cells. *Exp Neurol* 201(1):193–202.

Pulliam L, Herndier BG, Tang NM, and McGrath MS (1991). Human immunodeficiency virus–infected macrophages produce soluble factors that cause histological and neurochemical alterations in cultured human brains. *J Clin Invest* 87(2):503–512.

Pulliam L, Gascon R, Stubblebine M, McGuire D, and McGrath MS (1997). Unique monocyte subset in patients with AIDS dementia. *Lancet* 349(9053):692–695.

Qin L, Liu Y, Cooper C, et al. (2002). Microglia enhance beta-amyloid peptide-induced toxicity in cortical and mesencephalic neurons by producing reactive oxygen species. *J Neurochem* 83(4):973–983.

Rahmouni, S, Aandahl EM, Nayjib B, Zeddou M, Giannini S, Verlaet M, Greimers R, Boniver J, Tasken K, and Moutschen M (2004). Cyclo-oxygenase type 2-dependent prostaglandin E2 secretion is involved in retrovirus-induced T-cell dysfunction in mice. *Biochem J* 384:469–476.

Ranki A, Nyberg M, Ovid V, et al. (1995). Abundant expression of HIV Nef and Rev proteins in brain astrocytes in vivo is associated with dementia. *AIDS* 9(9):1001–1008.

Rappaport J, Joseph J, Croul S, et al. (1999). Molecular pathway involved in HIV-1-induced CNS pathology: role of viral regulatory protein, Tat. *J Leukoc Biol* 65(4):458–465.

Ribeiro RM, Hazenberg MD, Perelson AS, and Davenport MP (2006). Naive and memory cell turnover as drivers of CCR5-to-CXCR4 tropism switch in human immunodeficiency virus type 1: implications for therapy. *J Virol* 80(2):802–809.

Roberts ES, Zandonatti MA, Watry DD, et al. (2003). Induction of pathogenic sets of genes in macrophages and neurons in NeuroAIDS. *Am J Pathol* 162(6):2041–2057.

Roberts ES, Burudi EM, Flynn C, Madden LJ, Roinick KL, Watry DD, Zandonatti MA, Taffe MA, and Fox HS (2004). Acute SIV infection of the brain leads to upregulation of IL6 and interferon-regulated genes: expression patterns throughout disease

progression and impact on neuroAIDS. *J Neuroimmunol* 157:81–92.

Robertson K, Fiscus S, Kapoor C, et al. (1998). CSF, plasma viral load and HIV associated dementia. *J Neurovirol* 4(1):90–94.

Rozera C, Carattoli A, de Marco A, et al. (1996). Inhibition of HIV-1 replication by cyclopentenone prostaglandins in acutely infected human cells. Evidence for a transcriptional block. *J Clin Invest* 97(8):1795–1803.

Sacktor N, and McArthur J (1997). Prospects for therapy of HIV-associated neurologic diseases. *J Neurovirol* 3(2):89–101.

Sacktor N, Tarwater PM, Skolasky RL, et al. (2001). CSF antiretroviral drug penetrance and the treatment of HIV-associated psychomotor slowing. *Neurology* 57(3):542–544.

Sacktor N, Haughey N, Cutler R, et al. (2004). Novel markers of oxidative stress in actively progressive HIV dementia. *J Neuroimmunol* 157(1-2):176–184.

Saha RN, and Pahan K (2006). Regulation of inducible nitric oxide synthase gene in glial cells. *Antioxid Redox Signal* 8(5-6):929–947.

Sato H, Orenstein J, Dimitrov D, and Martin M (1992). Cell-to-cell spread of HIV-1 occurs within minutes and may not involve the participation of virus particles. *Virology* 186(2):712–724.

Schacker T, Collier AC, Hughes J, Shea T, and Corey L (1996). Cllinical and epidemiologic features of primary HIV infection. *Ann Intern Med* 125:257–264.

Schifitto G, Sacktor N, Marder K, et al. (1999). Randomized trial of the platelet-activating factor antagonist lexipafant in HIV-associated cognitive impairment. Neurological AIDS Research Consortium. *Neurology* 53(2):391–396.

Schifitto G, Kieburtz K, McDermott MP, et al. (2001). Clinical trials in HIV-associated cognitive impairment: cognitive and functional outcomes. *Neurology* 56(3):415–418.

Schifitto G, McDermott MP, McArthur JC, et al. (2005). Markers of immune activation and viral load in HIV-associated sensory neuropathy. *Neurology* 64(5):842–848.

Schmid P, Conrad A, Syndulko K, et al. (1994). Quantifying HIV-1 proviral DNA using the polymerase chain reaction on cerebrospinal fluid and blood of seropositive individuals with and without neurologic abnormalities. *J Acquir Immune Defic Syndr* 7(8):777–788.

Schmidtmayerova H, Nottet HS, Nuovo G, et al. (1996). Human immunodeficiency virus type 1 infection alters chemokine beta peptide expression in human monocytes: implications for recruitment of leukocytes into brain and lymph nodes. *Proc Natl Acad Sci U S A* 93(2):700–704.

Schmitt FA, Bigley JW, McKinnis R, et al. (1988). Neuropsychological outcome of zidovudine (AZT) treatment of patients with AIDS and AIDS-related complex. *N Engl J Med* 319(24):1573–1578.

Schmitz JE, Kuroda MJ, Santra S, et al. (1999). Control of viremia in simian immunodeficiency virus infection by CD8+ lymphocytes. *Science* 283(5403):857–860.

Schrier RD, McCutchan JA, and Wiley CA (1993). Mechanisms of immune activation of human immunodeficiency virus in monocytes/macrophages. *J Virol* 67(10):5713–5720.

Sharer L, Cho E, and Epstein LG (1985). Multinucleated giant cells and HTLV-III in AIDS encephalopathy. *Hum Pathol* 16:170–176.

Sharer LR, Baskin GB, Cho ES, et al. (1988). Comparison of simian immunodeficiency virus and human immunodeficiency virus encephalitides in the immature host. *Ann Neurol* 23(Suppl.):S108–S112.

Shi B, Raina J, Lorenzo A, Busciglio J, and Gabuzda D (1998). Neuronal apoptosis induced by HIV-1 Tat protein and TNF-alpha: potentiation of neurotoxicity mediated by oxidative stress and implications for HIV-1 dementia. *J Neurovirol* 4(3):281–290.

Shioda T, Levy JA, and Cheng-Mayer C (1992). Small amino acid changes in the V3 hypervariable region of gp120 can affect the T-cell-line and macrophage tropism of human immunodeficiency virus type 1. *Proc Natl Acad Sci U S A* 89(20):9434–9438.

Sidtis JJ, Gatsonis C, Price RW, et al. (1993). Zidovudine treatment of the AIDS dementia complex: results of a placebo-controlled trial. AIDS Clinical Trials Group. *Ann Neurol* 33(4):343–349.

Siliciano J, Kajdas J, Finzi D, Quinn TC, Chadwick K, Margolick JB, Kovacs C, Gange SJ, and Siliciano RF (2003). Long-term follow-up studies confirm the extraordinary stability of the latent reservoir for HIV-1 in resting CD4+ T cells. *Nat Med* 9:727–728.

Skolnik PR, Rabbi MF, Mathys JM, and Greenberg AS (2002). Stimulation of peroxisome proliferator-activated receptors alpha and gamma blocks HIV-1 replication and TNFalpha production in acutely infected primary blood cells, chronically infected U1 cells, and alveolar macrophages from HIV-infected subjects. *J Acquir Immune Defic Syndr* 31(1):1–10.

Smith D, Guillemin GJ, Pemberton L, Kerr S, Nath A, Smythe GA, and Brew BJ (2001). Quinolinic acid is produced by macrophages stimulated by platelet activating factor, Nef, and Tat. *J Neurovirol* 7(1): 56–60.

Snider WD, Simpson DM, Nielsen S, et al. (1983). Neurological complications of acquired immune deficiency syndrome: analysis of 50 patients. *Ann Neurol* 14(4):403–418.

Sodroski J, Goh WC, Rosen C, Campbell K, and Haseltine WA (1986). Role of the HTLV-III/LAV envelope in syncytium formation and cytopathicity. *Nature* 322(6078):470–474.

Song L, Nath A, Geiger JD, Moore A, and Hochman S (2003). Human immunodeficiency virus type 1 Tat protein directly activates neuronal N-methyl-D-

aspartate receptors at an allosteric zinc-sensitive site. *J Neurovirol* 9(3):399–403.

Sporer B, Missler U, Magerkurth O, et al. (2004). Evaluation of CSF glial fibrillary acidic protein (GFAP) as a putative marker for HIV-associated dementia. *Infection* 32(1):20–23.

Sriram K, Matheson JM, Benkovic SA, et al. (2002). Mice deficient in TNF receptors are protected against dopaminergic neurotoxicity: implications for Parkinson's disease. *FASEB J* 16(11):1474–1476.

Stamm WE, Handsfield HH, Rompalo AM, et al. (1988). The association between genital ulcer disease and acquisition of HIV infection in homosexual men. *JAMA* 260(10):1429–1433.

Stankoff B, Calvez V, Suarez S, et al. (1999). Plasma and cerebrospinal fluid human immunodeficiency virus type-1 (HIV-1) RNA levels in HIV-related cognitive impairment. *Eur J Neurol* 6(6):669–675.

Stern Y, McDermott MP, Albert S, et al. (2001). Factors associated with incident human immunodeficiency virus–dementia. *Arch Neurol* 58(3):473–479.

Stewart SA, Poon B, Jowett JB, and Chen IS (1997). Human immunodeficiency virus type 1 Vpr induces apoptosis following cell cycle arrest. *J Virol* 71(7):5579–5592.

Streit M, Ioannides AA, Liu L, et al. (1999). Neurophysiological correlates of the recognition of facial expressions of emotion as revealed by magnetoencephalography. *Brain Res Cogn Brain Res* 7(4): 481–491.

Strong M, and Rosenfeld J (2003). Amyotrophic lateral sclerosis: a review of current concepts. *Amyotroph Lateral Scler Other Motor Neuron Disord* 4(3):136–143.

Sui Y, Potula R, Pinson D, et al. (2003). Microarray analysis of cytokine and chemokine genes in the brains of macaques with SHIV-encephalitis. *J Med Primatol* 32(4-5):229–239.

Suparak S, Kespichayawattana W, Haque A, et al. (2005). Multinucleated giant cell formation and apoptosis in infected host cells is mediated by *Burkholderia pseudomallei* type III secretion protein BipB. *J Bacteriol* 187(18):6556–6560.

Swindells S, McConnell JR, McComb RD, and Gendelman HE (1995). Utility of cerebral proton magnetic resonance spectroscopy in differential diagnosis of HIV-related dementia. *J Neurovirol* 1(3-4):268–274.

Swindells S, Zheng J, and Gendelman HE (1999). HIV-associated dementia: new insights into disease pathogenesis and therapeutic interventions. *AIDS Patient Care STDS* 13(3):153–163.

Syndulko K, Singer EJ, Nogales-Gaete J, et al. (1994). Laboratory evaluations in HIV-1-associated cognitive/motor complex. *Psychiatr Clin North Am* 17(1): 91–123.

Takata K, Kitamura Y, Kakimura J, et al. (2000). Increase of bcl-2 protein in neuronal dendritic processes of cerebral cortex and hippocampus by the antiparkinsonian drugs, talipexole and pramipexole. *Brain Res* 872(1-2):236–241.

Tambuyzer BR, and Nouwen EJ (2005). Inhibition of microglia multinucleated giant cell formation and induction of differentiation by GM-CSF using a porcine in vitro model. *Cytokine* 31(4):270–279.

Tarkowski E, Andreasen N, Tarkowski A, and Blennow K (2003). Intrathecal inflammation precedes development of Alzheimer's disease. *J Neurol Neurosurg Psychiatry* 74(9):1200–1205.

Tassie JM, Szumilin E, Calmy A, et al. (2003). Highly active antiretroviral therapy in resource-poor settings: the experience of Medecins Sans Frontieres. *AIDS* 17(13):1995–1997.

Teismann P, Vila M, Choi DK, et al. (2003). COX-2 and neurodegeneration in Parkinson's disease. *Ann N Y Acad Sci* 991:272–277.

Thompson PM, Dutton RA, Hayashi KM, et al. (2005). Thinning of the cerebral cortex visualized in HIV/AIDS reflects CD4+ T lymphocyte decline. *Proc Natl Acad Sci U S A* 102(43):15647–15652.

Thurnher MM, Castillo M, Stadler A, et al. (2005). Diffusion-tensor MR imaging of the brain in human immunodeficiency virus–positive patients. *AJNR Am J Neuroradiol* 26(9):2275–2281.

Toborek M, Lee YW, Flora G, et al. (2005). Mechanisms of the blood–brain barrier disruption in HIV-1 infection. *Cell Mol Neurobiol* 25(1):181–199.

Tong N, Perry SW, Zhang Q, et al. (2000). Neuronal fractalkine expression in HIV-1 encephalitis: roles for macrophage recruitment and neuroprotection in the central nervous system. *J Immunol* 164(3):1333–1339.

Tracey I, Hamberg LM, Guimaraes AR, et al. (1998). Increased cerebral blood volume in HIV-positive patients detected by functional MRI. *Neurology* 50(6):1821–1826.

Tremolizzo L, Aliprandi A, Longoni M, Stanzani L, and Ferrarese C (2002). Glutamate may be the soluble cerebrospinal fluid factor that induces calcium dysregulation in cultured astrocytes in HIV dementia. *AIDS* 16(12):1691–1692; author reply 1692–1693.

Tu PH, Gurney ME, Julien JP, Lee VM, and Trojanowski J (1997). Oxidative stress, mutant SOD1, and neurofilament pathology in transgenic mouse models of human motor neuron disease. *Lab Invest* 76(4):441–456.

Tucker K, Robertson KR, Lin W, Smith JK, An H, Chen Y, Aylawrd SR, and Hall CD (2004). Neuroimaging in human immunodeficiency virus infection. *J Neuroimmunol* 157:153–162.

Tudor-Williams G, St Clair MH, McKinney RE, et al. (1992). HIV-1 sensitivity to zidovudine and clinical outcome in children. *Lancet* 339(8784):15–19.

Tyor WR, Glass JD, Griffin JW, et al. (1992). Cytokine expression in the brain during the acquired immunodeficiency syndrome. *Ann Neurol* 31(4):349–360.

Tyrer F, Walker AS, Gillett J, Porter K, for the UK Register of HIV Seroconverters (2003). The relationship between HIV seroconversion illness, HIV test interval and time to AIDS in a seroconverter cohort. *Epidemiol Infect* 131(3):1117–1123.

Valentine JS, and Hart PJ (2003). Misfolded CuZnSOD and amyotrophic lateral sclerosis. *Proc Natl Acad Sci U S A* 100(7):3617–3622.

Van den Bosch L, Van Damme P, Vlemincks V, et al. (2002). An alpha-mercaptoacrylic acid derivative (PD150606) inhibits selective motor neuron death via inhibition of kainate-induced Ca2+ influx and not via calpain inhibition. *Neuropharmacology* 42(5):706–713.

Vanhems P, Hirschel B, Phillips AN, Cooper DA, Vizzard J, Brassard J, and Perrin L (2000). Incubation time of acute human immunodeficiency virus (HIV) infection and duration of acute HIV infection are independent prognostic factors of progression to AIDS. *J Infect Dis* 182:334–337.

Vasilescu A, Heath SC, Diop G, et al. (2004). Genomic analysis of Fas and FasL genes and absence of correlation with disease progression in AIDS. *Immunogenetics* 56(1):56–60.

Veazey RS, DeMaria M, Chalifoux LV, et al. (1998). Gastrointestinal tract as a major site of CD4+ T cell depletion and viral replication in SIV infection. *Science* 280(5362):427–431.

Vesce S, Bezzi P, Rossi D, Meldolesi J, and Volterra A (1997). HIV-1 gp120 glycoprotein affects the astrocyte control of extracellular glutamate by both inhibiting the uptake and stimulating the release of the amino acid. *FEBS Lett* 411(1):107–109.

Vinters HV (2004). Infections and inflammatory diseases causing dementia. In MM Esiri, VY-M Lee, and JQ Trajanowski (eds.), *The Neuropathology of Dementia.* New York: Cambridge University Press.

Walensky RP, Paltiel AD, Losina E, et al. (2006). The survival benefits of AIDS treatment in the United States. *J Infect Dis* 194(1):11–19.

Wallace M, Nelson JA McCutchan JA, Wolfson T, Grant I, for the HNRC Group (HIV Neurobehavioral Reserach Center) (2001). Symptomatic HIV seroconverting illness is associated with more rapid neurlogical impairment. *Sex Transm Infect* 77:199–201.

Weber MS, Starck M, Wagenpfeil S, et al. (2004). Multiple sclerosis: glatiramer acetate inhibits monocyte reactivity in vitro and in vivo. *Brain* 127(Pt. 6):1370–1378.

Weed MR, and Steward DJ (2005). Neuropsychopathology in the SIV/macaque model of AIDS. *Front Biosci* 10:710–727.

Weidenheim KM, Epshteyn I, and Lyman WD (1993). Immunocytochemical identification of T-cells in HIV-1 encephalitis: implications for pathogenesis of CNS disease. *Mod Pathol* 6(2):167–174.

Weiss JM, Downie SA, Lyman WD, and Berman JW (1998). Astrocyte-derived monocyte-chemoattractant protein-1 directs the transmigration of leukocytes across a model of the human blood–brain barrier. *J Immunol* 161(12):6896–6903.

Wesselingh SL, and Thompson KA (2001). Immunopathogenesis of HIV-associated dementia. *Curr Opin Neurol* 14(3):375–379.

Weydt P, Hong S, Witting A, et al. (2005). Cannabinol delays symptom onset in SOD1 (G93A) transgenic mice without affecting survival. *Amyotroph Lateral Scler Other Motor Neuron Disord* 6(3):182–184.

Wie MB, Won MH, Lee KH, et al. (1997). Eugenol protects neuronal cells from excitotoxic and oxidative injury in primary cortical cultures. *Neurosci Lett* 225(2):93–96.

Wiley C, Schrier RD, Nelson JA, Lampert PW, and Oldstone MB (1986). Cellular localization of human immunodeficiency virus infection within the brains of acquired immune deficiency syndrome patients. *Proc Natl Acad Sci U S A* 83:7089–7093.

Wilkie FL, Goodkin K, Khamis I, et al. (2003). Cognitive functioning in younger and older HIV-1-infected adults. *J Acquir Immune Defic Syndr* 33(Suppl. 2): S93–S105.

Williams KC, and Hickey WF (2002). Central nervous system damage, monocytes and macrophages, and neurological disorders in AIDS. *Annu Rev Neurosci* 25:537–562.

Williams MA, Turchan J, Lu Y, Nath A, and Drachman DB (2005). Protection of human cerebral neurons from neurodegenerative insults by gene delivery of soluble tumor necrosis factor p75 receptor. *Exp Brain Res* 165(3):383–391.

Woelk CH, Ottones F, Plotkin CR, et al. (2004). Interferon gene expression following HIV type 1 infection of monocyte-derived macrophages. *AIDS Res Hum Retroviruses* 20(11):1210–1222.

Wojna V, Carlson KA, Luo X, et al. (2004). Proteomic fingerprinting of human immunodeficiency virus type 1–associated dementia from patient monocyte-derived macrophages: a case study. *J Neurovirol* 10(Suppl. 1):74–81.

Wolinsky JS (2006). The use of glatiramer acetate in the treatment of multiple sclerosis. *Adv Neurol* 98:273–292.

Wolters PL, and Brouwers P (2005). Evaluation of neurodevelopmental deficits in children with HIV-1 infection. In HE Gendelman, I Grant, IP Everall, SA Lipton, and S Swindells (eds.), *The Neurology of AIDS* (pp. 667–682). New York: Oxford University Press.

Woods SP, Childers M, Ellis RJ, et al. (2006). A battery approach for measuring neuropsychological change. *Arch Clin Neuropsychol* 21(1):83-89.

Worlein JM, Leigh J, Larsen K, et al. (2005). Cognitive and motor deficits associated with HIV-2(287) infection in infant pigtailed macaques: a nonhuman primate model of pediatric neuro-AIDS. *J Neurovirol* 11(1):34–45.

Wu DC, Teismann P, Tieu K, et al. (2003). NADPH oxidase mediates oxidative stress in the 1-methyl-4-phenyl-1,2,3,6-tetrahydropyridine model of Parkinson's disease. *Proc Natl Acad Sci U S A* 100(10): 6145–6150.

Wu DC, Re DB, Nagai M, et al. (2006). The inflammatory NADPH oxidase enzyme modulates motor neuron degeneration in amyotrophic lateral sclerosis mice. *Proc Natl Acad Sci U S A* 103(32):12132–12137.

Wu DT, Woodman SE, Weiss JM, et al. (2000). Mechanisms of leukocyte trafficking into the CNS. *J Neurovirol* 6(Suppl. 1):S82–S85.

Xiong H, Zeng YC, Lewis T, et al. (2000). HIV-1 infected mononuclear phagocyte secretory products affect neuronal physiology leading to cellular demise: relevance for HIV-1-associated dementia. *J Neurovirol* 6(Suppl. 1):S14–S23.

Yano S, Yano N, Rodriguez N, et al. (1998). Suppression of intracellular hydrogen peroxide generation and catalase levels in CD8+ T-lymphocytes from HIV+ individuals. *Free Radic Biol Med* 24(2):349–359.

Yoshihara T, Ishigaki S, Yamamoto M, et al. (2002). Differential expression of inflammation- and apoptosis-related genes in spinal cords of a mutant SOD1 transgenic mouse model of familial amyotrophic lateral sclerosis. *J Neurochem* 80(1):158–167.

Zeddou M, Greimers R, de Valensart N, Nayjib B, Tasken K, Boniver J, Moutschen M, and Rahmouni S (2005). Prostaglandin E2 induces the expression of functional inhibitory CD94/NKG2A receptors in human CD8+ T lymphocytes by a cAMP-dependent protein kinase A type I pathway. *Biochem Pharmacol* 70:714–724.

Zhang L, Ramratnam B, Tenner-Racz K, et al. (1999). Qunatifying residual HIV-1 replication in patients receiving combination antiretroviral therapy. *N Engl J Med* 340:1605–1613.

Zhang R, Fichtenbaum CJ, Hildeman DA, Lifson JD, and Chougnet C (2004). CD40 ligand dysregulation in HIV infection: HIV glycoprotein 120 inhibits signaling cascades upstream of CD40 ligand transcription. *J Immunol* 172(4):2678–2686.

Zhang W, Wang T, Pei Z, et al. (2005). Aggregated alpha-synuclein activates microglia: a process leading to disease progression in Parkinson's disease. *FASEB J* 19(6):533–542.

Zhang Z, Schuler T, Zupancic M, et al. (1999). Sexual transmission and propagation of SIV and HIV in resting and activated CD4+ T cells. *Science* 286(5443):1353–1357.

Zheng J, and Gendelman HE (1997). The HIV-1 associated dementia complex: a metabolic encephalopathy fueled by viral replication in mononuclear phagocytes. *Curr Opin Neurol* 10(4):319–325.

Zheng J, Thylin MR, Persidsky Y, et al. (2001). HIV-1 infected immune competent mononuclear phagocytes influence the pathways to neuronal demise. *Neurotox Res* 3(5):461–484.

Zhou B, Liu YY, Kim B, Xiao Y, and He JJ (2004). Astrocyte activation and dysfunction and neuron death by HIV-1 Tat expression in astrocytes. *Mol Cell Neurosci* 27(3):296–305.

Zink M, Coleman GD, and Mankowski JL (2001). Increased macrophage chemoattractant protein-1 in cerebrospinal fluid preceds and predicts simian immunodeficiency virus encephalitis. *J Infect Dis* 184:1015–1021.

Zink MC, Uhrlaub J, DeWitt J, et al. (2005). Neuroprotective and anti-human immunodeficiency virus activity of minocycline. *JAMA* 293(16):2003–2011.

Zink WE, Zheng J, Persidsky Y, et al. (1999). The neuropathogenesis of HIV-1 infection. *FEMS Immunol Med Microbiol* 26(3-4):233–241.

Zink WE, Anderson E, Boyle J, et al. (2002). Impaired spatial cognition and synaptic potentiation in a murine model of human immunodeficiency virus type 1 encephalitis. *J Neurosci* 22(6):2096–2105.

Chapter 20

Neurological Complications of HIV in the Spinal Cord and Peripheral Nervous System

Jessica Robinson Papp and David Simpson

Complications of HIV infection frequently arise in the nervous system. They occur at all stages of disease and are frequently underrecognized (Simpson et al., 1998). Many of these disorders have become more common as treatment with highly active anti-retroviral therapy (HAART) improves overall prognosis of HIV-infected patients. The etiologies of these complications are variable, including HIV itself, opportunistic infections, other comorbid illnesses, and HAART and other medications. Neurological disease leads to significant pain and disability, may exacerbate psychiatric disease, and makes compliance with treatment more difficult. Early recognition and treatment can significantly improve quality of life.

In order to diagnose neurological complications of HIV infection, the clinician must be alert to symptoms such as headache, dizziness, weakness, numbness, pain, visual changes, or gait abnormalities that may be harbingers of such conditions. When a patient is experiencing such symptoms, a detailed history and neurological examination are the first steps toward an accurate diagnosis. The examination will allow the clinician to begin to localize the origin of the symptom within the nervous system. This neuroanatomic localization then provides a framework with which to discern the etiology. Some symptoms, such as headache, may have a relatively clear localization, while others, like weakness, may be more difficult. It is helpful to think of the nervous system as a series of elements: cerebral hemispheres, brainstem, spinal cord (upper motor neuron), nerve roots (lower motor neuron), nerve plexuses, peripheral nerves, distal nerve, neuromuscular junction, and muscle.

Additional testing serves as confirmation of the clinically suspected anatomic source of the symptoms. Some of the more commonly employed diagnostic studies include blood tests, cerebrospinal fluid (CSF) examination, nerve conduction studies (NCS), electromyography (EMG), neuroimaging, including magnetic resonance imaging (MRI), and nerve and muscle biopsy.

In this chapter we address the effects of HIV and related complications on the spinal cord and peripheral nervous system (Table 20.1). Manifestations of HIV in the brain are discussed in Chapter 19. We review the most clinically important syndromes (Fig. 20.1): distal sensory polyneuropathy, inflammatory demyelinating polyneuropathy, mononeuropathy multiplex, progressive polyradiculopathy, myopathy, and myelopathy, with focus on diagnosis and treatment.

DISTAL SENSORY POLYNEUROPATHY

Epidemiology

Distal sensory polyneuropathy (DSP) is the most common neurological complication of HIV infection. Initial studies noted a prevalence of about 30% (So et al., 1988). Data from the Manhattan HIV Brain Bank suggest that the prevalence might be as high as 58% in cohorts of subjects with advanced HIV infection (Morgello et al., 2004). In the pre-HAART era, DSP was associated with advanced disease, low CD4 count, and high plasma HIV viral load. More recently DSP has become increasingly noted in patients with good virologic control and immune status (Morgello et al., 2004). DSP is more common in patients with additional risk factors for neuropathy, including diabetes mellitus, alcohol abuse, vitamin B12 deficiency, and poor nutritional status. Coinfection with hepatitis C may confer additional risk, although this issue requires further study (Brew, 2003).

Clinical Features

Distal sensory neuropathy presents with distal symmetric sensory symptoms. Patients typically complain of numbness, pain, or burning in the feet. They may notice that previously innocuous stimuli, such as the brush of bedsheets against their feet, are painful. Some patients have difficulty walking because of pain. As the disease progresses, symptoms proceed proximally up the lower extremities. The hands may ultimately be involved in advanced stages. There is usually no significant motor involvement, although weakness of the intrinsic muscles of the feet may be a feature of advanced disease (Cornblath and McArthur, 1988).

On physical examination, decreased pain, temperature, and vibratory sense, with relative preservation of proprioception, are typically seen. Deep tendon re-

flexes are reduced at the ankles compared to those at the knees (Lange et al., 1988). Hyperactive knee reflexes together with normal or reduced ankle jerks suggest the presence of combined central and peripheral nervous system disease. The skin on the distal lower extremities may appear shiny, hairless, or tight.

Pathogenesis

Distal sensory polyneuropathy occurs as a result of axonal injury to the most distal aspect of the sensory nerves, a process known as "dying back" (Pardo et al., 2001). The mechanism of this injury is not known and is likely multifactorial. HIV itself has been proposed as a contributing factor, although there is little evidence for direct HIV infection of peripheral nerves. Rather, HIV may cause neurotoxicity via secreted proteins such as the glycoprotein (gp) 120 subunit, or by leading to the release of neurotoxic, proinflammatory cytokines from infected glial cells (Keswani et al., 2003).

The antiretroviral agents didanosine (ddI), zalcitabine (ddC), and stavudine (d4T) are neurotoxins, which may exert their effects through mitochondrial toxicity (Simpson and Tagliati, 1995). In the course of treatment for other HIV-associated conditions, patients may be exposed to other neurotoxic agents, including chloramphenicol, cisplatin, ethambutol, isoniazid, metronidazole, paclitaxel, pyridoxine, thalidomide, vinca alkaloids, and interferon.

The loss of sensation in DSP follows directly from the loss of sensory axons. The mechanism by which the axonal damage causes pain is not understood. It is proposed that regardless of the initial mechanism, axonal injury leads to a common final pathway of gene expression changes that cause increased perception of pain. C-fibers, which are normally responsible for signaling pain, can become more excitable through upregulation of voltage-gated sodium channels. A-fibers, which conduct light touch, may express neuromodulators normally only expressed by C-fibers, in effect phenotypically switching to pain-conducting neurons, and causing light touch to be experienced as pain. This abnormal noxious sensory input from the periphery increases central sensitization, which further increases the perception of pain (Woolf, 2004).

Diagnosis

Blood testing, including that for glucose, renal and liver function, vitamin B12, folate, thyroid function,

TABLE 20.1. Summary of Major Complications of HIV in the Spinal Cord and Peripheral Nervous System

Disease	Time of Onset	Incidence	Clinical Features	Prognosis	Treatment
Distal sensory polyneuropathy	Anytime in disease course, may be more common in advanced cases	Common; 30%–58% of patients	Stocking and glove distribution sensory loss Parasthesias and pain beginning in feet	Non-life threatening; can significantly interfere with quality of life	Withdrawal of neurotoxic agents Nonspecific analgesia: NSAIDs, opioids Tricyclic antidepressants, duloxetine, gabapentin, lamotrigine Topical capsaicin, lidocaine
Inflammatory demyelinating polyneuropathy	Early infection	Rare	Ascending weakness Parasthesias	Good; major recovery within 4 weeks typical	IVIG, plasmapheresis
Mononeuropathy multiplex	Early and late forms	Rare	Early: sensorimotor deficits in 1–2 nerves Late: many nerves involved	Early: good; usually self-limited Late: poorer; may not recover fully	Early: steroids, IVIG, plasmapheresis Late: ganciclovir
Progressive polyradiculopathy	Advanced infection	Rare	Rapid-onset flaccid paraparesis	Poor; high mortality if untreated	Ganciclovir
Myopathy	Any stage	Moderate	Slowly progressive proximal weakness	Fair; course slow, may improve with treatment	Trial of ZDV withdrawl Steroids
Myelopathy	Any stage, more common in late disease	Common in autopsy studies, less so clinically	Slowly progressive spastic paraparesis Sensory loss, incontinence	Poor. Course progressive	Symptomatic: muscle relaxants, bladder management

IVIG, intravenous immunoglobulin; NSAIDs, nonsteriodal anti-in flammatories; ZDV, zidovudine.

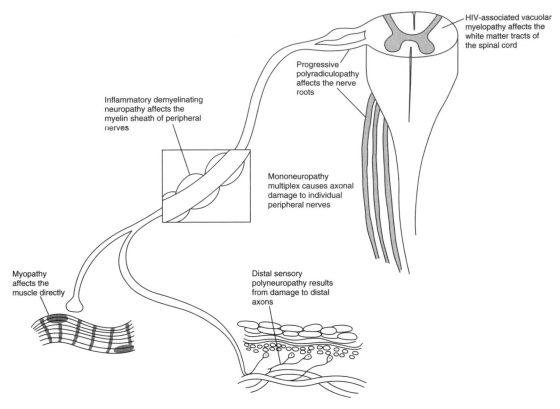

FIGURE 20.1. Localization of neurological complications of HIV in the spinal cord and peripheral nervous system.

rapid plasma reagin (RPR), erythrocyte sedimentation rate, anti-nuclear antibody, and serum protein electrophoresis, is helpful to exclude other causes of DSP. The diagnosis of DSP is based on clinical findings, and additional testing to confirm the diagnosis is usually unnecessary. In atypical cases, electrophysiological studies, specifically nerve conduction and EMG studies, may be helpful. The sural nerve, a sensory branch of the tibial nerve supplying the lateral calf, is the earliest to show abnormalities. A decrease in amplitude of the sural sensory nerve action potential (SNAP), with relative sparing of conduction velocity, is generally seen, consistent with axonal injury (Tagliati et al., 1999). EMG may show denervation in distal muscles. Additional diagnostic studies for DSP, done in atypical cases or as part of research protocols, may include nerve or skin biopsy and quantitative sensory testing (QST). QST allows measurement of sensory function, including large and small nerve fibers, by challenging the patient with small, repro-

ducible sensory stimuli. Skin biopsy reveals decreased intraepidermal nerve fiber density in the distal leg (Polydefkis et al., 2002).

Treatment

Comorbid factors, such as a history of diabetes or alcohol abuse, should be sought and modified as possible. If the patient is taking neurotoxic medications, discontinuation or dose reduction of these agents may improve or slow the progression of DSP. However, the clinician may choose to continue a neurotoxic antiretroviral if this drug is required for virologic control. This decision is based on a risk–benefit analysis, which should be addressed for each patient individually. If neurotoxic therapy is stopped the patient may experience a "coasting period" of 4 to 6 weeks, during which time symptoms persist despite cessation of the offending agents. After this period the patient will typically improve, to the extent that neuropathic symptoms are due to the neurotoxic medication (Berger et al., 1993). Regardless of whether neurotoxic treatment is continued, symptomatic management for DSP should be initiated, as discussed below.

There is no U.S. Food and Drug Administration (FDA)-approved treatment for HIV-related DSP. The treatment strategies outlined below are based on clinical trial results and clinical experience, some of which is derived from studies of other painful neuropathies, such as diabetic neuropathy and postherpetic neuralgia. The two treatment strategies for DSP are symptomatic control and neuroregenerative therapies. Unfortunately, regenerative treatments, such as recombinant human nerve growth factor, are not yet clinically available (Schifitto et al., 2001).

Pain management in the HIV-positive population is particularly challenging because of the high prevalence of substance abuse and comorbid psychiatric illness. Clinicians must be aware of their own biases toward these patient groups and how such bias may compromise effective pain management, particularly when opioid use is contemplated. Treatment of HIV-related DSP may require a multidisciplinary approach, involving neurologists, pain specialists, psychiatrists, and infectious disease clinicians. By understanding and effectively managing this common complica-tion of HIV, the practitioner can greatly enhance the patient's quality of life.

One may begin to approach the symptomatic treatment of HIV-related DSP by considering a more general approach to pain management, as outlined by the World Health Organization's (WHO) analgesic ladder. In this model, increasing severity of pain is treated accordingly with stronger analgesia, from non-steroidal anti-inflammatory drugs (NSAIDs), such as ibuprofen, and acetaminophen for mild pain, to combinations of NSAIDs with mild opiates for moderate pain, to potent opioids for severe pain (WHO, 1990). Adjuvant agents in combination with primary analgesics may provide added benefit (Table 20.2). These agents fall into two major categories, antidepressants and anticonvulsants. Of the former, the tricyclic antidepressants, such as amytriptiline and nortryptiline, have been most extensively studied (Max et al., 1987). These drugs are usually started as a single evening dose, as they may be sedating. Patients generally accommodate to this side effect and are then able to tolerate higher and more frequent doses. Tricyclic antidepressants with a lower anticholinergic toxicity profile, such as desipramine, may be better tolerated. A newer antidepressant, duloxetine, a selective serotoninergic noradrenergic reuptake inhibitor, has

TABLE 20.2. Summary of Adjuvant Treatment Options for Neuropathic Pain

Drug	Dosage	Most Common Side Effects	Comments
Amitriptyline/ nortriptyline	10 mg po qhs to start, titrate to 100 mg daily in divided doses	Initial sedation Dry mouth, dizziness, constipation, sexual and urinary dysfunction, weight gain, orthostatic hypotension, delirium	Desipramine may be better tolerated
Duloxetine	60 mg po qd	Nausea, dizziness, somnolence, fatigue	Side effects usually mild
Gabapentin	100 mg po tid to start, titrate to 800–1200 mg tid	Somnolence, dizziness, fatigue	Side effects usually mild
Lamotrigine	25 mg po daily to start, titrate to 300–400 mg daily	Dizziness, ataxia, somnolence, headache	Serious rash rare, but potentially fatal; slow titration reduces risk
Lidocaine patch	Apply patch to affected area for 12–24 hours	None	Rare local erythema
Pregabalin	150 mg po daily in divided doses to start, titrate to 300–600 mg daily in divided doses	Somnolence, dizziness	Side effects usually mild

recently been FDA approved for the treatment of painful diabetic neuropathy (Goldstein et al., 2005). Before widespread acceptance of its use in patients with HIV neuropathy, however, the metabolic interactions with protease inhibitors, also metabolized by cytochrome P450, should be better understood.

Several antiepileptic drugs (AEDs) may be used in the treatment of HIV-related DSP, including carbamazepine, phenytoin, gabapentin, and lamotrigine. Placebo-controlled trials have produced mixed results regarding the efficacy of phenytoin in the treatment of DSP, and carbamazepine has been studied mostly in the treatment of trigeminal neuralgia (McQuay et al., 1995). The mechanism of action of these agents is reduced neuronal excitability due to modification of sodium receptors. The newer AEDs, especially gabapentin, are more widely used. Placebo-controlled studies show that gabapentin is effective for treatment of DSP and is usually quite well tolerated even at high doses (Hahn et al., 2004). Many clinicians initiate treatment at 100 mg tid and rapidly titrate to an effective dose, sometimes to 3600 mg daily in divided doses. A related newer agent, pregabalin, is FDA approved for treatment of painful diabetic neuropathy and postherpetic neuralgia, and is under evaluation in HIV-related DSP in placebo-controlled trials (Freynhagen et al., 2005).

Lamotrigine has demonstrated efficacy in treating HIV-related DSP (Simpson et al., 2003). Although usually well tolerated, it must be initiated at low doses (e.g., 25 mg daily or every other day) and titrated slowly (over 6–8 weeks, to 300–400 mg/day) to avoid potentially serious rash. Two other newer AEDs, topiramate and oxcarbamazepine, may also have a role in the treatment of DSP, although they have yet to be well studied (Beydoun et al., 2004, Raskin et al., 2004). In practice, many clinicians find combinations of analgesics with different mechanisms of action to be the most effective treatment (Gilron et al., 2005).

Topical agents, including lidocaine gel and patch, and capsaicin, have been tried with some success and have the benefit of avoiding systemic effects (Estanislao et al., 2004). While currently available low-concentration topical capsaicin has marginal efficacy in DSP, a high-concentration capsaicin dermal patch shows promise in early clinical trials of HIV-related DSP (Simpson et al., 2004). A controlled trial demonstrated that acupuncture was ineffective in the treatment of painful HIV-related DSP (Shlay et al., 1998). Other nonpharmacologic methods, including hypno-

therapy, biofeedback, and physical therapy, may also be of benefit to some patients, although these complementary treatments have not been evaluated in controlled trials.

INFLAMMATORY DEMYELINATING POLYNEUROPATHY

Inflammatory demyelinating polyneuropathy (IDP) is a relatively uncommon complication of HIV infection, occurring most often in an acute form (AIDP) early in the course of infection or at the time of seroconversion (Cornblath et al., 1987). The manifestations of AIDP, also known as Guillan-Barre syndrome (GBS), seen in association with HIV are similar to those seen in HIV-negative patients. AIDP is characterized by rapidly progressive weakness, usually in an ascending pattern, with plateau of progression within 1 to 4 weeks (Asbury, 1981). The chronic form, CIDP, is characterized by prolonged or relapsing symptoms.

In addition to weakness and areflexia, there may be facial nerve or other cranial nerve involvement. Many patients report low back pain radiating to the legs, or dysesthetic or myalgic pain in the limbs. Although sensory complaints may be prominent, sensation is usually relatively spared on objective testing. Autonomic involvement is a rare but serious complication, which may lead to life-threatening dysregulation of heart rate and blood pressure.

AIDP is thought to be caused by an autoimmune attack of peripheral nerve myelin, which reduces conduction of impulses along the nerve and results in weakness. Axons are usually preserved, except in severe cases. AIDP may also be seen in advanced HIV infection as a manifestation of cytomegalovirus (CMV) infection (Morgello and Simpson, 1994).

The diagnosis of AIDP is usually suggested by the history and neurological examination. Ancillary studies may provide confirmation. Radiological studies are helpful to exclude compressive lesions of the spine, which may also present with low back pain and lower extremity weakness. Spinal MRI with gadolinium enhancement may reveal nerve root enhancement in IDP. Cerebrospinal fluid (CSF) lymphocytic pleocytosis (10–50 cells/mm^3) helps to distinguish IDP in HIV-positive from uninfected patients. Elevated CSF protein level (50–250 mg/dl) is present in both groups. Nerve conduction studies show features of a demyelinating process, including reduced conduction velocity, temporal dispersion, conduction block, and prolonged distal latency (Cornblath et al., 1987).

There have been no controlled clinical trials of treatment of AIDP or CIDP in HIV-positive patients. Thus treatment recommendations are derived from experience in treating HIV-negative patients. Most patients presenting with AIDP are initially managed in an inpatient setting to begin treatment and monitor for dangerous complications such as autonomic and respiratory failure. First-line management of AIDP includes either plasmapheresis or intravenous immunoglobulin (IVIG). Treatment options for CIDP are much the same as those for AIDP and include corticosteroids, but often these need to be administered on a chronic basis to avoid relapses.

MONONEUROPATHY MULTIPLEX

Mononeuropathy multiplex (MM) is an infrequent complication of HIV infection. There are two distinct forms, one presenting early in the course of disease, and the other in the setting of advanced AIDS. Both forms are characterized by impairment of sensory and motor function in the distribution of one or more peripheral nerves, nerve roots, or cranial nerves. Accordingly, the neurological deficits vary depending on the nerves involved and are typically asymmetric.

The early form of MM most often occurs in patients with CD4 counts >200 cells/mm^3. It typically manifests with acute onset of sensorimotor deficits, attributable to involvement of one or more peripheral or cranial nerves. Deficits are most often self-limited, resolving after several months either with or without treatment (Lipkin et al., 1985). In patients with advanced AIDS, particularly those with a CD4 count <50 cells/mm^3, MM takes a more extensive and rapidly progressive form, quickly involving multiple nerve distributions. These patients have a poorer prognosis for recovery (So and Olney, 1991).

Pathologically, axonal degeneration with inflammatory infiltrates is seen in both early- and late-onset MM. Demyelination may also occur in the late-onset form (Miller et al., 1988). The etiology of early-onset MM is thought to be autoimmune. MM in late-stage disease may be due to CMV infection (Said et al., 1991). If cranial neuropathies are a prominent presenting feature, CNS lymphoma, hepatitis C virus (HCV)-related cryoglobulinemia, cryptococcal meningitis, toxoplasmosis, and varicella zoster infection should also be considered. Rarely, pathological findings reveal a vasculitic neuropathy (Gherardi et al., 1989).

The diagnosis of MM is based predominantly on clinical findings, although electrodiagnostic studies and CSF examination may provide support and clarification. Decreased motor and sensory potentials consistent with axonal degeneration are most often seen on nerve conduction studies (Lange et al., 1988). Electromyography may show denervation. CSF analysis usually shows elevated protein and a mild mononuclear pleocytosis, which are nonspecific abnormalities in HIV-infected patients (Hollander, 1988). If these studies are unrevealing, nerve biopsy may be considered. In advanced patients, a positive CMV polymerase chain reaction (PCR) in CSF or evidence of CMV on nerve biopsy is diagnostic of primary CMV infection of peripheral nerve (Roullet et al., 1994).

MM in the relatively immunocompetent patient is usually self-limited. However in patients with inadequate spontaneous recovery, treatment with corticosteroids (e.g., 60–80 mg prednisone daily), plasmapheresis, or IVIG may provide benefit (Miller et al., 1988). Regardless of whether CMV is detected in CSF or nerve biopsy, empiric antiviral treatment with ganciclovir, cidofovir, or foscarnet should be considered for MM in the severely immunocompromised patient. Even with treatment, however, recovery is often incomplete and relapses may occur (Roullet et al., 1994).

PROGRESSIVE POLYRADICULOPATHY

Progressive polyradiculopathy (PP) usually occurs in advanced stages of AIDS, in patients with CD4 lymphocyte counts below 50 cells/mm^3 or in those with opportunistic infections (Miller et al., 1990). The incidence of PP has progressively declined in the HAART era.

Patients with PP generally present with a rapidly evolving cauda equina syndrome, starting with paresthesias and pain radiating to the lower extremities, associated with mild sensory loss and sphincter dysfunction. Neurological examination reveals flaccid paraparesis and lower extremity areflexia. The upper extremities and cranial nerves may be involved in advanced cases. Prognosis is poor, and death is expected within weeks in untreated individuals (Kim and Hollander, 1993).

Progressive polyradiculopathy is caused by inflammation and necrosis of lumbosacral nerve roots, usually due to CMV infection (Eidelberg et al., 1986). PP often coexists with other systemic signs of CMV infection such as retinitis, pneumonia, and gastroenteritis. Neurosyphilis and lymphomatous meningitis may also cause a similar syndrome, although these etiologies are less frequent (Lanska et al., 1988, Leger et al., 1992).

Radiological studies, such as gadolinium-enhanced MRI of the lumbosacral spine, are often the first diagnostic step in patients with suspected PP. Although these studies may be normal or show only meningeal enhancement in the cauda equina, they are needed to exclude focal compressive lesions of the cauda equine (Bazan et al., 1991). Lumbar puncture is also essential, as the diagnosis of CMV-related PP is confirmed by detection of CMV in the CSF with PCR techniques. Low glucose, elevated protein, and a prominent polymorphonuclear pleocytosis (as high as 2000 cells/mm^3) in the CSF are also suggestive of the diagnosis (Kim et al., 1993).

Electrodiagnostic studies show evidence of severe axonal polyradiculopathy, including low-amplitude compound muscle action potentials, and extensive denervation of lower extremity muscles, but relatively mild decrement in nerve conduction responses consistent with proximal axonal damage (Miller et al., 1990).

Most authors favor instituting empiric treatment with antiviral therapy, even before virologic studies have been completed, as the prognosis for untreated PP is poor, and damage to nerve roots becomes rapidly irreversible (Miller et al., 1990). Antiviral options include ganciclovir, foscarnet, or cidofovir, alone or in combination, although these regimens must be monitored for their toxic side-effect profile. Regardless of the agent chosen, treatment is often of several months duration and should be continued even if no clear improvement is seen, as stabilization may be the best possible outcome in some cases (Kim et al., 1993).

AUTONOMIC NEUROPATHY

The prevalence of autonomic neuropathy (AN) in HIV infection is unknown, as it is often subclinical (Villa et al., 1992). AN typically occurs late in the course of HIV infection, and may be characterized by sympathetic and parasympathetic dysfunction (Cohen and Laudenslager, 1989). Symptoms caused by parasympathetic dysfunction include tachycardia, impotence, and urinary dysfunction. Sympathetic dysfunction causes orthostatic hypotension, syncope, diarrhea, anhidrosis, and cardiac arrhythmia. The etiology of AN in HIV infection is unknown. There may be direct involvement of the descending hypothalamic tracts and the sympathetic ganglia (Esiri et al., 1993; Purba et al., 1993). These deficits may be exacerbated by medications, dehydration, and malnutrition.

Autonomic studies, including tilt-table and sudomotor testing, may be helpful in diagnosis. Treatment of AN is symptomatic and includes cessation of offending agents and increased fluid and salt intake. Fludrocortisone and midodrine are useful in attenuating orthostatic hypotension, as are mechanical techniques such as compressive stockings and avoiding the supine position. Anti-arrhythmics or implantation of a pacemaker or defibrillator may be necessary for cardiac arrhythmia.

MYOPATHY

Like many of the disorders discussed above, the prevalence of myopathy in HIV infection is unknown and may have changed in the HAART era (Tagliati et al., 1998). Myopathy occurs at all stages of HIV disease and is characterized by slowly progressive, proximal, and symmetric weakness (Simpson and Bender, 1988). The patient may report difficulty rising from a chair, climbing stairs, or brushing hair. Myalgias are often present but are not specific. Physical examination reveals proximal muscle weakness most prominent in hip and neck flexors. Myopathy may also present as a wasting syndrome with weight loss and weakness, or as acute rhabdomyolysis with myalgia, weakness, and elevated creatine kinase (CK) level (Simpson et al., 1990; Chariot et al., 1994).

The criteria used to define polymyositis in HIV-negative patients are also useful in the diagnosis of HIV-associated myopathy. These include objective muscle weakness, elevated serum CK, myopathic findings on EMG, and a myopathic muscle biopsy (Bohan and Peter, 1975). The presence of all four criteria leads to a definitive diagnosis; if three are met the diagnosis is probable.

The etiology of HIV-associated myopathy is unknown and is likely multifactorial. An immune-mediated mechanism has been proposed, supported by the presence of inflammatory infiltrates in some muscle biopsies from patients with HIV myopathy. Virus-infected inflammatory cells, especially macrophages, secrete toxic factors such as tumor necrosis factor, leading to muscle fiber damage (Illa et al., 1991). Mitochondrial toxicity, associated with nucleoside analogue antiretroviral agents, particularly zidovudine (ZDV, AZT), has also been implicated in HIV myopathy (Dalakas et al., 1990).

We have reported a rapidly progressive HIV-associated neuromuscular weakness syndrome in 69 patients, most of whom were receiving d4T therapy (HIV Neuromuscular Syndrome Study Group, 2004). The presence of lactic acidosis and pathological evidence of mitochondrial myopathy support a mitochondrial mechanism. These patients had variable combinations of severe axonal neuropathy and myopathy. Other less common causes of myopathy in HIV infection include toxoplasmosis, CMV, *Cryptococcus*, *Mycoplasma avium intracellulare*, and *Staphlococcus aureus*. Treatment of HIV myopathy includes withdrawal or dose reduction of AZT if applicable. Immunomodulating therapy includes corticosteroids or IVIG (Johnson et al., 2003). The patient may tolerate a rechallenge with AZT at a later time.

MYELOPATHY

HIV-associated myelopathy (HIVM, also known as vacuolar myelopathy) is the most common form of myelopathy seen in HIV-positive patients. Autopsy series have shown the characteristic pathological changes of HIVM in 17%–55% of HIV-infected patients, although clinically the syndrome is noted less frequently (Artigas et al., 1990; Henin et al., 1992). HIVM typically presents later in the course of HIV in the presence of AIDS-defining illnesses, but patients may have it at any time throughout the course of disease (Dal Pan et al., 1994). There has been speculation that as HAART continues to improve the overall prognosis for HIV-positive patients, the incidence of HIVM may increase.

HIV-associated myelopathy is characterized clinically by an insidious onset of symmetric weakness in the lower extremities and prominent spasticity. Patients may also complain of loss of bowel and bladder control as well as erectile dysfunction (Di Rocco and Simpson, 1998). Paresthesias and sensory loss may also be reported, although these are typically less promi-

nent. Neurological examination typically reveals hyperactive deep tendon reflexes, extensor plantar responses, diminished proprioception and vibratory sense, with relative preservation of pain and temperature, sensory ataxia, and a stiff, scissoring gait. Because the thoracic cord is the most frequently involved level, the arms are usually relatively spared. Unlike many other spinal cord lesions, a discrete sensory level, spinal tenderness, and back pain are typically absent.

The diagnosis of HIVM is made on clinical grounds, based on a typical history and physical examination. Diagnostic studies are performed largely to exclude other treatable causes of myelopathy. Gadolinium-enhanced MRI of the spine is performed to rule out structural etiologies, including intramedullary lesions, such as lymphoma, or extradural processes such as a compressive disc herniation.

Neuroradiological findings in HIVM are nonspecific. MRI may be normal or demonstrate spinal cord atrophy or nonspecific white matter hyperintensities on T2-weighted sequences (Chong et al., 1999). Several blood tests are indicated to rule out other, less common causes of myelopathy, including VDRL, toxoplasmosis, *Cryptococcus*, vitamin B12 level, and HTLV-I antibodies. Examination of the CSF is usually nonspecific, demonstrating mild pleocytosis and protein elevation, as found in most HIV-infected patients. Somatosensory-evoked potentials can help confirm the diagnosis of myelopathy, and nerve conduction studies may be used to define superimposed neuropathy.

The typical pathological change of HIVM is vacuoles concentrated in the white matter tracts of the thoracic lateral and posterior columns. The mechanism for these changes is not well defined. They do not appear to be a direct result of HIV infection, as HIV can be recovered from the spinal cord at autopsy in only a minority of patients. It is thought that macrophage activation and subsequent cytokine release may lead to the vacuolization (Petito et al., 1994).

There is no specific treatment for HIVM, and it is unclear that improvement of immune status with HAART is helpful (Yarchoan et al., 1987; Geraci and Di Rocco, 2000). On the basis of a possible immune-mediated pathogenesis, corticosteroids have been used without clear benefit (Dal Pan and Berger, 1997). We are pursuing studies of IVIG for HIVM, with preliminary evidence of efficacy. Since HIVM may have a metabolic etiology, L-methionine supplementation was tried with some success in a small open-label study

(Di Rocco et al., 1998). However, a larger controlled trial yielded negative results (Di Rocco et al., 2004). Treatment of HIVM is largely symptomatic, including management of bladder function and spasticity.

OTHER NEUROMUSCULAR DISEASES

Although not a disease specific to the HIV-infected population, herpes zoster virus (HZV) infection occurs with greater frequency in immunocompromised patients. HZV is a reactivation of latent varicella zoster infection characterized by pain, itching, and a vesicular rash in a dermatomal distribution. Treatment with antiviral medication and steroids may reduce the duration of disease. Following an episode of HZV, patients may develop a chronic pain syndrome in the same distribution, known as postherpetic neuralgia. Treatment of pain with anticonvulsants, tricyclic antidepressants, and topical lidocaine preparations may be tried (Rowbotham, 1994). The HZV vaccine currently in use employs a live attenuated virus and so is not recommended for immunocompromised patients. Vaccines using a varicella glycoprotein subunit are under development (Vafai and Berger, 2001).

There are several reports of motor neuron disease in HIV-positive patients, associated with response to antiretroviral therapy (Moulignier et al., 2001). It is unclear, however, if there is a true association between HIV and motor neuron disease, or if this reflects chance co-occurrence of two diseases (Verma et al., 1990). Myasthenia gravis has been reported in the course of HIV infection, but a causal relationship has not been shown (Nath et al., 1990). A primary sensory ataxia, termed sensory neuronopathy, has been described in several patients (Elder et al., 1986).

CONCLUSION

Diseases of the peripheral nervous system and spinal cord are common in the HIV-positive population. By becoming familiar with the more common entities and remaining alert for neurological signs and symptoms, clinicians caring for HIV-positive patients can improve the diagnosis of neurological disease and help patients receive the appropriate treatment. These strategies can reduce pain and disability, and lead to significant improvement in quality of life.

ACKNOWLEDGMENT The authors would like to thank Alejandro Campos, M.D., for his contributions to this chapter.

References

Artigas J, Grosse G, and Niedobitek F (1990). Vacuolar myelopathy in AIDS. A morphological analysis. Pathol Res Pract 186:228–237.

Asbury AK (1981). Diagnostic considerations in Guillain-Barre syndrome. Ann Neurol 9(Suppl.):1–5.

Bazan C 3rd, Jackson C, Jinkins JR, and Barohn RJ (1991). Gadolinium-enhanced MRI in a case of cytomegalovirus polyradiculopathy. Neurology 41:1522–1523.

Berger AR, Arezzo JC, Schaumburg HH, Skowron G, Merigan T, Bozzette S, Richman D, and Soo W (1993). 2′,3′-dideoxycytidine (ddC) toxic neuropathy: a study of 52 patients. Neurology 43:358–362.

Beydoun A, Kobetz SA, and Carrazana EJ (2004). Efficacy of oxcarbazepine in the treatment of painful diabetic neuropathy. Clin J Pain 20:174–178.

Bohan A, and Peter JB (1975). Polymyositis and dermatomyositis (first of two parts). N Engl J Med 292:344–347.

Brew BJ (2003). The peripheral nerve complications of human immunodeficiency virus (HIV) infection. Muscle Nerve 28:542–552.

Chariot P, Ruet E, Authier FJ, Levy Y, and Gherardi R (1994). Acute rhabdomyolysis in patients infected by human immunodeficiency virus. Neurology 44:1692–1696.

Chong J, Di Rocco A, Tagliati M, Danisi F, Simpson DM, and Atlas SW (1999). MR findings in AIDS-associated myelopathy. AJNR Am J Neuroradiol 20:1412–1416.

Cohen JA, and Laudenslager M (1989). Autonomic nervous system involvement in patients with human immunodeficiency virus infection. Neurology 39:1111–1112.

Cornblath DR, and McArthur JC (1988). Predominantly sensory neuropathy in patients with AIDS and AIDS-related complex. Neurology 38:794–796.

Cornblath DR, McArthur JC, Kennedy PG, Witte AS, and Griffin JW (1987). Inflammatory demyelinating peripheral neuropathies associated with human T-cell lymphotropic virus type III infection. Ann Neurol 21:32–40.

Dalakas MC, Illa I, Pezeshkpour GH, Laukaitis JP, Cohen B, and Griffin JL (1990). Mitochondrial myopathy caused by long-term zidovudine therapy. N Engl J Med 322:1098–1105.

Dal Pan G, and Berger J (1997). Spinal cord disease in human immunodeficiency virus infection. In J Berger and R Levy (eds.), AIDS in the Nervous System, second edition (p. 173). Philadelphia: Lippincott-Raven.

Dal Pan GJ, Glass JD, and McArthur JC (1994). Clinicopathologic correlations of HIV-1-associated vacuolar myelopathy: an autopsy-based case-control study. *Neurology* 44:2159–2164.

Di Rocco A, and Simpson DM (1998). AIDS-associated vacuolar myelopathy. *AIDS Patient Care STDS* 12: 457–461.

Di Rocco A, Tagliati M, Danisi F, Dorfman D, Moise J, and Simpson DM (1998). A pilot study of L-methionine for the treatment of AIDS-associated myelopathy. *Neurology* 51:266–268.

Di Rocco A, Werner P, Bottiglieri T, Godbold J, Liu M, Tagliati M, Scarano A, and Simpson D (2004). Treatment of AIDS-associated myelopathy with L-methionine: a placebo-controlled study. *Neurology* 63:1270–1275.

Eidelberg D, Sotrel A, Vogel H, Walker P, Kleefield J, and Crumpacker CS 3rd (1986). Progressive polyradiculopathy in acquired immune deficiency syndrome. *Neurology* 36:912–916.

Elder G, Dalakas M, Pezeshkpour G, and Sever J (1986). Ataxic neuropathy due to ganglioneuronitis after probable acute human immunodeficiency virus infection. *Lancet* 2:1275–1276.

Esiri MM, Morris CS, and Millard PR (1993). Sensory and sympathetic ganglia in HIV-1 infection: immunocytochemical demonstration of HIV-1 viral antigens, increased MHC class II antigen expression and mild reactive inflammation. *J Neurol Sci* 114: 178–187.

Estanislao L, Carter K, McArthur J, Olney R, Simpson D, for the Lidoderm-HIV Neuropathy Group (2004). A randomized controlled trial of 5% lidocaine gel for HIV-associated distal symmetric polyneuropathy. *J Acquir Immune Defic Syndr* 37:1584–1586.

Freynhagen R, Strojek K, Griesing T, Whalen E, and Balkenohl M (2005). Efficacy of pregabalin in neuropathic pain evaluated in a 12-week, randomised, double-blind, multicentre, placebo-controlled trial of flexible- and fixed-dose regimens. *Pain* 115:254–263.

Geraci AP, and Di Rocco A (2000). Anti-HIV therapy. *AIDS* 14:2059–2061.

Gherardi R, Lebargy F, Gaulard P, Mhiri C, Bernaudin JF, and Gray F (1989). Necrotizing vasculitis and HIV replication in peripheral nerves. *N Engl J Med* 321:685–686.

Gilron I, Bailey JM, Tu D, Holden RR, Weaver DF, and Houlden RL (2005). Morphine, gabapentin, or their combination for neuropathic pain. *N Engl J Med* 352:1324–1334.

Goldstein DJ, Lu Y, Detke MJ, Lee TC, and Iyengar S (2005). Duloxetine vs. placebo in patients with painful diabetic neuropathy. *Pain* 116:109–118.

Hahn K, Arendt G, Braun JS, von Giesen HJ, Husstedt IW, Maschke M, Straube ME, Schielke E, for the German Neuro-AIDS Working Group (2004). A placebo-controlled trial of gabapentin for painful HIV-associated sensory neuropathies. *J Neurol* 251: 1260–1266.

Henin D, Smith TW, De Girolami U, Sughayer M, and Hauw JJ (1992). Neuropathology of the spinal cord in the acquired immunodeficiency syndrome. *Hum Pathol* 23:1106–1114.

HIV Neuromuscular Syndrome Study Group (2004). HIV-associated neuromuscular weakness syndrome. *AIDS* 18:1403–1412.

Hollander H (1988). Cerebrospinal fluid normalities and abnormalities in individuals infected with human immunodeficiency virus. *J Infect Dis* 158: 855–858.

Illa I, Nath A, and Dalakas M (1991). Immunocytochemical and virological characteristics of HIV-associated inflammatory myopathies: similarities with seronegative polymyositis. *Ann Neurol* 29:474–481.

Johnson RW, Williams FM, Kazi S, Dimachkie MM, and Reveille JD (2003). Human immunodeficiency virus–associated polymyositis: a longitudinal study of outcome. *Arthritis Rheum* 49:172–178.

Keswani SC, Polley M, Pardo CA, Griffin JW, McArthur JC, and Hoke A (2003). Schwann cell chemokine receptors mediate HIV-1 gp120 toxicity to sensory neurons. *Ann Neurol* 54:287–296.

Kim YS, and Hollander H (1993). Polyradiculopathy due to cytomegalovirus: report of two cases in which improvement occurred after prolonged therapy and review of the literature. *Clin Infect Dis* 17:32 37.

Lange DJ, Britton CB, Younger DS, and Hays AP (1988). The neuromuscular manifestations of human immunodeficiency virus infections. *Arch Neurol* 45:1084–1088.

Lanska MJ, Lanska DJ, and Schmidley JW (1988). Syphilitic polyradiculopathy in an HIV-positive man. *Neurology* 38:1297–1301.

Leger JM, Henin D, Belec L, Mercier B, Cohen L, Bouche P, Hauw JJ, and Brunet P (1992). Lymphoma-induced polyradiculopathy in AIDS: two cases. *J Neurol* 239:132–134.

Lipkin WI, Parry G, Kiprov D, and Abrams D (1985). Inflammatory neuropathy in homosexual men with lymphadenopathy. *Neurology* 35:1479–1483.

Max MB, Culnane M, Schafer SC, Gracely RH, Walther DJ, Smoller B, and Dubner R (1987). Amitriptyline relieves diabetic neuropathy pain in patients with normal or depressed mood. *Neurology* 37:589–596.

McQuay H, Carroll D, Jadad AR, Wiffen P, and Moore A (1995). Anticonvulsant drugs for management of pain: a systematic review. *BMJ* 311:1047–1052.

Miller RG, Parry GJ, Pfaeffl W, Lang W, Lippert R, and Kiprov D (1988). The spectrum of peripheral neuropathy associated with ARC and AIDS. *Muscle Nerve* 11:857–863.

Miller RG, Storey JR, and Greco CM (1990). Ganciclovir in the treatment of progressive AIDS-related polyradiculopathy. *Neurology* 40:569–574.

Morgello S, and Simpson DM (1994). Multifocal cytomegalovirus demyelinative polyneuropathy associated with AIDS. *Muscle Nerve* 17:176–182.

Morgello S, Estanislao L, Simpson D, Geraci A, Di-Rocco A, Gerits P, Ryan E, Yakoushina T, Khan S, Mahboob R, Naseer M, Dorfman D, Sharp V, for the Manhattan HIV Brain Bank (2004). HIV-associated distal sensory polyneuropathy in the era of highly active antiretroviral therapy: the Manhattan HIV Brain Bank. *Arch Neurol* 61:546–551.

Moulignier A, Moulonguet A, Pialoux G, and Rozenbaum W (2001). Reversible ALS-like disorder in HIV infection. *Neurology* 57:995–1001.

Nath A, Kerman RH, Novak IS, and Wolinsky JS (1990). Immune studies in human immunodeficiency virus infection with myasthenia gravis: a case report. *Neurology* 40:581–583.

Pardo CA, McArthur JC, and Griffin JW (2001). HIV neuropathy: insights in the pathology of HIV peripheral nerve disease. *J Peripher Nerv Syst* 6:21–27.

Petito CK, Vecchio D, and Chen YT (1994). HIV antigen and DNA in AIDS spinal cords correlate with macrophage infiltration but not with vacuolar myelopathy. *J Neuropathol Exp Neurol* 53:86–94.

Polydefkis M, Yiannoutsos CT, Cohen BA, Hollander H, Schifitto G, Clifford DB, Simpson DM, Katzenstein D, Shriver S, Hauer P, Brown A, Haidich AB, Moo L, and McArthur JC (2002). Reduced intraepidermal nerve fiber density in HIV-associated sensory neuropathy. *Neurology* 58:115–119.

Purba JS, Hofman MA, Portegies P, Troost D, and Swaab DF (1993). Decreased number of oxytocin neurons in the paraventricular nucleus of the human hypothalamus in AIDS. *Brain* 116:795–809.

Raskin P, Donofrio PD, Rosenthal NR, Hewitt DJ, Jordan DM, Xiang J, Vinik AI, for the CAPSS-141 Study Group (2004). Topiramate vs. placebo in painful diabetic neuropathy: analgesic and metabolic effects. *Neurology* 63:865–873.

Roullet E, Assuerus V, Gozlan J, Ropert A, Said G, Baudrimont M, el Amrani M, Jacomet C, Duvivier C, and Gonzales-Canali G (1994). Cytomegalovirus multifocal neuropathy in AIDS: analysis of 15 consecutive cases. *Neurology* 44:2174–2182.

Rowbotham MC (1994). Postherpetic neuralgia. *Semin Neurol* 14:247–254.

Said G, Lacroix C, Chemouilli P, Goulon-Goeau C, Roullet E, Penaud D, de Broucker T, Meduri G, Vincent D, and Torchet M (1991). Cytomegalovirus neuropathy in acquired immunodeficiency syndrome: a clinical and pathological study. *Ann Neurol* 29:139–146.

Schifitto G, Yiannoutsos C, Simpson DM, Adornato BT, Singer EJ, Hollander H, Marra CM, Rubin M, Cohen BA, Tucker T, Koralnik IJ, Katzenstein D, Haidich B, Smith ME, Shriver S, Millar L, Clifford DB, McArthur JC, for the AIDS Clinical Trials Group Team 291 (2001). Long-term treatment with recombinant nerve growth factor for HIV-associated sensory neuropathy. *Neurology* 57:1313–1316.

Shlay JC, Chaloner K, Max MB, Flaws B, Reichelderfer P, Wentworth D, Hillman S, Brizz B, and Cohn DL (1998). Acupuncture and amitriptyline for pain due to HIV-related peripheral neuropathy: a randomized controlled trial. Terry Beirn Community Programs for Clinical Research on AIDS. *JAMA* 280:1590–1595.

Simpson DM, and Bender AN (1988). Human immunodeficiency virus–associated myopathy: analysis of 11 patients. *Ann Neurol* 24:79–84.

Simpson DM, and Tagliati M (1995). Nucleoside analogue-associated peripheral neuropathy in human immunodeficiency virus infection. *J Acquir Immune Defic Syndr Hum Retrovirol* 9:153–161.

Simpson DM, Bender AN, Farraye J, Mendelson SG, and Wolfe DE (1990). Human immunodeficiency virus wasting syndrome may represent a treatable myopathy. *Neurology* 40:535–538.

Simpson DM, Katzenstein DA, Hughes MD, Hammer SM, Williamson DL, Jiang Q, Pi JT (1998). Neuromuscular function in HIV infection: analysis of a placebo-controlled combination antiretroviral trial. AIDS Clinical Group 175/801 Study Team. *AIDS* 12:2425–2432.

Simpson DM, McArthur JC, Olney R, Clifford D, So Y, Ross D, Baird BJ, Barrett P, Hammer AE, for the Lamotrigine HIV Neuropathy Study Team (2003). Lamotrigine for HIV-associated painful sensory neuropathies: a placebo-controlled trial. *Neurology* 60:1508–1514.

Simpson D, Brown S, Sampson J, Estanislao L, Vilahu C, and Jermano J (2004). A single application of high-concentration trans-capsaicin leads to 12 weeks of pain relief in HIV-associated distal sensory polyneuropathy: results of an open label trial. Presented at the American Academy of Neurology 56th annual meeting, San Francisco.

So Y, and Olney R (1991). The natural history of mononeuritis multiplex and simplex in HIV infection. *Neurology* 41:375.

So YT, Holtzman DM, Abrams DI, and Olney RK (1988). Peripheral neuropathy associated with acquired immunodeficiency syndrome. Prevalence and clinical features from a population-based survey. *Arch Neurol* 45:945–948.

Tagliati M, Morgello S, and Simpson D (1998). Myopathy in HIV infection. In H Gendelman, S Lipton, L Epstein, and S Swindels (eds.), *Neurological and Neuropsychiatric Manifestations of HIV-1 Infection*. New York: Chapman and Hall.

Tagliati M, Grinnell J, Godbold J, and Simpson DM (1999). Peripheral nerve function in HIV infection: clinical, electrophysiologic, and laboratory findings. *Arch Neurol* 56:84–89.

Vafai A, and Berger M (2001). Zoster in patients infected with HIV: a review. *Am J Med Sci* 321:372–380.

Verma RK, Ziegler DK, and Kepes JJ (1990). HIV-related neuromuscular syndrome simulating motor neuron disease. *Neurology* 40:544–546.

Villa A, Foresti V, and Confalonieri F (1992). Autonomic nervous system dysfunction associated with

HIV infection in intravenous heroin users. *AIDS* 6:85–89.

Woolf CJ (2004). Dissecting out mechanisms responsible for peripheral neuropathic pain: implications for diagnosis and therapy. *Life Sci* 74:2605–2610.

[WHO] World Health Organization (1990). Cancer pain relief and palliative care. Report of a WHO expert committee. *World Health Organ Tech Rep Ser* 804:1–75.

Yarchoan R, Berg G, Brouwers P, Fischl MA, Spitzer AR, Wichman A, Grafman J, Thomas RV, Safai B, and Brunetti A (1987). Response of human-immunodeficiency-virus-associated neurological disease to 3′-azido-3′-deoxythymidine. *Lancet* 1:132–135.

Part VI

Risk Behaviors, HIV Transmission, and Adherence

Chapter 21

The Role of Psychiatric Disorders in HIV Transmission and Prevention

Christina S. Meade, Seth C. Kalichman, and David M. Stoff

Severe mental illness (SMI) describes a range of major psychiatric disorders that persist over time and cause extensive disability in social, occupational, and other important areas of functioning (Goldman et al., 1981; Schinnar et al., 1990). Such impairments are most often present in schizophrenia-spectrum disorders, bipolar disorders, and recurrent major depression. Common sequelae of SMI include substance abuse, unemployment, poverty, recurrent homelessness, and unstable relationships. An estimated 2.6% of American adults meet criteria for SMI during any 1-year period (Kessler et al., 1996).

Adults with SMI have been disproportionately affected by the HIV/AIDS epidemic. Comprehensive reviews of seroprevalence studies conducted throughout the 1990s revealed that approximately 8% of SMI adults living in large U.S. cities were HIV infected (Carey et al., 1995; Cournos and McKinnon, 1997). More recently, a multisite study reported HIV prevalence rates ranging from 2% to 5% in rural and large metropolitan sites, respectively (Rosenberg et al.,

2001a). The highest rates occur among persons with SMI who are also homeless and/or have a substance use disorder (Empfield et al., 1993; Silberstein et al., 1994; Rosenberg et al., 2001a). These rates are many times higher than the estimated HIV prevalence of 0.6% in the general U.S. population (UNAIDS, 2006). Persons with SMI are also at increased risk for other blood-borne and sexually transmitted diseases. For example, in a large sample of SMI adults, the prevalence rates of hepatitis B and C were 23% and 20%, respectively (Rosenberg et al., 2001a).

Adults with SMI engage in high rates of sexual and drug use behaviors associated with HIV transmission, including multiple sexual partnerships, unprotected intercourse in non-monogamous relationships, sex trade for money, drugs, or other survival resources, and injection drug use. As such, SMI is a risk factor for HIV risk behavior and infection. Conversely, psychiatric illness can also develop secondary to HIV infection, either directly through neurological changes or indirectly through psychosocial stressors (Treisman et al., 1998; Koutsilieri et al., 2002). Indeed, the majority of HIV-infected persons suffer from mental illness, including mood, anxiety, or psychotic disorders (Bing et al., 2001; Klinkenberg and Sacks, 2004). Given the high rate of HIV infection and HIV risk behavior among adults with SMI, the potential for spread of HIV in this population remains high. The objectives of this chapter are to (1) document the prevalence of HIV risk behavior among SMI adults; (2) discuss the ways in which psychiatric disorders directly and indirectly contribute HIV risk behavior, infection, and disease progression; (3) describe primary HIV prevention interventions; and (4) provide suggestions for clinical care.

PREVALENCE OF HIV RISK BEHAVIOR AMONG PERSONS WITH SEVERE MENTAL ILLNESS

In a systematic review of the literature, Meade and Sikkema (2005) identified 52 independent studies examining HIV risk behavior among SMI adults. Using weighted means to account for sample size, the prevalence of the following HIV risk factors were calculated: sexual activity, multiple partners, unprotected intercourse, sex trade, history of sexually transmitted infection, and injection drug use (see Table 21.1). Across U.S. studies, the majority of SMI adults had had sex in the past year. Approximately half of sexually active participants had been with multiple partners and never used condoms. Strikingly, nearly a quarter reported a history of sex trade, and a third had a history of sexually transmitted infection. Nearly a quarter had ever injected drugs; most injection drug users had shared needles, but only 4% were active within the past year. Based on six studies that included a comparison group, SMI adults were more likely than demographically similar adults without SMI to engage in certain behaviors that place them at risk for HIV, specifically multiple partners, sex trade, and injection drug use, but not necessarily sexual activity or unprotected intercourse. Elevated rates of HIV risk behavior have also been reported among SMI adults living in other countries, including Italy (Grassi et al., 1999), India (Chandra et al., 2003), and Australia (Davidson et al., 2001). It is notable, however, that the rate of HIV risk behavior reported in international samples was consistently lower than that in U.S. samples.

In the only study known to have examined the rates of HIV risk behavior among HIV-infected persons with SMI, 56% of participants had had sex in the past 6 months (Tucker et al., 2003). Among the sexually active, 48% had sex with multiple partners, 37% had unprotected intercourse, and 24% engaged in sex trade. Overall, 12% had injected drugs in the past 12 months. The prevalence of mental health problems among people living with HIV/AIDS, including those who continue to engage in high-risk practices, also suggests that these conditions often precede HIV infection and complicate subsequent behavior change. Thus, a substantial proportion of adults with SMI continue to engage in sexual and drug risk behaviors even after they are infected with HIV.

EFFECTS OF PSYCHIATRIC DISORDERS ON HIV RISK BEHAVIOR

Sexual and drug risk behaviors are influenced by multiple factors across several psychosocial domains, including psychiatric illness, substance use, traumatic experience, cognitive-behavioral factors, and social relationships. On the basis of empirical research, Meade and Sikkema (2005) developed a conceptual model of HIV risk behavior among SMI adults. Figure 21.1 represents an adaptation of this multifactorial and interactive model, with the five psychosocial domains representing mediating and moderating associations. In particular, psychiatric illness may contribute to HIV risk behavior directly through cognitive, emotional, social, and behavioral functioning, as well as indirectly through psychosocial sequelae such as substance abuse, trauma, and homelessness. Below we examine these direct and indirect effects.

Direct Effects of Psychiatric Disorders on HIV Risk Behavior

Table 21.2 lists a range of cognitive, emotional, social, and behavioral impairments associated with SMI, which can directly contribute to sexual risk behavior. For example, poor judgment and decision making may impair accurate risk assessment and promote sexual involvement with risky partners. Impaired decision making, negative view of the future, and decreased impulse control may reduce motivation to use condoms. Difficulty maintaining relationships may lead

TABLE 21.1. Self-Reported Prevalence Rates of HIV Risk Factors among Adults with Severe Mental Illness

Risk Factor	n	U.S. Studies Weighted Mean (range)	n	International Studies Weighted Mean (range)
Sexual Activity*				
Past year	14	60.07% (51%–74%)	7	47.05% (42%–73%)
Past 3 months	11	45.91% (32%–65%)	1	33%
Multiple (2+) Partners†				
Past year	12	43.24% (28%–69%)	5	34.99% (31%–46%)
Past 3 months	6	34.54% (23%–46%)	1	13%
Condom Use: Consistent†				
Past year	4	17.01% (8%–32%)	1	36%
Past 3 months	5	33.48% (20%–49%)	1	34%
Condom Use: Never†				
Past year	6	45.72% (29%–59%)	0	N/A
Past 3 months	4	41.76% (26%–66%)	0	N/A
Sex Trade				
Ever	5	22.43% (12%–45%)	3	4.60% (3%–12%)
Past year	12	13.66% (3%–42%)	3	7.12% (2%–11%)
History of Sexually Transmitted Infections				
Ever	17	32.94% (16%–54%)	2	6%–11%
Past year	4	8.02% (3%–10%)	1	5%
Injection Drug Use				
Ever	15	22.13% (15%–37%)	2	16.35% (14%–23%)
Past year	8	4.17% (1%–8%)	1	6%
Needle Sharing††				
Ever	3	64.91% (47%–73%)	2	38.46% (15%–53%)
Past year	2	55.56% (55%–57%)	1	38%

*Excluding studies with sexual activity as an eligibility criterion.

†Among sexually active participants only.

††Among injection drug users only.

to multiple partnerships, and poor relationship quality may lead to non-monogamous relationships. Poor negotiation skills may reduce the likelihood of using condoms with a resistant partner, and poor assertiveness skills and low self-esteem may lead to sexual exploitation. In a large sample of adults with SMI, greater psychiatric symptoms predicted HIV risk behavior (Rosenberg et al., 2001b). Among a sample of persons with schizophrenia, greater general psychopathology was associated with sexual activity (Cournos et al., 1994). Furthermore, those with multiple sex partners had lower levels of adaptive functioning, more positive psychotic symptoms, and a greater likelihood of delusions than did their monogamous and abstinent counterparts (Cournos et al., 1994). Among patients with mixed diagnoses, symptoms of behavioral disinhibition and fewer symptoms of disorganized thought predicted sexual activity (McKinnon et al., 1996). In addition, positive symptoms were associated with multiple partners, the subset of positive

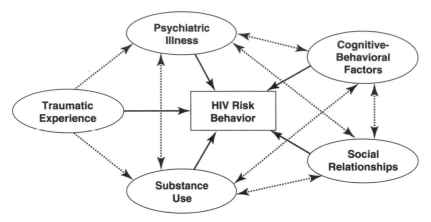

FIGURE 21.1. Conceptual model of HIV risk behavior among adults with SMI (adapted from Meade and Sikkema, 2005).

symptoms classified as excitement symptoms (e.g., mania) with sex trade, and depressed or anxious symptoms with a history of sexually transmitted diseases; there was no association between psychiatric symptoms and condom use (McKinnon et al., 1996). In an independent sample, positive symptoms were associated with injection drug use, but overall psychopathology and negative symptoms were not (Horwath et al., 1996). In sum, research supports a general association between severity of psychopathology and HIV risk behavior. However, there is still insufficient data to determine how certain symptom clusters (e.g., depression, mania, paranoia) or types of impairments (e.g., cognitive, social, behavioral) may relate to specific HIV risk behaviors among SMI adults.

Aspects of mood disorders in particular may directly impact sexuality. Hypersexuality is a common symptom of mania, which may lead to increased sexual activity and multiple partnerships. Manic episodes are also characterized by impulsivity, poor judgment, and excessive involvement in pleasurable and high-risk behaviors, which, when coupled with hypersexuality, may lead to sex with strangers or prostitutes and reduced condom use. In one study of patients with mood disorders, individuals with bipolar disorder were more likely to report increased sexual activity during emotional crises (Sacks and Dermatis, 1994). In contrast, depression commonly leads to diminished libido and sexual dysfunction, and therefore an overall reduction in sexual activity. Despite the commonly recognized association between mood symptoms and sexuality, however, there has been remarkably little research on HIV risk behavior among persons with mood disorders.

Consistently, persons with schizophrenia-spectrum disorders report lower rates of sexual activity and frequency of intercourse compared to those with other major psychiatric disorders (McKinnon et al., 1996; Carey et al., 2001, 2004b; Chandra et al., 2003). Negative symptoms (e.g., affective flattening, avolition, anergia) and other associated features (e.g., hypoactivity, depressed mood) may reduce sexual desire. In addition, grossly disorganized behavior and odd personality traits may impair an individual's ability to establish

TABLE 21.2. Characteristics of Severe Mental Illness Relevant to HIV Risk Behavior

Area of Functioning	Specific Impairments
Cognitive	Poor judgment
	Poor reality testing
	Poor decision making
	Negative view of the future
	Low self-esteem (e.g., worthlessness)
Emotional	Affective lability
	Generalized avolition and anergia
Social	Difficulty initiating and maintaining relationships
	Poor communication skills (e.g., assertiveness, negotiation)
	Poor relationship quality (e.g., high conflict, low intimacy)
Behavioral	Decreased impulse control
	Self-destructive tendencies
Sexual	Hypersexuality
	Decreased libido
	Sexual dysfunction

sexual partners. Previous research suggests that persons with psychotic disorders have social skills deficits, social anxiety, relationship difficulties, and loneliness that may impact sexual functioning (Mueser et al., 1991; Grant et al., 2001). Thus, persons with schizophrenia-spectrum disorders may benefit from adjunctive social skills training to help them develop satisfying and longer-lasting relationships. However, psychiatric diagnosis is generally unrelated to other HIV risk factors, such as multiple partners, condom use, history of sexually transmitted infection, or injection drug use (e.g., Kelly et al., 1995; Horwath et al., 1996; McKinnon et al., 1996; Susser et al., 1997; Levounis et al., 2002). This suggests that HIV prevention interventions might effectively target the SMI population broadly, rather than persons with specific diagnoses.

Approximately 30%–60% of adults with SMI have a comorbid personality disorder, including borderline and antisocial (Tyrer et al., 2000). Borderline personality disorder is characterized by emotional dysregulation, turbulent relationships, and impulsivity, each of which may lead to sexual risk behavior. In a study of women hospitalized for borderline personality disorder, nearly half reported that they had impulsively entered into sexual relationships with partners they did not know well (Hull et al., 1993). In another sample of inpatients diagnosed with borderline personality disorder, half reported sexual relationship difficulties (Zanarini et al., 2003). Antisocial personality disorder, which is characterized by a pervasive pattern of disregard for and violation of the rights of others, may also be associated with increased sexual risk behavior. In other populations, individuals with antisocial personality disorders were more likely to have multiple sex partners and less likely to use condoms (e.g., Biglan et al., 1990; Gill et al., 1992; Brooner et al., 1993; Kelley and Petry, 2000). Among SMI adults, co-occurring personality disorder was found to be associated with increased sexual risk behavior, including meeting partners in psychiatric clinics and sexual exploitation (Kalichman et al., 1994; Sacks and Dermatis, 1994).

Indirect Effects of Psychiatric Disorders on HIV Risk Behavior

Substance Use

Injection drug use serves as a direct route of transmission for HIV. Substance abuse in general can have indirect effects on sexual risk behavior through its impact on judgment and decision making. In addition, exchange of sex for crack and other drugs confers high risk for HIV transmission. Furthermore, substance abusers may be part of a social network comprised of high-risk partners and in which sexual risk behavior is normative.

Co-occurring substance use disorders are common among SMI adults, with estimates ranging from 25% to 65% across diagnoses (Regier et al., 1990). Rates of HIV infection among dually diagnosed patients are exceptionally high, ranging from 4% to 23% (Silberstein et al., 1994; Krakow et al., 1998; Rahav et al., 1998; Rosenberg et al., 2001a; Klinkenberg et al., 2003). In a large, multisite study, participants with current substance use disorder were nearly three times more likely than persons with no current substance use disorders to be HIV seropositive (4.3% vs. 1.5%) (Rosenberg et al., 2001). Individuals with lifetime substance use disorders are also more likely to have a history of sexually transmitted infection (McKinnon et al., 2001; Carey et al., 2004b).

Studies consistently find that non-injection substance use is associated with increased HIV risk behavior (e.g., Kalichman et al., 1994; Carey et al., 2001; Weinhardt et al., 2001; Chandra et al., 2003). However, the association between substance abuse and specific sexual risk behaviors is less clear. Sexual activity was associated with any substance use and greater substance abuse severity (Carey et al., 1999, 2001) but not lifetime substance use disorder (McKinnon et al., 2001). Another study found stepwise differences, with active substance abusers engaging in the highest rates of sexual activity, followed by persons with remitted substance use disorder, and finally those with no history of substance use disorder (Meade, 2006). Unprotected intercourse was associated with cocaine abuse but not alcohol abuse among homeless men (Susser et al., 1995) and with substance use before sex among men but not women (Menon and Pomerantz, 1997). An event-level analysis showed no association between alcohol use and condom use (Weinhardt et al., 2001). Furthermore, among substance abusers, neither drug of choice nor duration, quantity, or frequency of substance use was related to condom use (Kim et al., 1992; Levounis et al., 2002). Substance abuse before sex was associated with having a risky partner among men but not women (Menon and Pomerantz, 1997), but lifetime substance use disorder and substance abuse severity were not associated with number or risk of partners or with sex trade

(McKinnon et al., 2001; Carey et al., 2004b). A recent study found that lifetime substance use disorder predicted partner-related risk, whereas active substance abuse was associated with more unprotected intercourse (Meade, 2006). Finally, substance dependence was associated with injection drug use (Horwath et al., 1996), and needle sharing was more common among persons who reported cocaine as their drug of choice (Levounis et al., 2002). In sum, research suggests that persons dually diagnosed with SMI and substance use disorders are at particularly high risk for HIV infection, though the mechanisms through which substance abuse contributes to sexual risk behavior are yet to be delineated.

Traumatic Experience

Traumatic life experiences are common among persons with SMI, further exacerbating the impact of psychiatric illness on health. In one sample of SMI adults, 98% reported exposure to at least one traumatic event and 43% met criteria for posttraumatic stress disorder (Mueser et al., 1998). Sexual abuse is particularly common, with 31%–65% of women and 29%–35% of men with SMI self-reporting a childhood history (e.g., Goodman et al., 1995; Cloitre et al., 1996). Among adults with SMI, childhood sexual abuse was associated with multiple sexual partnerships, unprotected intercourse, and sex trade (Goodman and Fallot, 1998; Rosenberg et al., 2001b). One study found that childhood sexual abuse was indirectly related to HIV risk through drug use but not sexual risk behavior, and the effect of adult sexual abuse was mediated by childhood sexual abuse (Rosenberg et al., 2001b). Furthermore, greater trauma exposure of all types was related to increased HIV risk, but diagnosis of posttraumatic stress disorder was not (Rosenberg et al., 2001b). Childhood physical abuse was found to be unrelated to HIV risk behavior, suggesting specificity in the association between sexually traumatic experiences and subsequent sexual risk behavior (Goodman and Fallot, 1998; Rosenberg et al., 2001b).

Socioeconomic Factors

Many adults with SMI are socioeconomically disadvantaged, have transient living situations, and have small social support networks (Canton et al., 1995; Goldberg et al., 2003). These factors likely place persons with SMI in more high-risk situations than persons who are not comparatively disadvantaged. Indeed, persons with SMI who are homeless have particularly high rates of HIV infection (e.g., Empfield et al., 1993; Susser et al., 1996), and individuals living in urban settings appear to be at greater risk than those in rural areas (Brunette et al., 1999). Furthermore, persons with SMI who lack resources may experience significant pressure to trade sex for money or goods (Goodman and Fallot, 1998; Butterfield et al., 2003). A substantial proportion of SMI adults encounter high-risk situations, including sexual coercion, when relationships are connected with access to material resources (Otto-Salaj et al., 1998).

CONSEQUENCES OF PSYCHIATRIC DISORDERS ON HIV INFECTION AND DISEASE PROGRESSION

Psychiatric disorders can adversely impact HIV infection and disease progression. Immunological changes associated with depression affect HIV entry and replication, thereby increasing risk of infection among exposed individuals (Gorman et al., 1991; Clerici et al., 1997; Leserman, 2003). Among HIV-infected individuals, depression is associated with more rapid progression to AIDS and higher mortality rates (Burack et al., 1993; Leserman et al., 2000; Ickovics et al., 2001). In addition to the neuropsychiatric impact of depression on HIV disease progression, depression is associated with poor adherence to antiretroviral treatment and deterioration in psychosocial functioning (Starace et al., 2002). Psychosis may also alter the course of HIV infection by impairing immune functioning and influencing behavior (Sewell, 1996; Hinkin et al., 2001), though relatively less is known about the impact of psychosis on HIV infection and disease progression. Thus, treatment of psychiatric disorders among HIV-infected adults is critical for improving outcomes. Adults with SMI may also require specialized interventions to improve access to HIV treatment and adherence to both antiviral and psychiatric medications (Rosenberg et al., 2004).

PRIMARY HIV PREVENTION INTERVENTIONS FOR ADULTS WITH SEVERE MENTAL ILLNESS

Since the mid-1990s, a number of theory-based behavioral risk reduction interventions have been developed for adults with SMI. These interventions used cognitive-behavioral strategies to increase knowledge about HIV/AIDS and risk behaviors, enhance motivation for behavioral risk reduction, and strengthen self-efficacy and skills for behavioral risk reduction. Practice exercises and role-plays addressed personal triggers for HIV risk behavior, problem solving of risk reduction strategies, proper condom use and cleaning of injection drug equipment, and assertiveness and negotiation skills for communicating with sex partners. All interventions were delivered in small-group formats, with increasingly sophisticated designs.

The first randomized, controlled trial conducted among men and women with SMI compared a four-session HIV prevention intervention to a waitlist control (Kalichman et al., 1995). Participants in the HIV prevention intervention reported greater HIV-related knowledge, greater frequency of condom use, and stronger intentions to use condoms and insist on condom use with resistant partners. Within-subject comparisons showed gains in both HIV- and condom-related knowledge, as well as reduced frequency of unprotected intercourse and increased percentage of condom use.

Subsequently, a larger trial compared a seven-session HIV prevention intervention to a structurally equivalent health promotion intervention that focused on personal relationships, stress reduction, nutritional health, cancer and heart disease prevention, and general sexual health (Otto-Salaj et al., 2000). Participants in the HIV prevention intervention increased their frequency of condom use, had a higher percentage of protected vaginal intercourse occasions, and held more positive attitudes toward using condoms. Notably, there were large gender differences in response to the intervention. Men showed significant change only in HIV risk knowledge scores, while women showed significant changes in attitudes toward condom use, behavioral intentions of reducing risk, and sexual behavior.

Given possible gender differences, HIV prevention interventions may need to address the unique needs of women and men. A small pilot study sought to increase sexual assertiveness among women (Weinhardt et al., 1998). Participants were randomly assigned to either a 10-session assertiveness training intervention or a waitlist control condition. Compared with controls, women in the intervention group increased their assertiveness skill, HIV knowledge, and frequency of condom use. Thus, assertiveness training may be an important component of HIV prevention for women.

Another HIV prevention intervention was designed specifically for homeless men with SMI, using activities that are central to life in a shelter: competitive games, storytelling, and watching videos (Susser et al., 1998). This 15-session program was compared to a two-session control intervention. Among sexually active men, the mean score on a sexual risk index was three times lower for participants in the HIV prevention intervention than the score for those in the control intervention. However, participants in the intervention condition who had substance dependence demonstrated no reduction in sexual risk behavior compared to those in the control condition (Berkman et al., 2005), a finding suggesting the importance of substance abuse treatment for dually diagnosed patients.

In the most rigorous and statistically powered intervention trial with psychiatric patients to date, a 10-session HIV risk reduction intervention was tested against a structurally equivalent substance use reduction intervention (Carey et al., 2004a). The addition of the latter intervention is an important advance in intervention design because of the substantial moderating role that substance use can have on sexual risk behavior. Participants were randomly assigned to either the HIV prevention intervention, the substance use reduction intervention, or a standard-of-care group. Patients receiving the HIV prevention intervention reported less unprotected sex, fewer casual sex partners, fewer new sexually transmitted infections, more safer-sex communications, improved HIV knowledge, more positive attitudes toward condom use, stronger intentions to use condoms, and improved behavioral skills compared to patients in the other two conditions. Exploratory analyses found that female patients and patients diagnosed with major depressive disorder were more likely to benefit from the HIV risk reduction intervention.

Community-level interventions have become increasingly recognized as an important component of HIV prevention. Two innovative interventions have been developed for SMI adults. In the first, men and women were taught to become advocates for behavior change, in addition to receiving cognitive-behavioral skills for reducing individual HIV risk behaviors. Participants were randomly assigned to either a single-session HIV/AIDS education group, a seven-session cognitive-behavioral HIV risk reduction group, or a seven-session advocacy training group. Both the standard HIV risk reduction and the advocacy training interventions incorporated HIV/AIDS education and cognitive-behavioral risk reduction exercises. However, the advocacy training intervention consolidated these elements in the first half of the sessions, and added advocacy training in the remaining sessions. Compared to participants in the other two conditions, participants in the advocacy training intervention had fewer sex partners, used condoms more frequently, and had fewer occasions of unprotected sexual intercourse at follow-up. The second trial tested the feasibility of a community-level HIV prevention intervention for SMI adults living in supportive housing programs (Sikkema et al., 2007). The first component of this intervention consisted of six sessions of education and cognitive-behavioral skills building. Subsequent components involved the creation of peer norms and social-environmental reinforcement supportive of HIV risk reduction. Specifically, peer leaders were systematically identified and trained to communicate their HIV risk reduction messages, and to develop and implement activities within the supportive housing program to promote and reinforce efforts at behavior change. In addition, staff was trained to assess for HIV risk behavior, encourage risk reduction, and support efforts to change behavior. Results demonstrated significant improvements in condom use and self-efficacy in sexual communication, attitudes toward condom use, and behavioral intentions to use condoms following both the skills-building and community components, with improvements in HIV/AIDS knowledge and indications of sexual behavior change following the community component only.

In summary, a number of promising HIV prevention interventions have been developed for adults with SMI. Unfortunately, these interventions are limited by relatively modest and diminishing effects on sexual risk reduction (Johnson-Masotti et al., 2003). Moreover, they have not been widely disseminated from clinical trials into mental health care settings (Johnson-Masotti et al., 2003). Improvements are needed to promote more sustainable and meaningful behavior change. In addition to teaching HIV risk reduction skills, interventions must address substance abuse, sexual trauma, and other psychosocial risk factors. Interventions will likely need to occur on multiple levels and within the context of integrated services that address the full range of needs of SMI adults. The next phase of research should focus on the development and evaluation of structural, community, and social-network components that also have case management to promote more extensive risk reduction, and on trans-

lation of research results into ongoing mental health programs serving the SMI population.

SUGGESTIONS FOR CLINICAL PRACTICE

Given the high rate of sexual risk behavior among adults with SMI, routine HIV risk assessment for all psychiatric patients is indicated. Specifically, patients should be asked about sexual and drug use behaviors (e.g., current activity, number of partners, sex trade, condom use, injection drug use and needle sharing) and risk factors (e.g., sexual abuse, substance use, partner characteristics). All patients endorsing HIV risk behaviors should be offered HIV testing, ideally within the mental health agency to facilitate access and follow-up. Patients who test positive might then be referred for further medical evaluation, treatment, and secondary prevention services. Rosenberg and colleagues (2004) developed a best-practices intervention model for SMI adults that provides risk screening, testing for HIV and hepatitis, immunization for hepatitis A and B, risk reduction counseling, and treatment referral for infected persons. This brief intervention, which is delivered at community mental health centers by a mobile team of specialists, has been found to be both feasible and efficacious.

More intensive interventions are also needed to promote HIV risk reduction among SMI adults. To account for psychosocial risk factors, the most promising interventions will likely be multidimensional and occur at the individual, group, and community level. At the individual level, psychotherapy and medication are essential for treating psychiatric symptoms, intrapsychic barriers, and interpersonal difficulties that may underlie HIV risk behavior among adults with SMI. For example, mood stabilization, trauma recovery, and social-skills training may be essential precursors to risk reduction. Case management may be an important adjunctive service to facilitate and maintain behavior change. Given the high rates of HIV risk behavior among persons with substance use disorders and/or trauma histories, it may also be effective to integrate HIV prevention into existing treatments for substance abuse and trauma recovery. As discussed above, small-group interventions based on cognitive-behavioral change principles have been effective in promoting short-term behavioral change. Such group interventions should be integrated into ongoing mental health treatment settings. Community-level interventions delivered in supportive housing programs should also focus on maintenance of risk reduction, which may require booster sessions and/or a broader array of prevention services.

CONCLUSION

The high rates of HIV infection and HIV risk behavior among persons with SMI suggest the potential for rapid spread of HIV among this population, underscoring the need for targeted HIV risk reduction. Given the multiple psychiatric, medical, and psychosocial needs of persons with SMI, HIV prevention interventions should be integrated into existing services. This may not only improve outcomes but also increase participation and engagement, be resource efficient, and have wide dissemination potential. In addition, the effective treatment of substance abuse and sexual trauma should be prioritized. Mental health professionals are in an ideal position to assess HIV risk, encourage HIV testing, promote risk reduction, and thereby stem the HIV/AIDS epidemic among this vulnerable population.

ACKNOWLEDGMENTS   The opinions expressed herein are the views of the authors and do not necessarily reflect the official position of the National Institute of Mental Health or any other part of the U.S. Department of Health and Human Services.

References

Berkman A, Pilowsky DJ, Zybert PA, Leu C-S, Sohler N, and Susser E (2005). The impact of substance dependence on HIV sexual risk-reduction among men with severe mental illness. *AIDS Care* 17: 635–639.

Biglan A, Metzler CW, Wirt R, Ary D, Noell J, Ochs L, French C, and Hood D (1990). Social and behavioral factors associated with high-risk sexual behavior among adolescents. *J Behav Med* 13:245–261.

Bing EG, Burnam MA, Longshore D, Fleishman JA, Sherbourne CD, London AS, Turner BJ, Eggan F, Beckman R, Vitiello B, Morton SC, Orlando M, Bozzette SA, Ortiz-Barron L, and Shapiro M (2001). Psychiatric disorders and drug use among human immunodeficiency virus–infected adults in the United States. *Arch Gen Psychiatry* 58:721–728.

Brooner RK, Greenfield L, Schmidt CW, and Bigelow GE (1993). Antisocial personality disorder and HIV infection among intravenous drug abusers. *Am J Psychiatry* 150:53–58.

Brunette M, Rosenberg SD, Goodman LA, Mueser K, Osher FC, Vidaver R, Auciello P, Wolford G, and Drake R (1999). HIV risk factors among people with severe mental illness in urban and rural areas. *Psychiatr Serv* 50:556–558.

Burack JH, Barrett DC, Stall RD, Chesney MA, Ekstrand ML, and Coates TJ (1993). Depressive symptoms and CD4 lymphocyte decline among HIV-infected men. *JAMA* 270:2568–2573.

Butterfield MI, Bosworth HB, Meador KG, Stechuchak KM, Essock SM, Osher FC, Goodman LA, Swanson JW, Bastian LA, and Horner RD (2003). Gender differences in hepatitis C infection and risks among persons with severe mental illness. *Psychiatr Serv* 54:848–853.

Canton CL, Shrout PE, Dominguez B, Eagle PF, Opler LA, and Cournos F (1995). Risk factors for homelessness among women with schizophrenia. *Am J Public Health* 85:1153–1156.

Carey MP, Weinhardt LS, and Carey KB (1995). Prevalence of infection with HIV among the seriously mentally ill: review of research and implications for practice. *Prof Psychol Res Prac* 26:262–268.

Carey MP, Carey KB, Gleason JR, Gordon CM, and Brewer KK (1999). HIV-risk behavior among outpatients at a state psychiatric hospital: prevalence and risk modeling. *Behav Ther* 30:389–406.

Carey MP, Carey KB, Maisto SA, Gordon CM, and Vanable PA (2001). Prevalence and correlates of sexual activity and HIV-related risk behavior among psychiatric outpatients. *J Consult Clin Psychol* 69: 846–850.

Carey MP, Carey KB, Maisto SA, Gordon CM, Schroder KEE, and Vanable PA (2004a). Reducing HIV-risk behavior among adults receiving outpatient psychiatric treatment: results from a randomized controlled trial. *J Consult Clin Psychol* 72:252–268.

Carey MP, Carey KB, Maisto SA, Schroder KEE, Vanable PA, and Gordon CM (2004b). HIV risk behavior among psychiatric outpatients: association with psychiatric disorder, substance use disorder, and gender. *J Nerv Ment Dis* 192:289–296.

Chandra PS, Carey MP, Carey KB, Prasada Rao PSDV, Jairam KR, and Thomas T (2003). HIV risk behavior among psychiatric inpatients: results from a hospital-wide screening study in southern India. *Int J STD AIDS* 14:532–538.

Clerici M, Trabattoni D, Piconi S, Fusi ML, Ruzzante S, Clerici C, and Villa ML (1997). A possible role for the cortisol/anticortisols imbalance in the progression of human immunodeficiency virus. *Psychoneuroendocrinology* 22:S27–S31.

Cloitre M, Tardiff K, Marzuk PM, Leon AC, and Potera L (1996). Childhood abuse and subsequent assault among female inpatients. *J Trauma Stress* 9:473–482.

Cournos F, and McKinnon K (1997). HIV seroprevalence among people with severe mental illness in the United States: a critical review. *Clin Psychol Rev* 17:259–269.

Cournos F, Guido JR, Coomaraswamy S, Meyer-Bahlburg H, Sugden R, and Horwath W (1994). Sexual activity and risk of HIV infection among patients with schizophrenia. *Am J Psychiatry* 151:228–232.

Davidson S, Judd F, Jolley D, Hocking B, Thompson S, and Hyland B (2001). Risk factors for HIV/AIDS and hepatitis C among the chronically mentally ill. *Aust N Z J Psychiatry* 35:203–209.

Empfield M, Cournos F, Meyer I, McKinnon K, Horwath E, Silver M, Schrage H, and Herman R (1993). HIV seroprevalence among homeless patients admitted to a psychiatric inpatient unit. *Am J Psychiatry* 150:47–52.

Gill K, Nolimal D, and Crowley T (1992). Antisocial personality disorder, HIV risk behavior, and retention in methadone maintenance therapy. *Drug Alcohol Depend* 30:247–252.

Goldberg RW, Rollins AL, and Lehman AF (2003). Social network correlates among people with psychiatric disabilities. *Psychiatr Rehabil J* 26:393–402.

Goldman HH, Gattozzi AA, and Taube CA (1981). Defining and counting the chronically mentally ill. *Hosp Community Psychiatry* 32:21–27.

Goodman LA, and Fallot RD (1998). HIV risk-behavior in poor urban women with serious mental illness: association with childhood physical and sexual abuse. *Am J Orthopsychiatry* 68:73–83.

Gorman JM, Kertzner R, Cooper T, Goetz RR, Lagomasino I, Novacenko H, Williams JB, Stern Y, Mayeux R, and Ehrhardt AA (1991). Glucocorticoid level and neuropsychiatric symptoms in homosexual men with HIV infection. *Am J Psychiatry* 148:41–45

Grant C, Addington J, Addington D, and Konnert C (2001). Social functioning in first- and multiple-episode schizophrenia. *Can J Psychiatry* 46:746–749.

Grassi L, Pavanati M, Cardelli R, Ferri S, and Peron L (1999). HIV-risk behavior and knowledge about HIV/AIDS among patients with schizophrenia. *Psychol Med* 29:171–179.

Goodman LA, Dutton MA, and Harris M (1995). Episodically homeless women with serious mental illness: prevalence of physical and sexual assault. *Am J Orthopsychiatry* 65:468–478.

Hinkin CH, Castellon SA, Atkinson JH, and Goodkin K (2001). Neuropyschiatric aspects of HIV infection among older adults. *J Clin Epidemiol* 54:S44–S52.

Horwath W, Cournos F, McKinnon K, Guido JR, and Herman R (1996). Illicit drug injection among psychiatric patients without a primary substance use disorder. *Psychiatr Serv* 47:181–185.

Hull JW, Clarkin JF, and Yeomans F (1993). Borderline personality disorder and impulsive sexual behavior. *Hosp Community Psychiatry* 44:1000–1002.

Ickovics JR, Hamburger ME, Vlahov D, Schoenbaum EE, Schuman P, Boland RJ, and Moore J (2001). Mortality, CD4 cell count decline, and depressive symptoms among HIV-seropositive women: longitudinal analysis from the HIV epidemiology research study. *JAMA* 285:1466–1474.

Johnson-Masotti AP, Weinhardt LS, Pinkerton SD, and Otto-Salaj LL (2003). Efficacy and cost-effectiveness of the first generation of HIV prevention interventions for people with severe and persistent mental illness. *J Ment Health Policy Econ* 6:23–35.

Kalichman SC, Kelly JA, Johnson JR, and Bulto M (1994). Factors associated with risk for HIV infection among chronic mentally ill adults. *Am J Psychiatry* 151:221–227.

Kalichman SC, Sikkema KJ, Kelly JA, and Bulto M (1995). Use of a brief behavioral skills intervention to prevent HIV infection among chronic mentally ill adults. *Psychiatr Serv* 46:275–280.

Kelley JL, and Petry NM (2000). HIV risk behaviors in male substance abusers with and without antisocial personality disorder. *Subst Abuse Treat* 19:59–66.

Kelly JA, Murphy DA, Sikkema KJ, Somlai AM, Mulry GW, Fernandez MI, Miller JG, and Stevenson LY (1995). Predictors of high and low levels of HIV risk behavior among adults with chronic mental illness. *Psychiatr Serv* 46:813–818.

Kessler RC, Berglund PA, Zhao S, Leaf PJ, Kouzis AC, Bruce ML, Friedman RM, Grossier RC, Kennedy C, Narrow WE, Kuehnel TG, Laska EM, Manderscheid RW, Rosenheck RA, Santoni TW, and Schneier M (1996). The 12-month prevalence and correlates of serious mental illness. In RW Manderscheid and MA Sonnenschein (eds.), *Mental Health, United States, 1996* (pp. 59–70). Washington, DC: U.S. Government Printing Office.

Kim A, Galanter M, Castaneda R, Lifshutz H, and Franco H (1992). Crack cocaine use and sexual behavior among psychiatric inpatients. *Am J Drug Alcohol Abuse* 18:235–246.

Klinkenberg WD, and Sacks S (2004). Mental disorders and drug abuse in persons living with HIV/AIDS. *AIDS Care* 16:S22–S42.

Klinkenberg WD, Caslyn RJ, Morse GA, Yonker RD, McCudden S, Ketema F, and Constantine NT (2003). Prevalence of human immunodeficiency virus, hepatitis B, and hepatitis C among homeless persons with co-occurring severe mental illness and substance use disorders. *Compr Psychiatry* 44:293–302.

Koutsilieri E, Scheller C, Sopper S, ter Meulen V, and Riederer P (2002). Psychiatric complications in human immunodeficiency virus infection. *J Neurovirol* 8(Suppl. 2):S129–S133

Krakow DS, Galanter M, Dermatis H, and Westreich LM (1998). HIV risk factors in dually diagnosed patients. *Am J Addict* 7:74–80.

Leserman J (2003). HIV disease progression: depression, stress, and possible mechanisms. *Biol Psychiatry* 54:295–306.

Leserman J, Petito JM, Golden RN, Gaynes BN, Gu H, Perkins DO, Silva SG, Folds JD, and Evans DL (2000). Impact of stressful life events, depression, social support, coping, and cortisol on progression to AIDS. *Am J Psychiatry* 157:1221–1228.

Levounis P, Galanter M, Dermatis H, Hamowy A, and DeLeon G (2002). Correlates of HIV transmission risk factors and considerations for interventions for homeless, chemically addicted and mentally ill patients. *J Addict Dis* 21:61–72.

McKinnon K, Cournos F, Sugden R, Guido JR, and Herman R (1996). The relative contributions of psychiatric symptoms and AIDS knowledge to HIV risk behaviors among people with severe mental illness. *J Clin Psychiatry* 57:506–513.

McKinnon K, Cournos F, and Herman R (2001). A lifetime alcohol or other drug use disorder and specific psychiatric symptoms predict sexual risk and HIV infection among people with severe mental illness. *AIDS Behav* 5:233–240.

Meade CS (2006). Sexual risk behavior among persons dually diagnosed with severe mental illness and substance use disorders. *J Subst Abuse Treat* 30:147–157.

Meade CS, and Sikkema KJ (2005). HIV risk behavior among adults with severe mental illness: a systematic review. *Clin Psychol Rev* 25:433–457.

Menon AS, and Pomerantz S (1997). Substance use during sex and unsafe sexual behaviors among acute psychiatric inpatients. *Psychiatr Serv* 48:1070–1072.

Mueser KT, Bellack AS, Douglas MS, and Morrison RL (1991). Prevalence and stability of social skill deficits in schizophrenia. *Schizophr Res* 5:167–176.

Mueser KT, Goodman LB, Trumbetta SL, Roseberg SD, Osher FC, Vidaver R, Auciello P, and Foy DW (1998). Trauma and posttraumatic stress disorder in severe mental illness. *J Consult Clin Psychol* 66:493–499.

Otto-Salaj LL, Heckman TG, Stevenson LY, and Kelly JA (1998). Patterns, predictors, and gender differences in HIV risk among severely mentally ill men and women. *Community Ment Health J* 34:175–190.

Otto-Salaj LL, Kelly JA, Stevenson LY, Hoffman R, and Kalichman SC (2000). Outcomes of a randomized small-group HIV prevention intervention trial for people with severe mental illness. *Community Ment Health J* 37:123–144.

Rahav M, Nuttbrock L, Rivera JJ, and Link BG (1998). HIV infection risks among homeless, mentally ill, chemically misusing men. *Subst Use Misuse* 33:1407–1426.

Regier DA, Farmer ME, Rae DS, Locke BZ, Keith SJ, Judd LL, and Goodwin FK (1990). Comorbidity of mental disorders with alcohol and other drug abuse: results from the Epidemiological Catchment Area (ECA) Study. *JAMA* 264:2511–2518

Rosenberg SD, Goodman LA, Osher FC, Swartz MS, Essock SM, Butterfield MI, Constantine NT, Wolford GL, and Salyers MP (2001a). Prevalence

of HIV, hepatitis B, and hepatitis C in people with severe mental illness. *Am J Public Health* 91:31–37.

Rosenberg SD, Trumbetta SL, Muesser KT, Goodman LA, Osher FC, Vidaver RM, and Metzger DS (2001b). Determinants of risk behavior for human immunodeficiency virus/acquired immunodeficiency syndrome in people with severe mental illness. *Compr Psychiatry* 42:263–271.

Rosenberg S, Brunette M, Oxman T, Marsh B, Dietrich A, Mueser K, Drake R, Torrey W, and Vidaver R (2004). The STIRR model of best practices for blood-born diseases among clients with serious mental illness. *Psychiatr Serv* 55:660–664.

Sacks M, and Dermatis H (1994). Acute psychiatric illness: effects on HIV-risk behavior. *Psychosoc Rehabil J* 17:5–19.

Schinnar A, Rothbard A, Kanter R, and Jung Y (1990). An empirical literature review of definitions of severe and persistent mental illness. *Am J Psychiatry* 147:1602–1608.

Sewell DD (1996). Schizophrenia and HIV. *Schizophr Bull* 22:465–473.

Sikkema KJ, Meade CS, Doughty JD, Zimmerman SO, Kloos B, and Snow DL (2007). Community-level HIV prevention for persons with severe mental illness living in supportive housing programs: a pilot intervention study. *J Prev Interv Community* 33:121–135.

Silberstein C, Galanter M, Marmor M, Lifshutz H, Krasinski K, and Franco H (1994). HIV-1 among inner city dually diagnosed inpatients. *Am J Drug Alcohol Abuse* 20:101–114.

Starace F, Ammassari A, Trotta MP, Murri R, De Longis P, Izzo C, Scalzini A, d'Arminio Monforte A, Wu AW, and Antinori A (2002). Depression is a risk factor for suboptimal adherence to highly active antiretroviral therapy. *J Acquir Immune Defic Syndr* 31:S136–S139.

Susser E, Valencia E, Miller M, Tsai W-Y, Meyer-Bahlburg H, and Conover S (1995). Sexual behavior of homeless mentally ill men at risk for HIV. *Am J Psychiatry* 152:583–587.

Susser E, Miller M, Valencia E, Colson P, Roche B, and Conover S (1996). Injection drug use and risk of HIV transmission among homeless men with mental illness. *Am J Psychiatry* 153:794–798.

Susser E, Betne P, Valencia E, Goldfinger SM, and Lehman AF (1997). Injection drug use among homeless adults with severe mental illness. *Am J Public Health* 87:854–856.

Susser E, Valencia E, Berkman A, Sohler N, Conover S, Torres J, Betne P, Felix A, and Miller S (1998). Human immunodeficiency virus sexual risk reduction in homeless men with mental illness. *Arch Gen Psychiatry* 55:266–272.

Treisman G, Fishman M, Schwartz J, Hutton H, and Lyketsos C (2003). Mood disorders in HIV infection. *Depress Anxiety* 7:178–187.

Tucker JS, Kanouse DE, Miu A, Koegel P, and Sullivan G (2003). HIV risk behaviors and their correlates among HIV-positive adults with serious mental illness. *AIDS Behav* 7:29–40.

Tyrer P, Manley C, van Horn E, Leddy D, and Ukoumunne OC (2000). Personality abnormality in severe mental illness and its influence on outcome of intensive and standard case management: a randomized controlled trial. *Eur Psychiatry*15:7–10.

UNAIDS (2006). *Report on the Global HIV/AIDS Epidemic*. Geneva: UNAIDS.

Weinhardt LS, Carey MP, Carey KB, and Verdecias RN (1998). Increasing assertiveness skills to reduce HIV risk among women living with severe and persistent mental illness. *J Consult Clin Psychol* 66:680–684.

Weinhardt LS, Carey MP, Carey KB, Maisto SA, and Gordon CM (2001). The relation of alcohol use to HIV-risk sexual behavior among adults with severe and persistent mental illness. *J Consult Clin Psychol* 69:77–84.

Zanarini MC, Parachini EA, Frankenburg FR, Holman JB, Hennen J, Reich DB, and Silk KR (2003). Sexual relationship difficulties among borderline patients and Axis II comparison subjects. *J Nerv Ment Dis* 191:479–482.

Chapter 22

Psychiatric Aspects of Adherence to Medical Care and Treatment for HIV/AIDS

Jeffrey J. Weiss and David R. Bangsberg

Over the past decade, AIDS has been transformed from a fatal illness to a chronic one. This transformation began with the introduction of protease inhibitors in the mid-1990s and has accelerated with the continued development of new antiretroviral (ARV) medications. HIV-related hospitalizations and deaths in the developed world are largely limited to those who do not receive timely medical care or who are nonadherent (Riley et al., 2005; Sabin et al., 2006). Active drug use and mental illness are significant barriers to optimal care and treatment adherence among HIV-positive persons (Giordano et al., 2005b)

The prevalence estimates of lifetime psychiatric illness range from 38% to 88% in samples of HIV-positive persons as compared to 33% for the general population (Yun et al., 2005). In a representative probability sample of 2864 adults receiving HIV care in the United States in 1996, Bing and colleagues (2001) reported that 48% of the sample screened positive for a psychiatric disorder, 38% reported using an illicit drug other than marijuana, and 12% screened positive

for drug dependence during the prior year. The prevalence of current depression in this large representative sample of HIV-positive persons (36%) was three times higher than in the general population. In this same sample, 27% of the individuals were taking psychotropic medication, with antidepressants (21%) and anxiolytics (17%) being the most commonly prescribed (Vitiello et al., 2003).

HIV infection and psychiatric illness often exist in the context of complex social conditions, such as homelessness, poverty, unemployment, domestic violence, legal problems, discrimination, stigmatization, and a distrustful attitude toward traditional medicine. These social morbidities further complicate optimal and sustained adherence to medical care (Bouhnik et al., 2002; Palmer et al., 2003).

This chapter will focus on adherence to medical care and treatment among HIV-infected patients with psychiatric illness. Included in the broad category of psychiatric illness are substance use disorders and HIV-associated neurocognitive disorders. When the term "psychiatric illness" is used in this chapter, it refers to DSM-IV mental disorders, DSM-IV substance use disorders, and HIV-associated neurocognitive disorders (Minor Cognitive Motor Disorder and HIV-Associated Dementia).

In order to ground this discussion in a clinical context, consider the following two cases and what they have in common.

Case 1

The patient is a 47-year-old woman who has been attending the outpatient psychiatry clinic for the last 3 months. She is diagnosed with major depression, post-traumatic stress disorder, and cocaine dependence. Her attendance to outpatient appointments is sporadic and she is poorly adherent to her prescribed psychotropic medication. She is currently living in a single-room occupancy (SRO) hotel and is in a physically abusive relationship with a man. Her medical conditions include HIV infection, hypertension, and diabetes.

Case 2

The patient is a 47-year-old woman who has been attending the HIV outpatient clinic since being discharged from the inpatient medical service 5 months ago. During the admission she found out that she was HIV positive and has AIDS after *Pneumocystis carinii* pneumonia (PCP) was diagnosed. Her CD4+ cell count is 120 cells/microliter and her viral load is 500,000 copies/ml. She is nonadherent to her antiretroviral regimen and to her prophylactic medication. She has been referred to the outpatient psychiatric clinic for treatment of depression and substance use.

While these two vignettes appear to describe two different individuals, the first nonadherent to psychiatric care and the second nonadherent to HIV medical care, they are, in fact, the same person. The first case report is written by her outpatient psychiatrist, the second by her primary provider at the HIV outpatient clinic. The psychiatrist and primary provider understandably focus on different aspects of the patient's situation. The foreground for the psychiatrist is the background for the primary provider and vice versa. In this chapter we will thus seek to integrate the psychiatrist's and primary care provider's conceptuali-

zations of patients with complicated and interwoven social, psychiatric, and medical issues, with particular attention to how these factors impact adherence to medical care and treatment. The following sections of this chapter address (1) adherence to ARV medication and medical care, (2) determinants of medication adherence, (3) adherence interventions, and (4) implications of research findings for the medical and psychiatric clinical provider working with HIV-positive patients with psychiatric illness. "Primary provider" is used in this chapter to refer to the individual providing HIV care regardless of discipline (MD, DO, NP, PA). Similarly, discussion of the work of the psychiatrist is meant to be relevant to the work of other mental health professionals (psychologists, social workers, substance use counselors) as well.

ADHERENCE AMONG HIV-POSITIVE PERSONS WITH PSYCHIATRIC ILLNESS

The World Health Organization's Adherence to Long-term Therapies Project (WHO, 2003) defines adherence as "the extent to which a person's behavior—taking medication, following a diet, and/or executing lifestyle changes—corresponds with agreed recommendations from a health care provider." Most of the research on adherence among HIV-positive persons has focused on adherence to ARV therapy. Giordano and colleagues (2005a) argue for broadening the view of adherence to encompass a wide range of HIV health-related behaviors, including (1) receiving an HIV test, (2) entering quality health care services, and (3) starting ARV therapy. We will adopt this broader definition of adherence in our discussion of HIV-positive persons with psychiatric illness and their adherence to ARV therapy, their psychiatric treatment, and these broader health-related behaviors.

Adherence to Antiretroviral Therapy

The relationship between adherence to ARV therapy and virological suppression has been well documented (Bangsberg et al., 2000, 2001b; Low-Beer et al., 2000; Paterson et al., 2000). High levels of adherence to ARV regimens are needed to achieve complete and durable suppression of the HIV virus and to avoid the emergence of resistant strains of HIV virus (Bangsberg et al., 2003). While new, more potent regimens may lead to viral suppression in antiretroviral-naïve patients at moderate levels of adherence, optimal adherence remains between 95% and 100%. According to this standard, a patient on a twice-daily ARV regimen who missed one medication dose every 10 days would have 95% adherence. ARV medication thus demands a much higher level of adherence from patients than do treatments for most other medical conditions.

There are numerous methods of assessing adherence to ARV medication. They each have their strengths and weaknesses, and some are only feasible in the research but not clinical setting. We will discuss the most commonly used methods of assessing adherence in the clinical setting: (1) provider assessment, (2) structured self-report, and (3) use of pharmacy refill data, and briefly mention those used in the research setting: (4) medication event monitoring systems (MEMS), (5) pill counts, (6) biological indices, and (7) directly observed therapy (DOT).

Provider Assessment

Studies have consistently found that provider assessment of adherence is poor (Bangsberg et al., 2001d; Gross et al., 2002; and Miller et al., 2002). Generally, providers tend to overestimate medication adherence and are more accurate in their diagnosis of incomplete than complete adherence. Overestimation can in part be explained by patient awareness that nonadherence will be met with disappointment at best and possibly disapproval or judgment by their providers. Overestimation of adherence can also simply be due to the inherent difficulty in recalling something that had been forgotten. Regardless of the reason for nonadherence, patients often feel a sense of shame and failure when it comes time to see their provider and report this nonadherence. Some patients avoid this feared confrontation by failing to attend their appointment or attending but lying about or distorting their actual adherence behavior. Providers also tend to rely heavily on virologic treatment response to assess adherence. With fully suppressive ARV regimens, however, undetectable viral loads can be achieved at adherence levels that are less than optimal and still place patients at risk for the development of resistance. This scenario can result in the provider overestimating adherence. Alternatively, failure to achieve undetectable viral load in treatment-experienced patients with partially suppressive regimens may be due to drug resistance rather than to poor adherence, potentially resulting in the provider underestimating adherence.

Structured Self-Report

Structured self-report is the most commonly used method of assessing ARV medication adherence because of its low cost and ease of implementation. There are many self-report measures used, and they vary in terms of time frame assessed, dimensions assessed (number of pills taken, time of day taken, dietary restrictions followed), wording of questions, use of visual cues, and level of literacy and cognitive ability required to complete the measure. One of the most commonly used measures was developed by the Adult AIDS Clinical Trials Group (Chesney et al., 2000). This measure has been validated and continually modified to increase its sensitivity and accuracy and can be accessed at http://www.caps.ucsf.edu/tools/surveys/#8. Nieuwkerk and Oort (2005) conducted a meta-analysis of 65 studies and found that self-report is a valid method of assessing ARV medication adherence, based on its relationship to virologic treatment response.

In choosing a self-report measure of ARV adherence, providers should take into account the reading level and cognitive status of the patient completing the measure. A Visual Analogue Scale (VAS) has been developed and validated in urban (Walsh et al., 2002a; Giordano et al., 2004) and resource-poor settings (Oyugi et al., 2004). The VAS asks subjects to indicate a point on a line that shows their best guess about how much of each medication they have taken in a specified time period. The primary advantage of the VAS is that it is simpler to administer than a structured self-report questionnaire. For settings in which computers are available and patients are computer literate, computer-assisted self-interviewing programs have been developed and validated (Bangsberg et al., 2002) to assess ARV adherence.

Self-reported adherence measures often cover varying time intervals. The AIDS Clinical Trials Group (ACTG) measures usually cover 3-4 days while the VAS usually covers 30 days. Other measures (Mannheimer et al., 2002, 2005) may cover 7 days. The rationale for shorter intervals is that they may improve the accuracy of patient report; the rationale for longer intervals is that may detect more missed doses and thus reduce the ceiling effect of detecting 100% adherence in most individuals by self-report. While there is no consensus on the ideal interval, data presented by Liu and colleagues (2006) is that longer (30-day) intervals may be more closely associated with electronically monitored adherence than shorter (3-day) intervals.

Pharmacy Refill Data

Pharmacy refill records have been used to provide an objective and nonintrusive measure of adherence. This method tends to overestimate adherence but has been found in several studies to be related to virologic outcome (Low-Beer et al., 2000; Grossberg et al., 2004), drug resistance (Harrigan et al., 2005), and disease progression (Wood et al., 2003). It is best employed when patients use one pharmacy for all prescriptions, pharmacy data are easily accessible to the clinician by computer, and prescriptions are not automatically delivered without the patient needing to request them or pick them up. Because patients may accumulate an extra supply of medications by picking up medications a few days early over time, a single late refill may not necessarily indicate incomplete adherence. Picking up medications consistently late, however, can be an important marker of incomplete adherence and trigger further adherence assessment and intervention.

Medication Event Monitoring Systems

Medication event monitoring systems (MEMS) technology has been widely used in research studies of HIV medication adherence and is regarded by many as the most accurate method of assessing medication adherence. In this method, the medication bottle cap has a microchip which records all openings and closings of the bottle. This microchip provides the researcher with a precise record of the date and time of each bottle opening. While this method is closely associated with random home pill count (Bangsberg et al., 2001a), viral suppression (Bangsberg et al., 2000; Paterson et al., 2000; Arnsten et al., 2001; Walsh et al., 2002b; Moss et al., 2004), and drug resistance (Walsh et al., 2002b), it is generally used only in research settings. Potential problems associated with the use of MEMS caps are that patients can open the bottles without taking the medication, patients can take medication for multiple doses out of the bottle at one time, the bottle cannot be used in combination with pill box organizers, and they are expensive (over $100 per MEMS cap). More recently developed devices, however, have incorporated MEMS-like technology into a pillbox organizer that records the date and time of each dose (Brue et al. 2007).

Pill Counts

Patients in clinical research studies are often asked to bring their medication to study visits so that the change in the number of pills (accounting for refills) since the last visit can be used to assess adherence. Potential problems associated with these announced pill counts are that patients may forget to bring their medication to study visits, and nonadherent patients may throw out pills prior to the visit ("pill dumps") to avoid being labeled nonadherent. These problems have been avoided by using unannounced pill counts among marginally housed HIV-positive persons in San Francisco (Bangsberg et al., 2000). Members of the research staff visit research participants at their place of residence at an unannounced time to perform pill counts. The use of unannounced pill counts to monitor adherence requires trained staff who have been able to build trusting relationships, thus it is largely limited to research settings. Kalichman and colleagues (2007) have recently reported on an adaptation of the unannounced pill count assessment that is conducted over the telephone, allowing for the possibility of wider implementation of this assessment technique.

Biological Indices

Some researchers have used plasma concentrations of ARV drugs to assess adherence, most often to one particular ARV drug in a clinical trial. Plasma drug concentrations reflect both adherence behavior and the patient's individual pharmacokinetics. Liechty and colleagues (2004) observed that abnormally low drug levels were associated with incomplete adherence over the prior month, but normal drug levels did not confirm complete adherence. This discrepancy is likely due to the fact that drug levels are only to the last dose, and adherence behavior likely changes just prior to a clinical visit.

Directly Observed Therapy (DOT)

While directly observed therapy (DOT) provides a highly accurate assessment of adherence, the cost and intrusiveness of observing all doses of medication ingestion make it an impractical method of ARV adherence assessment, except in very specific settings (e.g., prisons or nursing homes). DOT will be discussed further as an adherence intervention later in this chapter.

Adherence in Patients with Psychiatric Disorders

In general, HIV-positive persons with psychiatric disorders and/or active substance use have lower levels of adherence than those of individuals without these problems (Tucker et al., 2003). It has been well documented that untreated or undertreated psychiatric disorders are associated with increased rates of medication nonadherence (Singh et al., 1996; Goodman and Fallot, 1998; Gordillo et al., 1999; Wagner et al., 2001; Starace et al., 2002; van Servellen et al., 2002; Carrieri et al., 2003). Nonetheless, HIV-positive persons with psychiatric illness are capable of medication adherence, particularly when the patient is well engaged in psychiatric care. In a large prospective study of the homeless population of HIV-infected persons in San Francisco (n = 148), Moss and colleagues (2004) assessed ARV adherence using unannounced pill counts and MEMS. This population had high rates of psychiatric illness (25% had been hospitalized for psychiatric treatment, 29% had current depressive symptomatology, 33% were injecting drugs, and 24% were using crack cocaine at time of study recruitment). While rates of discontinuation of therapy were high in this cohort (31%), the level of ARV adherence (74%) and HIV viral suppression (54%) among those who remained on ARV therapy was not dissimilar to that in other populations.

Engagement in Medical Care Predicts Outcome

To receive proper medical care the HIV-positive person needs to locate an appropriate and available medical provider and keep scheduled appointments with that provider. Giordano and colleagues' (2005a) model of adherence to engagement in the health system includes (1) receiving an HIV test; (2) entering quality health care services, and (3) provider initiation of ARV therapy. Berg and colleagues (2005) found that adherence to medical care predicts level of disease progression. They investigated the relationship between missed medical appointments and medical outcomes in a sample of almost 1000 persons receiving care in HIV primary care settings

during the era of highly active antiretroviral therapy (HAART). In multivariate models, the number of missed appointments was related to both having a CD4 cell count of <200 cells/microliter and having a detectable HIV viral load. These analyses accounted for the fact that patients who are more medically ill are likely to have more scheduled medical appointments.

Engagement in Psychiatric Care Predicts Outcome

Turner and colleagues (2001) found that HIV-positive persons who have psychiatric illness, in particular those who use illicit substances, are less likely to be prescribed ARV medication than those who do not have a psychiatric illness. Other studies found that engagement in mental health treatment increases the likelihood that ARV medication will be prescribed and mostly provides support for psychiatric and substance use treatment, improving adherence to ARV medication in this population. Sambamoorthi and colleagues (2000) analyzed Medicaid data on HIV-positive patients receiving services in New Jersey between 1991 and 1996 and found that depressed patients treated with antidepressants were almost twice as likely to receive ARV therapy than those not treated with antidepressants.

Turner and colleagues (2003) examined the relationship between medication adherence and mental health treatment (methadone clinic, psychiatric care, antidepressant medication) in a sample of over 5000 HIV-positive indigent drug users on ARV therapy. Only 22% of the patients in this sample had 95% adherence, based on pharmacy refill data over an 8-month period. Those patients diagnosed with depression (34% of the women and 29% of the men) had better medication adherence than those not diagnosed with depression. This finding runs counter to the larger literature demonstrating a strong relationship between depression and poorer adherence, perhaps because those diagnosed with depression in this study were also much more likely to be in drug treatment or psychiatric care. Among the patients with a diagnosis of depression, those who were in substance use treatment or psychiatric care (with or without antidepressants) had better adherence than those not under substance use or psychiatric care. This study found that psychiatric care had the most benefit on adherence for women, whereas substance use treatment had the most benefit on adherence for men.

Palepu and colleagues (2004) conducted a prospective study of 349 HIV-positive persons with a history of alcohol problems. They found that persons who engaged in substance use treatment were more likely to be placed on ARV medication than those who did not, although they did not find that substance use treatment conferred any benefit on adherence.

Several investigators have found a relationship between depression and level of disease progression (Burack et al., 1993; Page-Shafer et al., 1996; Ickovics et al., 2001). Cook and colleagues (2004) examined the relationship between depressive symptoms, treatment for depression, and mortality in a longitudinal cohort of over 2000 HIV-positive women. The mortality rate among women with chronic depression was double that for women with no or intermittent depression. While no data are reported on the relationship between mental health services and adherence, women who received mental health services were significantly less likely to die from AIDS-related causes during the study period. In a subsequent report on this cohort, Cook and colleagues (Cook et al., 2006) examined the temporal relationship between use of antidepressants and mental health therapy, individually and in combination, on subsequent use of HAART in the subset of women with depression. They found that women who received mental health therapy alone or the combination of mental health therapy and antidepressants had greater use of HAART than the depressed women who received no treatment. The use of antidepressants alone, however, did not increase the level of HAART use over that with no treatment for depression.

In a retrospective chart review study, Himelhoch and colleagues (2004) found that in a clinic setting with on-site psychiatric care, patients with a psychiatric disorder were 37% more likely to receive HAART, were 2.5 times more likely to remain on HAART for at least 6 months, and had a 40% reduction in mortality compared to those who did not have a psychiatric disorder. These subjects were receiving intensive psychiatric services colocated with their HIV primary care. While adherence was not assessed in this study, one plausible explanation for this unexpected finding is that the intensity of the psychiatric services and integration of psychiatric and medical care resulted in improved adherence among the patients with psychiatric illness.

DETERMINANTS OF MEDICATION ADHERENCE

Most research conducted on adherence among HIV-positive persons is focused on adherence to ARV medication. Determinants of medication adherence can be grouped into four categories: personal characteristics, characteristics of the treatment, characteristics of the relationship between the health professional and the client, and characteristics of the illness (Ickovics and Meisler, 1997; Reiter et al., 2000). In the population of HIV-positive persons with psychiatric illness, the personal characteristics shown to be most strongly and consistently predictive of degree of adherence are depression, active substance abuse, neurocognitive functioning, and self-efficacy. We will review the research findings on these individual determinants and discuss the literature on the impact of severe mental illness and posttraumatic stress disorder (PTSD) on ARV adherence. In addition, we will comment on determinants of adherence to psychotropic medication.

Depression

Most investigators examining the relationship between nonadherence to HIV therapy and psychiatric illness have focused on depression and have measured depression on continuous symptom scales rather than studying the diagnostic categories of depression. There is substantial evidence that depression is an independent risk factor for patient nonadherence to medical regimens in general and to HAART in particular (Singh et al., 1996; Gordillo et al., 1999; Tuldrà et al., 1999; Wagner et al., 2001; Starace et al., 2002; van Servellen et al., 2002; Carrieri et al., 2003; Ammassari et al. 2004; Gonzalez et al., 2004). Furthermore, there is evidence that affective disorders are even more strongly associated with discontinuation of HAART than other types of severe mental illness such as schizophrenia (Walkup et al., 2004).

The role of depression in effecting adherence is moderated by whether the person is receiving psychiatric treatment. In a recent meta-analysis of double-blinded, randomized controlled trials of antidepressant treatment among HIV-positive persons, Himelhoch and Medoff (2005) found that antidepressant medication is efficacious. They noted, however, that there was a significant underrepresentation of women and minorities in the samples studied. While to date there is no published data from large prospective studies or randomized controlled trials that directly addresses the relation between treatment for depression and adherence to ARV therapy (Davidson et al., 2006; Wilson and Jacobson, 2006), existing observational data suggest that depression treatment may be an important and relatively easily modified barrier to incomplete adherence to medical therapy. Highlighting that depression may be optimally treated prior to the initiation of ARV therapy, rather than during therapy, Balfour and colleagues (2006) conducted a randomized controlled psychosocial intervention trial which successfully reduced depressive symptoms in depressed, HIV-positive patients not currently on ARV therapy in order to improve readiness to begin therapy.

Substance Use Disorders

When assessing barriers to adherence, it is important to distinguish current substance use from past substance use. While *current* substance use is associated with incomplete adherence, a *history* of substance use is not. Studies have found a relationship between problem drinking and active illicit drug use and nonadherence among HIV-positive persons (Cook et al., 2001; Lucas et al., 2001; Wagner et al., 2001; Golin et al., 2002; Howard et al., 2002; Gebo et al., 2003; Tucker et al., 2003; Levine et al., 2005). Active cocaine use was found to be the strongest predictor of nonadherence in a study using electronic monitors to quantify adherence (Arnsten et al., 2002).

Neurocognitive Impairment and HIV Dementia

Four studies have investigated and found a relationship between neurocognitive functioning and medication adherence among HIV-positive adults. These studies examined the relationship between neuropsychological test data and adherence but did not look at the diagnostic categories of minor cognitive motor disorder or HIV dementia. Hinkin and colleagues (2002) found that deficits in executive function, memory, and attention were associated with poor medication adherence as measured by MEMS. Avants and colleagues (2001) found that deficits in executive functioning were related to nonadherence in a sample of HIV-positive, injection drug users beginning methadone maintenance. Albert and colleagues (2003) investigated the relationship between neurocognitive functioning and medication management skills in HIV-positive persons and found that persons with impairment on tests of executive function performed significantly poorer at pouring medicines in the Medication Management Test. Levine and colleagues (2005) categorized medication adherence behavior into five categories over a 4-week period and found that the subgroup with poor weekend adherence (relative to during the week) performed significantly worse on the global impairment index and the attention domain.

Self-Efficacy

Self-efficacy is a behavioral construct defined in social-cognitive theory (Bandura, 1997) as beliefs in one's capabilities to organize and execute the course of action required to perform a certain activity (e.g., adhering to a medication regimen). According to the theory, individuals who regard themselves as highly efficacious in their ability to adhere will set higher goals, be more firmly committed to them, and, therefore, exercise higher control over behavior that fosters adherence.

Self-efficacy has been shown to be consistently associated with medication adherence in HIV-positive persons (Eldred et al., 1998; Catz et al., 2000; Chesney et al., 2000; Gifford et al., 2000; Tuldrà et al., 2000; Safren et al., 2001; Kerr et al., 2004). Kalichman and colleagues (2005b) have developed and validated a pictographic VAS to assess medication self-efficacy among low-literacy patients.

Severe Mental Illness

Wagner and colleagues (2003) assessed adherence with electronic monitoring in a small sample of 47 HIV-positive persons with treated serious mental illness and found adherence rates comparable to those reported in general clinic and community samples (an average adherence rate of 66%; 40% of the sample achieved adherence levels of 90% or greater). In this sample of HIV-positive persons with severe mental illness, most of whom were engaged in psychiatric care, Wagner et al. (2004) found attendance to clinic appointments to be the one factor that most strongly predicted ARV medication adherence in a multivariate analysis. Individuals with higher rates of attendance had better adherence as measured by an electronic monitoring device.

Posttraumatic Stress Disorder

The higher rate of PTSD in patients with HIV than in the general population has been well documented. In the HIV-positive population PTSD may be caused by traumatic events that preceded infection with HIV and/or a traumatic response to the diagnosis of HIV. Clinical reports (Cohen et al., 2001; Ricart et al., 2002) have elucidated the dynamic processes by which PTSD can be related to nonadherence to care and treatment in HIV-positive persons. Given that PTSD is highly comorbid with depression and substance use disorders, it has been difficult for researchers to determine the independent impact of PTSD on adherence (Sledjeski et al., 2005).

Adherence to Psychotropic Medication

Wagner and colleagues (2003) found a significant correlation between ARV adherence and adherence to psychotropic medication among HIV-positive persons with serious mental illness. As would be expected, many of the determinants of ARV adherence are also determinants of adherence to psychotropic medication in the same population. There are, however, aspects of adherence to psychotropic medication that distinguish it from adherence to ARV medication. Most HIV-positive persons on ARV medication understand that HIV is a chronic illness for which they will likely always remain on medication. The positive outcomes of the medication (increased CD4+ cell count and decreased HIV viral load) are often motivators to continue taking ARV medication. The fear of death from HIV can serve to motivate patients to tolerate uncomfortable side effects of ARV medication. In contrast, effective psychotropic treatment removes the symptoms (e.g., of depression or psychosis) that the medication is targeting. This can result in patients perceiving that they no longer have a need for medication and in consequent poor adherence or self-discontinuation of medication. In addition, because of the perceived non-life-threatening nature of the psychiatric illness being treated, patients weigh the burden of side effects of psychotropic medication relative to the benefits in a different manner than that of weighing the costs of ARV medication side effects. Prospective studies of patient adherence to concomitant psychotropic medication and ARV medication are needed to elucidate the potential interrelated yet independent adherence patterns for psychotropic and ARV agents.

BEHAVIORAL INTERVENTIONS TO IMPROVE MEDICATION ADHERENCE

Continued simplification and improvement of ARV regimen tolerability have been important advances in improving adherence to ARV therapy. Decreases in the number of pills required, number of dosage times, food restrictions, storage restrictions, and medication side effects have all contributed to better adherence. While these advances lessen the adherence burden to patients, there are still many patients who, despite these improvements, have continued challenges with adherence.

In attempting interventions with nonadherent HIV-positive persons, it can be helpful to distinguish between intentional nonadherence and unintentional nonadherence. In the former, the patient does not intend to be adherent (e.g., a patient who decides not to take his medication on a night when he is going out because he wants to drink alcohol), while in the latter, the patient intends to be adherent but is having difficulty succeeding at this (e.g., a patient who forgets the afternoon dose because she is distracted by her child care responsibilities). There are numerous devices and tools available to help patients with medication adherence (information cards, pill organizers, alarms, pagers, medication diaries, visual medication schedules). These devices are particularly effective in improving adherence for patients who are nonadherent because of memory impairment (Andrade et al., 2005) and may be associated with modest improvements in the general population (Golin et al., 2002; Kalichman et al., 2005a). For many other patients, however, these supports are not sufficient to achieve optimal levels of adherence.

Many behavioral interventions have been developed to increase the level of HIV adherence by addressing adherence barriers and increasing motivation and self-efficacy. Some of these interventions have been formally evaluated in randomized controlled clinical trials.

In a meta-analysis of HIV adherence interventions, Simoni and colleagues (2006) identified 19 randomized, controlled clinical trials published from 1999 to 2005 that met the following three criteria: (1) described a behavioral intervention targeting individuals at least 18 years of age; (2) randomly assigned participants to intervention and control arms; (3) provided outcome data on adherence or HIV viral load.

Most of these 19 studies used samples drawn from HIV clinic settings that included patients both with and without psychiatric illness. Five of the studies excluded individuals with current psychiatric illness. When Simoni and colleagues examined all 19 studies, they identified four interventions that had the strongest effect on adherence (Knobel et al., 1999; Tuldrà et al., 2000; Safren et al., 2001; Rathbun et al., 2005). All four of these interventions consisted of one primary in-person session followed by varying intensities of follow-up either in person or by telephone. The interventions of Knobel and Tuldrà took place in Spain and were psychoeducational. In Knobel et al.'s study, a pharmacist conducted the initial educational session and offered follow-up telephone support. In Tuldrà et al.'s study, the intervention session was based on self-efficacy theory and conducted by a psychologist. Rathbun et al.'s psychoeducational intervention in Oklahoma was conducted by a pharmacist. Safren et al.'s study in Boston used an intervention that incorporated cognitive-behavioral, motivational interviewing, and problem-solving techniques. All of these studies demonstrate that brief, low-cost adherence interventions can be highly effective in improving adherence in diverse clinic settings. None of these studies, however, provided data on the prevalence of psychiatric illness in the samples.

Only 3 of the 19 studies in the meta-analysis chose subjects based on presence of current psychiatric illness, specifically substance use. In the first of these three studies, done by Margolin and colleagues (2003), 90 methadone-maintained injection drug users were recruited and randomly assigned, half of them to twice-weekly manual-guided group therapy sessions for 6 months in addition to the enhanced methadone maintenance program that the other half of the sample received. The group therapy program included adherence among other topics related to living with HIV. The 6-month group therapy intervention was found to have a significant impact on improving adherence relative to the control condition. The validity of the adherence data collected by structured interview was corroborated by corresponding changes in viral load.

In the second of these three studies, Rotheram-Borus and colleagues (2004) recruited 175 substance-using young people (ages 16–29) and randomly assigned them to a three-module intervention totaling 18 sessions over 15 months delivered by telephone, in person, or a delayed-intervention condition. Similar

to the Margolin intervention, adherence was one part of a broader intervention focused on physical, sexual, and emotional health. This study did not find that the intervention had any effect on ARV use or adherence to ARV use as measured by self-report.

In the third of these three studies, Samet and colleagues (2005) recruited 151 patients with a history of alcohol abuse and randomly assigned them to a four-session adherence intervention with a nurse or to usual medical care. The adherence intervention did not have an effect on self-reported adherence behavior (corroborated by use of MEMS).

One possible explanation for Margolin's intervention having an effect on adherence while Rotheram-Borus' and Samet's interventions did not is the greater intensity of Margolin's intervention than that of the other two (52 intervention sessions, as compared to 18 and 4). In contrast to the finding that brief adherence interventions are effective in general populations, it may be that for those with psychiatric illness, interventions of greater length are needed in order to be effective.

Directly observed therapy (DOT) has been shown to be an effective intervention to achieve optimal levels of adherence among HIV-positive persons with psychiatric illness in a residential care facility (de Socio et al., 2004). Mitty and colleagues (2005) investigated the effectiveness of a community-based, modified directly observed therapy (MDOT) program for HIV-positive persons with high rates of substance use (96% lifetime; 80% last 3 months). Although less than half of the participants remained in the study for 6 months, those who did remain and were still receiving MDOT had significant reductions in viral load, whereas those not still receiving MDOT showed little or no change. This study demonstrates the difficulties involved in applying a DOT approach in a real-world setting even with significant resources.

Altice and colleagues (2004) investigated the efficacy of a directly administered antiretroviral therapy (DAART) program for HIV-positive individuals currently using illicit drugs. The DAART intervention was integrated into services offered by an existing mobile syringe-exchange program. Preliminary data from this study show that adherence rates as measured by MEMS are significantly higher for supervised doses (76%) than for unsupervised doses (50%). By and large, DOT is an intensive intervention that should be directed at patients with advanced disease who have failed less intrusive and expensive attempts at improving adherence (Bangsberg et al., 2001c).

IMPLICATIONS OF RESEARCH FINDINGS FOR CLINICAL PRACTICE

As HIV-positive patients live longer and present with increasing numbers of comorbid medical conditions being treated, it is increasingly important to view and study adherence to ARV medication in the context of the entire medication regimen taken by the HIV-positive patient. It is important to understand whether and how patterns of adherence differ for ARV, psychotropic, and medication regimens for other non-HIV medical conditions in patients with multiple morbidities and to investigate the temporal associations among these patterns of adherence.

Patient adherence occurs in the context of a relationship with medical providers and the medical setting. As discussed earlier, providers do not precisely estimate adherence and often do not detect incomplete adherence of their patients. Even if patients are honest with their provider about their failure to adhere, they often leave the encounter feeling blamed for this failure. While a great deal of research has been conducted that attempts to change adherence by changing patient behavior, and studies have documented the impact of the quality of the physician–patient relationship on adherence to ARV therapy (Schneider et al., 2004; Ingersoll and Heckman, 2005; Lewis et al., 2006), there has been little research on interventions to change provider behavior and clinic characteristics to improve the adherence of HIV-positive patients. Wilson and colleagues (2007) did recently present findings from a randomized intervention trial targeting physician communication with HIV-positive patients about adherence. While the intervention did increase adherence related dialogue between physicians and patients, it did not improve medication adherence. There is an inherent conflict that must be taken into account and overcome when providers discuss nonadherent behavior with patients: Whereas providers are unambivalent about wanting their patients to adhere to treatment and are readily able to prioritize adherence above all other issues, patients are often struggling with significant barriers and competing priorities such as depression, substance use, memory problems, low self-esteem, unresolved trauma, pain, fatigue, nausea, discrimination, poverty, child and family care, abuse, housing problems, difficulty understanding health care instructions and the health care system, insurance problems, and treatment fatigue.

To further address the role of the provider, we return to the case of the nonadherent patient described by both her outpatient psychiatrist and her HIV provider. This patient was hospitalized, leading to her diagnosis of AIDS and referral to the HIV outpatient clinic upon discharge. Subsequently she was referred to an outpatient psychiatrist. Although she had had prior episodes of outpatient psychiatric treatment, she had never been referred for, or had, HIV testing. For patients with HIV and psychiatric illness, the inpatient unit, the HIV clinic, or the psychiatric clinic can all be the initial point of entry into care.

Psychiatrists seeing patients at risk for HIV should inquire about and recommend HIV testing. Some patients with known HIV infection and psychiatric illness are only able to eventually engage in medical care for HIV through initial engagement in psychiatric care and treatment. To facilitate this process, the psychiatrist might have to go beyond usual practice by, for example, ordering CD4+ and HIV viral load tests to document and help the patient understand the need for HIV medical treatment. For patients with CD4+ cell counts below 200 cells/microliter who are engaged in psychiatric care yet are not ready to seek medical care, the psychiatrist may consider prescribing prophylactic medication for opportunistic infections (particularly *Pneumocystis carinii* pneumonia) while working to help the patient overcome barriers to seeking HIV medical care.

Conversely, many patients engaged in primary HIV medical care may have undiagnosed and untreated mental illness, particularly depression. Depression can be easily screened for by asking two simple questions (Whooley and Simon, 2000). HIV primary care providers should screen for depression in their practice and may prescribe psychotropic medication to patients with uncomplicated depression or other psychiatric illness. Referral to a psychiatrist is usually made on the basis of availability of resources, the patient's openness to being referred, the complexity and severity of the psychiatric illness, and the need for psychotherapy.

Once patients are successfully engaged in both HIV and psychiatric care, communication and coordination of care between the HIV provider and psychiatrist are essential for achieving optimal adherence to and outcome of psychiatric and medical treatment.

ACKNOWLEDGMENTS   This work was supported by
NIMH grant MH071177 to J.J. Weiss.

References

Albert SM, Flater SR, Clouse R, Todak G, Stern Y,
Marder K, for the NEAD study group (2003). Medication management skill in HIV: I. Evidence for
adaptation of medication management strategies in
people with cognitive impairment. II. Evidence for
a pervasive lay model of medication efficacy. AIDS
Behav 7:329–338.

Altice FL, Mezger JA, Hodges J, Bruce RD, Marinovich
A, Walton M, Springer SA, and Friedland GH
(2004). Developing a directly administered antiretroviral therapy intervention for HIV-infected drug
users: implications for program replication. Clin Infect Dis 38:S376–S387.

Ammassari A, Antinori A, Aloisi MS, Trotta MP, Murri
R, Bartoli L, d'Arminio Monforte A, Wu AW, and
Starace F (2004). Depressive symptoms, neurocog-
nitive impairment, and adherence to highly active
antiretroviral therapy among HIV-infected persons.
Psychosomatics 45:394–402.

Arnsten JH, Demas PA, Farzadegan H, Grant RW,
Gourevitch MN, Chang CJ, Buono D, Eckholdt H,
Howard AA, and Schoenbaum EE (2001). Antiretroviral therapy adherence and viral suppression in
HIV-infected drug users: comparison of self-report
and electronic monitoring. Clin Infect Dis 33:1417–
1423.

Arnsten JH, Demas PA, Grant RW, Gourevitch MN,
Farzadegan H, Howard AA, and Schoenbaum EE
(2002). Impact of active drug use on antiretroviral therapy adherence and viral suppression in
HIV-infected drug users. J Gen Intern Med 17:377–
381.

Avants SK, Margolin A, Warburton LA, Hawkins KA, and
Shi J (2001). Predictors of nonadherence to HIV-
related medication regimens during methadone stabilization. Am Acad Addict Psychiatry 10:69–78.

Andrade ASA, McGruder HF, Wu AW, Celano SA,
Skolasky RL, Selnes OA, Huang IC, and McArthur
JC (2005). A programmable prompting device improves adherence to highly active antiretroviral therapy in HIV-infected subjects with memory impairment. Clin Infect Dis 41:875–882.

Balfour L, Kowal J, Silverman A, Tasca GA, Angel JB,
MacPherson PA, Garber G, Cooper CL, and
Cameron DW (2006). A randomized controlled
psycho-education intervention trial: improving psychological readiness for successful HIV medication
adherence and reducing depression before initiating HAART. AIDS Care 18:830–838.

Bandura A (1997). Self-Efficacy: The Exercise of Control
(pp. 79–115). New York: Freeman.

Bangsberg DR, Hecht FM, Charlebois ED, Zolopa AR,
Holodniy M, Sheiner L, Bamberger JD, Chesney MA,

and Moss A (2000). Adherence to protease inhibitors,
HIV-1 viral load, and development of drug resistance
in an indigent population. AIDS 14:357–366.

Bangsberg DR, Hecht FM, Charlebois E, Chesney M,
and Moss AR (2001a). Comparing objective methods of adherence assessment: electronic medication
monitoring and unannounced pill count. AIDS
Behav 5:275–281.

Bangsberg DR, Hecht FM, Clague H, Charlebois ED,
Ciccarone D, Chesney M, and Moss A (2001b).
Provider assessment of adherence to HIV antiretroviral therapy. J Acquir Immune Defic Syndr 26:435–
442.

Bangsberg DR, Mundy LM, and Tulsky JP (2001c). Expanding directly observed therapy: tuberculosis to
human immunodeficiency virus. Am J Med 110:
664–666.

Bangsberg DR, Perry S, Charlebois ED, Clark RA, Robertson M, Zolopa AR, and Moss A (2001d). Nonadherence to highly active antiretroviral therapy predicts progression to AIDS. AIDS 15:1181–1183.

Bangsberg DR, Bronstone A, Chesney MA, and Hecht FM
(2002). Computer-assisted self-interviewing (CASI)
to improve provider assessment of adherence in routine clinical practice. J Acquir Immune Defic Syndr
15:S107–S111.

Bangsberg DR, Charlebois ED, Grant RM, Holodniy
M, Deeks SG, Perry S, Conroy KN, Clark R,
Guzman D, Zolopa A, and Moss A (2003). High
levels of adherence do not prevent accumulation of
HIV drug resistance mutations. AIDS 17:1925–
1932.

Berg MB, Safren SA, Mimiaga MJ, Grasso C, Boswell S,
and Mayer KH (2005). Nonadherence to medical
appointments is associated with increased plasma
HIV RNA and decreased CD4 cell counts in a
community-based HIV primary care clinic. AIDS
Care 17:902–907.

Bing EG, Burnam A, Longshore D, Fleishman JA,
Sherbourne CD, London AS, Turner BJ, Eggan F,
Beckman R, Vitiello B, Morton SC, Orlando M,
Bozzette SA, Ortiz-Barron L, and Shapiro M
(2001). Psychiatric disorders and drug use among
human immunodeficiency virus–infected adults
in the United States. Arch Gen Psychiatry 58:721–
728.

Bouhnik AD, Chesney M, Carrieri P, Gallais H,
Moreau J, Moatti JP, Obadia Y, Spire B, and the
MANIF 2000 Study Group (2002). Nonadherence
among HIV-infected injecting drug users: the im-
pact of social instability. J Acquir Immune Defic
Syndr 31:S149–S153.

Brue V, Hahn J, Olmstead R, Grimes RM, Zielinski WL
and Simoni JM (2007). A novel technology to pro-
mote HAART adherence. Paper presented at the
NIMH/IAPAC Second International Conference on
HIV Treatment Adherence, 2007, Jersey City, New
Jersey.

Burack JH, Barrett DC, Stall RD, Chesney MA, Ekstrand MI, and Coates TJ (1993). Depressive symptoms and CD4 lymphcyte decline among HIV-infected men. *JAMA* 270:2568–2573.

Carrieri MP, Chesney MA, Spire B, Loundou A, Sobel A, Lepeu G, and Moatti JP (2003). Failure to maintain adherence to HAART in a cohort of French HIV-positive injecting drug users. *Int J Behav Med* 10:1–14.

Catz SL, Kelly JA, Bogart LM, Benotsch EG, and McAuliffe TL (2000). Patterns, correlates, and barriers to medication adherence among persons prescribed new treatments for HIV disease. *Health Psychol* 19:124–133.

Chesney MA, Ickovics JR, Chambers DB, Gifford AL, Neidig J, Zwickl B, Wu AW, for the Patient Care Committee and Adherence Working Group of the Outcomes Committee of the Adult AIDS Clinical Trials Group (AACTG) (2000). Self-reported adherence to antiretroviral medications among participants in HIV clinical trials: the AACTG adherence instruments. *AIDS Care* 12:255–266.

Cohen MA, Alfonso CA, Hoffman RG, Milau V, and Carrera G (2001). The impact of PTSD on treatment adherence in persons with HIV infection. *Gen Hosp Psychiatry* 23:294–296.

Cook JA, Grey D, Burke J, Cohen MA, Gurtman AC, Richardson JL, Wilson TE, Young MA, and Hessol NA (2004). Depressive symptoms and AIDS-related mortality among a multisite cohort of HIV-positive women. *Am J Public Health* 94:1133–1140.

Cook JA, Grey D, Burke-Miller J, Cohen MH, Anastos K, Gandhi M, Richardson J, Wilson T, and Young M (2006). Effects of treated and untreated depressive symptoms on highly active antiretroviral therapy use in a US multi-site cohort of HIV-positive women. *AIDS Care* 18:93–100.

Cook RL, Sereika SM, Hunt SC, Woodward WC, Erlen JA, and Conigliaro J (2001). Problem drinking and medication adherence among persons with HIV infection. *J Gen Intern Med* 16:83–88.

Davidson AJ, Yun L, and Maravi M (2006). In response to Wilson and Jacobson. *J Acquir Immune Defic Sydr* 41:255.

de Socio GVL, Fanelli L, Longo A, and Stagni G (2004). Adherence to antiretroviral therapy in HIV patients with psychiatric comorbidity. *J Acquir Immune Defic Syndr* 36:1109–1110.

Eldred LJ, Wu AW, Chaisson RE, and Moore RD (1998). Adherence to antiretroviral and pneumocysttis prophylaxis in HIV disease. *J Acquir Immune Defic Syndr Hum Retrovirol* 18:117–125.

Gebo KA, Keruly J, and Moore RD (2003). Association of social stress, illicit drug use, and health benefits with nonadherence to antiretroviral therapy. *J Gen Intern Med* 18:104–111.

Gifford AL, Bormann JE, Shively MJ, Wright BC, Richman DD, and Bozzette SA (2000). Predictors of self-reported adherence and plasma HIV concentrations in patients on multidrug antiretroviral regimens. *J Acquir Immune Defic Syndr* 23:386–395.

Giordano TP, Guzman D, Clark R, Charlebois ED, and Bangsberg DR (2004). Measuring adherence to antiretroviral therapy in a diverse population using a visual analogue scale. *HIV Clin Trials* 5:74–79.

Giordano TP, Suarez-Almazor ME, and Grimes RM (2005a). The population effectiveness of highly active antiretroviral therapy: are good drugs good enough? *Curr HIV/AIDS Rep* 2:177–183.

Giordano TP, Visnegarwala F, White AC Jr, Troisi CL, Frankowski RF, Hartman CM, and Grimes RM (2005b). Patients referred to an urban HIV clinic frequently fail to establish care: factors predicting failure. *AIDS Care* 17:773–783.

Golin CE, Liu H, Hays RD, Miller LG, Beck CK, Ickovics J, Kaplan AH, and Wenger NS (2002). A prospective study of predictors of adherence to combination antiretroviral medication. *J Gen Intern Med* 17:756–765.

Gonzalez JS, Penedo FJ, Antoni MH, Durán RE, Fernandez MI, McPherson-Baker S, Ironson G, Klimas NG, and Fletcher MA (2004). Social support, positive states of mind and HIV treatment adherence in men and women living with HIV/AIDS. *Health Psychol* 23:413–418.

Goodman LA, and Fallot RD (1998). HIV risk-behavior in poor urban women with serious mental disorders: association with childhood physical and sexual abuse. *Am J Orthopsychiatry* 68:73–83.

Gordillo V, del Amo J, Soriano V, and Gonzales-Lahoz J (1999). Sociodemographic and psychological variables influencing adherence to antiretroviral therapy. *AIDS* 13:1763–1769.

Gross R, Bilker WB, Friedman H, Coyne JC, and Strom BL (2002). Provider inaccuracy in assessing adherence and outcomes with newly initiated antiretroviral therapy. *AIDS* 16:1835–1837.

Grossberg R, Zhang Y, and Gross R (2004). A time-to-prescription-refill measure of antiretroviral adherence predicted changes in viral load in HIV. *J Clin Epidemiol* 57:1107–1110.

Harrigan PR, Hogg RS, Dong WW, Yip B, Wynhoven B, Woodward J, Brumme CJ, Brumme ZL, Mo T, Alexander CS, and Montaner JS (2005). Predictors of HIV drug-resistance mutations in a large antiretroviral-naïve cohort initiating triple antiretroviral therapy. *J Infect Dis* 191:339–347.

Himelhoch S, and Medoff DR (2005). Efficacy of antidepressant medication among HIV-positive individuals with depression: a systematic review and meta-analysis. *AIDS Patient Care STDS* 19:813–822.

Himelhoch S, Moore RD, Treisman G, and Gebo KA (2004). Does the presence of a current psychiatric disorder in AIDS patients affect the initiation of antiretroviral treatment and duration of therapy? *J Acquir Immune Defic Syndr* 37:1457–1463.

Hinkin CH, Castellon SA, Durvasula RS, Hardy DJ, Lam MN, Mason KI, Thrasher D, Goetz MB, and Stefaniak M (2002). Medication adherence among HIV+ adults: effects of cognitive dysfunction and regimen complexity. *Neurology* 59:1944–1950.

Howard AA, Arnsten JH, Lo Y, Vlahov D, Rich JD, Schuman P, Stone VE, Smith DK, Schoenbaum EE, for the HER Study Group (2002). A prospective study of adherence and viral load in a large multi-center cohort of HIV-infected women. *AIDS* 16: 2175–2182.

Ickovics JR, and Meisler AW (1997). Adherence in AIDS clinical trials: a framework for clinical research and clinical care. *J Clin Epidemiol* 50:385–391.

Ickovics JR, Hamburger ME, Vlahov D, Schoenbaum EE, Schuman P, Boland RJ, and Moore J (2001). Mortality, CD4 cell count decline, and depressive symptoms among HIV-seropositive women: longitudinal analysis from the HIV Epidemiology Research Study. *JAMA* 285:1466–1474.

Ingersoll KS, and Heckman CJ (2005). Patient–clinician relationships and treatment system effects on HIV medication adherence. *AIDS Behav* 9:89–101.

Kalichman SC, Amaral CM, Stearns H, White D, Flanagan J, Pope H, Cherry C, Cain D, Eaton L, and Kalichman MO (2007). Adherence to antiretroviral therapy assessed by unannounced pill counts conducted by telephone. *J Gen Intern Med* (in press).

Kalichman SC, Cain D, Cherry C, Kalichman M, and Pope H (2005a). Pillboxes and antiretroviral adherence: prevalence of use, perceived benefits, and implications for electronic medication monitoring devices. *AIDS Patient Care STDS* 19:833–839.

Kalichman SC, Cain D, Fuhrel A, Eaton L, Di Fonzo K, and Ertl T (2005b). Assessing medication adherence self-efficacy among low-literacy patients: development of a pictographic visual analogue scale. *Health Educ Res* 20:24–35.

Liu M, Rogers W, Coady W, Safren S, Skolnik P, Hardy H, and Wilson I (2006). What is the optimal recall period for self-report (SR) of antiretroviral (ARV) adherence (ADH)? Evidence from comparisons of SR and the Medication Event Monitoring Systems (MEMS). Paper presented at the NIMH/IAPAC International Conference on HIV Treatment Adherence, 2006, Jersey City, New Jersey.

Kerr T, Palepu A, Barnes G, Walsh J, Hogg R, Montaner J, Tyndall M, and Wood E (2004). Psychosocial determinants of adherence to highly active antiretroviral therapy among injection drug users in Vancouver. *Antiretrovir Ther* 9:407–414.

Knobel H, Carmona A, Lopez JL, Gimeno JL, Saballs P, Gonzalez A, Guelar A, and Diez A (1999). Adherence to very active antiretroviral treatment: Impact of individualized assessment. *Enferm Infecc Microbiol Clin* 17:78–81.

Levine AJ, Hinkin CH, Castellon SA, Mason KI, Lam MN, Perkins A, Robinet M, Longshore D, Newton T, Myers H, Durvasula RS, and Hardy DJ (2005).

Variations in patterns of highly active antiretroviral therapy (HAART) adherence. *AIDS Behav* 9:355–362.

Lewis MP, Colbert A, Erlen J, and Meyers M (2006). A qualitative study of persons who are 100% adherent to antiretroviral therapy. *AIDS Care* 18:140–148.

Liechty CA, Alexander CS, Harrigan PR, Guzman JD, Charlebois ED, Moss AR, and Bangsberg DR (2004). Are untimed antiretroviral drug levels useful predictors of adherence behavior? *AIDS* 18:127–129.

Low-Beer S, Yip B, O'Shaughnessy MV, Hogg RS, and Montaner JSG (2000). Adherence to triple therapy and viral load response. *J Acquir Immune Defic Syndr* 23:360–361.

Lucas GM, Cheever LW, Chaisson RE, and Moore RD (2001). Detrimental effects of continued illicit drug use on the treatment of HIV-1 infection. *J Acquir Immune Defic Syndr* 27:251–259.

Mannheimer S, Friedland G, Matts J, Child C, and Chesney M (2002) The consistency of adherence to antiretroviral therapy predicts biologic outcomes for human immunodeficiency virus–infected persons in clinical trials. *Clin Infect Dis* 34:1115–1121.

Mannheimer SB, Matts J, Telzak E, Chesney M, Child C, Wu AW, and Friedland G (2005). Quality of life in HIV-infected individuals receiving antiretroviral therapy is related to adherence. *AIDS Care* 17:10–22.

Margolin A, Avants SK, Warburton LA, Hawkins KA, and Shi J (2003). A randomized clinical trial of a manual-guided risk reduction intervention for HIV-positive injection drug users. *Health Psychol* 22: 223–228.

Miller LG, Liu H, Hays RD, Golin CE, Beck CK, Asch SM, Ma Y, Kaplan AH, and Wenger NS (2002). How well do clinicians estimate patients' adherence to combination antiretroviral therapy? *J Gen Intern Med* 17:1–11.

Mitty JA, Macalino GE, Bazerman LB, Loewenthal HG, Hogan JW, MacLeod CJ, and Flanigan TP (2005). The use of community-based modified directly observed therapy for the treatment of HIV-infected persons. *J Acquir Immune Defic Syndr* 39: 545–550.

Moss AR, Hahn JA, Perry S, Charlebois ED, Guzman D, Clark RA, and Bangsberg DR (2004). Adherence to highly active antiretroviral therapy in the homeless population in San Francisco: a prospective study. *Clin Infect Dis* 39:1190–1198.

Nieuwkerk PT, and Oort FJ (2005). Self-reported adherence to antiretroviral therapy for HIV-1 infection and virologic treatment response: a meta-analysis. *J Acquir Immune Defic Syndr* 38:445–448.

Oyugi JH, Byakika-Tusiime J, Charlebois ED, Kityo C, Mugerwa R, Mugyenyi P, and Bangsberg DR (2004). Multiple validated measures of adherence indicate high levels of adherence to generic HIV antiretroviral therapy in a resource-limited setting. *J Acquir Immune Defic Syndr* 36:1100–1102.

Page-Shafer K, Delorenze GN, Satariano WA, and Win-
kelstein W Jr (1996). Comorbidity and survival in
HIV-infected men in the San Francisco Men's
Health Survey. *Ann Epidemiol* 6:420–430.

Palepu A, Horton NJ, Tibbetts N, Meli S, and Samet JH
(2004). Uptake and adherence to highly active antiretroviral therapy among HIV-infected people with alcohol and other substance use problems: the impact
of substance use treatment. *Addiction* 99:361–368.

Palmer NB, Salcedo J, Miller AL, Winiarski M, and
Arno P (2003). Psychiatric and social barriers to
HIV medication adherence in a triply diagnosed
methadone population. *AIDS Patient Care STDS*
17:635–644.

Paterson DL, Swindells S, Mohr J, Brester M, Vergis
EN, Squier C, Wagener MM, and Singh N (2000).
Adherence to protease inhibitor therapy and out-
comes in patients with HIV infection. *Ann Intern
Med* 133:21–30.

Rathbun RC, Farmer KC, Stephens JR, and Lockhart
SM (2005). Impact of an adherence clinic on behavioral outcomes and virologic response in the
treatment of HIV infection: a prospective, randomized, controlled pilot study. *Clin Ther* 27:199–209.

Reiter GS, Stewart KE, Wojtusik L, Hewitt R, Segal-
Maurer S, Johnson M, Fisher A, Zackin R, Masters
H, and Bangsberg DR (2000). Elements of success
in HIV clinical care: multiple interventions that
promote adherence. *Topics HIV Med* 8:21–30.

Ricart F, Cohen MA, Alfonso CA, Hoffman RG,
Quiñones N, Cohen A, and Indyk D (2002). Understanding the psychodynamics of non-adherence
to medical treatment in persons with HIV infection.
Gen Hosp Psychiatry 24:176–180.

Riley ED, Bangsberg DR, Guzman D, Perry S, and
Moss AR (2005). Antiretroviral therapy, hepatitis C
virus, and AIDS mortality among San Francisco's
homeless and marginally housed. *J Acquir Immune
Defic Syndr* 38:191–195.

Rotheram-Borus MJ, Swendeman D, Comulada WS,
Weiss RE, Lee M, and Lightfoot M (2004).
Prevention for substance-using HIV-positive young
people: telephone and in-person delivery. *J Acquir
Immune Defic Syndr* 37:S68–S76.

Sabin CA, Smith CJ, Youle M, Lampe FC, Bell DR,
Puradiredja D, Lipman MCI, Bhagani S, Phillips
AN, and Johnson MA (2006). Deaths in the era of
HAART: contribution of late presentation, treat-
ment exposure, resistance and abnormal laboratory
markers. *AIDS* 20:67–71.

Safren SA, Otto MW, Worth JL, Salomon E, Johnson
W, Mayer K, and Boswell S (2001). Two strategies
to increase adherence to HIV antiretroviral medication: life-steps and medication monitoring. *Behav
Res Ther* 39:1151–1162.

Sambamoorthi U, Walkup J, Olfson M, and Crystal S
(2000). Antidepressant treatment and health services
utilization among HIV-infected Medicaid patients

diagnosed with depression. *J Gen Intern Med* 15:
311–320.

Samet JH, Horton NJ, Meli S, Dukes K, Tripps T,
Sullivan L, and Freedberg KA (2005). A randomized
controlled trial to enhance antiretroviral therapy adherence in patients with a history of alcohol problems. *Antivir Ther* 10:83–93.

Schneider J, Kaplan SH, Greenfield S, Li W, and
Wilson IB (2004). Better physician–patient relationships are associated with higher reported adherence to antiretroviral therapy in patients with HIV
infection. *J Gen Intern Med* 19:1096–1103.

Simoni JM, Pearson CR, Pantalone DW, Marks G, and
Crepaz N (2006). Efficacy of interventions in improving highly active antiretroviral therapy adherence and HIV-1 RNA viral load. A meta-analytic
review of randomized controlled trials. *J Acquir
Immune Defic Syndr* 43:S23–S35.

Singh N, Squier C, Sivek C, Wagener M, Nguyen MH,
and Yu VL (1996). Determinants of compliance
with antiretroviral therapy in patients with human
immunodeficiency virus: prospective assessment with
implications for enhancing compliance. *AIDS Care*
8:261–269.

Sledjeski EM, Delahanty DL, and Bogart LM (2005).
Incidence and impact of posttraumatic stress disor-
der and comorbid depression on adherence to
HAART and CD4+ counts in people living with
HIV. *AIDS Patient Care STDS* 19:728–736.

Starace F, Ammassari A, Trotta MP, Murri R, de Longis
P, Izzo C, Scalzini A, d'Arminio Monforte A, Wu
AW Antinori A, AdICoNA and the Neuro IcoNA
Study Groups (2002). Depression is a risk factor for
suboptimal adherence to highly active antiretrovi-
ral therapy. *J Acquir Immune Defic Syndr* 31:S136–
S139.

Tucker JS, Burnam MA, Sherbourne CD, Kung FY,
and Gifford AL (2003). Substance use and mental
health correlates of nonadherence to antiretroviral
medications in a sample of patients with human
immunodeficiency virus infection. *Am J Med* 114:
573–580.

Tuldrà A, Ferrer MJ, Fumaz CR, Bayes R, Paredes R,
Burger DM, and Clotet B (1999). Monitoring adherence to HIV therapy. *Arch Intern Med* 159:
1376–1377.

Tuldrà A, Fumz CRr, Ferrer MJ, Bayés R, Arnó A,
Balagué M, Bonjoch A, Jou A, Negredo E, Paredes
R, Ruiz L, Romeu J, Sirera G, Tural C, Burger D,
and Clotet B (2000). Prospective randomized two-
arm controlled study to determine the efficacy of a
specific intervention to improve long-term adherence to highly active antiretroviral therapy. *J Acquir
Immune Defic Syndr* 25:221–228.

Turner BJ, Fleishman JA, Wenger N, London AS,
Burnam MA, Shapiro MF, Bing EG, Stein MD,
Longshore D, and Bozzette SA (2001). Effects of
drug abuse and mental disorders on use and type of

antiretroviral therapy in HIV-infected persons. *J Gen Intern Med* 16:625–633.

Turner BJ, Laine C, Cosler L, and Hauck WW (2003). Relationship of gender, depression, and health care delivery with antiretroviral adherence in HIV-infected drug users. *J Gen Intern Med* 18:248–257.

van Servellen G, Chang B, Garcia L, and Lombardi E (2002). Individual and system level factors associated with treatment nonadherence in human immunodeficiency virus–infected men and women. *AIDS Patient Care STDS* 16:269–281.

Vitiello B, Burnam MA, Bing EG, Beckman R, and Shapiro MF (2003). Use of psychotropic medications among HIV-infected patients in the United States. *Am J Psychiatry* 160:547–554.

Wagner GJ, Kanouse DE, Koegel P, and Sullivan G (2003). Adherence to HIV antiretrovirals among persons with serious mental illness. *AIDS Patient Care STDS* 17:179–186.

Wagner GJ, Kanouse DE, Koegel P, and Sullivan G (2004). Correlates of HIV antiretroviral adherence in persons with serious mental illness. *AIDS Care* 16:501–506.

Wagner JH, Justice AC, Chesney M, Sinclair G, Weissman S, Rodriquez-Barradas M, for the VACS 3 Project Team (2001). Patient and provider-reported adherence: toward a clinically useful approach to measuring antiretroviral adherence. *J Clin Epidemiol* 54:S91–S98.

Walkup JT, Sambamoorthi U, and Crystal S (2004). Use of newer antiretroviral treatments among HIV-infected Medicaid beneficiaries with serious mental illness. *J Clin Psychiatry* 65:1180–1189.

Walsh JC, Mandalia, S, and Gazzard BG (2002a). Responses to a 1 month self-report on adherence to antiretroviral therapy are consistent with electronic data and virological treatment outcome. *AIDS* 16:269–277.

Walsh JC, Pozniak AL, Nelson MR, Mandalia S, and Gazzard BG (2002b). Virologic rebound on HAART in the context of low treatment adherence is associated with a low prevalence of antiretroviral drug resistance. *J Acquir Immune Defic Syndr* 30:278–287.

Whooley MA, and Simon GE (2000). Managing depression in medical outpatients. *N Engl J Med* 343:1942–1950.

Wilson IB, and Jacobson D (2006). Regarding "Antidepressant treatment improves adherence to antiretroviral therapy among depressed HIV-infected patients." *J Acquir Immune Defic Syndr* 41:254–255.

Wilson IB, Lu M, Safren SA, Coady W, Skolnik PR, Hardy H, Laws MB, and Rogers WH (2007). Results of a physician-focused intervention to improve antiretroviral medication adherence. Paper presented at the NIMH/IAPAC Second International Conference on HIV Treatment Adherence, 2007, Jersey City, New Jersey.

Wood E, Hogg RS, Yip B, Harrigan PR, O'Shaughnessy MV, and Montaner JS (2003). Effect of medication adherence on survival of HIV-infected adults who start highly active antiretroviral therapy when the CD4+ cell count is .200 to 0.350 × 10(9) cells/L. *Ann Intern Med* 139:810–816.

[WHO] World Health Organization (2003). *Adherence to Long-Term Therapies: Evidence for Action*. Geneva: World Health Organization.

Yun LWH, Maravi M, Kobayashi JS, Barton PL, and Davidson AJ (2005). Antidepressant treatment improves adherence to antiretroviral therapy among depressed HIV-infected patients. *J Acquir Immune Defic Syndr* 38:432–438.

Chapter 23

Homelessness and HIV Risk and Prevention

Naomi Adler, Daniel B. Herman, Alan Berkman, and Ezra S. Susser

Homelessness is associated with poorer health and higher risk of morbidity and mortality (Barrow et al., 1999; Culhane et al., 2001; Cheung and Hwang, 2004). Mortality in the homeless population ranges from 3.5 times to greater than 8 times that of the housed population (Hibbs et al., 1994; Hwang, 2000), and HIV prevalence rates are significantly higher than those of their housed counterparts (Culhane et al., 2001; Robertson et al., 2004). The elevated prevalence of infection combined with lack of access to treatment and poor living conditions have contributed to HIV/AIDS becoming a leading cause of death in homeless people (Cheung and Hwang, 2004).

In this chapter we will examine the issue of HIV risk and prevention in the homeless population. We first provide a brief overview of the problem of homelessness in the United States and of the characteristics of specific subgroups within the homeless population. We then discuss the possibilities for HIV prevention and treatment among people who are homeless.

HOMELESSNESS IN THE UNITED STATES

Homelessness is a significant problem in the United States and has recently been prioritized as an important issue by the federal government. In the past, single men made up the vast majority of the homeless population, but since the 1980s the number of homeless families has increased dramatically. The causes of homelessness include poverty, a lack of affordable housing, and inadequate community supports for persons with serious mental health and substance use problems. It is important to bear in mind that although individual-level factors may increase the risk of certain individuals becoming homeless, the overall prevalence of homelessness in the United States is determined primarily by poverty and an inadequate supply of affordable housing.

Because of the transient nature of homelessness, it is difficult to obtain accurate estimates of the number of individuals who are currently homeless.

Furthermore, there is no universally accepted defini- tion of homelessness: some include only those who are currently literally homeless while others may in- clude those who are marginally or unstably housed or who have been homeless in the past. As a result, es- timates of the number of homeless individuals vary greatly from one study to the next and are often dif- ficult to compare. Nonetheless, the most reliable re- cent reports suggest that on any given day there are more than 800,000 persons homeless in the United States, while over the course of a year there are be- tween 2.3 and 3.5 million individuals who experience a period of homelessness (Burt et al., 2001). It has been found that 14% of the population, or 26 million people, have experienced a period of homelessness at some point in their lives (Link et al., 1994).

The homeless population is quite heterogeneous and is generally seen as comprising four major groups: single adult men, single adult women, members of homeless families (typically a single parent with one or more children), and youth. According to a recent report from the U.S. Conference of Mayors (2004), single women make up 14% of the homeless popu- lation, single adult men 41%, families about 40%, and unaccompanied youth 5% (U.S. Conference of Mayors, 2004). Each of these groups possesses its own social and clinical characteristics, service needs, and reasons for homelessness (Caton et al., 1994, 1995; Bassuk et al., 1996).

Homelessness impacts ethnic minorities more than any other population (Burt et al., 2001) and particu- larly individuals of African-American descent. It is estimated that 49% of the homeless population is Af- rican American, 13% are Hispanic, and 35% are white (U.S. Conference of Mayors, 2004).

HIV PREVALENCE IN
THE HOMELESS POPULATION

Although the prevalence of HIV/AIDS among home- less persons is thought to exceed that of the non- homeless population, reliable data are difficult to ob- tain. In studies carried out in Los Angeles and New York City, the prevalence of HIV infection in home- less samples ranged between 1.5% and 19% (Susser et al., 1993; Herndon et al., 2003). A recent study in San Francisco reported an overall HIV prevalence of 10.5% for currently homeless and marginally housed adults, which is five times higher than that of the general San Francisco population (Robertson et al., 2004). In other studies the prevalence of HIV among the homeless has been found to be nine times that of the general population (Culhane et al., 2001). When comparing HIV prevalence estimates it is important to keep in mind that the prevalence of HIV infection has changed significantly over time, making it espe- cially difficult to accurately assess the number of cur- rently homeless HIV-positive individuals.

The association between homelessness and HIV appears to be a two-way street. HIV-positive persons are at greater risk of homelessness because of discrim- ination and the high costs of housing and medical care. At the same time, homelessness has been shown to increase risk-taking behavior leading to an elevated likelihood of contracting HIV (Galea and Vlahov, 2002; Metraux et al., 2004). Furthermore, homeless persons are in transient living situations, typically in impoverished communities with high HIV prevalence. Thus, risky behaviors they may engage in are also more likely to result in infection.

It is well understood that HIV/AIDS dispropor- tionately affects ethnic minorities and that minority women are at particularly high risk compared to white women (Cargill and Stone, 2005). Men and women of minority descent are both highly represented in the homeless population. Prevention of HIV infection and care for ethnic minorities who are HIV positive are further complicated by their disproportionate ex- perience of adverse social factors that contribute to poor health (Galea and Vlahov, 2002), as well as by their unequal access to health care services (Cargill and Stone, 2005).

RISK FACTORS FOR HIV TRANSMISSION
IN THE HOMELESS POPULATION

A number of conditions generally associated with homelessness increase the overall risk of adverse health outcomes in this population. These include lack of access to basic resources such as shelter, nutrition, and appropriate physical and mental health care, as well as discrimination and social exclusion. While some of the risk factors for HIV transmission are common to the overall homeless population, a number of these factors vary by subpopulation. In this section we con- sider four main homeless subgroups—single women, families, adolescents, and single men—and discuss risks that are particularly salient in each respective group.

Single Women

Homeless persons are more likely to evidence drug and alcohol abuse than the general population. In a cross-sectional study, 43% of currently homeless individuals were found to have either a mental illness or substance abuse disorder (Burt et al., 2001). By another estimate in 2000, 69% of homeless single women had either a drug, alcohol, or mental disorder (North et al., 2004). Furthermore, female injection drug users were more likely to engage in risky behaviors, such as needle sharing, than were their male counterparts (Evans et al., 2003).

Nearly one-fourth of the single-adult homeless population suffers from severe and persistent mental illness (Burt et al., 2001). Most of these cases of mental illness are accounted for by major depression (North et al., 2004). However, they also include schizophrenia and other psychotic disorders. Severely mentally ill individuals are a subpopulation with disproportionately high HIV seroprevalence (Rosenberg et al., 2003). The prevalence of substance abuse disorders and severe mental illness has important implications for both the prevention and transmission of HIV. The impulsivity and impaired judgment often associated with substance abuse and mental illness can contribute to risky behaviors such as unprotected sex, having multiple sexual partners, sharing needles, or exchanging sex for drugs.

Homeless women frequently report physical and sexual traumas in childhood (Goodman and Aman, 1990; Shinn et al., 1991; North et al., 1994) and are more likely to have experienced childhood abuse than their housed counterparts (Wechsberg et al., 2003). Research has shown that a history of either abuse or neglect during childhood places both women and men at greater risk for adult homelessness (Herman et al., 1997). It is also well documented that adverse childhood experiences are associated with greater risk-taking behaviors later in life, such as having multiple sex partners, leading to increased transmission of sexually transmitted disease (STD), higher rates of adolescent pregnancy (Hillis et al., 2000, 2001, 2004), and potentially a greater likelihood of HIV transmission.

Intimate partner violence is known to be a characteristic associated with risk factors such as unsafe sex or injection practices that increase the risk of contracting HIV and other sexually transmitted diseases, especially when substance abuse is involved (El-Bassel et al., 2005). Homeless women report higher rates of substance abuse (North et al., 2004) and partner violence than those of their housed counterparts. There is significant evidence that alcohol abuse increases a woman's likelihood of being abused (Miller, 1990; Miller et al., 1993; Abbott et al., 1995; El-Bassel et al., 2003) and that women with a history of childhood sexual and physical abuse often turn to drugs or alcohol as a coping mechanism (Yegidis, 1992; Miller et al., 1993; Zierler and Krieger, 1997). Current homelessness combined with substance use in turn increases a woman's risk of both partner violence and HIV infection.

Homeless Families

Homeless families are one of the largest and fastest growing groups in the homeless population (U.S. Conference of Mayors, 2003). They are the end users of 34% of all services for the homeless nationally (Burt et al., 2001).

Single homeless mothers have many of the same characteristics that have been associated with increased risk factors for HIV transmission among single homeless women. These characteristics include childhood physical and sexual abuse (Burt et al., 2001; North et al., 2004), sexual assault, partner violence, substance abuse (Goering, 1998; Burt et al., 2001), and poor social support (Bassuk et al., 1996; Herman et al., 1997).

Among homeless mothers approximately two-thirds have experienced severe physical violence as a child, 42% report sexual abuse during childhood, and 61% have experienced partner violence in adulthood (Browne and Bassuk, 1997). Partner violence among homeless mothers has been widely documented (Bassuk et al., 1996; Hien and Bukszpan, 1999). Rates of severe physical and sexual assault over the lifespan of homeless and marginally housed mothers has been found to exceed 80% (Bassuk et al., 1996). Homeless mothers typically have diminished social networks and few social supports (Shinn et al., 1991; Bassuk et al., 1996).

In one study more than 70% of homeless mothers reported symptoms of psychological distress or substance abuse and yet only 15% had access to mental health services of any sort (Zima et al., 1996). Research has shown that homeless mothers are not well integrated into primary health care services and must rely instead on emergency departments for health care (Duchon et al., 1999). Many homeless mothers demonstrate misconceptions about HIV transmission (Weinreb et al., 1999) and appear to have access to few resources for improved information.

Homeless Youth

Homeless youth are a group at exceptionally high risk for HIV. They are 6 to 12 times more likely to become HIV positive than other youth (Rotheram-Borus et al., 2003). Although HIV/AIDS is not a leading cause of death among homeless youth, it has been shown that during periods of homelessness risk of death increases significantly for this population, particularly death by suicide (Roy et al., 2004). Injection drug use, alcohol use, and HIV infection are also independent predictors of mortality among homeless youth (Roy et al., 2004).

African Americans account for 56% of all HIV cases in youth between the ages of 13 and 24 (CDC, 2005) and make up a significant proportion of the homeless youth. Young men under the age of 25 who have sex with men and who are of African-American or Latino descent are at particular risk for HIV infection (Celentano et al., 2005).

Substance use among homeless youth is more widespread than among housed youth. In 2004, 69% of homeless youth reported alcohol use and approximately three-quarters of surveyed youth reported the use of ecstasy, ketamine, and other hallucinogens at least one to three times a month (Van Leeuwen et al., 2004). Club drugs can increase potential HIV transmission by lowering inhibitions, increasing sexual endurance, and leading to high risk sexual behavior such as unprotected sex (Swanson and Cooper, 2002). Other risky behaviors such as trading sex for drugs and sharing needles have also been reported by many homeless youth (Van Leeuwen et al., 2004).

Single Homeless Men

Single homeless men are more likely than single housed men to have a substance abuse disorder or mental illness. By one estimate, 88% of homeless single men show evidence of drug, alcohol, or mental disorders (North et al., 2004). Single homeless men, like homeless women, also report significant histories of abuse. Nearly 27% of homeless men report an incident of physical assault within the past year (Kushel et al., 2003).

It has been demonstrated that among single men and adolescents, longer periods of homelessness are associated with a greater likelihood of risk-taking behaviors (Rahav et al., 1998; Ennett et al., 1999) such as unprotected sex or sharing needles. Among single homeless men, those men who have sex with men (MSM) or who are injection drug users (IDUs) are more likely to be HIV positive. A recent study in San Francisco reported that in the homeless MSM population, 30% tested positive for HIV and of homeless IDUs, 8% tested positive for HIV (Robertson et al., 2004). It has also been shown that among IDUs, those who are currently homeless are more likely to test positive for HIV than those who are housed (Reyes et al., 2005).

Injection drug use is a significant problem in this population. Injection drug use among homeless men with a severe mental illness ranges from 16% to 26% (Susser et al., 1997; Linn et al., 2005). Homelessness has been shown to increase injection drug use risk-taking behavior and adverse health outcomes, with approximately 70% of homeless IDUs reporting practices such as sharing needles and participating in shooting galleries (Galea and Vlahov, 2002; Linn et al., 2005). It has been found that the majority of homeless mentally ill men who are IDUs engage in both unsafe injection practices and sexual behaviors (Susser et al., 1996).

HIV/AIDS TREATMENT AND PREVENTION IN THE HOMELESS POPULATION

The relationship between homelessness and health outcomes is complex. Nonetheless, the research shows clearly that homelessness contributes to poorer health, higher mortality (Hibbs et al., 1994; Hwang, 2000), and reduced access to health care services. For currently homeless individuals, prioritizing daily needs such as food, shelter, and work typically takes precedence over less urgent matters such as health care. Even when health services are actively sought, they are difficult to access with issues such as payment, documentation, transportation, obtaining and storing medications, and continuity of care posing major barriers.

In our view, in order for HIV prevention efforts to be most effective, basic survival needs such as shelter and food must be tended to first. It has been shown that simply providing homeless individuals with housing and cash benefits can effectively reduce risk-taking behavior such as unprotected sex, drug use, and needle sharing (Aidala et al., 2005; Riley et al.,

2005). Shorter periods of homelessness are associated with recent employment, reliable income source, family support, and substance abuse treatment (Caton et al., 2005). For persons with severe mental illness, approaches such as critical time intervention (CTI) may help prevent recurrent homelessness by enhancing continuity of care during periods of transition from institutional care to community living (Susser et al., 1997b).

A common misconception is that the greatest barrier to delivering prevention and treatment services to homeless persons is finding them. The reality, however, is that homeless people are often visible by living or working in the streets and/or are readily accessible in shelters. The forming of trusting relationships, consistent contact over time, and use of already existing social networks can help in finding and retaining homeless persons for follow-up and services. In one HIV testing program for homeless persons with severe mental illness, nearly 90% of those tested returned for their results. The greatest predictor of returning for results was good social support (Desai and Rosenheck, 2004).

Characteristics and behaviors associated with HIV risk factors, such as unsafe sexual or drug use practices, vary from one subgroup of the homeless population to another, thus programs must be tailored to each group's individual needs. For example, nearly 28% of homeless male youth report trading sex to meet their basic survival needs (Haley et al., 2004). Thus in addition to HIV prevention education outreach and support services, programs to address basic survival needs, substance abuse, and other underlying mental health issues are particularly needed for homeless youth (Woods et al., 2003).

Behavioral HIV prevention interventions show promising results for reducing HIV transmission among currently homeless individuals. One such example is the Sex, Games and Videotapes intervention carried out in a New York City homeless shelter. Sex, Games and Videotapes is a program designed for homeless mentally ill men in a New York City shelter that is built around activities central to shelter life: competitive games, storytelling, and watching videos. For many of these men sex is conducted in public spaces, revolves around drug use, and must be conducted quickly. The program allows for sex issues to be brought up in a nonjudgmental way. In a randomized trial, the program successfully reduced sexual risk behavior threefold (Susser et al., 1998).

Many homeless individuals currently receive much of their medical care in emergency rooms. Nearly 40% of homeless persons reported one or more visits to the emergency room in the past year (Kushel et al., 2002). This is a clear indication of the need for improved, ongoing medical care in the homeless population; it may also present an opportunity for identifying potentially HIV-infected individuals, now that testing in emergency departments, even in low-prevalence areas, has been shown to be effective (Lyons et al., 2005).

Traditionally the homeless population has been thought to be a group that is likely to have poor adherence to medication regimens and thus be at high risk for the development of drug-resistant strains of HIV. Despite difficulties in accessing ongoing medical care, a recent study found that nearly one-third of homeless HIV-positive individuals were able to maintain their medication regimens (Moss et al., 2004).

To improve the ability of currently homeless HIV-positive individuals to adhere to their medication, comprehensive programs are needed to help provide for basic needs. An example of one such program is Housing Works in New York City. Housing Works is an AIDS service organization that specializes in providing comprehensive care to HIV-positive homeless persons. Their services include housing, health care, job training and placement, and a variety of other advocacy services for homeless HIV-positive persons (Housing Works, 2006).

Coordinated care networks that provide homeless persons with comprehensive care and that allow staff to link individuals quickly and easily to the services they need have been shown to be more successful in retaining individuals in care (Woods et al., 2003; Hwang et al., 2005). For example, Boston HAPPENS provides coordinated health education, case management, basic medical care, HIV testing, counseling, and mental health care for HIV-positive at-risk youth, many of whom are homeless. Through persistent outreach, individualized case management, and a large, coordinated group of providers, HAPPENS retains homeless at-risk youth in care (Harris et al., 2003).

HIV prevention activities and coordination of care for the homeless are frequently restricted by institutional barriers and settings. Staffing at shelters is often only adequate to provide basic needs, and shelters may be reluctant to allow outside HIV prevention program staff to talk explicitly about sex and drugs or to distribute condoms because those activities are forbidden in most shelters. While institutions may find it necessary to forbid these activities on their premises, it is also clear that in order to encourage homeless individuals to practice safe sex, they also need to be given private space where they can do so. A lack of private space can also be a serious barrier for counseling and education around sensitive topics. There is an ongoing need to deliver effective prevention activities in the service settings that homeless persons use, such as soup kitchens, shelters, residential hotels, and clinics. Staff of these organizations should be trained in HIV prevention education methods that recognize specific risk factors related to homelessness, employ realistic expectations for change, and give homeless people concrete goals that they can accomplish.

Ultimately homelessness is characterized by two factors: a lack of a permanent place to live and extreme poverty. Long-term efforts to provide homeless individuals with the resources to remedy these two needs will go a long way toward both decreasing the growing prevalence of chronic homelessness and reducing the likelihood of HIV transmission.

References

Abbott J, Johnson R, Koziol-McLain J, and Lowenstein SR (1995). Domestic violence against women. Incidence and prevalence in an emergency department population. *JAMA* 273(22):1763–1767.

Aidala A, Cross JE, Stall R, Harre D, and Sumartojo E (2005). Housing status and HIV risk behaviors: implications for prevention and policy. *AIDS Behav* 9(3):251–265.

Barrow SM, Herman DB, Cordova P, and Struening EL (1999). Mortality among homeless shelter residents in New York City. *Am J Public Health* 89(4): 529–534.

Bassuk EL, Weinreb LF, Buckner JC, Browne A, Salomon A, and Bassuk SS (1996). The characteristics and needs of sheltered homeless and low-income housed mothers. *JAMA* 276(8):640–646.

Browne A, and Bassuk SS (1997). Intimate violence in the lives of homeless and poor housed women: prevalence and patterns in an ethnically diverse sample. *Am J Orthopsychiatry* 67(2):261–278.

Burt M, Laudan Y, and Lee E (2001). *Helping America's Homeless: Emergency Shelter or Affordable Housing?* Washington, DC: Urban Institute Press.

Cargill VA, and Stone VE (2005). HIV/AIDS: a minority health issue. *Med Clin North Am* 89(4):895–912.

Caton CL, Shrout PE, Eagle PF, Opler LA, Felix A, and Dominguez B (1994). Risk factors for homelessness among schizophrenic men: a case–control study. *Am J Public Health* 84(2):265–270.

Caton CL, Shrout PE, Dominguez B, Eagle PF, Opler LA, and Cournos F (1995). Risk factors for homelessness among women with schizophrenia. *Am J Public Health* 85(8 Pt. 1):1153–1156.

Caton CL, Dominguez B, Schanzer B, Hasin DS, Shrout PE, Felix A, et al. (2005). Risk factors for long-term homelessness: findings from a longitudinal study of first-time homeless single adults. *Am J Public Health* 95(10):1753–1759.

[CDC] Centers for Disease Control and Prevention (2005).*HIV Prevention in the Third Decade*. Atlanta: US Department of Health and Human Services, CDC

Celentano D, Sifakis F, Hylton J, Torian L, Guillin V, and Koblin B (2005). Race/ethnic differences in HIV prevalence and risks among adolescent and young adult men who have sex with men. *J Urban Health*. 82(4):610–621.

Cheung AM, and Hwang SW (2004). Risk of death among homeless women: a cohort study and review of the literature. *CMAJ* 170(8):1243–1247.

Culhane D, Gollub E, Kuhn R, and Shpaner M (2001). The co-occurrence of AIDS and homelessness: results from the integration of administrative databases for AIDS surveillance and public shelter utilization in Philadelphia. *J Epidemiol Community Health* 55(7):515–520.

Desai MM, and Rosenheck RA (2004). HIV testing and receipt of test results among homeless persons with serious mental illness. *Am J Psychiatry* 161(12): 2287–2294.

Duchon LM, Weitzman BC, and Shinn M (1999). The relationship of residential instability to medical care utilization among poor mothers in New York City. *Med Care* 37(12):1282–1293.

El-Bassel N, Gilbert L, Witte S, Wu E, Gaeta T, Schilling R, et al. (2003). Intimate partner violence and substance abuse among minority women receiving care from an inner-city emergency department. *Womens Health Issues* 13(1):16–22.

El-Bassel N, Gilbert L, Wu E, Go H, and Hill J (2005). HIV and intimate partner violence among methadone-maintained women in New York City. *Soc Sci Med* 61(1):171–183.

Ennett ST, Federman EB, Bailey SL, Ringwalt CL, and Hubbard ML (1999). HIV-risk behaviors associated with homelessness characteristics in youth. *J Adolesc Health* 25(5):344–353.

Evans JL, Hahn JA, Page-Shafer K, Lum PJ, Stein ES, Davidson PJ, et al. (2003). Gender differences in sexual and injection risk behavior among active young injection drug users in San Francisco (the UFO Study). *J Urban Health* 80(1):137–146.

Galea S, and Vlahov D (2002). Social determinants and the health of drug users: socioeconomic status, homelessness, and incarceration. *Public Health Rep* 117(Suppl. 1):S135–145.

Goering P (1998.). Pathways to homelessness. Toronto, Ontario, Canada: Health Systems Research Unit,

Clarke Institute of Psychiatry, Department of Psychiatry, University of Toronto.

Goodman GS, and Aman C (1990). Children's use of anatomically detailed dolls to recount an event. *Child Dev* 61(6):1859–1871.

Haley N, Roy E, Leclerc P, Boudreau JF, and Boivin JF (2004). HIV risk profile of male street youth involved in survival sex. *Sex Transm Infect* 80(6):526–530.

Harris SK, Samples CL, Keenan PM, Fox DJ, Melchiono MW, and Woods ER (2003). Outreach, mental health, and case management services: can they help to retain HIV-positive and at-risk youth and young adults in care? *Matern Child Health J* 7(4):205–218.

Herman DB, Susser ES, Struening EL, and Link BL (1997). Adverse childhood experiences: are they risk factors for adult homelessness? *Am J Public Health* 87(2):249–255.

Herndon B, Asch SM, Kilbourne AM, Wang M, Lee M, Wenzel SL, et al. (2003). Prevalence and predictors of HIV testing among a probability sample of homeless women in Los Angeles County. *Public Health Rep* 118(3):261–269.

Hibbs JR, Benner L, Klugman L, Spencer R, Macchia I, Mellinger A, et al. (1994). Mortality in a cohort of homeless adults in Philadelphia. *N Engl J Med* 331(5):304–309.

Hien D, and Bukszpan C (1999). Interpersonal violence in a "normal" low-income control group. *Women Health* 29(4):1–16.

Hillis SD, Anda RF, Dube SR, Felitti VJ, Marchbanks PA, and Marks JS (2004). The association between adverse childhood experiences and adolescent pregnancy, long-term psychosocial consequences, and fetal death. *Pediatrics* 113(2):320–327.

Hillis SD, Anda RF, Felitti VJ, and Marchbanks PA (2001). Adverse childhood experiences and sexual risk behaviors in women: a retrospective cohort study. *Fam Plann Perspect* 33(5):206–211.

Hillis SD, Anda RF, Felitti VJ, Nordenberg D, and Marchbanks PA (2000). Adverse childhood experiences and sexually transmitted diseases in men and women: a retrospective study. *Pediatrics* 106(1):E11.

Housing Works (2006). *Campaign to end AIDS*. Retrieved November 15, 2005, from http://www.housing works.org/home_c2ea.html

Hwang SW (2000). Mortality among men using homeless shelters in Toronto, Ontario. *JAMA* 283(16):2152–2157.

Hwang SW, Tolomiczenko G, Kouyoumdjian FG, and Garner RE (2005). Interventions to improve the health of the homeless: a systematic review. *Am J Prev Med* 29(4):311–319.

Kushel MB, Evans JL, Perry S, Robertson MJ, and Moss AR (2003). No door to lock: victimization among homeless and marginally housed persons. *Arch Intern Med* 163(20):2492–2499.

Kushel MB, Perry S, Bangsberg D, Clark R, and Moss AR (2002). Emergency department use among the homeless and marginally housed: results from a community-based study. *Am J Public Health* 92(5):778–784.

Link BG, Susser E, Stueve A, Phelan J, Moore RE, Struening E. (1994) Lifetime and five-year prevalence of homelessness in the United States. *Am J Public Health* 84(12):1885–1886.

Linn JG, Brown M, and Kendrick L (2005). Injection drug use among homeless adults in the southeast with severe mental illness. *J Health Care Poor Underserved* 16(4A):83–90.

Lyons MS, Lindsell CJ, Ledyard HK, Frame PT, and Trott AT (2005). Emergency department HIV testing and counseling: an ongoing experience in a low-prevalence area. *Ann Emerg Med* 46(1):22–28.

Metraux S, Metzger DS, and Culhane DP (2004). Homelessness and HIV risk behaviors among injection drug users. *J Urban Health* 81(4):618–629.

Miller BA (1990). The interrelationships between alcohol and drugs and family violence. *NIDA Res Monogr* 103:177–207.

Miller BA, Downs WR, and Testa M (1993). Interrelationships between victimization experiences and women's alcohol use. *J Stud Alcohol Suppl* 11:109–117.

Moss AR, Hahn JA, Perry S, Charlebois ED, Guzman D, Clark RA, et al. (2004). Adherence to highly active antiretroviral therapy in the homeless population in San Francisco: a prospective study. *Clin Infect Dis* 39(8):1190–1198.

North CS, Eyrich KM, Pollio DE, and Spitznagel EL (2004). Are rates of psychiatric disorders in the homeless population changing? *Am J Public Health* 94(1):103–108.

North CS, Smith EM, and Spitznagel EL (1994). Violence and the homeless: an epidemiologic study of victimization and aggression. *J Trauma Stress* 7(1):95–110.

Rahav M, Nuttbrock L, Rivera JJ, and Link BG (1998). HIV infection risks among homeless, mentally ill, chemical misusing men. *Subst Use Misuse* 33(6):1407–1426.

Reyes JC, Robles RR, Colon HM, Matos TD, Finlinson HA, Marrero CA, et al. (2005). Homelessness and HIV risk behaviors among drug injectors in Puerto Rico. *J Urban Health* 82(3):446–455.

Riley ED, Moss AR, Clark RA, Monk SL, and Bangsberg DR (2005). Cash benefits are associated with lower risk behavior among the homeless and marginally housed in San Francisco. *J Urban Health* 82(1):142–150.

Robertson MJ, Clark RA, Charlebois ED, Tulsky J, Long HL, Bangsberg DR, et al. (2004). HIV seroprevalence among homeless and marginally housed adults in San Francisco. *Am J Public Health* 94(7):1207–1217.

Rosenberg SD, Swanson JW, Wolford GL, Osher FC, Swartz MS, Essock SM, et al. (2003). The five-site health and risk study of blood-borne infections among persons with severe mental illness. *Psychiatr Serv* 54(6):827–835.

Rotheram-Borus MJ, Song J, Gwadz M, Lee M, Van Rossem R, and Koopman C (2003). Reductions in HIV risk among runaway youth. *Prev Sci* 4(3):173–187.

Roy E, Haley N, Leclerc P, Sochanski B, Boudreau JF, and Boivin JF (2004). Mortality in a cohort of street youth in Montreal. *JAMA* 292(5):569–574.

Shinn M, Knickman JR, and Weitzman BC (1991). Social relationships and vulnerability to becoming homeless among poor families. *Am Psychol* 46(11): 1180–1187.

Susser E, Betne P, Valencia E, Goldfinger SM, and Lehman AF (1997). Injection drug use among homeless adults with severe mental illness. *Am J Public Health* 87(5):854–856.

Susser E, Valencia E, and Conover S (1993). Prevalence of HIV infection among psychiatric patients in a New York City men's shelter. *Am J Public Health* 83(4): 568–570.

Susser E, Miller M, Valencia E, Colson P, Roche B, and Conover S (1996). Injection drug use and risk of HIV transmission among homeless men with mental illness. *Am J Psychiatry* 153(6):794–798.

Susser E, Valencia E, Conover S, Felix A, Tsai WY, and Wyatt RJ (1997). Preventing recurrent homelessness among mentally ill men: a "critical time" intervention after discharge from a shelter. *Am J Public Health* 87(2):256–262.

Susser E, Valencia E, Berkman A, Sohler N, Conover S, Torres J, et al. (1998). Human immunodeficiency virus sexual risk reduction in homeless men with mental illness. *Arch Gen Psychiatry* 55(3):266–272.

Swanson J, and Cooper A (2002). Dangerous liaison: club drug use and HIV/AIDS. *IAPAC Monthly* 8:1–15.

U.S. Conference of Mayors (2003). A *Status Report on Hunger and Homelessness in America's Cities: 2003*. Retrieved January 25, 2006, from http://www.usmayors.org/uscm/hungersurvey/2003/onlinereport/HungerAndHomelessnessReport2003.pdf

U.S. Conference of Mayors (2004). A *Status Report on Hunger and Homelessness in America's Cities: 2004*. Retrieved January 25, 2006, from http://www.usmayors.org/uscm/hungersurvey/2004/onlinereport/HungerAndHomelessnessReport2004.pdf

Van Leeuwen JM, Hopfer C, Hooks S, White R, Petersen J, and Pirkopf J (2004). A snapshot of substance abuse among homeless and runaway youth in Denver, Colorado. *J Community Health* 29(3):217–229.

Wechsberg WM, Lam WK, Zule W, Hall G, Middlesteadt R, and Edwards J (2003). Violence, homelessness, and HIV risk among crack-using African-American women. *Subst Use Misuse* 38(3-6): 669–700.

Weinreb L, Goldberg R, Lessard D, Perloff J, and Bassuk E (1999). HIV-risk practices among homeless and low-income housed mothers. *J Fam Pract* 48(11): 859–867.

Woods ER, Samples CL, Melchiono MW, and Harris SK (2003). Boston HAPPENS Program: HIV-positive, homeless, and at-risk youth can access care through youth-oriented HIV services. *Semin Pediatr Infect Dis* 14(1):43–53.

Yegidis B (1992). Clinical care update, family violence: Contemporary research findings and practice issues. *Community Mental Health J* 28(6):519–530.

Zierler S, and Krieger N (1997). Reframing women's risk: social inequalities and HIV infection. *Annu Rev Public Health* 18:401–436.

Zima BT, Wells KB, Benjamin B, and Duan N (1996). Mental health problems among homeless mothers: relationship to service use and child mental health problems. *Arch Gen Psychiatry* 53(4):332–338.

Part VII

AIDS Psychiatry through the Life Cycle

Chapter 24

Childhood and Adolescence

Maryland Pao and Lori Wiener

Since the use of highly active antiretroviral therapy (HAART) in the United States became widespread, issues in the psychosocial and psychiatric management of HIV-infected children and adolescents have evolved from a bereavement and family stabilization model to one promoting quality of life in chronic illness. While issues related to the medical management of HIV infection remain important, preparing for long-term survival, achieving academic success, living independently, and preventing secondary infection have become primary goals in the care of HIV-infected youth. For most HIV-infected young persons and their caregivers, complex social and psychiatric needs driven by familial substance abuse, histories of trauma and family disruption, mental illness, socioeconomic stressors, and urban violence complicate provision of care.

Young people are affected by HIV (1) through perinatally acquired pediatric HIV/AIDS, (2) as adolescents with HIV/AIDS acquired through their risky sexual behavior and drug use, or (3) as children of parents with HIV. While many topics addressed in this chapter are also covered in other chapters in this textbook, this chapter specifically addresses the issues as they relate to children and adolescents with HIV and AIDS. Epidemiology is covered in Chapter 4, psychiatric disorders are covered in Chapters 3 through 13, neurological issues in Chapters 19 and 20, adherence in Chapter 22, psychopharmacologic issues in Chapter 32, end-of-life issues in Chapter 39, and ethical issues in Chapter 40. This chapter reviews the epidemiology of HIV/AIDS in these groups and presents an overview of the sequelae of HIV infection as it influences psychological and psychiatric well-being. The chapter also presents a comprehensive approach to psychiatric assessment and management of HIV-infected youth, ethical considerations, secondary prevention, and resources available to meet the needs of pediatric HIV/AIDS survivors.

EPIDEMIOLOGY

There have been dramatic shifts in the fight against HIV/AIDS since the mid-1980s. The variety of treatments now available in the United States for HIV-infected individuals has transformed the disease from certain death to a chronic medical illness (Donenberg and Pao, 2005). Significant reduction in mother-to-child transmission has led to a steadily decreasing number of perinatally acquired AIDS cases among children (Cooper et al., 2002), but new groups are now at the forefront of the disease, including adolescents and women, especially women of color (CDC, 2000). There has been a steady rise in the number of persons infected with HIV in the 15- to 24-year age group (CDC, 2005).

Parental Substance Use

In the United States, AIDS in women and children represents a convergence of two major epidemics plaguing American cities: HIV infection and substance abuse (Wiener et al., 2003). By the end of 2005, an estimated 988,376 persons in the United States were living with AIDS (CDC, 2005). Of the estimated 182,822 female adults and adolescents living with AIDS, 56% were exposed through heterosexual contact, and 40% were exposed through injection drug use (CDC, 2005). In the United States, over half of children with AIDS are born to women with HIV acquired through intravenous drug use (CDC, 2004). Thus an understanding of the mental health problems common in families affected by substance abuse is essential for clinicians working with HIV-infected children and their caregivers (Wiener et al., 2003).

Perinatal HIV Infection

Nearly all new HIV infections in children are acquired through mother–infant transmission. HIV can be transmitted from women to their children during pregnancy, at the time of labor and delivery, and postnatally during the period of breastfeeding (Kourtis et al., 2001). The widespread use of antiretroviral interventions for the prevention of mother-to-child transmission during pregnancy, labor, and the newborn period has reduced the risk of transmission to below 2% in the United Statues and other resource-rich settings (UNAIDS, 2004). The Centers for Disease Control and Prevention (CDC) reports that between 1992 and 2002, perinatally acquired AIDS cases declined 90% in the United States from 912 cases to 90 cases (CDC, 2007).

Acquired Adolescent HIV Infection

As a result of heterosexual transmission, men having sex with men, substance use, and lack of awareness of safer sexual practices, young people in the United Statues are at high risk for HIV infection. An estimated 38,490 persons between the ages of 13 and 24 received a diagnosis of AIDS through 2003. This accounts for about 4% of the 929,985 total estimated AIDS diagnoses (CDC, 2006). An estimated 3897 young people received a diagnosis of HIV/AIDS in the year 2003 alone, with 78% of those being between the ages of 13 and 14 years (CDC, 2003b). Many young adults aged 21 to 29 who present with AIDS almost certainly acquired their infection as adolescents. Also, a growing number of pregnancies have been reported in vertically infected adolescent females in the United States and Puerto Rico (CDC, 2003b), highlighting the importance of promoting HIV prevention strategies.

Children Affected by HIV

The impact of the HIV/AIDS epidemic on children has been and will continue to be devastating. By 2003, worldwide, AIDS had left 15 million children under the age of 18 orphaned, with more than 320,000 living in the United States. Most of these children are currently in the care of their grandparents or other caregivers, while in Africa many live in orphanages or on the street (UNICEF, 2004, 2005). The majority of children who survive the death of a parent or sibling from AIDS are not themselves HIV-infected.

CDC DEFINITION IN CHILDREN AND ADOLESCENTS

The CDC AIDS case definition for children is used for surveillance and reporting and is similar to the one for adults, with several exceptions. Lymphoid interstitial pneumonia/pulmonary lymphoid hyperplasia (LIP/PLH) and multiple or recurrent serious bacterial infections are AIDS defining for children, but not for adults. Additionally, certain types of cytomegalovirus

(CMV), herpes simplex virus infections, and toxoplasmosis of the brain are AIDS defining only for adults and for children greater than one month of age. An expanded definition for AIDS in adolescents and adults, amended in 1993, does not apply to children less than 13 years old.

A separate classification system has been developed to describe the spectrum of HIV disease to include HIV-exposed infants with undetermined infection status. Categories and clinical manifestations are well described in the Baylor International Pediatric AIDS Initiative Education Resources (Kline, 2007) (Tables 24.1 and 24.2). The system employs two axes that are mutually exclusive to indicate severity of clinical signs and symptoms and degree of immunosuppression. Degree of immunosuppression is defined on the basis of age-adjusted CD4+ lymphocyte counts and percentages. As is the case for an adult, once classified, an infant or child may not be reclassified in a less severe category even if improvement in clinical or immunological status occurs (Kline, 2007).

DIAGNOSIS OF PEDIATRIC HIV INFECTION

HIV antibody detection is not useful for neonatal diagnosis of HIV infection. If vertical HIV transmission is suspected, virologic tests to identify antibody to the virus or components including DNA polymerase chain reaction (PCR) and RNA PCR are made within 48 hours of birth, at 1 to 2 months, and at 3 to 6 months to distinguish decreasing maternal antibody from infant antibody. Other tests include enzyme-linked immunosorbent assay (ELISA) or enzyme immunoassay, Western blot, p24 antigen capture assay, and culture. CD4 count and HIV RNA provide additional complementary and independent information about prognosis and may later help determine when to start or change antiretroviral therapy. In children who are older than 18 months of age, serologic tests such as ELISA and Western blot remain the most cost-effective methods for HIV-1 detection (Krogstad, 2006).

In vertically acquired HIV infection, clinical manifestations do not usually appear in the neonatal period and in infants and children are varied and often nonspecific. Lymphadenopathy, often in association with hepatosplenomegaly, can be an early sign of infection. During the first year of life, oral candidiasis, failure to thrive, and developmental delay are other common presenting features of HIV infection. Table 24.2 lists the most common AIDS-defining conditions observed among children in the United States with vertically acquired HIV infection.

NEUROCOGNITIVE DEVELOPMENT

Mental Health Risk Factors Associated with Parental Substance Abuse

Most studies of children of substance-using mothers are conducted among young children exposed to prenatal cocaine, despite the fact that most substance-using mothers ingest multiple substances (Lester et al., 2001). Some investigators have not found an association between prenatal cocaine exposure and cognitive performance (Chasnoff et al., 1998), academic achievement, or attention or teacher-rated classroom behavior (Richardson et al., 1996), while others have found that exposure may be associated with behavior problems (Chasnoff et al., 1998), decreased task persistence, attention problems (Bandstra et al., 2001), poorer language performance (Bandstra et al., 2004), and mental health problems (Linares et al., 2006). Recent studies have also demonstrated that many

TABLE 24.1. 1994 Revised HIV Pediatric Classification System: Immune Categories Based on Age-Specific CD4+ T-Lymphocyte Count and Percentage

	Less than 12 Months	1–5 Years	6–12 Years
Immune category	N/L (%)	N/L (%)	N/L (%)
Category 1: no suppression	>1500 (>25%)	>1000 (>25%)	>500 (>25%)
Category 2: moderate suppression	750–1499 (15%–24%)	500–999 (15%–24%)	200–499 (15%–24%)
Category 3: severe suppression	<750 (<15%)	<500 (<15%)	<200 (<15%)

Source: From the Centers for Disease Control. *Morbidity and Mortality Weekly Report*, 1994;43(no. RR-12):1–10.

TABLE 24.2. 1994 Revised HIV Pediatric Classification System: Clinical Categories

---

Category N: Not Symptomatic

Children who have no signs or symptoms considered to be the result of HIV infection or who have only one of the conditions listed in category A

Category A: Mildly Symptomatic

Children with two or more of the following conditions but none of the conditions listed in categories B and C:

Lymphadenopathy (>0.5 cm at more than two sites; bilateral—one site)
Hepatomegaly
Splenomegaly
Dermatitis
Parotitis
Recurrent or persistent upper respiratory infection, sinusitis, or otitis media

Category B: Moderately Symptomatic

Children who have symptomatic conditions other than those listed for category A or category C that are attributed to HIV infection. Examples of conditions in clinical category B include but are not limited to the following:

Anemia (<8 g/dl), neutropenia (<1000/mm^3), or thrombocytopenia (<100,000/mm^3) persisting >30 days
Bacterial meningitis, pneumonia, or sepsis (single episode)
Candidiasis, oropharyngeal (i.e., thrush) persisting for >2 months
Cardiomyopathy
Cytomegalovirus infection with onset before age 1 month
Diarrhea, recurrent or chronic
Hepatitis
Herpes simplex virus (HSV) stomatitis, recurrent (i.e., more than two episodes within 1 year)
HSV bronchitis, pneumonitis, or esophagitis with onset before age 1 month
Herpes zoster (i.e., shingles) involving at least two distinct episodes
  or more than one dermatome
Leiomyosarcoma
Lymphoid interstitial pneumonia (LIP) or pulmonary lymphoid
  hyperplasia (PLH) complex
Nephropathy
Nocardiosis
Fever lasting >1 month
Toxoplasmosis with onset before age 1 month
Varicella, disseminated (i.e., complicated chickenpox)

Category C: Severely Symptomatic

Children who have any condition listed in the 1987 surveillance case definition
  for acquired immunodeficiency syndrome, with the exception of LIP
  (which is a category B condition)

Source: From the Centers for Disease Control. *Morbidity and Mortality Weekly Report*, 1994;43(no. RR-12):1–10. Accessed from Kline (2007).

of the effects originally thought to be specific to prenatal drug exposure were due to the quality of the child's environment (Frank et al., 2001; Brown et al., 2004). This finding highlights the importance of considering the contributions of contextual factors such as poverty, caregiver stability, caregiver psychiatric illness, and ongoing drug use on child development, regardless of prenatal drug exposure and HIV disease status (Coles and Black, 2006). Such factors suggest multiple points of entry for possible psychiatric interventions.

HIV Encephalopathy

It has been well documented that children infected with HIV-1 are at risk for developing central nervous system (CNS) disease characterized by impairments in cognitive, language, motor, and behavioral functions (Wolters and Brouwers, 2005). The clinical presentation of pediatric HIV-1 CNS disease varies among patient subgroups in the time of onset, rate of deterioration, severity of deficits, and number of domains affected (Rausch and Stover, 2001). Manifestations range from mild impairments in select domains of cognitive functioning to the most severe form, referred to as HIV encephalopathy, in which children exhibit global and debilitating neurodevelopmental deficits with possible loss of previously acquired skills (Belman, 1994).

During the first decade of the disease, 50% to 90% of young children were estimated to exhibit encephalopathy (Epstein, 1986; Belman et al., 1988). The current prevalence of severe HIV encephalopathy, characterized by brain atrophy, motor abnormalities, and cognitive delays, is estimated to be approximately 13% to 23% (Lobato et al., 1995; Blanche et al., 1997; Cooper et al., 1998; Tardieu et al., 2000). This decrease is thought to be the result of improved treatment such as combination antiretroviral therapy (ART), including HAART (Brodt et al., 1997; Palella et al., 1998; d'Arminio et al., 2000; Tardieu and Boulet, 2002; Shanbhag et al., 2005), which reduces systemic viral replication (Deeks et al., 1997) and in turn lowers the number of HIV-infected cells entering the CNS (Tardieu, 1999).

In the past, HIV encephalopathy was associated with computed tomography (CT) findings showing increased basal ganglia calcifications, brain atrophy, enlarged ventricles, and enlarged cortical sulci (Brouwers et al., 1994). Neurocognitive deficits in expressive language were affected more severely than receptive language in children with vertically transmitted HIV (Wolters et al., 1995). Longer-term follow-up from the Women and Infants Transmission Study group suggests that scores on the Bayley Scales of Infant Development independently predicted mortality even after adjusting for age, viral load, CD4 counts, and treatment

(Llorente et al., 2003). Recent data also suggest that severity of cortical atrophy is reflective of viral load in the cerebrospinal fluid (CSF) and does not correlate with intracerebral calcifications (Brouwers et al., 2000).

Susceptibility to developing HIV CNS disease is a critical concern throughout development. Many adolescents and young adults are nonadherent to their HAART regimens, and suboptimal drug levels in the CSF may lead to the emergence of drug-resistant virus in the CNS (Gisslen and Hagberg, 2001). Moreover, the CNS may be a key anatomical reservoir for persistent HIV-1 replication (Enting et al., 1998; Schrager and D'Souza, 1998; Sonza and Crowe, 2001) since many antiretroviral agents, including protease inhibitors (PIs), have poor CNS penetration (Swindells, 1998; Aweeka et al., 1999).

Neuroimaging, such as brain magnetic resonance imaging (MRI) screening, has been recommended in otherwise asymptomatic children with progressive neurocognitive dysfunction (Patsalides et al., 2002). In addition to detecting mass lesions such as those seen in toxoplasmosis or CNS lymphoma, brain MRI is useful for detecting cerebrovascular complications in HIV-infected children, who have of a higher incidence of ischemic strokes and cerebral artery aneurysms than that seen in adults (Civitello, 2003). One positron emission tomography (PET) study showed diffuse hypometabolism in some children with severe encephalopathy (Depas et al., 1995); PET and functional MRI (fMRI) are not useful at this time, however, for early detection for neurocognitive deficits. A preliminary proton MR spectroscopy study showing cerebral metabolites such as N-acetylaspartate (NAA), a marker of neuronal activity, may eventually be useful in assessing cerebral changes in HIV-infected subjects (Keller et al., 2006).

Recent concerns have arisen that exposure to nucleoside reverse transcriptase inhibitor (NRTIs) in utero may contribute to neurologic toxicity including progressive encephalopathy, peripheral neuropathy, and myopathy via depletion of mitochondria and lactic acidemia (Church et al., 2001; Alimenti et al., 2003). Even HIV-uninfected children exposed to zidovudine in utero may develop transient mitochondrial dysfunction with unexplained neurologic symptoms and demonstrate cerebral MR changes (Tardieu et al., 2005).

Adults with AIDS have specific patterns of brain damage linked to the degree of immune system deterioration on which the use of antiretroviral therapy does not seem to have a significant effect (Thompson et al., 2005). Frontal cortical thinning has been strongly linked with cognitive impairment and may underlie the commonly observed HIV-related decline in frontal lobe functions such as attention, executive function, and working memory in survivors (Thompson et al., 2005). These cognitive impairments could significantly affect academic success in HIV-infected long-term survivors. Consequently, serial neurodevelopmental assessments are recommended (1) every 6 months for children under 2 years because of a higher risk of developing CNS disease, (2) once a year for children between the ages of 2 and 8 years (unless they exhibit neurodevelopmental deficits), and (3) every 2 years for children over 8 years of age who exhibit stable functioning in the average range (Wolters and Brouwers, 2005).

LIVING WITH HIV/AIDS: DEVELOPMENTAL AND PSYCHOSOCIAL ISSUES

Infants and Toddlers

Often the biological mother learns of her own infection during routine HIV testing during pregnancy or mandatory HIV testing to her newborn. A positive test result is a crisis point and an essential time for psychosocial intervention and education. Common immediate questions include how and when the mother became infected, and with whom the diagnosis can be shared. When the mother learns of her own infection during her pregnancy, she is counseled to begin antiretroviral therapy to treat her own infection, choose an elective cesarean birth, and avoid breastfeeding to help prevent mother–infant transmission. Becoming educated about the disease and the complex medical regimens associated with treatment of the infection can be overwhelming as mothers anxiously await confirmatory tests to learn whether their newborn infant is also HIV infected. When the child is indeed positive, learning to administer medication to the infant and finding a way to balance hope with fear of illness and dying are the first major hurdles for the mother to overcome. The complexity of problems associated with caring for a child with HIV infection clearly extends far beyond the medical issues associated with infection, and these mothers benefit from medical outreach and support (Faithfull, 1997).

The psychological trauma of the diagnosis falls primarily on the child's caregiver, as children younger than the age of 2 years are unable to grasp the concept of a diagnosis of a life-threatening disease. Toddlers and young children do not understand the concept of chronic illness. They experience episodes of HIV-related illness as discrete events rather than as part of an ongoing process (Wiener et al., 1998b). They do benefit, however, from ongoing and developmentally appropriate explanations of illness and treatment.

School-Age Children

How the school-age child copes with his or her illness depends on many factors, including age and developmental stage, parental adaptation, social skills, and his or her psychological makeup (Wiener et al., 2003). When possible, an assessment should include information about the child's ability to trust, to use and/or reach out for help, tolerate pain or frustration, make and maintain friendships, and cope with change and separation. It should also state whether support from family and others is available. Similarly, it is important to assess the child's cognitive abilities, disclosure status, and stage of illness. These factors determine the meaning the illness carries for the child and the kind of psychological and intellectual resources available to cope with the disease and to meet each challenge.

For the child this is a period of developmental inquiry, so universal questions that begin with "why," "what," "when," "how," and "what if" need to be anticipated. Along with trust between the parent and child, a bond between the physician and child will often enhance understanding and compliance, further reducing anxiety (Wiener et al., 1998b). This trust is essential, as almost all parents struggle for at least 2 years before feeling that they are ready to disclose information about the infection to the child (Wiener et al., 1996).

Disclosure

One of the greatest areas of psychological stress for children, adolescents, and parents and caregivers is the question of when and how to disclose the HIV diagnosis to one's child and others. Early in the epidemic, few children were predicted to survive past their fifth birthday (CDC, 1993), thus little attention was given to diagnosis disclosure. Today, well into the third decade of the AIDS epidemic, most HIV-infected children in the United States and developed world will live into older adolescence and beyond, with the hope of leading an independent life as an adult. Furthermore, as HIV-infected children reach adolescence, issues such as maintaining adherence to complex medication regimens and sexual behavior are of critical concern and are likely influenced by the knowledge of having a chronic, life-threatening, stigmatized, sexually transmissible illness. The potential negative individual and public health risks of nonadherence and risky sexual behavior substantively add a sense of urgency to the issue of disclosure of HIV status.

Models that address ways to communicate with children about their illness have focused primarily on cancer (Spinetta, 1980; Katz and Jay, 1984) and suggest that diagnostic disclosure to children with chronic illness is generally most successful if accurately mapped to the child's cognitive and emotional development (Bibace and Walsh, 1980). Moreover, investigations of children with cancer consistently show that open communication about cancer diagnoses improves child psychological adjustment, with the effects of open communication lasting into adulthood for both the child and his or her family members (Spinetta and Maloney, 1978; Slavin et al., 1982; Katz and Jay, 1984, Chesler et al., 1986). Although the positive effects of open communication and full disclosure of a cancer diagnosis are well documented, one cannot easily apply the oncology model of disclosure to pediatric HIV disease, given significant differences in the epidemiology and the unique social stigma surrounding HIV transmission (Lipson, 1994). Additionally, disclosure of a child's HIV diagnosis often leads to disclosure of other family secrets, including paternity, history of parental sexual behavior, and substance abuse (Havens et al., 2005). The fact that the majority of children acquired the virus from their mothers and the ensuing parental guilt about transmission also distinguish this disease from cancer and other life-threatening pediatric illnesses.

In 1999, the American Academy of Pediatrics (1999) published guidelines that endorsed disclosure of HIV to older children and adolescents as beneficial and ethically appropriate. Several reports followed that reviewed factors associated with a parent's decision to disclose the HIV diagnosis to his or her child, predictors of disclosure, and the psychological impact of disclosure (Wiener et al., 1998a; Howland et al.,

2000; Instone, 2000; Nehring et al., 2000; Sherman et al., 2000; Bachanas et al., 2001; Gerson et al., 2001; Lester et al., 2002; Mellins et al., 2002). Some studies have suggested positive outcomes associated with disclosure, including the promotion of trust, improved adherence, enhanced support services, open family communication, and better long-term health and emotional well-being (Walker, 1991; Lipson, 1994; Funck-Brentano et al., 1997; Wiener et al., 1998a; Mellins et al., 2002, Ng et al., 2004). Increased internalizing-behavior problems (Bachanas et al., 2001) and closed and isolating communication (Hardy et al., 1994) are reported when disclosure did not take place. Other studies have reported that knowledge of serostatus may contribute to depression, anxiety, and behavioral problems (Bennett, 1994; Lester et al., 2002; New et al., 2003) and increased risk of psychiatric hospitalizations (Gaughan et al., 2004). While no relationship has been found between timing of disclosure and psychological adjustment, social support, or the adolescent's own decision to disclose his or her HIV status to others (Wiener and Battles, 2006), a caregiver's intuition must be respected, as one report found 65% of children felt the right person told them (who in almost all cases was the child's parent[s]) and 86% felt the disclosure was at the right time (Wiener et al., 1996).

Disclosure of an HIV diagnosis to children is an individualized and dynamic process. Patterns of disclosure vary from full disclosure (the name of the virus, ways to treat the disease, and transmission routes) to partial disclosure (a child is given a description of symptoms and treatment but the exact name of the illness is not revealed), with patterns of nondisclosure varying from deception (the illness is hidden behind another condition) to complete nondisclosure (no communication about the illness at all) (Funck-Brentano et al., 1997). Disclosure should take place in a supportive atmosphere of cooperation between health professionals and parents (Wiener, 1998). It should be conceived of as a process rather than as a single event and may need to occur on several visits (Lipson, 1993, 1994). See Table 24.3 for a guide to helping parents through the disclosure process.

In order for culturally competent care to be provided, it is important to obtain a clear understanding of the family's cultural background and the factors that might influence responses to an HIV diagnosis or disclosure of the diagnosis to the child (Mason et al., 1995; Mettler et al., 1997). Clear and effective lan-

TABLE 24.3. Disclosure Process

Step 1. Preparation

- Have a meeting with the parent or caregivers involved in the decision-making process. Staff members that the family trusts should be present.

- Address the importance of disclosure and ascertain whether the family has a plan in mind. Respect the intensity of feelings about this issue. Obtain feedback on the child's anticipated response. Explore the child's level of knowledge and his or her emotional stability and maturity.

- If the family is ready to disclose, guide them in various ways of approaching disclosure (Step 2).

- If the family is not ready, encourage them to begin using words that they can build on later, such as immune problems, virus, or infection. Provide books for the family to read with the child on viruses. Strengthen the family through education and support and schedule a follow-up meeting. Let the family know that you will meet with them on a regular basis to help guide them through the disclosure process and to support the child and family after disclosure. Respect the family's timing, but strongly encourage the family not to lie to the child if he or she asks directly about having HIV, unless significant, identifiable safety concerns render the decision to disclose inadvisable. Also remind the family to avoid disclosure during an argument or in anger.

Step 2. Disclosure

- In advance, have the family think through or write out how they want the conversation to go. They need to give careful consideration to what message they want their child to walk away with. Encourage the family to begin with "Do you remember . . .", to include information about the child's life, medications, and/or procedures so that the child is reminded of past events before introducing new facts.

- Have the family choose a place where the child will be most comfortable to talk openly.

- Provide the family with questions the child may ask so they are prepared with answers. Such questions include "How long have you known this?" "Who else has the virus?" "Will I die?" "Can I ever have children?" "Who can I tell?" "Why me?" and "Who else knows?"

- Encourage having present only the people with whom the child is most comfortable. The health care provider may offer to facilitate this meeting, but if at all possible, preparation should be done in advance so that the family can share the information on their own.

- Medical facts should be kept to a minimum (immunology, virology, the effectiveness of therapy) and hope should be reinforced. Silence as well as questions need to be accepted. The child should be told that nothing has changed except a name is now being given to what they have been living with. The child also needs to hear that they didn't do or say anything to cause the disease and that their family will be always remain by their side.

- If the diagnosis is to be kept a secret, it is important that the child be given the names of people they can talk to, such as a health care provider, another child living with HIV, and/or a family friend. By stating "you can't tell anyone," makes the child feel ashamed and guilty.

- Provide the child with a journal or diary to record their questions, thoughts, and feelings. If appropriate, provide books about children living with HIV.

- Schedule a follow-up meeting.

Step 3. After Disclosure

- Provide individual and family follow-up 2 weeks after disclosure and again every 2–4 weeks for the first 6 months to assess impact of disclosure, answer questions, and to help foster support between the child and family.

- Ask the child to tell you what they have learned about their virus. This way misconceptions can be clarified. Writing and art may be useful techniques.

- Asses changes in emotional well-being and provide the family with information about symptoms that could indicate the need for more intensive intervention.

- Support parents for having disclosed the diagnosis and, if interested and available, refer them to a parents support group. Encourage them to think about the emotional needs of the other children in the family in the disclosure process.

- Remind parents that disclosure is not a one-time event. Ongoing communication will be needed. Ask parents what other supports they feel would be helpful to them and their child. Provide information about HIV camp programs for HIV-infected and HIV-affected children and families.

Source: From Wiener LS, and Battles HB. Untangling the web: a close look at diagnosis disclosure among HIV-infected adolescents. *J Adolesc Health* 38(3):307–9. Copyright (2006), with permission from Elsevier.

guage interpretation services are essential when delivering a diagnosis, reviewing treatment options, or talking to a family about disclosure-related issues (Munet-Vilaro, 2004). Cognitive impairment must be considered as well. Although the adolescent may be able to meet "mature minor" criteria for "competence," observations of adolescent-onset dementia or impairment of executive abilities, combined with the observation of deteriorating function in adolescence, point to the need for careful consideration of earlier disclosure and development of new models for comprehension support of HIV-related information as children mature (Armstrong et al., 2002).

Being prepared for the emotional reactions following disclosure is critical. While the child's disclosure reaction tends to be consistent with previous responses to a crisis, it is essential for a child's parent to be aware of the scope of emotions that might follow. The reactions can commonly range from no reaction at all to acute panic or anxiety. Delayed reactions are also often seen. Parents may report the onset of new psychosomatic complaints, nightmares, emotional lability, and regressive behavior. Other children present with an adult-like acceptance (Wiener et al., 2003). In spite of what appears to be acceptance of the illness, it is important to help parents be sensitive to a profound sense of shame and personal defectiveness often exacerbated by the stigma and need for secrecy associated with the diagnosis (Hays et al., 1993).

Post-disclosure counseling can be enormously helpful. Artwork often reveals confusion, guilt, or a sense of damage that the child may have internalized. Yet, with time and support, most children demonstrate considerable pride with mastery of information, increased knowledge about the illness, reduction of guilt, and the ability to tolerate procedures such as blood draws and pill swallowing (Wiener and Battles, 2002; Wiener et al., 2003). By inquiring into the inner world of children and helping them to put understanding and meaning into their plight, psychological movement, growth, and healing can be facilitated (Wiener and Figueroa, 1998).

School Issues

Because of the stigma associated with this disease, parents' anxiety associated with informing school personnel about their child's diagnosis remains tremendous (Cohen et al., 1997). Most parents remain anon-

ymous and keep an HIV/AIDS diagnosis from the school for as long as possible. If the family decides it is in the child's best interest to share the diagnosis with the school, the health care team can assist families with the school process. Possible interventions include (a) informing parents of a child's right to an education; (b) meeting with school officials and school personnel to educate them about HIV infection and apprise them of the individual needs of a specific child; (c) accompanying parents to a school board meeting when they feel this would be of support; (d) providing consultation to teachers and principals in talking to the other classmates about HIV and AIDS; and (e) providing up-to-date information to the school about the child's progress if the child has been out ill for a period of time (Armstrong et al., 1993; Cohen et al., 1997; Wiener et al., 1998b).

Balancing academic expectations for the child and flexibility in terms of what the child can keep up with (e.g., in light of frequent clinic visits or cognitive deficits) is a challenge for both parents and teachers. Nevertheless, this balance is of great importance in terms of preparing the child for the responsibilities of adolescence and young adulthood (Wiener et al., 2003).

Adolescents at Risk for HIV

Developmental tasks of adolescence such as risk taking, struggles for independence, experimenting with adult behaviors, impulsivity, and a sense of invulnerability, coupled with awakening sexuality, put adolescents at particular risk for acquiring HIV (Samples et al., 1998). The primary risk for acquiring HIV/AIDS during adolescence comes from drug use and high-risk sexual behavior. Youth with mental health problems may be at greater risk of exposure to HIV (Brown et al., 1997a; Donenberg et al., 2001). Gay and lesbian youth may be at increased risk for mental health concerns (Fergusson et al., 1999) and for sexual risk-taking behaviors that place them at particular risk for acquiring HIV (Garofalo et al., 1998). Compared to community samples, psychiatrically hospitalized adolescents are twice as likely to be sexually active, twice as likely not to use condoms, and more than twice as likely to have used intravenous drugs (DiClemente and Ponton, 1993). Teens in outpatient mental health care have higher rates of sexual activity and pregnancy, with sexually active youth reporting earlier sexual debut, higher incidence of sexually transmitted diseases (STDs), higher use of alcohol or drugs during sex, and less condom use (Donenberg et al., 2001; 2003). Early sexual debut increases risk of HIV infection because of the increased number of sexual contacts and partners. Additionally, up to 30% of adolescents admit to comorbid substance abuse (Arrufo et al., 1994), which may interfere with safe decision making and effective management of affective arousal (Donenberg and Pao, 2005).

A sociopersonal model that highlights the processes associated with HIV transmission in youth with mental health problems in a broad contextual framework has been described (Donenberg and Pao, 2005). Four factors in this model include (1) personal attributes (cognitions about HIV, affect dysregulation, mental health problems, personality traits); (2) family context (affective characteristics, parental monitoring, parent–teen communication); (3) peer and partner relationships (relationship concern, peer influence, partner communication); and (4) environmental circumstances (neighborhood disadvantage, stressful events). These factors can be identified and allow multiple opportunities for mental health interventions.

Adolescents with HIV

Levels of stress in coping with HIV appear to increase over time, beginning with the onset of adolescence — when the need for a change in therapy may develop, when dating begins, when future goals are being considered, and when decisions about informing friends or potential romantic partners need to be made. Throughout adolescence, pubertal development and sexuality, fear of contagion and transmissibility, and a need to promote adherence to complex and often toxic regimens become primary concerns (Grubman et al., 1995). The effect of peer pressure should not be underestimated. It is important for the care provider to talk openly to adolescents about their peer relationships, sexuality, and sexual practices and explore their underlying fears of stigmatization and rejection to facilitate open discussion and behavior change (Lightfoot and Rotheram-Borus, 1998). As these adolescents and young adults age, pregnancy will occur (CDC 2003b), so health care providers should review safer sexual behaviors and make barrier protection available.

Many of the adolescents living with HIV have already experienced significant hardships prior to their diagnosis, including poverty, violence, abandonment, and living environments with constant threats and dangers (Falloon et al., 1989), and experience additional negative life events after learning their diagnosis (Moss et al., 1998; Lester et al., 2002). Regardless of how the teenager acquired his or her infection, the most damaging result is its effect on the formation of relationships outside the family (Wiener et al., 1998b). These adolescents often fear social rejection more than they fear dying from the disease.

The Montefiore Adolescent AIDS Program has identified four key time points for intervention with HIV-positive adolescents: when (1) receiving an HIV diagnosis, (2) disclosing HIV status to parents, partner, and others, (3) coping with HIV illness, and (4) preparing for death (Kunins et al., 1993). Frequent staff phone calls to youth at these crisis moments are helpful, as symptoms of maladaptation may go unnoticed or be perceived as "normal adolescent behavior" until a major episode, such as a suicidal gesture, failing grades, acute illness resulting from nonadherence to medications, or an episode with the law, brings the symptoms to attention (Wiener et al., 2003). Without ongoing psychosocial intervention, the mental health outcome of these teens could be seriously jeopardized, especially as they are transferred to adult clinics, where the change in staff and routines can be experienced as traumatic and follow-up may be absent. Medical care centers and their HIV health care providers are frequently the most consistent part of these adolescents' lives.

Adherence

There are only a few studies examining adherence among children and adolescents living with HIV (Van Dyke et al., 2002, Hammami et al., 2004; Wiener et al., 2004; Murphy et al., 2005; Marhefka et al., 2006), and they suggest that adherence is a significant clinical issue. Side effects of treatment such as diarrhea, nausea, skin rashes, and unusual deposits of body fat and lipodystrophy are additional barriers to adherence (Santos et al., 2005; Heath et al, 2002). Other factors that contribute to poor adherence include impulsivity, shorter attention spans, and a desire to fit in with peers' schedules and eating habits. Adolescents with advanced HIV disease who are out of school, have higher alcohol use, and have depression appear to be less likely to be adherent (Wiener et al., 2004; Murphy et al., 2005; Sternhell and Corr, 2002). A social crisis such as a death, a breakup with a girlfriend or boyfriend, a family fight, or a problem in school or on the job can lead to a period of nonadherence. Teenagers in crisis or teenagers who are depressed may stop taking their medications, no longer eat well, or invest less energy into having protected sex. Oppositional behavior is common and many teenagers are "tired" of obeying parents' and doctors' orders; they feel that the decision of whether they take their medication is an event that they can control. Teens also express concern that their medications may no longer be effective against the virus and decide to discontinue their medications. Those who are the most adherent are usually well informed about their treatment and feel that taking medications is their own decision (Lewis et al., 2006; Wiener et al., 2003). There is an urgent need for better interventions to assist adolescents infected with HIV to stick to their medication regimens. These interventions include (1) helping adolescents with problem solving, (2) assessing for psychological distress, and (3) treating depression (Murphy et al., 2005).

With the increased risks of HIV viral resistance in teens who are nonadherent, it may be wise to wait to begin treatment with a protease inhibitor until the treatment team believes the teen will be able to adhere to the regimen. Including the teen in therapeutic decisions and listening to what he or she has to say about treatment-related body changes will contribute to greater adherence to proposed interventions and may improve the patient's quality of life (Santos et al., 2005).

Transition to Young Adulthood and Long-Term Survivors

A significant number of children with HIV live into their late adolescent years and are now graduating from high school, attending trade schools or colleges, and holding down part-time or full-time jobs. The goals for these young adults with HIV/AIDS is to increase self-care behaviors such as medical adherence and health-related interactions, to reduce secondary transmission, and to enhance their quality of life (Rotheram-Borus and Miller, 1998). The psychological transition of anticipating an early death to planning for one's future, however, with uncertainty about the effectiveness of HIV drug regimens and fears of losing health insurance or disability insurance can result in significant anxiety. The cumulative effects of multiple losses can also lead to increased anxiety and depression.

Multiple losses or "loss overload" are phrases frequently heard when describing the psychological impact of HIV/AIDS. As many HIV-positive youngsters age, they find themselves grieving for parents, siblings, and/or close friends who did not live long enough to benefit from currently available drug treatments. Others have been shuffled between care providers, households, schools, neighborhoods, and social service agencies. It is often not until late adolescence that the impact of these losses "hits home." This distress often occurs at a time when transition from pediatric care providers to adult programs or centers is required, and this move is experienced as yet another loss. Unresolved and complicated grief reactions can mask difficulty making decisions, feeling "lost," guilt surrounding survival, oppositional behavior, or depression and anxiety, each of which can lead to disabling mental health problems. Assessing for grief reactions needs to be a part of the mental health care provided for each HIV-positive child, adolescent, and surviving young adult.

Many teens are reluctant to seek mental health services or attend traditional support groups, though such interventions have the potential to offer tremendous benefit. Support groups can offer a sense of belonging for these teens; a place where they don't need to lie about their illness, where fears can be shared, experiences validated, isolation reduced, trauma understood, and where a deeper connection with other teens can be made. Overnight camping programs for teens can also provide this effect, and within specialty camps (for children infected or affected by HIV, or immunology sessions) many teens have the opportunity to obtain counselor training and find summer employment. See Table 24.4 for a list of such summer camps. Community-based service providers often hire HIV-positive youth to serve as peer leaders. Peer empowerment programs provide HIV-positive young men and women the opportunity to deliver HIV prevention messages to other youth (Luna and Rotheram-Borus, 1999). Being HIV-positive themselves, their message is often perceived as more credible and powerful than that of a seronegative educator. While close supervision and guidance is necessary, these teens learn to articulate their own life experiences, gain access to resources, meet new friends, and receive employment in return.

Teens who are able to keep themselves mentally active, believe their life has purpose, have a sense of humor, adapt to loss and change, and create a backup

TABLE 24.4. Summer Camps

Arizona

Camp Hakuna Matata
Contact: AIDS Project Arizona
Phoenix, AZ
Phone: (602) 253-2437

California

Camp Arroyo: year-round camp serving children with
life-threatening diseases and disabilities
Contact: Camp Arroyo, Taylor Family Foundation
5555 Arroyo Rd.
Livermore, CA 94550
Phone: (925) 455-5118

Camp Care: support for women, children, and families
infected and affected by HIV/AIDS
Contact: All About Care
4974 Fresno Street, PMB #156
Fresno, CA 93726
Phone: (559) 222-9471

Camp Dream Street: serves children with cancer, blood
disorders, and other life-threatening illnesses
Contact: Dream Street Foundation
9536 Wilshire Blvd. Suite 310
Beverly Hills, CA 90212
Phone (310) 274-7227

Camp Pacific Heartland: full-service summer camp for
children and adolescents infected and affected
by HIV/AIDS
Contact: Hollywood Heart
3310 W Vanowen St.
Burbank, CA 91505
Phone: (818) 260-0372

Camp Kindle: summer camp serving children infected
and affected by HIV/AIDS
PO Box 803220
Santa Clarita, CA 91380
Phone: 1-877-800-CAMP (2267)

Camp Laurel: serves children infected and affected
HIV/AIDS
75 South Grand Avenue
Pasadena, CA 91105
Phone: (626) 683-0800

Camp Sunburst: long-term residential camp for
children living with HIV/AIDS
Contact: Sunburst Projects
2 Padre Parkway, Suite 106
Rohert Park, CA 94928
Phone: (707) 588-9477

Colorado

Camp Ray-Ray: short-term residential camp for families
affected by AIDS
Contact: Angels Unaware
6370 Union Street
Arvada, CO 80004
Phone: (303) 420-6370

Connecticut

Association of Hole in the Wall Camps: serves children
with cancer and other serious blood conditions
who, because of their disease, its treatment, or its
complications, cannot attend an ordinary summer
camp. They have a special immunology session.
They offer a 1-week session for brothers and sisters.
The Hole In The Wall Gang Camp
565 Ashford Center Road
Ashford, CT 06278
Phone (860) 429-3444

Camp AmeriKids: serves children ages 7–15 infected
and affected with HIV/AIDS
88 Hamilton Avenue
Stamford, CT 06902
Phone: 1-800-486 HELP (4357)

Camp Meechimuk: long-term residential camp for
children affected by HIV/AIDS
Contact: Hispanos-Unidos
116 Sherman Avenue, 1st floor
New Haven, CT 06511
Phone: (203) 781-0226

Camp Totokett: non-denominational summer camp for
children ages 5–16 whose families are affected by
HIV/AIDS
Contact: First Congregational Church of Branford
1009 Main Street
Branford, CT
Phone: (203) 481-4339

Washington, DC

Camp Safe Haven: Maryland long-term residential
camp for children infected or affected by HIV/AIDS
Contact: Lutheran Social Services of the National
Capitol Area
4406 Georgia Ave, N.W.
Washington, DC 20011
Phone: (202) 723-3000

Florida

The Boggy Creek Gang Part of the Association of Hole
in the Wall Camps
30500 Brantley Branch Road
Eustis, FL 32736
Phone: (352) 483-4200

Georgia

Camp High Five: serving children infected and
affected by HIV/AIDS
www.camphighfive.org
Contact: The ROCK, Inc.
Decator, GA
Phone: (773) 394-7063

Illinois

Camp Getaway: long-term residential camp for families
affected by HIV/AIDS

TABLE 24.4. (*continued*)

Access Community Health Network
1501 South California Ave.
Chicago, IL 60608
Phone: (773) 394-7063

Children's Place: serves children and families affected
by HIV with a variety of programming
Contact: The Children's Place Association
3059 West Agusta Blvd.
Chicago, IL 60622
Phone: (773) 826-1230

Indiana

Tataya Mato: long-term residential camp for children
infected or affected by HIV/AIDS
Contact: Jameson, Inc.
PO Box 31156
2001 S. Bridgeport, RD
Indianapolis, IN 46231
Phone: (317) 241-2661

Kentucky

Camp Heart to Heart: free summer camp for children
(ages 5–12) living with HIV/AIDS
Lions Camp Crescendo, Inc.
PO Box 607
Lebanon Junction, KY 40150
Phone: Daniel Coe (502) 969-0336, Teresa Davis (502)
456-6385

Massachusetts

Camp Safe Haven: serves children infected and
affected by HIV/AIDS. Family events, community-
based camps and retreat experiences and year-long
programs are held.
Contact: The Safe Haven Project, Inc.
PO Box 24
Vineyard Haven, MA 02568
Phone: (508) 693-1767

Michigan

Camp Rainbear: short-term residential camp for
families affected by HIV/AIDS
Rainbow Alliance, Inc.
8569 Stonegate Dr.
Northville, MI 48167
Phone: (248) 486-3872

Minnesota

Camp Knutson: serves families in which any member is
infected with HIV/AIDS for a 1-week residential
camp.
Contact: Camp Knutson and Knutson Point Retreat
Center
11169 Whitefish Ave.

Crosslake, MN 56442
Phone: (218) 543-4232

Missouri

Camp Hope: weekend-long camp for HIV-infected
children and their families
Contact: Project Ark (AIDS/HIV Resources &
Knowledge)
4169 Laclede Avenue
St. Louis, MO 63108
Phone: (314) 535-7275

Nebraska

Camp Knutson: serves families in which any member is
infected with HIV/AIDS for a 1-week residential
camp.
Contact: Camp Knutson and Knutson Point Retreat
Center
Nebraska Address
PO Box 81147
Lincoln, NE 68501
Phone: 1-877-800-CAMP (2267)

New Jersey

Camp Bright Feathers: long-term residential camp for
children affected by HIV/AIDS
Contact: YMCA Camp Ockanickon, Inc.
1303 Stokes Rd.
Medford, NJ 08055
Phone: (856) 428-5688

New York

The Birch Family Camp
Herbert G. Birch Services
275 Seventh Ave, Nineteenth Floor
New York, NY 10001
Phone: (212) 741-6522, ext. 208

The Double "H"–Hole in the Woods Ranch
Part of the Association of Hole in the Wall Camps
97 Hidden Valley Road
Lake Luzerne, NY 12846
Phone (518) 696-5676

Camp Courage: serves children between the ages
of 7 and 17 who are living with AIDS. The sister
camp, TLC, serves children who have a parent or
sibling who has AIDS or who has died from the
disease.
Contact: Camp Good Days and Special Times, Inc.
1332 Pittsford-Mendon Road
Mendon, NY 14506-9732
Phone: (585) 624-5555

Camp S.O.A.R.: camping and recreational activities for
children infected or affected by HIV/AIDS
Contact: Catholic Charities Community Services

(*continued*)

TABLE 24.4. (*continued*)

1945 E. Ridge Rd., Suite 24
Rochester, NY 14622
Phone: (585) 339-9800

Camp Viva: 1-week camp and after-camp follow-up program serving children and families with HIV/AIDS
Contact: Family Services of Westchester, White Plains Office
One Summit Avenue
White Plains, NY 10606
Phone: (914) 948-8004

Pact Weekend Camp
Children's Hospital of Buffalo, PACT Program
218 Bryant Street
Buffalo, NY 14222
Phone: (716) 878-7666

North Carolina

Agape Summer Camp: day camp for children affected by AIDS
Contact: Agape Family Center, Metrolina AIDS Project
PO Box 32662
Charlotte, NC 28232
Phone: (704) 333-1435

Camp Kaleidoscope: summer program open to all Duke University Medical Center pediatric patients ages 7–16.
Box 3417
DUMC
Durham, NC 27710
Phone (919) 681-4349

Victory Junction Camp: year-round camp for children (ages 8–13) living with HIV/AIDS. Includes disease-specific summer camp sessions, family retreat weekends, specialized programs, sibling weekends, and camper reunion. A sister camp to the Hole in the Wall Gang Association.
4500 Adam's Way
Randleman, NC 27317
Phone: (336) 498-9055

Ohio

Camp Sunrise: residential camp for children impacted by HIV/AIDS
1160 N. High Street
Columbus, OH 43201
Phone: (614) 297 – 8404

Oregon

Camp Starlight
Program of the Cascade AIDS Project
620 SW 5th Ave, Suite 300
Portland, OR 97204
Phone: (503) 238-4420

Pennsylvania

Camp Dreamcatcher: year-round programs for children infected or affected by HIV/AIDS
110 East State Street, Suite C
Kennett Square, PA 19348
Phone: (610) 925-2998

South Carolina

Camp for Kids: short-tern camp for children living with HIV/AIDS
Contact: Sue Kulen Camp for Kids, Inc.
Columbia, SC
Phone: (803) 957-7814

Virginia

Camp Funshine: serves children with HIV/AIDS and their families for a weekend camping program
Contact: Special Love
117 Youth Development Court
Winchester, VA 22602
Phone: (540)-667-3774

Camp Wakonda: serves children and families infected and affected by HIV/AIDS in a day-camp environment
Contact: Diocesan Center, Frances Barber
600 Talbot Hall Road
Norfolk, VA 23505
Phone: (757) 461-3595

Texas

Camp Firelight: day camp for children affected by HIV/AIDS
Contact: AIDS Outreach Center
Fort Worth, TX
Phone: (817) 335–1994

Camp Hope: serving children ages 6–15 with HIV/AIDS
Contact: AIDS Foundation Houston, Inc.
3202 Weslayan Annex
Houston, TX 77027
Phone: (713) 623-6796

Camp H.U.G. (Hope, Understanding, Giving): weekend camp for families and children with HIV/AIDS
Contact: AIDS Foundation Houston, Inc.
3202 Weslayan Annex
Houston, TX 77027
Phone: (713)-623-6796

Jennifer's Camp: long-term residential camp for children infected and affected by HIV/AIDS
www.aarcsa.com
Alamo Area Resource Center
San Antonio, TX
Phone: (210) 358-9995

TABLE 24.4. (*continued*)

Vermont

Twin States Kids Camp: short-term residential camp
 for children infected and affected by
 HIV/AIDS
Twin States Network
Bellow Falls, VT
Phone: (888) 338-8796

Washington

Northwest Reach Camp: long-term residential camp for
 children and families infected and affected by HIV/
 AIDS
Contact: REACH Ministries
419 Martin Luther King Jr. Way

Tacoma, WA 98405
Phone: (253) 383-7616

Rise N' Shine Camp: long-term residential camp for
 children infected and affected by HIV/AIDS
Contact: Rise N' Shine Foundation, Inc.
417 23rd Avenue South
Seattle, WA 98144
Phone: (206) 628-8949

Wisconsin

Camp Heartland: serves children infected and affected
 by HIV/AIDS
1845 North Farwell Ave., Suite 310
Milwaukee, WI 53202
Phone: 1-800-724-4673

plan in case they become ill appear to thrive under the continued uncertainties associated with this disease (Wiener et al., 2003). Despite the many stresses inherent in living with HIV/AIDS, these young adults should be given the opportunity to develop and pursue individual aspirations and goals. If recognized and nurtured, they have the potential to contribute significantly to society (Wiener et al., 1998b).

ASSESSMENT OF PSYCHOLOGICAL ADJUSTMENT AND FUNCTIONAL IMPAIRMENT

Despite the tremendous stress associated with living with HIV, early (pre-HAART) evidence suggested that most school-age HIV-positive children (6–11 years) exhibit stable psychological functioning (Bose et al., 1994; Wiener et al., 1999). However, with age, maladaptive responses appear to increase on measures of social function, anxiety, depressive symptomatology, and conduct problems, and there is a decline in positive social self-concept (Wiener et al., 1999; Battles and Wiener, 2002; New et al., 2003). Prevalence rates of behavioral and psychiatric symptoms including depression, anxiety, conduct disorders, hyperactivity, and behavioral and social problems have been described in 12% to 44% children and adolescents with HIV infection (Hopkins et al., 1989; Lifschitz et al., 1989; Esposito et al., 1999; Battles and Wiener, 2002; Mellins et al., 2003; Wiener and Battles, 2006). Additional investigations have found negative life events (Moss et al., 1998), limited social support (Battles and

Wiener, 2002), disclosure, (Battles and Wiener, 2002; Lester et al., 2002; Gaughan et al., 2004), and maternal loss (Battles and Wiener, 2002) to be associated with adverse psychologic and behavioral outcomes. Increased but similar levels of emotional and psychiatric problems have been found when comparing HIV-infected children to HIV-exposed but uninfected children (Havens et al., 1994; Mellins et al., 2003) and/or to a demographically matched non-HIV-exposed control group (Havens et al., 1994; Bachanas et al., 2001). These findings suggest that some behavior problems are not related to HIV variables (e.g., severity of CNS disease, length and type of antiretroviral therapy) but rather may be attributed to other etiologies such as environmental conditions (parent or primary caregiver mental health, substance abuse, family stability, and the cumulative effects of poverty), biological factors (maternal or paternal mental illness), or other psychosocial difficulties (Wolters and Brouwers, 2005). Whatever the ultimate etiology of the CNS impairment, we can anticipate that HIV-infected youth will remain at high risk for psychological distress and at greater risk for comorbid psychiatric symptoms. Therefore, providers from multiple disciplines will need to work together to maximize the child's function and quality of life.

Belman and colleagues (1992) classified the stress associated with HIV infection in children and adolescents into three primary categories: (1) medical factors (complex medical regimens, side effects of therapy); (2) psychological stressors (secrecy, fear of ostracism, death, guilt, uncertainties of future, sexual activity); and (3) social stressors (concerns surrounding disclosure, dating, insurance, academic success, neurocognitive impairment). These categories are helpful in deciphering changes in a child's behavior and affect and should be incorporated into a comprehensive psychosocial assessment obtained soon after presentation to a medical center. The psychosocial assessment is a critical part of a comprehensive multidisciplinary evaluation and has the benefit of anticipating family adaptation and high-risk factors for psychiatric distress, maladaptive coping, and signs of neurodevelopmental deficits. Information about the child's premorbid personality, specifically interpersonal relationships, academic functioning in school and play, coping abilities, prior losses, knowledge of and reaction to the diagnosis, recent stressful life events, and energy level and mood are very useful to include in the assessment (Wiener et al., 1998b).

PSYCHIATRIC DISORDERS AND TREATMENT IN HIV/AIDS

Investigations of psychiatric disorders in pediatric HIV/AIDS have been limited by small and diverse demographic samples, lack of consistent testing measurements, frequent subthreshold DSM-IV diagnoses, lack of appropriate control groups, pre-HAART exposure, and a paucity of available child and adolescent AIDS psychiatrists (Lourie et al., 2005). A recent review of reported DSM psychiatric diagnoses in pediatric HIV/AIDS found average prevalence rates of attention deficit hyperactivity disorder at 28.6%, anxiety disorders at 24.3 %, and depression at 25% (Scharko, 2006), but the analysis did not distinguish between populations by age or mode of transmission and may have missed important determinants of specific psychopathology. Included in the review is a study of HIV-infected youth ages 6–15 that suggests that depression (47%) and attentional disorders (29%) are common and that depression may be associated with encephalopathy and worsening immune function (Misdrahi et al., 2004). A small study of HIV-positive adolescents with sexually acquired HIV, assessed with the Kiddie Schedule for Affective Disorders and Schizophrenia (K-SADS), found high rates of mood disorder and substance abuse (Pao et al., 2000). In a recent sample of adolescents with perinatally acquired HIV who underwent the Diagnostic Interview Schedule for Children (DISC-IV), investi-

gators found high rates of anxiety and other disorders (Mellins et al., 2006).

There is sparse literature on the treatment of psychiatric disorders in medically ill children; the research literature on children with HIV is limited to case reports. A higher rate of psychotropic medication use and psychiatric hospitalizations among HIV-infected children compared with HIV-uninfected controls has been reported (Gaughan et al., 2004). In addition, a high rate of psychotropic medication use (45%) in an HIV clinic cohort (N = 64, mean age 15.3 years) has been reported, with psychostimulants and antidepressants being most commonly prescribed, and 30% of the sample on two or more psychotropic medications (Wiener et al., 2006).

GENERAL CONSIDERATIONS FOR PSYCHOPHARMACOLOGIC TREATMENT IN CHILDREN

While the full gamut of developmental and childhood psychiatric disorders are seen in children and adolescents with HIV/AIDS, only the most commonly seen clinical disorders will be highlighted here. Adult psychiatric syndromes of adjustment disorder, major depression, anxiety, and delirium apply to children as well. As in adults, treatment of psychiatric syndromes may improve outcomes (Angelino and Triesman, 2001). A thorough psychiatric assessment based on multiple brief examinations of the child and information gathered from additional sources including family, staff, and teachers is needed to make the best diagnosis and institute treatment. A child's biologic predisposition to depression and anxiety is suggested by (1) a family history of a mood or anxiety disorder or other psychiatric disorder and (2) previous psychiatric symptoms or psychiatric treatment. Precipitating and perpetuating factors for psychiatric disorders should also be identified.

Although many children cope well and adapt to their illness and treatment, symptoms of depression such as fatigue, cognitive impairment, decreased social interaction and exploration, and anorexia may in part derive from a cytokine or immunologic response to HIV and its treatments. Psychotropic medications do not replace comprehensive, multidisciplinary care and multimodal treatment, but they may improve the quality of life for pediatric HIV/AIDS patients by decreasing discomfort and increasing the functioning of medically ill children. Important determining factors for pharmacologic intervention are severity and duration of psychiatric symptoms and overall level of functional impairment. While there have been no well-controlled antidepressant trials in depressed medically ill children, and dosing of psychiatric medications in children with HIV/AIDS has not been systematically studied, off-label use of antidepressants has been helpful for treating anxiety and depression in other medically ill pediatric populations (Shemesh et al., 2002, 2005).

Factors such as body weight, Tanner staging, clinical status, and potentially interacting medications should be weighed when determining doses. Therefore, specific doses will not be described here. Table 24.5 lists U.S. Food and Drug Administration (FDA)-approved uses of common psychotropic medications in children.

Developmental Disorders

In addition to the neurocognitive deficits associated with HIV encephalopathy described earlier, children need to be assessed for language and communication disorders as well as pervasive developmental disorders, including autism, an impairment in reciprocal social interaction.

Behavioral Disorders

Attention Deficit Hyperactivity Disorder

Attention deficit hyperactivity disorder (ADHD) is a childhood-onset (before age 7 years) disorder characterized by sustained impulsivity, poor attention, and hyperactivity (APA, 1994). It is frequently diagnosed in children with HIV/AIDS. Forgetfulness, disorganization, and difficulty staying seated are often described, while on neuropsychological tests, poor processing speed is frequently noted. The differential diagnoses include anxiety, cognitive disorders, language disorders, medication toxicity, psychosocial stressors, and progressive HIV disease.

Psychostimulants are frequently used to treat ADHD in children with HIV, though dosage has not been established. Often, higher doses of stimulants are required to achieve scholastic benefit; these need to be balanced against appetite loss, growth retardation, and insomnia. Novel antidepressants such as bupropion and atomoxetine have been used as well. A case report found that clonidine was tolerated in three

children with HIV for behavioral problems (Cesena et al., 1995).

Oppositional Defiant Disorder and Conduct Disorder

Oppositional defiant disorder (ODD) is characterized by a recurrent pattern of losing one's temper, frequent arguing with adults or authority, refusal to follow rules, blaming others for one's mistakes, and being angry or vindictive for at least 6 months and of sufficient severity to cause impairment (APA, 1994). These behaviors are often seen in children from disrupted or unstable environments and must be distinguished from underlying cognitive or language difficulties as well as from mood and anxiety disorders. Conduct disorder is a repetitive and persistent pattern of aggressive behaviors, serious violation of rules, and destruction of property. New onset of conduct-disordered behaviors in an adolescent should lead to screening for mood, learning, and substance abuse disorders first.

Treatment for these behavioral disorders is initially directed at behavioral and parenting interventions. Low doses of atypical antipsychotics or mood stabilizers can be considered if behavioral dyscontrol is severe.

Mood Disorders

Major Depression

Major depression is marked by depressed mood or irritability in children daily for at least 2 weeks' duration (APA, 1994). Vegetative symptoms such as decreased appetite, difficulty sleeping, and poor energy are difficult to assess in youth with HIV because they may be secondary to HIV and its treatment. Increased somatic complaints such as headaches and fatigue as well as withdrawal from peers and family are commonly seen among depressed children. Anhedonia, or the lack of enjoyment of activities, may also be seen. A diagnosis of major depression occurs with increasing frequency during adolescence. Whether this is due to developmental aspects of mood neurobiology or to increased cognitive abilities in understanding one's situation is not clear. Differential diagnoses include worsening medical status, nonadherence (age-appropriate), bereavement, adjustment disorder, and dysthymia.

In one study a depressed adolescent with hemophilia and AIDS was treated for depression and pain

TABLE 24.5. Psychotropic Medications with FDA-Approved Uses in Children and Adolescents

Class	Medications	FDA-Labeled Use in Children
Antidepressants	Fluoxetine	7–17 years, for depression, OCD
	Sertraline	6–17 years, for OCD
	Paroxetine	No
	Citalopram	No
	Escitalopram	No
	Fluvoxamine	8 years and older, for OCD
	Venlafaxine	No
	Mirtazapine	No
	Bupropion	No
	Trazodone	No
	Amitriptyline	12 years and older, for depression
	Desipramine	No
	Nortriptyline	No
Anxiolytics	Clonazepam	Up to 10 years of age or 30 kg, for epilepsy
	Alprazolam	No
	Lorazepam	12 years and older, for insomnia (oral), anesthesia premed (oral)
Mood stabilizers	Lithium	12 years and older, for bipolar disorder
	Valproate	10 years and older, for migraine
		Prophylaxis epilepsy
	Carbamazepine	Pediatric, for epilepsy
	Oxcarbazepine	4–16 years, for epilepsy
	Gabapentin	3–12 years, for partial seizures
	Lamotrigine	2 years and older, for partial seizures
Antipsychotics	Haloperidol	3 years and older, for delirium, Tourette's, severe problematic behavior
	Risperidone	No
	Olanzapine	No
	Quetiapine	No
	Ziprasidone	No
	Aripiprazole	No
	Droperidol	2 years of age and older, for postoperative nausea and vomiting, prophylaxis
	Chlorpromazine	6 months and older, for anxiety about presurgery
		1–12 years, for behavioral syndrome
	Thioridazine	Pediatric, for nausea and vomiting, tetanus
		2 years and older, for schizophrenia
Stimulants	Methylphenidate	6 years and older, for ADHD, narcolepsy
	Dextroamphetamine	3 years and older, for ADHD, narcolepsy
Other	Atomoxetine	6 years and older, for ADHD
	Clonidine	Pediatric, for epidural for pain relief
	Guanfacine	12 years and older, for hypertension
	Propranolol	Pediatric, for hypertension
	Doxepin	12 years and older, for mixed anxiety and depressive disorder

ADHD, attention deficit disorder; OCD, obsessive-compulsive disorder.

with methylphenidate, which may also potentiate opiate treatment (Walling and Pfefferbaum, 1990). Tricyclic antidepressants (TCAs), novel antidepressants, and selective serotonin reuptake inhibitors (SSRIs) have been used empirically in youth with HIV. There is no clear evidence that one SSRI is more effective than another in youth. Citalopram or mirtazapine are used because they have fewer side effects and drug–drug interactions, or to promote weight gain and treat insomnia.

Fluoxetine is the only FDA-approved SSRI for depression in children older than 6 years of age.

Fluoxetine and sertraline are approved for obsessive-compulsive disorder in children older than 6 years, while fluvoxamine is approved for those age 8 years and older. Fluoxetine has an active metabolite, norfluoxetine, and fluvoxamine, which are potent inhibitors of CYP 3A3 and 3A4. They are contraindicated with macrolide antibiotics, azole antifungal agents, and several other medications. Amitriptyline is approved for depression in patients 12 years of age and older. TCAs are useful for treating insomnia, weight loss, anxiety, and some pain syndromes. Because of recent evidence that antidepressants may contribute to suicidal thinking in children and adolescents, suicidality should be assessed prior to initiation of antidepressant medications and carefully monitored during ongoing treatment (Rosenstein et al., 2005).

Bipolar Disorder

Bipolar disorder, characterized by elevated mood, grandiosity, decreased sleep requirement, racing thoughts, and hypersexuality, can also be seen in prepubertal youth (Geller et al., 2002). Pediatric bipolar disorder is sometimes difficult to distinguish from ADHD and is frequently comorbid with ADHD and substance abuse disorder. There is no evidence that there are higher rates of pediatric bipolar disorder associated with pediatric HIV infection, as is seen in adults. Treatment options are similar to those used in adults and include depakote, other mood stabilizers, and, rarely, lithium (Kowatch and DelBello, 2006). Similarly, drug–drug interactions and hepatotoxicity are clinical management concerns.

Anxiety Disorders

Anxiety symptoms are developmentally appropriate at particular ages, as with stranger anxiety at 9–12 months.

Separation Anxiety

Separation anxiety, or anxiety that is developmentally inappropriate and excessive around separation from home or from those to whom the child is attached, is usually seen at school entry and again in middle school. Children often report difficulty sleeping, a desire to be at home, fears that harm may befall attachment figures, and somatic complaints of stomachaches and headaches so as not to attend school or other social functions. Such anxiety is frequently precipitated by a life stress such as moving or death of a pet. Cognitive-behavioral therapy is useful. In severe cases of school refusal, treatment with SSRIs and TCAs has been reported.

Posttraumatic Stress Disorder

Posttraumatic stress disorder from traumatic events, including those arising from the hospital environment and invasive medical treatments, may be seen in children with HIV/AIDS.

Benzodiazepines, such as lorazepam, used in low doses in conjunction with nonpharmacologic distraction techniques and psychotherapy may be appropriate for procedures that provoke significant anxiety in children. Clonazepam is longer acting and may be helpful with more pervasive and prolonged anxiety symptoms. Benzodiazepines can cause sedation, confusion, and behavioral disinhibition and should be carefully monitored, especially in those patients with CNS dysfunction. Benzodiazepine withdrawal precipitated by abrupt discontinuation occurs most frequently on transfer out of intensive care settings.

Antihistamines have been used to sedate anxious children but are not recommended for treatment-persistent anxiety and their anticholinergic properties can precipitate or worsen delirium. Intravenous diphenhydramine may be sought by teens because of the "high" or euphoria experienced when given by intravenous push (Dinndorf et al., 1998); very high doses can provoke seizures.

Delirium

As in adults, the hallmark of delirium is impaired attention and fluctuating consciousness. Disorientation, sleep disturbance, irritability, confusion, apathy, agitation, exacerbation at night, and impaired responsiveness are also seen. In younger children, hallucinations or other perceptual disturbances, paranoia, and memory impairment are less common (Turkel and Tavaré, 2003). Underlying medical causes, especially medication intoxication, should be evaluated. Certain antiviral agents, especially efavirenz, have been associated with a number of significant CNS effects including dizziness, sleep disturbances, and mood alterations, which often resolve after the first few weeks of therapy but may also persist (Treisman and Kaplin, 2002).

Treatment is directed at reorienting children in developmentally appropriate ways and by enhancing environmental cues (lights on during the day, off at night; or by positioning near a window). Benzodiazepines and anticholinergic agents should be avoided. Very small doses of an atypical antipsychotic medication may be considered. However, Scharko et al. (2006) described a case in which risperidone was not effective, and haloperidol was required to treat delirium in the context of HIV dementia.

Dementia

The above case report (Scharko et al., 2006) suggests that HIV-associated dementia (HAD), well described in adults (McArthur, 2004), may also be seen in HIV-positive adolescents who become treatment resistant or discontinue treatment. This clinical picture is becoming more common, and low-dose atypical antipsychotic medications can be useful.

Substance Abuse Disorders

Clinicians need to be aware that adolescents with HIV/AIDS are at risk for developing substance abuse disorders, despite their medical condition. What may begin as experimentation can develop into a disorder as youth find substances that help them escape the reality of having a chronic life-threatening illness. These substances may treat underlying pain, anxiety, or mood disorders. In addition, the patient may have a learned and genetic predisposition to substance abuse. Treatment needs to be initiated immediately and monitored closely.

FAMILY TREATMENT CONSIDERATIONS

HIV-Positive Mothers

Clinicians should be vigilant to assess for substance abuse, depression, and anxiety disorders as well as posttraumatic stress disorder in HIV-positive mothers (Regier et al., 1990; Haller et al., 1993, Wiener et al., 1994, 1995; Mellins et al., 1997; Najavitz et al., 1997). Appropriate identification of and intervention in these mental health problems at the time of presentation is essential for optimizing a woman's adaptation to her own HIV illness and illness in her family members (Havens et al., 1996).

One of the most difficult tasks for parents with HIV is to face planning for the placement of their children after their death. Optimally, HIV-positive mothers begin the communication and permanency planning process prior to the final stage of their illness and have identified adults to provide care and support for their children. However, those struggling unsuccessfully with mental illness and/or substance abuse may not have taken care of these matters. In these families, special attention to the mental health needs of the children and adolescents is essential, as such lack of preparation suggests increased risk for mental health problems in these children (Wiener et al., 2003).

When a parent reaches the final phase of HIV illness, the care of younger children may be left to older adolescents or young adult family members, who are themselves facing the impending loss of a parent. In cases where parents develop AIDS-related delirium or dementia, mental status changes and disinhibited or disorganized behavior can not only be frightening but also dangerous to the children in their care (Wiener et al., 2003).

Many parents find legacy and remembrance projects therapeutic and exceptionally helpful. These activities help people express their thoughts, experiences, hopes, and dreams, and provide lasting, tangible evidence of their love for family members. Examples of such activities include writing letters to their children, and making audiotapes of their child's favorite stories, memory boxes, memory books, or videotapes. Parents have found these interventions invaluable and can provide a vivid and lasting sense of intimacy that is cherished by the family for generations to come (Taylor-Brown and Wiener, 1993).

Fathers

The role of fathers within the HIV/AID epidemic has taken on new significance. Women are the predominant caregivers of children infected with the virus, and most children live within single-parent families. Consequently, most of the attention, programs, interventions, and research initiatives have focused on women and children. There is very limited psychosocial information available on fathers, despite the fact that these individuals may outlive their partners. As the mother becomes increasing symptomatic or after she dies, some of these men become the sole caregivers of their infected children (Wiener et al., 2003). Just as for mothers, appropriate identification of and intervention in mental health problems as they present are essential to optimizing a father's adaptation to HIV illness in family members. When the father is HIV positive, custody planning is essential, regardless of the father's current health status.

In one of the few studies designed to explore the psychosocial adjustment, parenting stress, and identified needs associated with fathering a child with HIV infection, Wiener and colleagues (2001) demonstrated that fathers of children living with HIV are at risk for elevated levels of psychological distress, with one-third of a cohort meeting criteria for needed psychological intervention. The fathers also exhibited clinically significant increases in parenting stress compared to normative fathers. These findings support the need for paternal assistance in parenting training, in obtaining medical information for their child(ren), and accessing social support services. Mental health professionals need to be cognizant of the paternal adjustment process and the stresses associated with being a parent of a child who is not only living with HIV but has most probably suffered the loss of his or her mother (Wiener et al., 2001).

Other Caregivers

HIV-infected children whose parents are unable to care for them because of the physical demands of their own HIV/AIDS disease, substance use, emotional dysfunction, or death are often cared for by extended-family members. The Pediatric Spectrum of Disease project (1992) collected data on the primary caregiver of 1683 children born to HIV-infected mothers in six geographic locations through 1990 and found that 55% were living with a biologic parent and 10% with another relative, 28% were in foster care, 3% had been adopted, and 4% lived in group settings or with other caregivers. In all locations and for all racial and ethnic groups, children of mothers who used intravenous drugs were more likely to be living with an alternative caregiver than were children of mothers who had not used intravenous drugs. While regional differences in alternative-care placement exist, maternal drug use appeared to be the most important factor determining whether a child lived with a biologic parent (Caldwell et al., 1992).

When a mother dies of AIDS, infected and affected children often go to live with aunts, grandparents, and great-grandmothers (Minkler and Rose, 1993). These family members have the daunting task

of dealing with the loss of their own child or sibling while at the same time helping the surviving generation of children endure the loss of a parent (Wiener et al., 1998b). While sharing of caregiving with other family members is often preferable to placement outside of the family, several risks are inherent. No matter how willing and devoted these individuals are, many find themselves unable to bear the escalating burdens because of their own health care needs, emotional exhaustion, poverty, or the severity of the children's health, behavior, or academic problems (Levine, 1995).

Despite extensive efforts to find family members as caregivers, in some cases no appropriate relatives are identified and children end up in foster care. For the most part, foster parents, who have made a commitment to care for medically challenged children, have been courageous and excellent care providers. Nevertheless, foster home placement can present psychosocial challenges. If the child has been removed from the biological home due to abuse or neglect, the foster family has the challenge of helping the child cope with the trauma and sudden removal from their parent's home. Children placed in foster care after the death of their parents have significant losses, including the loss of relationships within the family and loss of neighborhood friends and teachers (Wiener et al., 1998b). Separation of siblings in foster care is also a critical concern (Groce, 1995). Mental health services for all care providers that address these issues are essential. Engaging community resources for in-home support, respite care, and financial assistance is critical to keep the family together. It is important to help the caregiver anticipate stressful events, such as disclosure to school, friends, and romantic partners. Caregivers should also be assessed for psychological distress, especially depression, anxiety, and disordered sleep.

Siblings: Uninfected Children in Affected Households

The social, psychological, and legal implications for the "well" children in the household are immense. Since many of these children have likely had a series of preexisting and long-standing family disruptions prior to the HIV diagnosis, these children suffer from widespread anxieties about future losses, who will care for them if all family members die, and concerns about their own health. It is the pervasive threat of death and fear of being left alone that constitutes chronic trauma for child survivors of HIV infection

(Mendelsohn, 1997). With no voice to represent them, these "well" or "affected" children are the silent victims of the HIV/AIDS pandemic (Fair et al., 1995).

It is common for some of these youngsters to become "parentified," a term used to describe children who are prematurely forced to take on adult responsibilities and roles before they are emotionally or developmentally able to manage these roles successfully (Bekir et al., 1993; Valleau et al., 1995). The greater the severity of their parents' illness, the more these children assume inappropriate adult role behaviors. Those who report more parental role behaviors also report more externalizing dysfunctional behaviors, including sexual behavior, alcohol and marijuana use, and conduct problems (Stein et al., 1999). A recent study found that 40% of young adolescents (ages 11–15) with an HIV-positive parent reported ever using tobacco, alcohol or drugs, thus interventions that promote family functioning and address social-influence factors are essential (Rosenblum et al., 2005). Psychotherapeutic interventions for the well children in HIV-affected households must concentrate on assessing for children acting as parents, providing respite child and parental care, assisting with permanency planning, and building legacies, social-support networks, and ongoing mental health services (Wiener et al., 2003). Special attention must also be given to the envy and rivalry that might arise in the well child when the HIV-infected child is receiving special medical care and parental attention (Fanos and Wiener, 1994).

The process of losing a sibling to AIDS may take place in the context of the illness or death of one or both parents and may be the harbinger of a still more frightening future (Walker, 1991), leaving these youth at high risk for psychologic distress and posttraumatic symptoms. Survivor guilt, guilt over the reaction to the death, guilt over past feelings about AIDS, and guilt over not being able to make the parents feel better can all contribute to anxiety and poor self-esteem. Earlier studies found among non-HIV-infected children externalizing behavior problems and somatic symptoms related to their parents' health status (Rotheram-Borus and Stein, 1999).

Globally, more than 15 million children have been orphaned by AIDS (UNAIDS, 2007) and it is estimated that by the year 2010, 18 million children in sub-Saharan Africa alone will be orphaned as a result of AIDS (UNAIDS, 2006) Almost half of orphaned children are between 11 and 17 years old (UNICEF, 2004). In a recently published study examining the impact of HIV-related parental death on 414 adolescents over a period of 6 years (Rotherum-Borus et al., 2005) bereaved adolescents had significantly more emotional distress, negative life events, and contact with the criminal justice system than non-bereaved youths. Depressive symptoms, passive problem solving, and sexual risk behaviors increased soon after parental death, compared with those of non-bereaved adolescents. One year after parental death, these levels were similar to those of nonbereaved peers, a finding suggesting the importance of early family intervention soon after parental HIV diagnosis, prior to parental death, and sustained over time. Recent work suggests that behavioral difficulties in pre-orphans may begin before the mother's death and may emerge more fully after 1–2 years rather than at 6 months (Pelton and Forehand, 2005).

Within medical centers and community-based programs, screening and family-based intervention for these siblings is needed. These children must be allowed to grieve, feel appropriate anger for the tragedies in their life, and find ways of channeling these emotions. Eth and Pynoos (1985) have stressed that traumatized individuals cannot mourn until the traumatic elements of the loss have been resolved. The hallmarks of posttraumatic stress disorder are common in cases of sibling loss from other chronic illnesses. Camps geared for the HIV- affected family members have been helpful for many of these children (Table 24.4), providing the opportunity to share their family's plight, meet others facing similar challenges, and often reach out and, if interested, be trained to be a spokesperson for adolescents at risk for HIV infection.

LIVING WITH HIV: OTHER CONSIDERATIONS

Pain

Children living with HIV commonly experience pain (Hirshfield et al., 1996; Gaughan et al., 2002; Lolekha et al., 2004), including abdominal pain of unclear etiology, myositis, and tension headaches, and difficulty managing neuropathic pain. Discomfort related to invasive procedures, toxicities and adverse drug reactions, invasive secondary infections, pancreatitis, and erosive esophagitis are more easily addressed and treated pharmacologically. Pain has been found to be associated with more severe immunosuppression and increased likelihood of death (Gaughan et al., 2002).

There are no published studies examining the relationship between chronic pain and psychological distress in HIV-infected children. Children fear pain and pain is made worse by emotional distress. The treatment goal must be freedom from pain with as little sedation as possible. Sound pediatric pain management principles of age-appropriate assessment of all developmental ages should be applied. This includes a repertoire of nonpharmacologic (such as distraction, relaxation, psychotherapy, and hypnosis) and pharmacologic treatments, although drug–drug interactions are a major concern (Duff, 2003, Greco and Berde, 2005).

Symptoms of dying children include fatigue, sedation, pain, and irritability, as well as gastrointestinal symptoms such as nausea, vomiting, or constipation (Wolfe et al., 2000). Yet pain management for youth is significantly less comprehensive than that provided to adults. Barriers to adequate treatment of pain include fear of harming children and adolescents with opiates; side effects, particularly respiratory depression; fears of addiction and abuse or diversion of opiates; ethical and legal concerns about pain relief versus euthanasia; and staff reluctance to ask for assistance from experts in managing pain medications in terminal settings (Galloway and Yaster, 2000). Psychotropic medications given in this setting such as benzodiazepines for anxiety and opiates for pain can be very sedating and induce significant confusion. Specific psychopharmacologic recommendations exist to manage terminal sedation while maximizing children's ability to interact. Comfort care consultations have resulted in fewer medical procedures and more supportive services to families (Galloway and Yaster, 2000; Himmelstein et al., 2004).

Ethical and Legal Issues

Knowledge of a psychiatrist's obligation to hold HIV-positive patients' diagnosis confidential and an understanding of a provider's responsibilities to warn and protect the rights of others from harm are essential. As laws differ from state to state, practitioners have an obligation to know the law in the state in which they practice and to be aware that the law may differ greatly even within a small geographical area. Additional information on treatment of adolescents with psychiatric conditions in terms of respective

consent, confidentiality, and competence, which may also vary from state to state, is described by Campbell (2006).

Providers working with HIV-positive adolescents and young adults in clinical practice benefit from having a working model as proposed by The American Psychological Association (APA) curricula, *Ethical Issues and HIV/AIDS: A Multi-Disciplinary Mental Health Services Curriculum* (Jue et al., 2000), when addressing HIV-related issues of disclosure.

For practitioners, the issue of partner notification is critical. The scholarly work of Gostin and Hodge (2002) provides guidelines for handling willful exposure cases, i.e., when an HIV-positive person intends to cause harm by intentionally infecting another person. The article also discusses HIV partner counseling and referral services, reviews the CDC and other governmental policies and procedures, issues of privacy and the right to know from a legal and ethical perspective, as well as the powers and duties to protect individuals and the public health.

Legal and ethical issues may also arise when it comes to school disclosure, employment, and reproductive decisions. School staff are now required to protect the privacy of students and to practice universal precautions. A position paper from The National Association of School Psychologists includes recommendations pertaining to disclosure in the school setting (National Association of School Psychologists, 2005). The book *Someone at School Has AIDS: A Guide to Developing Policies for Student and School Staff Members Who are Infected with HIV* (Bodgen et al., 2001) provides a guide to helping schools develop or revise existing policies to deal effectively with HIV in the school setting.

On June 25, 1998, the U.S. Supreme Court ruling in *Bragdon v. Abbott* stated that HIV disease falls within the scope of the Americans with Disabilities Act (ADA) for protection from discrimination. General and technical questions can be answered at http://www.usdoj.gov/crt/ada/adahom1.htm. Legal experts state that the ADA does offer protection to HIV-infected workers and these employees should seek reasonable accommodation at their workplace whenever possible and necessary (AIDS Alert, 2001). Regardless of the law, some HIV-infected patients have postponed antiretroviral treatment or taken early leave from their work, fearing loss of benefits and/or employment, rather than face disclosure of their HIV status (Wiener and Lyons, 2006).

End-of-Life Issues

The point at which treatments are unlikely to be successful is typically another crisis point for the family. Unlike cancer or other diseases in which there is a clear point when treatment has failed, in HIV, end of life usually presents as a result of an overwhelming opportunistic infections in the face of severe immunosuppression. Adolescents who often have not been adherent with their medication may present with severe wasting, chronic diarrhea, and poor quality of life. Meetings with the family to discuss options and to explore palliative care are often helpful, especially if staff members who have been most intimately involved with the child can be present.

As parents begin the process of accepting that their child will die, they may experience preparatory (anticipatory) grief. Many of their thoughts focus on preparing for death (this may include rehearsing the funeral in their imagination) while continuing to hope for a cure or recovery (Komp and Crocket, 1977). Hope can be redefined by redirecting energies toward providing as good a quality of life as possible for as long as possible, followed by a good quality of death (absence of anxiety and pain, combined with the presence of loved ones). The success of comprehensive care is dependent on open discussions ahead of time that addresses painful decisions, including home versus hospital care for the dying child, do not resuscitate (DNR) status, autopsy, and funeral arrangements. Once these logistics have been discussed, the family can reinvest energy in supporting their child. Open communication, pain control, involvement with friends and family, distractions, and the maintenance of familiar routines all convey a sense of security that is important in reassuring the dying child (Wiener et al., 2005).

Talking to the Dying Child

Struggling with their own anticipations and fears of separation and death, many parents and staff find it very difficult to discuss the imminence of death with their child (Frantz, 1983, Field and Behrman, 2003). Waechter (1971) conducted a study of hospitalized and fatally ill children and found that giving a child the opportunity to discuss issues related to death does not heighten anxiety. In a recent study of parents who had recently lost a child to cancer, many parents who did not speak with their children about death later regretted it; none of the parents who did speak with their children about dying had regrets (Kreicbergs et al., 2004). These findings suggest that permission to discuss any aspect of the illness decreases feelings of isolation and alienation from parents and other meaningful adults and communicates to the child that his or her illness is not too terrible to discuss. Hurwitz and colleagues (2004) provide staff examples of developmentally appropriate conversations with dying children.

While most children understand that a cure for HIV/AIDS does not exist, telling a child that there are no treatments that can stop the progression of his or her disease is the most difficult but also the most important message to convey. In doing so, one must also allow room for hope by redirecting the child's energy from active treatment to comfort interventions. Comfort includes having loved ones around, being free of further diagnostic or treatment procedures, if possible, not being in a hospital isolation room, and, most importantly, having controlled pain (Wiener et al., 2005). Providing comfort also involves acknowledgment and acceptance of a range of feelings, including feeling confused, sad, or angry. One of the greatest fears of young patients is being abandoned by or separated from family and friends; children need repeated reassurances that they will not be left alone. When given the opportunity, children frequently ask what will death be like, what will happen to them after they die, whether their parents will be all right after their death, whether they will experience much pain while dying, or whether they will be punished for the "bad" things they have thought, said, or done. Through play, art, drama, and therapeutic conversation, mental help professionals can ascertain the child's private perceptions and concerns and can correct distortions, dispel fantasies, and promote self-esteem through mastery of fears (Adams-Greenly, 1984; Wiener and Battles, 2002; Stuber and Houskamp, 2004). Spiritual ministry professionals can be of enormous support for both the child and family during this time as well.

As death approaches, families often need assurance that they have done all they could for their child. Often emotionally and physically exhausted and trying to hold on to whatever control they have, parents may appear less cooperative, irritable, easily frustrated, and annoyed. Health care providers need to respect each family's readiness, delicately balancing life issues with those related to palliative care, death, and loss (Wiener et al., 2005). The medical team's participation and investment in caring for the dying child is extremely important to and greatly appreciated by all families, even those who appear to be coping well on their own.

Talking to the Dying Adolescent

The timing and pace of conversations about advance care planning between adolescents and their families are not known, but the Institute of Medicine has recommended that such conversations commence at the time of diagnosis (Field and Behrman, 2003). In a survey of healthy and chronically ill adolescents (HIV, cancer, sickle cell, asthma), chronically ill adolescents said that they wanted to share in decision making about end-of-life care and that they wanted to have these conversations before they were hospitalized or dying (Lyon et al., 2004). It is easier to have some of these conversations when patients are medically stable, but often adolescents may not disclose their preferences to their families to protect them, by choosing what they think their family or doctor wants. Or they may wish to avoid letting their families know that they are dying (Lyon and Pao, 2006).

Before initiating discussions about end-of-life care with adolescents, it is important to evaluate for depression, bereavement, anxiety, pain, and even unrecognized delirium. In adults, cognitive impairment in patients with advanced AIDS has been reported to increase the desire for hastened death (Pessin et al., 2003). Psychiatric illnesses such as depression and anxiety disorders can be identified even in the midst of terminal illnesses, and treatment may alleviate many symptoms and improve quality of life.

The Initiative for Pediatric Palliative Care (2003) has developed a model curriculum for health care professionals that includes a module on adolescents' decision making. Such modules provide a base for training professionals to be more comfortable in helping families openly discuss how to make hard choices. Health care providers need to explicitly state the steps of the advance care–planning process to ensure that adolescents' wishes are honored (Lyon and Pao, 2006).

HIV PREVENTION STRATEGIES IN TEENS

The most viable strategy to reduce the spread of infection remains behavioral prevention. Over the past decade, many prevention programs have been delivered in a variety of settings with variable emphases on risk reduction. There is considerable evidence that comprehensive sexuality and HIV education programs that encourage abstinence, discuss correct condom use, educate adolescents about STDs, and teach sexual communication skills lead to reduced risk taking even among HIV-positive youth (Rotheram-Borus et al., 2001; Kirby, 2002b). There is no evidence to suggest that these programs hasten sexual activity (Office of the Surgeon General, 2001), but they are effective at reducing sexual risk taking among sexually experienced youth (Mullen et al., 2002).

Current HIV prevention efforts for adolescents are less focused on HIV/AIDS knowledge and more focused on behavior change strategies through practical suggestions for adolescents in real-life situations. Although there are few reports of HIV prevention intervention for youth in psychiatric care (Ponton et al., 1991; Brown et al., 1997b), recent programs have focused on strengthening parent–adolescent relationships and communication about sexual topics and teaching teens in therapeutic day schools to manage their negative emotional arousal to decrease unsafe behaviors (Donenberg and Pao, 2005).

CONCLUSION

Mental health clinicians can play a significant role in improving the lives of youth with HIV/AIDS. Early interventions addressing psychosocial and psychiatric needs can improve the overall health and quality of life for these youth and their caregivers.

ACKNOWLEDGMENTS   This research was supported in part by the National Institute of Mental Health and the National Cancer Institute. The views expressed by the authors are their views and do not necessarily represent the views of the NIMH, NCI, NIH, HHS, or the United States Government.

References

Adams-Greenly M (1984). Helping children communicate about serious illness and death. *J Psychosoc Oncol* 2:133–138.
AIDS Alert (2001). How much does the ADA (Americans With Disabilities Act) protect workers with HIV? *AIDS Alert* 16:23–24.

Alimenti A, Burdge D, Ogilvie A, et al. (2003). Lactic academia in HIV infants exposed to perinatal antiretroviral therapy. *Pediatr Inf Dis J* 22:782–789.

American Academy of Pediatrics Committee on Pediatrics AIDS (1999). Disclosure of illness status to children and adolescents with HIV infection. *Pediatrics* 103:164–166.

[APA] American Psychiatric Association (1994). *Diagnostic and Statistical Manual of Mental Disorders*, fourth edition (DSM-IV). Washington DC: American Psychiatric Association.

Angelino AF, and Treisman GJ (2001). Management of psychiatric disorders in patients infected with human immunodeficiency virus. *Clin Infect Dis* 33: 847–856.

Armstrong FD, Seidel JF, and Swales TP (1993). Pediatric HIV infection: a neuropsychological and educational challenge. *J Learn Disabil* 26:92–103.

Armstrong DWE, Levy J, Briery B, Vazquez, E, Jensen M, Miloslavich K, and Mitchell C (2002). Merging of neuroscience, psychosocial functioning, and bioethics in pediatric HIV. Presented at the 110th Annual American Psychological Association, Chicago, Illinois.

Arrufo JF, Gottleib A, Webb R, and Neville B (1994). Adolescent psychiatric inpatients: alcohol use and HIV risk-taking behavior. *Psychiatr Rehab J* 17: 150–156.

Aweeka F, Jayewaardene A, Staprana S, Bellibas SE, Kearney B, Lizak P, et al. (1999). Failure to detect nelfinavir in the cerebrospinal fluid of HIV-1-infected patients with and without AIDS dementia complex. *J Acquir Immune Defic Syndr Hum Retrovirol* 20:39–43.

Bachanas P, Kullgren K, Schwartz K, Lanier B, McDaniel S, Smith J, et al. (2001). Predictors of psychological adjustment in school-age children infected with HIV. *J Pediatr Psychol* 26:343–352.

Bandstra ES, Morrow CE, Anthony JC, Accornero VH, and Fried PA (2001). Longitudinal investigation of task persistence and sustained attention in children with prenatal cocaine exposure. *Neurotoxicol Teratol* 23:545–559.

Bandstra ES, Vogel AL, Morrow CE, Xue L, and Anthony JC (2004). Severity of prenatal cocaine exposure and child language functioning through age seven years: a longitudinal latent growth curve analysis. *Subst Use Misuse* 39:25–59.

Battles HB, and Wiener LS (2002). From adolescence through young adulthood: psychosocial adjustment associated with long-term survival of HIV. *J Adolesc Health* 30:161–168.

Bekir P, McLellan T, Childress AR, and Gariti P (1993). Role reversals in families of substance abusers: A transgenerational phenomenon. *Int J Addict* 28: 613–630.

Belman AL (1994). HIV-1 associated CNS disease in infants and children. In RW Price and SW Perry (eds.), *HIV, AIDS and the Brain* (p. 289). New York: Raven Press.

Belman AL, Diamond G, Dickson D, Horoupian D, Llena J, Lantos G, et al. (1988). Pediatric acquired immunodeficiency syndrome: neurologic syndromes. *Am J Dis Child* 142:29–35.

Belman A, Brouwers P, and Moss H (1992). HIV-1 and the central nervous system. In DM Kaufman, GE Solomon GE, and CR Pfeffer (eds.), *Child and Adolescent Neurology for Psychiatrists* (p. 238). Baltimore: Williams & Wilkins.

Bennett DS (1994). Depression among children with chronic medical problems: a meta-analysis. *J Pediatr Psychol* 19:149–169.

Bibace R, and Walsh ME (1980). Development of children's concepts of illness. *Pediatrics* 66:912–917.

Blanche S, Newell M, Mayaux M, Dunn D, Teglas J, Rouzioux C, et al. (1997). Morbidity and mortality in European children vertically infected by HIV-1. *J Acquir Immune Defic Syndr Hum Retrovirol* 14: 442–450.

Bodgen JK, Fraser C, Veg J, and Aschcroft J (2001). *Someone at School Has AIDS: A Complete Guide to Education Policies Concerning HIV Infection.* Alexandria, VA: National Association of State Boards of Education.

Bose S, Moss H, Brouwers P, Pizzo P, and Lorion R (1994). Psychologic adjustment of human immunodeficiency virus–infected school-age children. *J Dev Behav Pediatr* 15:S26–S33.

Brodt HR, Kamps BS, Gute P, Knupp B, Staszewski S, and Helm EB (1997). Changing incidence of AIDS-defining illnesses in the era of antiretroviral combination therapy. *AIDS* 11:1731–1738.

Brouwers P, DeCarli C, Tudor-Williams G, et al. (1994). Interrelations among patterns of change in neurocognitive, CT brain imaging and CD4 measures associated with anti-retroviral therapy in children with symptomatic HIV infection. *Adv Neuroimmunol* 4:223–231.

Brouwers P, Civitello L, DeCarli C, Wolters P, and Sei S (2000). Cerebrospinal fluid viral load is related to cortical atrophy and not to intracerebral calcifications in children with symptomatic HIV disease. *J Neurovirol* 6:390–397.

Brown JV, Bakeman R, Coles CD, Platzman KA, and Lunch WE (2004). Prenatal cocaine exposure: a comparison of 2-year-old children in parental and nonparental care. *Child Dev* 75:1282–1296.

Brown LK, Danovsky MB, Lourie KJ, et al. (1997a). Adolescents with psychiatric disorders and the risk of HIV. *J Am Acad Child Adolesc Psychiatry* 36:1609–1617.

Brown LK, Reynolds LA, and Lourie KJ (1997b). A pilot HIV prevention program for adolescents in a psychiatric hospital. *Psychiatr Serv* 48:531–533.

Caldwell MB, Mascola L, Smith W, Thomas P, Hsu HW, Maldonado Y, Parrott R, Byers R, Oxtoby M, and The Pediatric Spectrum of Disease Clinical

Consortium (1992). Biologic, foster, and adoptive parents: care givers of children exposed perinatally to human immunodeficiency virus in the United States. *Pediatrics* 90:603–607.

Campbell AT (2006). Consent, competence, and confidentiality related to psychiatric conditions in adolescent medical practice. *Adolesc Med* 17:25–47.

[CDC] Centers for Disease Control and Prevention (1993). U.S. AIDS cases reported through June 1993. *HIV/AIDS Surveill Rep* 5:1–19.

[CDC] Centers for Disease Control and Prevention (1994). Revised classification system for human immunodeficiency virus infection in children less than 13 years of age. *MMWR Morb Mortal Wkly Rep* 43(RR-12):1–10.

[CDC] Centers for Disease Control and Prevention (2000). *Young People at Risk: HIV/AIDS among America's Youth.* Retrieved April 3, 2007, from http://www.cdc.hiv/pubs/facts/youth.pdf.

[CDC] Centers for Disease Control and Prevention (2003a). *HIV/AIDS Surveillance Report, 2003,* Vol. 15, pp. 1–46. Atlanta: U.S. Department of Health and Human Services, CDC.

[CDC] Centers for Disease Control and Prevention (2003b). Pregnancy in perinatally HIV-infected adolescents and young adults—Puerto Rico, 2002. *MMWR Morb Mortal Wkly Rep* 52:149–151.

[CDC] Centers for Disease Control and Prevention (2004). *HIV/AIDS Surveillance Report, 2004.* Retrieved April 3, 2007, from http://www.cdc.gov/hiv/topics/surveillance/resources/reports/2004report/default.htm.

[CDC] Centers for Disease Control and Prevention (2005). *HIV/AIDS Surveillance Report: HIV Infection and AIDS in the United States and Dependent Areas, 2005. Retrieved April 12, 2007.* http://www.cdc.gov/HIV/topics/surveillance/basic.htm#exposure

[CDC] Centers for Disease Control and Prevention (2006). *HIV/AIDS among Youth, 2006.* Retrieved April 3, 2007, from http://www.cdc.gov/hiv/resources/factsheets/youth.htm.

[CDC] Centers for Disease Control and Prevention (2007). *Pregnancy and Childbirth.* Retrieved April 3, 2007, from http://www.cdc.gov/HIV/projects/perinatal/background.htm.

Cesena M, Lee DO, Cebollero AM, et al. (1995). Behavioral symptoms of pediatric HIV-1 encephalopathy successfully treated with clonidine. *J Am Acad Child Adolesc Psychiatry* 34:302–306.

Chasnoff IJ, Anson A, Hatcher R, Stenson H, Laukea K, and Randolph LA (1998). Prenatal exposure to cocaine and other drugs: outcome at four to six years. *Ann N Y Acad Sci* 846:314–328.

Chesler MA, Paris J, and Barbarin OA (1986). "Telling" the child with cancer: parental choices to share information with ill children. *J Pediatr Psychol* 11: 497–516.

Chesney M (2003). Adherence to HAART regimens. *AIDS Patient Care STDS* 17:169–177.

Church JA, Mitchell WG, Gonazalez-Gomez I, et al. (2001). Mitochondrial DNA depletion, near fatal metabolic acidosis and liver failure in an HIV-infected child treated with combination antiretroviral therapy. *J Pediatr* 138:748–751.

Civitello L (2003). Neurologic aspects of HIV infection in infants and children: therapeutic approaches and outcomes. *Curr Neurol Neurosci Rep* 3:120–128.

Cohen J, Reddington C, Jacobs D, et al. (1997). School-related issues among HIV-infected children. *Pediatrics* 100:e8.

Coles CD, and Black MM (2006). Impact of prenatal substance exposure on children's health, development, school performance, and risk behavior. *J Pediatr Psychol* 31:1–4.

Cooper ER, Hanson C, Diaz C, Mendez H, Abboud R, Nugent R, et al. (1998). Encephalopathy and progression of human immunodeficiency virus disease in a cohort of children with perinatally acquired human immunodeficiency virus infection. Women and Infants Transmission Study Group. *J Pediatr* 132:808–812.

Cooper ER, Charurat M, Mofenson L, et al. (2002). Combination antiretroviral strategies for the treatment of pregnant HIV-1 infected women and prevention of perinatal HIV-1 transmission. *J Acquir Immune Defic Syndr Hum Retrovirol* 29:484–494.

d'Arminio Monforte A, Duca PG, Vago L, Grassi MP, and Moroni M (2000). Decreasing incidence of CNS AIDS-defining events associated with antiretroviral therapy. *Neurology* 54:1856–1859.

Deeks SG, Smith M, Holodniy M, and Kahn JO (1997). HIV-1 protease inhibitors. *JAMA* 277:145–153.

Depas G, Chiron C, Tardieu M, et al. (1995). Functional brain imaging in HIV-1-infected children born to seropositive mothers. *J Nucl Med* 36:2169–2174.

DiClemente RJ, and Ponton LE (1993). HIV-related risk behaviors among psychiatrically hospitalized adolescents and school-based adolescents. *Am J Psychiatry* 150:324–325.

Dinndorf P, McCabe MA, and Frierdich C (1998). Risk of abuse of diphenhydramine in children and adolescents with chronic illnesses. *J Pediatr* 133:293–295.

Donenberg GR, and Pao M (2005). Youths and HIV/AIDS: psychiatry's role in a changing epidemic. *J Am Acad Child Adolesc Psychiatry* 44:728–747.

Donenberg GR, Bryant F, Emerson E, Wilson H, Pasch K (2003). Tracing the roots of early sexual debut among adolescents in psychiatric care. *J Am Acad Child Adolesc Psychiatry* 42:594–608.

Donenberg GR, Emerson E, Bryant FB, et al. (2001). Understanding AIDS-risk behavior among adolescents in psychiatric care: links to psychopathology and peer relationships. *J Am Acad Child Adolesc Psychiatry* 40:642–653.

Duff AJA (2003). Incorporating psychological approaches into routine paediatric venipuncture. *Arch Dis Child* 88:931–937.

Enting RH, Hoetelmans RMW, Lange JMA, Burger DM, Beijnen JH, and Portegies P (1998). Antiretroviral drugs and the central nervous system. *AIDS* 12:1941–1955.

Epstein LG (1986). Neurologic manifestations of HIV infection in children. *Pediatrics* 78:678–687.

Esposito S, Musetti L, Musetti MC, et al. (1999). Behavioral and psychological disorders in uninfected children aged 6 to 11 years born to human immunodeficiency virus–seropositive mothers. *J Dev Behav Pediatr* 20:411–417.

Eth S, and Pynoos RS (1985). Post-traumatic stress disorder in children. In D Spiegel (ed.), *The Progress in Psychiatry Series*. Washington, DC: American Psychiatric Press.

Fair C, Dupont-Spencer E, Wiener L, and Riekert K (1995). Healthy children in families with AIDS: epidemiological and psychosocial considerations. *Child Adolesc Social Work J* 12:165–181.

Faithfull J (1997). HIV positive and AID infected women: challenges and difficulties of mothering. *Am J Orthopsychiatry* 67:144–151.

Falloon J, Eddy J, Wiener L, and Pizzo PA (1989). Human immunodeficiency virus infection in children. *J Pediatr* 114:1–30.

Fanos JH, and Wiener L (1994). Tomorrow's survivors: siblings of HIV-infected children. *J Dev Behav Pediatr* 15:S43–S48.

Fergusson DM, Horwood J, and Beautrais AL (1999). Is sexual orientation related to mental health problems and suicidality in young people? *Arch Gen Psychiatry* 56:876–880.

Field MJ, and Behrman RE (eds.) (2003). *When Children Die: Improving Palliative and End-of-Life Care for Children and Their Families.* Washington, DC: The National Academies Press.

Frank DA, Augustyn M, Knight WG, Pell T, and Zuckerman B (2001). Growth, development, and behavior in early childhood following prenatal cocaine exposure: a systematic review. *JAMA* 285: 1613–1625.

Frantz T (1983). When Your Child has a Life-Threatening Illness. Washington, DC: Association for the Care of Children's Health and the Candlelighters Foundation.

Funck-Brentano I, Costagliola D, Seibel N, Straub E, Tardieu M, and Blanche S (1997). Patterns of disclosure and perceptions of the human immunodeficiency virus in infected elementary school-age children. *Arch Pediatr Adolesc Med* 151:978–985.

Galloway KS, and Yaster M (2000). Pain and symptom control in terminally ill children. *Pediatr Clin North Am* 47:711–746.

Garofalo R, Wolf RC, Kessel S, Palfrey J, and DuRant RH (1998). The association between health risk behaviors and sexual orientation among a school-based sample of adolescents. *Pediatrics* 101:895–902.

Gaughan DM, Hughes MD, Seage GR 3rd, Selwyn PA, Carey VJ, Gortmaker SL, and Oleske JM (2002). The prevalence of pain in pediatric human immunodeficiency virus/acquired immunodeficiency syndrome as reported by participants in the Pediatric Late Outcomes Study (PACTG 219). *Pediatrics* 109:1144–1152.

Gaughan DM, Hughes MD, Oleske JM, Malee K, Gore CA, Nachman S, for the Pediatric AIDS Clinical Trials Group 219C Team (2004). Psychiatric hospitalizations among children and youths with human immunodeficiency virus infection. *Pediatrics* 113:e544–e551.

Geller B, Zimerman B, Williams M, Delbello MP, Frazier J, Beringer L (2002). Phenomenology of prepubertal and early adolescent bipolar disorder: examples of elated mood, grandiose behaviors, decreased need for sleep, racing thoughts and hypersexuality. *J Child Adolesc Psychopharmacol* 12(1): 3–9.

Gerson AC, Joyner M, Fosarelli P, et al. (2001). Disclosure of HIV diagnosis to children: when, where, why, and how. *J Pediatr Health Care* 15:161–167.

Gisslen M, and Hagberg L (2001). Antiretroviral treatment of central nervous system HIV-1 infection: a review. *HIV Med* 2:97–104.

Gostin LO, and Hodge JG (2002). HIV partner counseling and referral services—handling cases of willful exposure. Georgetown/Johns Hopkins Program on Law & Public Health.

Greco C, and Berde C (2005). Pain management for the hospitalized pediatric patient. *Pediatr Clin N Am* 52:995–1027.

Groce NE (1995). Children and AIDS in a multicultural perspective. In S Geballe, J Gruendel, and W Andiman (eds.), Forgotten Children of the AIDS Epidemic (p. 95). New Haven: Yale University Press.

Grubman S, Gross E, Lerner-Weiss N, et al. (1995). Older children and adolescents living with perinatally acquired human immunodeficiency virus infection. *Pediatrics* 95:657–663.

Haller DL, Knisely JS, Dawson KS, et al. (1993). Perinatal substance abusers: psychological and social characteristics. *J Nerv Ment Dis* 181:509–513.

Hammami N, Nostlinger C, Hoeree T, et al. (2004). Integrating adherence to highly active antiretroviral therapy into children's daily lives: a qualitative study. *Pediatrics* 114:591–597.

Hardy MS, Armstrong FD, Routh DK, Albrecht J, and Davis J (1994). Coping and communication among parents and children with human immunodeficiency virus and cancer. *J Dev Behav Pediatr* 15: S49–S53.

Havens J, Whitaker A, Feldman J, and Ehrhardt A (1994). Psychiatric morbidity in school-age children with congenital human immunodeficiency virus infection: a pilot study. *J Dev Behav Pediatr* 15:S18–S25.

Havens J, Mellins CA, and Pilowski D (1996). Mental health issues in HIV-affected women and children. *Int Rev Psychiatry* 8:217–225.

Havens JF, Mellins CA, and Ryan S (2005). Child psychiatry: psychiatric sequalae of HIV and AIDS. In B Sadock and V Sadock (eds.), *Kaplan & Sadock's Comprehensive Textbook of Psychiatry*, eighth edition (p. 3434). Philadelphia: Lippincott Williams & Wilkins.

Hays RB, McKusick L, Pollack L, Hilliard R, Hoff C, and Coates TJ (1993). Disclosing HIV seropositivity to significant others. *AIDS* 7:425–431.

Heath KV, Singer J, O'Shaughnessy MV, Montaner JS, and Hogg RS (2002). Intentional nonadherence due to adverse symptoms associated with antiretroviral therapy. *J Acquir Immun Definc Syndr* 31: 211–217.

Himelstein BP, Hilden JM, Boldt AM, and Weissman D (2004). Pediatric palliative care. *N Engl J Med* 350:1752–1762.

Hirschfeld S, Moss H, Dragisic K, Smith W, and Pizzo PA (1996). Pain in pediatric human immunodeficiency virus infection: incidence and characteristics in a single-institution pilot study. *Pediatrics* 98(3 Pt. 1):449–452.

Hopkins KM, Crosz J, Cohen H, Diamond G, and Nozyce M (1989). The developmental and family services unit—a model AIDS project serving developmentally disabled children and their families. *AIDS Care* 1(3):281–285.

Howland LC, Gortmaker SL, Mofenson LM, et al. (2000). Effects of negative life events on immune suppression in children and youth infected with human immunodeficiency virus type 1. *Pediatrics* 106:540–546.

Hurwitz CA, Duncan J, and Wolfe J (2004). Caring for the child with cancer at the close of life. *JAMA* 292:2141–2149.

Instone SL (2000). Perceptions of children with HIV infection when not told for so long: implications for diagnosis disclosure. *J Pediatr Health Care* 14:235–243.

Initiative for Pediatric Palliative Care (2003). *Pediatric Palliative Care Curricula*. Newton, MA: Education Development Center.

Jue S, Eversole T, and Anderson JR (2000). *Ethical Issues and HIV/AIDS Mental Health Services*. Washington, DC: American Psychological Association.

Katz ER, and Jay SM (1984). Psychological aspects of cancer in children, adolescents, and their families. *Clin Psychol Rev* 4:525–542.

Keller MA, Venkatraman TN, Thomas MA, Deveikis A, LoPresti C, Hayes J, Berman N, Walot I, Ernst T, and Chang L (2006). Cerebral metabolites in HIV-infected children. *Neurology* 66:874–879.

Kirby D (2002a). Impact of schools and school programs upon adolescent sexual behavior. *J Sex Res* 39: 27–33.

Kirby D (2002b). Effective approaches to reducing adolescent unprotected sex, pregnancy, and childbearing. *J Sex Res* 39:51–57.

Kline MW (2007). *Pediatric HIV Infection. Baylor International Pediatric AIDS Initiative*. Retrieved April 3, 2007, from http://bayloraids.org/resources/pedaids/manifestations.shtml.

Komp D, and Crocket J (1977). Educational needs of the child with cancer. Presented at the American Cancer Society Second National Conference on Human Values and Cancer, Chicago.

Kourtis AP, Bulterys M, Nesheim SR, and Lee FK (2001). Understanding the timing of HIV transmission from mother to infant. *JAMA* 285:709–712.

Kowatch RA, and DelBello MP (2006). Pediatric bipolar disorder: emerging diagnostic and treatment approaches. *Child Adolesc Psychiatr Clin N Am* 15: 73–108.

Kreicbergs U, Valdimarsdottir D, Onelov E, Henter JI, and Steineck G (2004). Talking about death with children who have severe malignant disease. *N Engl J Med* 351:1175–1186.

Krogstad D (2006). Diagnosis of HIV infection in children. In SL Zeichner SL and JS Read (eds.), *Handbook of Pediatric HIV Care*, second edition. Cambridge, UK: Cambridge University Press.

Kunins H, Hein K, Futterman D, Tapley E, and Elliot ES (1993). Guide to adolescent HIV/AIDS program development. *J Adolesc Health* 14(Suppl):S1–S140.

Lester BM, ElSohly M, Wright LL, Smeriglio VL, Verter J, Bauer CR, et al. (2001). The maternal lifestyle study: drug use by meconium toxicology and maternal self-report. *Pediatrics* 107:309–317.

Lester P, Chesney M, Cooke M, Weiss R, Whalley P, Perez B, Glidden D, Petru A, Dorenbaum A, and Wara D (2002). When the time comes to talk about HIV: factors associated with diagnostic disclosure and emotional distress in HIV-infected children. *Acquir Immune Defic Syndr* 31:309–317.

Levine C (1995). Today's challenges, tomorrow's dilemmas. In S Geballe, J Gruendel, and W Andiman (eds.), *Forgotten Children of the AIDS Epidemic* (p. 190). New Haven: Yale University Press.

Lewis MP, Colbert A, Erlen J, and Meyers M (2006). A qualitative study of persons who are 100% adherent to antiretroviral therapy. *AIDS Care* 18:140–148.

Lifschitz M, Hanson C, Wilson G, and Shearer WT (1989). Behavioral changes in children with human immunodeficiency virus (HIV) infection. Proceedings of the V International Conference on AIDS 1:316.

Lightfoot M, and Rotheram-Borus MJ (1989). Negotiating behavior change with HIV-positive adolescent girls. *AIDS Patient Care STDS* 12:395–401.

Linares TJ, Singer LT, Kirchner HL, Short EJ, Min MO, Hussey P, and Minnes S (2006). Mental health outcomes of cocaine-exposed children at 6 years of age. *J Pediatr Psychol* 31:85–97.

Lipson M (1993). What do you say to a child with AIDS? *Hastings Cent Rep* 23:6–12.

Lipson M (1994). Disclosure of diagnosis to children with human immunodeficiency virus or acquired immunodeficiency syndrome. *J Dev Behav Pediatr* 15:S61–S65.

Llorente A, Brouwers P, Charurat M, et al., for the Women and Infant Transmission Study Group. Early neurodevelopmental markers predictive of mortality in infants infected with HIV-1. *Dev Med Child Neurol* 45:76–84.

Lobato MN, Caldwell MB, Ng P, and Oxtoby MJ (1995). Encephalopathy in children with perinatally acquired human immunodeficiency virus infection. *J Pediatr* 126:710–715.

Lolekha R, Chanthavanich P, Limkittikul K, Luangxay K, Chotpitayasunodh T, and Newman CJ (2004). Pain: a common symptom in human immunodeficiency virus–infected Thai children. *Acta Paediatr* 93:891–898.

Lourie KJ, Pao M, Brown LK, and Hunter H (2005). Psychiatric issues in pediatric HIV/AIDS. In K Citron, MJ Brouillette, and A Beckett (eds.), *HIV and Psychiatry. A Training and Resource Manual,* second edition (pp. 181–195). Cambridge, UK: Cambridge University Press.

Luna GC, and Rotheram-Borus MJ (1999). Youth living with HIV as peer leaders. *Am J Community Psychol* 27:1–23.

Lyon M, and Pao M (2006). When all else fails: end-of-life care for adolescents.In ME Lyon M and LJ D'Angelo (eds.), *Teenagers, HIV, and AIDS: Insights from youths living with the virus.* (pp. 213–233). Westport, CT: Praeger Publishers,

Lyon ME, McCabe MA, Patel K, and D'Angelo LJ (2004). What do adolescents want? An exploratory study regarding end-of-life decision-making. *J Adolesc Health* 35:e1–e6.

Marhefka SL, Tepper VT, Brown JL, and Farley JJ (2006). Caregiver psychosocial characteristics and children's adherence to antiretroviral therapy. *AIDS Patient Care STDS* 20(6):429–437.

Mason HRC, Marks G, Simoni JM, Ruiz MS, and Richardson JL (1995). Culturally sanctioned secrets: Latino men's nondisclosure of HIV infection to family, friends, and lovers. *Health Psychol* 14:6–12.

McArthur J (2004). HIV dementia: an evolving disease. *J Neuroimmunol* 157:3–10.

Mellins CA, Ehrhardt AA, and Grant WF (1997). Psychiatric symptomatology and psychological functioning in HIV infected women. *AIDS Behav* 1(4): 233–245.

Mellins CA, Brackis-Cott E, Dolezal C, Richards A, Nicholas SW, and Abrams EJ (2002). Patterns of status disclosure to perinatally HIV-infected children and subsequent mental health outcomes. *Clin Child Psychol Psychiatry* 7:101–114.

Mellins CA, Smith R, O'Driscoll P, Magder LS, Brouwers P, Chase C, et al. (2003). High rates of behavioral problems in perinatally HIV-infected children are not linked to HIV disease. *Pediatrics* 111:384–393.

Mellins CA, Brackis-Cott E, Dolezal C, and Abrams E (2006). Psychiatric disorders in youth with perinatally acquired human immunodeficiency virus infection. *Pediatr Infect Dis J* 25:432–437.

Mendelsohn A (1997). Pervasive traumatic loss from AIDS in the life of a 4-year-old African boy. *J Child Psychother* 23:399–415.

Mettler MA, Borden K, Lopez E, et al. (1997). Racial and ethnic patterns of disclosure to children with HIV. Presented at the American Psychological Association's Annual Conference, Chicago, IL.

Minkler M, and Rose KM (1993). *Grandmothers as Caregivers. Raising Children of the Cocaine Epidemic.* Newbury Park, CA: Sage Publications.

Misdrahi D, Vila G, Funk-Brentano I, Tardieu M, Blanche S, and Mouren-Simeoni MC (2004). DSM-IV mental disorders and neurological complications in children and adolescents with human immunodeficiency virus type 1 infection (HIV-1). *Eur Psychiatry* 19:182–184.

Moss H, Bose S, Wolters P, and Brouwers P (1998). A preliminary study of factors associated with psychological adjustment and disease course in school-age children infected with the human immunodeficiency virus. *J Dev Behav Pediatr* 19:18–25.

Mullen PD, Ramirez G, Strouse D, Hedges LV, and Sogolow E (2002). Meta-analysis of the effects of behavioral HIV prevention interventions on the sexual risk behaviors of sexually experienced adolescents in controlled studies in the United States. *J Acquir Immune Defic Syndr* 30: S94–S105.

Munet-Vilaro F (2004). Delivery of culturally competent care to children with cancer and their families—the Latino experience. *J Pediatr Oncol Nurs* 21:155–159.

Murphy DA, Belzer M,. Durako SJ, Sarr M, Craig M., Wilson CM, and Muenz LR (2005). Longitudinal antiretroviral adherence among adolescents infected with human immunodeficiency virus. *Arch Pediatr Adolesc Med* 159:764–770.

Najavits LM, Weiss RD, and Shaw SR (1997). The link between substance abuse and posttraumatic stress disorder in women: a research review. *Am J Addict* 6:273–283.

National Association of School Psychologists (2005). *Position Statement on HIV/AIDS.* http://www.nasponline.org/information/pospaper_aids.html.

Nehring WM, Lashley FR, and Malm K (2000). Disclosing the diagnosis of pediatric HIV infection: mother's views. *J Soc Pediatr Nurs* 5:5–14.

New M, Lee S, and Pao M (2003). Prevalence of mental health in pediatric HIV: a family perspective. Presented at the NIMH Conference on the Role of Families in Preventing and Adapting to HIV/AIDS, Washington, DC.

Ng WYK, Mellins CA, and Ryan S (2004). The mental health treatment of children and adolescents perinatally infected with HIV. In E Abrams (ed.), Topic of the Month, 2004. http://web.archive.org/web/20040214070503/hivfiles.org/index.html.

Office of the Surgeon General (2001). The Surgeon General's Call to Action to Promote Sexual Health and Responsible Sexual Behavior. Rockville, MD: U.S. Department of Public Health Service.

Palella FJ, Delaney KM, Moorman AC, Loveless MO, Fuhrer J, Satten GA, et al. (1998). Declining morbidity and mortality among patients with advanced human immunodeficiency virus infection. N Engl J Med 338:853–860.

Pao M, Lyon M, D'Angelo L, Schuman W, Tipnis T, and Mrazek D (2000). Psychiatric diagnoses in adolescents seropositive for the human immunodeficiency virus. Arch Pediatr Adolesc Med 154:240–244.

Patsalides AD, Wood LV, Atac GK, et al. (2002). Cerebrovascular disease in HIV-infected pediatric patients: neuroimaging findings. AJR AM J Roentgenol 179:999–1003.

Pelton J, and Forehand R (2005). Orphans of the AIDS epidemic: an examination of clinical level problems of children. J Am Acad Child Adolesc Psychiatry 44:585–591.

Pessin HB, Burton RL, and Breitbart W (2003). The role of cognitive impairment in desire for hastened death: a study of patients with advanced AIDS. Gen Hosp Psychiatry 25:194–199.

Ponton LE, DiClemente RJ, and McKenna S. (1991). An AIDS education and prevention program for hospitalized adolescents. J Am Acad Child Adolesc Psychiatry 30:729–734.

Rausch DM, and Stover ES (2001). Neuroscience research in AIDS. Prog Neuropsychopharmacol Biol Psychiatry 25:231–257.

Regier DA, Farmer ME, Rae DS et al. (1990). Comorbidity of mental disorders with alcohol and other drugs of abuse. JAMA 264:2511–2518.

Richardson GA, Conroy ML, and Day NL (1996). Prenatal cocaine exposure: effects on the development of school-age children. Neurotoxicol Teratol 18:627–634.

Rosenblum A, Magura S, Fong C, Cleland C, Norwood C, Casella D, Truell J, and Curry P (2005). Substance use among young adolescents in HIV-affected families: resiliency, peer deviance, and family functioning. Subst Use Misuse 40:581–560.

Rosenstein DR, Pao M, and Cai J (2005). Psychopharmacologic management in oncology. In J Abraham, CJ Allegra, and J Gulley (eds.), Bethesda Handbook of Clinical Oncology, second edition (pp. 521–528). Philadelphia: Lippincott Williams and Wilkins.

Rotheram-Borus MJ, Wiess R, Alber S, and Lester P (2005). Adolescent adjustment before and after HIV-related parental death. J Consult Clin Psychol 73:221–228.

Rotheram-Borus MJ, and Miller S (1998). Secondary prevention for youths living with HIV. AIDS Care 10:17–34.

Rotheram-Borus MJ, and Stein JA (1999). Problem behavior of adolescents whose parents are living with AIDS. Am J Orthopsychiatry 69:228–239.

Samples CL, Goodman E, and Woods E (1998). Epidemiology and medical management of adolescents. In PA Pizzo and C Wilfert (eds.), Pediatric AIDS, third edition (p. 615). Baltimore: Lippincott Williams and Wilkins.

Santos CP, Felipe YX, Braga PE, Ramos D, Lima RO, and Segurado AC (2005). Self-perception of body changes in persons living with HIV/AIDS: prevalence and associated factors. AIDS 19:S14–S21.

Scharko AM, Baker E, Kothari P, Khattak H, and Lancaster D (2006). Case study: delirium in an adolescent girl with human immunodeficiency virus–associated dementia. J Am Acad Child Adolesc Psychiatry 45:104–108.

Scharko AM (2006). DSM psychiatric disorders in the context of pediatric HIV/AIDS. AIDS Care 18:441–445.

Schrager LK, and D'Souza MP (1998). Cellular and anatomical reservoirs of HIV-1 in patients receiving potent antiretroviral combination therapy. JAMA 280:67–71.

Shanbhag MC, Rutstein RM, Zaoutis J, Zhao H, Chao D, and Radcliffe J (2005). Neurocognitive functioning in pediatric human immunodeficiency virus infection: effects of combined therapy. Arch Pediatr Adolesc Med 159:651–656.

Shemesh E, Bartell A, Newcorn JH (2002). Assessment and treatment of depression in medically ill children. Curr Psychiatry Rep 4:88–92.

Shemesh E, Yehuda R, Rockmore L et. al. (2005). Assessment of depression in medically ill children presenting to pediatric specialty clinics. J Am Acad Child Adolesc Psychiatry 44:1249–1257.

Sherman BF, Bonanno GA, Wiener L, and Battles HB (2000). When children tell their friends they have AIDS: possible consequences for psychological well-being and disease progression. Psychosom Med 62:238–247.

Slavin LA, O'Malley JE, Koocher GP, and Foster DJ (1982). Communication of the cancer diagnosis to pediatric patients: impact on long-term adjustment. Am J Psychiatry 139:179–183.

Sonza S, and Crowe S (2001). Reservoirs for HIV infection and their persistence in the face of undetectable viral load. AIDS Patient Care STDS 15:511–518.

Spinetta JJ, and Maloney LJ (1978). The child with cancer: patterns of communication and denial. J Consult Clin Psychol 46:1540–1541.

Spinetta JJ (1980). Disease-related communication: how to tell. In J Kellerman (ed.), Psychological Aspects of Childhood Cancer (p. 257). Springfield, IL: Charles C. Thomas.

Stein JA, Riedel M, and Rotheram-Borus MJ (1999). Parentification and its impact on adolescent children of parents with AIDS. *Fam Process* 38:193–208.

Sternhell PS, and Corr MJ (2002). Psychiatric morbidity and adherence to antiretroviral medication in patients with HIV/AIDS. *Aust N Z J Psychiatry* 36: 528–533.

Stuber M, and Houskamp BM (2004). Spirituality in children confronting death. *Child Adolesc Psychiatr Clin N Am* 13:127–136.

Swindells S (1998). *Therapy of HIV-1 Infection: A Practical Guide for Providers*. New York: Chapman & Hall.

Tardieu M, Chenadec JL, Persoz A, Meyer L, Blanche S, and Mayaux MJ (2000). HIV-1-related encephalopathy in infants compared with children and adults. *Neurology* 54:1089–1095.

Tardieu M, and Boutet A (2002). HIV-1 and the central nervous system. *Curr Top Microbiol Immunol* 265:183–195.

Tardieu M (1999). HIV-1-related central nervous system disease. *Curr Opin Neurol* 12:337–381.

Tardieu M, Brunelle F, Raybaud C, et al. (2005). Cerebral MR imaging in uninfected children born to HIV-seropositive mothers and perinatally exposed to zidovudine. *AJNR Am J Neuroradiol* 26:695–701.

Taylor-Brown S, and Wiener L (1993). Making videotapes of HIV-infected women for their children. *Fam Soc* 74:468–480.

Thompson PM, Dutton RA, Hayashi KM, et al. (2005). Thinning of the cerebral cortex visualized in HIV/AIDS reflects CD4+ T lymphocyte decline. *Proc Natl Acad Sci U S A* 102(43):15647–15652.

Treisman GL, and Kaplin AI (2002). Neurologic and psychiatric complications of antiretroviral agents. *AIDS* 16:1201–1215.

Turkel SB, and Tavaré CJ (2003). Delirium in children and adolescents. *J Neuropsychiatry Clin Neurosci* 15:431–435.

UNAIDS (2004). *2004 Report on the Global AIDS Epidemic*. Retrieved April 4, 2007, from http://www.unaids.org/bangkok2004/GAR2004_html/GAR2004_00_en.htm.

UNAIDS (2006). World Not Doing Nearly Enough to Protect Children Affected by AIDS. Retrieved April 12, 2007, http://www.unaids.org/en/Media Centre/PressMaterials/FeatureStory/GlobalPartners Forum.asp.

UNAIDS (2007). Orphans. Retrieved April 12, 2007, http://www.unaids.org/en/Issues/Affected_communities/orphans.asp

UNICEF (2005). *State of the World's Children 2005*. Retrieved April 4, 2007, from http://www.unicefusa.org/site/c.duLRI8O0H/b.1300301/k.4D04/State_of_the_Worlds_Children__Publications__Media_Center__US_Fund_for_UNICEF.htm

UNICEF (2004). *Global Summary of the HIV and AIDS Epidemic*, December 2004. http://www.thebody.com/whatis/global_statistics.html

Valleau MP, Bergner RM, and Horton CB (1995). Parentification and caretaker syndrome: an empirical investigation. *Fam Ther* 22:157–164.

Van Dyke RB, Lee S, Johnson GM, et al. Reported adherence as a determinant of response to highly active antiretroviral therapy in children who have human immunodeficiency virus infection. *Pediatrics* 109:e61.

Waechter E (1971). Children's awareness of fatal illness. *Am J Nurs* 71:1168–1172.

Walker G (1991). *In the Midst of Winter: Systematic Therapy with Families, Couples and Individuals with AIDS Infection*. New York: Norton.

Walling VR, and Pfefferbaum B (1990). The use of methylphenidate in a depressed adolescent with AIDS. *J Dev Behav Pediatr* 11:195–197.

Wiener L (1998). Helping a parent with HIV tell his or her children. In D Aronstein and B Thomspon (eds.), *HIV and Social Work: A Practitioner's Guide* (pp. 327–338). Binghamton, NY: Haworth Press.

Wiener L, and Battles H (2002). Mandalas as a therapeutic technique for HIV-infected children and adolescents. *J HIV/AIDS Soc Work* 1:27–39.

Wiener L, and Battles H (2006). Untangling the web: a close look at diagnosis disclosure among HIV-infected adolescents. *J Adoles Health* 38(3):307–309.

Wiener L, and Lyons M (2006). *HIV disclosure: who knows? Who needs to know? Clinical and ethical considerations*. In M Lyons and L D'Angelo (eds.), *Teenagers, HIV and AIDS: Insights from Youths Living with the Virus (Sex, Love, and Psychology)*. Westport, CT: Praeger.

Wiener L, and Figueroa V (1998). Children speaking with children and families about HIV infection. In P Pizzo and K Wilfert (eds.), *Pediatric AIDS: The Challenge of HIV Infection in Infants, Children, and Adolescents*, third edition (p. 729). Baltimore: Williams and Wilkins.

Wiener L, Theut S, Steinberg S, Reikert K, and Pizzo P (1994). The HIV-infected child: parental responses and psychosocial implications. *Am J Orthopsychiatry* 64:485–492.

Wiener L, Reikert K, Theut S, Steinberg S, and Pizzo PA (1995). Parental psychological adaptation and children with HIV: a follow-up study. *AIDS Patient Care* 9:233–239.

Wiener L, Battles H, Heilman N, Sigelman C, and Pizzo PA (1996). Factors associated with disclosure of diagnosis to children with HIV/AIDS. *Pediatr AIDS HIV Infect* 7:310–324.

Wiener L, Battles H, and Heilman N (1998a). Factors associated with parents decision to disclose their HIV diagnosis to children. *Child Welfare* LXXVII: 115–135.

Wiener L, Septimus A, and Grady C (1998b). Psychosocial support and ethical issues for the child and family. In P Pizzo and K Wilfert (eds.), *Pediatric AIDS: The Challenge of HIV Infection in Infants,*

Children, and Adolescents, third edition (p. 703). Baltimore: Williams and Wilkins.

Wiener L, Battles H, and Riekert K (1999). Longitudinal study of psychological disturbances in HIV-infected, school aged children. *J HIV/AIDS Prev Ed Adolesc Child* 3:13–36.

Wiener L, Vasquez MJP, and Battles HB (2001). Brief report: fathering a child with HIV/AIDS: psychosocial parenting stress. *J Pediatr Psychol* 26:353–358.

Wiener L, Havens J, and Ng W (2003). Psychosocial problems in pediatric HIV infection. In WT Shearer WT (ed.), *Medical Management of AIDS in Children*. Philadelphia: W.B. Saunders.

Wiener L, Riekert K, Ryder, C, and Wood L (2004). Assessing medication adherence in adolescents with HIV when electronic monitoring is not feasible. *AIDS Patient Care STDS* 18:31–43.

Wiener L, Hersh SP, and Kazak A (2005). Psychiatric and psychosocial support for child and family. In PA Pizzo and DG Poplack DG (eds.), *Principles and Practice of Pediatric Oncology*, fifth edition. Philadephia: Lippincott.

Wiener L, Battles H, Ryder C, and Pao M (2006). Psychotropic medication use in HIV-infected youth receiving treatment in a single institution. *J Child Adolesc Psychopharmacol* 16(6):744–753.

Wolfe J, Grier HE, Klar N, et al. (2000). Symptoms and suffering at the end of life in children with cancer. *N Engl J Med* 342:326–333.

Wolters PI, Brouwers P, Moss HA, Pizzo P (1995). Differential receptive and expressive language functioning of children with asymptomatic HIV disease and relation to CT scan brain abnormalities. *Pediatrics* 95:112–119.

Wolters PL, and Brouwers P (2005). Neurobehavioral function and assessment of children and adolescents with HIV-1 infection. In SL Zeichner and JS Read (eds.), *Textbook of Pediatric Care*. Cambridge, UK: Cambridge University Press.

Chapter 25

Young Adulthood and Serodiscordant Couples

Marshall Forstein

Since the beginning of the AIDS epidemic, HIV has significantly affected the physical and mental health of individuals, couples, their children, extended families, and social support networks. Transmitted primarily by sexual behavior and injecting drug use, the HIV pandemic carries more symbolic meaning than other infectious diseases. In the United States and other developed nations, the initial reports focused on the impact of a disease called "gay-related immunodeficiency syndrome" (GRID) in men who had sex with men, and then among intravenous drugs users, interpreted to mean that "immoral" behavior had overwhelmed the immune system.

As the epidemiology unfolded, HIV was diagnosed in hemophiliacs receiving clotting factor and in Haitians recently immigrated to the United States. Scientists began searching for what epidemiologically appeared to be an infectious agent rather than a consequence of "lifestyle." Except for the "innocent victims" receiving tainted blood, the die had been cast to stigmatize HIV as a disease associated with non-

normative sexual and drug-using behaviors. In developing nations, heterosexual behavior was associated from the very beginning of the epidemic with the increasing transmission of HIV, requiring a complex examination of cultural mores, sexual practices, and social structures. This stigmatization of AIDS deriving from sexual and drug-using behaviors not only had profound effects on the sociopolitical environment in which the epidemic developed but also fostered the psychological substrates of guilt and shame that continue to impede coping with HIV on an individual, familial, community, and national level (Zich and Temoshok, 1987; Moore, 1993; Remien et al., 1995; van der Straten et al., 1998).

Couples of same- or opposite-sex orientation initially discovered that one or both of them were HIV infected when symptomatic illness appeared. Several years passed before it was possible to test whether the non-ill partner was also infected. Once the antibody test became available, couples that had been thrust into the turmoil of dealing with one partner having a life-threatening illness had to make decisions about the other partner (and children) getting tested, even when there was no available intervention.

Research has shown that same- or opposite-gender coupling within and across cultures is dynamic and diverse. Couples do not all share the same beliefs about what constitutes commitment, fidelity, or individual rights and privileges within the relationship. All couples affected by HIV, however, have to manage information about how the infection entered the relationship, decide what to disclose and to whom, and learn how to cope with a life-threatening illness and, often, how to face death and loss. The way in which HIV is similar to and different from other medical illnesses that couples face is an important and ongoing area of research.

This chapter will focus on the particular aspects of HIV's impact on discordant couples in which only one member is infected. After reviewing some of the extant literature, clinical issues that emerge in evaluating and treating couples will be presented. The author has been assessing and treating individuals and couples affected by HIV since the very beginning of the epidemic.

IMPACT OF MEDICAL ILLNESS ON FAMILIES AND COUPLES

Many studies have reported on the increased psychosocial stress in families experiencing a major medical illness (Cohen and Lazarus, 1979; Coyne and Fiske, 1992; Lippman et al., 1993). Most early studies of stress in families examined the impact of illnesses such as chronic arthritis or heart disease, or that of progressive neurological illness such as amyotrophic lateral sclerosis or multiple sclerosis. The psychological distress of families dealing with HIV/AIDS includes the added factor of the potential for transmission of the disease to one of the members of the family who serves as a primary support for the person infected (Britten et al., 1993; McShane et al., 1994). Other investigators have analyzed the distress experienced by HIV-positive individuals. Social support correlates highly with improved quality of life (Folkman et al., 1993; Chesney and Folkman, 1994; Pakenham et al., 1994). The literature on stress and distress in HIV-positive individuals clearly shows the impact of stigma, poor physical health, lower perceived social support, decreased functional capacity, loss of control over one's life, and loss of friends and loved ones (Rabkin et al., 1991; Catalan et al., 1992; Gluhoski et al., 1997; Rabkin et al., 1997).

Little has been written, however, about the aspects of HIV disease that make coping with it different from coping with other chronic fatal illnesses, in terms of types of psychological defensive structures. Medical factors alone rarely account for how people function psychosocially when facing a significant illness (Meyerowitz et al., 1983). Although other chronic, fatal illnesses (i.e., advanced cardiac disease, emphysema due to smoking, diabetes due to obesity) may result from "lifestyle" choices, there is little moral outcry about the behaviors involved. Sex and drugs, however, represent powerful human drives that evoke blame, retaliation, and withholding on many personal and societal levels. Management of HIV individually or within a couple may be significantly affected by conscious and unconscious forces that play out in the social context in which the couple lives.

Much has been written about the relationship between social support, coping mechanisms, and psychosocial functioning. Self-disclosure of HIV status, (Mandel, 1986), having an active coping strategy (Namir et al., 1989) and the capacity to use social support (Zich and Temoshok, 1987; Ostrow et al., 1989), and minimizing the impact of HIV symptoms on function have all been associated with increased quality of life for individuals infected with HIV (Peterson et al., 1996). There are fewer long-term studies of couples with similar (seroconcordant) or dissimilar (discordant) serologic status (also referred to as mixed HIV status). While several newer studies have looked at the risks for seroconversion in mixed-status couples (Freeman and Glynn, 2004; Remien et al., 2005) and at the impact of interventions for couples on adherence to antiretroviral medications (Remien et al., 2005) there is a paucity of research examining the psychological impact of mixed status on couples after a decade of antiretroviral therapy.

Pakenham and colleagues (1994) reviewed some of the literature that frames two types of coping that may be relevant to understanding how individuals deal with HIV/AIDS. Problem-focused strategies are deployed when there is a sense of control over the source of potential stress. Such strategies include changing behavior to prevent infection or, perhaps, to prevent transmission if the person is infected (Lazarus and Folkman, 1984). Under circumstances (such as already being infected, progression of illness) where there may be little to control but much to be endured, emotion-focused coping may predominate (Auerbach, 1989).

Applying the above precepts, one could imagine that in discordant couples, the infected person might be more likely to employ emotion-focused coping while the HIV-negative member might tend toward problem solving, to take care of the infected member and remain uninfected. As the epidemic has progressed through several stages (see below) in terms of the available scientific understanding and the possibilities for intervention, these coping mechanisms can shift both within individuals and within couples. Other factors, such as the strength of the relationship, the capacity for self-care in the face of sadness and grief, the capacity to remain individuated within a relationship, and personality styles and temperament, make coping unique in each case. Cultural precepts that proscribe how men and women act in relationships are also relevant to the process of coping with a life-threatening illness that is transmitted by the very intimate behaviors that help to define the relationship itself.

Keegan and colleagues (2005) have examined the impact of living longer on antiretroviral therapy on sexuality and relationships and concluded that difficulties with sexual functioning, low libido, fears of HIV disclosure and of infecting partners, and problems in negotiating safer sex continue to be major issues among women living with HIV and may not have been mitigated by a more optimistic future outlook. Little research exists describing the intrapsychic or dyadic experience of members of mixed-status couples from either point of view, in the context of greater social awareness of HIV, increased possibilities for longevity, bearing children, or reaching previously unexpected developmental stages. As the HIV pandemic has progressed from the early 1980s to the present, couples have formed in a variety of ways that inform the issues they face medically, psychologically, and socially. As Staten and colleagues (1998) state, "HIV sero-discordant relationships . . . are unique in that the threat of transmission and disease progression co-occur within the same dyad, forcing partners to develop strategies along the continuum from HIV prevention to care."

TEMPORAL FRAMEWORK OF THE EPIDEMIC

Conceptually, there are several phases of the HIV epidemic that inform our understanding of the impact of HIV on individuals infected with HIV and their sexual partners. The time frame below provides an approximate demarcation of these phases.

Phase I: During this phase, sexual behavior and coupling took place prior to the recognition of HIV as a sexually transmitted disease (prior to 1981).

Phase II: This phase starts after the epidemiological evidence for sexual and blood transmission was gathered, but before there was clear identification of HIV as the causative agent (1981–1985).

Phase III: This phase starts after HIV was identified and serologic testing became available, but nothing but prophylaxis for opportunistic infections was available. Prevention of further transmission required difficult discussions of sexual and drug behavior within varied cultural and ethnic and racial populations.

Phase IV: The first phase of antiretroviral monotherapy changed the importance of testing, raising ethical issues of access to care and the role of discrimination in sustaining health disparities (1987–1995).

Phase V: The discovery of rapid resistance to monotherapy led to highly active antiretroviral therapy (HAART) with the development of multiple biological classes of agents effective to prevent resistance. For some individuals (in nations that can afford and distribute HAART), HIV infection (1995–) can be seen as a chronic, manageable disease rather than as an acute, irrevocably fatal illness. The vast majority of the world's HIV-infected population, however, remains without access to basic health care and prophylaxis against opportunistic infections, much less HAART, essentially remaining in phase II or III above.

Studies from other countries that examine mixed- or similar-status couples incorporate data from widely disparate cultures with varying degrees of access to medical and antiretroviral medication. Comparison of studies across cultures and phases of the epidemic illustrates the inconsistency of even the definition of what constitutes a couple, a union, or a marriage. In this chapter, the word "couple" will be used to refer to any two people who identify themselves as being primarily committed to each other, independent of legal, social, or cultural parameters.

Seroconcordant and serodiscordant couples may share many of the same concerns, related to the impact of the disease process itself on the person(s) infected. Both types of couples face the problems of access to medical care and sustained adherence to antiretroviral medication, as well as the uncertainty of the response to medications and the course of illness. In families with children in which both parents are ill, permanency placement is a significantly stressful concern.

Couples with similar or mixed serostatus almost universally report greater levels of stigma, stress in relationships, and difficulty in maintaining sexual and emotional intimacy from discovery of HIV infection throughout the course of illness, including death. In discussing relationships affected by HIV, it is helpful to know the phase of the epidemic in which an individual acquired HIV, as this may imply complex psychological, behavioral, and social substrates that inform the particular experience and meaning of infection for the dyad as well as for the individual. To understand how couples manage serostatus and their relationship, it is useful to know what each member knew about their own and their partner's serostatus prior to and throughout their relationship.

GAY MALE COUPLES

The few studies of gay male couples with serodiscordance are based on data gathered prior to the widespread use of HAART, which may significantly change some of the psychological and social issues facing couples of similar or mixed status in the present (Carpenter et al., 1997).

Early on (phase I), before the illness was even identified, gay men were forging relationships as one or both men were infected but unaware of this. The development of illness could be quite sudden with the onset of an opportunistic infection, often heralding a rapid demise, before antiretroviral treatment became available. Having emerged from the long-standing social disapprobation and pathologizing of homosexuality into the Gay Liberation era, celebrating sexuality as part of asserting an "out" lifestyle, a generation of gay men instead found themselves burying their friends and partners. Often for those couples in which both men were infected, the less ill member saw his own demise foreshadowed in the horrible, painful, wasting illness of AIDS. Men who had finally found a life partner saw their future wrenched from them

because of a virus that they never saw coming. Functional couples stayed together, with the negative or less ill partner providing the care and support for the one with the more advanced illness. Dysfunctional couples often broke apart. HIV-negative men in relationship with a man with AIDS sometimes used the partner's illness as a reason to pull away, while others, out of guilt or sense of responsibility to care for their dying partner, stayed, knowing that it would be simply a matter of time before death freed them. Serosimilar couples, though strained by illness and social stigmatization and less concerned with transmission of the virus, faced the stress of maintaining emotional and sexual intimacy as they confronted mortality at a developmentally unanticipated time (Forstein, 1994).

In the early stages of the epidemic, it was not uncommon for gay men to lose an entire network of friends, their "chosen families," leaving them as individuals or couples to face the stigma and isolation that AIDS represented in the larger society. In the urban gay communities, social service agencies arose to provide much needed support, with the development of groups for HIV-positive gay men. But the divide between those who were seropositive and those who were seronegative continued to grow, with serodiscordant couples often caught in the middle. Nothing had prepared a generation of gay men for the developmental crisis that a sexually transmitted disease could bring during the prime of life.

As the epidemiology suggested that HIV was sexually transmitted, efforts to control the spread of HIV began with assumptions that protection against other sexually transmitted diseases (STDs) might be effective in preventing the transmission of HIV as well. Prior to the advent of serologic testing for HIV antibodies, the denial that one might be infected or be at risk for becoming infected informed decisions about sexual behaviors. Gay men, having struggled to make sexuality a celebrated part of life, saw efforts to limit intercourse, or to use protection as ploys by the government and social structures to once again pathologize homosexuality and limit same-sex behavior and enforce a "moral monogamy." As a result, some men fearing HIV retreated into a self-imposed sexual celibacy. Others struggled with how to negotiate safer sex and relationships according to HIV status. The already complex world of finding same-sex partners became almost universally more anxiety provoking, affecting the decisions made in almost all encounters, consciously or not. Many gay men experienced once again the "coming out process," often emotionally and socially traumatizing as someone who was HIV infected.

Men of color, particularly in the African-American population, where prevalence rates among men who had sex with men (MSM) were rising out of proportion to their representation in society, were often driven deeper into social isolation because of the condemnation of homosexuality by many African-American religious denominations. As a consequence, access to HIV testing and medical and mental health care continues to lag behind what is available to other MSM.

Remien and colleagues (2003) have summarized the challenges facing serodiscordant same-sex couples: disclosing positive HIV status to friends and families, coping with the uncertainty of illness progression and anticipated death, planning for the future, experiencing social isolation and social stigma, making reproductive decisions, facing the ongoing risk of HIV transmission to the negative partner, and maintaining a safe and satisfying sexual intimacy. Role definitions within a relationship may also change in the event of declining health. Of note are findings that both seronegative and seropositive members of the serodiscordant couple have similar rates of distress, as with heterosexual couples dealing with a significant chronic medical illness.

In Remien et al.'s study, the results of data collected from 1994 to 1995 were presented, revealing factors associated with distress in male couples that were serodiscordant before the advent of HAART. Analysis of 75 male discordant couples "demonstrated that measures of dyadic satisfaction, sexual satisfaction, avoidance and self-blaming coping style, and support from one's partner are associated with levels of psychological distress among individuals in HIV discordant relationships" (Remien et al., 2003, p. 533). The authors report that a primary relationship can serve as both a buffer and a source of the distress, depending on whether there is a perception of "consensus and cohesion" and sexual satisfaction with one's partner or a sense of avoidance and lack of sexual intimacy. The issue of sexual satisfaction correlating with level of distress illustrates the importance of understanding the meaning of protected versus unprotected sexual behavior to each member of the couple.

At that time, serodiscordance was clearly associated with higher levels of psychological distress for individuals and couples than that of the general population. Sexual satisfaction and intimacy were associated with greater risk-taking behaviors within the relationship, even when safer sex practices were observed with outside sexual partners.

Since the advent of antiretroviral treatment, gay men have increased their quality of life, general health, and expectations for a future that had previously been foreclosed. With the awareness that the infected member of the couple might live for many years with the advent of HAART, couples face the future with more, but often less certain, prospects. Many questions remain unanswered. How will serodiscordant couples cope with the ongoing stress of potential infection? As the time course potentially changes, how will the dynamic issues within each couple change? What are the factors that might help or hinder couples manage the ongoing stress of serodiscordance? How will couples develop strategies to manage serodiscordance and emotional concordance at the same time?

Studies of distress in HIV-negative caretakers have shown stigma, the burden of illness in a loved one, the uncertainty of the future, and potential loss to be important factors (Folkman et al., 1993; Pakenham et al., 1994). The extent to which these factors remain significant since the advent of HAART is currently under study. The long-term impact of multidrug treatment is yet to be seen, as there is some concern that long-term adherence to such regimens may be difficult for some HIV-positive persons, and that despite the long-term use of HAART, the prevalence of HIV-related cognitive impairment may increase with longevity (Sacktor et al., 2002; Bell, 2004; Stoff, 2004; Parsons et al., 2006). In the context of increasing physical health and social function, the slow decline of subcortical mental function will present significant challenges to both serosimilar and seromixed couples. For example, whereas hope that the future is possible may have decreased suicidal ideation in some individuals, the specter of cognitive decline even in the face of generally improved health may precipitate new crises for individuals and couples.

HETEROSEXUAL COUPLES

Most of the research on heterosexual couples dealing with HIV in one or both partners in the developed nations has been published prior to the impact of HAART on health, quality of life, and longevity (Lippman et al., 1993; Straten et al., 1998; Moore et al., 1998; Van Devanter et al., 1999). In the developing nations, where HAART is still not available to most of the population, the literature is focused on prevention efforts to decrease risky sexual behaviors and consequently partner transmission rates, and on procreative intentions to prevent maternal infant transmission. Thus the majority of studies of serodiscordant couples focus on sexual behavior risk, the survival of the union, and the emotional, economic, and physical impact on children and families (Tangmunkongvoralakul et al., 1999).

The impact of parental HIV serodiscordance on families is dynamic and significant for all members. Concerns may be different for parents (depending on which parent is seropositive), both in terms of how each member of the family is affected and how decisions about the future are managed. One retrospective study in the United Kingdom reported on over 200 families who had children referred to a pediatric HIV service or family clinic between 1991 and 1996 (White et al., 1997). Some of the children were themselves infected while others had infected mothers. In the analysis of the data the authors compared HIV-positive children who had an HIV-positive mother and HIV-negative father, a positive mother, or an untested or unavailable father, and HIV-negative children who had an HIV-negative mother and HIV-positive father or unknown father. Several findings emerged. A diagnosis during pregnancy could put women in a difficult position in terms of maintaining a relationship, particularly if the partner was seronegative and she feared she would be left for a seronegative person. It also implied that partners should be tested, raising issues about how the woman got infected, particularly if the partner was found to be seronegative. In spite of coming from cultures that encourage large families, many seropositive women had single children. Some went on to have additional children over time, perhaps as they became better able to manage their infection. Women often found meaning in life in their role as mother, although the study suggested that a positive diagnosis affected not only her role in the relationship but also that of her seronegative partner, as well as the future expectations for seropositive or seronegative children. Women who were seropositive were concerned about abandonment, and could feel isolated and lonely if they were the only one infected. They might find it hard to cope with role of caregiver and parent if suffering from HIV without having a partner or family support. Inevitably, concerns about care for children when the mother is sick or has died leads to increased emotional stress.

In one of the few prospective studies of discordant couples, Van Dervanter and colleagues (1999) reported on 41 sexually active heterosexual couples who participated in a 10-week support group between 1992 and 1994. Analysis of the data revealed four areas of concern: (1) dealing with the emotional and sexual impact of HIV serodiscordance on relationships, (2) confronting reproductive decisions, (3) planning for the future of children and the surviving partner, and (4) disclosing HIV status to friends and family.

Among heterosexuals, coupling that occurred prior to the awareness of HIV brought to light past sexual behaviors or intravenous drug use as HIV appeared clinically in one or both of the partners. How much did one know about one's partner's past? How much did one know about the continued behaviors that put the negative partner at risk? These unexpected revelations, occurring in the context of one partner becoming sick, often created tremendous strains and fractures in the relationship. Even when couples managed to survive the initial diagnosis with the awareness that an imminent death might be likely, anger and betrayal were common reactions. When both partners were infected, questions of who infected whom sometimes led to vitriolic rage, and domestic violence was not uncommon. Others found illness to be a binding force, forgiving past discretions and making the virus a common enemy to be fought against. During the earlier phases of the epidemic, heterosexual couples struggled to manage the impact of a sudden, catastrophic illness on them, their children, and their families. Facing deterioration and death, couples were propelled into confronting the strengths and vulnerabilities of their relationship and renegotiating emotional, physical, and sexual intimacy. The specter of death and issues related to the surviving partner's needs presented great challenges to the normal development of couples, including questions of reproduction. Finding out that children born to the couple were infected as well presented yet another challenge to the couple.

Sometimes it was only after the death of one member of the couple that the surviving partner could begin dealing with either the implications of their own infection or, in the case of the uninfected partner, deal with the emotional consequences of loss and the meaning of the relationship. When children were involved, fears of leaving orphaned children behind brought families into the fray, exacerbating preexisting dynamics.

Among presumably monogamous heterosexual couples, suggesting the use of condoms in the context of an established relationship was tantamount to a statement of distrusting the fidelity of one's partner. The previous sexual history of one's partner, or sexual indiscretions that had previously been overlooked, brought new meaning of personal risk for infection into the relationship. Often this scenario created emotional and physical alienation, leading to difficulties with sexual intimacy and trust. Alternatively, some partners eschewed the use of condoms, putting themselves at high risk for acquiring HIV from their partner. Intense emotional bonding, guilt, anxiety about being alone upon the death of the partner, or a belief that getting infected would simply mean having to take medications are all rationalizations that have been explored in the clinical setting. Other partners, believing that antiretrovirals and "undetectable viral loads" reduce the actual risk of transmission (Castilla et al., 2005), make calculated choices to have unprotected intercourse to fulfill the emotional and physical needs for intimacy.

Alternatively, some studies have examined the use of condoms in committed relationships of mixed HIV status (Buchacz et al., 2001). Decreased condom use was associated with lower educational and socioeconomic level, recent unemployment, and being African American. Cultural factors continue to be important when adjusting for other factors. Current drug use and previous experience with high-risk behavior were also predictors of decreased condom use.

In a cross-sectional analysis of 104 serodiscordant heterosexual couples, over two-thirds of the couples' members reported having unprotected sex with their partner in the past 6 months. Most respondents stated that viral load testing and awareness of post-exposure prevention had no effect on condom use. Knowledge that their partner had an undetectable viral load was associated with greater use of condoms in the seronegative partner. Almost 33% of HIV-infected members and 40% of HIV-negative couple members admitted decreased concern about transmission, in the context of HIV treatments. Seronegative partners were more likely to report risk-taking sexual behaviors than their seropositive partners (van der Straten et al., 2000). Whether these behaviors or socioeconomic factors correlate with internal sense of agency to control one's health and well-being is less clear.

DISCORDANT COUPLE RELATIONSHIPS IN NON-WESTERN COUNTRIES

Cultural and religious issues around the world affect similar- and mixed-status couples in significant ways. Space prohibits an in-depth analysis here of each culture's and nation's concerns about HIV. The epidemiology of HIV in Western nations is similar, varying by degree of intravenous drug abuse, same sex risk, and heterosexual transmission. Western nations in which antiretroviral therapy is more accessible may have more extant programs for HIV testing and prevention efforts targeted to particular communities at risk.

In developed or developing non-Western nations, many issues affect couples in terms of HIV, such as public (governmental) policies about HIV testing, access to primary medical care and antiretrovirals, overt and covert sexual beliefs and practices, and gender roles and power dynamics within a particular culture and society. While homosexual behavior is extant throughout the world and every culture, same-sex couples occur most overtly in Western developed countries and covertly in most other nations, particularly those where sexuality is not discussed openly.

There is little in the literature about same-sex couples in most non-Western nations, where homosexuality is less well described or socially discussed. Among Asian cultures, for example, acceptance of homosexuality varies tremendously. Terminology is itself inconsistent: what defines homosexual behavior may be more certain than how men define their sexual orientation or sexual identity role. The way in which same-sex couples define themselves may also vary.

Cultural factors that affect homosexual men in Asia are inferred from studying the impact of HIV on Asian men living in Western countries, such as Canada, Australia, or the United States. One study of homosexual Asian men living in Australia used social psychological research methodology to analyze several aspects of culture that may be relevant to understanding same-sex behavior, coupling, and HIV risk among this population: "1) the impact of collectivistic cultural ideologies on self-conception and self esteem; 2) self-identity related to the status of Asians as numerical and status minorities; 3) the existence of stereotypes of Asians in the gay communities and their consequences on individual Asians; and 4) issues related to self-esteem of gay Asian men as determined by their identification with the Asian and/or gay communities and acculturation to the dominant Australian Anglo-Celtic culture" (Sanitioso, 1999).

A literature search for same-sex couples in African nations revealed almost nothing about same-sex coupling (much less serodiscordance). The heteronormative and "macho" culture of Lesotho, for example, is described as having reconciled in the early 1900s with the homosexual behavior of the Basotho men in the South African mines. In 1941, reports indicated that Basotho men were not only engaging in homosexual behavior but in public cross dressing and same-sex marriage ceremonies (Epprect, 2002).

According to UNAIDS, fewer than 5% of AIDS cases in Kenya result from male–male sex. Data on STDs suggest that truck drivers engage in homosexual activity with boys ages 12 to 16. Since homosexual activity is a criminal offense, data are difficult to come by, and the meaning of the behavior even more elusive to research. Most same-sex behavior is secretive, although along the Kenyan coast homosexuality is more accepted and there are "marriages" among men. The degree to which HIV infection occurs in serosimilar or dissimilar relationships is unknown (Africa Health, 1998).

Several studies have examined the factors influencing seroconcordance or discordance in African cultures, but focus on physiological parameters as indicators for HIV transmission, rather than the complex social, psychological, and developmental issues (Teunis, 1991; Freeman and Glynn, 2004; Malamba et al., 2005; Modjarrad et al., 2005). Most studies of discordant couples report that maintaining sexual intimacy is one of the greatest struggles and is manifested by ambivalence about consistent condom use, conflicts about extramarital sexual relationships, and mythology about the way in which HIV is transmitted (Bunnell et al., 2005).

A study in Haiti (Deschamps et al., 1996) showed that provision of condoms increased safer sex practices to 45% of discordant heterosexual couples, meaning that 55% remained inconsistent users of condoms. Studies vary widely in terms of condom use in varying cultures; few of them offer psychological explanations for the motivation behind the decisions that discordant couples make in using safer sex strategies, abstaining from sex, or dissolving the couple as a means of avoiding infection to the negative partner (Mehendale et al., 2006). Many studies were conducted before the widespread use of antiretrovirals, when the usual outcome of a discordant couple was that the HIV-positive member became sick and died. How couples manage that probability individually and as a couple must be factored into a dynamic understanding of how discordant couples make decisions about staying together, sexual intimacy, using condoms, and facing the inevitable course of illness. Clinically, ambivalence, denial, and reaction formation are not uncommon defenses used in coping with the discordant status. What is not clear from the research is whether the greater availability of antiretroviral medications has significantly influenced the complex psychological coping mechanisms used by discordant couples.

While these factors may help elucidate the complex impact of cultural values, interpersonal customs, and mores, they do not provide a psychodynamic understanding of how same-sex oriented men or couples manage, understand, and negotiate ongoing "couple" relationships. Understanding of serodiscordance in male couples around the world continues to rely on case studies, clinical experience, and ethnographic narratives.

Since heterosexual transmission of HIV accounts for 90% of HIV infections worldwide, the medical and social science literature continues to expand in addressing this significant issue. Most of the extant studies review how couples engage in acquiring knowledge about HIV, proceed with HIV testing to assess risk and infection, partner notification, and the impact of serostatus on sexual decision making, condom use, and risk-taking behaviors in the context of dissimilar status. Studies also explore the impact of HIV on partnership stability, sexual intimacy, fears of stigmatization by families and society, and on the welfare of children who are born HIV infected (Tangmunkongvorakul et al., 1999; Porter et al., 2004; Brunnell et al., 2005; Mehendale et al., 2006).

In each cultural setting, the role of marriage and the expected obligations of men and women affect how prevention and treatment proceeds. In all countries, HIV has forced a confrontation with traditional roles that men and women play in relationships. Many experience role reversals and changes in autonomy and dependency within the relationship as illness occurs. Economic constraints often contribute to the changing stability of relationships.

REPRODUCTIVE ISSUES

Reproductive issues arise among concordant and discordant couples throughout the world. In 2003 an estimated 700,000 children were newly infected with HIV, with 90% of these infections occurring in sub-Saharan Africa. More than 90% of them were born to HIV-infected mothers, acquiring the infection before or during birth or through breastfeeding (UNAIDS, 2003). In resource-rich nations, mother-to-infant transmission has been significantly reduced by voluntary testing and counseling, access to antiretroviral therapy, safe delivery practices including caesarean delivery when appropriate, and the availability of breast milk substitutes (De Cock et al., 2000; Cooper et al., 2002; UNAIDS, 2006). Overall, rates of mother-to-infant transmission have been reduced from 30% to 45% with breastfeeding and no antiretroviral therapy, 25% to 30% with no breast feeding and no therapy, and to less than 2% where antiretroviral therapy and breast milk substitutes are available (Brocklehurst and Volmink, 2002; Tuomala et al., 2002; CDC, 2006; Gilling-Smith et al., 2006).

In developed nations, as HIV-infected people live longer, discordant couples may stabilize and inquire about the prospect of conceiving a child. For many couples, as the crises of acute illness gives way to a sense of chronic illness, the desire to have children may emerge. Underlying reasons include wanting to fulfill a sense of role as mother or father, leaving a child as legacy, or believing that with the current state of treatment the child will likely be born uninfected.

When the man is HIV negative, alternative methods of insemination rather than unprotected intercourse are safer for facilitating conception. However, serodiscordant couples who intend to become pregnant do not always use protection. While studies have reported rates of unprotected intercourse among serodiscordant couples (Remien et al., 2005), the underlying motivations and meaning of the sexual behavior in that context have not been well studied.

When the male partner is HIV positive, two options have been described. The safest is sperm washing, which involves centrifuging the sperm from the seminal fluid and associated non-sperm cells. Follow-up tests for viral RNA and proviral DNA further reduce the risk of infected sperm from being introduced into the HIV-negative female partner (Gilling-Smith et al., 2006). Counseling must include awareness that sperm washing is a risk-reducing but not risk-free enterprise.

Alternatively, couples in which the male is positive may limit their unprotected intercourse to the fertile window, although in one study (Mandelbrot et al.,

1997) 4% of the women seroconverted with this technique. Studies have estimated the HIV-negative female partner has a 0.1%–0.5% risk of acquiring HIV per act of unprotected intercourse, assuming a stable and monogamous relationship with no intravenous drug use and no other high-risk sexual behaviors (De Vincenzi, 1994; Gray et al., 2003). Viral load in semen correlates poorly with serum viral load, and men with undetectable viral loads may still transmit HIV in semen (Zhang et al., 1998).

Although not explored in depth here, there is a growing literature about the medical and psychological aspects of reproductive technologies that are changing the way we think about pregnancy and parenting among HIV-affected couples (VanDevanter et al., 1998; Gilling-Smith, 2000; Panozzo et al., 2003; Gilling-Smith et al., 2006). The possibility of creating a family may enhance the capacity and motivation to adhere to antiretroviral regimens. Adherence to antiretrovirals over a lifetime of infection, however, may be imbued with significant and changing meaning as different stresses and developmental issues arise. Adherence, like safer sex, is best understood as a complex matrix of conscious and unconscious forces filtered through the reality of the changing landscape of HIV disease and societal stigma.

PSYCHOLOGICAL ISSUES

Since the beginning of the epidemic, volumes have been written about the psychological issues engendered by the AIDS virus. As mentioned above, it is impossible to consider HIV as just another epidemic or medical illness, given its social, political, and economic implications. But as with any social problem, illness, or catastrophic event, ultimately it is the core issues of human attachment and loss that inform our understanding of how to cope with and make meaning out of any threat to existence. Psychological development and emotional health or illness, while significantly mediated in the case of HIV by medical and psychiatric disorders, is dependent on balancing the need for connection to others and the capacity to defend against the inevitability of mortality. Sexuality and identity are fundamental aspects of those parts of the self that work to maintain psychological and physiological homeostasis. Because humanity depends on procreation for its continuation, sexual behavior is hard wired into our basic drives. Unlike other species, however, humans do not have estrous cycles, and thus have to manage the complex meanings of sexuality throughout the entire life cycle. Culture and religion have been powerful mediators of sexuality and gender identity, but ultimately, each individual and his or her partner have to figure out the particular dance of intimacy.

For some heterosexual and homosexual couples, the risk of getting infected may increase the intensity of the sexual experience, and a subculture of "barebacking" (intercourse without protection) has evolved, along with a variety of conscious and unconscious substrates. These may include fear of abandonment, existential anxiety about death, feelings of failure, and unacceptable rage leading to reaction formation. The capacity to verbalize the desire to use condoms in an intimate relationship may represent a variety of motivations and deeply held beliefs, and may be experienced differently by the HIV-negative and HIV-positive partners. The HIV-negative partner who actively encourages protection may feel as though he or she is acknowledging a fact of life that separates the couple at the most intimate level: one partner will survive, one may not. It is an assertion of the desire to live while someone they love faces the alternative possibility. This may be experienced as a form of conscious abandoning. To do so requires a capacity for self-protection as a higher priority than commitment to another. Does one rush to the edge of the cliff if one doesn't have to? The HIV-positive person who insists on using protection must also be acknowledging at some level the need to differentiate from the other partner, and may feel an obligation to protect them. Whether this can be consciously acknowledged or manifests as a decrease in sexual interest or provoking conflict with the partner may depend on how self-aware and psychologically minded the individuals are. Only in the exploration of the meaning of the behaviors in the therapeutic setting can issues of motivation and unconscious fears and anxieties be understood on an individual basis (Forstein, 2002).

With the advent of multidrug therapy, and consequently the transformation of a lethal disease into a potentially chronic illness, couples whose physical quality of life improves can begin to incorporate strategies into their daily lives that allow some sense of a future together. However, stresses that existed prior to illness might again emerge. HIV-negative partners who have stayed in the relationship out of guilt from leaving an ill partner, or positive partners who no

longer believe that they will not be better off alone have to face the greater sense of uncertainty that antiretroviral treatment now brings to the natural course of HIV infection.

Couples may also have to deal with the loss of others who are HIV infected. It is not uncommon for discordant couples to have other HIV-positive people in their social network. Discovering that a friend or acquaintance progressed to death while on the same combination of medications may engender a sense of capriciousness and inequity that undermines the sense of stability in those who survive. Dealing with the progression of disease or death of others can precipitate crises in the discordant couple. Grief and bereavement, extant or anticipated, have emotional implications for couples trying to see the future with hope.

CLINICAL ASSESSMENT

Working with HIV-concordant or HIV-discordant couples requires a comprehensive biopsychosocial approach. The best principles of psychological assessment, psychiatric diagnosis, and therapeutic strategies for individuals, couples, and families are necessary. Assessment should include, for each member of the couple, a review of the complete medical and psychiatric history as well as psychological structures and defenses, and an appreciation of cultural and individual beliefs and expectations about what the illness means and what the future is likely to bring. Understanding the cultural expectations for couples and the meaning of the illness is also essential. The following questions may be useful in the assessment of couples affected by HIV. The assessment should include questions about not only the context and facts but also the meaning of the behavior, anxieties, fears, and the coping mechanisms involved.

1. What are the initial issues that have brought the couple for treatment? (Couples may present with non-HIV-related issues; it is important to explore those issues and at the same time inquire about the impact of their HIV discordance on the relationship.)
2. Is the major focus of the couple's decision to come for therapy to stay together or find ways of separating? Is the goal the same for both members of the relationship?

3. When historically (given the above phases of the HIV epidemic) did the couple become a couple? What is the customary nature of unions within the cultural background of each member? What is the relationship history of each person? Had either one been in a relationship prior to this one with someone HIV negative or positive?

4. What did each member of the couple know at that time about their own and the other's serologic status? What assumptions were made? What factors contributed to a realistic or unrealistic set of assumptions?

5. What is the current medical status of the HIV-positive person? What is the viral load, CD4 count, level of health? Does the HIV-negative person have any medical problems?

6. Is there a history of mental illness or current psychiatric disorder for which either member is being treated? Is there a history of substance use? Is there present use? Do both members of the couple agree on the impact of the substances on the relationship?

7. If there has been a major episode of illness, how has the individual and the couple coped?

8. What does each member of the couple know about the other's sexual and/or intravenous drug use history?

9. How does each person understand his or her own risk for HIV?

10. To whom else has the HIV-positive person disclosed their status? What was the response? If there are children, what is their status, and what is their knowledge of the parent's HIV status?

11. What are the nature and level of support in the couple's social and familial network? Are there resources that can be called upon to help with economic burdens, child care, or respite care when needed?

12. How has the HIV-positive person's illness changed expectations about role identity in the relationship? What specific changes have occurred and how has each member of the couple managed to deal with those changes?

13. How does the stage of illness in the HIV-infected partner affect their beliefs about what is happening? Is the assessment by the couple about the medical status realistic?

14. What is the nature of how each person feels about the other's status? Is there guilt? Shame? Envy?

15. How has each member of the couple managed other non-HIV-related experiences that have challenged the integrity of the self and its relationship to others? What are the individual coping strengths and how does the couple use the strengths of each to support the stability of the relationship?

Developing a trusting, nonjudgmental relationship with providers allows the couple to reflect on a dynamic individual and relationship process that is often unpredictable for providers and patients alike.

THERAPEUTIC ISSUES

Mental health clinicians have been involved in treating HIV-positive persons and their partners and families since the beginning of the epidemic. Understanding the changes in the social meaning of the epidemic, the availability of treatments, and the cultural response to illness has made clinical work conceptually and emotionally challenging.

Clinical work with HIV-discordant couples may elicit strong countertransference feelings in the therapist. People who are both HIV infected or negative do not always act in a way that an outside observer would deem "rational"—e.g., wanting to avoid condoms to preserve intimacy, or avoiding confronting a partner who is suspected of having sex outside the relationship. But most issues that individuals or couples face in therapy that induce stress or distress are not rational. Indeed, rational thinking often gives way to more deeply seated anxieties or to beliefs that are overdetermined by history, personality, and unconscious substrates. For example, almost all couples know cognitively how to protect the uninfected partner, yet they find it difficult over the long term to maintain safer sex behaviors. Ambivalence may be seen as a component of a psychological, emotionally homeostatic mechanism in a complex and often confusing context of a life-threatening disease over time.

Therapists often experience frustration and anxiety when witnessing the continued risk associated with discordant couples. Power differentials and cultural norms of gender role and autonomy that differ from the therapist's experience and beliefs may elicit countertransference that can affect how each member of the couple participates in the therapy. Managing the conflicting feelings of guilt and entitlement on the part of the HIV-positive person to remain intimate with the HIV-negative partner and the failure of the couple to make the choices that might be considered "rational" can challenge even experienced therapists.

Powerful emotional reactions may occur when HIV-affected couples begin talking about wanting to have a child. Therapists can find themselves quite stirred by the worry about bringing a baby into the world. Although the risk of having an infected child is significantly reduced by the new medical technologies mentioned above, therapists often think about the impact of HIV illness over time on the child's development. More difficult is how to raise and work through the issues of what the impact of pregnancy may mean for the HIV-infected partner, given the enormous energy and focus that a baby would bring into the family. With limited coping resources, some couples find the burden of parenting overwhelming when there is a significant medical illness. Although parents with other non-HIV progressive illnesses often conceive and parent, HIV may elicit a deeper unconscious hesitation on the part of the therapist to support the HIV-discordant couple in having a child. The impact of the possible death of the HIV-infected parent on the child often emerges, and therapists may experience hostile, resentful feelings toward the couple, sometimes manifesting an unconscious belief about the behavior that led to the HIV infection in the first place.

For some women, even the prospect of giving birth to an HIV-infected baby may not impede the decision to go forward with pregnancy. I have provided care for more than one HIV-infected pregnant woman who has explained that although she realizes that the child might be born infected and not have a long life, the child would have a soul, thus fulfilling the meaning and purpose of the mother's own existence. Therapists may find themselves having to examine their own religious, spiritual, and existential beliefs, as well as their countertransferential feelings in such situations. Therapists are faced with many reactions with sero-discordant couples, but little research has been done in this area. Supervision may be very helpful in facing the ambivalence and beliefs that emerge.

Clinically, discordant couples come for therapy for many concerns. In my experience, it is never easy to predict which issues will emerge or which couples will learn how to cope better and which will split apart with the stress of dealing with HIV. Since both the infected and noninfected members of the couple are at risk for premorbid or comorbid psychiatric disorders, a thorough evaluation of the individuals as well as of the couple is important. Couples are often dealing with unresolved issues that existed before the couple met or arose because of the discordant status. They are also dealing with issues that all couples face under the stress of a chronic and potentially life-threatening illness.

Deeply entrenched behaviors, beliefs, and maladaptive coping mechanisms may not respond to a cognitive behavioral approach alone. There is almost no research in the literature that provides long-term intervention outcome data on any particular methodology since the advent of antiretroviral treatment that can guide the therapeutic process. We are in the middle of a unique sociological experiment with a world pandemic that is changing rapidly. As medical technologies develop to help contain HIV as a chronic illness, many questions remain, such as long-term outcomes of decades of antiretroviral therapy, the emergence of new strains of virus, and the changing social structures that result from and affect how societies deal with sexually transmitted diseases.

As the second decade of antiretroviral therapy continues in the developed nations, a growing concern is the possibility of increasing risks for mild and moderate cognitive disorders that emerge even in the context of fully suppressed peripheral viral replication. Still unclear is the long-term implication of less than adequate penetration into the central nervous system of currently available anti-HIV medications (Sacktor et al., 2002; Letendre et al., 2004).

Experience suggests that medical advances alone will not ameliorate all of the uncertainty about how individuals and couples live with a disease so fraught with meaning that derives from the core issues we face as humans. In my experience, the process of working with discordant couples may be ongoing, with stages of illness, normative life stage developmental issues, and individual internal conflicts often emerging as different aspects of the relationship bring into focus sources of ambivalence and interpersonal conflicts.

As more HIV-infected people get access to anti-retrovirals, those who are able to respond and maintain adherence to the medications are identifying more with a chronic rather than lethal illness. Many are searching to find ways to move forward in changing careers, having children, and reentering the social world. Application of therapeutic strategies that incorporate the specific issues relevant to the meaning of discordance to couples of any sexual orientation requires assessment of the complex factors and underlying strengths and vulnerabilities that confront discordant couples trying to remain alive and connected in the face of a terrible illness. Over time, couples may find that issues of intimacy, fears of transmission, adherence, and the many emotional aspects of coping with an unpredictable chronic disease will fluctuate in the normal course of development. Health care providers should maintain a dynamic view of the medical and mental health concerns of individuals and of the couple over time.

In spite of growing technologies and rapid advances in our understanding of the pathophysiology of the virus, the HIV pandemic rages out of control. Each new generation confronts the dilemmas and joys of emerging sexuality and the pursuit of pleasure. Humans strive for intimacy in complex individual and social contexts that have been brought into focus by the HIV pandemic. Increasingly, in terms of prevention and treatment, we are asked to think rationally about the most irrational aspects of the human condition.

References

Africa Health (1998). HIV and Kenya's homosexuals. *Africa Health* 20(6):48.

Auerbach SM (1989). Stress management and coping research in the health care setting: an overview and methodological commentary. *J Consult Clin Psychol* 57:388–395.

Bell JE (2004). An update on the neuropathology of HIV in the HAART era. *Histopathology* 45(6):549–559.

Britten PJ, Zarski JJ, and Hobfoll SE (1993). Psychological distress and the role of significant others in a population of gay/bisexual men in the era of HIV. *AIDS Care*, 5(1):43–54.

Brocklehurst P, and Volmink J (2002). Antiretrovirals for reducing the risk of mother-to-child transmission of HIV infection. *Cochrane Database Syst Rev* 2: CD003510.

Buchacz, van der Straten A, Saul J, Shiboski SC, Gomez CA, and Padian N (2001). Sociodemographic, behavioral, and clinical correlates of inconsistent condom use in HIV-serodiscordant heterosexual couples. J Acquir *Immune Defic Syndr* 28(3):289–297.

Bunnell RE, Nassozi J, Marum E, Mubangizi J, Malamba S, Dillon B, et al. (2005). Living with discordance: knowledge, challenges, and prevention strategies of HIV discordant couples in Uganda. *AIDS Care* 17(8):999–1012.

Carpenter CC, Fischl MA, Hammer SM, Hirsch MS, Jacobsen DM, Katzenstein DA, et al. (1997). Antiretroviral therapy for HIV infection. *JAMA* 277:1962–1969.

Castilla J, Del Romero J, Hernando V, Marincovich B, García S, and Rodríguez C (2005). Effectiveness of highly active antiretroviral therapy in reducing heterosexual transmission of HIV. *J Acquir Immune Defic Syndr* 40(1):96–101.

Catalan J, Klimes I, Bond A, Day A, Garrod A, and Rizza C (1992). The psychosocial impact of HIV infection in men with haemophilia: controlled investigation and factors associated with psychiatric morbidity. *J Psychosom Res.* 36(5):409–416.

[CDC] Centers for Disease Control and Prevention (2006). Achievements in public health. Reductions in perinatal transmission of HIV infection—United States 1985–2005. *MMWR Morb Mortal Wkly Rep* 55(21):592–597.

Chesney M, and Folkman S. (1994). Psychological impact of HIV disease and implications for intervention. *Psychiatr Manifestations HIV Dis* 17(1): 163–182.

Cohen F, and Lazarus RS (1979). Coping with the stresses of illness. In GC Stone, F Cohen, and NE Adler (eds.), *Health Psychology* (pp. 217–254). San Francisco: Josey Bass.

Cooper ER, Charurat M, Mofenson, L, Hanson, IC, Pitt, J, Diaz, C, et al. (2002). Combination antiretroviral strategies for the treatment of pregnant HIV-1-infected women and prevention of perinatal HIV-1 transmission. *J Acquir Immune Defic Syndr* 29(5):484–494.

Coyne JC, and Fiske V (1992). Couples coping with chronic and catastrophic illness. In TJ Akamatsu, MAP Stephens, SE Hobfoll, and J Crowther (eds.), *Family Health Psychology* (pp. 129–149). Washington, DC: Hemisphere.

De Cock KM, Fowler MG, Mercier E, de Vincenzi I, Saba J, Hoff E, et al. (2000). Prevention of mother-to-child HIV transmission in resource-poor countries: translating research into policy and practice. *JAMA* 283(9):1175–1182.

Deschamps MM, Pape JW, Hafner A, and Johnson WD Jr (1996). Heterosexual transmission of HIV in Haiti. *Ann Intern Med* 125(4):324–330.

de Vincenzi I (1994). A longitudinal study of human immunodeficiency virus transmission by heterosexual partners. *N Engl J Med* 331:341–346.

Epprecht M (2002). Male-male sexuality in Lesotho: two conversations. *J Men's Studies* 10(3):373–389.

Folkman S, Chesney M, Pollack I, and Coates T (1993). Stress, control, coping and depressive mood in human immunodeficiency virus positive and negative gay men in San Francisco. *J Nerv Ment Dis* 181: 409–416.

Forstein M (1994). Psychotherapy with gay male couples: loving in the time of AIDS. In: S Cadwell, R Burnham, and M Forstein (eds.), *Therapists on The Front Line: Challenges in Psychotherapy with Gay Men in the Age of AIDS* (pp. 293–315). Washington, DC: American Psychiatric Press.

Forstein M (2002). Commentary on Cheuvront's "High risk sexual behavior in the treatment of HIV-negative patients." *J Gay Lesbian Psychother* 6(3):35–43.

Freeman EE, and Glynn JR, for the Study Group on Heterogeneity of HIV Epidemics in African Cities (2004). Factors affecting HIV concordancy in married couples in four African cities. *AIDS* 18(12): 1715–1721.

Gilling-Smith C (2000). HIV prevention. Assisted reproduction in HIV-discordant couples. *AIDS Read* 10(10):581–587.

Gilling Smith C, Nicopoullos JD, Semprimi AE, and Frodsham LC (2006). HIV and reproductive care—a review of current practice. *BJOG* 113(8): 869–878.

Gluhoski VL, Fishman B, and Perry SW (1997). The Impact of multiple bereavement in a gay male sample. *AIDS Educ Prev* 9(6):521–531.

Gray RH, Wawer MJ, Brookmeyer R, Sewankambo NK, Serwadda D, Wabwire-Mangen F, et al. (2001). Probability of HIV-1 transmission per coital act in monogamous, heterosexual, HIV-1-discordant couples in Rakai, Uganda. *Lancet* 357(9263):1149–1153.

Keegan A, Lambert S, and Petrak J (2005). Sex and relationships for HIV-positive women since HAART: a qualitative study. *AIDS Patient Care STDS* 19(10):645–654.

Lazarus RS, and Folkman S. (1984). *Stress, Appraisal, and Coping.* New York: Springer.

Letendre SL, McCutchan JA, Childers ME, Woods SP, Lazzaretto D, Heaton RK, et al. (2004). Enhancing antiretroviral therapy for human immunodeficiency virus cognitive disorders. *Ann Neurol* 56(3):416–423.

Lippmann SB, James WA, and Frierson RL (1993). AIDS and the family: implications for counseling. *AIDS Care* 5:71–78.

Malamba SS, Mermin JH, Bunnell R, Mubangizi J, Kalule J, Marum E, Hu DJ, Wangalwa S, Smith D, and Downing R (2005). Couples at risk: HIV-1 concordance and discordance among sexual partners receiving voluntary counseling and testing in Uganda. *J Acquir Immune Defic Syndr* 39(5):576–580.

Mandel JS (1986). Psychosocial challenges of AIDS and ARC: clinical and research observations. In L McKusick (ed.), *What to Do about AIDS: Physicians and Mental Health Professionals Discuss the Issues* (pp. 75–86). Berkeley: University of California Press.

Mandelbrot L, Heard I, Henrion-Geant R, and Henrion R (1997). Natural conception in HIV negative women with HIV infected partners. *Lancet* 349: 850–851.

McShane RE, Bumbalo JA, and Patsdaughter CA (1994). Psychological distress in family members living with human immunodeficiency virus/acquired immune deficiency syndrome. *Arch Psychiatr Nurs* 8(3):209.

Mehendale SM, Ghate MV, Kishore Kumar B, Shay S, Gamble TR, Godbole SV, Thakar MR, Kulkarni SS, Gupta A, Gangakhedkar RR, Divekar AD, Risbud AR, Paranjape RS, and Bollinger RC (2006). Low HIV-1 incidence among married serodiscordant couples in Pune, India. *J Acquir Immune Def Syndr* 41(3):371–373.

Meyerowitz BE, Heinrich RL, and Schag CA (1983). Competency-based approach to coping with cancer. In TG Burish and LA Bradley (eds.), *Coping with Chronic Disease: Research and Applications* (pp. 137–158). San Diego: Academic Press.

Modjarrad K, Zulu I, Karita E. Kancheya N, Funhouser E, and Allen S (2005). Predictors of HIV serostatus among discordant couples in Lusaka, Zambia and female antenatal clinic attendants in Kigali, Rwanda. *AIDS Res Hum Retroviruses* 21(1):5–12.

Moore J, Harrison JS, Vandevanter N, Kennedy C, Padian N, Abrams J, Lesondar IM, and O'Brien T (1998). Factors influencing relationship quality of HIV serodiscordant heterosexual couples. In VJ Derlega and AP Barbee (eds.), *HIV and Social Interaction.* Thousand Oaks, CA: Sage Press.

Moore LD (1993). The Social Context of Sexual Risk Taking and HIV Prevention in a Cohort of Heterosexuals: A Qualitative Investigation. Doctoral Dissertation, University of California at Berkeley.

Namir S, Alumbaugh MJ, Fawzy IF, and Wolcott DL (1989). The relationship of social support to physical and psychological aspects of AIDS. *Psychol Health* 3:77–86.

Ostrow DG, Monjan A, Joseph J, VanRaden M, Fox R, Kingsley L, Dudley J, and Phair J (1989). HIV-related symptoms and psychological functioning in a cohort of homosexual men. *Am J Psychiatry* 146: 737–741.

Pakenham KI, Dadds MR, and Terry DJ (1994). Relationships between adjustment to HIV and both social support and coping. *J Consult Clin Psychol* 62(6):1194–1203.

Panozzo L, Battegay M, Friedl A, Vernazza PL (2003). Swiss Cohort Study: high risk behavior and fertility desires among heterosexual HIV positive patients with a serodiscordant partner—two challenging issues. *Swiss Med Wkly* 133(7–8):124–127.

Parsons TD, Braaten AJ, Hall CD, and Robertson KR (2006). Better quality of life with neuropsychological improvement on HAART. *Health Qual Life Outcomes* 4:11.

Peterson JL, Folkman S, and Bakeman R (1996). Stress, coping, HIV status, psychosocial resources, and depressive mood in African American gay, bisexual, and heterosexual men. *Am J Commun Psychol* 24: 461–487.

Porter L, Hao L, Bishai D, Serwadda D, Wawer M, Lutalo T, and Gray R (2004). HIV status and union dissolution in Sub Saharan Africa: the case of Rakai, Uganda. *Demography* 41(3):465–482.

Rabkin JG, Williams JBW, Remien RH, Goetz R, Kertzner R, and Gorman JM (1991). Depression, distress, lymphocyte subsets, and human immunodeficiency virus symptoms on two occasions in HIV-positive homosexual men. *Arch Gen Psychiatry* 48:111–119.

Rabkin JG, Goetz RR, Remien RH, Williams JBW, Todak G, and Gorman JM (1997). Stability of mood despite HIV illness progression in a group of homosexual men. *Am J Psychiatry* 154(2):231–238.

Remien RH, Carballo-Dieguez A, and Wagner G (1995). Intimacy and sexual risk behaviour in serodiscordant male couples. *AIDS Care* 4:429–438.

Remien RH, Wagner G, Colezal C, and Carballo-Dieguez A (2003). Levels and correlates of psychological distress in male couples of mixed HIV status. *AIDS Care* 15(4):525–538.

Remien RH, Stirratta MS, Dolezala C, Dogninb JS, Wagner GJ, Carballo-Dieguez A, El-Basselc N, and Jung TM (2005). Couple-focused support to improve HIV medication adherence: a randomized controlled trial. *AIDS* 19:807–814.

Sacktor N, McDermott MP, Marder K, Schifitto G, Selnes OA, McArthur JC, Stern Y, Albert S, Palumbo D, Kieburtz K, De Marcaida JA, Cohen B, and Epstein L (2002). HIV-associated cognitive impairment before and after the advent of combination therapy. *J Neurovirol* 8(2):136–142.

Sanitioso R (1999). A social psychological perspective on HIV/AIDS and gay or homosexually active Asian men. *J Homosex* 36(3–4):69–85.

Stoff DM (2004). HIV/AIDS and aging. *AIDS* 18(1):S3–S10.

Tangmunkongvoralakul A, Celentano DD, Burke JG, DeBoer MA, Wongpan P, and Suriyanon V (1999). Factors influencing marital stability among HIV discordant couples in northern Thailand. *AIDS Care* 11(5):511–524.

Teunis N (2001). Same-sex sexuality in Africa: a case study from Senegal. *AIDS Behav* 5(2):173–178.

Tuomala RE, Shapiro DE, Mofenson LM, et al. (2002). Antiretroviral therapy during pregnancy and the risk of an adverse outcome. *N Engl J Med* 346:1863–1870.

UNAIDS (2003). *2003 AIDS Epidemic Update*, December 2003. Geneva: Joint United Nations Programme on HIV/AIDS.

UNAIDS (2006). http://www.unaids.org/en/HIV_data/epi2006/default.asp.

Van Devanter N, Cleary P, Moore J, Stuart Thacker A, and O'Brien T (1998). Reproductive behaviors among discordant heterosexual couples: implications for counseling. *AIDS Patient Care STDS* 12:43–49.

Van Devanter N, Thacker AS, Bass G, and Arnold M (1999). Heterosexual couples confronting the challenges of HIV infection. *AIDS Care* 11(2):181–193.

van der Straten A, Vernon KA, Knight KR, Gomez CA, and Padian NS (1998). Managing HIV among serodiscordant heterosexual couples: serostatus, stigma and sex. *AIDS Care* 10(5):533–549.

van der Straten A, Gomez CA, Saul J, Quan J, and Padian N (2000). Sexual risk behaviors among heterosexual HIV serodiscordant couples in the era of post-exposure prevention and viral suppressive therapy. *AIDS* 14(4):F47–F54.

White J, Melvin D, Moore C, and Crowley S (1997). Parental HIV discordancy and its impact on the family. AIDS Care 9(5):609–615.

Zhang H, Domadula G, Beumint M, Livornese L Jr, Van Uitert B, Henning K, et al. (1998). Human immunodeficiency virus type 1 in the semen of men receiving highly active antiretroviral therapy. *N Engl J Med* 339:1803–1809.

Zich J, and Temoshok L (1987). Perceptions of social support in patients with ARC and AIDS. *J Appl Soc Psychol* 17:193–215.

Chapter 26

Older Age and HIV Infection

Karl Goodkin and David Stoff

A widely held misconception about older age and HIV infection is based on the definition of terms— that is, "older" is not equivalent to the term "elderly" (≥65 years of age). In the domain of HIV/AIDS, 50 years of age has been the designated cutoff for "older age" originally promulgated by the Centers for Disease Control and Prevention (CDC) and most frequently cited in the literature. Predominantly, HIV-infected persons fall into the 50- to 59-year-old age range, with fewer cases in the 60- to 65-year-old range and very few in the over-65 age range. Hence, it is the latter part of middle age that is intended by the term "older age," and use of the term "elderly" remains premature in the setting of HIV infection. Yet, over the coming decade there will likely be increasing numbers of HIV-infected persons older than 65 and there will be a need to extend the research discussed here to determine generalizability to that age range.

In this chapter, we will review the extant literature on older HIV-infected individuals in terms of epidemiology, primary and secondary prevention techniques, systemic disease progression, immunological disease progression, neurocognitive manifestations (including HIV-associated dementia, HIV-associated minor-cognitive motor disorder, and subclinical neuropsychological impairment), and HIV-related and -unrelated comorbidities. We will also address issues facing those affected by HIV through their relationship with an older HIV-infected individual. This chapter updates and expands on an earlier review on the topic (Stoff, 2004).

OLDER AGE AND THE EPIDEMIOLOGY OF HIV INFECTION

Earlier in the epidemic, older age and HIV infection were thought to be non-overlapping issues. By the late 1990s, the cumulative prevalence of all persons with AIDS in the United States who were 50 years of age or older was 10%. Between 1991 and 2001, newly reported AIDS cases among older persons increased by 22%.

While an increased incidence of AIDS among older adults had occurred, AIDS incidence among younger persons had declined. Meanwhile, the "true elderly" accounted for a total of only about 2% of AIDS cases in the United States, despite the fact that there had been an increase of 13% for those over 65 during the same time period (CDC, 2004). Since the late 1990s, the number of persons living with AIDS in the United States in the 50 and older age range increased from 59,649 in 2000 to 112,147 in 2004 (up to nearly 17% for that year). This represents a change of nearly twofold over those 4 years—with approximately equal increases throughout the age range (CDC, 2005). The CDC currently predicts that by 2015, 50% of all cases of HIV/AIDS in the United States will be in persons ≥50 years of age. There are two subpopulations contributing to the rapid increase in HIV prevalence among this age group: (1) those surviving into older age because of the efficacy of highly active antiretroviral combination therapy (HAART) in reducing mortality, and (2) those newly infected by HIV in older age. Yet, very little is currently known about these specific subpopulations in the United States. Moreover, epidemiological information on the entire population of those with AIDS who are at least 50 years old is largely confined to resource-rich countries.

Regarding particular regions within the United States, the cumulative number of AIDS patients 50 years of age or older increases, consecutively, from the national level (12%), to the state of Florida (15%), to Miami-Dade County (where the cumulative percentage is now 16.4%, with 5.1% over 60) (Miami-Dade County Health Department, 2006). Florida has been ranked third nationally in total number of AIDS cases since early in the epidemic. Of the patients with AIDS over 50 years of age in Florida, 65% reside in three counties—Miami-Dade (34%), Broward (20%), and Palm Beach (11%). Thus, the Miami-Dade County area represents an epidemiological area of special concentration.

Another area of concentration of HIV infection among older persons is the state of Hawaii, where the overall per-capita AIDS prevalence is 22nd among the 50 states. Yet, for the subpopulation of older persons, the percentage of those age 50 and over with AIDS doubled there from the 1983–1999 time period to 2005 (increasing from 12% to 24%) (Hawaii State Department of Health, 2006). The large majority of AIDS cases (72%) have been diagnosed in Honolulu County,

followed by Hawaii County (13%), Maui County (10%), and Kauai County (4%).

This epidemiological change may relate to the composition of the population of older HIV-infected persons. One of the factors linking the Miami and Honolulu areas is that older persons tend to migrate to these areas after retirement, contributing to a type of "sun belt" migration. This effect might well include both older HIV-infected persons as well as older persons at risk to contract HIV infection. With regard to the latter, the advent of the cGMP-specific phosphodiesterase type 5 (PDE5) inhibitors (sildenafil [Viagra], tadalafil [Cialis], and vardenafil [Levitra]) and the relative lack of knowledge of safer sex techniques in the older population could account for a specific increase in the newly infected older subpopulation. However, the risk factor distribution in Honolulu continues to be predominated by men who have sex with men (MSM) (65% of AIDS cases in Hawaii over the years 2001–2005), with heterosexual risk at only 7%, whereas in Miami heterosexual risk predominated (34%) over MSM as a risk factor (25%) in the years 2003–2005. Hence, there are epidemiological differences between these groups that should be further explored, specifically among those 50 years of age or older.

Much less information is available about aging and HIV infection internationally. In Western Europe, nearly 10% of new infections declared between January 1997 and mid-June 2000 were among the group age 50 or older. Specifically, in Italy, similar increases in HIV infection among older persons have been reported, with the mean age at diagnosis increasing from 26 in 1985 to 38 in 2002 (Manfredi, 2004). The Western European prevalence of HIV infection in older age is similar to that in the United States and compares to only 4.3% in Central Europe and 0.7% in Eastern Europe. More international studies of HIV infection in older age are needed, particularly in resource-limited countries.

OLDER AGE AND PRIMARY AND SECONDARY HIV DISEASE PREVENTION

The distribution of risk factors for HIV infection has changed considerably since the early stages of the epidemic. Ten years ago, the distribution of HIV risk factors among those 50 years of age or older reflected the HIV risk factor distribution in the general population in the very beginning of the epidemic, as if the "clock had been turned back" in this age range. At that point in the epidemic in the United States, a significant percentage of HIV-seropositive older persons were transfusion recipients—15% of those 50 or older and 64% of those 70 or older (Ship et al., 1991). This risk factor was later reduced to a very low level following the institution of routine HIV antibody test screening of the nation's blood banks that had begun in March of 1985 and was subsequently further reduced by autologous donor procedures, minimization of blood loss during surgery, and development of additional alternatives to transfusion. As was true for transfusion recipients, among those 50 or older, there was also a large number of MSM cases earlier in the epidemic. At the present time, there has been a considerable decrease in HIV-positive MSM in this age group and a proportionate decrease of injection substance users, whereas heterosexual contact has increased as a source of infection in the older age range, consistent with the demographic shift in more recent HIV infections among younger persons nationally (CDC, 2005). Similarly, the more current HIV risk factor distribution reflects a demographic shift away from Caucasians to one in which more than 50% of those 50 or older are of African-American or Hispanic-American ethnicity. This change indicates the greater risk today among older persons in minority groups (McGinnis et al., 2003). Likewise, consonant with these changes, the risk for older women has increased. During a recent 5-year period the number of new cases in older women increased by 40%. Risk factor research for older women suggests that lack of knowledge of the risk of the male partner, mental health issues (particularly physical and sexual abuse and life crises), and taking risks for the sake of preserving relationships might be specific contributors to the risk in this group (Neundorfer et al., 2005). Finally, many older persons with HIV infection today are categorized as "no identified risk factor." This may reflect the level of fear of the consequences of disclosure of HIV risk factor and/or serostatus among this group.

Older people tend to view condoms primarily as a contraceptive measure. Postmenopausal women no longer fear unwanted pregnancy and may not insist on condom use. The National AIDS Behavioral Surveys study showed that the prevalence of one or more risk factors for HIV transmission was 8.8% for Americans aged 50 years or older, including 0.8% with multiple risk factors (Stall and Catania, 1994). This study also documented that persons at risk for HIV infection in this age range were one-sixth as likely to use condoms and one-fifth as likely to seek HIV antibody testing as younger at-risk persons (in their 20s). Women also undergo physical changes with aging that increase their vulnerability to HIV infection. Thinning and decreased lubrication of the vagina secondary to atrophic vaginitis in this age range results in increased exposure to the blood during intercourse, increasing the risk to contract HIV infection.

Many other factors contribute to a higher order of risk for HIV infection among older people. Older persons generally have less HIV/AIDS knowledge than younger persons (Zablotsky, 1998). Supporting this finding, older persons have largely been neglected in HIV education and prevention interventions (Linsk, 2000). Moreover, older persons tend to avoid conversations about HIV risk factors with their primary medical care providers, who typically themselves have an unrealistically low index of suspicion for HIV infection in this age group. This has resulted in significant delays in making the diagnosis of HIV infection in this population, so much so that, in the past decade, diagnoses of HIV infection were frequently being made within the month of death. Hence, interventions are also necessary with primary care providers to dismantle ageism and promote active screening discussion of HIV high-risk sexual and substance use behaviors among their older patients.

Furthermore, older people frequently mistake the symptoms of HIV infection for age-associated changes or symptoms of comorbid illnesses, such as type 2 diabetes mellitus (DM) or arthritis (described in detail below in Older Age and Comorbidities in HIV Infection). In fact, it has been demonstrated that older persons have increased symptom ambiguity so that recognizing symptoms due to HIV infection becomes a more difficult task (Siegel et al., 1999). This, in turn, further mitigates against appropriate HIV antibody testing in this population. A recent study suggests that laboratory screening for a decreased albumin:globulin ratio (<1.0), especially in patients with a history of alcohol abuse or sexually transmitted diseases, should prompt the primary care provider to consider HIV infection (Szerlip et al., 2005). Once identified as HIV seropositive, newly infected older persons still face negative social responses related to misinformation, social isolation, fear of the consequences of serostatus disclosure, ageism, and HIV/AIDS stigma.

Primary prevention interventions directly targeted to older adults at risk for HIV infection are sadly lacking at this stage of the epidemic (Coon et al., 2003). Interventions building upon successes with younger populations while considering modifications tailored to the needs of older populations are required. In addition, research into the situations and sociocultural settings that increase risk taking among older adults is specifically needed (Levy et al., 2003). Strategies for targeting deficits in HIV/AIDS knowledge and improving it, for combating ageism, and for reducing the stigma of discussing sexual and substance use–related risk behaviors are organizing principles for this population. In the future, planning for dissemination of successful interventions for this population, maximizing sustainability, and translating intervention principles developed for older persons for use in different settings are likely to become the major concerns.

Regarding secondary prevention, a focus of concern has been the stigmatization and social isolation experienced by older HIV-infected individuals. Some data have suggested that it may be possible to enhance the coping efforts and quality of life of older adults living with HIV/AIDS through coping skills enhancement programs (Chesney et al., 1996). When age-appropriate coping improvement interventions are delivered in group settings, older HIV-infected adults may be enabled to discuss their emotions, expand their social support availability, and enhance the efficacy of their coping strategies. In examining relationships of psychosocial context on distressed mood (as well as neuroendocrine, immune, and physical heath outcomes), we have employed a "stressor-support-coping" theoretical model (Goodkin et al., 2003). This model predicts that high life stressors, low social support, and more passive, maladaptive than active coping strategies are associated with increases in distressed mood. In line with this model, it has been reported that reductions in life stressor burden and improvements in social support and use of adaptive coping strategies occur after participating in face-to-face coping skills enhancement interventions (Heckman et al., 2001). With modifications for teleconference delivery technology, this intervention may be particularly helpful for older HIV-infected adults, who are often socially isolated and disenfranchised (Heckman et al., 2006).

Such interventions can provide a basis for secondary prevention of psychopathology, particularly depressive-spectrum disorders.

OLDER AGE AND SYSTEMIC PROGRESSION OF HIV DISEASE

Although the incidence of HIV infection among older adults has increased in recent years, it is clear that this does not account for the entire shift being observed toward older age among HIV-seropositive individuals at the national level. As previously discussed, a completely separate cohort of older HIV-seropositive persons derives from the successful treatment of HIV infection after the introduction of HAART in 1996. The issue of survival has re-entered the forefront of HIV/AIDS studies, but this time in a positive light, compared to the negative focus on survival during the pre-antiretroviral therapy era (1981–1987). While HAART has increased survival time for the entire population of HIV-seropositive persons, studies of the subgroup of older HIV-seropositive persons predominantly show decreased survival time compared to that of their younger counterparts after the diagnosis of positive HIV serostatus or of AIDS (Baillergeon et al., 1999; Inungu et al., 2001). However, some studies have not shown this deleterious aging effect (Keller et al., 1999). Discrepancies in research on the effects of aging may be accounted for by a number of factors. Zingmond and colleagues (2001) studied a nationally representative sample of HIV-infected adults under care in the United States from the HIV Cost and Service Utilization Study (HCSUS). They showed that older "non-Whites" had fewer symptoms and were less likely to have AIDS than "older Whites;" yet, the same group showed a trend toward shorter survival time. Potential explanations offered for this confusing finding were that older non-Whites might show decreased survival time once developing AIDS or that older non-Whites receive less effective antiretroviral therapy. In a subsequent study, this same HCSUS sample was compared to the Veterans Aging Cohort 3 Site Study (VACS3) (Zingmond et al., 2003). Overall, older VACS3 participants were less likely to report depressive symptoms, consistent with Goodkin et al.'s (2003) findings, but were more likely to report peripheral neuropathy, consistent with results found by Simpson et al. (1998) and Watters et al. (2004), as well as weight loss. Regarding ethnicity, the results of the VACS3 study supported those of the HCSUS study, showing a yet stronger effect for older "non-Whites" to report fewer symptoms than "older Whites," "younger non-Whites," or "younger Whites." Hence, it might be concluded that ethnicity is one factor accounting for discrepancies in this area of research.

Another factor of import regarding survival time appears to be the higher rate of non-HIV-related comorbidity among older HIV-seropositive patients (see Older Age and Comorbidities in HIV Infection, below, and Chapters 33–37). In an early report on the impact of comorbidity on survival in older patients with HIV infection, Skiest and colleagues (1996) used a case-control study to compare an older cohort (age >55 years) with a matched younger cohort (age <45 years). They found that the older cohort had significantly lower CD4 cell counts (205 vs. 429 cells/mm^3) and a significantly higher Charlson comorbidity index (39.5 vs. 10.5%), indicating a high prevalence of non-HIV-related comorbid conditions among older HIV-seropositive patients. A higher comorbidity index was a predictor of mortality in that study. One earlier report from the Multi-Center AIDS Cohort Study (MACS) on survival time after onset of AIDS also addressed the issue of comorbidity (Saah et al., 1994) in a sample of 886 homosexual men who had developed AIDS. The multivariate relative hazard of older age (>37 years) for earlier mortality was 1.28 ($p = .019$) and that of having "multiple diagnoses" was 1.64 ($p = .008$). While this study did not focus on the impact of comorbidity, *per se*, data nevertheless strongly supported comorbidity as a factor of prominence. More studies of comorbidity issues and disease progression are needed in the HAART era, particularly in the setting of older age.

OLDER AGE AND IMMUNOLOGICAL DISEASE PROGRESSION

Older age has been suggested to lead to more rapid immunological disease progression in HIV infection (see Chapter 3 for a general discussion). Regarding age and the response to HAART, a long-term study of immune reconstitution has reported on immune status at 4 years following treatment initiation (Kaufmann et al., 2002). This study showed that greater immune reconstitution was associated with younger age, a higher baseline CD4 count at treatment initi-

ation, and a higher CD4 nadir as well as with less advanced clinical stage. Only younger age and higher CD4 cell nadir remained predictive in a multivariate model, supporting a primary focus on aging. Another study of clinical outcome after four years of HAART treatment focused upon virological versus immunologic responses to HAART (Nicastri et al., 2005). This study showed that older age was associated with an increased likelihood of a virological response without a concomitant immunological response. A clinical risk for older age (10-year increment) with a new AIDS-defining illness or mortality was also reported. One study evaluated the opposite type of a change — the decay in CD4 cell count among patients achieving complete viral suppression and subsequently discontinuing HAART (N = 72) (Tebas et al., 2002). The slope of the CD4 cell decay was inversely correlated with age. This was likewise the case for the extent of increase of CD4 T cells during HAART, baseline viral load, CD4 cell count upon HAART discontinuation, and duration of nondetectable plasma viral load. Multiple regression analysis again supported the aging association, showing that older age and the extent of increase of CD4 cell count during HAART were independently associated with the rate of CD4 cell decay after HAART discontinuation. This work suggests the import of a contribution by the functional adult thymus to thymic emigrants responsible for the long-term rise in the naive subset of CD4 cells after HAART initiation. This function may now be easily measured by a marker of episomal DNA circles generated by excisional rearrangement of T cell receptor genes (T-cell receptor excision circles, or TRECs) (Douek et al., 1998).

Outside of HAART treatment, aging itself is associated with a CD4 cell loss disproportionate from the naive subset of CD4 cells to the memory subset of CD4 cells (Saule et al., 2006). This phenomenon may explain, at least in part, a potential for an age-associated decreased ability to respond to novel pathogens associated with the secretion of IL-2 (a Th1 cytokine originally described as T-cell growth factor). Moreover, as noted above, the recovery of naive CD4 cells among older HIV-infected individuals is related to thymic function and is delayed following the initiation of HAART (Powderly et al., 1998). Therefore, age-related thymic functional changes may directly exacerbate immunological decrements of concern known to be associated with HAART treatment among older HIV-infected persons.

OLDER AGE AND NEUROCOGNITIVE
MANIFESTATIONS OF HIV INFECTION

Older Age and HIV-Associated Dementia

In addressing aging and neurocognitive disorders in HIV infection, we would expect to examine relationships with both HIV-associated minor cognitive-motor disorder (MCMD) and HIV-associated dementia complex (HAD), as originally defined by the American Academy of Neurology (AAN, 1991) (although these criteria are now in the process of being revised following the Frascati Conference [Heaton et al., 2005]). More research in this area has been conducted on HAD than on MCMD (also see Chapters 10 and 19).

Janssen and colleagues (1992) reported on CDC data in an early study, showing a linear increase in HAD with increasing age (15–34 years, 6%; 35–54 years, 8%; 55–74 years, 12%; >75 years, 19%). These findings were based on the rate of HAD as an AIDS-defining illness (ADI), which could have underestimated the actual frequency of HAD because the vast majority of HAD cases occur after the diagnosis of another ADI. A second source of underestimation arises from the very low physician index of suspicion for HIV infection among older persons, leading to the assumption of another etiology for dementia and the decreased likelihood that these patients would be tested for HIV prior to their death (Weiler et al., 1988). In another pre-HAART study, McArthur and colleagues (1993) reported that after a diagnosis of AIDS, HAD developed at an annual rate of 7%. Older age at AIDS onset was a risk factor of 1.60 per decade of age, while constitutional symptoms were also associated with an increased risk. In a confirmatory study, Chiesi and colleagues (1996) reported the results of a large epidemiological study (N = 6548) in Europe, which showed an increased risk of HAD of 14% as an ADI and of 19% per 5-year age increment afterward for those not diagnosed with HAD as an ADI.

After the introduction of HAART, the incidence of HAD has been reduced by approximately 50%. In one of the few studies of aging and HAD conducted after the introduction of HAART, Valcour and colleagues (2004) showed that a risk factor of 2.13 applied, adjusting for race, education, substance dependence, antiretroviral medication status, viral load, CD4 cell count, and depressed mood level. Hence, for HAD, it appears that there is consistent evidence for age as a contributory factor.

Older Age and Minor
Cognitive-Motor Disorder

With respect to neurocognitive disorders and aging, significantly less is known about the relation of MCMD to age than that of HAD. In our current study of older and younger HIV-seropositive and HIV-seronegative individuals, we have examined the frequency of MCMD symptoms by age (see Fig. 26.1). MCMD symptoms per the AAN (1991) criteria included the following six symptoms: (1) impaired attention or concentration, (2) impaired memory, (3) mental slowing, (4) motor slowing, (5) incoordination, and (6) irritability, lability, and/or personality change. Only two of these symptoms occurring for at least 1 month in association with a mild functional status deficit are needed for the diagnosis of MCMD. In our study comparing older (≥50-year-old) and younger (18- to 39-year-old) HIV-seropositive and HIV-seronegative individuals, we found a statistically significant age effect. Older HIV-seropositive individuals had a higher mean MCMD symptom frequency than that of younger HIV-seropositive individuals (Goodkin et al., 2001). Hence, the impact of aging on cognitive-motor disorder in HIV infection may apply to this less severe disorder, MCMD, as well as to HAD. Moreover, older HIV-seronegative individuals showed a higher MCMD symptom frequency than that of younger HIV-seronegative individuals, documenting that aging is associated with greater MCMD symptom frequency outside of HIV infection and suggesting that a true synergism may exist on a pathophysiological level. This synergism could be due to any one of a number of potential mechanisms, including increased quinolinic acid production, increased oxidative stress, decrements in dopaminergic transmission, increased neuronal apoptosis, and decreased synaptic protein turnover through the proteasome. Although the clinical significance of MCMD for progression to HAD had been questioned previously, subsequent controlled evidence has shown that MCMD is, indeed, associated with an increased risk for progression to HAD (Stern et al., 2001). Thus, the clinical significance of the impact of older age is likely to apply across the two HIV-related neurocognitive disorders—MCMD and HAD.

Linkage of the impact of aging with MCMD and HAD may contribute to the broader, established link of older age and HIV infection to an increased mortality risk. The risk of HAD for mortality has been well established since the early stages of the epidemic,

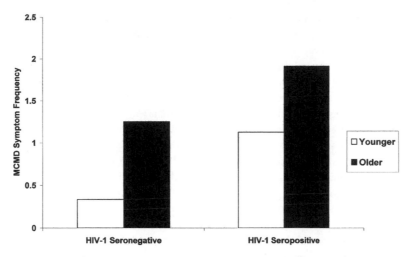

FIGURE 26.1. Older age and minor cognitive-motor disorder (MCMD) symptom frequency.

when it was associated with an expected mean survival time of 6 months. Ellis and colleagues (1997) demonstrated that MCMD, likewise, is associated with an increased risk for mortality (RR = 2.2). However, it remains unclear the extent to which the age-associated risks for MCMD and HAD mediate an increased risk for early mortality independently of the broader, established age-associated risk for systemic disease progression. By some researchers the age-associated risk for neurocognitive disorder is thought to be mediated through immunological decrements associated with aging (too early to refer to as "immunosenescence") that might compound the immunodeficiency due to HIV itself. Delay in diagnosis known to occur among older HIV-seropositive persons and the resulting delay in access to HAART might also mediate impacts on mortality through neurocognitive disorder. In these two cases, the age-associated risk for MCMD and HAD may merge with that for mortality. However, other researchers believe that entirely independent age-associated effects may play a role, such as decreased cerebral vasomotor reactivity associated with the dyslipidemia known to occur as a toxicity of long-term HAART. Moreover, the impact of neurocognitive disorders on decreased antiretroviral medication adherence may also be an independent effect of neurocognitive disorder on survival time among the HIV infected. To date, the literature on antiretroviral adherence among older HIV-infected patients is mixed, with some studies showing higher adherence (Maggiolo et al., 2002; Hinkin et al., 2004) while

others do not show higher adherence in this group (Goodkin et al., 2004; Manfredi, 2004). Future research is needed to tease apart a specific contribution of such a neurocognitive disorder–mediated effect on mortality. Given the pending change in nomenclature of MCMD to mild neurocognitive disorder (MND) and the changes of diagnostic criteria anticipated for both MCMD and HAD with publication of the results of the Frascati Conference (Heaton et al., 2005), additional complications will be introduced into research tracking the long-term impact of aging and neurocognitive disorder on mortality.

Older Age and Subclinical Neuropsychological Impairment

While one might predict that the relation of older age to subclinical neuropsychological impairment would parallel that with MCMD and HAD, this may not be the case. The latter two are medical disorders, whereas the former is a disease manifestation. With respect to MCMD, the diagnosis is specifically based on the presence or absence of the AAN-defined symptoms (American Academy of Neurology, 1991). Hence, there is a dysjunction in defining criteria among these levels of the spectrum of HIV-associated neurocognitive disturbance, which may interfere with comparative analyses for an association with aging.

The results of studies examining the relationship between aging ands neurocognitive performance and impairment have been mixed (van Gorp et al., 1994; Hardy et al., 1999; Hinkin et al., 2001; Wilkie et al., 2003; Becker et al., 2004; Cherner et al., 2004), although the findings generally support the view that an interaction is more likely to occur in late-stage HIV disease (AIDS) rather than during the early symptomatic or asymptomatic stage of HIV disease. These mixed findings may be related to a number of factors that complicate such studies at this level, including the greater likelihood that subclinical neurocognitive impairment may spontaneously revert to normal functioning (when compared with that same likelihood for MCMD or HAD). Another issue is that studies have been variable in how they attempt to differentiate between subclinical and clinical impairment, the latter of which overlaps with the diagnoses of MCMD or HAD. This issue is particularly relevant given the lack of consistent identification of MCMD against subclinical impairment and HAD.

In addition, the likelihood of finding an effect relates to the sensitivity of the domains sampled for neurocognitive deficits due to both HIV infection and older age, as well as to the specific tests incorporated to represent each domain. Moreover, these studies are highly variable in the controls employed for the impact of factors other than older age on neurocognitive performance or impairment. While most studies do address ethnicity and stage of HIV disease progression, few also address antiretroviral medication use variables (e.g., number of failures, regimens with CSF penetration, length of treatment, presence of resistance, and level of adherence), alcohol and substance use and disorder, fatigue, pain level, depressed mood level and disorder, comorbidities (type 2 DM, hypertension, hepatitis C coinfection), prescribed medication toxicities (efavirenz, interferon-alpha), test motivation, nutritional deficiencies, cognitive reserve, and bilingualism. Hence, future research in this area should address methodological issues as well as the consistency of the definition of the condition of subclinical neurocognitive impairment. It is likely that this goal will be supported by addition of the defining criteria for the similar condition of asymptomatic neurocognitive impairment to the revised criteria for the HIV-associated neurocognitive disorders derived at the Frascati Conference.

Regarding the relationship of neurocognitive impairment to mortality, a sample with participants predominantly in the CDC-defined asymptomatic clinical disease stage has been investigated (Wilkie et al.,

1998). It was observed there that deficits in information processing speed and in long-term verbal memory retrieval accuracy significantly increased mortality risk, controlling for CD4 cell count, clinical stage of HIV disease progression, and antiretroviral medication use. The relative risk for mortality, compared to the non-impaired, was 6.4 for information processing–speed deficits and 3.5 for verbal memory deficits. Hence, defining older HIV-infected individuals with subclinical neurocognitive impairment as at-risk has established clinical relevance, although this is more clearly demonstrated in survival time than by the association of older age with the level or pattern of the impairment itself.

OLDER AGE AND COMORBIDITIES IN HIV INFECTION

Two overarching types of comorbidities may be associated with HIV infection: (1) those due to the complications of immunosuppression caused by HIV infection itself and occurring only in the presence of HIV infection (often referred to as HIV-related comorbidities) and (2) comorbid illnesses that are either unrelated to HIV infection or are due to the therapies prescribed for HIV infection and occur independently of HIV infection itself (often referred to as non-HIV-related comorbidities) (see Chapters 33–37). For the HIV-related type, multiple research groups have reported dramatically lower incidences of the previously most common HIV-related complications of immunosuppression after the introduction of HAART (e.g., *Pneumocystis carinii* pneumonia, Kaposi's sarcoma, and *Mycobacterium avium* complex infection). For the non-HIV-related type, an example is herpes simplex virus (HSV) type 2 infection, which in many cases occurs prior to HIV infection (along with other sexually transmitted diseases). Certainly, type 2 DM occurs commonly as an illness in the general population and may be present prior to HIV infection (like HSV type 2 infection).

It should be noted that these two types of comorbidities may overlap. For example, HSV type 2 infection, particularly recurrences, may be caused by the immunosuppression associated with HIV infection. The occurrence of cancer may also be either HIV related or unrelated. Biggar and colleagues (2004) identified cancer in 8828 older patients (>60 years of age) with AIDS (1142 of whom developed cancer) and found that the AIDS-defining cancers (Kaposi's sarcoma, non-Hodgkin's lymphoma, and invasive cervical cancer) among older patients occurred at similar rates to those for younger patients. However, a higher rate of non-AIDS-defining cancer incidence (1.2-fold) was found in older HIV-infected patients compared to that found in their younger counterparts (both groups demonstrated the same cancer types). This relatively small but significant effect lends some support to the concern about the impact of an increase in non-HIV-related cancers among older HIV-infected patients (to the extent that these non-AIDS-defining cancers are, indeed, also non-HIV-related). At the larger level, it is noteworthy that in recent years a much higher incidence has been reported for the type of comorbidities unrelated to HIV infection.

As is the case with cancer, the occurrence of neurological diseases may be either HIV related or unrelated. The most common neuro-AIDS condition among HIV-infected patients in the HAART era is peripheral neuropathy, with distal sensory polyneuropathy (DSP) being the most common type. DSP can be induced by HIV infection itself (i.e., HIV related) or by the toxicity of the dideoxynuclcoside antiretroviral medications (ddI, ddC, and d4T; i.e., non-HIV related) (see Chapter 20). The non-HIV-related issue of aging is associated with deterioration in light touch sensation in the foot in humans, and peripheral neuropathy has been associated with aging in animal studies. The sensory symptoms of DSP can be pain, numbness, and/or paresthesias and may be disabling. Motor deficits are minimal, and there are reduced or absent ankle reflexes. After initial progression, the sensorimotor symptoms may plateau and cease to progress further but persist despite ongoing attempts at treatment. An association of age with presence of DSP has been shown in HIV-infected individuals clinically (Simpson et al., 1998; Watters et al., 2004). Because peripheral neuropathy is known to be a true risk factor for falls and HIV-infected patients are exposed to other factors causing decreased balance (such as efavirenz toxicity), falls, a well-known risk for morbidity and mortality among older persons generally, might be expected to present a yet higher risk for older HIV-infected persons. Furthermore, the pain associated with DSP might relate to decreased adherence to HAART regimens, threatening control of systemic disease progression as well.

Another neuro-AIDS condition of concern to older patients is progressive multifocal leukoencephalopathy (PML), an HIV-related comorbidity due to severe immunosuppression. PML is a devastating, demyelinating neurological disease that without effective treatment is estimated to arise in 2% to 7% of HIV-infected individuals. It results from lytic infection of oligodendrocytes (which produce myelin) by JC virus (JCV). JCV may be frequently present in the brains of immunocompetent elderly patients. Given that JCV is transactivated by HIV, it is likely that JCV is reactivated relatively early in HIV disease progression and to a greater extent among older HIV-infected individuals.

A third neuro-AIDS condition of particular concern for older patients is cerebrovascular accident (CVA), generally agreed upon as a non-HIV-related comorbidity associated with antiretroviral medication toxicity and aging. CVA is the third most common cause of death in the United States, and the risk for vascular disease increases significantly with age. With the long-term toxicities from the protease inhibitors and nucleoside reverse transcriptase inhibitors resulting in decreased cerebral vasomotor reactivity, along with increased intima-media thickness and a higher prevalence of plaques in the internal carotid arteries, the risk for CVA now represents a common treatment focus. In fact, the higher risk for both myocardial infarction (MI) and CVA among older HIV-infected patients may represent the first signs of a convergence between the morbidity and mortality risks for the general population with those of the HIV infected. Moreover, it is likely that this convergence will increase further in the coming years. These three examples demonstrate that neurological diseases run the gamut of illnesses from those that are HIV related, those that overlap the two types, to those that are non-HIV related. Given the increased likelihood of the neuro-AIDS conditions of PML, DSP, and CVA, respectively, among older HIV-infected patients, they might appropriately be considered candidates for more aggressive screening techniques than normal to identify these illnesses.

Non-HIV-related comorbidities are actually more common than the HIV-related comorbidities reviewed above among HIV-seropositive people in primary medical care today (Brown et al., 2005; Sulkowski and Thomas, 2005; Sax, 2006). Recent data show that since the introduction of HAART, the proportion of deaths caused by liver failure, renal failure (unrelated to HIV associated nephropathy), cardiac disease, non-HIV-associated malignancy, chronic obstructive pulmonary disease, and drug overdose in patients with

HIV infection is increasing (Jain et al., 2003). Some of these conditions cause an increased risk of future cardiovascular events, may be exacerbated by HAD, or (as previously noted) are caused by the complications of long-term exposure to certain antiretroviral therapies (e.g., insulin resistance, dyslipidemia, type 2 DM, atherosclerosis, lipodystrophy syndrome, MI, and CVA). With increased survival time due to the success of HAART as well as (to a lesser extent) the rise in new infections among older individuals, non-HIV-related medical conditions have increased in importance (Sheth et al., 2006). This is true not only because they constitute a disease burden at least equivalent to HIV-related comorbidities in this group (Kilbourne et al., 2001) but also because they carry their own independent risks for morbidity and mortality among older HIV-infected persons.

Recent trends have been noted for an increasing prevalence of neuropsychiatric non-HIV-related comorbidities (i.e., excluding the neurocognitive disorders directly referable to HIV) as well as of the general medical non-HIV-related comorbidities discussed above. Neuropsychiatric comorbidities are key complicating factors that must be addressed because they affect HIV disease progression among older persons living with HIV/AIDS. Such comorbidities may not only decrease immunologic function but more generally impair one's ability to carry out the more demanding activities of daily living (e.g., antiretroviral medication adherence, maximal occupational function). In one study analyzing longitudinal employment status among HIV-seropositive persons (N = 141), the major factors associated with unemployment or partial employment, in order of influence, were noted to be financial status (disability benefits), neuropsychiatric comorbidity (past or current diagnosis of major depression and/or dysthymia), general medical comorbidity (physical limitations), neurocognitive impairment (executive function, specifically), and education (Rabkin et al., 2004b). Interestingly, age (mean = 40, standard deviation = 8) itself did not predict employment status, suggesting that treatment efficacy specifically for comorbidities may be critical to maximization of functional status among older HIV-infected persons. Moreover, a study of HIV-infected persons and their driving ability demonstrated an association between visual inattention (by the Usual Field of View test) and increased motor vehicle accidents, as well as a trend for such an association with the comorbidity of neurocognitive impairment (Marcotte et al., 2006).

These results suggest that clinicians should actively screen older HIV-infected patients for visual inattention as well as for neurocognitive impairment in evaluating their risk for driving impairment. It should also be noted that seizures occur with increased frequency in HIV infected persons and may create a driving risk. When one examines the impact of primary comorbidities of HIV infection due to immunosuppression, that of general medical comorbidities unrelated to HIV infection that are more frequent in older age, and that of neuropsychiatric comorbidities, the current concern for the level of impact of comorbidity on functional status in daily life for older HIV-infected persons becomes clear.

Extending this concern beyond functional status, a study using a national administrative database of 25- to 84-year-olds suggested that the decreased survival time experienced by minority HIV-seropositive veterans (of about a 40% compared to white HIV-seropositive veterans) may derive from differences in non-HIV-related medical and neuropsychiatric comorbid conditions and in the severity of illness of HIV-related complications due to immunosuppression (McGinnis et al., 2003). One study has shown that HIV-infected individuals over age 55 have approximately four times the percentage with non-HIV-1-related comorbidities compared to HIV infected individuals below age 45 years of age, and that non-HIV-related comorbidities are associated with increased mortality (independent of age) (Skiest et al., 1996).

Non-HIV-related comorbidity requires the use of medications other than the antiretrovirals, and these other medications often contribute to increases in morbidity and mortality among older HIV-infected patients (Shah et al., 2002; Gebo and Moore, 2004). Emerging evidence clearly indicates that metabolic, cardiovascular, and neuropsychiatric comorbidites could be exacerbated by the use of antiretroviral medications (e.g. efavirenz; Clifford et al., 2005). Tenofovir and indinavir should be used less frequently with older patients because of their nephrotoxicity in patients who may already have decreased creatinine clearance. Because of both decreased renal and hepatic metabolism in older HIV-infect patients, comorbidities due to drug–drug interactions are a greater concern for these patients. Regimens containing ritonavir should be avoided because of its frequent association with dyslipidemia. When treating hypercholesterolemia and hyperlipidemia, lovastatin and simvastatin may achieve toxic levels in combination with antiretroviral medication regimens because of their metabolism by the cytochrome P450 isoenzyme microsomal oxidase system in the liver, thus pravastatin and fluvastatin are preferred. The PDE5 inhibitors also interact with antiretroviral medications, so their dose should be decreased accordingly. Likewise, a number of benzodiazepine medications interact with antiretroviral medications on this same basis. Thus, oxazepam, lorazepam and temazapam, which are primarily conjugated (by hepatic glucoronidation) and thus bypass cytochrome P450 3A4 metabolism, are generally preferred (though conjugation reactions are also subject to drug–drug interactions).

These pharmacological considerations argue for the modification of antiretroviral guidelines (DHHS, 2005) specifically for the needs of older HIV-infected patients. Metabolic, cardiovascular, and neuropsychiatric comorbidities could also be exacerbated by HIV infection itself (Casau, 2005). Thus, additional research in this area is needed to optimize the care of older HIV-infected patients. With the increasing frequency of comorbidities seen among older patients with HIV infection, routine general health maintenance and appropriate diagnosis, treatment, and prevention of non-HIV-related medical and neuropsychiatric conditions are becoming prominent in providing optimal care to patients with HIV infection.

Since it is the neuropsychiatric comorbidities that are of prime relevance to mental health clinicians and researchers, we present the literature from this area in tabular form, which covers comorbidities of neuropsychiatric symptoms and disorders from studies of HIV risk and disease (see Table 26.1). These comorbidities may occur either in the subpopulation of newly infected older persons (emerging as consequences of recent HIV infection) or among the subpopulation of older adults who have successfully survived into older age with HIV infection through the efficacy to HAART (allowing more time for aging-associated comorbidities to develop). To date, this research has not differentiated between neuropsychiatric comorbidites in these two distinctly different subpopulations. The sparse literature in this area for older adults devolves from the longstanding preponderance of attention focused on neuropsychiatric conditions as a risk for or consequence of HIV infection among younger adults. There is increasing evidence in the younger HIV-infected population that the prevalence of HIV infection is greater among the severely mentally ill (Blank et al., 2002); that those with comorbid HIV infection and severe

mental illness (such as schizophrenia) are more likely to be substance users (Walkup et al., 1999); and that alcohol use, substance use, and the presence of psychiatric disorders among HIV-infected and at-risk persons are each associated with increased levels of high-risk sexual behaviors (Remien and Johnson, 2004; Stein et al., 2005). In the younger population, alcohol and substance use disorders and other psychopathology not only increase the risk of contracting HIV infection but also are associated with decreased HAART utilization as well as decreased adherence (upon utilization) and a lack of suppression of viral replication.

Parallel research of this nature in older HIV-infected adults is limited and conflicting, as can be seen from Table 26.1. For example, we expect that both general medical and neuropsychiatric comorbidities may be of special concern in the older age group. Yet one recent study in Australia confirmed that older patients living with HIV/AIDS were less likely to describe good or excellent health and had a higher percentage of general medical comorbidities but showed no significant difference in neuropsychiatric comorbidities (Pitts et al., 2005). Nevertheless, it is clear that neuropsychiatric disorders decrease the functional status and endanger the survival of older HIV-infected individuals. Likewise, it is clear that concurrent alcohol and/or psychoactive substance use, abuse, or dependence compound the deleterious impact of the presence of other neuropsychiatric disorders in this population. More research is needed to better define and measure the impact of neuropsychiatric comorbidities among older HIV-infected persons, particularly when alcohol and substance abuse or dependence is present.

Reliable and valid statewide and national epidemiological data are not yet available on the incidence, prevalence, course, and phenomenology of neuropsychiatric disorders among older HIV-infected adults. As has occurred in the area of HIV-related neurocognitive disorders, with the HIV-related neuropsychiatric disorders it will also prove ultimately to be essential for research on functional status measures and instrumental activities of daily living to establish norms for use in standardized diagnosis, assessment of impact, and determination of meaningful change with treatment. Prospective studies of epidemiological comorbidity should examine the incidence and prevalence rates of neuropsychiatric disorders to determine whether the age-related decline in psychopathology in the general population holds for the older HIV-infected patient population as well. Such research should

TABLE 26.1. Comorbid Neuropsychiatric Symptoms and Disorders in HIV Risk and Disease

Study	Population	Measures of Psychopathology and/or Alcohol/Drug Use	Findings
Braithwaite et al. (2005)	N = 2352 HIV-seropositive and HIV-seronegative veterans 50 years mean age	Alcohol consumption (self-report) Depressive symptoms (PRIME-MD)	Alcohol consumption has temporal and dose-dependent relationship to poor antiretroviral medication adherence; no effects occurred for depression severity on adherence.
Catz et al. (2001)	N = 113 HIV seropositive 47–69 years old	Psychological distress (SCL-90-R) Depressive symptomatology (BDI) Alcohol use (self-report)	One-third of older adults had inconsistent antiretroviral adherence (skipping medication doses) related to greater alcohol use, increased anxiety, somatization, and life stressors; depressive symptoms were unrelated to adherence problems.
Cherner et al. (2004)	N = 67 HIV seropositive 50+ years	SCID, PRISM, and depression symptoms (BDI)	Neither lifetime nor 12-month diagnosis of depressive disorder nor history of recent substance use disorders predicted the rate of HIV-related neuropsychological impairment among young and old participants.
Goodkin et al. (2003) (Cohort 1—of Heckman et al.)	N = 113 Older HIV-seropositive persons (47 years and older)	Depressed mood level (BDI) Anxious mood level and somatization from the SCL-90-R	For depressed mood, higher stressors due to family, finances, and lack of social support were related to mood level. For anxious mood, older age within this older sample was related to lower anxious mood level and distancing and escape/avoidant coping were related to higher levels. For somatization, AIDS bereavement stressors and distancing and escape/avoidant coping were related to higher levels, while family support was related to lower levels.
Goodkin et al. (2003) (Cohort 2—of Goodkin et al.)	N = 128 Older HIV seropositive = 27 Younger HIV seropositive = 49 Older HIV seronegative = 28 Younger HIV seronegative = 24	Depressed mood (HRSD) Anxious mood (HARS)	HIV-seropositive older adults (predominantly long-term infected) had lower depressed and anxious mood levels than those of their younger counterparts (controlling positive serostatus duration), while HIV-seronegative older adults had higher depressed and anxious mood levels than those of their younger counterparts. Both effects remained with exclusion of somatic items.
Heckman et al. (2002)	N = 83 HIV seropositive 50+ years	Depressive symptoms (BDI) Psychological symptoms (GSI, SCL-90-R)	25% of participants had moderate or severe levels of depressed mood; an elevated number of somatic symptoms and increased psychological symptomatology occurred in those with high levels of HIV-related life stressor burden, less social support, and reduced health care access.

TABLE 26.1. *(continued)*

Study	Population	Measures of Psychopathology and/or Alcohol/Drug Use	Findings
Heckman et al. (2006)	$N = 90$ HIV seropositive 54.3 years mean age	Psychological symptoms (SCL-90-R) Depressive symptoms (GDS) PRIME-MD	Telephone-delivered coping skills enhancement intervention-produced decreases in global psychological symptoms (and life stressor burden) mediated by increases in coping self-efficacy; intervention did not reduce depressive symptoms.
Hinkin et al. (2004)	$N = 148$ HIV seropositive 26–69 years (mean age 44.2 years, 26% 50+ years)	DSM-IV psychoactive substance abuse/dependence disorder module	Older participants had improved antiretroviral adherence compared to younger participants, and current drug abuse/dependence (primarily with cocaine) was associated with lower adherence.
Justice et al. (2004)	$N = 50$ HIV seronegative (49 years, median) and seropositive (51 years median) veterans	Depressive symptoms (PHQ-9 and provider reported); alcohol abuse or dependence (AUDIT, ICD-9 codes) and drug abuse or dependence (DAST-10)	Higher prevalence of depressive symptoms, alcohol abuse or dependence, and drug abuse or dependence in HIV-seropositive persons (than HIV-seronegative persons) with increasing age; depressive symptoms and alcohol abuse or dependence decrease with age among HIV-negative persons but do not decrease with age among HIV-seropositive persons.
Kwiatkowski and Booth (2003)	$N = 1508$ HIV at-risk injection drug users (IDUs) and crack smokers 50+ years of age	Drug use, sexual behaviors, and health/medical history (RBA)	Older HIV at-risk individuals were more likely to be IDUs than younger individuals but were less risky in needle-sharing practices. The older cohort was less likely to consume alcohol or smoke crack but those who did smoke crack were extremely risky. Among the older cohort high-risk sex behavior was more than twice as frequent as smoking crack.
Pitts et al. (2005)	$N = 894$ Respondents to the HIV Futures Survey 23% age 50 or older	Anonymous questionnaire with items on health, well-being, presence of major health condition, presence of mental health condition	Older HIV-infected patients reported their health and well-being as significantly less likely than younger HIV-infected patients to be good or excellent; they were more likely to have additional health conditions. No significant difference was shown for mental health conditions.
Rabkin et al. (2004b)	$N = 42$ HIV seropositive 50+ years	SCID	36% of older HIV-seropositive persons (50+ years of age) had a lifetime diagnosis of major depressive disorder compared to only 20% of HIV-seronegative younger persons; 33% of older HIV-seropositive persons had a lifetime diagnosis of substance dependence compared to only 5% of older HIV-seronegative persons. Of note, rates for older HIV-seropositive persons were nonsignificantly higher than those of younger HIV-seropositive persons. However, there was no parallel decline *(continued)*

TABLE 26.1. *(continued)*

Study	Population	Measures of Psychopathology and/or Alcohol/Drug Use	Findings
			in rates of major depressive disorder and substance use disorder for older HIV-seropositive adults—unlike the decline seen in older HIV-seronegative adults with respect to younger HIV-seronegative adults. They concluded that a larger epidemiological study was necessary.
Valcour et al. (2004)	N = 103 HIV seropositive 50+ years	Depressive symptoms (BDI); DSM-IV-based substance abuse/dependence inventory	HIV-associated dementia (HAD) was unrelated to depressive disorder or drug dependence: odds of HAD was 2.13 times greater than that in younger cohort (20–39 years), adjusting for race, education, substance dependence, antiretroviral medication status, viral load, CD4 cell count, and depressed mood level.

AUDIT, Alcohol Use Disorders Identification Test; BDI, Beck Depression Inventory; DAST-10, Drug Abuse Screening Test; GDS, Geriatric Depression Scale; GSI, Global Severity Index; HARS, Hamilton Anxiety Rating Scale; HRSD, Hamilton Rating Scale for Depression; ICD-9, International Classification of Disease, 9th edition; PHQ-9, Patient Health Questionnaire, 9 item; PRIME-MD, Primary Care Evaluation of Mental Disorders; PRISM, Psychiatric Research Interview for Substance and Mental Disorders; RBA, Risk Behavior Assessment; SCID, Structured Clinical Interview for DSM-IV; SCL-90-R, Symptom Checklist-90-Revised.

address the differentiation of the newly infected older subpopulation from the long-term infected older subpopulation. Additionally, future epidemiological research on these neuropsychiatric comorbidities will need to clarify whether the statistical relevance of the results also has physiological and clinical relevance. For example, older HIV-infected individuals with past major depressive episodes may be more vulnerable to future episodes and associated immunosuppression that could potentiate immunological HIV disease progression. Epidemiological studies should be carefully designed and interpreted not only to simply uncover the existence of comorbidities but also to determine whether such comorbidities have specific research or clinical impact that warrants further study.

Treatment research targeted toward neuropsychiatric comorbidities requires an understanding of the mechanisms that combine to produce neuropsychiatric symptoms and disorders in this population. Both HIV infection itself and antiretroviral therapy toxicities are involved. Progress in this area has been notably lacking. Much research in the younger population has demonstrated ways in which the challenges of treating mental health and substance use disorders are inextricably intertwined with the challenges of treating the HIV infected. These studies show that when

comorbidities are treated, individuals benefit as a result of more consistent treatment of their HIV infection (Sambamoorthi et al., 2000; Palepu et al., 2004). Yet, little parallel research targeting neuropsychiatric comorbidities in older adults has been reported to date. It is important to note a caveat that the impact of mental health or substance abuse treatment alone on sexual and substance use risk behaviors may be limited, thus highlighting the importance of comprehensive care models that integrate behavioral health services with medical treatment for HIV disease.

A key consideration in understanding the etiology and impact of non-HIV-related comorbidities in older adults involves distinguishing and understanding the etiology and impact of the concomitant and overlapping conditions associated with HIV infection risk and/or HIV disease. The non-HIV-related comorbidities include the physiological processes of normal aging and the etiological factors of age-associated diseases. For example, older Americans have their own population-specific health challenges, such as Alzheimer disease, Parkinson disease, type 2 DM, hypertension, MI, CVA, osteoporosis, and prostrate cancer. It will be necessary to distinguish the impact of such age-associated diseases from the effects of the aging process itself among older HIV-infected persons.

The sequelae of HIV infection (and its antiretroviral treatment) must be differentiated from conditions caused by the normal aging process per se and from age-associated medical disorders that occur independently of HIV infection. Many of the latter may have a significant impact on the immune system and overlap with HIV-associated immunologic decrements. Virtually nothing is known about whether the age-related risk of modifying the complications of HIV infection itself (or its antiretroviral therapy) depends on the presence of relevant comorbidities. It may be that the shorter survival time observed in older HIV-infected adults is significantly related to the effects of these comorbid conditions. Further, age-related dementia syndromes that mimic HAD must now be examined as part of the differential diagnosis of HIV-associated neurocognitive disorders. Therefore, research will have to determine not only how age-related physiologic changes (e.g., immunologic decline, metabolic changes, and hormonal alterations) affect the course and treatment of HIV-associated neuropsychiatric and neurocognitive disorders but also how HIV-associated medical conditions (e.g., hepatitis, renal disease, antiretroviral medication–induced toxicities, and psychotropic–antiretroviral drug interactions) impact these disorders.

The challenges of differential diagnosis may be even more complicated among older HIV-infected individuals because of the misattribution by patients of the symptoms of HIV infection as being due to normal aging, the difficulty in discriminating depressive symptoms from cognitive symptoms, and the underdiagnosis of depressive-spectrum disorders generally among the HIV infected (a challenge in common with many other medical illnesses). Future research will need to determine whether these neuropsychiatric comorbidities are synergistic with advancing age (and with age-associated physiologic changes), with peripheral and central neuro-AIDS disorders, and/or with age-associated general medical comorbidities. Such research should also address the mechanisms involved that might drive this synergism when it is demonstrated.

OLDER AGE AND THE HIV AFFECTED

Up to 100,000 adult Americans with AIDS receive help from older caregivers. One-half of adults with HIV-associated illness depend on older relatives for financial, physical, medical, or emotional support (Allers, 1990). In addition, a growing population of AIDS orphans exists. After a caregiving parent with AIDS has died, many patients are cared for by older persons. In the United States, most of these children are cared for by grandparents through standby adoption or guardianship. Because most of those orphaned by HIV/AIDS are of minority ethnicity, most of the older caregivers are disproportionately of minority ethnicity as well. The differential likelihood of AIDS-related caregiver burden (mental and physical) contributes another source of health care disparities among minority groups that needs to be addressed in the United States.

An American Association of Retired Persons study estimated that 70% of HIV caregivers are women, with 31% being between 45 and 64 years old and 35% over 65 (Ogu and Wolfe, 1994). Older minority women face multiple disadvantages, including compromised health, poverty, and sexism. One recent study gathered survey data from 135 dyads in which the caregiver was a middle-aged or older mother or wife, and the care recipient was her HIV-infected adult son or husband. Stigma was higher among HIV-infected patients than among caregivers, higher among caregiving wives than mothers, and similar between patients who are husbands and sons. The stigma of the caregiving dyad was influenced by the caregiver's HIV serostatus, the ethnicity of the dyad, caregiving duration, and household income (Wight et al., 2006).

Scant research explores the problems encountered by older parents and grandparents when caring for younger family members who are (or whose parents are) infected by HIV. Forehand and colleagues (1998) showed children of HIV-seropositive mothers to have psychosocial adjustment problems in several domains—social withdrawal, attention deficits, and depressed mood. In another study of a sample of older female, HIV-affected African-American caregivers, most of the caregivers had not disclosed the family member's HIV serostatus to anyone to avoid unwanted social reactions, leading to inadequate social support (Poindexter and Linsk, 1999). Linsk and Mason (2004) studied caregivers of HIV-affected children receiving Aid to Dependent Children and Families entitlement support in the Chicago metropolitan area. The caregivers were predominantly African-American males, averaging 48.5 years of age and completing 11.6 years of education. Caregiving commonly took place in the context of caregiver illness self-management (most commonly for arthritis). Most did not show depressed mood elevations, although there was a depressed subgroup. Other studies show that HIV-affected caregivers generally may delay seeking help for their own needs because of the associated stigma. The same association has been supported by international studies — in Thailand (Kespichayawattana and Van Landingham, 2003), Botswana (Lindsey et al., 2003), and Zimbabwe (Howard et al., 2006).

Another Thai study (Knodel et al., 2001) examining older caregivers of HIV-infected persons included a total of 963 HIV-seropositive (older and younger) adults who were either symptomatic or dying from an HIV-related illness. The frequencies of HIV-seropositive patients co-residing with a parent and having a parent as one's main caretaker were noted to decrease with age, especially for the oldest patients (though only <5% are 50 years old or older). For the entire age range of the HIV-seropositive patient sample, two-thirds of all of those dying moved back to their home community, and 70% of them received care from a parent or older relative (many over age 60). It was concluded that older caregivers are more common in Thailand than in the United States, which is likely to be true of other resource-limited countries as well. More international research of this type is needed in the future.

Research studies on interventions specific to older family members who are caregivers for persons with HIV/AIDS are very limited and mixed in results. Hansell and colleagues (1998) measured the effects of a modified case management approach, showing increased caregiver social support but unchanged stressor levels and coping strategies. Burnette (1997) used a school-based, group intervention with grandparents that focused on specific psychosocial topics and showed improved depressed mood level and service knowledge but unchanged social support.

SUMMARY

Nationally and internationally there is a steadily increasing prevalence of HIV-infected patients over age 50. They represent two subpopulations: patients newly HIV infected in older age, and patients who were HIV infected previously and survived into older age through the success of HAART. Newly infected older persons are more likely to be psychologically distressed, socially isolated, and in need of educational interventions about appropriate access to care and health maintenance strategies. In contrast, longer-term HIV-infected older persons are more likely to be psychologically accommodated and connected to social agencies addressing HIV infection. These individuals need nonetheless to be prepared for addressing the longer-term effects of HIV infection as well as the long-term toxicities of antiretroviral medications. These subpopulations differ significantly and should be analyzed separately in the future.

Many barriers exist to identifying newly infected older persons, including misinformation, ageism, and HIV/AIDS stigma. HIV/AIDS knowledge remains relatively limited among older people, and HIV primary prevention interventions have not yet been sufficiently tailored to the needs of this group. Secondary prevention interventions aimed at psychopathology, particularly for depressive-spectrum disorders, appear promising in this population and merit further study.

Older persons have also been noted to have an increased risk for systemic HIV disease progression and for decreased survival time. Hence, identification of HIV infection among older persons as early as possible is a priority, and interventions with primary care providers need to be developed to achieve this goal. Yet, research on immunological aspects of HIV disease progression suggests that older HIV-seropositive persons may well remain at risk for more rapid clinical disease progression, regardless of a reduction in lead-time diagnostic bias. Thus immunostimulant therapies need to be developed to supplement antiretroviral therapies for older HIV-infected persons.

Regarding neurocognitive disorders, older age has been associated for some time with an increased risk for HAD and, more recently, with an increased risk for MCMD. The risk of older age for HIV-related subclinical neurocognitive impairment is less well established. Nevertheless, early identification of neurocognitive impairment in older HIV-infected persons should be considered a high priority in that such screening could be used to forestall the eventual development of neurocognitive disorders. A particularly important aspect of research in this area involves the unique predominance of comorbid illnesses among older HIV-infected persons. This population faces comorbidities due not only to complications of HIV-related immunosuppression but also to non-HIV-related illnesses common to older persons in the general population (e.g., DM, hypertension, arthritis, and coronary artery disease). The presence of non-HIV-related comorbidities may play a major role in exacerbating HIV disease progression (by accelerating HIV-related immunologic decrements and/or by reducing antiretroviral medication adherence). When these aspects of comorbidities have been addressed, the consideration remains of how to ensure that these comorbidities do not add to HIV-induced decrements in activities of daily living. The neurological comorbidities of particular concern include DSP, which may increase the rate of falls among older HIV-infected persons, and CVA, which is now an increased risk due to the long-term toxicities of the antiretroviral medications themselves. Finally, neuropsychiatric comorbidities of importance include major depressive disorder and alcohol and psychoactive substance use disorders in this patient subpopulation.

Linking the epidemic among older persons back to health issues faced by the older population generally is an issue of HIV-related caregivers (regardless of caregiver HIV serostatus). The caregiving burden of HIV infection continues to increase nationally and internationally. Unfortunately, all too frequently it is borne by those least able to respond to the burden, particularly older persons. Older persons are further compromised by having to face other caregiver demands, stigma, ageism, lack of HIV/AIDS knowledge among the general public, their own medical burdens, fear of serostatus disclosure, social isolation, and low socioeconomic resources. Further research is sorely needed to address the needs of older caregivers of the HIV infected. With the more rapid progression of the pandemic at the global level, the call must go out for more international research on the issues of older age and HIV infection generally. Additional commitment to research on aging and HIV infection at this time may prove quite beneficial in the not-too-distant future when it will become commonly necessary to address yet more prominent age-related issues among the true elderly with HIV infection.

ACKNOWLEDGMENTS The opinions expressed herein are the views of the authors and do not necessarily reflect the official position of the National Institute of Mental Health or any other part of the U.S. Department of Health and Human Services.
We acknowledge NIMH grants R01 MH58532 and R01 MH/AG61629 to K. Goodkin.

References

Allers CT (1990). AIDS and the older adult. *Gerontologist* 30:405-407.

American Academy of Neurology (1991). Nomenclature and research case definitions for neurological manifestations of human immunodeficiency virus type-1 (HIV-1) infection. *Neurology* 41:778–785.

Baillargeon J, Borucki M, Black SA, and Dunn K (1999). Determinants of survival in HIV-positive patients. *Int J STD AIDS* 10:22–27.

Becker JT, Lopez OL, Dew MA, and Aizenstein HJ (2004). Prevalence of cognitive disorders differs as a function of age in HIV virus infection. *AIDS* 18(Suppl. 1):S27–S34.

Biggar RJ, Kirby KA, Atkinson J, McNeel TS, and Engels E, for the AIDS Cancer Match Study Group (2004). Cancer risk in elderly persons with HIV/AIDS. *J Aquir Immune Defic Syndr* 36(3):861–868.

Blank MB, Mandell DS, Aiken L, and Hadley TR (2002). Co-occurrence of HIV and serious mental illness among Medicaid recipients. *Psychiatr Serv* 53(7): 868–873.

Braithwaite RS, McGinnis KA, Conigliaro J, Maisto SA, Crystal S, Day N, Cook RL, Gordon A, Bridges MW, Seiler JFS, and Justice AC (2005). A temporal and dose–response association between alcohol consumption and medication adherence among veterans in care. *Alcohol Clin Exp Res* 29(7):1190–1197.

Brown TT, Cole SR, Li X, Kingley LA, Palella FJ, Riddler SA, Visscher BR, Margolick JB, and Dobs AS (2005). Antiretroviral therapy and the prevalence of diabetes mellitus in the multicenter AIDS cohort study. *Arch Intern Med* 165:1179–1184.

Burnette D (1997). Grandparents raising grandchildren in the inner city. Families in society. *J Contemp Hum Serv* 78:489–499.

Casau NC (2005). Perspective on HIV infection and aging: emerging research on the horizon. *Clin Infect Dis* 41:855–863.

Catz SL, Heckman TG, Kochman A, and DiMarco M (2001). Rates and correlates of HIV treatment adherence among late middle-aged and older adults living with HIV disease. *Psychol Health Med* 6:47–58.

[CDC] Centers for Disease Control and Prevention (2005). *HIV/AIDS Surveillance Report, 2004* (16:1–46). Atlanta: U.S. Department of Health and Human Services, Centers for Disease Control and Prevention.

Centers for Disease Control and Prevention (2004). *HIV/AIDS Surveillance Report, 2003* (15:1–46). Atlanta: U.S. Department of Health and Human Services, Centers for Disease Control and Prevention.

Cherner M, Ellis RJ, Lazzaretto D, Young C, Rivera-Mindt M, Atkinson H, Grant I, Heaton RK, and the HNRC Group (2004). Effects of HIV-1 Infection and aging on neurobehavioral functioning: preliminary findings. *AIDS* 18(Suppl. 1):S27–S34.

Chesney M, Folkman S, and Chambers D (1996). Coping effectiveness training for men living with HIV: preliminary findings. *Int J STD AIDS* 7(Suppl. 2): 75–82.

Chiesi A, Vella S, Dally LG, Pedersen C, Danner S, Johnson AM, Schwander S, Goebel FD, Glauser M,

Antunes F, and Lundgren JD (1996). Epidemiology and AIDS dementia complex in Europe. *J Aquir Immune Defic Syndr Hum Retrovirol* 11(1): 39–44.

Clifford DB, Evans S, Yang Y, Acosta EP, Goodkin K, Tashima K, Simpson D, Dorfman D, Ribaudo H, Gulick RM, for the A5097s Study Team (2005). Impact of efavirenz on neuropsychological performance and symptoms in HIV-infected individuals. *Ann Intern Med* 143(10):714–721.

Coon DW, Lipman PD, and Ory MG (2003). Designing effective HIV/AIDS social and behavioral interventions for the population of those age 50 and older. *J Aquir Immune Defic Syndr* 33(Suppl. 2):S194–S205.

[DHHS] U.S. Department of Health and Human Services (2005). *Guidelines for the Use of Antiretroviral Agents in HIV-1-Infected Adults and Adolescents.* October, 2005.

Douek DC, McFarland RD, Keiser PH, Gage EA, Massey JM, Haynes BF, Polis MA, Haase AT, Feinberg MB, Sullivan JL, Jamieson BD, Zack JA, Picker LJ, and Koup RA (1998). Changes in thymic function with age and during the treatment of HIV infection. *Nature* 396(6712):690–695.

Ellis RJ, Deutsch R, Heaton RK, Marcotte T, McCutchan JA, Nelson J, Abramson I, Thal LJ, Atkinson JH, Wallace MR, Grant I, for the HNRC Group (1997). Neurocognitive impairment is an independent risk factor for death in HIV infection. *Arch Neurol* 54:416–424.

Forehand R, Steele R, Armistead L, Morse E, Simon P, and Clark L (1998). The family health project: psychosocial adjustment of children whose mothers are HIV infected. *J Consult Clin Psychol* 77:513–520.

Gebo KA, and Moore RD (2004). Treatment of HIV infection in the older patient. *Expert Rev Anti Infect Ther* 2(5)733–743.

Goodkin K, Wilkie FL, Concha M, Hinkin CH, Symes S, Baldewicz TT, Asthana D, Fujimura RK, Lee D, van Zuilen MH, Khamis I, Shapshak P, and Eisdorfer C (2001). Aging and neuro-AIDS conditions: a potential interaction with the changing spectrum of HIV-1 associated morbidity and mortality in the era of HAART? *J Clin Epidemiol* 54:S35–S43.

Goodkin K, Heckman T, Siegel K, Linsk N, Khamis I, Lee D, Lecusay R, Poindexter CC, Mason SJ, Suarez P, and Eisdorfer C (2003). "Putting a face" on HIV infection/AIDS in older adults: a psychosocial context. *J Aquir Immune Defic Syndr* 33 (Suppl. 2):S171–S184.

Goodkin K, Shapshak P, Asthana D, Zheng W, Concha M, Wilkie FL, Molina R, Lee D, Suarez P, Symes S, and Khamis I (2004). Older age and plasma viral load in HIV-1 infection. *AIDS* 18(Suppl. 1):S87–S98.

Hansell PS, Hughes CB, Clinadro G, Russo P, Budin WC, Hartman B, and Hernandez OC (1998). The effect of a social support boosting intervention on stress, coping, and social support in caregivers of children with HIV/AIDS. *Nurs Res* 47:79–86.

Hardy, DJ, Hinkin CH, Satz P, Stenquist PK, van Gorp WG, and Moore LH (1999). Age differences and neurocognitive performance in HIV-infected adults. *N Z J Psychol* 28:94–101.

Hawaii State Department of Health (2006). *HIV/AIDS Surveillance Semi-Annual Report.* Retrieved April 5, 2007, from www.state.hi.us/health/healthy-lifestyles/std-aids/aboutus/prg-aids/aids_rep/index.html.

Heaton R, Antinori A, Goodkin K, Joseph J, Marder K, and Marra C (2005). Algorithm for classifying HIV-related neurocognitive disorders. In *HIV Infection and the Central Nervous System: Developed and Resource Limited Settings* (p. 50). Pavia: Edizioni Internazionali.

Heckman TG, Kochman AR, Kalichman SC, Masten J, and Catz S (2001). A coping improvement intervention for middle-aged and older adults living with HIV/AIDS. *AIDS Care* 12:613–624.

Heckman TG, Heckman BD, Kochman A, Sikkema KJ, Suhr J, and Goodkin K (2002). Psychological symptoms among persons 50 years of age and older living with HIV disease. *Aging Ment Health* 6(2):121–128.

Heckman TG, Barcikowski R, Ogles B, Suhr J, Carlson B, Holroyd K, and Garske JA (2006). Telephone-delivered coping improvement group intervention for middle-aged and older adults living with HIV/AIDS. *Ann Behav Med* 32(1):343–354.

Hinkin CH, Castellon SA, Atkinson JH, and Goodkin K (2001). Neuropsychiatric aspects of HIV-infection among older adults. *J Clin Epidemiol* 54:S44–S52.

Hinkin CH, Hardy DJ, Mason JI, Castellon SA, Durvasula RS, Lam MN, and Stefaniak M (2004). Medication adherence in HIV-infected adults: effect of patient age, cognitive status, and substance abuse. *AIDS* 18(Suppl. 1):S19–S26.

Howard BH, Phillips CV, Matinhure N, Goodman KJ, McCurdy SA, and Johnson CA (2006). Barriers and incentives to orphan care in a time of AIDS and economic crisis: a cross-sectional survey of caregivers in rural Zimbabwe. *BMC Public Health* 6:27.

Inungu JN, Mokotoff ED, and Kent JB (2001). Characteristics of HIV infection in patients fifty years or older in Michigan. *AIDS Patient Care STDS* 15:567–573.

Jain MH, Skiest DJ, Cloud JW, Jain CL, Burns D, and Berggren RE (2003). Changes in mortality related to human immunodeficiency virus infection: comparative analysis of inpatient deaths in 1995 and in 1999–2000. *Clin Infect Dis* 36:1030–1038.

Janssen RS, Nwanyanwu OC, Selik RM, and Stehr-Green JK (1992). Epidemiology of human immunodeficiency virus encephalopathy in the United States. *Neurology* 42:1472–1476.

Justice AC, McGinnis DA, Atkinson JH, Heaton RK, Young C, Sadek J, Madenwald T, Becker J, Conigliaro J, Brown ST, Rimland D, Crystal S, Simberkoff M, for the VACS 5 Project Team (2004). Psychiatric and neurocognitive disorders among HIV-positive and negative veterans in care: veterans aging cohort five-site study. *AIDS* 18(Suppl. 1):S49–S60.

Kaufmann GR, Bloch M, Finlayson R, Zaunders J, Smith D, and Cooper DA (2002). The extent of HIV-1-related immunodeficiency and age predict the long-term CD4 T lymphocyte response to potent antiretroviral therapy. *AIDS* 16(3):359–367.

Keller MJ, Hausdorff JM, Kyne L, and Wei JY (1999). Is age a negative prognostic indicator in HIV infection or AIDS? *Aging (Milano)* 11(1):35–38.

Kespichayawattana J, and VanLandingham M (2003). Effects of coresidence and caregiving on health of Thai parents of adult children with AIDS. *J Nurs Scholarsh* 35(3):217–224.

Kilbourne AM, Justice AC, Rabeneck L, Rodriguez-Barrada M, Weissman S, for the VACS 3 Project Team (2001). General medical and psychiatric comorbidity among HIV-infected veterans in the post-HAART era. *J Clin Epidemiol* 54:S22–S28.

Knodel J, VanLandingham M, Saengtienchai C, and Im-em W (2001). Older people and AIDS: quantitative evidence of the impact in Thailand. *Soc Sci Med* 52(9):1313–1327.

Kwiatkowski CF, and Booth RE (2003). HIV risk behaviors among older American drug users. *J Acquir Immune Defic Syndr* 33(Suppl. 2):S131–S137.

Levy JA, Ory MG, and Crystal S (2003). HIV/AIDS interventions for midlife and older adults: current status and challenges. *J Acquir Immune Defic Syndr* 33(Suppl. 2):S59–S67.

Lindsey E, Hirschfeld M, and Tlou S (2003). Home-based care in Botswana: experiences of older women and young girls. *Health Care Women Int* 24(6):486–501.

Linsk NL (2000). HIV among older adults: age-specific issues in prevention and treatment. *AIDS Read* 10(7):430–440.

Linsk NL, and Mason S (2004). Stresses on grandparents and other relatives caring for children affected by HIV/AIDS. *Health Soc Work* 29(2):127–136.

Maggiolo F, Ripamonti D, Arici C, Gregis G, Quinzan G, Camacho GA, Ravasio L, and Suter F (2002). Simpler regimens may enhance adherence to antiretrovirals in HIV-infected patients. *HIV Clin Trials* 3(5):371–378.

Manfredi R (2004). HIV infection and advanced age. Emerging epidemiological, clinical, and management issues. *Ageing Res Rev* 3:31–54.

Marcotte TD, Lazzaretto D, Scott JC, Roberts E, Woods SP, Letendre S, for the HNRC Group (2006). Visual attention deficits are associated with driving accidents in cognitively impaired HIV-infected individuals. *J Clin Exp Neuropsychol* 28(1):13–28.

McArthur JC, Hoover DR, Bacellar H, Miller EN, Cohen BA, Becker JT, Graham NMH, McArthur JH, Selnes OA, Jacobson LP, Visscher BR, Concha M, and Saah A (1993). Dementia in AIDS patients: incidence and risk factors. *Neurology* 43:2245–2252.

McGinnis KA, Fine MJ, Sharma RK, Skanderson M, Wagner JH, Rodriguez-Barradas MC, Rabeneck L, and Justice AC (2003). Understanding racial disparities in HIV using data from the veterans aging cohort 3-site study and VA administration data. *Am J Public Health* 93:1728–1733.

Miami-Dade County Health Department (2006). *HIV/AIDS Surveillance Report.* Retrieved March 1, 2006, from http://www.dadehealth.org/downloads/MAR-06.pdf.

Neundorfer MM, Harris PB, Britton PJ, and Lynch DA (2005). HIV-risk factors for midlife and older women. *Gerontologist* 45(5):617–625.

Nicastri E, Chiesi A, Angeletti C, Sarmati L, Palmisano L, Geraci A, Andreoni M, and Vella S (2005). Italian Antiretroviral Treatment Group (IATG). Clinical outcome after 4 years follow-up of HIV-seropositive subjects with incomplete virologic or immunologic response to HAART. *J Med Virol* 76(2):153–160.

Ogu C, and Wolfe LR (1994). *Midlife and Older Women and HIV/AIDS.* Washington, DC: AARP.

Palepu A, Horton NJ, Tibbetts N, Meli S, and Samet JH (2004). Uptake and adherence to highly active antiretroviral therapy among HIV-infected people with alcohol and other substance use problems: the impact of substance abuse treatment. *Addiction* 99:361–368.

Pitts M, Grierson J, and Misson S (2005). Growing older with HIV: a study of health, social and economic circumstances for people living with HIV in Australia over the age of 50 years. *AIDS Patient Care STDS* 19(7):460–465.

Poindexter CC, and Linsk NL (1999). HIV-related stigma in a sample of HIV-affected older female African-American caregivers. *Soc Work* 44:46–61.

Powderly WG, Landay A, and Lederman MM (1998). Recovery of the immune system with antiretroviral therapy: the end of opportunism? *JAMA* 280(1):72–77.

Rabkin JC, McElhiney, and Ferrando S (2004a). Mood and substance use disorders in older adults with HIV/AIDS: methodological issues and preliminary evidence. *AIDS* 18(Suppl. 1):S43–S48.

Rabkin JG, McElhiney M, Ferrando SJ, Van Gorp W, and Lin SH (2004b). Predictors of employment of men with HIV/AIDS: a longitudinal study. *Psychosom Med* 66(1):72–78.

Remien RH, and Johnson JG (2004). Psychiatric disorders and symptoms associated with sexual risk behavior. *Psychiatr Times* 2004:21.

Saah AJ, Hoover DR, He Y, Kingsley LA, and Phair JP (1994). Factors influencing survival after AIDS: report from the Multicenter AIDS Cohort Study (MACS). *J Acquir Immune Defic Syndr* 7(3):287–295.

Sambamoorthi U, Walkup J, Olfson M, and Crystal S (2000). Antidepressant treatment and health services utilization among HIV-infected Medicaid patients diagnosed with depression. *J Gen Intern Med* 15:311–320.

Sax PE (2006). Strategies for management and treatment of dyslipidemia in HIV/AIDS. *AIDS Care* 18(2): 149–157.

Saule P, Trauet J, Dutriez V, Lekeux V, Dessaint JP, and Labalette M (2006). Accumulation of memory T cells from childhood to old age: central and effector memory cells in CD4(+) versus effector memory and terminally differentiated memory cells in CD8(+) compartment. *Mech Ageing Dev* 127(3):274–281.

Shah SS, McGowan JP, Smith C, Blum S, and Klein RS (2002). Co-morbid conditions, treatment, and health maintenance in older persons with HIV infection in New York City. *Clin Infect Dis* 35:1238–1243.

Sheth AN, Moore RD, and Gebo K (2006). Provision of general and HIV-specific health maintenance in middle aged and older patients in an urban HIV clinic. *AIDS Patient Care STDS* 20(5):318–325.

Ship JA, Wolff A, and Selik RM (1991). Epidemiology of acquired immune deficiency syndrome in persons aged 50 years or older. *J Acquir Immune Defic Syndr* 4:84–88.

Siegel K, Schrimshaw EW, and Dean L (1999). Symptom interpretation: implications for delay in HIV testing and care among HIV-infected late middle-aged and older adults. *AIDS Care* 11(5):525–535.

Simpson DM, Katzenstein DA, Hughes MD, Hammer SM, Williamson DL, Jiang Q, and Pi JT (1998). Neuromuscular function in HIV infection: analysis of a placebo-controlled combination antiretroviral trial. AIDS Clinical Trial Group 175-801 Study Team. *AIDS* 12(18):2425–2432.

Skiest DJ, Rubinstein E, Carley N, Gioiella L, and Lyons R (1996). The importance of comorbidity in HIV-infected patients over 55. A retrospective case-control study. *Am J Med* 101:605–611.

Stall R, and Catania J (1994). AIDS risk behaviors among late middle-aged and elderly Americans. *Arch Intern Med* 154(1):57–63.

Stein M, Herman DS, Trisvan E, Pirraglia P, Engler P, and Anderson BJ (2005). Alcohol use and sexual risk behavior among human immunodeficiency virus–positive persons. *Alcohol Clin Exp Res* 29: 837–843.

Stern Y, McDermott MP, Albert S, Palumbo D, Selnes OA, McArthur J, Sacktor N, Schifitto G, Kieburtz K, Epstein L, Marder KS. Dana Consortium on the Therapy of HIV-Dementia and Related Cognitive Disorders (2001). Factors associated with incident human immunodeficiency virus-dementia. *Arch Neurol* 58(3):473–479.

Stoff DM (2004). Mental health research in HIV/AIDS and aging: problems and prospects. *AIDS* 18 (Suppl.):S3–S10.

Sulkowski MS, and Thomas DL (2005). Perspectives on HIV/hepatitis C virus co-infection, illicit drug use and mental illness. *AIDS* 19(Suppl. 3):S8–S12.

Szerlip MA, Desalvo KB, and Szerlip HM (2005). Predictors of HIV-infection in older adults. *J Aging Health* 17(3):293–304.

Tebas P, Henry K, Mondy K, Deeks S, Valdez H, Cohen C, and Powderly WG (2002). Effect of prolonged discontinuation of successful antiretroviral therapy on CD4+ T cell decline in human immunodeficiency virus–infected patients: implications for intermittent therapeutic strategies. *J Infect Dis* 186(6): 851–854.

Valcour V, Shikuma C, Shiramizu B, Walters M, Poff P, Selnes O, Holck P, Grove J, and Sacktor N (2004). Higher frequency of dementia in older HIV-1 individuals. *Neurology* 63:822–827.

van Gorp WG, Miller EN, Marcotte TD, Dixon W, Paz D, Selnes O, Wesch J, Becker JT, Hinkin CH, Mitrushina M, Satz P, Weisman JD, Buckingham SL, and Stenquist PK (1994). The relationship between age and cognitive impairment in HIV-1 infection: findings from Multicenter AIDS Cohort Study and clinical cohort. *Neurology* 44:94–101.

Walkup J, Crystal S, and Samabamoorthi U (1999). Schizophrenia and major affective disorder among Medicaid recipients with HIV/AIDS in New Jersey. *Am J Public Health* 89:1101–1103.

Watters MR, Poff PW, Shiramizu BT, Holck PS, Fast KMS, Shikuma CM, and Valcour VG (2004). Symptomatic distal polyneuropathy in HIV after age 50. *Neurology* 62:1378–1383.

Weiler PG, Mungas D, and Pomerantz S (1988). AIDS as a cause of dementia in the elderly. *J Am Geriatr Soc* 36:139–141.

Wight RG, Aneshensel CS, Murphy DA, Miller-Martinez D, and Beals KP (2006). Perceived HIV stigma in AIDS caregiving dyads. *Soc Sci Med* 62(2):444–456.

Wilkie FL, Goodkin K, van Zuilen MH, Lee D, Lecusay R, Khamis I, Concha M, and Symes S (2003). The cognitive effects of HIV-1 infection in younger and older adults. *J Acquir Immune Defic Syndr Hum Retrovirol* 33(Suppl. 2):S93–S105.

Wilkie FL, Goodkin K, Eisdorfer C, Morgan R, Feaster D, Fletcher MA, Symes S, and Blaney N (1998). Mild cognitive impairment and risk of mortality in HIV-1 infection. *J Neuropsychiatry Clin Neurosci* 10:125–132.

Zablotsky DL (1998). Overlooked, ignored and forgotten: older women at risk for HIV infection and AIDS. *Res Aging* 20:760–766.

Zingmond DS, Wenger NS, Crystal S, Joyce GF, Liu H, Sambamoorthi U, Lillard LA, Leibowitz AA, Shapiro MF, and Bozzette SA (2001). HCSUS Consortium. Circumstances at HIV diagnosis and progression of disease in older HIV-infected Americans. *Am J Public Health* 91(7):1117–1120.

Zingmond DS, Kilbourne AM, Justice AC, Wenger NS, Rodriguez-Barradas M, Rabeneck L, Taub D, Weissman S, Briggs J, Wagner J, Smola S, and Bozzette SA (2003). Differences in symptom expression in older HIV-positive patients: the Veterans Aging Cohort 3 Site Study and HIV Cost and Service Utilization Study experience. *J Acquir Immune Defic Syndr* 33(Suppl. 2):S84–S92.

Part VIII

AIDS Psychiatric Treatment and Psychotherapeutic Modalities

Chapter 27

Psychiatric Interventions

Karin Dorell, Jocelyn Soffer,
and Jack M. Gorman

Psychosocial interventions for patients with HIV are treatments aimed to alleviate psychological distress associated with medical and psychiatric illness, including depression and anxiety, in people with HIV. These treatments have been shown to enhance adaptive coping strategies, provide social support, improve a patient's sense of purpose and self-esteem, and help with overall adjustment to living with HIV infection. Psychosocial interventions can occur in individual or group formats, such as informal support groups or groups that target specific populations (e.g., women, men, mothers, or caregivers). Interventions might target specific concerns, such as HIV risk reduction or treatment adherence (Aversa and Kimberlin, 1996). Potential psychosocial interventions span the spectrum from individual to family or group psychotherapy and include psychodynamic/psychoanalytic, interpersonal, behavioral, and supportive approaches. Because of the spectrum of social, psychological, and neuropsychiatric consequences of HIV infection, the psychiatrist needs to consider the range of possible treatment modalities, choosing an appropriate intervention or combination of treatments for each individual.

Psychological distress in persons with HIV infection has been associated with disease progression, mortality, and quality of life. Considering a biopsychosocial model, emotional distress in HIV can be viewed as secondary to one or more of the following:

1. Medical aspects: physical symptoms, pain, and compromised energy level.
2. Psychological and psychiatric aspects: comorbid psychiatric disorders; difficulty coping with severe medical illness; shame and guilt; bereavement and loss; conflicts over sexuality, dependency, meaning of life and spirituality; cultural-specific issues.
3. Social aspects: negotiation of social and intimate relationships, disclosure, stigma and acceptance by the community, unemployment, finances, benefits, access to care, and housing.

Psychological distress and quality of life have been shown to affect immunological measures in HIV-infected patients (Goodkin et al., 1992b; Burack et al., 1993; Kertzner et al., 1993; Sahs et al., 1994: Evans et al., 1995; Kemeny et al., 1995; Theorell et al., 1995). Depressed mood and stressful life events have been linked to lower CD4 cell counts (Goodkin et al., 1992b; Burack et al., 1993; Evans et al., 1995; Kemeny et al., 1995), lymphocyte proliferation to phytohemagglutinin (Kemeny et al., 1995; Goodkin et al., 1996), natural killer cell cytotoxicity (Goodkin et al., 1996), and increased serum neopterin levels (Kemeny et al., 1995). Kemeny and Dean (1995) found that while grief reactions were unrelated to CD4 decline and symptom onset, aspects of depression such as self-reproach were predictive of CD4 loss (Goodkin et al., 1996).

Social support and active coping with stressful life events have been associated with higher CD4 cell counts (Goodkin et al., 1992a; Theorell et al., 1995), with effects observed for up to 4 years in follow-up (Kemeny et al., 1995). These social interventions have been shown to lower anxiety and HIV risk behaviors among HIV-positive adults (Leserman et al., 1992; Linn et al., 1993; Hall, 1999) Evidence for a positive effect of behavioral interventions on immunity in individuals infected with HIV is still somewhat scattered and comes from a limited number of controlled trials. Hence, while improving immunological status should be thought of as a potential benefit of psychosocial treatment for people with HIV infection, relieving the suffering inherent to psychiatric illness and improving quality of life remain the primary goals.

INDIVIDUAL PSYCHOTHERAPY

Cognitive Behavioral Psychotherapy

Considerable interest has developed in the role that cognitive-behavioral techniques might play in ameliorating the stress and distress commonly experienced by patients with HIV infection. Originally developed by Aaron Beck and traditionally used for patients with depression, cognitive-behavioral therapy (CBT) has been demonstrated in the last decade to be useful in conjunction with other stress management techniques for some of the psychological challenges and problems that patients with HIV face. In CBT, the patient learns to identify emotions and actions that coincide with particular negative behaviors, and to develop adaptive emotional and behavioral responses to stressors that lead to those behaviors.

In a recent pilot project, CBT was combined with motivational interviewing in an intervention consisting of eight weekly individual sessions with a trained therapist. Significant reductions in substance use were found among the HIV-positive individuals studied (Parsons et al., 2005). There were positive trends toward increased HIV medication adherence that did not reach statistical significance. The authors cited the 73% retention rate over the 8 weeks as evidence of the feasibility of such interventions for this population.

Some studies have suggested that ethnicity might play a role in the outcomes of psychotherapy interventions in patients with HIV. Markowitz et al. (2000) randomized 101 patients to 16 weeks of interpersonal psychotherapy, CBT, supportive psychotherapy, or imipramine plus supportive psychotherapy. African-American subjects in this study who were assigned to CBT had significantly poorer outcomes.

Other studies have compared CBT to contingency management (CM) interventions. CM strategies employ behavioral reinforcement techniques in which a patient receives a tangible reward (such as a voucher for goods or services) for refraining from negative behaviors (such as drug use) or demonstrating positive behaviors. One study of changes in HIV risk behaviors among patients receiving combined pharmacological and behavioral interventions for heroin and cocaine dependence demonstrated positive effects in all treatment groups, consisting of CBT alone, CM alone, combination CBT and CM, and a group therapy control group (Schroeder et al., 2006). The observed behavioral risk reductions were largely unrelated to treatment modality. Some measures of HIV risk behaviors, however, were significantly reduced in the group receiving both CBT and CM, such as the reported cessation of unprotected sex.

Despite the studies cited above, the bulk of the literature on CBT for patients with HIV pertains to group rather than individual settings for the intervention; information on individual CBT in this population remains sparse.

Psychodynamic Psychotherapy

Most psychological interventions in the HIV population focus on supporting and counseling to enhance adjustment to living with HIV. Psychodynamically oriented psychotherapies can be used when the functioning of the self is compromised by HIV illness. The use of such an approach to further an understanding of the conflicts and struggles of the HIV-positive patient has been described by multiple authors (Rogers, 1989; Allers and Benjack, 1991; Weiss, 1997; Cohen et al., 1998; Cohen, 1999; Ricart et al., 2002). Core themes that can be effectively addressed with psychodynamically oriented approaches include acceptance of illness and decreasing conflicts surrounding sexuality (Weiss, 1997). With the advent of new antiretroviral treatments, new psychotherapy themes have emerged, such as living with a chronic illness, maintaining a sense of life purpose, and negotiating relationships (Selwyn et al., 1998; Farber and McDaniel, 1999).

Studies have shown a strong association of childhood sexual abuse, HIV risk behavior, and nonadherence to HIV treatment (Allers and Benjack, 1991; Lodico and DiClemente, 1994; James and Meyerding, 1997; Lenderking et al., 1997; Thompson et al., 1997; Wingood and DiClemente, 1997; Goodman et al., 1998; Hutton et al., 2001). Addressing childhood trauma in psychodynamically oriented psychotherapy can improve psychiatric symptoms, decrease risk behaviors, and increase adherence (Ricart et al., 2002). Controlled studies of psychodynamically oriented psychotherapies remain of difficult design; therefore, conclusive evidence of the efficacy of this modality is still missing.

Interpersonal Psychotherapy

The primary goal of interpersonal psychotherapy is to treat a depressive episode by helping patients link the depression to specific interpersonal stresses and then facilitating resolution of those stresses. In extensive research examining the role of environmental influences on mood, several common problem areas were identified, including unresolved grief following the death of a loved one, role transitions (difficulty adjusting to changed life circumstances), interpersonal role disputes (conflicts with a significant other), and interpersonal deficits (impoverished social networks).

Interpersonal psychotherapy has been studied in the treatment of patients with coronary disease (Koszycki et al., 2004) and is linked with significant reduction in scores on both the Hamilton Depression Scale and the Beck Depression Inventory II. Medicated and unmedicated patients responded similarly

to interpersonal psychotherapy, a finding suggesting this modality to be an effective alternative to medication. Studies specifically addressing the HIV population have reported similar positive results. One study found better outcomes with interpersonal psychotherapy as compared to both supportive psychotherapy alone and supportive psychotherapy with imipramine (Markowitch et al., 1995, 1998). In another study, Catalán et al. (1999) found that interpersonal psychotherapy was more effective than CBT or supportive therapy alone, and was comparable to supportive psychotherapy plus pharmacotherapy for treating depressive symptoms in HIV-positive patients.

COUPLE THERAPY

The psychological well-being of the HIV patient will inevitably affect the social systems in which he or she is involved. Both parties in a couple face significant challenges in managing the relationship and the role each person plays. Relationships are always affected by illness of one of the individuals. Issues involving role dynamics as well as uncertainty about the future commonly present challenges to the relationship. Because of the sexual nature of HIV transmission, other themes are likely to emerge. Mixed-status couples will need to negotiate satisfying and safe sexual practices. The AIDS-infected person can lose interest in sexual relations or feel unattractive because of the progressive nature of the illness. The couple is further affected by the proximity of death; some people may emotionally distance themselves to protect their partner or themselves. Guilt and blame are common in serodiscordant and seroconcordant couples.

Therapists can help couples manage the emotional complexities and psychological impact of HIV infection. Studies evaluating the efficacy of psychiatric interventions in this domain have largely focused on the ability of couple therapy to reduce unprotected sex within discordant couples. A number of studies have demonstrated that providing intervention sessions jointly to both members of a dyad is efficacious in promoting HIV counseling and testing, as well as for increasing condom use. El Bassel and colleagues (2003) examined the efficacy of a six-session relationship-based intervention provided to women and their sexual partners in a population displaying high-risk sexual behaviors. The intervention significantly reduced the number of unprotected sexual acts at 12 months post-intervention compared with a control group. No significant differences were observed when comparing couples receiving the intervention together or separately (El-Bassel et al., 2005).

GROUP PSYCHOTHERAPY

Group psychotherapy addressing the psychological distress associated with medical illness has been an accepted form of psychotherapy for over 50 years. The efficacy of such treatment has been most frequently examined in studies with cancer patients. There is compelling evidence that group interventions are effective in reducing mood disturbance and pain and in improving quality of life for patients with cancer. Furthermore, there is some evidence that psychotherapy may extend the survival of cancer patients (Blake-Mortimer et al., 1981; Telch and Telch, 1986; Leszcz et al., 2004), although not all studies have confirmed this finding.

HIV psychotherapy groups can be peer led or therapist led, educational or therapeutic, and general or focused on a specific theme such as bereavement, parenting, or discordant couples. Groups can also address particular concerns such as spirituality or target particular populations such as youths. Among the different types of group treatments, those that have been more thoroughly studied are the cognitive behavioral groups, the supportive groups, and the emotive expressive groups (Zisook et al., 1998).

Support Groups

Sikkema and colleagues (2004a) demonstrated the efficacy of an AIDS-related bereavement coping intervention for men and women living with HIV/AIDS. The intervention significantly improved general health-related quality of life and health issues specific to HIV/AIDS compared to community standard of care. The women in the group intervention exhibited more improvement than men in health-related quality of life.

Goodkin and colleagues (1998) reported on a randomized controlled trial of a bereavement support group intervention conducted with HIV-positive and negative homosexual men who had lost a close friend or intimate partner within the previous 6 months. The group receiving the intervention demonstrated a de-

crease in psychological distress and grief level. There was also an improvement of immunological factors in the intervention group compared to the control group, the clinical relevance of which was supported by a decrement in health care use at 6 months post-intervention. Because bereavement is an example of a severe life stressor, this conclusion may also hold for stressor management interventions generally.

Group therapy has been widely advocated for victims of abuse (Van der Kolk et al., 1993). Feelings of mistrust, isolation, and anxiety in abuse victims frequently result in emotional and/or physical detachment from others. Group therapy appears to be well suited for the treatment of traumatized individuals who might otherwise maintain stances of isolation and avoidance.

HIV-positive individuals are often victims of childhood physical and sexual trauma. Psychotherapy groups for HIV-positive individuals who experienced trauma and abuse are particularly indicated. Sikkema and colleagues (2004b) reported that more than 75% of those who participated in trauma-focused group intervention showed some improvement in mood.

As Sikkema points out, given the chaotic and stressful life situations of trauma survivors, an overemphasis on exposure and trauma could be more detrimental than beneficial. The focus should be on skills building, coping tools, and practical learning of the application of these modalities in everyday life.

Cognitive Behavioral Groups

A considerable literature supports the efficacy of CBT group interventions for patients with HIV infection. A study in 2002 assessed a 16-week cognitive-behavioral group psychotherapy intervention for HIV-infected patients, finding that patients improved both on measures of depression (Beck Depression Inventory) and anxiety (State/Trait Anxiety Inventory), with effects that persisted at 3-month follow-up (Blanch et al., 2002). Patients with higher levels of anxiety at baseline showed the greatest improvement on anxiety subscale scores, thus such techniques may be particularly helpful in certain subgroups of patients.

Lee and colleagues (1999) examined cognitive-behavioral group therapy in combination with antidepressant use in HIV-infected patients; 13 out of 15 patients completed the 20-week course of therapy, attending an average of 15 sessions. The authors found decreased depression scores compared to baseline in the intervention group, with further decreases in measures of depression observed at 1-year follow-up.

Only a few published controlled trials comparing group psychotherapy and medication treatment are available, with inconsistent results. In a randomized, double-blind, placebo-controlled study comparing the efficacy and safety of fluoxetine plus group psychotherapy versus group psychotherapy alone in HIV-positive men, Zisook and colleagues (1998) reported the efficacy of fluoxetine over and above group psychotherapy for the treatment of HIV-associated major depression.

Studies comparing the efficacy of CBT interventions with that other types of psychotherapeutic modalities have similarly yielded mixed results. Some have demonstrated CBT to be superior to other modalities. For example, a pilot study of Chinese patients with symptomatic HIV disease compared the effects of cognitive-behavioral group therapy and peer support/counseling on psychological distress and quality of life (Molassiotis et al., 2002). Both groups met weekly for 12 weeks and were compared to a control group with no psychosocial intervention. Mood and quality of life were assessed before and after the intervention and at 3-month follow-up, with greater improvement of mood and quality of life in the CBT group than in the other two groups.

Other studies have shown CBT techniques to be as effective as other psychotherapy modalities. A study comparing CBT and experiential group psychotherapy for HIV-infected gay men found that after 17 sessions, both groups had significantly decreased distress levels compared to a waiting-list control group. However, there were no significant changes in coping styles, social support, or emotional expression (Mulder et al., 1995).

Kelly and colleagues (1993) examined 68 depressed men with HIV who were randomly assigned to eight sessions of a cognitive-behavioral group, social support group, or comparison condition, measuring distress symptoms, substance use, and sexual practices. Both treatment groups relative to the control group had decreased depression, hostility, and somatization after the intervention. The authors reported some benefit of each treatment group in reducing negative behaviors at 3-month follow-up; the cognitive-behavioral group had less frequent illicit drug use, whereas the

social support group had overall reduced psychiatric symptoms and decreased unprotected sex.

A recent prospective, multisite, phase III clinical trial examined a group intervention combining CBT with stress management, relaxation techniques, and expressive-supportive therapeutic strategies (Laperriere et al., 2005). The authors reported significantly decreased depression scores on the Beck Depression Inventory for women immediately following the intervention, with maintenance of these decreased levels at 1-year follow-up.

A fascinating line of research has explored the effect of CBT interventions on immunological parameters, positing that through stress reduction, such interventions might alter the hypothalamic-pituitary-adrenal axis, shown to be altered in many patients with HIV infection. Mulder and colleagues (1995) studied CD4 counts and T-cell response in asymptomatic HIV-infected homosexual men treated with a 15-week CBT or experiential group therapy program. While neither group had a significant change in the measured parameters, it was noteworthy that CD4 counts declined less in subjects (in both groups) whose distress levels were more decreased.

Along these theoretical lines, researchers have conducted a number of studies examining the effects of a cognitive-behavioral stress management (CBSM) intervention on various immunological, psychological, and endocrine factors. The treatment protocol in these studies consisted of 10 weekly group sessions of three to six men, led by two facilitators. Each session was divided into 45 minutes of relaxation techniques (including muscle relaxation, autogenic training, guided imagery, meditation, and breathing exercises) and 90 minutes of stress management (included increasing awareness of the effects of stress, identifying automatic thoughts, using cognitive restructuring, increasing coping skills and assertiveness, and enhancing strategies for anger management and use of social supports) (Antoni et al., 2005). Patients were instructed to practice relaxation exercises twice daily between sessions and were assigned cognitive homework exercises. The studies used a wait-list comparison group as a control. Compared to the control group, the CBSM group showed significantly lower post-treatment levels of self-reported depressed affect, anxiety, anger, and confusion—that is, a general decrease in psychological distress. Multiple endocrine changes were observed to be associated with these effects. The treatment group had lower levels of urinary cortisol, with decreases in depressed mood paralleling cortisol decreases in urine. The CBSM group also had decreased urinary norepinephrine (NE) output, with anxiety decreases correlating with NE reduction (Antoni et al., 2000a). Cruess and colleagues (2000) also found statistically significant increases in testosterone in the CBSM group, with altered free testosterone inversely related to changes in measures of distress. There were immunological benefits seen in the CBSM group as well, with greater numbers of T-cytotoxic/suppressor cells (CD3+CD8+) found at 6- to 12-month follow-up compared to the control group. A greater NE decrease and greater frequency of relaxation home practice during the intervention predicted higher CD3+CD8+ counts at follow-up (Antoni et al., 2000b). Men in the CBSM group at 6- to 12-month follow-up also had higher transitional naïve T-cell counts than those in control subjects, independent of initial number of naïve T cells and HIV virus load (Antoni et al., 2002).

More recently, Sherman and colleagues (2004) as well as Leszcz and colleagues (2004) reported a positive impact of group intervention on immunological and endocrine measures as well as on mood at different phases of illness in HIV and cancer patients. Collectively, these results provide promising evidence that stress management may be associated with improved immunological reconstitution in this population of men. Further research needs to be done to replicate these findings.

In the past decade, researchers have also examined whether CBT methods might help reduce common risk behaviors in HIV-positive populations, again with somewhat mixed results. One study examined the efficacy of a cognitive-behavioral intervention to reduce HIV risk behaviors in crack and injection drug users, comparing a two-session standard drug counseling and testing protocol developed by the National Institute on Drug Abuse (NIDA) to a more intensive nine-session intervention with both group and individual sessions that included the standard counseling and testing (Herschberger et al., 2003). The researchers measured cessation and/or reduction of drug use (through urine tests and self-report), entry into drug treatment, and increased condom use, concluding that the theory-based cognitive-behavioral intervention had limited advantages over the standard one.

Other studies have compared CBT to contingency management (CM) interventions. As described above,

CM strategies employ behavioral reinforcement techniques in which a patient receives a reward for refraining from negative behaviors or demonstrating positive behaviors. Shoptaw and colleagues (2005) recently demonstrated better results for CM treatment alone and CM combined with CBT than for standard CBT alone, in a population of urban gay and bisexual men, assessed for methamphetamine use and HIV-related sexual risk behaviors.

Expressive Emotive Groups

Although fewer reports assess the efficacy of expressive emotive group psychotherapy, available studies confirm the clinical utility of this group modality (Weiss et al., 2003). Different intervention styles aiming to reduce emotional distress through psychoeducation and coping styles training have also been proposed. Chesney and colleagues (2003) compared the effects of a theory-based coping effectiveness training (CET) intervention with an active informational control and a wait-list control on psychological distress and positive mood in HIV-positive gay men. The CET participants showed significantly greater decreases in perceived stress and burnout as well as decreases in anxiety. Treatment group differences for positive morale were maintained at 6 and 12 months.

Spiritually Focused Groups

More recently, attention to the spiritual well-being of the medically ill has added a different dimension to the psychological treatment of these patients. The literature is generally supportive of the positive role of spirituality in coping with serious illness and dying (Chibnall et al., 2002; McClain et al., 2003; Newlin et al., 2003). Spirituality can help to counteract the negative effects of depression and emotional distress on health-related quality of life and illness morbidity (McClain et al., 2003; Newlin et al., 2003). Facing terminal illness is an inherently spiritual dilemma because of questions regarding life meaning and purpose as well as separation anxieties. Therefore, medical care that recognizes and supports the spiritual nature of human beings can help promote the spiritual well-being that many patients seek at the end of life. Very few studies have evaluated the efficacy of addressing spirituality in group psychotherapy. Miller and colleagues (2005) found that patients receiving such an intervention had significantly fewer symptoms of depression and death-related feelings of meaninglessness and had significantly better spiritual well-being as compared to control patients. More substantial research assessing the efficacy of spirituality in group treatment should be forthcoming.

Group Treatment in Pediatric Population

Youths with HIV sometimes have additional risk factors, including disrupted home life, family history of mental illness and substance abuse, experience of death, fear of disclosure, and danger of rejection (Frederick et al., 2000; Bachanas et al., 2001). A high incidence of psychiatric symptoms has been reported in children and adolescents affected by HIV (Gaugham et al., 2004; Misdrahi et al., 2004). Social, psychological, and treatment issues are age specific and usually involve difficulties with peers, self-image, sexuality, and planning for life as an adult. Nonadherence is also a common problem in this population. The efficacy of group treatment modalities in children affected by HIV was reported by Funck-Brentano and colleagues (2005). This pilot study suggests that a peer support group intervention is associated with an improvement in adolescents' emotional well-being, which can have a positive influence on medical outcomes.

Family Therapy

Medically ill parents who care for their children while simultaneously coping with ongoing physical symptoms face particular challenges and are especially vulnerable to psychosocial stressors that may affect their health. These parents often struggle with social and financial difficulties that have a great impact on their children's well-being. If the children themselves are HIV positive, maintaining healthy family dynamics can be especially difficult to achieve. Issues around disclosure, emotional reactions to the HIV diagnosis, fear of death, role adjustments, loss and bereavement, and social stigma are all examples of challenges to families with HIV. Pressure to reduce risky behaviors also commonly presents as a struggle. Multiple studies have reported increased adherence, improved well-being, and improved health measures in families receiving family group support (Kmita et al., 2002; Lyon et al., 2003; Mitrani et al., 2003; Rotheram-Borus et al., 2003; McKay et al., 2004).

COMPLEMENTARY AND ALTERNATIVE MODALITIES

Many patients with HIV infection seek complementary and alternative modalities (CAM) of treatment. These include use of substances such as herbal supplements, nutritional supplements, and marijuana, as well as nontraditional therapeutic activities such as massage, acupuncture, hypnosis, prayer, meditation, and yoga. Complementary therapies can be passive (massage therapy, acupuncture), while others emphasize active patient participation (yoga, meditation). Patients usually choose a modality on the basis of others' experience, through word of mouth, or according to personal preference.

In the past few years, a large study funded by the National Institutes of Health (NIH), the Office of Alternative Medicine (OAM), and the National Institute of Allergy and Infectious Diseases (NIAID) has evaluated the extent of the use of these modalities among 1675 HIV-positive men and women (Standish et al., 2001). The most frequently reported substances used were vitamin C (63%), multiple vitamin and mineral supplements (54%), vitamin E (53%), and garlic (53%). Providers most commonly consulted by the cohort were massage therapists (49%), acupuncturists (45%), nutritionists (37%), and different forms of counseling (35%). The activities most commonly used were aerobic exercise (63%), prayer (58%), massage (53%), and meditation (46%). The choice of therapies did not appear to be based on scientific evidence of efficacy of individual therapies.

Despite inadequate scientific literature confirming their efficacy, many individuals report benefit from CAM therapy, and large amounts of money are spent yearly on such treatments. Many reports show positive effects (Deng and Cassileth, 2005), but controlled studies are still limited. Clinical trials of frequently used CAM are needed to inform physicians and patients about therapies that may have measurable benefit or measurable risk (Fairfield et al., 1998). The majority of subjects in the NIH study mentioned above consulted with both conventional and CAM providers and used both conventional and CAM treatments, suggesting the utility of a model of integrated medicine. It is unfortunately rare for conventional and CAM providers to work as a team, however. Further research would be helpful to support and promote such models for integration of care.

Mind–body interventions, acupuncture, massage therapy, and music therapy have all been studied as treatments for mood disturbance in cancer patients. Relaxation techniques, guided imagery, and meditation were investigated in several oncology randomized, controlled trials and were linked with improvements in anxiety, depression, and other symptoms of distress (Speca et al., 2000; Petersen et al., 2002; Targ and Levine, 2002).

While there are fewer published reports of relaxation interventions in patients with HIV, some studies are promising. Fukunishi and colleagues (1997) compared the efficacy of relaxation techniques in a sample of HIV patients to that of use of an ordinary supportive psychotherapy group or a nonpsychiatric treatment group. Scores for anxiety, fatigue, depression, and confusion were significantly lower after the relaxation intervention than scores for the other groups. Taylor (1995) evaluated the effects of a behavioral stress-management program on anxiety, mood, self-esteem, and T-cell count in a group of asymptomatic HIV-positive men. The program consisted of 20 biweekly sessions of progressive muscle relaxation and electromyography biofeedback-assisted relaxation training, meditation, and hypnosis. The treatment group showed significant improvement on all dependent measures compared to the control group.

Mindfulness meditation seeks to focus attention and objectively acknowledge thoughts, emotions, sensations, and perceptions as they arise. The cognitive skills learned through the meditation process are transferred from a focus on breathing to attention in all activities of life.

A small body of evidence has emerged over the past two decades suggesting that mindfulness-based stress reduction (MBSR) may be an effective adjunctive treatment for a variety of physical and psychological conditions. Robinson and colleagues (2003) examined the effects of a structured, 8-week MBSR program on perceived stress, mood, endocrine function, immunity, and functional health outcomes in individuals infected with HIV. Natural killer cell activity and number increased significantly in the MBSR group compared to the comparison group. No significant changes or differences were found, however, for psychological, endocrine, or functional health variables.

A considerable literature addresses the role of hypnosis in helping cancer patients. Liossi and Hatira (1999) reported similar pain relief for both hypnosis and CBT used with pediatric cancer patients. Both therapies also reduced anxiety and distress, with hypnosis showing greater effectiveness. Among the small number of studies evaluating use of hypnosis in the HIV population, Langenfeld and colleagues (2002) showed significant improvement, with decreased pain and medication requirements in patients receiving hypnosis.

Massage therapy or reflexology (foot massage) may be beneficial for patients with chronic cancer pain as well as patients suffering from neuropathic pain. Reduction of pain and anxiety has been demonstrated in randomized, controlled trials evaluating this therapy in cancer patients (Ahles et al., 1999; Stephenson et al., 2000; Wilkie et al., 2000; Smith et al., 2002; Cassileth and Vickers, 2004). There are currently no controlled studies showing similar effects for HIV-positive patients.

Acupuncture therapy involves the insertion of needles along specific pathways targeted by the problem or body organ involved. It is sometimes used in conjunction with heat, acupressure, or electric stimulation. Several single-arm studies found reduction of cancer pain, although the lack of controls limited their conclusions (Filshie and Redman, 1985; Leng, 1999). In a recent randomized, single-blinded, placebo-controlled trial, Alimi and colleagues (2003) tested auricular acupuncture for cancer patients who still experienced pain despite stable analgesic treatment. Pain intensity decreased by 36% at 2 months from baseline in the treatment group, a significant difference compared with the two control groups. There is currently no evidence of a similar effect among HIV-positive patients. There are currently no studies of use of acupuncture in HIV-positive patients.

The use of herbal supplements is becoming increasingly widespread. Herbal supplement products including vitamins, proteins, herbs, and other over-the-counter substances can be found in capsule, tablet, liquid, or dried forms. Among the most widely used herbal supplements by HIV patients for their reputed mood-altering effects are kava, for its anxiolytic effect; ephedra (Mahuang), for the stimulant effect; and St. John's wort, for its antidepressant effect. Valerian and passionflower are both used as a sleep aid, while ginkgo biloba is reported to have cognitive-enhancing effects. Control trials to demonstrate beneficial effects of these herbal supplements are still lacking.

CONCLUSIONS

The past two decades have witnessed an exciting expansion of psychological treatment options for the HIV-infected population, which can be integrated with and complement the medical and pharmacological care of persons with HIV/AIDS. The psychological needs of HIV-positive persons are complex and multilayered and require a multidisciplinary approach. Traditionally, the psychological treatment provided has depended more on available resources and theoretical background of the providers. Evidence-based treatment choices are becoming more common, however, as more reliable research is growing on the effectiveness of different treatment modalities.

As described in this chapter, despite current research limitations, a considerable literature supports the feasibility and utility of various treatment modalities for reducing psychological distress in persons with HIV infection. Both group and individual treatments have been shown to be effective, including psychodynamic/psychoanalytic, interpersonal, behavioral, and supportive approaches. In some cases, psychosocial interventions have been associated with improved immunological parameters.

While many different therapeutic modalities have been studied, the field would benefit from further research to provide more consistent evidence in support of various treatment approaches. This is especially true of the less widely used modalities, for which evidence of efficacy is still largely lacking. More research is also needed to discern what aspects of a patient's psychological and medical condition might predict positive response to particular treatment modalities. This would help clinicians with the ultimate goal of forming the best individualized treatment plan for each patient.

There is growing literature on patient-focused research (Howard et al., 1996; Lambert et al., 2001). Whereas traditional psychotherapy research has tended to focus on the general efficacy of an intervention, patient-focused research assesses the efficacy of an intervention as it relates to a specific patient. The goal of patient-focused research is to increase the clinical utility of research findings, providing tools that clinicians can use to evaluate individual patient response to treatment. Although this methodology is gaining some momentum in psychotherapy research (Lambert et al., 2003), it has yet to gain significant attention

in HIV treatment and research. The future of psychosocial interventions for patients with HIV will depend on and benefit greatly from further study of the various available treatment modalities, using traditional, evidence-based, and patient-focused research.

References

Ahles TA, Tope DM, Pinkson B, et al. (1999). Massage therapy for patients undergoing autologous bone marrow transplantation. *J Pain Symptom Manage* 18:157–163.

Alimi D, Rubino C, Pichard-Leandri E, et al. (2003). Analgesic effect of auricular acupuncture for cancer pain: a randomized, blinded, controlled trial. *J Clin Oncol* 21:4120–4126.

Allers CT, and Benjack KJ (1991). Connection between childhood abuse, and HIV infection. *J Counsel Dev* 70:309–313.

Antoni MH, Cruess S, Cruess DG, Kumar M, Lutgendorf S, Ironson G, Dettmer E, Williams J, Klimas N, Fletcher MA, and Schneiderman N (2000a). Cognitive-behavioral stress management reduces distress and 24-hour urinary free cortisol output among symptomatic HIV-infected gay men. *Ann Behav Med* 22(1):29–37.

Antoni MH, Cruess DG, Cruess S, Lutgendorf S, Kumar M, Ironson G, Klimas N, Fletcher MA, and Schneiderman N (2000b). Cognitive-behavioral stress management intervention effects on anxiety, 24-hr urinary norepinephrine output, and T-cytotoxic/suppressor cells over time among sympomatic HIV-infected gay men. *J Consult Clin Psychol* 68(1):31–45.

Antoni MH, Cruess DG, Klimas N, Maher K, Cruess S, Kumar M, Lutgendorf S, Ironson G, Schneiderman N, and Fletcher MA (2002). Stress management and immune system reconstitution in symptomatic HIV-infected gay men over time: effects on transitional naive T cells (CD4(+)CD45RA(+) CD29(+)). *Am J Psychiatry* 159(1):143–145.

Antoni MH, Cruess DG, Klimas N, Carrico AW, Maher K, Cruess S, Lechner SC, Kumar M, Lutgendorf S, Ironson G, Fletcher MA, and Schneiderman N (2005). Increases in a marker of immune system reconstitution are predated by decreases in 24-h urinary cortisol output and depressed mood during a 10-week stress management intervention in symptomatic HIV-infected men. *J Pscyhosom Res* 58:3–13.

Aversa SL, and Kimberlin C (1996). Psychosocial aspects of antiretroviral medication use among HIV patients. *Patient Educ Couns* 29:207–219.

Bachanas PJ, Kullgren KA, Schwartz KS, Lanier B, McDaniel JS, Smith J, et al. (2001). Predictors of psychological adjustment in school-age children infected in HIV. *J Pediatr Psychol* 26:343–352.

Blake-Mortimer C, Gore-Felton R, Kimerling J, Turner-Cobb M, and Spiegel D (1981). Improving the quality and quantity of life among patients with cancer a review of the effectiveness of group psychotherapy. *Eur J Cancer* 11:1581–1586.

Blanch J, Rousaud A, Hautzinger M, Martínez E, Peri J-M, Andrés S, Cirera E, Gatell JM, and Gastó C (2002). Assessment of the efficacy of a cognitive-behavioural group psychotherapy programme for HIV-infected patients referred to a consultation-liaison psychiatry department. *Psychother Psychosom* 71:77–84.

Burack JH, Barrett DC, Stall RD, et al. (1993). Depressive symptoms and CD4 lymphocyte decline among HIV-infected men. *JAMA* 270:2568–2573.

Cassileth BR, and Vickers AJ (2004). Massage therapy for symptom control: outcome study at a major cancer center. *J Pain Symptom Manage* 28:244–249.

Catalán J (1999). Interpersonal therapy alone and supportive therapy plus antidepressant drugs were most effective for depression in HIV positive patients. *Evid Based Ment Health* 2:14–14.

Chesney MA, Chamber DB, Taylor JM, Johnson LM, and Folkman S (2003). Coping effectiveness training for men living with HIV: results from a randomized clinical trial testing a group-based intervention. *Psychosom Med* 65(6):1038–1046.

Chibnall JT, Videen SD, Duckro PN, and Miller DK (2002). Psycho-social-spiritual correlates of death distress in patients with life-threatening medical conditions. *Palliat Med* 16:331–338.

Cohen MA (1998). Psychiatric care in an AIDS nursing home. *Psychosomatics* 39:154–161.

Cohen MA (1999). Psychodynamic psychotherapy in an AIDS nursing home. *J Am Acad Psychoanal* 27(1):121–133.

Cruess DG, Antoni MH, Schneiderman N, Ironson G, McCabe P, Fernandez JB, Cruess SE, Klimas N, and Kumar M (2000). Cognitive-behavioral stress management increased free testosterone and decreases psychological distress in HIV-seropositive men. *Health Psychol* 19(1):12–20.

Deng G, and Cassileth BR (2005). Integrative oncology: complementary therapies for pain, anxiety, and mood disturbance. *CA Cancer J Clin* 55(2):109–116.

El-Bassel N, Witte S, Gilbert L, Wu E, Chang M, Hill J, and Steinglass P (2003). The efficacy of a relationship-based HIV/STD prevention program for heterosexual couples. *Am J Public Health* 93(6):963–969.

El-Bassel N, Witte S, Gilbert L, Wu E, Chang M, Hill J, and Steinglass P (2005). Long-term effects of an HIV/STI sexual risk reduction intervention for heterosexual couples. *AIDS Behav* 9(1):1–13.

Evans DL, Leserman J, Perkins DO, et al. (1995). Stress-associated reductions of cytotoxic T lymphocytes and natural killer cells in asymptomatic HIV infection. *Am J Psychiatry* 152:543–550.

Fairfield K, Eisenberg D, Davis R, Libman H, and Phillips R (1998). Patterns of use, expenditures,

and perceived efficacy of complementary and alternative therapies in HIV-infected patients. *Arch Intern Med* 158:2257–2264.

Farber EW, and McDaniel JS (1999). Assessment and psychotherapy practice implications of new combination antiviral therapies in HIV disease. *Prof Psychol Res Pract* 30:173–179.

Filshie J, and Redman D (1985). Acupuncture and malignant pain problems. *Eur J Surg Oncol* 11:389–394.

Frederick T, Thomas P, Mascola L, Hsu HW, Rakusan T, Mapson C, et al. (2000). Human immunodeficiency virus–infected adolescents: a descriptive study of older children in New York City, Los Angeles County, Massachusetts and Washington DC. *Pediatr Infect Dis* 19:551–555.

Fukunishi I, Hosaka T, Matsumoto T, Hayashi M, Negishi M, and Moriya H (1997). Liaison psychiatry and HIV infection (II): Application of relaxation in HIV positive patients. *Psychiatry Clin Neurosci* 51(1):5–8.

Funck-Brentano I, Dalban C, Veber F, Quartier P, Hefez S, Costagliola D, and Blanche S (2005). Evaluation of a peer support group therapy for HIV-infected adolescents. *AID* 19(14):1501–1508.

Gaugham DM, Hughes MD, Oleske JM, Malee K, Gore CA, and Nachman S (2004). Pediatric AIDS. Psychiatric hospitalizations among children and youths with human immunodeficiency virus infection. *Pediatrics* 113:e544–e551.

Goodkin K, Blaney NT, Feaster D, et al. (1992a). Active coping style is associated with natural killer cell cytotoxicity in asymptomatic HIV-1 seropositive homosexual men. *J Psychosom Res* 36:635–650.

Goodkin K, Fuchs I, Feaster D, et al. (1992b). Life stressors and coping style are associated with immune measures in HIV-1 infection: a preliminary report. *Int J Psychiatry Med* 22:155–172.

Goodkin K, Feaster DJ, Tuttle R, et al. (1996). Bereavement is associated with time-dependent decrements in cellular immune function in asymptomatic HIV-1 seropositive homosexual men. *Clin Diagn Lab Immunol* 3:109–118.

Goodkin K, Feaster DJ, Asthana D, et al. (1998). A bereavement support group intervention is longitudinally associated with salutary effects on CD4 cell count and on number of physician visits. *Clin Diagn Lab Immunol* 5:382–391.

Goodman LA, and Fallot RD (1998). HIV risk-behavior in poor urban women with serious mental disorders: association with childhood physical, and sexual abuse. *Am J Orthopsychiatry* 68:73–83.

Hall VP (1999). The relationship between social support and health in gay men with HIV/AIDS: an integrative review. *J Assoc Nurses AIDS Care* 10:74–86.

Hershberger SL, Wood MM, and Fisher DG (2003). A cognitive-behavioral intervention to reduce HIV risk behaviors in crack and injection drug users. *AIDS Behav* 7(3):229–243.

Howard KI, Moras K, Brill PL, Martinovich Z, Lutz W (1996). Evaluation of psychotherapy: efficacy, effectiveness, and patient progress. *Am Psychologist* 51:1059–1064.

Hutton HE, Treisman JD, Fishman M, et al. (2001). HIV risk behaviors and their relationship to post-traumatic stress disorder among women prisoners. *Psychiatr Serv* 52:508–513.

James J, and Meyerding J (1997). Early sexual experience, and prostitution. *Am J Psychiatry* 134:1381–1385.

Kelly JA (1998). Group psychotherapy for persons with HIV and AIDS-related illnesses. *Int J Group Psychother* 48(2):143–162.

Kelly JA, Murphy DA, Bahr GR, Kalichman SC, Morgan MG, Stevenson LY, Koob JJ, Brasfield TL, and Bernstein BM (1993). Outcomes of cognitive-behavioral and support group brief therapies for depressed, HIV-infected persons. *Am J Psychiatry* 150(11):1679–1686.

Kemeny ME, and Dean L (1995). Effects of AIDS-related bereavement on HIV progression among New York City gay men. *AIDS Educ Prev* 7(s):36–47.

Kemeny ME, Weiner H, Duran R, et al. (1995). Immune system changes after the death of a partner in HIV-positive gay men. *Psychosom Med* 57:547–554.

Kertzner RM, Goetz R, Todak G, Cooper T, Lin SH, Reddy MM, Novacenko H, Williams JB, Enhardt AA and Gorman JM (1993). Cortisol levels, immune status, and mood in homosexual men with and without HIV infection. *Am J Psychiatry* 150(11):1674–1678.

Kmita G, Baranska M, and Niemiec T (2002). Psychosocial intervention in the process of empowering families with children living with HIV/AIDS—a descriptive study. *AIDS Care* 14(2):279–284.

Koszycki D, Lafontaine S, Frasure-Smith N, Swenson R, and Lesperance F (2004). An open-label trial of interpersonal psychotherapy in depressed patients with coronary disease. *Psychosomatics* 45(4):319–324.

Lambert MJ, Hansen NB, and Finch AE (2001). Patient-focused research: using patient outcome data to enhance treatment effects. *J Consult Clin Psychol* 69(2):159–172.

Lambert MJ, Whipple JL, Hawkins EJ, Vermeersch DA, Nielsen, SL, and Smart, DW (2003). Is it time for clinicians to routinely track patient outcome? A meta-analysis. *Clin Psychol Sci Pract* 10:288–301.

Langenfeld MC, Cipani E, and Borckardt JJ (2002). Hypnosis for the control of HIV/AIDS-related pain. *Int J Clin Exp Hypn* 50(2):170–188.

Laperriere A, Ironson GH, Antoni MH, Pomm H, Jones D, Ishii M, Lydston D, Lawrence P, Grossman A, Brondolo E, Cassells A, Tobin JN, Schneiderman N, and Weiss SM (2005). Decreased depression up to one year following CBSM+ intervention in depressed women with AIDS: the smart/EST women's project. *J Health Psychol* 10(2):223–231.

Lee MR, Cohen L, Hadley SW, and Goodwin FK (1999). Cognitive-behavioral group therapy with medication for depressed gay men with AIDS or symptomatic HIV infection. *Psychiatr Serv* 50:948–952.

Lenderking WR, Wold D, Mayer KH, et al. (1997). Childhood sexual abuse among homosexual men. Prevalence and association with unsafe sex. *J Gen Intern Med* 12:250–253.

Leng G (1999). A year of acupuncture in palliative care. *Palliat Med* 13:163–164.

Leserman J, Perkins DO, and Evans DL (1992). Coping with the threat of AIDS: the role of social support. *Am J Psychiatry* 149:1514–1520.

Leszcz M, Sherman A, Mosier J, Burlingame GM, Cleary T, Ulman KH, Simonthon S, Latif U, Strauss B, and Hazelton L (2004). Group interventions for patients with cancer and HIV disease: part IV. Clinical and policy recommendations. *Int J Group Psychother* 54(4):539–556; discussion, 557–562, 563–568, 569–574.

Linn JG, Lewis FM, Cain VA, and Kimbrough GA (1993). HIV-illness, social support, sense of coherence, and psychosocial well-being in a sample of help-seeking adults. *AIDS Educ Prev* 5:254–262.

Liossi C, and Hatira P (1999). Clinical hypnosis versus cognitive behavioral training for pain management with pediatric cancer patients undergoing bone marrow aspirations. *Int J Clin Exp Hypn* 47:104–116.

Lodico MA, and DiClemente RJ (1994). The association between childhood abuse, and prevalence of HIV-related risk behaviors. *Clin Pediatr* 33:498–502.

Lyon ME, Trexler C, Akpan-Townsend C, Pao M, Selden K, Fletcher J, Addlestone IC, and D'Angelo LJ (2003). A family group approach to increasing adherence to therapy in HIV-infected youths: results of a pilot project. *AIDS Patient Care STDS* 17(6):299–308.

Markowitz JC, Klerman GL, Clougherty KF, Spielman LA, Jacobsberg LB, Fishman B, Frances AJ, Kocsis JH, and Perry SW (1995). Individual psychotherapies for depressed HIV-positive patients. *Am J Psychiatry* 152:1504–1509.

Markowitz JC, Kocsis JH, Fishman B, et al. (1998). Treatment of depressive symptoms in human immunodeficiency virus–positive patients. *Arch Gen Psychiatry* 55:452–457.

Markowitz JC, Spielman LA, Sullivan M, and Fishman B (2000). An exploratory study of ethnicity and psychotherapy outcome among HIV-positive patients with depressive symptoms. *J Psychother Pract Res* 9(4):226–231.

McClain CS, Rosenfeld B, and Breitbart W (2003). Effect of spiritual well-being on end-of-life despair in terminally ill cancer patients. *Lancet* 361:1603–1607.

McKay MM, Chase KT, Paikoff R, McKinney LD, Baptiste D, Coleman D, Madison S, and Bell CC (2004). Family-level impact of the CHAMP Family Program: a community collaborative effort to support urban families and reduce youth HIV risk exposure. *Fam Process* 43(1):79–93.

Miller DK, Chibnall JT, Videen SD, and Duckro PN (2005). Supportive-affective group experience for persons with life-threatening illness: reducing spiritual, psychological, and death-related distress in dying patients. *J Palliat Med* 8(2):333–343.

Misdrahi D, Vila G, Funck-Brentano I, Tardieu M, Blanche S, and Mouren-Simeoni MC (2004). DSM-IV mental disorders and neurological complications in children and adolescents with human immunodeficiency virus type 1 infection (HIV-1). *Eur Psychiatry* 19:182–184.

Mitrani VB, Prado G, Feaster DJ, Robinson-Batista C, and Szapocznik J (2003). Relational factors and family treatment engagement among low-income, HIV-positive African American mothers. *Fam Process* 42(1):31–45.

Molassiotis A, Callaghan P, Twinn SF, Lam SW, Chung WY, and Li CK (2002). A pilot study of the effects of cognitive-behavioral group therapy and peer support/counseling in decreasing psychological distress and improving quality of life in Chinese patients with symptomatic HIV disease. *AIDS Patient Care STDS* 16(2):83–96.

Mulder CL, Antoni MH, Emmelkamp PM, Veugelers PJ, Sandfort TG, van de Vijver FA, and de Vries MJ (1995). Psychosocial group intervention and the rate of decline of immunological parameters in asymptomatic HIV-infected homosexual men. *Psychother Psychosom* 63(3–4):185–192.

Newlin K, Melkus GD, Chyun D, and Jefferson V (2003). The relationship of spirituality and health outcomes in Black women with type 2 diabetes. *Ethnic Dis* 13:61–68.

O'Leary A (2000). Women at risk for HIV from a primary partner: balancing risk and intimacy. *Annu Rev Sex Res* 11:191–234.

Padian NS, O'Brien TR, Chang YC, Glass S, and Francis D (2003). Prevention of heterosexual transmission of human immunodeficiency virus through couple counseling. *J Acquir Immune Defic Syndr* 6:1043–1048.

Parsons JT, Rosof E, Punzalan JC, and Di Maria L (2005). Integration of motivational interviewing and cognitive behavioral therapy to improve HIV medication adherence and reduce substance use among HIV-positive men and women: results of a pilot project. *AIDS Patient Care STDS* 19(1):31–39.

Petersen RW, and Quinlivan JA (2002). Preventing anxiety and depression in gynaecological cancer: a randomised controlled trial. *Br J Obstet Gynaecol* 109:386–394.

Ricart F, Cohen MA, Alfonso CA, Hoffman RG, Quinone N, Cohen A, and Indyk D (2002). Understanding the psychodynamics of non-adherence to medical treatment in persons with HIV infection. *Gen Hosp Psychiatry* 24(3):176–180.

Robinson FP, Mathews HL, and Witek-Janusek L (2003). Psycho-endocrine-immune response to mindfulness-based stress reduction in individuals infected with the human immunodeficiency virus: a quasiexperimental study. *J Altern Complement Med* 9(5):683–694.

Rogers RR (1989). Beyond morality: the need for psychodynamic understanding and treatment of responses to the AIDS crisis. *Psychiatr J Univ Ott* 14(3):456–459.

Rotheram-Borus MJ, Lee M, Leonard N, Lin YY, Franzke L, Turner E, Lightfoot M, and Gwadz M (2003). Four-year behavioral outcomes of an intervention for parents living with HIV and their adolescent children. *AIDS* 17(8):1217–1225.

Sahs J, Goetz R, Reddy M, Rabkin JG, Williams JB, Kertzner R, and Gorman JM (1994). Psychological distress and natural killer cells in gay men with and without HIV infection. *Am J Psychiatry* 151(10):1479–1484.

Schroeder JR, Epstein DH, Umbricht A, and Preston KL (2006). Changes in HIV risk behaviors among patients receiving combined pharmacological and behavioral interventions for heroin and cocaine dependence. *Addict Behav* 31(5):868–879.

Selwyn PA, and Arnold R (1998). From fate to tragedy: the changing meanings of life, death, and AIDS. *Ann Intern Med* 129:899–902.

Sherman AC, Leszcz M, Mosier J, Burlingame GM, Cleary T, Ulman KH, Simonton S, Latif U, Strauss B, and Hazelton L (2004). Group interventions for patients with cancer and HIV disease: Part II. Effects on immune, endocrine, and disease outcomes at different phases of illness. *Int J Group Psychother* 54(2):203–233.

Sherman AC, Mosier J, Leszcz M, Burlingame GM, Ulman KH, Cleary T, Simonton S, Latif U, Hazelton L, and Strauss B (2004c). Group interventions for patients with cancer and HIV disease: Part III. Moderating variables and mechanisms of action. *Int J Group Psychother* 54(3):347–387.

Shoptaw S, Reback CJ, Peck JA, Yang X, Rotheram-Fuller E, Larkins S, Veniegas RC, Freese TE, and Hucks-Ortiz C (2005). Behavioral treatment approaches for methamphetamine dependence and HIV-related sexual risk behaviors among urban gay and bisexual men. *Drug Alcohol Depend* 78:125–134.

Sikkema KJ, Hansen NB, Kochman A, et al. (2004a). Outcomes from a randomized controlled trial of a group intervention for HIV positive men and women coping with AIDS-related loss and bereavement. *Death Stud* 28:187–209.

Sikkema KJ, Hansen NB, Tarakeshwar N, Kochman A, Tate DC, and Lee RS (2004b). The clinical significance of change in trauma-related symptoms following a pilot group intervention for coping with HIV-AIDS and childhood sexual trauma. *AIDS Behav* 8(3):277–291.

Smith MC, Kemp J, Hemphill L, and Vojir CP (2002). Outcomes of therapeutic massage for hospitalized cancer patients. *J Nurs Scholarsh* 34:257–262.

Speca M, Carlson LE, Goodey E, and Angen M (2000). A randomized, wait-list controlled clinical trial: the effect of a mindfulness meditation-based stress reduction program on mood and symptoms of stress in cancer outpatients. *Psychosom Med* 62:613–622.

Standish LJ GK, Bain S, Reeves C, Sanders F, Wines RC, Turet P, Kim JG, and Calabrese C (2001). Alternative medicine use in HIV-positive men and women: demographics, utilization patterns and health status. *AIDS Care* 13:197–208.

Stephenson NL, Weinrich SP, and Tavakoli AS (2000). The effects of foot reflexology on anxiety and pain in patients with breast and lung cancer. *Oncol Nurs Forum* 27:67–72.

Targ EF, and Levine EG (2002). The efficacy of a mind–body–spirit group for women with breast cancer: a randomized controlled trial. *Gen Hosp Psychiatry* 24:238–248.

Taylor DN (1995). Effects of a behavioral stress-management program on anxiety, mood, self-esteem, and T-cell count in HIV positive men. *Psychol Rep* 76(2):451–457.

Telch CF, and Telch MJ (1986). Group coping skills instruction and supportive group therapy for cancer patients: a comparison of strategies. *J Consult Clin Psychol* 54:802–808.

Theorell T, Blomkvist V, Jonsson H, et al. (1995). Social support and the development of immune function in human immunodeficiency virus infection. *Psychosom Med* 57:32–36

Thompson NJ, Potter JS, Sanderson CA, and Maibach EW (1997). The relationship of sexual abuse, and HIV risk behaviors among heterosexual adult female STD patients. *Child Abuse Neglect* 21:149–156.

Van der Kolk, B (1993). Group psychotherapy with posttraumatic stress disorder. In HI Kaplan and BJ. Sadock (eds.), *Comprehensive Group Psychotherapy, third edition* (pp. 550–560). Baltimore: Williams & Wilkins.

Weiss JJ, (1997). Psychotherapy with HIV-positive gay men: a psychodynamic perspective. *Am J Psychother* 51(1):31–44.

Weiss JJ, Mulder CL, Antoni MH, de Vroome EM, Garssen B, and Goodkin K (2003). Effects of a supportive-expressive group intervention on long-term psychosocial adjustment in HIV-infected gay men. *Psychother Psychosom* 72(3):132–140.

Wilkie DA, Kampbell J, Cutshall S, et al. (2000). Effects of massage on pain intensity, analgesics and quality of life in patients with cancer pain: a pilot study of a randomized clinical trial conducted within hospice care delivery. *Hosp J* 15:31–53.

Wingood GM, and DiClemente RJ (1997). Child sexual abuse, HIV sexual risk, and general relations of African-American women. *Am J Prev Med* 13:380–384.

Zisook S, Peterkin J, Goggin KJ, et al. (1998). Treatment of major depression in HIV-seropositive men. HIV Neurobehavioral Research Center Group. *J Clin Psychiatry* 59:217–224.

Chapter 28

Social Service Interventions

Mary Ann Malone

AIDS is a medical illness that can be seen as having biological, psychological, social, and cultural aspects. The biopsychosocial approach to AIDS was first described and defined (Cohen and Weisman, 1986) early in the epidemic. The need for a coordinated approach was also specified (Cohen, 1987): "The acquired immunodeficiency syndrome (AIDS) may be thought of as a medical problem that requires a coordinated, humane, comprehensive, holistic, and biopsychosocial approach." Patients benefit greatly from this collaborative care since it also (Cohen, 1992) "maintains a view of each patient as a member of a family, community, and culture who deserves coordinated compassionate care and treatment with dignity." A social worker plays a vital role in this approach as a fully integrated member of the treatment team.

This chapter will present the role of hospital social work in this biopsychosocial approach to the treatment of patients with AIDS. Persons with AIDS often require help with concrete services and varying de-grees of psychological or psychiatric support in order to cope at different times during the course of their illness. The current medical, psychiatric, and social service needs of AIDS patients have been altered by the changing climate in the treatment of AIDS over the last decade. The introduction of new and more effective medications has led to a change in perception of the illness from being fatal to chronic. The pressures within the hospital system for increased productivity and expeditious discharges add to this changing climate. This chapter will shed light on how these changes affect hospital social work. The first section of the chapter will discuss the collaborative relationship between psychiatry and social work. The second section will highlight the past and present role of the hospital social worker as it relates to AIDS. The final section will summarize practical social work interventions used to assist AIDS patients deal with the challenges of their everyday lives during this time of change.

PSYCHIATRY AND SOCIAL WORK:
A COLLABORATIVE RELATIONSHIP

The professions of psychiatry and social work have been working side by side for many years. Mental health, which both professions address, is an important aspect of the care of people with AIDS. There are similarities between the two professions, the strongest of which is the skill of the practitioner to help patients generate within themselves the strength to promote their own healing and resulting positive action. Professional values that guide social work and psychiatry are also similar. A non-discriminatory attitude, professional expertise, and self-understanding guide the work of the practitioners in both disciplines. There are many opportunities for psychiatry and social work to work together collaboratively within the hospital setting. Working in conjunction with other disciplines is a necessary component of the care of patients with HIV/AIDS. Psychiatry and social work need to be an integral part of a multidisciplinary team that includes medical doctors, nurses, psychologists, dieticians, and other infectious disease specialists. Each patient is unique and brings a unique set of needs. The coordinated effort of the team is to create a plan tailored to the needs of the individual (Forstein and McDaniel, 2001). Although each discipline specializes in a specific aspect of the patient's care, emphasis should always be on collaboration. The objective is to provide the most comprehensive and compassionate treatment possible. All individuals involved in the patient's care need to work side by side toward this end. For example, topics around end-of-life issues require input from the patient, significant others, and members of the whole team with emphasis on communication and shared decisions.

Within the framework of the team, helping patients adhere to psychiatric and AIDS medications is another area where psychiatry and social work coordinate services. When assessing for problems with adherence, the social worker can determine what factors hinder the patient from keeping up with the regimen. Reasons for patients' problems with adherence can include side effects of the medications. Very often patients feel that the cure is worse than the illness; they were feeling relatively well before starting the medications and now they are sick. Patients need encouragement by members of the team to continue taking the medicine, as very often the side effects will subside over time.

Another reason for lack of adherence can be illicit drug use, which often takes precedence over medication regimens. Sometimes active use of alcohol or other drugs may become overwhelming. A person with AIDS may be unable to continue to adhere to medical care, keep appointments, and follow complex regimens of medications and diet, especially when intoxicated, withdrawing from, or engaging in drug- or alcohol-related activities. It is important for team members to be alert to any drug-related problems. In this case it may be necessary to stop the regimen entirely, since medications taken sporadically or not at all lose their effectiveness. Many patients who have illicit drug-related problems are already being seen by a psychiatrist and receiving guidance on issues with adherence.

Sometimes patents will tire of the AIDS medication regimen or feel so much better that they stop taking the antiretroviral medications without informing their doctor. Stopping and starting antiretroviral medications can result in the emergence of resistant viral strains, resistance to antiretrovirals, and the need for an entirely different medication regimen. Patients who keep up with scheduled appointments with their doctor and psychiatrist are less likely to encounter this problem. Once the reasons for an individual patient's lack of adherence are known, professionals from psychiatry and social work, along with the other disciplines, can work together on an approach that can assist the patient to get back on track.

Support groups in which topics discussed center around both psychiatric and psychosocial issues can be facilitated by individuals from both disciplines. Many psychiatric and psychological disorders for which AIDS patients are treated come from problems related to the progression of the illness and/or the side effects of the AIDS medications. Support groups often help patients find solutions to AIDS-related concerns and problems. After a patient is diagnosed HIV positive or develops an opportunistic infection, anxiety and depression often appear and need treatment. Topics important to the patients can be springboards for group discussions.

The availability of psychiatrists as part of the team in a hospital AIDS clinic is an advantage. In this setting the patient can usually get an appointment with a psychiatrist sooner than when patients are referred to specialists outside the clinic, where there is often an extended wait for an appointment. Also, the patient naturally feels more at home in the familiar clinic surroundings and is often already aware of the psychiatrist's presence there.

An example of social work and psychiatric collaboration is demonstrated in the following vignette. Recently, one of the AIDS psychiatrists at our hospital and I had the opportunity to work together to coordinate services for a patient. The patient was a recovering cocaine-dependent woman who, after attaining sobriety, had acquired a full-time job and custody of her young son. She was doing very well and was receiving much encouragement and support from her psychiatrist, who arranged her visits with the patient around the patient's work schedule. Members of the team were concerned about anything that might interfere with the patient's excellent progress. Abruptly, the patient lost her insurance coverage. Rapid social work intervention was needed. Since I was not available when the patient was seen by psychiatry, coordination with her for needed information and help had to be done by phone and fax with the patient and appropriate agencies. Ultimately, the situation was resolved and her life resumed smoothly. Subsequently, through a social work referral to a community-based organization, she was able to receive the help she needed to obtain more adequate housing for herself and her family and avoid eviction from her former apartment.

All disciplines, particularly social work and psychiatry, need to work together to assist patients with adjustments like these during the course of their illness.

SOCIAL WORK AND HIV/AIDS: MEETING THE CURRENT PROFESSIONAL CHALLENGES

When I started my professional career in social work 15 years ago, I wanted to work with the most disenfranchised population. I chose the field of AIDS, eager to learn about the illness and help persons with HIV and AIDS in any way I could. I wanted to work in a hospital where I thought I could be closer to the heart of what was happening in the field. My work with my patients over the years has been both challenging and rewarding. As a frontline AIDS hospital social worker, I feel it is my responsibility to learn about the new developments and changes in the field that are most relevant to social work practice. In

keeping up with these changes and the latest resources, I can help patients save time developing the skills they require to adjust.

Since the needs of AIDS patients have changed over the last two decades, the approaches that social work employs have also changed. (Strug et al., 2002) The early 1980s saw the beginning of the epidemic. Everyone was shocked at the rapid progression to death for those with AIDS. In many areas during the first years of the epidemic, AIDS was primarily an illness of gay white men. During that time, social workers helped patients, partners, and families face the inevitability of the death of their loved ones. Health care proxies, living wills, family meetings, connecting patients with long lost relatives, burial arrangements, and helping partners and families handle grief made up the social worker's list of ongoing services.

In the mid-1980s HIV spread to intravenous drug users and heterosexual women and children, leading to another shift in the AIDS social work perspective. Again, social workers needed education. Education about drug addiction and the resources available for help was particularly important. As AIDS spread to African-American and Hispanic communities, the numbers of newly diagnosed patients in persons of color far outnumbered those in the white community (Strug et al., 2002). Social workers had to develop a better understanding of the African-American and Hispanic cultures and attitudes toward AIDS within those cultures. Many patients brought multiple layers of family problems that needed to be addressed. Grandparents caring for children of their sick children, relationship problems, and disclosure issues were among the many concerns that patients needed help with.

In 1985 zidovudine was introduced along with other reverse transcriptase inhibitors and used until a decade later in 1995, when the combination therapies were introduced and came to be known as highly active antiretroviral therapy (HAART). This remarkable change in therapies brought a rapid improvement in the health of many AIDS patients. Patients' quality of life improved and they began to live longer with watchful enthusiasm. Now, in the public eye, the topic of AIDS seems to be diminishing. Other medical issues and current world events are now in the spotlight.

Working in an infectious disease clinic in a hospital, it is remarkable to see how the faces of so many of our patients have changed from gaunt and worried to full and peaceful. This is most noticeable in the waiting room in the clinic. Not so long ago, the majority of the patients waiting to be seen by their doctors looked like cadavers and seemed to hang onto life by a thread. As new therapies were gradually introduced, faces began to fill out. Patients came with more energy and the prospect of death did not seem inevitable. This change has sometimes been referred to as "the Lazarus syndrome," describing Jesus' good friend in the Bible whom he raised from the dead (Tucker, 2003). The work with these revitalized patients has changed as well. In many cases, instead of helping them accept their death, the work now focuses on helping them move on with their lives. Many patients need time to get used to feeling well again, remaining in a state of shock for a period of time. One patient, who is a war veteran, compared the feeling to being shell shocked, waiting for the next bomb to drop—in his case, for the next opportunistic infection that might bring an end to his life.

The number of newly infected people has decreased very little over the years, and there is still no cure. Many people are still dying with AIDS. However, the prevailing attitude toward AIDS is similar to the reaction to living with a chronic illness, like diabetes. The dominant themes are no longer loss and grief, but survival and ways of living with the disease. Many patients with AIDS are returning to school and reentering the work force (Arns et al., 2004). There are also ethical dilemmas to consider as we see more and more undocumented immigrants with AIDS coming to our clinics. Providers often feel conflicted when these patients present with a serious illness and there is no insurance to cover the cost of their treatment. Sometimes medical services can be provided without charge, but this is rare.

The response to all of these changes requires a diverse range of social work skills. AIDS social workers face new professional challenges at this time in the history of the disease. Now that people with AIDS are living longer and healthier lives, there is an increased burden on health and social systems. Even now, Medicaid and Medicare are beginning to set limits on medical coverage for our patients. The type of work that we do in the future could also change. Looking ahead, social work efforts may become more concentrated on secondary prevention. The future of the epidemic may require that social workers provide

prevention education as well, to reduce the likelihood of transmission in the general population and further infection in those with AIDS (Strug et al., 2002.)

It is necessary to have an understanding of the constantly changing systems within the hospital (Mizrahi and Berger, 2001). The field of social work needs to adjust to changes in billing, admitting, diagnostic procedures, and patient relations and to the changing functions of doctors, nurses, and other specialists. Most hospitals today are driven by monetary considerations. Social work departments in many hospitals have been downsized, combined with other disciplines, or eliminated altogether. The social work department in the hospital where I work has been able to remain intact and maintain a strong presence, mainly because of strong social work leadership, an idea consistent with Pockett (2003). This entails making every effort to work with the changing hospital system and not against it, providing ideas needed to achieve the current goals of the hospital administration. Integrating and coordinating programs with other discipline also needs to take place in order to maintain a social work presence (Globerman et al., 2002). Through these and other efforts to promote our valuable contributions the voice of social work will continue to be heard.

Many hospital social workers thrive on the challenges that they meet daily. The work is always stimulating, but at times frustrating and physically and emotionally draining. Social workers must be adept at handling their own emotions in order to deal with the many emotionally charged situations they encounter in their work (Nelson and Merighi, 2003) No two days are ever the same, and adjustments to unforeseen circumstances are the order of the day. One can come to work in the morning with a plan for the day and an unexpected crisis can change the focus for the whole day. The work needs to be done quickly and autonomously, since patients, staff members, and the hospital organization's requirements are constantly imposing demands on the social worker's expertise. How does the individual social worker survive on a day-to-day basis in this setting? I derive my energy from the patients themselves. Almost daily I am affected in a positive way by the courage of the patients with whom I work. There are always opportunities to ask questions of colleagues and staff in other disciplines to learn more about specific illnesses and treatments. The support of colleagues who share this difficult work is important. Strong bonds are sometimes formed between workers. Wade (1993) concludes, "Peer support can moderate the effects of stress and reduce the likelihood of burnout." Lending support and validating similar daily experiences of one's colleagues can help sustain a collegial atmosphere. For some, peer support groups can be helpful. It is salutary to go about one's work maintaining a sense of equilibrium in the midst of a highly charged environment. Above all, the willingness to work as a team player is the most essential skill for the social worker to develop in this setting. Sometimes taking on tasks that others would prefer not to do is necessary to promote teamwork. Speaking of clinical social workers in a hospital setting, Gregorian (2005) has said, "Called upon to use a full range of diagnostic and treatment skills in an atmosphere of change and shifting priorities, the strongest of them is self-aware, self confident and constantly seeking new knowledge."

SOCIAL WORK INTERVENTIONS WITH HIV/AIDS PATIENTS: PRACTICAL APPROACHES

Persons with AIDS have a broad array of needs aside from medical and psychiatric care. Assistance with obtaining financial and insurance benefits, housing, home care, counseling, and drug treatment are among the most prevalent issues that social work addresses. The clinic setting in which I work is conducive to meeting these needs through case management services. Here the social worker assumes the role of case manager, who is in charge of coordinating the various disciplines around the patients' needs. Case management services have proven to be effective in assisting patients with meeting needs that improve their quality of life (Katz et al 2000). This is very much in keeping with the biopsychosocial approach to the treatment of patients. The social worker/case manager has the responsibility to become knowledgeable about the most up-to-date and cost-effective resources available to the patients. To keep abreast of what is happening in social work and the health care field, it is necessary to attend workshops, seminars, and conferences on relevant topics held both inside and outside the hospital. As a case manager armed with knowledge and skills, what are the basic tools needed to provide the best help to the patient?

Establishing a Relationship with the Patient

Forming a therapeutic relationship with a patient while assisting with multiple concrete service needs at the same time is a formidable challenge. A good relationship with the patient is the foundation on which effective work can be accomplished. Felix Biestek (1957) defines the patient–caseworker relationship as "the dynamic interaction of attitudes and emotions between caseworker and client, with the purpose of helping the client achieve a better adjustment between himself (sic) and his environment." When patients are working with someone they trust, they will work harder and come closer to their goals more quickly. Sometimes a short-term intervention is needed. Such is the case when social workers coordinate discharges for hospital patients, as there are multiple details that need to be taken care of when helping a patient get ready to leave the hospital. Relationships with patients are often developed when helping them with these needed discharge services, even in a climate where budgets and efficiency propel the work. Conveying an unrushed attitude of concern and acceptance of the patient while helping with even the smallest detail can go a long way toward establishing a therapeutic connection.

Knowing a patient's interests can also often be a vehicle for connecting. I remember being able to establish a connection using a patient's avid interest in basketball; I was "okay" because I knew the game and had some recognition of the players. In some cases a sense of humor can help bring normalcy and relaxation to a stressful situation, providing a means by which patient and worker can meet each other on common ground. Also, sensitivity to the appropriate timing of humor and spontaneity is essential.

Social workers also need to be sensitive to the complex emotions that the patient may be experiencing, including anger, fear, shame, and guilt. Helping patients find the words to express painful emotions can assist in creating a therapeutic relationship. Sometimes these emotions are stuck in the patient's throat, waiting for the right moment to be expressed. Often the patient simply needs permission to express them. The social worker, being sensitive to this, can grant that permission.

When appropriate, creating hopefulness can help patients cope with progressing illness and strengthen the relationship between the social worker and the patient; "imparting hope during counseling is the most important beneficial treatment" (Westburg and Guindon, 2004). Some ways that have been useful for me in developing and maintaining hope in the patient include anticipating medical breakthroughs in the future; helping maintain any religious or spiritual beliefs that the patient may have; providing opportunities for the patient to become involved in absorbing and interesting hobbies or work that can often help to take one's mind off problems; and encouraging the development of supportive relationships with family and friends.

These efforts are just a few ways in which a relationship with the patient can be developed and maintained. Once it is established, almost any help the social worker gives the patient can have a therapeutic effect. Realistically, we all know that we cannot make this connection with every patient we try to help. Different personalities, and sometimes resistance on the part of the patient, can interfere with these efforts. In those cases we hope that the person can relate therapeutically to someone else, and we can continue assisting the patient on a concrete level, always with an open mind and an outstretched hand.

Assisting with Adherence to Medical Regimen

Through collaboration, advocacy, education and resource referrals, health social workers are challenged to meet the social support needs of clients and compliance expectations that medical staff have of clients. (Cox, 2002)

As mentioned earlier in this chapter, the social worker is a key player in guiding a patient to full adherence to a medical regimen, with both keeping appointments and taking prescribed medications. Adherence to a specific regimen is important for anyone dealing with an illness, but it is vital for those with AIDS. The effectiveness of the medications depends on taking them according to a prescribed schedule. Nonadherence can result in failure of the medications to be effective, and the choice of regimens available at this time is limited. Patients present many barriers to adherence. Sometimes patients are too embarrassed to tell their doctor that they have not been faithful to taking their medications. Only when the CD4 count goes down and the viral load goes up is there evidence of nonadherence. The social worker needs to support

the physician in assessing the patient's adherence and communicate with the doctor if there are any problems. A good patient–doctor relationship is strongly associated with adherence (Ingersol and Heckman, 2005). The ability to communicate well with a provider can help towards improving one's health (Adamian et al., 2004). Access to the same provider over a long period of time seems to have a positive effect on general well-being and health (Knowlton et al., 2005).

There are as many reasons for, as there are solutions to, problems with adherence. Some patients are simply too busy or forget to take the medications. Often patients feel sick from the side effects of the medications or report that they don't have the medications with them when they were scheduled to take them. One patient said she often missed the bedtime dose because she fell asleep before the time she was scheduled to take it. After the social worker conferred with the doctor and the patient it was decided that the patient could take the medication an hour or so earlier so the dose would not be missed.

Factors that present difficulties with adherence can include demographic characteristics of the patient (gender, age, ethnicity, socioeconomic status), life crises, alcohol or drug use, lack of adequate housing, and depression (Remien et al., 2003) Very often, assisting with stabilizing a patient's daily life can mean better adherence. For example, help with finding more adequate housing for an ill AIDS patient living in a four-story walkup can mean better adherence with both follow-up clinic visits and medication. There is no easy answer, no single strategy that works for every patient. An individualized approach to finding a solution works best, and success is sometimes achieved simply by trial and error. Often all that is needed is interest and determination on the part of the patient to take responsibility for his or her care.

Recently, a more scientific step-by-step approach to promoting adherence was conceived and initiated for people living with HIV/AIDS in substandard conditions (Boyer and Indyk, 2006). The HIV Cluster of Tools (HIVCOT) is used to determine the current level of adherence and helps the individual create a plan for reaching higher levels of adherence in increments tailored to his or her needs. Whetten et al. (2005) developed a screening tool for persons with HIV to determine how mental illness and substance abuse can negatively affect medication adherence.

Studies have shown that depression can diminish adherence of patients (DiMatteo et al., 2000), thus social workers need to be alert to signs of depression. Depression can be one of the side effects of the AIDS medications, and a referral to a psychiatrist for evaluation may be needed.

Sometimes the regimens are complicated, with many pills to be taken frequently, some with water and some with or without food. Efforts are being made in the field of pharmacology to streamline the regimens so that the taking of medications is more tolerable. The social worker, in coordination with the doctor and the patient, can find ways to ease the patient's burden and arrange a regimen with fewer side effects that fits in better with the patient's daily schedule. The goal, in the not too distant future, is to have the patient take one pill once a day. Adherence may then not be the major problem that it is today.

Nurses play a vital role in helping patients with adherence. Social workers and nurses work closely in their efforts on behalf of the patients (Oliver and Dykeman, 2003). Nurses instruct patients on how to take their medications properly and what side effects, if any, they can expect. Some pharmaceutical companies have produced colored charts with the names and pictures of the various medications, providing a helpful visual guide for the patient. Patients will often be given pillboxes that they are asked to bring to the clinic nurse to fill with daily doses of their medications for the week. If a patient is receiving home care services, the nurse who visits the patient weekly can do this. An electronic reminder device, sold in drug stores, is an effective way for some patients to remember to take their medications at specific times. Social workers need to be familiar with the medications, side effects, and regimen schedules in order to assist nurses. When social workers see an adherence problem they can call on nursing staff to evaluate the patient's need for their help.

As soon as a patient begins a new regimen, social work follow-up at each clinic visit to evaluate adherence is a necessity. Any problems can then be brought to the attention of the medical and nursing staff. Positive reinforcement and support by all team members of patient's efforts to be adherent are also essential. These coordinated efforts by the team to assist patients with adherence need to continue until the regimens are simplified. Adherence is another area of AIDS patient care that demonstrates the biopsychosocial approach to treatment. The patient, doctors, psychiatrists, nurses, social workers, and other staff members all work together to achieve the needed adherence.

Believing that the show rate of patients for medical appointments in our clinic could improve, I initiated a program of calling clinic patients the day before to remind them of their appointments. This resulted in a 10% increase in the number of patients who were seen in the clinic (unpublished data).

Support Groups

Support groups can often relieve the loneliness associated with AIDS. Being with others can be revitalizing. Group interaction for AIDS patients has been described "as an effective means to provide support, an outlet for feelings, a common bond, and a relief of societal stigma" (Cohen and Alfonso, 2004). Groups can provide companionship, help lighten the weight of heavy burdens, and create feelings of optimism. They can help put life in perspective and create a more positive outlook on life. From their research Fontaine et al. (1997) concluded that gay HIV+ white males felt they had more control of their lives as a result of belonging to a support group. Kalichman et al. (1996) found that HIV positive people "who had not attended support groups reported more emotional distress, including depression, than those who had attended." Simoni and Cooperman (2000) discovered that HIV+ women in New York City had less depression and more physical well-being when they had social support. Results of a study by Serovich et al. (2001) found that even perceived social support resulted in reduced emotional distress. On the other hand, people with AIDS can sometimes feel disconnected from family and friends. This is especially true with older persons who are experiencing the loss of others who are not HIV positive who have become ill and died from other conditions. Many older people with AIDS are also coping with several age related illnesses at the same time. Groups can give them the opportunity to form new and sometimes very strong relationships (Kornhaber and Malone, 1996). For example, in a group I facilitate for HIV/AIDS patients over 50, (Malone, 1998) an 82-year-old woman developed a relationship with a 65-year-old woman. The friendship gave each of them the strength they needed to face the challenges of their illness. If one was sick, the other was at her side. They also had fun together. They attended shows and dances and were very excited as they related stories of these events during group sessions. It became a truly therapeutic experience for each of them and for other group members as well.

Groups are formed and develop on the basis of various needs of the AIDS population. Groups can be created for patients of different ages and backgrounds, for adolescents, young adults, adults, and older people. Our clinic has five active support groups for those infected and affected by HIV/AIDS: an HIV support group that meets once a week and consists mainly of former drug users; a women's support group for any HIV-positive woman of any age; a hepatitis C–HIV support group for those who are coinfected with HIV and hepatitis C; a 50+ support group for those people who are HIV positive and over the age of 50; and a group called Fathers Helping Fathers, for those who are infected themselves or have children who are HIV infected. There is a group into which almost any patient in our clinic can fit.

Sometimes people are reluctant or, because of scheduling, cannot attend groups. The 50+ support group mentioned above has developed a telephone "buddy" system giving people the opportunity to exchange phone numbers and set up a supportive relationship without having to come to a formal group session. Groups are not for everyone, but they have proven to be effective for many patients.

Assisting with Concrete Services

Patients with AIDS need assistance with multiple concrete services. Some patients readily express their need for services and others need to be encouraged to express these needs. The most prevalent needs are for housing, financial benefits, insurance, clothing, food, transportation, home care services, and referrals for drug treatment. Since a hospital-based social worker cannot go into the community to offer services to the patient, referrals are very frequently made to agencies that provide case management services in the community. The services these workers provide are invaluable. They can guide patients through the system to obtain benefits, and often accompany them to the various local and state agencies when they cannot manage to get to these places on their own. These workers remind the patients of their clinic visits and often come with them to make sure they don't miss these appointments. This community support is so important for patients' adherence to medical care. In a recent article, Indyk and Reir (2006) talk about the importance of coordination of services for inner city populations: "Not only academic researchers, but also community-based clinicians and service providers,

and clients/patients as well, possess unique expertise that makes them vital participants in generating, disseminating and applying knowledge for fighting the AIDS epidemic."

Patients often need immediate help with referrals to detoxification or rehabilitation programs for treatment of drug and alcohol use. Sometimes these programs are able to accept the patient immediately and even provide transportation to bring the patient to the rehabilitation or detoxification site. This immediate service is very helpful as it takes advantage of the patient's commitment to go for help right at that moment. So often when patients needing this help are given a referral to follow up with a program in a day or two they don't get there because the temptation to revert back to substance use is too strong.

Up until a few years ago, the providers in the AIDS unit at this hospital worked under a continuity-of-care model. A doctor, nurse, and social worker followed a specific panel of patients from the time of their diagnosis to their death, both on the inpatient and outpatient service. This coordination of care was a model for the biopsychosocial approach to treatment. When budget and staffing considerations at the hospital did not allow for this approach to continue, each discipline cared for the patient separately. This restructuring has contributed to the changing climate in AIDS patient care referred to earlier in this chapter. Now inpatient and outpatient social work, although coordinated, are separate functions.

There is a difference in the focus of concrete services offered by inpatient and outpatient hospital social workers. Inpatient social workers are involved with assisting patients and families adjust to the hospital routine. More important, because of the current climate in most hospitals, from the day of admission, emphasis is given to discharge planning and the services needed to get the patient out of the hospital in a timely manner and meet the hospital demands for length of stay. An inpatient worker's first thought upon reviewing the chart before meeting the patient is what options are available for the patient's discharge–nursing home, home care services, transportation, referrals for benefits or insurance, methadone maintenance, or drug rehabilitation. If the patient will be receiving follow-up medical care in the clinic at the same hospital, conferring with the outpatient social worker in the clinic is necessary.

Outpatient social workers provide many of the same services as those provided by inpatient workers.

However, these services are for the patient who is already living in the community. The focus is different and often without the pressure of meeting deadlines. Referrals for drug detoxification, as mentioned above, are fairly straightforward. Like inpatients, outpatients can receive home care through a referral to a nursing service and, if the patient is determined appropriate, services are in place in a few days. Nursing home placement takes a little longer for outpatients because most nursing homes admit patients directly from an inpatient setting, giving priority to more acutely ill patients.

Most of the outpatient social work interventions are concentrated on the patients' needs in the community. Referrals for case management services through community-based organizations are made frequently. It is in the outpatient setting that most of the referrals are made to community-based organizations. Referrals to Legal Aid and other advocacy agencies for legal assistance are frequent. Help with benefit eligibility, custody planning for children, resolution of debt incurred from unpaid bills and immigration status relative to benefits are some of the issues for which patients require legal assistance.

The present climate also necessitates providing referrals and resources for services that can assist patients in being educated and trained to enter the work force. Since so many patients have improved health because of the effective treatments for AIDS, there is generally an eagerness and enthusiasm among patients to move on with their lives. Referrals are often made to resources that provide opportunities for social interaction as well. Generally, in this author's experience, those patients who have strong family/friend support require fewer social work services. This conclusion is consistent with a study on this topic by Sanders and Burgoyne (2001).

Both inpatient and outpatient social workers work very closely with the psychiatry staff. The medical needs of AIDS patients take priority, but mental health is also vitally important. So often the patient's mental status helps or hinders the effectiveness of medical treatment. Social workers are keenly aware of this and make appropriate referrals to psychiatry for patients to be evaluated if there is a perceived mental health issue. Psychiatry staff, in turn, depend on social workers to participate in and support the psychiatric treatment plan by monitoring the patient's behavior and mental state during social work encounters. Social workers and psychiatrists confer frequently, especially when working with persons with multiple and complex problems.

Additional Social Work Services

Many other issues are addressed in a social worker's encounters with patients. Some are considered very tough subjects that need to be discussed for patients to consider all aspects of how AIDS relates to them. Topics surrounding disclosure of HIV-positive status to family and friends are often discussed. The necessary secrecy involved with the inability to disclose can cause stress and anxiety in the patient. The perceptions that patients have of the consequences of disclosing their status are often unrealistic and the result of creating the "worst-case" scenario. Guiding patients through different aspects of this difficult process is challenging.

Conversations about risk reduction and safe sex practices are also a necessary part of social workers' communications with AIDS patients. It is important to help patients understand the need to protect those who are not infected, as well as prevent further infection in those who are.

Mending relationships with family members, partners, and friends is an area in which some patients need guidance and support. So often when these problems are resolved, patients can cope better and concentrate on things they need to do to take care of themselves. More often than not they end up having the support of the people with whom they have reconciled.

Planning for the care of dependent children is a topic that many patients do not want to address. It is usually very difficult for patients to face the possibility of leaving their children. Once a patient agrees to seek legal help for this issue and the planning is in place, the patient usually feels very relieved.

CONCLUSIONS

At the present time, social work plays an even greater role in the management of patients with AIDS than at almost any other time in the history of the illness. Our responsibility now extends beyond the usual provision of basic concrete services and counseling. The scope of our practice has broadened to include an obligation to become knowledgeable about the most up-to-date resources that can help patients deal with the fast-paced changes in their medical care (Kaplan et al., 2004). Social workers should be able to direct patients to the resources they need to adjust to the challenges of their changing lives and obtain help with dealing with a world outside that of AIDS that is experiencing tremendous turmoil. What kind of a framework for this challenging work makes the most sense for both worker and patient?

The basic guidelines should include the following:

- Keep focused on what is best for the patient.
- Respond as a team player at all times, despite the constant demands and pressures of the job.
- Maintain equanimity, and don't allow yourself to react hastily as you are pulled in many different directions.
- Develop a healthy confidence in your ability to get the job done.
- Be willing to learn and try new and sometimes difficult approaches.
- Find opportunities to laugh, and take your work seriously, but not yourself.

References

Adamian MS, Golin CE, Shain LS, and DeVellis B (2004). Brief motivational interviewing to improve adherence to antiretroviral therapy: development and qualitative pilot assessment of an intervention. AIDS Patient Care STDS 18:229–238.

Arns PG, Martin DJ, and Chernoff RA (2004). Psychosocial needs of HIV positive individuals seeking workforce re-entry. AIDS Care 16:377–386.

Biestek F (1957). The Casework Relationship. Chicago: Loyola University Press.

Boyer A, and Indyk D (2006). Shaping garments of care: tools for maximizing adherence potential. Soc Work Health Care 42:151–166.

Cohen MA, and Alfonso CA (2004). AIDS psychiatry: psychiatric and palliative care and pain management. In GP Wormser (ed.), AIDS and Other Manifestations of HIV Infection, fourth edition (pp. 537–576). San Diego: Elsevier Academic Press.

Cohen MA (1992). Biopsychosocial aspects of the HIV epidemic. In GP Wormser (ed.), AIDS and Other Manifestations of HIV Infection, second edition (pp. 349–371). New York: Raven Press.

Cohen MA (1987). Psychiatric aspects of AIDS: a biopsychosocial approach. In GP Wormser, RE Stahl, EJ Bottone (eds.), AIDS-Acquired Immune Deficiency Syndrome and Other Manifestations of HIV Infection (pp. 579–622). Park Ridge, NJ: Noyes Publishers.

Cohen MA, and Weisman HW (1986). A biopsychosocial approach to AIDS. Psychosomatics 27:245–249.

Cox L (2002). Social support medication compliance and HIV/AIDS. Soc Work Health Care 35:425–460.

DiMatteo MR, Lepper HS, and Croghan TW (2000). Depression is a risk factor for noncompliance with medical treatment: meta-analysis of the effects of anxiety and depression on patient adherence. Arch Intern Med 160:2101–2107.

Fontaine K, McKenna L, and Cheskin L (1997). Support group membership and perceptions of control over health in HIV+ men. J Clin Psychol 53:249–252.

Forstein M, and McDaniel JS (2001). Medical overview of HIV infection and AIDS. Psychiatr Ann 31:16–20.

Globerman J, White J, and McDonald G (2002). Social work in restructuring hospitals: program management five years later. Health Soc Work 27:274–284.

Gregorian C (2005). A career in hospital social work: do you have what it takes? Soc Work Health Care 40:1–14.

Indyk D, and Reir DA (2006). Requisites, benefits and challenges of sustainable HIV/AIDS system-building: where theory meets practice. Soc Work Health Care 42:93–110.

Ingersoll KS, and Heckman CJ (2005). Patient–clinician relationships and treatment system effects on HIV medication adherence. AIDS Behav 9:89–101.

Kalichman SC, Sikkema KJ, and Somlai A (1996). People living with HIV infection who attend and do not attend support groups: a pilot study of needs, characteristics and experiences. AIDS Care 8:589–599.

Kaplan LE, Tomaszewski E, and Gorin S (2004). Current trends and the future of HIV/AIDS services: a social work perspective. Health Soc Work 2:153–160.

Katz MH, Cunningham WE, Mor V, Andersen RM, Kellogg T, Zierler S, Crystal SC, Stein MD, Cylar K, Bozzette SA, and Shapiro MF (2000). Prevalence and predictors of unmet need or supportive services among HIV-infected persons: impact of case management. Med Care 38:58–69.

Knowlton AR, Hua W, and Latkin C (2005). Social support networks and medical service use among HIV-positive injection drug users: implications to intervention. AIDS Care 17:479–492.

Kornhaber B, and Malone MA (1996). Creating a support group. In KM Nokes (ed.), HIV/AIDS and the Older Adult (pp. 47–60). Washington, DC: Taylor and Francis.

Malone MA (1998). HIV-Positive women over fifty: how they cope. AIDS Pt Care 12:639–643.

Mizrahi T, and Berger CS (2001). Effect of a changing health care environment on social work leaders: obstacles and opportunities in hospital social work. Soc Work 46:170–182.

Nelson KR, and Merighi JR (2003). Emotional dissonance in medical social work practice. Soc Work Health Care 36:63–79.

Oliver C, and Dykeman M (2003). Challenges to HIV service provision: the commonalities for nurses and social workers. AIDS Care 15:649–663.

Pockett R (2003). Staying in hospital social work. Soc Work Health Care 36:1–24.

Remien RH, Hirky A, Johnson E, Mallory O, Weinhardt LS, Whittier D, and Le GM (2003). Adherence to medication treatment: a qualitative study of facilitators and barriers among a diverse sample of HIV+ men and women in four U.S. cities. *AIDS Behav* 7:61–72.

Saunders DS, and Burgoyne RW (2001). Help-seeking patterns in HIV/AIDS outpatients. *Social Work Health Care* 32:65–80.

Serovich JM, Kimberly JA, Mosack KE, and Lewis TL (2001). The role of family and friend social support in reducing emotional distress among HIV-positive women. *AIDS Care* 13:335–341.

Simoni JM, and Cooperman NA (2000). Stressors and strengths among women living with HIV/AIDS in New York City. *AIDS Care* 12:291–297.

Strug DL, Grube BA, and Beckerman NL (2002). Challenges and changing roles in HIV/AIDS social work: implications for training and education. *Soc Work Health Care* 35:1–19.

Tucker M (2003). Revisiting the 'Lazarus syndrome'. In A Rice and BI Willinger (eds.), *A History of AIDS Social Work in Hospitals: A Daring Response to an Epidemic* (pp. 255–261). New York: Haworth Press.

Wade K, and Simon EP (1993). Survival bonding: a response to stress and work with AIDS. *Soc Work Health Care* 19:77–89.

Westburg NG, and Guindon MH (2004). Hopes, attitudes, emotions and expectations in healthcare providers of services to patients infected with HIV. *AIDS Behav* 8:1–8.

Whetten K, Reif S, Swartz M, Stevens R, Ostermann J, Hanisch L, and Eron J (2005). A brief mental health and substance abuse screener for persons with HIV. *AIDS Patient Care STDS* 19:89–99.

Chapter 29

Nursing Support

Carl Kirton

Nurses have a long history of working in the delivery of health services to individuals with acute and chronic illnesses. With the emergence of the HIV epidemic in the 1980s, nursing professionals stepped up to the challenge to care for those infected with this rare illness in our hospitals, nursing homes, community centers, and private practices, and sometimes in very nontraditional health care settings.

To competently care for people with HIV or AIDS, nurses have to provide care that is advanced and specialized. Nurses have needed to obtain advanced knowledge of virology and infectious disease to address the needs of persons with HIV-related illness. Nurses have had to learn about drugs with new and novel therapeutic actions. They must be knowledgeable about politics and public policy. Nurses have had to learn how to be strong advocates with and sometimes alongside their patients. For many nurses, the realities of mental health disorders and substance use have materialized as significant comorbidities that they were initially unprepared to address. As a result of these complex-

ities, new models of care and new roles for nurses have emerged from the epidemic.

Clinical case management is a collaborative, multidisciplinary model that appoints the nurse as a care coordinator and facilitator who conducts patient assessment, provides education, coordinates community involvement, and manages patient-centered care. The clinical case management approach emerged as a predominant model of care early in the epidemic (Morrison, 1993). This model was most appropriate because it provides coordinated services ranging from care provided in the patient's home to acute care and even palliative care when indicated.

To meet the ongoing needs of nurses involved in the care of persons with HIV and AIDS, a small group of nurses banded together in the fall of 1987. The goal of this group was to promote the individual and collective professional development of nurses involved in the delivery of health care to persons infected or affected by HIV. From this group has evolved the Association of Nurses in AIDS (ANAC). ANAC is a specialty organization with members from around the United States and the world and remains the leading voice in matters related to HIV/AIDS nursing. The mission and goals of ANAC are outlined in Table 29.1. To demonstrate their specialized knowledge, skill, and experience in AIDS care, nurses can obtain certification in this specialty. Board certification in HIV/AIDS is highly valued and provides formal recognition of HIV/AIDS nursing knowledge. Nurses who meet eligibility requirements and pass the certification examination in HIV/AIDS nursing are eligible to use the registered credential of ACRN (HIV/AIDS Certified Registered Nurse) after their name. Nurses with advanced educational preparation (master's degree or higher) who function in advanced practice roles, such as clinical nurse specialist or nurse practitioner, and have pass the advanced certification examination may use the registered credential of AACRN (Advanced HIV/AIDS Certified Registered Nurse).

The HIV epidemic also saw the growth of nurse practitioners (NPs) as primary care providers in both acute and outpatient settings. The number of NPs that work as HIV specialists is unknown. A recent study of the quality of care provided by NPs and physicians

TABLE 29.1. Association of Nurses in AIDS Care Mission Statement

The Association of Nurses in AIDS Care (ANAC) is a nonprofit professional nursing organization committed to fostering the individual and collective professional development of nurses involved in the delivery of health care to persons infected or affected by the HIV and to promoting the health, welfare, and rights of all HIV-infected persons.

Association Goals

The members of ANAC strive to achieve the mission by

- Creating an effective network among nurses in HIV/AIDS care
- Studying, researching, and exchanging information, experiences, and ideas leading to improved care for persons with HIV/AIDS infection
- Providing leadership to the nursing community in matters related to HIV/AIDS infection
- Advocating for HIV infected persons
- Promoting social awareness concerning issues related to HIV/AIDS

Inherent in this mission is an abiding commitment to the prevention of further HIV infection.

assistants (PAs) at 68 HIV care sites in 30 different states for 6651 persons with HIV or AIDS estimated that 20% of patients received most of their HIV care from NPs and PAs. This national study was also important in that it was designed to compare the quality of care provided by non-physician providers (NPs and PAs) with that of physician providers. The study found that the quality of HIV care provided by NP and PA HIV specialists was similar to that of physician HIV specialists and generally better than that of non-HIV physicians (Wilson et al., 2005).

In the beginning of the AIDS epidemic, most nursing was provided in the general hospital acute care setting. Early in the epidemic, in hospitals where persons with AIDS occupied a large proportion of beds, two predominant models of care delivery emerged. The first was a cluster model in which all persons with AIDS were hospitalized in AIDS-dedicated units (ADUs). The other model was a scatter-bed approach where persons with AIDS were admitted to beds throughout general acute care. San Francisco General Hospital established the first ADU in 1983. Many nurses chose to work on this and other ADUs because they had friends or family members with AIDS. Others chose AIDS care as a personal response to the discrimination against AIDS patients by other health professionals that they bore witness to (Pascreta and Jacobsen, 1989; Sherman, 2000).

AIDS-dedicated units provided high-acuity care for the acutely ill AIDS patient. Generally, the level of care provided was not the type of care seen on a general medical unit; it was not atypical for nurses to provide care to patients on ventilators, with central access and medicated infusions. The ADUs tended to be characterized by nurses as offering an unusual level of professional autonomy (Aiken et al., 1997). These nurses were not only skilled in the technical aspects of care but also had to be knowledgeable about symptom assessment and palliation, crisis intervention, and grief work (Kirton, 2001). Nurses working on ADUs also, for the first time, had to assist clients with disclosure around their illness. They often had to resolve conflicts among friends and families and prepare patients for the stigma, isolation, and rejection they might encounter in the community. They also had to assist clients, family, and friends with mourning and prepare clients, family, and friends for the reality of death.

Advances in the pharmacotherapeutics for HIV, prophylaxis of opportunistic infections, and an emphasis on healthy living has shifted AIDS care primarily from inpatient settings to predominantly ambulatory settings. The number of hospital admissions for HIV infection in the United States declined from a high of 149,000 in 1995 to 70,000 admissions in 2003 (Agency for Healthcare Research and Quality, 2005). During the same period, the percentage of AIDS patients who died in the hospital dropped by 32%—from a death rate of 12.5% in 1995 to 8.5% in 2003 (Agency for Healthcare Research and Quality, 2005). Despite the major advances in the care of persons with HIV and AIDS and the profound changes in the numbers of hospital admissions and death rates, there are still patients who are becoming severely ill, dying of AIDS-related opportunistic infections and cancers as they did early in the epidemic, as a result of lack of access or nonadherence to care. Although the setting of nursing care has changed, the goal of nursing practice remains the same—the provision of educational, therapeutic, and supportive interventions to patients, families, and communities.

This chapter addresses the key aspects of nursing care of the HIV-infected adult throughout the spectrum of HIV illness. The chapter will focus on the nurse's role in minimizing risk, preventing HIV transmission, caring for persons with HIV, helping individuals to cope with illness, and negotiating the health care system.

NURSING CARE AS PART OF PRIMARY PREVENTION

In 2005 nearly five million people globally were newly infected with HIV. The need for education related to HIV transmission and safer sexual practices continues to grow (UNAIDS, 2005). In the United States nearly 900,000 to one million persons are living with HIV. The number of new infections remains stable at approximately 40,000 per year, with a rise in the number of new infections occurring among certain groups, especially adolescents (CDC, 2004). It has been estimated that one-quarter to one-third of persons with HIV, particularly younger and black men who have sex with men (MSM), are not aware of their HIV status, and as a result of this lack of awareness may contribute to the continued spread of HIV (CDC, 2005). Investigators have developed models suggesting that although undiagnosed persons with HIV may constitute 20%–30% of persons infected, they may cause 50% or more of new infections (Rhodes and Glynn, 2005). *Primary HIV prevention* refers to activities or strategies directed at abating the further spread of HIV to those currently not infected. The Centers for Disease Control and Prevention, as a strategy to advance HIV prevention, recommends that all health care providers include HIV testing, when indicated, as part of routine medical care on the same voluntary basis as other diagnostic and screening tests (CDC, 2003).

Every nurse–patient encounter should be seen as an opportunity to integrate prevention messages into care. Although many patients believe that discussing sexual health is an important part of a physician– or nurse–patient health care encounter, few health care providers routinely discuss HIV transmission and prevention with their patients (Edne et al., 1984; Gott et al., 2004; Makadon and Silin, 1995). It is estimated that provider assessment for HIV risk occurs in only 10%–36% of appropriate encounters (Carney and Ward, 1998). In an effort to understand the perceived barriers to sexual health discussions, Gott and colleagues (2004) conducted semistructured interviews with 22 general practitioners and 35 practicing nurses to identify perceived barriers. Gott's work identified that health care providers found it most difficult to discuss sexual topics with patients of the opposite gender, patients from African-American and ethnic minority groups, middle-aged and older patients, and non-heterosexual patients. The investigators provide potential strategies to improve communication about sexual health within the primary care encounter. These strategies include training providers how to discuss sexual health during the health care encounter, training patients to ask their health care provider questions, and expanding the role of the nurse in sexual health discussions.

Contrary to provider belief, prevention education need not take extensive amounts of time. Findings from a 1995-96 study indicated that a comprehensive evaluation of a patient at risk or concerned about HIV took approximately 5–7 minutes (Epstein et al., 1998). Components of the primary prevention brief intervention are outlined in Table 29.2.

Primary Prevention in the Mentally Ill

Persons with severe mental illness are at increased risk for contracting HIV. The prevalence of HIV is alarmingly high among persons with serious mental illness, and severely mentally ill adults frequently engage in

TABLE 29.2. Components of Primary Prevention Brief Intervention

Primary HIV Risk Assessment (Suggested Questions)

Sexual Behaviors

Tell me about your current sexual relationship or relationships.

Tell me about your sexual activity in the past (ask about same-sex and cross-sex encounters).

How old were you the first time you had a sexual experience with another person?

HIV/STI Risk

What are you doing now to protect yourself from HIV and other sexually transmitted infections? How about in the past?

Have you ever had a sexually transmitted infection, such as chlamydia, trichomoniasis or "trich," herpes, HPV or warts, gonorrhea, syphilis?

Have you ever been tested for HIV?

Substance Use History

Have you ever felt that alcohol or drugs were a problem for you?

How many times in the past week have you used alcohol or other drugs?

Have you ever injected drugs?

To your knowledge, have any of your sexual partners injected drugs?

How has drinking or using drugs affected your sexual behavior?

Sexual Functioning and Relationship Issues

How satisfied are you with your sexual relationship(s)?

Has your partner ever tried to hurt you?

Domestic Violence and Sexual Assault or Abuse

Have you ever been forced to have sex when you didn't want to?

Other HIV-Related Risks

Since 1977, have you had a blood transfusion?

Have you had sex with someone who has had a blood transfusion?

Do you have hemophilia? Have you had sex with someone who has hemophilia?

Have you shared equipment for tattoo, body piercing?

Options for Reducing risk (Prevention Messages)

• Monogamy with an uninfected partner
• Limiting the number of sex partners
• Not engaging in anal or vaginal sex
• Using extra lubrication if engaging in anal or vaginal sex (extra lubricant will help decrease tears and abrasions)
• Always using condoms (male or female, latex or polyurethane)
• Not using spermicides with nonoxynol-9 (it can cause irritation and increase risk)
• Not engaging in oral sex. If engaging in oral sex, always using latex condoms, dental dams, or plastic wrap
• Not brushing, flossing, or using mouthwash prior to or just after performing oral sex. This can cause tears, cuts, and irritation to the mucous membranes.
• Avoiding ejaculation inside the mouth, vagina, or rectum
• Avoiding swallowing of ejaculate
• Not using needles
• Only using clean needles and "works"
• Cleaning needles, syringes, and "works" before and after use with bleach
• Not sharing inkwells or piercing equipment
• Limiting the number of needle sharing partners

Nursing Interventions

• Provide educational material about STD symptoms
• Provide advice on how to obtain STD diagnostic and treatment services (if not readily available from HIV care provider, use local STD clinic)
• Educate about sexual behavior changes and safer sex methods
• Screen for drug and alcohol abuse when appropriate
• Educate about high-risk substance-use behaviors and harm reduction practices
• Offer HIV testing and counseling if indicated
• Develop and record a risk reduction plan
• Provide referral to risk reduction programs as needed

high-risk behaviors. Early studies conducted in mostly large metropolitan areas provided prevalence estimates that ranged from 4% to 23% (Carey et al., 1995). More recently, Rosenberg and colleagues (2001) assessed 931 psychiatric patients undergoing inpatient or outpatient treatment in four states and reported that 3.1% were infected with HIV. Blank and colleagues (2002) examined a Medicaid population in Philadel-phia (n = 391,454) who also were receiving public assistance. In this population, 4.1% of persons who were treated for HIV infection were also treated for schizophrenia, and 8.8% were treated for a major affective disorder, compared to 2.8% of the rest of the population. Factors contributing to HIV risk among persons with severe mental illness include sexual activity with multiple, casual, or high-risk partners; low levels of condom use; sex trading; and unprotected intercourse occurring between male partners. Sequelae of severe psychopathology such as deficits in problem solving, impulse control, and social and assertiveness skills can also serve to increase HIV risk (Otto-Salaj et al., 2001). Additionally, persons living with mental illness are at increased risk for substance use, and substance use is often associated with increased risk for HIV infection.

Nurses working in mental health or with patients with severe mental illness should incorporate HIV risk reduction into their practice. Although HIV risk reduction assessment and education in the severely mentally ill can be challenging, researchers have demonstrated that severely ill psychiatric patients can be recipients of prevention messages (Kelly, 1997; Carey et al., 2004). Carey (2004) used a 10-session theory-based prevention program designed to help clients reduce their risk sexual behaviors and/or substance use. At the end of the prevention program, patients receiving the HIV risk reduction intervention reported less unprotected sex, fewer casual sex partners, fewer new sexually transmitted infections, more safer sex communications, improved HIV knowledge, more positive attitudes toward condom use, stronger condom use intentions, and improved behavioral skills.

In helping clients reduce their risk for HIV and modify risky behaviors, the nurse uses the behavioral nursing process to assess the client's current behavior and related contingencies, specify the behavioral problem, formulate a treatment plan, implement a treatment program, and evaluate the results of the intervention.

NURSING CARE DURING HIV INFECTION

The morbidity and mortality from HIV infection has declined dramatically since the introduction of potent protease inhibitors into the antiretroviral regimen. Despite improvements in the reduction of medical diseases associated with HIV infection, psychiatric and substance abuse disorders are common in the population and may prevent persons with HIV from adhering to risk reduction and medical care. It is estimated that 50% of HIV-infected patients receiving medical care in the United States suffer from symptoms indicative of mood or anxiety disorders (Bing

et al., 2001). Drug use and drug dependence among people with HIV is also high; again, approximately 50% of patients from the HIV Cost and Services Utilization Study (HCSUS), a national probability survey of HIV-infected adults receiving medical care in the United States, in early 1996 (N = 2864: 2017 men, 847 women), reported using an illicit drug during the previous 12 months of the study period (Bing et al., 2001). Alcohol consumption is common among people receiving treatment for HIV, with rates of heavy drinking almost twice those found in the general population. Heavy drinking is especially high among individuals with lower educational levels and among users of cocaine or heroin (Galvan et al., 2002).

Psychiatric illness, including substance use disorders, impacts HIV illness in many ways. Psychiatric illness may adversely affect medical outcomes and quality of patient life, interfere with access to health services, and undermine adherence to antiretroviral therapy. Because of the impact of psychiatric illness on HIV and AIDS, mental health clinicians are an important part of the HIV treatment team. The need for mental health services is high. Data from the HCSUS mental health survey (n = 1489) conducted in 1997–1998 showed that 70% of persons in this cohort needed mental health care. Of these, 30% had received no mental health services in the previous 6 months, 16% received services from general medical providers (GMPs) only, and 54% used mental health specialists (Taylor et al., 2004). In the Human Immunodeficiency Virus Epidemiology Research Study (HERS) study, 38% of HIV-positive women and 35% of high-risk HIV-negative women reported needing mental health services in the prior 6 months and, of those, only 67% of HIV-positive and 65% of HIV-negative women actually received services (Schuman et al., 2001). One conclusion to be drawn from this and other studies is that access to mental health services may be limited by the number of mental health providers that specialize in treating patients with HIV.

Clinical nurses can serve important roles as screeners for substance use and other psychiatric disorder in comprehensive HIV care settings. Although there is wide support for screening in primary care settings, very little screening actually takes place (Arthur, 1998). There is growing evidence to support the effectiveness of nurse-led brief interventions in both hospital and primary care settings (Werch, et al., 1996; Haddock and Burrows, 1997; Tomson et al., 1998). Thus clinical nurses are a greatly underused resource within primary care settings for screening and brief interventions (Deehan et al., 1998). Early identification of psychiatric illness and prompt psychiatric intervention can be lifesaving and are a critical part of comprehensive care. However, several obstacles impede processes of screening for psychiatric illness. These obstacles have been documented and include organization of care (i.e., access to professional nursing, access to appropriately trained nurses), staffing skill mix (e.g., the number of professional to nonprofessional staff), and time spent with each patient. The lack of available providers for immediate referral for those with a positive screen has been identified as another major barrier for at-risk patients. The lack of staff training and lack of adequate screening instruments for the primary care setting have also been identified as barriers (Barry et al., 2004; Nkowane and Saxena, 2004; Johansson et al., 2005).

An effective nurse screening program must be able to overcome many if not all of these obstacles if an effective screening program is to be incorporated into routine clinical practice. Screening tools must be brief, easy to score, and sensitive across diverse patient populations if they are to gain widespread acceptance in clinical work. Several brief, valid tools have been designed to screen for alcohol and other drug use as well as mood disorders. Brown and colleagues (2001) reported on the criterion validity of a two-item conjoint screen (TICS) for alcohol and other drug abuse or dependence for a sample of primary care patients. At least one positive response to the TICS ("In the last year, have you ever drunk or used drugs more than you meant to?" and "Have you felt you wanted or needed to cut down on your drinking or drug use in the last year?") detected current substance use disorders with nearly 80% sensitivity and specificity. The TICS was particularly sensitive to polysubstance use disorders. Respondents who gave 0, 1, and 2 positive responses had a 7.3%, 36.5%, and 72.4% chance, respectively, of a current substance use disorder; likelihood ratios were 0.27, 1.93, and 8.77. Rost and colleagues (1993) reported on a two-item screener to detect depression or dysthymia within the last year and three-item screeners for lifetime drug disorders and alcohol disorders. The sensitivity of the depression screener ranged between 83% and 94%. The sensitivity of the drug screener ranged between 91% and 94%, excluding one site with an extremely low prevalence of drug problems. The sensitivity of the alcohol screener ranged between 87% and 92%. These tools have not been validated in subsequent studies and have not been tested in HIV-infected populations. More importantly, no brief questionnaire will be able to detect the whole host of mental health problems that are present in the HIV-infected population.

Whetten and colleagues (2005) developed a tool that screens for both mental illness and substance use in the HIV-infected population and can be used by persons differing in educational and experiential background. This tool, the Substance Abuse and Mental Illness Symptom Screener (SAMISS), is a 16-item questionnaire and was created from existing and tested instruments (Table 29.3). The substance use screening items include the following: (1) questions from the Alcohol Use Disorders Identification Test (AUDIT) regarding frequency and amount of alcohol use; (2) questions from the Two Item Conjoint Screen for Alcohol and Other Drug Problems (see above); (3) one question regarding use of illicit drugs, such as heroin or cocaine; and (4) one question about abuse of prescription drugs. The questions about illicit drug use and prescription drug use were developed by the investigators.

Eight mental health screening questions are from the Composite International Diagnostic Interview (CIDI). The CIDI items query for symptoms of manic and depressive episodes, generalized anxiety disorder, panic disorder, posttraumatic stress disorder, and adjustment disorder. An additional question inquires about use of antidepressant medications in the past year. The question on adjustment disorder references the preceding 3 months, whereas all others reference the past year (Whetten et al., 2005).

The tool is administered verbally to patients and takes about 5–10 minutes to complete. The definition of a positive screen for a probable substance use disorder consists of any of the following: a total score of ≥ 5 on questions 1–3; a response of "weekly" or "daily or almost daily" to question 4 or 5; or any response other than "never" to questions 6 or 7. The definition of a positive screen for a probable mood or anxiety disorder consists of an affirmative response to any of questions 8–16.

Pence and colleagues (2005) validated the SAMISS using the reference standard tool, the Structured Clinical Interview for DSM-IV (*Diagnostic and Statistical Manual of Mental Disorders*, fourth edition) SCID to determine test characteristics (see Table 29.4). The SAMISS demonstrates high sensitivity and

TABLE 29.3. The Substance Abuse and Mental Illness Symptom Screener (SAMISS)

Substance Use Items

Patient considered positive for substance use symptoms if any of the following criteria are met:
a) The sum of responses for Questions 1–3 is ≥ 5
b) The sum of responses for Questions 4–5 is ≥ 3
c) The sum of responses for Questions 6–7 is ≥ 1

1. How often do you have a drink containing alcohol?

   0 [ ] Never
   1 [ ] Monthly or less
   2 [ ] 2–4 times a month
   3 [ ] 2–4 times a week
   4 [ ] ≥4 times a week

2. How many drinks do you have on a typical day when you are drinking?

   0 [ ] None
   1 [ ] 1 or 2
   2 [ ] 3 or 4
   3 [ ] 5 or 6
   4 [ ] 7–9
   5 [ ] ≥10

3. How often do you have four or more drinks on one occasion?

   0 [ ] Never
   1 [ ] Less than monthly
   2 [ ] Monthly
   3 [ ] Weekly
   4 [ ] Daily or almost never

4. In the past year, how often did you use non-prescription drugs to get high or to change the way you feel?

   0 [ ] Never
   1 [ ] Less than monthly
   2 [ ] Monthly
   3 [ ] Weekly
   4 [ ] Daily or almost never

5. In the past year, how often did you use drugs prescribed to you or to someone else to get high or change the way you feel?

   0 [ ] Never
   1 [ ] Less than monthly
   2 [ ] Monthly
   3 [ ] Weekly
   4 [ ] Daily or almost never

6. In the past year, how often did you drink or use drugs more than you meant to?

   0 [ ] Never
   1 [ ] Less than monthly
   2 [ ] Monthly
   3 [ ] Weekly
   4 [ ] Daily or almost never

7. How often did you feel you wanted or needed to cut down on your drinking or drug use in the past year, and not been able to?

   0 [ ] Never
   1 [ ] Less than monthly
   2 [ ] Monthly
   3 [ ] Weekly
   4 [ ] Daily or almost never

Mental Health Items

Patient considered positive for symptoms of mental illness if he or she responded yes to any mental health question

Mood Disorder

8. In the past year, when not high or intoxicated, did you ever feel extremely energetic or irritable and more talkative than usual?

   1 YES
   2 NO

9. During the past 12 months, were you ever on medication or antidepressants for depression or nerve problems?

   1 YES
   2 NO

10. During the past 12 months, was there ever a time when you felt sad, blue, or depressed for 2 weeks or more in a row?

    1 YES
    2 NO

11. During the past 12 months, was there ever a time lasting 2 weeks or more when you lost interest in most things like hobbies, work, or activities that usually give you pleasure?

    1 YES
    2 NO

Panic Disorder

12. During the past 12 months, did you ever have a period lasting more than 1 month when most of the time you worried or anxious?

    1 YES
    2 NO

13. In the past year, did you have a spell or an attack when all of a sudden you felt frightened, anxious, or very uneasy when most people would not be afraid or anxious?

    1 YES
    2 NO

14. During the past 12 months, did you ever have a spell or an attack when for no reason your heart suddenly started to race, you felt faint, or you couldn't catch your breath? [If respondent volunteers "only when having a heart attack or due to physical causes," mark NO.]

    1 YES
    2 NO

(*continued*)

TABLE 29.3. (*continued*)

Posttraumatic Stress Disorder

15. During your lifetime, as a child or adult, have you experienced or witnessed traumatic event(s) that involved harm to yourself or others? [If YES: in the past year, have you been troubled by flashbacks, nightmares, or thoughts of the trauma?]

1   YES

2   NO

16. In the past 3 months, have you experienced any event(s) or received information that was so upsetting it affected how you cope with everyday life?

1   YES

2   NO

Source: Pence, B.W., Gaynes, B.N., Whetten, K., Eron, J.J., Jr., Ryder, R.W., & Miller, W.C. Validation of a brief screening instrument for substance abuse and mental illness in HIV-positive patients. *J Acquir Immune Defic Syndr*, 40(4), 434–444. Copyright (2005), with permission from Lippincott Williams and Wilkins.

moderate specificity for both substance abuse and mental illness, making it an effective screening instrument. Because of the limited specificity, patients who screen positive will require a more rigorous mental health assessment. There are several limitations to this tool, but because of its brevity and ease in administration, it is worthy of consideration for use in a routine clinical practice with limited mental health resources.

NURSING SUPPORT FOR THE HIV-INFECTED INDIVIDUAL

The purpose of HIV/AIDS nursing practice is to provide educational, therapeutic, and supportive interventions that prevent illness, promote client, family, and community adaptation to HIV infection and its sequelae, and ensure continuity of quality care by collaborating with other professionals (HIV/AIDS Nursing Certification Board, Definition of Nursing Practice). A brief overview of the key minimum standards of nursing practice typically found in any HIV practice follows.

Patient and Family Education: Support by Nurses

Persons with HIV and AIDS need assistance with understanding health situations, making appropriate health care decisions, and changing health-related behaviors. Patient education begins at the initial visit and continues throughout the entire patient–provider experience. In most settings, various personnel may take on the responsibilities of providing health education to patients. They may include primary care providers, nurses, social workers, case managers, and pharmacists. Some settings have designated health educators whose role is to provide this type of support for patients. Even when a formal health educator is available, a collaborative, multidisciplinary approach to patient education serves both patients and providers optimally. However, it is important to ensure that patient edu-

TABLE 29.4. Test Characteristics of the Substance Abuse and Mental Illness Symptom Screener (SAMISS)

Screening Module	Diagnosis*	No Diagnosis	Sensitivity (95% CI)	Specificity (95% CI)	LR+	LR−
SA	29	119	86.2 (68.3–96.1)	74.8 (66.0–82.3)	3.4	0.18
MI	59	84	94.9 (85.9–98.9)	48.8 (37.7–60.0)	1.9	0.10
Combined†	68	75	97.1 (89.8–99.6)	44.0 (32.5–55.9)	1.7	0.067

CI, confidence interval; LR+, positive likelihood ratio; LR−, negative likelihood ratio; MI, mental illness; SA, substance abuse; SCID, Structured Clinical Interview for DSM-IV.

*From SCID.

†Positive screen on either SA or MI module, compared with any SCID diagnosis.

From: Pence, B.W., Gaynes, B.N., Whetten, K., Eron, J.J., Jr., Ryder, R.W., & Miller, W.C. Validation of a brief screening instrument for substance abuse and mental illness in HIV-positive patients. *J Acquir Immune Defic Syndr*, 40(4), 434–444. Copyright (2005), with permission from Lippincott Williams and Wilkins.

cation messages are coordinated and that patients are receiving consistent information. Patient education must be provided in a language and at a literacy level appropriate for the patient. Patient education should be conducted in the patient's primary language, if possible; otherwise, skilled medical interpreters should be involved (United States Department of Veterans Affairs, 2005).

What Does Patient Education Involve?

The nurse should assess the patient's understanding of the following elements of HIV illness and begin patient education at the initial evaluation. The content and number of items discussed are dependent on a number of factors, including time appropriated for education, resources and tools available, and the literacy level of the patient. Suggested content includes: the following:

- How HIV is transmitted
- Natural history of HIV illness and consequences of immune system destruction
- The meaning of the viral load and CD4 count
- The beneficial impact of antiretroviral drugs
- Early signs and symptoms of opportunistic illnesses
- The role of prophylactic agents
- The critical role of the patient in his or her own care

Educating Patients before Beginning Antiretroviral Therapy

Although the initiation of antiretroviral therapy is not the only focus of the clinic encounter, it is an important aspect of HIV care. Before initiating antiretroviral therapy, patients must be fully aware of the following:

- The importance of adhering completely to the treatment regimen
- The possibility of drug resistance and loss of treatment options
- The proper timing of pills and coordinating pill-taking with meals
- Possible side effects and long-term drug toxicities
- The critical need for adherence to medical follow-up to prevent life-threatening side effects

During the course of treatment, if adherence problems are identified, the nurse can provide counseling for the patient on strategies and techniques to improve adherence. The nurse assesses the factors that contribute to decreased adherence, plans a course of action with the patient to improve adherence, and assists the patient with the implementation of the plan. An evaluation of that plan is achieved by assessing adherence at each clinic visit by any and all providers. For a more extensive review of medication adherence and adherence strategies see Chapter 22.

Symptom Management: Support by Nurses

Symptom management refers to how the person with HIV illness makes day-to-day decisions regarding aspects of symptoms experienced as a direct or indirect result of HIV-related illness or its treatments. Symptom management is a complex science shaped by demographics, culture, perceived risk, stage of illness, treatments, provider relationships, social support, access, and the extent of the patient's education about HIV and AIDS.

While symptoms may be related to comorbidities and opportunistic infections, medication side effects are growing sources of patient symptoms. Medication side effects such as nausea, diarrhea, increased fatigue, headache, and sleep disturbances are ever-present and are an important source of poor adherence. Preparing the patient and anticipating potential side effects is an important role for the nurse in HIV care. Some of the more common side effects from antiretroviral agents are described in Table 29.5, along with some suggested nursing interventions.

Nursing Telephone Triage

A nurse telephone triage serves an important role in the delivery of HIV services. Telephone triage nurses provide an important link for patients to their clinic and to their health care providers. Managing HIV illness on a day-to-day basis can be both challenging and daunting, and having a readily available resource is an important connection. The scope of telephone nursing practice includes the provision of health counseling, primary care advice, routine health assessments, utilization control, and illness triage. Telephone nurses can also coordinate care among external agencies that provide services to HIV patients. These services

TABLE 29.5. Managing Common Symptoms from Antiretroviral Therapy

Side Effect	Etiology/Patient Counseling	Clinical Interventions	Nonpharmacologic Interventions
Nausea	Avoid known triggers (e.g., the smell of certain foods). Teach patient to use deep breathing and relaxation at first onset of feeling nauseated. Ensure proper room ventilation.	Antiemetics as prescribed	Use of crystallized ginger has been helpful for some patients.
Fatigue	HIV-related fatigue can be multifactorial. It can be related to HIV itself, zidovudine-related anemia, or anemia of chronic disease, among others. Ask the patient at what time of the day the fatigue occurs and look for treatable patterns.	Assess hemoglobin, hematocrit, liver function tests, thyroid function, or possible opportunistic infection. Treat any underlying abnormal finding.	If not contraindicated, counsel patient on the use of a light, progressive exercise program
Dyspnea	Shortness of breath can be caused by anxiety, opportunistic infections, anemia, or other respiratory conditions.	Perform a comprehensive respiratory assessment.	Maintain adequate fluid intake to lessen any secretions Review proper positioning to promote ease of respiration. Avoid toxic stimulants such as smoke, perfume, and heavily scented flowers.
Difficulty in swallowing	Assess for any oral lesions or airway obstruction. Ask patient about any possible triggers (e.g., food, antiretrovirals, large pills, etc.)	Treat any pathology such as lesions or exudate.	Encourage the use of soft or pureed foods. Eat foods at room temperature. Avoid "dense" foods such as peanut butter, milk, and candy.

Source: From Willard S. Managing Side Effects and Promoting Adherence in Patients with HIV Disease: The Nurse's Role. C.E. Available at: http://www.medscape.com/viewprogram/4573. Accessed January 29, 2006. With permission from Medscape.

generally place calls to the telephone line to report symptoms or to gain patient information.

Wess and Bronaugh (2003) have described telephone triage as an excellent vehicle in identifying and promoting self-management and adherence; it is an important and necessary component of any HIV program.

SUMMARY

Despite the therapeutic advances that have occurred since the epidemic began more than 20 years ago, HIV infection continues to affect individuals, families, and communities at the alarming rate of approximately five million new infections worldwide. Much has been learned about caring for patients in a constantly changing, complex epidemic, but much is yet to be learned about supporting a chronic illness and providing primary and secondary prevention. Nursing practice is multifaceted and occurs in an array of settings, including primary care, acute care facilities, communities, and schools. HIV/AIDS nursing practice can be defined as the provision of educational, therapeutic, and supportive interventions to promote client, family, and community adaptation to HIV infection. Nurses in HIV care are constantly challenged by the complexities of the disease. Persons with HIV and AIDS who are actively engaged in substance use present major challenges to nurses who are trying to promote adherence to care and risk reduction. Mental illness may emerge or be exacerbated by HIV illness and its treatments. Mental illness and substance use may go untreated and interfere with HIV illness or contribute to its transmission. Nurses are an important resource in the process of screening for substance use and psychiatric illness. They are also an important part of the multidisciplinary team that includes mental health providers. Although nursing research has contributed to the elucidation of the complex combination of both medical and psychiatric issues that constitute the dynamics of HIV illness, there is still much more to be understood. Nurses have contributed to and will continue to contribute to the HIV/AIDS knowledge base in professional, scientific, and personal ways that have served to enhance the lives of persons infected with HIV.

References

Agency for Healthcare Research and Quality (2005). *Hospital Admissions of HIV Patients Have Fallen By More Than Half Since 1995.* Press release, December 1, 2005. Retrieved April 5, 2007, from http://www.ahrq.gov/news/press/pr2005/hivadmispr.htm.

Aiken LH, Sloane DM, and Lake ET (1997). Satisfaction with inpatient acquired immunodeficiency syndrome care. A national comparison of dedicated and scattered-bed units. *Med Care* 35(9):948–962.

Arthur D (1998). Alcohol-related problems: a critical review of the literature and directions in nurse education. *Nurse Educ Today* 18(6):477–487.

Barry KL, Blow FC, Willenbring ML, McCormick R, Brockmann LM, and Visnic S (2004). Use of alcohol screening and brief interventions in primary care settings: implementation and barriers. *Subst Abus* 25(1):27–36.

Bing EG, Burnam MA, Longshore D, Fleishman JA, Sherbourne CD, London AS, et al. (2001). Psychiatric disorders and drug use among human immunodeficiency virus–infected adults in the United States. *Arch Gen Psychiatry* 58(8):721–728.

Blank MB, Mandell DS, Aiken L, and Hadley T (2002). Co-occurrence of HIV and serious mental illness among Medicaid recipients. *Psychiatr Serv* 53(7):868–873.

Brown RL, Leonard T, Saunders LA, and Papasouliotis O (2001). A two-item conjoint screen for alcohol and other drug problems. *J Am Board Fam Pract* 14(2):95–106.

Carey M, Weinhardt L, and Carey K (1995). Prevalence of infection with HIV among the seriously mentally ill: review of research and implications for practice. *Prof Psychol Res Pract.* 26:262–268.

Carey MP, Carey KB, Maisto SA, Gordon CM, Schroder KE, and Vanable PA (2004). Reducing HIV-risk behavior among adults receiving outpatient psychiatric treatment: results from a randomized controlled trial. *J Consult Clin Psychol* 72(2):252–268.

Carney P, and Ward D (1998). Using unannounced standardized patients to assess the HIV preventive practices of family nurse practitioners and family physicians. *Nurse Practitioner* 23:56–58, 63, 67–68.

[CDC] Centers for Disease Control and Prevention (2003). Advancing HIV prevention: new strategies for a changing epidemic—United States, 2003. *MMWR Morb Mortal Wkly Rep* 52(15):329–332.

[CDC] Centers for Disease Control and Prevention (2004). *HIV/AIDS Surveillance Report.* Retrieved April 5, 2007 from www.cdc.gov/HIV/topics/surveillance/resources/reports/index.htm#surveillance.

[CDC] Centers for Disease Control and Prevention (2005). HIV prevalence, unrecognized infection, and HIV testing among men who have sex with men—five U.S. Cities, June 2004–April 2005. *MMWR Morb Mortal Wkly Rep* 54(24):597–601.

Deehan A, Templeton L, Taylor C, Drummond C, and Strang J (1998). Are practice nurses an unexplored resource in the identification and management of alcohol misuse? Results from a study of practice nurses in England and Wales in 1995. *J Adv Nurs* 28(3):592–597.

Edne J, Rockwell S, and Glasglow M (1984). The sexual history in general medicine practice. *Arch Intern Med* 144:558–561.

Epstein RM, Morse DS, Frankel RM, Frarey L, Anderson K, and Beckman HB (1998). Awkward moments in patient–physician communication about HIV risk. *Ann Intern Med* 128(6):435–442.

Galvan FH, Bing EG, Fleishman JA, London AS, Caetano R, Burnam MA, et al. (2002). The prevalence of alcohol consumption and heavy drinking among people with HIV in the United States: results from the HIV Cost and Services Utilization Study. *J Stud Alcohol* 63(2):179–186.

Gott M, Galena E, Hinchliff S, and Elford H (2004). "Opening a can of worms": GP and practice nurse barriers to talking about sexual health in primary care. *Fam Pract* 21(5):528–536.

Haddock J, and Burrows C (1997). The role of the nurse in health promotion: an evaluation of a smoking cessation programme in surgical pre-admission clinics. *J Adv Nurs* 26(6):1098–1110.

Johansson K, Akerlind I, and Bendtsen P (2005). Under what circumstances are nurses willing to engage in brief alcohol interventions? A qualitative study from primary care in Sweden. *Addict Behav* 30(5):1049–1053.

Kelly JA (1997). HIV risk reduction interventions for persons with severe mental illness. *Clin Psychol Rev* 17(3):293–309.

Kirton C (2001). Hospitalized clients with HIV/AIDS. In C Kirton, D Tallota, and K Zwolski (eds.), *Handbook of HIV/AIDS Nursing* (pp. 157–166). St. Louis: Mosby.

Makadon HJ, and Silin JG (1995). Prevention of HIV infection in primary care: current practices, future possibilities. *Ann Intern Med* 123:715–719.

Morrison C (1993). Delivery systems for the care of persons with HIV infection and AIDS. *Nurs Clin North Am* 28(2):317–333.

Nkowane AM, and Saxena S (2004). Opportunities for an improved role for nurses in psychoactive substance use: review of the literature. *Int J Nurs Pract* 10(3):102–110.

Otto-Salaj LL, Kelly JA, Stevenson LY, Hoffmann R, and Kalichman SC (2001). Outcomes of a randomized small-group HIV prevention intervention trial for people with serious mental illness. *Community Ment Health J* 37(2):123–144.

Pascreta J, and Jacobsen P (1989). Addressing the need for staff support among nurses caring for the AIDS population. *Oncol Nurs Forum* 16(5):659–663.

Pence BW, Gaynes BN, Whetten K, Eron JJ Jr, Ryder RW, and Miller WC (2005). Validation of a brief screening instrument for substance abuse and mental illness in HIV-positive patients. *J Acquir Immune Defic Syndr* 40(4):434–444.

Rhodes P, and Glynn K. (2005). Modeling the HIV Epidemic. Presented at the National HIV Prevention Conference, Atlanta, Georgia, June 12–15, 2005. From http://www.aegis.com/conferences/NHIVPC/2005/T1-B1102.html.

Rosenberg SD, Goodman LA, Osher FC, Swartz MS, Essock SM, Butterfield MI, et al. (2001). Prevalence of HIV, hepatitis B, and hepatitis C in people with severe mental illness. *Am J Public Health* 91(1):31–37.

Rost K, Burnam MA, and Smith GR (1993). Development of screeners for depressive disorders and substance disorder history. *Med Care* 31(3):189–200.

Schuman P, Ohmit SE, Moore J, Schoenbaum E, Boland R, Rompalo A, et al. (2001). Perceived need for and use of mental health services by women living with or at risk of human immunodeficiency virus infection. *J Am Med Womens Assoc* 56(1):4–8.

Sherman DW (2000). AIDS-dedicated nurses: what can be learned from their perceptions and experiences. *Appl Nurs Res* 13(3):115–124.

Taylor SL, Burnam MA, Sherbourne C, Andersen R, and Cunningham WE (2004). The relationship between type of mental health provider and met and unmet mental health needs in a nationally representative sample of HIV-positive patients. *J Behav Health Serv Res* 31(2):149–163.

Tomson Y, Romelsjo A, and Aberg H (1998). Excessive drinking—brief intervention by a primary health care nurse. A randomized controlled trial. *Scand J Prim Health Care* 16(3):188–192.

UNAIDS (2005). *AIDS Epidemic: 2005.* Retrieved February 3, 2006, from http://data.unaids.org/Publications/IRC-pub06/epi_update2005_en.pdf.

United States Department of Veterans Affairs (2005). *Clinical Management of the HIV- Infected Patient, AIDS Education and Training Centers Date: November 28, 2005.* Retrieved January 25, 2005, from http://www.hiv.va.gov/vahiv?page=cm-901_patiented.

Werch CE, Carlson JM, Pappas DM, and DiClemente CC (1996). Brief nurse consultations for preventing alcohol use among urban school youth. *J Sch Health*, 66(9):335–338.

Wess Y, and Bronaugh M (2003). *Telephone Triage for People with HIV/AIDS: You Make the Call.* Philadelphia: Hanley & Belfus Medical Publishers.

Whetten K, Reif S, Swartz M, Stevens R, Ostermann J, Hanisch L, et al. (2005). A brief mental health and substance abuse screener for persons with HIV. *AIDS Patient Care STDS* 19(2):89–99.

Willard S (2005). *Managing Side Effects and Promoting Adherence in Patients With HIV Disease: The Nurse's Role.* Medscape Nurses. 2005. Retrieved January 29, 2006, from http://www.medscape.com/viewprogram/4573.

Wilson IB, Landon BE, Hirschhorn LR, McInnes K, Ding L, Marsden PV, et al. (2005). Quality of HIV care provided by nurse practitioners, physician assistants, and physicians. *Ann Intern Med* 143(10): 729–736.

Chapter 30

Palliative and Spiritual Care of Persons with HIV and AIDS

Anna L. Dickerman, William Breitbart, and Harvey Max Chochinov

The meaning and role of palliative and spiritual care have evolved over the last decade, along with the dramatically changing clinical picture of AIDS. Advances in antiretroviral therapy and appropriate medical care have allowed individuals with AIDS to live longer and healthier lives. Death rates from AIDS decreased dramatically after 1996 (CDC, 2003). Despite this, a variety of barriers prevent many persons with AIDS in the United States and throughout the world from receiving adequate care (Sanei, 1998; Cohen and Alfonso, 2004; Harding et al., 2005). AIDS-related deaths in the United States have plateaued in the past decade; similarly, new diagnoses of HIV infection have not decreased significantly (CDC, 2005). As the number of patients living with HIV continues to grow, there is an increased need for comprehensive symptom management, including psychosocial and family support.

The ideal model for the comprehensive care of patients with HIV is not one that can be readily dichotomized into disease-specific "curative" and symptom-specific "palliative" approaches, unlike incurable cancers that may be treated in hospice (Selwyn and Forstein, 2003). The curative versus palliative dichotomy has become less relevant now that persons with AIDS live longer, have a high incidence of cancer and other comorbidities, and continue to have an ongoing need for supportive care. Rather, curative and palliative approaches must be integrated in a multidisciplinary fashion to meet the challenges of advanced HIV illness (O'Neill et al., 2000; Selwyn and Forstein, 2003; Selwyn et al., 2003; Alexander and Back, 2004). Skilled and expert psychiatric care is integral to optimal HIV/AIDS palliative care delivery (O'Neill et al., 2003). Psychosomatic medicine psychiatrists in particular, with their expertise in the interface of medicine and psychiatry, are in the unique position to play a major role in the development of psychiatric, psychosocial, and existential aspects of palliative care for AIDS patients.

This chapter reviews basic concepts and definitions of palliative and spiritual care, as well as the distinct challenges facing the psychosomatic medicine practitioner involved in HIV palliative care. Finally, issues such as bereavement, cultural sensitivity, communication, and psychiatric contributions to common physical symptom control are also reviewed.

DEFINING PALLIATIVE CARE

The terms *palliative care* and *palliative medicine* are often used interchangeably. Palliative medicine refers to the medical discipline of palliative care. Modern palliative care has evolved from the hospice movement into a more expansive network of clinical care delivery systems with components of home care and hospital-based services (Butler et al., 1996; Stjernsward and Papallona, 1998).

Palliative care must meet the needs of the "whole person," including the physical, psychological, social, and spiritual aspects of suffering (World Health Organization, 1990). The definition of palliative care set forth by the World Health Organization is one that encompasses the requirements of body, mind, and spirit. According to this definition, palliative care (1) affirms life and regards dying as a normal process; (2) views the dying process as a valuable experience; (3) neither hastens nor postpones death; (4) provides relief from pain and other symptoms; (5) integrates psychological and spiritual care; (6) offers a support system to help patients live as actively as possible until death; (7) helps family cope with illness and bereavement; and, finally, (8) is multidisciplinary, and includes a caregiver team of physicians, nurses, mental health professionals, clergy, and volunteers (World Health Organization 1990, 1998). The Canadian Palliative Care Association (1995) states that palliative care must strive to meet the physical, psychological, social, and spiritual expectations and needs of patients, while also remaining sensitive to personal, cultural, and religious values, beliefs, and practices. Thus, the control of pain and other symptoms, as well as management of psychological, social, and spiritual problems, is essential. The goal of palliative care is to alleviate suffering and maximize quality of life for patients and their families.

The nature and focus of palliative care have evolved over the century, expanding beyond the concept of comfort care only for the dying. This care may begin with the onset of a life-threatening illness and proceeds beyond death to include bereavement interventions for family and others. Indeed, for persons with HIV/ AIDS, many aspects of palliative care are applicable at every stage of illness, from initial diagnosis to the end of life (Cohen and Alfonso, 2004). Persons with a severe illness such as AIDS should not have to wait until the end of their lives to experience relief from suffering and distress. Though palliative care does not merely consist of providing comfort at the end of life, comfort does take on greater importance when cure becomes less feasible. Ideally, as illness proceeds, gradual movement from curative approaches to palliation takes place along a smooth continuum (Cohen and Alfonso, 2004). Table 30.1 summarizes the comprehensive, biopsychosocial approach, recommended for AIDS palliative care. The biopsychosocial approach to AIDS psychiatry is also reviewed in Chapter 1 of this text.

PALLIATIVE CARE ISSUES AND CHALLENGES IN AIDS

AIDS is a chronic illness with exacerbations and remissions, a growing disease burden, medical and psychological comorbidities, and toxic side effects from treatment (Selwyn and Forstein, 2003). The uncertain prognosis of many AIDS patients, as well as the limitations and promise of rapidly evolving therapies,

TABLE 30.1. AIDS Palliative Care: A Biopsychosocial Approach

Biological	Psychological	Social
Pain	Depression	Alienation
Dyspnea	Anxiety	Social isolation
Insomnia	Confusion	Stigma
Fatigue	Psychosis	Spirituality
Nausea	Mania	Financial loss
Vomiting	Withdrawal	Job loss
Diarrhea	Intoxication	Loss of key roles
Blindness	Substance	Loss of independence
Paralysis	dependance	
Weakness	Existential anxiety	
Cachexia	Bereavement	
Incontinence	Suicidality	
Pruritus		
Hiccups		

Source: From Cohen MA and Alfonso CA. AIDS psychiatry: Psychiatric and palliative care, and pain management. In GP Wormser (ed.), *AIDS and Other Manifestations of HIV Infection*, 4th edition (pp. 537–576). Copyright (2004), with permission from Elsevier.

makes decision making about advance care planning and end-of-life issues more complex and elusive than before the advent of highly active antiretroviral therapy (HAART). For patients with AIDS, the World Health Organization's definition of palliative care as "active total care" includes use of antiretroviral therapy, prevention and management of opportunistic infections, as well as a palliative approach of offering symptomatic and supportive care at all stages of disease (Foley and Flannery, 1995; Stephenson et al., 2000).

Pain and Symptom Management

There is a high prevalence of pain, side effects related to antiretroviral therapy, and other symptoms throughout the HIV disease trajectory, which may be underrecognized and undertreated (Moss, 1990; O'Neill and Sherrard, 1993; Singer et al., 1993; Filbet and Marceron, 1994; Foley, 1994; LaRue et al., 1994; Breitbart et al., 1996b, 1998, 1999; Fantoni et al., 1997; Kelleher et al., 1997; LaRue and Colleau, 1997; Wood et al., 1997; Fontaine et al., 1999; Vogl et al., 1999; Mathews et al., 2000; Selwyn and Rivard, 2002; Selwyn et al., 2003).

Pain Management

The deleterious influence of uncontrolled pain on a patient's psychological state is often intuitively understood and recognized. Yet pain is dramatically undertreated in persons with HIV (Schofferman, 1988; Breitbart et al., 1992; Rosenfeld et al., 1997). The World Health Organization (1986) recommends a stepwise process for the pharmacological treatment of pain related to cancer. This model has been adopted by clinicians treating AIDS patients with pain (Newshan and Wainapel, 1993; Reiter and Kudler, 1996) and consists of (1) non-opioid prescription, with or without an adjuvant; (2) prescription of a weak opioid, with or without and adjuvant; and (3) prescription of a strong opioid, with or without a non-opioid with or without an adjuvant. This analgesic "ladder" is more effective for the treatment of nociceptive than for neuropathic pain (Cohen and Alfonso, 2004). Neuropathic pain related to HIV can be treated with adjuvant or coanalgesic agents, such as tricyclic antidepressants and anticonvulsants (Cornblath and McArthur, 1988; Newshan and Wainapel, 1993; Reiter and Kudler, 1996). Acute and chronic pain is best treated on an around-the-clock schedule (Goldberg,

1993; Newshan and Wainapel, 1993), rather than on an as-needed or p.r.n. basis, regardless of the etiology of pain.

Most pain syndromes associated with AIDS respond to pharmacotherapy (Cohen and Alfonso, 2004). Nonetheless, nonpharmacologic analgesic modalities such as surgical procedures, radiation therapy, and neurological stimulatory approaches can provide effective adjuvant therapy (Carmichael, 1991; Geara et al., 1991; Jonsson et al. 1992; Tosches et al., 1992; Newshan and Wainapel 1993; Portenoy, 1993; Jacox et al., 1994). International guidelines also suggest the importance of incorporating psychosocial and behavioral approaches into an opioid management plan (Maddox et al., 1997; Ontario Workplace Safety and Insurance Board, 2000; Kalso et al., 2003; Pain Society and Royal Colleges of Anaesthetists, 2004). Behavioral interventions such as hypnosis, biofeedback, and multicomponent cognitive-behavioral interventions have been shown to be effective in the management of acute, procedurally related cancer pain (Hilgard and LeBaron, 1982; Kellerman et al., 1983; Jay et al., 1986). Typically, behavioral interventions used in the management of acute procedure related pain employ the basic elements of relaxation and distraction or diversion of attention.

Behavioral interventions are also effective as an adjunct treatment for chronic pain, both related and unrelated to cancer (Morley et al., 1999; Guzman et al., 2001; Adams et al., 2006). In chronic cancer pain, cognitive-behavioral techniques are most effective when they are employed as part of a multimodal, multidisciplinary approach (Breitbart, 1989). These techniques can provide much needed respite from pain. Even short periods of relief from pain can break the vicious pain cycle that entraps many cancer patients.

A recent review by Breitbart and colleagues (2004b) addresses in detail the use of behavioral, psychotherapeutic, and psychopharmacologic interventions in pain control.

Management of Other Physical Symptoms

Physical symptoms other than pain can often go undetected and cause significant emotional distress. These symptoms must be assessed by the psychologist or psychiatrist concerned with the evaluation and treatment of psychiatric syndromes. Aggressive treatment of troublesome physical symptoms is necessary to enhance the patient's quality of life (Bruera et al.,

1990; Harding et al., 2005). In addition to providing physical, psychological, and emotional comfort for the patient, symptom management may also improve adherence to antiretroviral therapy (Selwyn and Forstein, 2003).

A comprehensive review of pharmacologic and nonpharmacologic interventions for common physical symptoms encountered in the terminally ill can be found in the *Oxford Textbook of Palliative Medicine*, third edition (Doyle et al., 2003) and the *Handbook of Psychiatry and Palliative Medicine* (Chochinov and Breitbart, 2000). The management of insomnia and fatigue in AIDS is discussed Chapters 15 and 16, respectively, of this text.

Psychiatric Complications

Patients with advanced AIDS are at risk for the development of major psychiatric disturbances (Breitbart et al., 2004a). Indeed, psychiatric complications such as depression and anxiety occur as frequently if not more so than pain and other physical symptoms (Portenoy et al., 1994; Vogl et al., 1999). Thus, palliative care must encompass psychiatric as well as pain and physical symptom management. Psychiatric interventions for the treatment of negative emotional states can in fact complement palliative symptom management strategies (Cohen and Alfonso, 2004). Table 30.2 summarizes some of these interventions. The management of a variety of psychiatric disturbances is also discussed in Chapters 8–13 of this text. Unique psychiatric manifestations of HIV infection are discussed in Chapters 14–18.

TABLE 30.2. Palliative Care and Symptom Management

Symptom	Treatment
Intractable hiccups	Chlopromzine; olanzapine
Dyspnea	Oxygen; morphine; fan; relaxation
Nausea	Ondansetron; olanzapine
Pruritus	Doxepin
Pain (nociceptive)	Strong opioid analgesics (e.g., fentanyl, morphine sulfate)
Pain (neuropathic)	Adjuvant analgesics (e.g., antidepressants, anticonvulsants, stimulants, antihistamines)

Source: Cohen MA and Alfonso CA. AIDS psychiatry: psychiatric and palliative care, and pain management. In GP Wormser (ed.), *AIDS and Other Manifestations of HIV Infection*, 4th edition (pp. 537–576). Copyright (2004), with permission from Elsevier.

Treatment Failure

Despite the promise of new antiretroviral regimens, viral suppression with HAART may not be feasible. Failure of HAART can be caused by drug–drug interactions resulting in suboptimal drug levels, poor adherence, or preexisting drug resistance (Easterbrook and Meadway, 2001).

Polypharmacy is common in persons with AIDS. Newer antiretroviral medications are substantially safer than their predecessors, but the side effects of these agents still pose diagnostic and management challenges (Department of Health and Human Services, 2006). The expanding number of drugs taken by AIDS patients can be problematic, especially since many of these medications are substrates for cytochrome p450 drug-metabolizing enzymes in the liver. Nonnucleoside reverse transcriptase inhibitors and ritonavir-boosted regimens of protease inhibitors in particular have several important drug interactions with other medications, including HIV-related medications (Department of Health and Human Services, 2006). The potential for pharmacokinetic drug interactions can be circumvented by modifying the dose of one or several drugs (Easterbrook and Meadway, 2001). Table 30.3 summarizes the potential interactions between common HIV and palliative care medications.

Patients may have difficulty complying with treatment regimens because of high pill burdens, dietary restrictions, or unacceptable side effects. Psychiatric comorbidities and cognitive impairment can also impact adherence (Ellis, 1997; Goodkin, 1997; Lopez et al., 1998; Evans et al., 2002); the psychiatric aspects of adherence to medical care and antiretrovirals are discussed in Chapter 22 of this text. Studies suggest that 20% of patients do not comply with therapy at all, and the remaining 80% probably comply only about 60% of the time (Easterbrook and Meadway, 2001). Thus, there is a great need for more potent and simplified antiretroviral regimens. The more physicians become frustrated with patients' difficulties in adhering to recommended HAART regimens or with their own inability to reverse the disease course, the less effective they may be in accompanying the patient through the illness (Selwyn and Forstein, 2003).

There is an ongoing debate about the viral fitness of HIV and the possible benefit of continued antiretroviral therapy despite high viral load (Deeks

TABLE 30.3. Potential Drug Interactions Between Common HIV and Palliative Care Medications*

Cytochrome P450 Inhibitors		Antimycobacterials
HIV Medication	**Palliative Care Medication**	Rifampin Rifabutin
Protease Inhibitors Ritonivir† Indinavir Nelfinavir Saquinavir Amprenavir	**Antidepressants** Fluoxetine Paroxetine Sertraline	*Cytochrome P450 Substrates*
		Palliative Care Medication
Nonnucleoside Reverse Transcriptase Inhibitors Delavirdine		**Opioids** Meperidine‡ Methadone Codeine Morphine Fentanyl
Antifungals Ketoconazole Fluconazole Itraconazole		**Appetite Stimulants or Antiemetics** Dronabinol
		Benzodiazepines Clonazepam Diazepam Triazolam‡ Midazolam‡
Cytochrome P450 Inducers		
HIV Medication	**Palliative Care Medication**	**Hypnotics** Zolpidem
Nonnucleoside Reverse Transcriptase Inhibitors Efavirenz Nevirapine	**Anticonvulsants** Carbamazepine Phenytoin Phenobarbital	**Antihistamines** Terfenadine‡ Astemizole

*The palliative care medications listed may require careful monitoring due to potential drug interactions with certain HIV medications. Multiple pathways and feedback loops may exist, especially when multiple P450 active medications are combined and net effects are not always predictable. Most agents are active through the CYP3A4 isoform of the P450 system, but other isoforms are involved to a lesser degree (CYP206, CYP2D19).

†The most potent P450 inhibitor among the protease inhibitors.

‡Not recommended for use with ritonavir or indinavir.

Source: From Selwyn PA, and Forstein M. Overcoming the false dichotomy of curative vs. palliative care for late-stage HIV/AIDS: "Let me live the way I want to live, until I can't." 290(6):806–814. Copyright (2003), with permission from JAMA/Archives Journals.

et al., 2001; Frenkel and Mullins, 2001). The potential risks and benefits of continuing HAART in late-stage HIV illness are summarized in Table 30.4. No guidelines currently exist for the cessation of HAART after treatment failure; this is an important consideration for clinical trials and for the development of the best practices for advanced HIV disease (Selwyn and Forstein, 2003). Failure to cure should not cause the physician to withdraw emotionally because of a perceived or unconscious sense of futility; rather, it is a signal to reiterate the commitment to the patient and to stay with him or her throughout the course of illness (Selwyn and Forstein, 2003).

Multiple Medical Problems and Coexisting Diagnoses

Though HAART has increased the life expectancy of patients with HIV and reduced the incidence of AIDS-related illnesses (Huang et al., 2006), the frequency of pulmonary, cardiac, gastrointestinal, and renal diseases that are often not directly related to underlying HIV disease has increased (Morris et al., 2002; Casalino et al., 2004; Narasimhan et al., 2004; Vincent et al., 2004). A substantial number of persons with AIDS have comorbidities that may complicate their management. Hepatitis B and C, for example, are common in individuals who become infected with

TABLE 30.4. Potential Benefits and Risks of Highly Active Antiretroviral Treatment in Late-Stage Human Immunodeficiency Virus Disease

*Potential Benefits**

Selection for less fit virus (i.e., less pathogenic than wild type), even in the presence of elevated viral loads
Protection against HIV encephalopathy or dementia
Relief or easing of symptoms possibly associated with high viral loads (e.g., constitutional symptoms)
Continued therapeutic effect, albeit attenuated
Psychological and emotional benefits of continued disease-combating therapy

Potential Risks

Cumulative and multiple drug toxic effects in the setting of therapeutic futility (including certain rare, potentially life-threatening toxic effects)
Diminished quality of life from demands of treatment regimen
Therapeutic confusion (i.e., use of future-directed, disease-modifying therapy in a dying patient)
Distraction from end-of-life and advance care planning issues, with narrow focus on medication adherence and monitoring

*Evidence is lacking for some of these potential benefits, although they are commonly considered in clinical decision making.

Source: From Selwyn PA, and Forstein M. Overcoming the false dichotomy of curative vs. palliative care for late-stage HIV/AIDS: "Let me live the way I want to live, until I can't." 290(6):806–814. Copyright (2003), with permission from JAMA/Archives Journals.

HIV via intravenous drug use. Coinfection with HIV is a strong risk factor for progression to end-stage liver disease (Easterbrook and Meadway, 2001). Treatment of both of these viral infections is also associated with greater risk of adverse events, and management of coinfection poses challenges for palliative care. In addition, such patients are likely to have limited access to health care and limited support networks, and are likely to be estranged from their families as well (Easterbrook and Meadway, 2001). Comorbid medical conditions are discussed further in Chapters 33–37 of this text.

Fluctuation in Condition and Difficulty Determining Terminal Stage

Determining the prognosis of patients with advanced HIV disease can be difficult, as responses to therapy are often unpredictable. Identification of the predic-

tors of mortality and prognostic variables for patients with advanced illness in the era of HAART can help inform planning and coordination of care (Shen et al., 2005).

In 1996, short-term mortality predictors promulgated by the National Hospice Organization included CD4 cell count, viral load, and certain opportunistic infections (National Hospice Organization, 1996). These traditional HIV prognostic markers, however, no longer accurately predict death in late-stage patients because of the impact of HAART. Shen and colleagues (2005) studied a heterogeneous population of 230 patients in a palliative care program. Of 120 deaths, the most frequent causes were end-stage AIDS (36%), non-AIDS-defining cancers (19%), bacterial pneumonia or sepsis (18%), and liver failure or cirrhosis (13%). Thus, AIDS patients in the United States are now living long enough that they may experience morbidity and mortality from non-AIDS-defining illnesses. These may in fact pose more of an acute risk than that of HIV-related factors (Sansone and Frengley, 2000; Selwyn et al., 2000; Puoti et al., 2001; Valdez et al., 2001; Welch and Morse, 2002). Shen and colleagues also found that death was not predicted by gender, baseline symptoms on the Memorial Symptom Assessment Scale, HIV risk behavior, HIV disease stage, baseline CD4+ count, or baseline HIV viral load. The only significant predictors of mortality were age greater than 65 years and total ADL impairments or Karnofsky performance score. Thus, as previously suggested by Justice et al. (1996), functional status may be a useful means of predicting mortality in AIDS patients.

COMMUNICATION ABOUT END-OF-LIFE ISSUES

Because of the nonlinear progression of late-stage AIDS, advance care planning and goals of care should be addressed repeatedly during the course of illness (Selwyn and Forstein, 2003). This is especially true because AIDS patients are less likely to discuss advance directives and life-limiting interventions than are other patient populations (Curtis and Patrick, 1997; Mouton et al., 1997; Wenger et al., 2001). Persons with AIDS may also experience doubt and ambivalence as their clinical condition fluctuates; this demands flexibility, patience, and tolerance on the part of the clinician. Regular and direct inquiry into how patients are handling the uncertainty of their lives provides support and indicates that the clinician is ready to hear the patient's concerns (Selwyn and Forstein, 2003). Possible barriers to discussions about end-of-life issues include physicians' reluctance to discuss death (Curtis and Patrick, 1997) and cross-cultural concerns. Chapters 39 and 40 of this text review end-of-life issues, ethical issues, advance directives, and surrogate decision-making.

Cross-Cultural Issues in the Care of the Dying

Ethnicity and culture strongly influence a person's attitude toward death and dying. Although there is a "universal fear of cancer [and other terminal diseases] that results from its [cancer's] association with images of extreme debility and pain and the fear of death" (Butow et al., 1997, p. 320), individuals from Western cultures use different coping strategies to deal with serious illness than those of individuals from non-Western cultures (Barg and Gullate, 2001). These differences likely exist because of variations in basic values and cultural norms among these broad cultural groupings, such as reliance on the family and others for social support, and spiritual or religious beliefs (Mazanec and Tyler, 2003).

Blackhall and colleagues (1995) studied ethnic attitudes toward patient autonomy regarding disclosure of the diagnosis and prognosis of a terminal illness and toward end-of-life decision making. They found that different ethnic, racial, and cultural groups feel differently about how much information physicians should provide concerning diagnoses and prognoses. The investigators determined that African Americans (63%) and European Americans (69%) are more likely than Korean Americans (35%) and Mexican Americans (48%) to believe that a patient should be informed of a terminal prognosis and should be actively involved in decisions concerning use of life-sustaining technology. African Americans are also less likely to consider withdrawal or cessation of life-prolonging measures than certain other racial or ethnic groups (Blackhall et al., 1995; Crawley et al., 2000; Kagawa-Singer and Blackhall, 2001; Candib, 2002). Blackhall and colleagues (1995) concluded that physicians should ask their patients whether they wish to be informed of their diagnoses and prognoses and whether they wish to be involved in treatment decisions or prefer to let family members or caregivers handle such matters.

A similar study of Navajo Indian beliefs about autonomy in patient diagnosis and prognosis found that in the Navajo culture, physicians and patients must speak in only a positive way, avoiding any negative thought or speech (Carrese and Rhodes, 1995). Because Navajos believe that language can "shape reality and control events," informing patients of a negative diagnosis or prognosis is considered disrespectful, as well as physically and emotionally dangerous (Carrese and Rhodes, 1995).

An exhaustive review of the literature on cultural and ethnic differences in the face of life-threatening illness is beyond the scope of this chapter. Nonetheless, as these two studies indicate, patients' cultural beliefs should be considered when disclosing the diagnosis and prognosis of a terminal illness, during evaluation of the patient, and during intervention. Koenig and Gates-William (1995) present a framework for such culturally sensitive evaluation, termed the "ABCDE" model (see Table 30.5). Such a model may provide an effective template for clinicians to incorporate cultural issues into their evaluation and treatment of culturally diverse patients.

Doctor–Patient Communication

Doctor–patient communication is an essential component of caring for a dying patient (Buckman 1993, 1998; Smith, 2000; Baile and Beale, 2001; Parker et al., 2001; Fallowfield, 2004). Despite the recognized importance of caregiver–patient communication, many physicians are not adequately trained in communication skills (Fallowfield et al., 1998). Improved training

TABLE 30.5. "ABCDE" Model for Culturally Sensitive Evaluation

Attitudes about illness, family and related responsibilities

Beliefs about religion and spirituality, with special sensitivity to potential expectations of "miracles"

Cultural context in which both the patient and their family operate

Decision-making style and how cultural beliefs and practices might affect it

Environment and any key features of it that may impact the patient during the course of their illness

Source: Koenig BA, and Gates-William J. Understanding cultural difference in caring for dying patients. West J Med 163:244–249, Copyright (1995), with permission from BMJ Publishing Group.

in doctor–patient communication can help ease anxiety on both sides and improve health outcomes (Simpson et al., 1991). Suchman and colleagues (1997) found that improving physicians' empathic responses to patients in medical interviews can improve the doctor–patient relationship, improve quality of care, and increase both physician and patient satisfaction. On the basis of their findings, Suchman et al. (1997) defined basic empathic skills, necessary for meaningful communication with patients, such as "recognizing when emotions may be present but not directly expressed, inviting exploration of these unexpressed feelings, and effectively acknowledging these feelings so that the patient feels understood" (p. 680).

Buckman (1993, 1998) proposed a guide for communication and empathy in caring for the dying patient. He asserted that the important elements of communication in palliative care are basic listening skills, the breaking of bad news, therapeutic dialogue, and communicating with the family and with other professionals. He acknowledged several sources of difficulty in communicating with a dying patient, including the social denial of death, a lack of experience of death in the family, high expectations of health and life, materialism, and the changing role of religion. The patient's fear of dying is also significant, as are factors originating in the health care professional (e.g., sympathetic pain, fear of receiving blame, fear of the untaught, fear of expressing emotions, and fear of one's own illness and death). However, Buckman (1993) emphasized the importance of teaching and practicing listening skills, using comforting body language, responding empathically to patients, and engaging in therapeutic and supportive dialogue. He also advocated improved communication with patients' families and friends and among medical caregivers.

Buckman (1998) as well as Baile and Beale (2001) have promoted what is commonly referred to as the six-step protocol for breaking bad news (see Table 30.6), which many clinicians find extremely useful and which can be used by psychosomatic medicine specialists when they teach communication skills to physicians in the palliative care setting. Most recently, several intensive training programs in doctor–patient communication have been demonstrated to have both short-term and long-term efficacy in improving communication skills among physicians (Maguire, 1999; Fallowfield, 2004). These programs use a variety of teaching methods, including role-playing, videotaped feedback, experiential exercises, and didactics.

TABLE 30.6. Six Step Protocol for Breaking Bad News

1. Getting the physical context right
2. Finding out how much the patient knows
3. Finding out how much the patient wants to know
4. Sharing information (aligning and educating)
5. Responding to the patient's feelings
6. Planning and following through

Sources: Baile W, and Beale E (2001). Giving bad news to cancer patients: matching process and content. *J Clin Oncol* 19(9):2575–2577 and Buckman R (1998). Communication in palliative care: a practical guide. In D Doyle, GWC Hanks, and N MacDonald (eds.), *Oxford Textbook of Palliative Medicine*, 2nd edition (pp. 141–156). Copyright (1998), with permission from Oxford University Press.

PROGRAMS AND MODELS OF HIV PALLIATIVE CARE DELIVERY

Even end-stage AIDS patients can be restored to independence and good quality of life (Rackstraw et al., 2000; Stephenson et al., 2000). Fully developed, ideal palliative care programs offer control of symptoms and provision of support to those living with chronic, life-threatening illnesses such as AIDS. Such programs optimally include all of the following components: (1) a home care program (e.g., hospice program); (2) a hospital-based palliative care consultation service; (3) a day care program or ambulatory care clinic; (4) palliative care inpatient unit (or dedicated palliative care beds in hospital); (5) a bereavement program; (6) training and research programs; and (7) Internet-based services.

Of HIV patients who express a preference for location of their death, less than 10% wish to die in hospital (Goldstone et al., 1995). The disadvantages of hospitals for dying patients include variable quality of palliative care in acute medical settings, and focus on management of acute problems in a person who may in fact be dying slowly (Easterbrook and Meadway, 2001).

The merits of specialized hospices versus nonspecialized hospices for the delivery of HIV palliative care have been reviewed (Schofferman, 1987; Mansfield et al., 1992). Staff at specialized hospices are experienced in the management of HIV-related problems, and as a result are particularly sensitive to the social and psychological issues associated with HIV illness. Moreover, the environment of the specialized hospice provides patients with the opportunity to meet and gain encouragement from other patients in similar settings (Easterbrook and Meadway, 2001).

Patients in the later stages of AIDS commonly express the desire to die at home (Easterbrook and Meadway, 2001). Where available, hospital support teams and community HIV nurse specialists can be helpful. Rather than merely practicing traditional approaches to care, it is important to take into consideration the direction and needs of those who choose to die at home (Johnson, 1995).

For further review of special settings such as psychiatric facilities, nursing homes, correctional facilities, and homeless outreach, please see Chapter 31 of this text.

SPIRITUAL CARE

Issues of spirituality are essential elements of quality palliative care. The need to address the spiritual domains of supportive care has been identified as a priority by medical practitioners and patients alike (Singer et al., 1999). Palliative care practitioners in particular have begun to recognize the importance of spiritual suffering in their patients and have begun to design interventions to address it (Puchalski and Romer, 2000; Rousseau, 2000).

Defining Spirituality

Puchalski and Romer (2000) define spirituality as that which allows a person to experience transcendent meaning in life. Karasu (1999) views spirituality as a construct that involves concepts of faith and/or meaning. Faith is a belief in a higher transcendent power, not necessarily identified as God. It need not involve participation in the rituals or beliefs of a specific organized religion. Indeed, the transcendent power may be identified as external to the human psyche or internalized; it is the relationship and connectedness to this power, or spirit, that is an essential component of the spiritual experience and is related to the concept of meaning. Meaning, or having a sense that one's life has meaning, involves the conviction that one is fulfilling a unique role and purpose in a life that is a gift; a life that comes with a responsibility to live to one's full potential as a human being. In so doing, one is able to achieve a sense of peace, contentment, or even transcendence through connectedness with something greater than oneself (Frankl, 1959). The "faith" component of spirituality is most often associated with religion and religious belief, while the "meaning" com-

ponent of spirituality appears to be a more universal concept that can exist in individuals who do, or do not, identify themselves to be religious.

The FACIT Spiritual Well-Being Scale, or FACITSWBS (Peterman et al., 1996), is a widely used measure of spiritual well-being that consists of both a faith and meaning component of spirituality. The FACITSWBS generates a total score as well as two subscale scores: one corresponding to "Faith," and a second corresponding to "Meaning/Peace". Other measures commonly used to measure aspects of spirituality include the Daily Spiritual Experiences Scale, or DSES (Underwood and Teresi, 2002), and the Spiritual Beliefs Inventory, or SBI-15 (Baider et al., 2001).

Assessing Spirituality

A spiritual history should be taken as early in the treatment as possible, as it provides an opportunity to give more comprehensive care and serves in building a relationship with a patient. Several general communication strategies should help to elicit patient concerns around spiritual concerns. These include the use of open-ended questions, asking patients follow-up questions to elicit more detail about their concerns, acknowledging and normalizing patient apprehension and distress, the use of empathetic comments in response to patient concerns, and inquiring about patient's emotions around these issues (Lo et al., 2003).

There are several methods of taking a spiritual history. Puchalski and Romer (2000) recommend the acronym FICA to structure a spiritual history, which stands for Faith and belief, Importance, Community, and Address. A good spiritual assessment should include the questions outlined in Table 30.7 (Koenig, 2002; Pulchalski and Romer, 2000).

In addition to these more open-ended questions, several formal assessment tools exist for the assessment of spirituality (Maugans, 1996). Most importantly, a detailed spiritual assessment should not be regarded as a one-time discussion but rather as the beginning of a dialogue that continues throughout a patient's care. This type of assessment should serve to let the patient know that the provider is open to these discussions and that the patient's concerns regarding spiritual issues will be met in a supportive and respectful manner (Post et al., 2000). Simply being present, actively listening, offering empathetic responses, and trying to understand the patient's point of view will foster a productive dialogue and offer great comfort to the patient.

TABLE 30.7. Questions to Ask When Performing a Spiritual Assessment

1. Do you consider yourself a spiritual or religious person?
2. What gives your life meaning?
3. Do the religious or spiritual beliefs provide comfort and support or cause stress?
4. What importance do these beliefs have in your life?
5. Could these beliefs influence your medical decisions?
6. Do you have beliefs that might conflict with your medical care?
7. Are you part of a spiritual or religious community? Are they important to you or a source of support?
8. What are your spiritual needs that someone should address? How would you like these needs to be addressed as part of your health care?

Sources: Koenig HG: Religion, spirituality, and medicine: how are they related and what does it mean? *Mayo Clin Proc* 2002; 12:1189–1191; Puchalski C, and Romer AL: Taking a spiritual history allows clinicians to understand patients more fully. *J Palliat Med* 3:129–137. Copyright (2000), with permission from Mary Ann Liebert, Inc.

Spirituality and Life-Threatening Medical Illness

There has been great interest in spirituality, faith, and religious beliefs with regard to their impact on health outcomes and their role in palliative care (Koenig et al., 1992, 1998; Baider et al., 1999; McCullough and Larson, 1999; Sloan et al., 1999). Some researchers theorize that religious beliefs may play a role in helping patients construct meaning out of the suffering inherent to illness, in turn facilitating acceptance of their situation (Koenig et al., 1998). Importantly, recent studies have found that religion and spirituality generally play a positive role in patients' coping with illnesses such as HIV and cancer (Peterman et al., 1996; Baider et al., 1999; Nelson et al., 2002).

Several studies (Breitbart et al., 2000; Nelson et al., 2002; McClain et al., 2003) have demonstrated a central role for spiritual well-being and meaning as a buffer against depression, hopelessness, and desire for hastened death among advanced cancer patients. These findings are significant in the face of what we have come to learn about the consequences of depression and hopelessness in palliative care patients. Depression and hopelessness are associated with poorer survival among cancer patients (Watson et al., 1999), as well as dramatically higher rates of suicide, suicidal ideation, desire for hastened death, and interest in physician-assisted suicide (Chochinov et al.,

1994, 1995, 1998; Breitbart et al., 1996a, 2000). Such findings point to the need for the development of interventions in palliative patients that address depression, hopelessness, loss of meaning, desire for death, and what many practitioners (Rousseau, 2000) refer to as "spiritual suffering." Several recently developed interventions are reviewed below.

Treatment of Spiritual Suffering

Rousseau (2000) has developed an approach to the treatment of spiritual suffering that centers on (1) controlling physical symptoms; (2) providing a supportive presence; (3) encouraging life review to assist in recognizing purpose value and meaning; (4) exploring guilt, remorse, forgiveness, and reconciliation; (5) facilitating religious expression; (6) reframing goals; (7) encouraging meditative practices; and (8) focusing on healing rather than cure. This approach to spiritual suffering encompasses a blend of several basic psychotherapeutic principles common to many psychotherapies. It should be noted that this intervention contains a heavy emphasis on facilitating religious expression and confession that may be extremely useful to many patients, but not all patients or clinicians will feel comfortable with this approach.

Meaning-Centered Interventions

In contrast, Breitbart and colleagues (Greenstein and Breitbart, 2000; Breitbart, 2002; Breitbart and Heller, 2003; Gibson and Breitbart, 2004) have attempted to apply the work of Viktor Frankl and his concepts of meaning-based psychotherapy (Frankl, 1955) to address spiritual suffering. While Frankl's logotherapy was not designed for the treatment of patients with life-threatening illness, his concepts of meaning and spirituality clearly have applications in psychotherapeutic work with advanced medically ill patients, many of whom seek guidance and help in dealing with issues of sustaining meaning, hope, and understanding in the face of their illness, while avoiding overt religious emphasis. This "meaning-centered group psychotherapy" (Greenstein and Breitbart, 2002) uses a mixture of didactics, discussion, and experiential exercises that focus on particular themes related to meaning and advanced cancer. It is designed to help patients with advanced cancer sustain or enhance a sense of meaning, peace, and purpose in their lives, even as they approach the end of life.

Gibson and Breitbart (2004) have manualized an individual form of this therapy, and are currently conducting outcome studies to determine the feasibility and efficacy of both the group and individual forms of this therapy.

Treatment of Demoralization

Kissane and colleagues (2001) have described a syndrome of "demoralization" in the terminally ill, distinct from depression. Demoralization syndrome consists of a triad of hopelessness, loss of meaning, and existential distress expressed as a desire for death. It is associated with life-threatening medical illness, disability, bodily disfigurement, fear, loss of dignity, social isolation, and feelings of being a burden. Because of the sense of impotence and hopelessness, those with the syndrome predictably progress to a desire to die or commit suicide. Kissane and colleagues (2001) have formulated a treatment approach for demoralization syndrome (see Table 30.8).

Dignity-Conserving Care

Finally, ensuring dignity in the dying process is a critical goal of palliative care. Despite use of the term *dignity* in arguments for and against a patient's self-governance in matters pertaining to death, there is little empirical research on how this term has been used by patients who are nearing death. Chochinov and colleagues (2002a, 2002b) examined how dying

TABLE 30.8. Multidisciplinary Model for Treatment of Demoralization Syndrome

1. Ensure continuity of care and active symptom management
2. Ensure dignity in the dying process
3a. Use various types of psychotherapy to help sustain a sense of meaning
3b. Limit cognitive distortions and maintain family relationships (i.e., via meaning–based, cognitive-behavioral, interpersonal, and family psychotherapy interventions.
4. Use life review and narrative, giving attention to spiritual issues
5. Use pharmacotherapy for comorbid anxiety, depression, or delirium

Source: Kissane D, Clarke DM, and Street AF. Demoralization syndrome: a relevant psychiatric diagnosis for palliative care. *J Palliat Care* 17:12–21. Copyright (2001), with permission from Mary Ann Liebert, Inc.

patients understand and define the term *dignity* to develop a model of dignity in the terminally ill. A semistructured interview was designed to explore how patients cope with their illness and their perceptions of dignity. Three major categories emerged: (1) illness-related concerns (concerns that derive from or are related to the illness itself and threaten to or actually do impinge on the patient's sense of dignity); (2) dignity-conserving repertoire (internally held qualities or personal approaches or techniques that patients use to bolster or maintain their sense of dignity); and (3) social dignity inventory (social concerns or relationship dynamics that enhance or detract from a patient's sense of dignity). These broad categories and their carefully defined themes and sub-themes form the foundation for an emerging model of dignity among the dying. The concept of dignity and the notion of dignity-conserving care offer a way of understanding how patients face advancing terminal illness. They also present an approach that clinicians can use to explicitly target the maintenance of dignity as a therapeutic objective.

Accordingly, Chochinov (2002) has developed a short-term dignity therapy for palliative patients that incorporates those facets from this model that are most likely to bolster the dying patient's will to live, lessen the desire for death or overall level of distress, and improve quality of life. The dignity model establishes the importance of "generativity" as a significant dignity theme. As such, the sessions are taped, transcribed, and edited, and the transcription is returned within 1 to 2 days to the patient. The creation of a tangible product that will live beyond the patient acknowledges the importance of generativity as a salient dignity issue. The immediacy of the returned transcript is intended to bolster the patient's sense of purpose, meaning, and worth by tangibly experiencing that their thoughts and words continue to be valued. In most instances, these transcripts are left for family or loved ones and form part of a personal legacy that the patient has actively participated in creating and shaping. In a study of 100 terminally ill cancer patients, Chochinov et al. (2005) reported that 91 participants were satisfied with dignity therapy, 76% reported a heightened sense of dignity, 68% reported an increased sense of purpose, 67% reported a heightened sense of meaning, 47% reported an increased will to live, and 81% reported that it had been or would be of help to their family. Measures of suffering and depression also showed significant improvement, suggesting that dignity therapy is a novel therapeutic intervention for suffering and distress at the end of life.

Communicating about Spiritual Issues

There may be several factors that inhibit effective communication with patients about spirituality in a palliative care setting (Ellis et al., 1999; Sloan et al., 1999; Clayton, 2000; Post et al., 2000). Promoting religion, faith, or specific religious beliefs or rituals (e.g. prayer, belief in an afterlife) in an effort to deal with patients' spiritual concerns or suffering at the end of life has limited acceptance among health care providers and is not universally applicable to all patients. Maugans and Wadland (1991) suggest that there is a great discrepancy between physicians and patients on such issues as belief in God, belief in an afterlife, regular prayer, and feeling close to God, with physicians endorsing such beliefs or practices less than half as often as patients (none greater than 40%).

Several additional factors have been cited as contributing to the avoidance of these discussions, including a lack of time on the part of the provider, a lack of training in this area, fear of projecting one's own beliefs onto the patient, and concerns about patient autonomy (Ellis et al., 1999). Finally, providers may feel that these discussions are inappropriate, as they are outside of their area of expertise or intrusive to the patient's privacy, and may experience some discomfort in pursuing these topics (Ellis et al., 1999; Sloan et al., 1999; Post et al., 2000; Cohen et al., 2001). However, most studies have demonstrated that in fact the opposite is true, as patients welcome these discussions (Anderson et al., 1993; King and Bushwick, 1994; Maugans 1996). Therefore, discussions about spiritual, religious, or existential concerns— that is, finding out what matters to the patient in terms of being imbued with continued meaning and purpose, regardless of its source—should not be avoided, but rather, may simply require more time and consideration on the part of the provider.

Communicating about spirituality with patients effectively requires comfort in several domains: (1) a basic knowledge of common spiritual concerns and sources of spiritual pain for patients; (2) the principles and beliefs of the major religions common to the patient populations one treats; (3) basic clinical communication skills, such as active and empathetic listening, with an ability to identify and highlight spiritually relevant issues; and (4) the ability to remain present while patients struggle with spiritual issues in light of their mortality (Storey and Knight, 2001). This final domain is often the most trying, especially for clinicians early in their career.

The American Academy of Hospice and Palliative Medicine offers the following guidelines for clinicians when communicating about spiritual issues (Doyle, 1992; Hay, 1996; Storey and Knight, 2001). First, it is important to recognize that every patient is an individual and has a unique belief system that should be honored and respected. A patient's spiritual views may or may not incorporate religious beliefs, as spirituality is considered the more inclusive category. Therefore, initial discussions should focus on broad spiritual issues and then, when appropriate, on more specific religious beliefs. Caregivers should maintain appropriate boundaries and avoid discussions of their own religious beliefs, as it is usually not relevant. Finally, fostering hope and integrating meaning into a patient's life is often a more important aspect of providing spiritual healing than any adherence to a particular belief system or religious affiliation.

Pathways of Spiritual Care

Spirituality can help patients and families cope with life-threatening medical illness and its ensuing stressors. By understanding and respecting their beliefs, clinicians may allow their patients to believe in their own abilities to cope. Psychosomatic medicine clinicians can seek both specialized training and referrals to appropriate sources to help them deal more effectively with the often complicated and painful spiritual issues their patients present.

It is essential to effectively use an interdisciplinary team approach that incorporates members of pastoral care services. The chaplain is the spiritual care specialist on the health care team and has the training necessary to treat spiritual distress in all its forms (Handzo and Koenig, 2004). Referrals to chaplains ought to be approached just as referrals to any other specialist would be; such referrals are an essential part of comprehensive care (Thiel and Robinson, 1997). The role of the physician is to assess spiritual needs as they relate to health care (i.e., briefly screen) and then refer to a professional pastoral caregiver as indicated (i.e., to address those needs). Seeing the physician as the generalist in spiritual care and the chaplain as the specialist is a helpful model (Handzo and Koenig, 2004). Finally, the doctor or nurse needs to be able to recognize and appreciate how a given patient's religious and cultural beliefs impact the way in which that patient makes health care decisions. This ensures a more effective path toward agreement with patients on those decisions.

ROLE OF THE PSYCHOSOMATIC CLINICIAN AT TIME OF DEATH AND AFTERWARDS

The physician plays a key role as someone who can accompany the patient and family through a complex process that extends far beyond medical treatment. Spending time with the dying patient is crucial. At the end of life, it can be extremely helpful to talk, hold hands, and surround the patient with loved ones, if available (Cohen and Alfonso, 2004). This may alleviate any fears of abandonment or of dying alone.

Grief and Bereavement

Bereavement care is an integral dimension of palliative care. Knowledge of and competence in assessing grief is essential to recognize the 20% of the bereaved who need additional assistance. Routine assessment of the bereaved for risk factors associated with complicated grief provides a method by which psychosomatic medicine specialists can preventatively intervene to reduce unnecessary morbidity. Effective therapies are available to assist in the management of complicated grief (Kissane, 2004). Grief is an inevitable dimension of our humanity, an adaptive adjustment process, and one that, with adequate support, can eventually be traversed.

Although words such as "grief," "mourning," and "bereavement" are commonly used interchangeably, the following definitions may be helpful:

- *Bereavement* is the state of loss resulting from death (Parkes, 1998).
- *Grief* is the emotional response associated with loss (Stroebe et al., 1993).
- *Mourning* is the process of adaptation, including the cultural and social rituals prescribed as accompaniments (Raphael, 1983).
- *Anticipatory grief* precedes the death and results from the expectation of that event (Raphael, 1983).
- *Complicated grief* represents a pathological outcome involving psychological, social, or physical morbidity (Rando, 1983).

- *Disenfranchised grief* represents the hidden sorrow of the marginalized, where there is less social permission to express many dimensions of loss (Doka, 1989).

Anticipatory Grief

As the patient and family journey through palliative care, the clinical phases of grief progress from anticipatory grief through to the immediate news of the death, to the stages of acute grief and, potentially for some, the complications of bereavement. Anticipatory grief generally draws the supportive family into a configuration of mutual comfort and greater closeness as the news of the illness and its proposed management is tackled. For a time this perturbation advantages the care of the sick, until the pressures of daily life draw the family back toward their prior constellation. Movement back and forth is evident thereafter, as news of illness progression unfolds. Periods of grief can become interspersed with phases of contentment and happiness. When the family is engaged in home care of their dying member, their cohesion may increase as they share their fears, hopes, joy, and distress. In some families, the stress of loss may result in further divisiveness and the accentuation of previously contentious dynamics.

Difficulties can emerge for some families as they express their anticipatory grief. Impaired coping manifests itself via protective avoidance, denial of the seriousness of the threat, anger, or withdrawal from involvement. Sometimes family dysfunction is glaring. More commonly, however, subthreshold or mild depressive or anxiety disorders develop gradually as individuals struggle to adapt to unwelcome changes. While anticipatory grief was historically suggested to reduce postmortem grief (Parkes, 1975), intense distress is now well recognized as a marker of risk for complicated grief. During this phase of anticipatory grief, clinicians can help the family that is capable of effective communication by encouraging them to openly share their feelings as they go about the instrumental care of their dying family member or friend. Saying goodbye is a process that evolves over time, with opportunities for reminiscence, celebration of the life and contribution of the dying person, expressions of gratitude, and completion of any unfinished business (Meares, 1981). These tasks have the potential to generate creative and positive emotions out of what is otherwise a sad time for all.

Grief of Family and Friends Gathered Around the Death Bed

When relatives or close friends gather to keep watch by the bed of a dying person, they not only support the sick but also help their own subsequent adjustment. For years to come, these poignant moments will be recalled in immense detail; thus, the sensitivity and courteous respect of health professionals is crucial (Maguire, 1985). Clinicians can helpfully comment on the process of dying, explaining the breathing patterns and commenting on any noises, secretions, patient reactions, and comfort measures. Moreover, the physician can empathically normalize the experience and reassure the family whenever concern develops. Discussions about pain, reasons for medications, and skilled prediction of events will assuage worry and build a collaborative approach to the care of the dying.

Religious rituals warrant active facilitation, including appropriate notification of a religious minister or pastoral care worker. Respect for the body remains paramount once death has occurred, and the expression of sympathy from clinicians is greatly appreciated. The family will be invariably grateful for time spent alone with the deceased, and regard for cultural approaches to the laying out of the body is essential (Parkes, 1997). Sometimes staff will have concerns about the emotional response of the bereaved. If there is uncertainty about its cultural appropriateness, consultation with an informed cultural intermediary may prove helpful. The prescription of short-acting benzodiazepines will help some, while others will prefer to manage without medication. A follow-up telephone call soon after the death is worthwhile to check on coping and identify the need for continued support.

Caution is warranted in settings where grief could be marginalized, well exemplified by ageism (Doka, 1989). If a death is normalized because it appears in step with the life cycle, family members can be given less support and reduced permission to express many aspects of their loss. In the process, the disenfranchised can be ignored in their sorrow.

Acute Grief and Time Course of Bereavement

The bereaved move through sequences of phases over time; these phases are never rigidly demarcated, but rather, merge gradually one into the other (Raphael, 1983; Parkes, 1998). The time course of mourning is shaped by the nature of the loss, the context within such loss took place, as well as a multitude of factors ranging from personal resilience to cultural, social and ethnic affiliations. There is no sharply defined end point to grief. The clinical task is to differentiate those that remain with the spectrum of normalcy from those that cross the threshold of complicated grief.

Complicated Grief

Normal and abnormal responses to bereavement span a spectrum. Intensity of reaction, presence of a range of related grief behaviors, and time course all factor into the differentiation between normal and abnormal grief. Common psychiatric disorders resulting from grief include clinical depression, anxiety disorders, alcohol abuse or other substance abuse and dependence, and, less commonly, psychotic disorders and posttraumatic stress disorder. When frank psychiatric disorders complicate bereavement, their recognition and management is straightforward. Subthreshold states, however, present a greater clinical challenge.

Studies of the bereaved indicate groups in which clusters of intense grief symptoms are distinct from uncomplicated grief (Parkes, 1983; Prigerson et al., 1995). Their recognition calls for an experienced clinical judgement that does not normalize the distress as understandable. Risk factors for complicated grief should be assessed at entry to the service and upgraded during the phase of palliative care. This includes revision shortly after the death. Completion of the family genogram presents an ideal time for such assessment as relationships, prior losses, and coping are considered. Some palliative care services have developed checklists based on such risk factors to generate a numerical measure of risk. To date, there has been insufficient validation of such scales, but the presence of any single factor signifies greater risk. Continued observation of the pattern of grief evolution over time is appropriate whenever such concern exists.

Grief Therapies

Because loss is so ubiquitous in the palliative care setting, psychosomatic medicine clinicians need skill in the application of grief therapies. For most of the bereaved, personal resilience ensures normal adaptation in the face of their painful situation. As such, there is no justification for routine intervention, as grief is not a disease. Those considered at risk of maladaptive outcome, however, can be treated preventatively.

Those who later develop complicated bereavement need active treatments.

The spectrum of interventions spans individual, group, and family-oriented therapies, and encompasses all schools of psychotherapy as well as appropriately indicated pharmacotherapies. Adoption of any model, or parts thereof, is based on the clinical issues and their associated circumstances. Thus, variation will be influenced by age, perception of support, the nature of the death, the personal health of the bereaved, and the presence of comorbid states. Most interventions consist of six to eight sessions over several months. In this sense, grief therapy is focused and time limited. Multimodal therapies, however, are commonplace. Thus, group and individual therapies better support the lonely so that socialization interpersonally complements any intrapersonal support.

Pharmacotherapies are widely used to support the bereaved. Nonetheless, judicious prescription is important. Benzodiazepines allay anxiety and assist sleep, but words of caution should be offered about intermittent use to avoid tachyphylaxis and dependence. Antidepressants are indicated whenever bereavement is complicated by the development of depressive disorder, panic attacks, and moderate to severe adjustment disorders (Jacobs et al., 1987; Pasternak et al., 1991). If insomnia is prominent, tricyclics (e.g., nortriptyline, desipramine) are beneficial. Otherwise, selective serotonergic reuptake inhibitors (e.g., sertraline, paroxetine, citalopram, fluvoxamine, fluoxetine) or combined noradrenergic and serotonergic reuptake inhibitors (e.g., venlafaxine, mirtazepine) are indicated. Occasionally, antipsychotics are needed for hypomania or other forms of psychosis.

Family therapists have long recognized the importance of family processes in mourning, as well as their systemic influence on outcome (Kissane and Bloch, 1994). Exploration of the association between family functioning and bereavement morbidity highlights the manner in which family dysfunction predicts increased rates of psychosocial morbidity in the bereaved (Kissane et al., 1996). Family-centered care that focuses on the well-being of the family during palliative care is uniquely placed to reduce rates of morbidity in those subsequently bereaved.

A family approach to grief intervention is exemplified by family-focused grief therapy (FFGT), developed by Kissane and Bloch (2002). Such a model aims to improve family functioning while also supporting the expression of grief. As previously mentioned, this approach can be applied preventatively to those families judged through screening to be at high risk of complicated outcomes (Kissane and Bloch, 2002). Thus, FFGT commences during palliative care and includes the ill family member. It continues throughout the early phases of bereavement until there is confidence that morbidity has been prevented or appropriately treated. This approach invites the family to identify and work on aspects of family life that they specifically recognize as a cause of concern. Through enhancing cohesion, promoting open communication of thoughts and feelings, and teaching effective problem solving, conflict is reduced and tolerance of different opinions is optimized. The improved functioning of the family as a unit becomes the means to accomplish adaptive mourning.

CONCLUSION

Palliative care for patients with advanced AIDS requires a biopsychosocial approach consistent with the patient's expressed goals of care. As the possibility of a cure or prolongation of life becomes less remote in the care of the patient with advanced AIDS, the focus of treatment shifts to symptom control and enhanced quality of life. Patients are uniquely vulnerable to both physical and psychiatric complications. The role of the psychosomatic medicine psychiatrist in the care of the terminally ill or dying AIDS patient is critical to both adequate symptom control and integration of the medical, psychological, and spiritual dimensions of human experience in the last weeks of life. To be most effective in this role, the psychiatrist must have specialized knowledge of not only the psychiatric complications of terminal illness and the existential issues confronting those at the end of life but also the common physical symptoms that plague the patient with advanced AIDS and contribute so dramatically to their suffering.

References

Adams N, Poole H, and Richardson C (2006). Psychological approaches to chronic pain management: Part 1. *J Clin Nurs* 15:290–300.

Alexander CS, and Back A (eds.), for the Workgroup on Palliative and End-of-Life Care in HIV/AIDS (2004). *Integrating Palliative Care into the Continuum of HIV Care.* Missoula, MT: Robert Wood Johnson Foundation.

Anderson JM, Anderson LJ, and Felsenthal G (1993). Pastoral needs for support within an inpatient rehabilitation unit. *Arch Phys Med Rehabil* 74:574–578.

Baider L, Holland JC, Russak SM, and Kaplan De-Nour A (2001). The system of belief inventory (SBI-15). *Psycho-Oncology* 10:534–540.

Baider L, Russak SM, Perry S, Kash K, Gronert M, Fox B, Holland J, and Kaplan-Denour A (1999). The role of religious and spiritual beliefs in coping with malignant melanoma: an Israeli sample. *Psycho-oncology* 8:27–35.

Baile W, and Beale E (2001). Giving bad news to cancer patients: matching process and content. *J Clin Oncol* 19:2575–2577.

Barg FK, and Gullate MM (2001). Cancer support groups: meeting the needs of African Americans with cancer. *Semin Oncol Nurs* 17:171–178.

Blackhall LJ, Murphy ST, Frank G, Michel V, and Azen SP (1995). Ethnicity and attitudes toward patient automony. *JAMA* 274:820–825.

Breitbart W (1989). Psychiatric management of cancer pain. *Cancer* 63(11):2336–2342.

Breitbart W (2002). Spirituality and meaning in supportive care: spirituality and meaning-centered group psychotherapy interventions in advanced cancer. *Support Care Cancer* 10(4):272–280.

Breitbart W, and Heller KS (2003). Reframing hope: meaning-centered care for patients near the end-of-life. *J Palliat Med* 6:979–88.

Breitbart WS, Passik S, Eller KC, and Sison A (1992). Suicidal ideation in AIDS: the role of pain and mood [NR 267 (abstract)]. Presented at the 145th Annual Meeting of the American Psychiatric Association, Washington, DC.

Breitbart W, Rosenfeld BD, and Passik SD (1996a). Interest in physician-assisted suicide among ambulatory HIV-infected patients. *Am J Psychiatry* 153:238–242.

Breitbart W, Rosenfeld B, Passik SD, McDonald MV, Thaler H, and Portenoy RK (1996b). The undertreatment of pain in ambulatory AIDS patients. *Pain* 65:243–249.

Breitbart W, McDonald MV, Rosenfeld B, Monkman ND, and Passik S (1998). Fatigue in ambulatory AIDS patients. *J Pain Symptom Manage* 15:159–167.

Breitbart W, Kaim M, and Rosenfeld B (1999). Clinicians' perceptions of barriers to pain management in AIDS. *J Pain Symptom Manage* 18:203–212.

Breitbart W, Rosenfeld B, Pessin H, Kaim M, Funesti-Esch J, Galietta J, Nelson CJ, and Brescia R (2000). Depression, hopelessness, and desire for death in terminally ill patients with cancer. *JAMA* 284:2907–2911.

Breitbart W, Chochinov H, and Passik S (2004a). Psychiatric symptoms in palliative medicine. In D Doyle, G Hanks, N Cherny, and K Calman (eds.), *Oxford Textbook of Palliative Medicine*, third edition (pp. 746–771). New York: Oxford University Press.

Breitbart W, Payne D, and Passik S (2004b). Psychological and psychiatric interventions in pain control. In D Doyle, G Hanks, N Cherny, and K Calman (eds.), *Oxford Textbook of Palliative Medicine*, third edition (pp. 424–437). New York: Oxford University Press.

Bruera E, MacMillan K, Pither J, and MacDonald RN (1990). Effects of morphine on the dyspnea of the terminal cancer patients. *J Pain Sympton Manage* 5:1–5.

Buckman R (1993). *How to Break Bad News: A Guide for Healthcare Professionals*. London: Macmillan Medical.

Buckman R (1998). Communication in palliative care: a practical guide. In D Doyle, GWC Hanks, and N MacDonald (eds.), *Oxford Textbook of Palliative Medicine*, second edition (pp. 141–156). New York: Oxford University Press.

Butler RN, Burt R, Foley KM, Morris J, and Morrison RS (1996). Palliative medicine: providing care when cure is not possible. A roundtable discussion: Part I. *Geriatrics* 51:33–36.

Butow P, Tattersall M, and Goldstein D (1997). Communication with cancer patients in culturally diverse societies. *Ann N Y Acad Sci* 809:317–329.

Canadian Palliative Care Association (1995). *Palliative Care. Towards a Consensus in Standardized Principles of Practice*. Ottawa, ON: Canadian Palliative Care Association.

Candib L (2002). Truth telling and advance planning at the end-of-life: problems with autonomy in a multicultural world. *Fam Syst Health* 20:213–228.

Carmichael JK (1991). Treatment of herpes zoster and postherpetic neuralgia. *Am Fam Physician* 44:203–210.

Carrese J, and Rhodes L (1995). Western bioethics on the Navajo reservation. *JAMA* 274:826–829.

Casalino E, Wolff M, Ravaud P, Choquet C, Bruneel F, and Regnier B (2004). Impact of HAART advent on admission patterns and survival in HIV-infected patients admitted to an intensive care unit. *AIDS* 18:1429–1433.

[CDC] Centers for Disease Control and Prevention (2005). *HIV/AIDS Surveillance Report 2005*, Vol. 16. Retrieved April 5, 2007, from www.cdc.gov/hiv/topics/surveillance/resources/reports/index.htm#surveillance.

[CDC] Centers for Disease Control and Prevention (2003). Summary of notifiable disease: United States. 2001. *MMWR Morb Mortal Wkly Rep* 50:1–22.

Chochinov HM (2002). Dignity-conserving care: a new model for palliative care: helping the patient feel valued. *JAMA* 287(17):2253–2260.

Chochinov HM, and Breitbart W (eds.) (2000). *Handbook of Psychiatry and Palliative Medicine*. New York: Oxford University Press.

Chochinov HM, Wilson KG, Enns M, and Lander S (1994). Prevalence of depression in the terminally ill: effects of diagnostic criteria and symptom threshold judgments. *Am J Psychiatry* 151(4):537–540.

Chochinov HM, Wilson KG, Enns M, Mowchun N, Lander S, Levitt M, and Clinch JJ (1995). Desire for death in the terminally ill. *Am J Psychiatry* 152: 1185–1191.

Chochinov H, Wilson K, Enns M, and Lander S (1998). Depression, hopelessness, and suicidal ideation in the terminally ill. *Psychosomatics* 39(4):366–370.

Chochinov HM, Hack T, Hassard T, Kristjanson LJ, McClement S, and Harlos M (2002a). Dignity in the terminally ill: a cross-sectional, cohort study. *Lancet* 360:2026–2030.

Chochinov HM, Hack T, McClement S, Harlos M, and Kristjanson L (2002b). Dignity in the terminally ill: an empirical model. *Soc Sci Med* 54:433–443.

Chochinov HM, Hack T, Hassard T, Kristjanson LJ, McClement S, and Harlos M (2005). Dignity therapy: a novel psychotherapeutic intervention for patients near the end of life. *J Clin Oncol* 23(24): 5520–5525.

Clayton CL (2000). Barriers, boundaries and blessings: ethical issues in physicians' spiritual involvement with patients. *Med Humanities Rpt* 21:234–256.

Cohen MA, and Alfonso CA (2004). AIDS psychiatry: psychiatric and palliative care, and pain management. In GP Wormser (ed.), *AIDS and Other Manifestations of HIV Infection*, fourth edition (pp. 537–576). San Diego: Elsevier Academic Press.

Cohen CB, Wheeler SE, and Scott DA (2001). Walking a fine line: physician inquiries into patients' religious and spiritual beliefs. *Hastings Cent Rep* 31: 29–39.

Cornblath DR, and McArthur JC (1988). Predominantly sensory neuropathy in patients with AIDS and AIDS-related complex. *Neurology* 38:794–796.

Crawley LV, Payne R, Bolden J, Payne T, Washington P, and Williams S (2000). Initiative to improve palliative and end-of-life care in the African-American community. *JAMA* 284:2518–2521.

Curtis JR, and Patrick DL (1997). Barriers to communication about end-of-life care in AIDS patients. *J Gen Intern Med* 12:736–741.

Deeks S, Wrin T, Liegler T, Hoh R, Hayden M, Barbour JD, Hellmann NS, Petropoulos CJ, and McCune JM (2001). Virologic and immunologic consequences of discontinuing combination antiretroviral-drug therapy in HIV-infected patients with detectable viremia. *N Engl J Med* 344:472–480.

Department of Health and Human Services. *Guidelines for the Use of Antiretroviral Agents in HIV-1-Infected Adults and Adolescents*. Retrieved June 16, 2006, from http://www.AIDSinfo.nih.gov.

Doka K (1989). Disenfranchised grief. In K Doka (ed.), *Disenfranchised Grief: Recognizing Hidden Sorrow* (pp. 3–11). Lexington, MA: Lexington Books.

Doyle D (1992). Have we looked beyond the physical and psychosocial? *J Pain Symptom Manage* 7(5): 302–311.

Doyle D, Hanks G, Cherny N, and Calman K (eds.) (2003). *Oxford Textbook of Palliative Medicine*, third edition. New York: Oxford University Press.

Easterbrook P, and Meadway J (2001). The changing epidemiology of HIV infection: new challenges for HIV palliative care. *J R Soc Med* 94(9):442–448.

Ellis M, Vinson D, and Ewigman B (1999). Addressing spiritual concerns of patients: family physicians' attitudes and practices. *J Fam Pract* 48:105–109.

Ellis R (1997). Neurocognitive impairment is an independent risk factor for death in HIV infection. *Arch Neurol* 6:416–424.

Evans D, Ten Have T, Douglas SD, Gettes DR, Morrison M, Chiappini MS, Brinker-Spence P, Job C, Mercer DE, Wang YL, Cruess D, Dubé B, Dalen EA, Brown T, Bauer R, and Petitto JM (2002). Association of depression with viral load, CD8 T lymphocytes, and natural killer cells in women with HIV infection. *Am J Psychiatry* 159:1752–1759.

Fallowfield L (2004). Communication and palliative medicine. In D Doyle, G Hanks, N Cherny, and K Calman (eds.), *Oxford Textbook of Palliative Medicine*, third edition (pp. 101–107). New York: Oxford University Press.

Fallowfield L, Lipkin M, and Hall A (1998). Teaching senior oncologists communication skills: results from phase I of a comprehensive longitudinal program in the United Kingdom. *J Clin Oncol* 16:1961–1968.

Fantoni M, Ricci F, Del Borgo C, Izzi I, Damiano F, Moscati AM, Marasca G, Bevilacqua N, and Del Forna A (1997). Multicentre study on the prevalence of symptoms and symptomatic treatment in HIV infection. *J Palliat Care* 13:9–13.

Filbet M, and Marceron V (1994). A retrospective study of symptoms in 193 terminal inpatients with AIDS [abstract]. *J Palliat Care* 10:92.

Foley F (1994). AIDS palliative care [abstract]. *J Palliat Care* 10:132.

Foley F, and Flannery S (1995). AIDS palliative care: challenging the palliative paradigm. *J Palliat Care* 11:34–37.

Fontaine A, LaRue F, and Lassauniere JM (1999). Physicians' recognition of the symptoms experienced by HIV patients: how reliable? *J Pain Symptom Manage* 18:263–270.

Frankl VF (1955). *The Doctor and the Soul*. New York: Random House.

Frankl VF (1959). *Man's Search for Meaning*, fourth edition. Boston: Beacon Press.

Frenkel L, and Mullins J (2001). Should patients with drug-resistant HIV-1 continue to receive antiretroviral therapy? *N Engl J Med* 344:520–522.

Geara F, Le Bourgeois JP, Piedbois P, Pavlovitch JM, and Mazeron JJ (1991). Radiotherapy in the management of cutaneous epidemic Kaposi's sarcoma. *Int J Radiat Oncol Biol Phys* 21:1517–1522.

Gibson CA, and Breitbart W (2004). Individual meaning-centered psychotherapy treatment manual. Unpublished.

Goldberg RJ (1993). Acute pain management. In A Stoudemire and BS Fogel (eds.), *Psychiatric Care of the Medical Patient* (pp. 323–340). New York: Oxford University Press.

Goldstone I, Kuhl D, Johnson A, Le R, and McLeod A (1995). Patterns of care in advanced HIV disease in a tertiary treatment centre. *AIDS Care* 7(Suppl. 1): S47–S56.

Goodkin K (1997). Subtle neuropsychological impairment and minor cognitive-motor disorder in HIV-1 infection. *Neuroimaging Clin N Am* 6:561–580.

Greenstein M, and Breitbart W (2000). Cancer and the experience of meaning: a group psychotherapy program for people with cancer. *Am J Psychother* 54: 486–500.

Guzman J, Esmail R, Karjalainen K, Malmivaara A, Irvin E, and Bombardier C (2001). Multidisciplinary rehabilitation for chronic low back pain: systematic review. *BMJ* 322:1511–1516.

Handzo G, and Koenig HG (2004). Spiritual care: whose job is it anyway? *South Med J* 97(12):1242–1244.

Harding R, Easterbrook P, Higginson IJ, Karus D, Raveis VH, and Marconi K (2005). Access and equity in HIV/AIDS palliative care: a review of the evidence and responses. *Palliat Med* 19(3):251–258.

Hay MW (1996). Developing Guidelines for Spiritual Caregivers in Hospice: Principles for Spiritual Assessment. Presented at the National Hospice Organization Annual Sympsium and Exposition, November 6–9, Chicago, IL.

Hilgard E, and LeBaron S (1982). Relief of anxiety and pain in children and adolescents with cancer: quantitative measures and clinical observations. *Int J Clin Exp Hypn* 30:417–442.

Huang L, Quartin A, Jones D, and Havlir DV (2006). Intensive care of patients with HIV infection. *N Engl J Med* 355:173–181.

Jacobs S, Nelson J, and Zisook S (1987). Treating depressions of bereavement with antidepressants: a pilot study. *Psychiatr Clin North Am* 10:501–510.

Jacox AJ, Carr DB, and Payne R (1994). New clinical-practice guidelines for the management of pain in patients with cancer. *N Engl J Med* 330:651.

Jay SM, Elliott C, and Varni JW (1986). Acute and chronic pain in adults and children with cancer. *J Consult Clin Psychol* 54:601–607.

Johnson AS (1995). Palliative care in the home? *J Palliat Care* 11(2):42–44.

Jonsson E, Coombs DW, Hunstad D, Richardson JR Jr, von Reyn CF, Saunders RL, and Heaney JA (1992). Continuous infusion of intrathecal morphine to control acquired immunodeficiency syndrome–associated bladder pain. *J Urol* 147:687–689.

Justice AC, Aiken LH, Smith HL, and Turner BJ (1996). The role of functional status in predicting inpatient mortality with AIDS: a comparison with current predictors. *J Clin Epidemiol* 49:193–201.

Kagawa-Singer M, and Blackhall LJ (2001). Negotiating cross-cultural issues at the end-of-life: "You got to go where he lives." *JAMA* 286:2993–3001.

Kalso E, Allan L, Dellemijn PL, Faura CC, Ilias WK, Jensen TS, Perrot S, Plaghki LH, and Zenz M (2003). Recommendations for using opioids in chronic non-cancer pain. *Eur J Pain* 7:381–386.

Karasu BT (1999). Spiritual psychotherapy. *Am J Psychother* 53:143–162.

Kearney M, and Mount B (2000). Spiritual care of the dying patient. In HM Chochinov and W Breitbart (eds.), *Handbook of Psychiatry in Palliative Medicine* (pp. 357–371). New York: Oxford University Press.

Kelleher P, Cox S, and McKeogh M (1997). HIV infection: the spectrum of symptoms and disease in male and female patients attending a London hospice. *Palliat Med* 11:152–158.

Kellerman J, Zeltzer L, Ellenberg L, and Dash J (1983). Adolescents with cancer: hypnosis for the reduction of acute pain and anxiety associated with medical procedures. *J Adolesc Health Care* 4:85–90.

King DE, and Bushwick B (1994). Beliefs and attitudes of hospital inpatients about faith healing and prayer. *J Fam Pract* 39:349–352.

Kissane DW (2004). Bereavement. In D Doyle, G Hanks, N Cherny, and K Calman (eds.), *Oxford Textbook of Palliative Medicine*, third edition (pp. 1135–1154). New York: Oxford University Press.

Kissane D, and Bloch S (1994). Family grief. *Br J Psychiatry* 164:728–740.

Kissane D, and Bloch S (2002). *Family Focus Grief Therapy: A Model of Family-centered Care during Palliative Care and Bereavement.* Buckingham: Open University Press.

Kissane D, Bloch S, Dowe D, et al. (1996). The Melbourne family grief study I & II. *Am J Psychiatry* 153:650–658, 659–666.

Kissane D, Clarke DM, and Street AF (2001). Demoralization syndrome: a relevant psychiatric diagnosis for palliative care. *J Palliat Care* 17:12–21.

Koenig BA, and Gates-William J (1995). Understanding cultural difference in caring for dying patients. *West J Med* 163:244–249.

Koenig HG (2002). Religion, spirituality, and medicine: how are they related and what does it mean? *Mayo Clinic Proc* 12:1189–1191.

Koenig HG, Cohen HJ, Blazer DG, et al. (1992). Religious coping and depression among elderly, hospitalized medically ill men. *Am J Psychiatry* 149:1693–1700.

Koenig HG, George, LK, and Peterson BL (1998). Religiosity and remission of depression in medically ill older patients. *Am J Psychiatry* 155(4):536–542.

LaRue F, and Colleau SM (1997). Underestimation and undertreatment of pain in HIV disease: multicentre study. *BMJ* 314:23–28.

LaRue F, Brasseur L, Musseault P, Demeulemeester R, Bonifassi L, and Bez G (1994). Pain and symptoms in HIV disease: a national survey in France [abstract]. *J Palliat Care* 10:95.

Lo B, Kates LW, Ruston D, Arnold RM, Cohen CB, Puchalski CM, Pantilat SZ, Rabow MW, Schreiber RS, and Tulsky JA (2003). Responding to requests regarding prayer and religious ceremonies by patients near the end-of-life and their families. *J Palliat Med* 3:409–415.

Lopez OL, Wess J, Sanchez J, Dew MA, and Becker JT (1998). Neurobehavioral correlates of perceived mental and motor slowness in HIV infection and AIDS. *J Neuropsychiatry Clin Neurosci* 10:343–350.

Maddox JD, Joranson D, and Angarola RT (1997). The use of opioids for the treatment of chronic pain (position statement). *Clin J Pain* 167:30–34.

Maguire P (1985). Barriers to psychological care of the dying. *BMJ* 291:1711–1713.

Maguire P (1999). Improving communication with cancer patients. *Eur J Cancer* 35:2058–2065.

Mansfield S, Barter G, and Singh S (1992). AIDS and palliative care. *Int J STD AIDS* 3:248–50.

Mathews WC, McCutcheon JA, Asch S, Turner BJ, Gifford AL, Kuromiya K, Brown J, Shapiro MF, and Bozzette SA (2000). National estimates of HIV-related symptom prevalence from the HIV Cost and Services Utilization Study. *Med Care* 38:750–762.

Maugans TA (1996). The SPIRITual history. *Arch Fam Med* 5:11–16.

Maugans TA, and Wadland WC (1991). Religion and family medicine: a survey of physicians and patients. *J Fam Pract* 32:210–213.

Mazanec P, and Tyler MK (2003). Cultural considerations in end-of-life care. *Am J Nursing* 103(3): 50–58.

McClain CS, Rosenfeld B, and Breitbart W (2003). Effect of spiritual well-being on end-of-life despair in terminally-ill cancer patients. *Lancet* 61:1603–1607.

McCullough ME, and Larson DB (1999). Religion and depression: a review of the literature. *Twin Res* 2: 126–136.

Meares R (1981). On saying goodbye before death. *JAMA* 246:1227–1229.

Morley S, Eccleston C, and Williams A (1999). Systematic review and meta-analysis of randomized controlled trials of cognitive behaviour therapy for chronic pain in adults, excluding headache. *Pain* 80:1–13.

Morris A, Creasman J, Turner J, Luce JM, Wachter RM, and Huang L (2002). Intensive care of human immunodeficiency virus–infected patients during the era of highly active antiretroviral therapy. *Am J Respir Crit Care Med* 166:262–267.

Moss V (1990). Palliative care in advanced HIV disease: presentation, problems, and palliation. *AIDS* 1990; 4(Suppl. 1):S235–S242.

Mouton C, Teno JM, Mor V, and Piette J (1997). Communications of preferences for care among human

immunodeficiency virus–infected patients: barriers to informed decisions? *Arch Fam Med* 6:342–347.

Narasimhan M, Posner AJ, DePalo VA, Mayo PH, and Rosen MJ (2004). Intensive care in patients with HIV infection in the era of highly active antiretroviral therapy. *Chest* 125:1800–1804.

National Hospice Organization (1996). *Guidelines for Determining Prognosis for Selected Non-Cancer Diagnoses*. Alexandria, VA: National Hospice Organization.

Nelson CJ, Rosenfeld B, Breitbart W, et al. (2002). Spirituality, religion, and depression in the terminally ill. *Psychosomatics* 43:213–220.

Newshan GT, and Wainapel SF (1993). Pain characteristics and their management in persons with AIDS. *J Assoc Nurses AIDS Care* 4:53–59.

O'Neill W, and Sherrard J (1993). Pain in human immunodeficiency virus disease: a review. *Pain* 54:3–14.

O'Neill JF, Marconi K, Surapruik A, and Blum N (2000). Improving HIV/AIDS services through palliative care: an HRSA perspective. *J Urban Health* 77:244–254.

O'Neill JF, Selwyn PA, and Schietinger H (eds.) (2003). *A Clinical Guide to Supportive & Palliative Care for HIV/AIDS*. Washington DC: U.S. Department of Health and Human Services, Health Resources and Services Administration, HIV/AIDS Bureau.

Ontario Workplace Safety and Insurance Board (2000). *Report of the Chronic Pain Expert Advisory Panel*. Ontario: Ontario Workplace Safety and Insurance Board.

Pain Society and Royal Colleges of Anaesthetists (2004). Consensus Statement from the Pain Society and Royal Colleges of Anaesthetists. General Practitioners and Psychiatrists: Recommendations. London: The Royal College of Anaesthetists.

Parker B, Baile W, deMoor C, et al. (2001). Breaking bad news about cancer: patients' preferences for communication. *J Clin Oncol* 19(7):2049–2056.

Parkes C (1975). Determinants of outcome following bereavement. *Omega* 6:303–323.

Parkes C (1998). *Bereavement: Studies of Grief in Adult Life*, third edition. Madison: International Universities Press.

Parkes C, Laungani P, and Young B (eds.) (1997). *Death and Bereavement Across Cultures*. London: Routledge.

Pasternak R, Reynolds C, and Schlernitzauer M (1991). Acute open-trial nortriptyline therapy of bereavement-related depression in late life. *J Clin Psychiatry* 52:307–310.

Peterman AH, Fitchett G, and Cella DF (1996). Modeling the relationship between quality of life dimensions and an overall sense of well-being. Presented at the Third World Congress of Psycho-Oncology, New York, NY.

Portenoy RK (1993). Chronic pain management. In A Stoudemire and BS Fogel (eds.), *Psychiatric Care of the Medical Patient*. New York: Oxford University Press.

Portenoy RK, Thaler HT, Kornblith AB, et al. (1994). The Memorial Symptom Assessment Scale: an instrument for the evaluation of symptom prevalence, characteristics, and distress. *Eur J Cancer* 30A: 1326–1336.

Post SG, Puchalski CM, and Larson DB (2000). Physicians and patient spirituality: professional boundaries, competency, and ethics. *Ann Intern Med* 132: 578–583.

Prigerson H, Maciejewski P, Newson J, et al. (1995). Inventory of complicated grief. *Psychiatry Res* 59: 65–79.

Puchalski C, and Romer AL (2000). Taking a spiritual history allows clinicians to understand patients more fully. *J Palliat Med* 3:129–137.

Puoti M, Spinetti A, Ghezzi A, et al. (2001). Mortality from liver disease in patients with HIV infection: a cohort study. *J Acquir Immune Defic Syndr* 24:211–217.

Rackstraw S, Conley A, and Meadway J (2000). Recovery from progressive multifocal leukoencephalopathy following directly observed highly active antiretroviral therapy (HAART) in a specialized brain impairment unit. *AIDS* 14(Suppl. 4):S129.

Rando T (1983). *Treatment of Complicated Mourning.* Champaign, IL: Research Press.

Raphael B (1983). *The Anatomy of Bereavement.* London: Hutchinson.

Reiter GS, and Kudler NR (1996). Palliative care and HIV: systemic manifestations and late-stage issues. *AIDS Clin Care* 8:27–36.

Rosenfeld B, Breitbart W, McDonald MV, Passik SD, Thaler H, and Portenoy RK (1997). Pain in ambulatory AIDS patients: impact of pain on physiological functioning and quality of life. *Pain* 68:323–328.

Rousseau P (2000). Spirituality and the dying patient. *J Clin Oncol* 18:2000–2002.

Sanei L (1998). *Palliative Care for HIV/AIDS in Less Developed Countries.* Arlington, VA: Health Technical Services (HTS) Project for USAID.

Sansone RG, and Frengley JD (2000). Impact of HAART on causes of death of persons with late-stage AIDS. *J Urban Health* 77:165–175.

Schofferman J (1987). Hospice care of the patient with AIDS. *J Hospice* 3:51–74.

Schofferman J (1988). Pain: diagnosis and management in the palliative care of AIDS. *J Palliat Care* 4:46–49.

Selwyn PA, and Forstein M (2003). Overcoming the false dichotomy of curative vs. palliative care for late-stage HIV/AIDS: "Let me live the way I want to live, until I can't." *JAMA* 290:806–814.

Selwyn PA, and Rivard M (2002). Palliative care for AIDS: challenges and opportunities in the era of highly active anti-retroviral therapy. *Innovations in End-of-Life Care* 4(3). Retrieved April 6, 2007, from www.edc.org/lastacts

Selwyn PA, Goulet JL, Molde S, Constantino J, Fennie KP, Wetherill P, Gaughan DM, Brett-Smith H, and Kennedy C (2000). HIV as a chronic disease: long-term care for patients with HIV at a dedicated skilled nursing facility. *J Urban Health* 77:187–203.

Selwyn PA, Rivard M, Kapell D, Goeren B, LaFosse H, Schwartz C, Caraballo R, Luciano D, and Post LF (2003). Palliative care for AIDS at a large urban teaching hospital: program description and preliminary outcomes. *J Palliat Med* 6(3):461–474.

Shen JM, Blank A, and Selwyn PA (2005). Predictors of mortality for patients with advanced disease in an HIV palliative care program. *J Acquir Immune Defic Syndr* 40(4):445–447.

Simpson M, Buckman R, Stewart M, Maguire P, Lipkin M, Novack D, and Till J (1991). Doctor-patient communication: the Toronto consensus statement. *BMJ* 303 (6814):1385–1387.

Singer JE, Fahy-Chandon B, Chi S, Syndulko K, and Tourtellotte WW (1993). Painful symptoms reported by ambulatory HIV-infected men in a longitudinal study. *Pain* 54:15–19.

Singer PA, Martin DK, and Kelner M (1999). Quality end-of-life care: patients' perspective. *JAMA* 281: 163–168.

Sloan RP, Bagiella E, and Powell T (1999). Religion, spirituality, and medicine. *Lancet* 353:664–667.

Smith TJ (2000). Tell it like it is. *J Clin Oncol* 18:3441–3445.

Stephenson J, Woods S, Scott B, and Meadway J (2000). HIV-related brain impairment: from palliative care to rehabilitation. *Int J Palliat Nurs* 6:6–11.

Stjernsward J, and Papallona S (1998). Palliative medicine: a global perspective. In D Doyle, GWC Hanks, and N MacDonald (eds.), *Oxford Textbook of Palliative Medicine,* second edition (pp. 1227–1245). New York: Oxford University Press.

Storey P, and Knight C (2001). *American Academy of Hospice and Palliative Medicine UNIPAC Two: Alleviating Psychological and Spiritual Pain in the Terminally Ill.* Larchmont, NY: Mary Ann Liebert.

Stroebe M, Stroebe W, and Hansson R (eds.) (1993). *Handbook of Bereavement.* Cambridge, UK: Cambridge University Press.

Suchman AL, Markakis K, Beckman HB, et al. (1997). A model of empathic communication in the medical interview. *JAMA* 277:678–681.

Thiel MM, and Robinson MR (1997). Physicians' collaboration with chaplains: difficulties and benefits. *J Clin Ethics* 8:94–103.

Tosches WA, Cohen CJ, and Day JM (1992). A pilot study of acupuncture for the symptomatic treatment of HIV-associated peripheral neuropathy [8:14 abstract]. Presented at the VIIIth International Conference on AIDS, Amsterdam, the Netherlands.

Underwood LG, and Teresi JA (2002). The daily spiritual experience scale. *Ann Med* 24:22–33.

Valdez H, Chowdhry TK, Asaad R, Woolley IJ, Davis T, Davidson R, Beinker N, Gripshover BM, Salata RA, McComsey G, Weissman SB, and Lederman MM

(2001). Changing spectrum of mortality due to HIV: analysis of 260 deaths during 1995–1999. *Clin Infect Dis* 32:1487–1493.

Vincent B, Timsit JF, Auburtin M, Schortgen F, Bouadma L, Wolff M, and Regnier B (2004). Characteristics and outcomes of HIV-infected patients in the ICU: impact of the highly active antiretroviral treatment era. *Intensive Care Med* 30:859–866.

Vogl D, Rosenfeld B, Breitbart W, Thaler H, Passik S, McDonald M, and Portenoy RK (1999). Symptom prevalence, characteristics and distress in AIDS outpatients. *J Pain Symptom Manage* 18:253–262.

Watson M, Haviland JJ, Greer S, et al. (1999). Influence of psychological response on survival in breast cancer population-based cohort study. *Lancet* 354:1331–1336.

Welch K, and Morse A (2002). The clinical profile of end-state AIDS in the era of highly active anti-retroviral therapy. *AIDS Patient Care STDS* 16:75–81.

Wenger NS, Kanouse DE, Collins RL, Liu H, Schuster MA, Gifford AL, Bozzette SA, and Shapiro MF (2001). End-of-life discussions and preferences among persons with HIV. *JAMA* 22:2880–2887.

Wood CG, Whittet S, and Bradbeer CS (1997). ABC of palliative care: HIV infection and AIDS. *BMJ* 315:1433–1436.

World Health Organization (1986). *Cancer Pain Relief.* Geneva: World Health Organization.

World Health Organization (1990). *Cancer Pain Relief and Palliative Care: Report of a WHO Expert Committee* (Technical Bulletin 804). Geneva: World Health Organization.

World Health Organization (1998). *Symptom Relief in Terminal Illness.* Geneva: World Health Organization.

Chapter 31

Special Settings: Psychiatric Facilities, Nursing Homes, Correctional Facilities, and Homeless Outreach

Mary Ann Cohen, Karin Dorell, Julio Riascos, and David Chao

At the beginning of the AIDS pandemic, persons who were infected experienced discrimination in many settings including psychiatric facilities, nursing homes, correctional facilities, shelters for the homeless, and even hospitals. In 1981, persons with AIDS were often refused admission to nursing homes, hospices, hospitals, and even homeless shelters. There have been many changes in the past quarter century since 1981, when the first descriptions of the illness appeared in the literature. These changes have involved many significant medical and scientific advances as well as codification of legal protections against discrimination, some societal changes, and social and political efforts to improve both care and access to care for persons with HIV and AIDS. These improvements have enabled more persons with AIDS to be treated with dignity and to obtain adequate care and support services in some resource-rich and resource-limited areas. For most persons with HIV infection who have access to care, this has meant a profound change in the course and outcome of the illness, with AIDS evolving from being a rapidly progressive and fatal illness to becoming a chronic illness such as diabetes mellitus. However, AIDS has also magnified the disparities in health care delivery, as exemplified by the lack of access to care for many patients in both resource-rich (Rastegar et al., 2001) and resource-limited countries throughout the world.

Psychiatric factors including severe mental illness and psychiatric illnesses such as substance use disorders contribute to major disparities in access to health care. The social factors of stigma, discrimination, and racial disparities combine with poverty and political issues to compromise access to care for many individuals. In this chapter, we explore the treatment of persons with HIV and AIDS in the settings of psychiatric facilities, nursing homes and other long-term care facilities, addiction treatment programs, community treatment programs, and correctional facilities. Although issues related to care of persons with

HIV and AIDS in these special settings is addressed in other chapters in this textbook, we thought it important to link the special settings in one chapter. Psychiatric care is covered in chapters throughout this book particularly in Chapters 4 through 13. Substance use disorders are explored in detail in Chapter 8, homelessness in Chapter 23, and stigma in Chapter 1. One particularly complex special setting, the correctional facility, is covered in depth in Chapter 5 of this textbook. We feel that these special settings are places where persons with HIV and AIDS may be the most fragile and vulnerable. Despite the many changes and mitigation of some of the stigma and discrimination, care in special settings remains complex and deserving of special attention.

PSYCHIATRIC FACILITIES

Many individuals with diagnosed or undiagnosed HIV infection are not receiving adequate medical care (Bozette et al., 1998). Persons with HIV/ AIDS as well as individuals with serious mental illness may not have a regular source of care. Persons with both HIV and serious mental illness are even less likely to be receiving adequate care (Swartz et al., 2003; Joyce et al., 2005; Stoskopf et al., 2001). Homelessness, substance abuse, and poor social support, often associated with HIV and serious mental illness, together constitute an additional barrier to regular care (Bosworth et al., 2004; Lundgren et al., 2005). Distrust, prejudice, and the inexperience of health care providers in the treatment of HIV-infected persons with severe mentally illness and substance abuse can constitute a barrier to getting appropriate treatment (Miller et al., 2001).

Despite inadequate access to care, the medical and psychiatric needs of patients with these illnesses are very high (Bosworth et al., 2004). Persons with comorbid serious mental illness and HIV infection or AIDS have the highest annual medical and behavioral health treatment expenditures, followed by persons with HIV infection or AIDS only (Bosworth et al., 2004). The integration of HIV prevention into ongoing case management for persons with serious mental illness who are at risk of infection may prove to be a cost-effective intervention strategy (Rothbard et al., 2003). An integrated system of care that identifies and addresses patient needs in a comprehensive and coordinated way not only improves care (Cournos et al., 2005) but also lowers the cost of care (Schaedle et al., 2002).

Emergency Rooms

Access to care through emergency evaluation can occur when a medical or a psychiatric complication occurs. Psychiatric emergencies affecting the HIV-positive individual can be associated with the direct effect of the virus on the brain, psychiatric symptoms secondary to medical illness, psychological distress related to the infection, or other factors such as substance abuse or homelessness (Lyketsos et al., 1995; Cunningham et al., 2005). The high frequency of comorbid psychiatric symptoms in HIV-positive individuals often prompts psychiatric consultations when the patient presents for a medical emergency. The uncertain etiology of the presenting symptoms also requires a higher level of collaboration between the medical and psychiatric teams.

Patients who lack a regular source of medical care often gain access to care through emergency care settings (Swartz et al., 2003; Joyce et al., 2005). HIV status, drug use, and marginal housing have been associated with higher use of emergency services (Palepu et al., 1999; Kagay et al., 2004). Frequent use of emergency services has also been linked to higher mortality (Hansagi et al., 1990). In a large sample of drug users, Lundgren and colleagues (2005) found that emergency room use was strongly associated with mental health status and severity of drug use, while homelessness, HIV status, and sociodemographic factors were not.

Cunningham and colleagues (2005) evaluated utilization patterns of a highly marginalized population in New York City and found high measures of access to and use of ambulatory care services, along with high use of acute care services. Knowlton and colleagues (2005) found that persons with HIV and AIDS who had larger numbers of drug users in their support networks were more likely to have suboptimal emergency room use as compared to persons with fewer drug users in their support systems. Improvement of the support networks of HIV-positive individuals may lead to improvement in medical service utilization among underserved populations.

Leserman and colleagues (2005) found that patients with a history of trauma, recent stressful events, and posttraumatic stress disorder (PTSD) are more likely to require emergency room visits. Patients with history of abuse had twice the risk of having an overnight stay in the hospital or an emergency room visit compared to those without a history of abuse.

Despite availability for appropriate treatment, utilization of emergency care remains high especially by populations struggling to maintain ongoing and stable treatment, such as active drug users and the homeless. The development of case management teams in HIV clinics is likely to facilitate stability and continuity of care (Okin et al., 2000; Witbeck et al., 2000).

Psychiatric Outpatient Clinics

Psychiatrists and other mental health professionals are in an ideal position to prevent HIV transmission, encourage behavior change, and ensure adherence to care in persons with HIV and AIDS. Psychiatrists routinely take detailed and thorough substance use and sexual histories. They may be able to recognize risky behaviors and encourage not only behavior change but also HIV testing. They also have long-term, trusting relationships with patients and routinely work with patients to identify and alter self-destructive behavior patterns. The ambulatory psychiatric setting may be an ideal place to provide education for prevention of transmission as well as adherence to medical care for persons with HIV and AIDS. The introduction of antiretroviral therapies has shifted most of the care for HIV-positive individuals from inpatient care to outpatient settings. There are several different models for delivery of HIV ambulatory medical and mental health care.

The HIV virus can affect every organ and every system in the human body. The expertise of a wide range of professionals is therefore needed to address both the medical and the psychosocial needs of the patients (Cohen, 1992). Different settings are often compartmentalized and isolated from each other. Traditionally, mental health clinics, substance abuse clinics, and infectious disease or HIV clinics have been separate and isolated in general hospitals. Specialized professionals often lack the ability to identify patients' needs that are not related to their particular expertise (Rosenheck and Lam, 1997).

Persons with HIV/AIDS and especially persons who are coinfected with hepatitis C often have multiple coexisting problems such as psychiatric and addictive disorders as well as housing and financial instability that interfere with successful management of their care (Goldberg, 2005). Because these different issues are often addressed by different disciplines, fragmentation of care often leads to difficulty with entry into care as well as easy disengagement. Although the fragmentation of care may occur with any combina-

tion of disabilities that cut across system boundaries, it is more likely to occur when psychiatric and substance use disorders are involved (Budin et al., 2004; Klinkenberg et al., 2004). Psychiatric disorders, in fact, cause disability in themselves, which, through effects on cognition, mood, and motivation, may have a disproportionate impact on the ability to negotiate a complex care system (Scheft and Fontenette, 2005; Willenbring, 2005).

Some innovative hospitals are able and willing to integrate medical, mental health, and substance abuse treatment within their programs. This integrated treatment approach enables staff to identify and treat individuals who are often falling through the cracks in non-integrated programs and therefore provide care to an even more impaired population (Batki, 1990; Gomez et al., 1999; American Psychiatric Association, 2000).

Integrated care can be based in HIV clinics, infectious disease clinics, mental health centers, substance abuse treatment centers, or community-based centers. Integrated models vary in the degree and quality of the different services provided. These differences are often secondary to organizational constraints (Friedmann et al., 1999). The most common model in the United States is based in a medical clinic and uses a mental health case manager to identify needs and refer patients to psychiatric treatment (Gomez et al., 1999; Brunettte et al., 2003). More specialized centers offer psychiatric treatment within the medical clinic identifying psychiatric and psychological needs at a very early stage. A different approach designates a psychiatrist in a mental health center as primary provider. Having a psychiatrist as primary treatment provider can furthermore facilitate the coordination of the medical and psychiatric care with the addiction treatment. In the United Kingdom, the National Health System designates a general practitioner to provide both medical and psychiatric care, with referral to specialist care provided only for the more complicated cases. Placing a medical provider in a mental health agency is another approach that may prove effective (Brunette et al., 2003).

While an integrated medical, psychiatric, and substance abuse treatment approach is crucial for basic care, integration of a fourth component addressing community outreach, able to engage the individuals who are not able to access the system, would significantly optimize the care delivered to this population. Most evidence supporting integrated care is from observational data. Outcomes most often found to improve are process of care outcomes and patient satisfaction (Budin et al., 2004). Most randomized, controlled trials do not demonstrate the superiority of integrated care. The poor quality of available evidence is probably a result of the difficulty in conceptualizing, planning, funding, and conducting large randomized, controlled trials for patients with multiple, complex problems. However, preliminary results from available studies appear very promising (Taylor, 2005). Clearly, much more needs to be done to identify effective strategies for improving outcomes in these populations. Until this treatment modality is validated, integration may be desirable on a pragmatic basis alone (Willenbring, 2005).

Direct Observation Treatment

Directly observed therapy (DOT) has been historically used in the treatment of tuberculosis (TB), for which DOT programs have improved cure rates in hard-to-reach populations and have proved to be highly cost-effective (Gourevitch et al., 1998). HIV and TB are both infectious diseases that affect similar populations. Both populations are poorly connected with the health system, thus it is very difficult to prevent, treat, and contain the spread of the infection. For both infections poor adherence increases the likelihood of the development of resistant strains, thus increasing the likelihood of the development of significant and resistant epidemics. As with TB, DOT may benefit certain HIV-infected people who have difficulty adhering to highly active antiretroviral therapy (HAART). DOT for management of HIV infection has been effective among prisoners and in pilot programs in Haiti, Rhode Island, and Florida (Mitty et al., 2002).

Many HIV-positive individuals are injection drug users who receive agonist treatment in methadone maintenance therapy programs. These programs require individuals to attend daily and receive methadone under direct observation. Such programs provide a unique opportunity to administer HAART to HIV-infected persons in conjunction with their methadone therapy (Clarke et al., 2002).

Directly observed therapy has been tested in several pilot programs either in the administration of HAART alone or in combination with methadone maintenance. These published observational accounts suggest that DOT may be effective (Teplin, 1990; Searight and

Pound, 1994; Witbeck et al., 2000; Clarke et al., 2002; McCance-Katz et al., 2002; Mitty et al., 2002; CDC, 2003; Conway et al., 2004; Kagay et al., 2004; Lucas et al., 2004; Macalino et al., 2004; Scheft and Fontanette, 2005), but a more definitive answer awaits the publication of randomized, controlled trials. As far as prisons are concerned, long-term studies will need to assess the long-term outcome following release from prisons and the ability to keep these individuals connected with the health system. The correctional setting may provide an opportunity to safely treat patients with comorbid HCV and HIV (Reindollar, 2005). DOT could potentially be combined with pharmacotherapy for psychiatric and addictive disorders in addition to methadone, greatly improving adherence to medications in this population (Willenbring, 2005).

Psychiatric Inpatient Units

The percentage of psychiatric inpatients affected by HIV varies between 5% and 10% (Sacks et al., 1995; Rosenheck and Dennis, 2001). HIV-infected patients can be admitted to a psychiatric hospital for many reasons, including psychiatric complications of the virus, psychological distress associated with the HIV diagnosis, or psychiatric symptoms related to an underlying psychiatric disorder such as substance dependence. Often an interaction of two or more of these factors is present (Wiener, 1994). AIDS-phobic, HIV-bereaved, and factitious HIV-positive admissions are also HIV-related admissions encountered in psychiatric ward. The introduction of HAART has greatly decreased the frequency of neurological complications in these patients as well as the distress experienced in dealing with this infection (Sacks et al., 1995).

The psychiatric patient with known HIV infection is as likely to be a man as a woman and is frequently a member of an ethnic minority group. HIV-positive patients with psychiatric disorders have multiple risks for HIV infection including injecting drug use and unprotected sex. Most patients are at a late stage of HIV infection, typically with CD4+ cell counts of 400 or less. A recent stressful event, especially in the more vulnerable population, such as the pediatric one, is often a trigger for admission (McCance-Katz et al., 2002; Gaughan et al., 2004). Discharge plans are usually complicated by HIV illness, and most HIV-positive patients have a longer length of hospital stay than persons who are not infected with HIV (Meyer et al., 1995; Hoover et al., 2004).

NURSING HOMES AND LONG-TERM CARE FACILITIES

During the beginning of the AIDS epidemic, most persons with AIDS did not survive long enough to require long-term care. Just as medical advances have enabled more people in the general population to survive to older ages, persons with AIDS are surviving and living longer with their illnesses (Cohen, 1998). Admission of HIV-infected patients to nursing homes in the initial phase of the HIV epidemic was difficult because of lack of knowledge and prejudice (Gentry et al., 1994). During the first decade of the HIV epidemic these nursing homes provided end-of-life and palliative care for patients whose life expectancy was very limited. With the advent of HAART, life expectancy greatly increased and many patients were able to return to a functioning and overall healthy life in the community. Most of the medical and psychiatric care shifted from the general hospital and nursing homes to the community.

In the last decade, the role of nursing homes in the treatment of the HIV patient has changed, to meet the needs of a different reality. Many HIV nursing homes closed, while others started to integrate HIV treatment with non-HIV treatment. The number of nursing homes specifically treating HIV patients is limited worldwide. The vast majority of nursing homes in the United States do not provide any specialty areas for HIV/AIDS care. As our population ages and the life span of those diagnosed with HIV/AIDS continue to increase, nursing homes will see more and more patients diagnosed with HIV/AIDS among those seeking care (Pearson and Heuston, 2004).

The average person with HIV admitted to a nursing home in the United States is between age 40 and 60, male, and more likely to be African American or Latino American. It is estimated that the prevalence of psychiatric disorders in nursing homes for older adults ranges from 80% to 90%. Comorbid psychiatric diagnoses (especially dementia) as well as substance dependence and poor social support are prevalent among nursing home patients who are HIV infected (Cohen, 1998; Shin et al., 2002). HIV residents with dementia are significantly more likely to have other diseases, in-

fections, and other health care conditions then other residents with HIV (Buchanan et al., 2001). Despite the multiple complications secondary to psychiatric comorbidities, patients with AIDS who have a psychiatric condition are found to have more favorable admission characteristics and have a better prognosis. These patients are likely to be admitted earlier in their disease course for reasons not due to HIV infection. Once admitted, these patients have fewer discharge options in the community and therefore are more likely to stay in the nursing home until they die (Gentry et al., 1994; Goulet et al 2000).

During their stay in the nursing home, patients' physical and psychological state greatly improves if specialized care is provided. The physical status of the residents improves as evidenced by an increase in body weight, increased CD4 count, and lowered viral loads. Furthermore, there is evidence of improved self-acceptance and self-confidence coupled with diminished levels of psychopathology (Carroll et al., 2000; McGovern et al., 2002). A comprehensive psychiatric program should include individual, couple, family, and group psychotherapy; bereavement interventions; pain management; and support for staff. An educational program can prevent violence and create innovative ways to maximize residual cognitive function and coping strategies. By creating a supportive and accepting environment and addressing pain and psychological distress, individuals with late-stage AIDS can live more comfortable lives, die more dignified and comfortable deaths, and have less need for hastened death (Cohen, 1998, 1999).

Despite the great improvement of treatment available, long-term nursing home care for people with AIDS has a significant role in the care of patients with advanced disease, acute convalescence, long-term care, and terminal care (Blustein et al., 1992; Dore et al., 1999). The need for long-term care may continue to grow for patients who do not respond fully to current antiretroviral therapies and/or have significant neuropsychiatric comorbidities (Selwyn et al., 2000). By creating a bridge between acute hospital care and the community, these facilities can provide a cost-effective alternative when people with HIV can no longer receive appropriate care using home and community-based services (McGovern et al., 2002). The prospect of increasing prevalence of HIV-associated dementia in people with advanced HIV disease similarly increases the role for the nursing home in the treatment of HIV (Cohen, 1999; Carroll et al., 2000). Finally, nursing homes may be the best and last option for the nonadherent patient with late-stage AIDS to have DOT with antiretrovirals that may prove to be both a lifesaving and life-changing experience.

SUBSTANCE ABUSE TREATMENT

Methadone Maintenance Treatment Programs

Substance abuse programs address physical and psychological treatment of individuals who are abusing alcohol, cocaine, opioids, and/or other substances. While treatment of most addictions includes short-term physical detoxification followed by long-term psychiatric and psychological care, treatment of opioid addiction most frequently consists of therapy with opioid or mu-receptor agonists such as methadone administered in methadone maintenance treatment programs.

There is a high prevalence of infection with blood-borne organisms in individuals who are injection drug users, and many clients are monoinfected or coinfected with HIV and hepatitis C virus. HIV infection is frequently transmitted by the sharing of contaminated needles, syringes, and other drug paraphernalia. HIV infection is also transmitted through unprotected sexual activity that may have occurred as a result of disinhibition during intoxication or the exchange of sex for drugs. More than 35% of new HIV cases are among injection drug users, their sexual partners, and their offspring (CDC, 2006).

Methadone maintenance treatment programs provide a significant opportunity for both preventing and diagnosing HIV infection. Clients come on a regular basis and are usually required to have a counselor and to attend groups as well as 12-step programs. Staff members at these programs are in an ideal position to educate about reduction of risky behaviors and provide access to barrier contraception by making free condoms available. The effectiveness of methadone maintenance treatment has been well established (NIH, 1998). Maintenance treatment reduces risky behavior, diminishes consequent infection with HIV, and increases life expectancy (Cooper, 1989; Hartel and Schoenbaum, 1998; Brugal et al., 2005). Barriers to methadone maintenance deny injection drug users access to a cost-effective intervention that generates significant health benefits for the general population (Zaric et al., 2000). Expansion of methadone maintenance programs or even the continuation of existing programs is nonetheless controversial (NIH, 1998).

Integrated Opioid Agonist Maintenance Treatment

In the United States policies that would allow physicians and private group practices to provide opioid agonist treatment have been under consideration. This would entail prescribing opioid agonist treatment outside the traditional setting of methadone maintenance treatment programs. Because of the current federal restrictive regulations on methadone prescribing, the U.S. experience with integrating methadone maintenance treatment with primary care has been limited, compared to that in other countries. Both physicians and policymakers in the United States have significant concerns about this treatment integration. Physicians are generally concerned about taking responsibility for "difficult patients" and for the management of controlled substances, and lack clinical expertise in addiction treatment. Political concerns involve the voters' perception of a liberal policy in a generally conservative culture. The absence of rigorous, large-scale evaluations of the comparative safety and efficacy of traditional methadone clinics and primary care–based opioid agonist treatment programs amplifies these concerns (Weinrich and Stewart, 2000).

Positive experiences in Glasgow and Edinburgh, Scotland, demonstrate that integrating methadone treatment into primary care increases the availability of an important treatment modality, increases access to medical care of marginalized populations, and decreases HIV seroprevalence and drug-related crime (Gruer et al., 1997). Medical clinics offering HIV specialty care are still limited. Clinics that provide specialist HIV care are more likely to provide methadone or buprenorphine than clinics without HIV care. Greater expertise in HIV treatment and enhanced funding appear to be related to an increased willingness of primary care clinics to sustain maintenance programs within their facilities. Access to addiction and psychiatric expertise greatly enhances the willingness of medical clinics to provide substance maintenance programs among their services (Gruer et al., 1997; Weinrich and Stewart, 2000; Turner et al., 2005).

The introduction of buprenorphine maintenance treatment will probably facilitate integration between HIV care and addiction treatment. Medical providers can now prescribe buprenorphine within their facilities after appropriate training (Basu, 2006). Preliminary studies about the provision of buprenorphine maintenance for heroin dependence in primary care settings appear promising (O'Connor et al., 1998). The Health Resources and Service Administration recently awarded 5-year grants to 10 U.S. programs to study the impact of integrating buprenorphine maintenance therapy with HIV medical care. Data from these sites will be available in the next few years (USDHHS, 2005).

Needle Exchange Programs

Syringe exchange programs (SEPs) in the United States and elsewhere were developed in response to the spread of hepatitis B virus, hepatitis C virus, and HIV among injection drug users. These programs limit one of the main vectors of blood-borne infectious diseases, the sharing of contaminated needles and syringes. Through these programs clean needles and syringes are exchanged for used ones free of charge. This also promotes harm reduction (Kaplan and Heimer, 1994; Normand et al., 1995). While there is scientific and individual consensus that SEPs are an important part of infectious disease prevention, there is political debate about providing injections drug users access to clean needles at no cost.

Grau and colleagues (2005) compared psychosocial and behavioral differences among intravenous drug users who used or did not use syringe exchange programs and found no demographic or psychosocial differences between the two groups. The most significant factor distinguishing the two groups was self-efficacy.

Supervised Injecting Centers

Medically supervised injecting centers (SICs) are "legally sanctioned and supervised facilities designated to reduce the health and public order problems associated with illegal injection drug use" (Wright and Tompkins, 2004). The primary objectives of the these centers are reduction of fatal and nonfatal overdose, reduction of risk of infection disease, and increased access to medical, addiction, and psychiatric care (Wright and Tompkins, 2004).

Injection drug users attending SICs are provided with a safe and clean environment, medical care, and referral resources. Supervised injecting centers are also referred to as health rooms, supervised injecting rooms, drug consumption rooms, and safer injecting rooms. They operate in over 26 European cities, Australia, and Canada. In the only comprehensive evaluation of SICs (conducted in Sydney, Australia) a reduction of injecting-related problems was reported (Dolan et al., 2000). Recent reports confirm the decrease in drug-related death rates as well as of drug users in countries where there is a comprehensive policy addressing harm reduction programs through use of SICs, such as Switzerland (Kerr et al., 2005) and the Netherlands (Wood et al., 2004). The UN International Narcotics Control Board, however, views the SIC as violating international drug conventions, and public opinion remains controversial about these centers.

COMMUNITY TREATMENT

Many factors are involved in nonadherence to medical and psychiatric care of patients affected by HIV, including drug use, cognitive disorders associated with HIV, history of PTSD (Cohen et al., 2001; Kerr et al., 2004), poor financial and social support, psychiatric diagnoses, and poor access to care. Health care plans focusing solely on the delivery of medical and psychiatric care within hospital settings are unable to provide services to the most vulnerable patients affected by HIV, mental illness, and substance abuse at the same time. Community-based services with intensive case management that provide a wide array of services and are tailored to each patient's needs have a significant impact on providing access to care as well as retention in care. These ancillary services include case management, mental health and substance abuse treatment and counseling, advocacy, respite and buddy or companion services, food, housing, and emergency financial assistance, and transportation.

Assertive Community Treatment and Intensive Case Management

Community-based treatment can be delivered through an assertive community treatment (ACT) or intensive case management. Both modalities are patient focused and attempt to create a link between the patient and medical services by addressing the specific additional needs of each patient. Assertive community treatment has a special emphasis on a team approach. These multidisciplinary teams share caseloads and meet frequently. Intensive case management, by contrast, encompasses a variety of community-based programs involving individual caseloads and a less defined structure. Assertive community treatment teams mirror the medical model of care in which psychiatrists and nurses have critical roles, and its goal is the provision of comprehensive treatment and rehabilitation that do not broker services. In contrast, the principal function of intensive case management is to link and coordinate services as well as increase community integration (Schaedle et al., 2002).

In recent years, ACT services have expanded to target the homeless population (Burnam et al., 1995; Rosenheck and Dennis, 2001). Studies examining the impact of these services on medical care show improved adherence and retention in primary care of the patients receiving multiple services. The number of services provided seems to be significantly associated with improved adherence, improved retention, and a decreased number of hospitalizations and emergency visits. These findings suggest that receipt of case management and ancillary services is associated with improvement in multiple outcomes for HIV-infected patients. (Braucht et al., 1995; Rahav et al., 1995; Lin et al., 1998; Thompson et al., 1998; Magnus et al., 2001; Ashman et al., 2002; Sherer et al., 2002; Harris et al., 2003; Woods et al., 2003).

Homeless Adolescents

Studies examining the impact of community services on homeless adolescents infected and affected by HIV suggest that outreach is not only important in initially connecting hard-to-reach young persons to services but also necessary for retention in care (Woods et al., 2000, 2002). The impact of these services on the well-being of adolescents infected and affected with HIV seems to be significantly related to the number of contacts with the community team. This higher threshold level suggests that establishing a relationship between the service provider and the client may be critical to client retention in care (Baldwin et al., 1996; Woods et al., 1998). Regardless of the way these supportive services are provided, they represent an extraordinary link between vulnerable adolescents and medical and psychiatric care.

CORRECTIONAL FACILITIES

HIV in Prison

The incarcerated population in the United States has increased dramatically over the past two decades and is currently over two million individuals (Rich et al., 2005). The United States now has the highest per-capita incarceration rate in the world. This phenomenon has been fueled in large part by the "war on drugs," which has led to an increase in drug-related arrests coupled with strict mandatory sentencing requirements. Over the past 20 years, the number of people incarcerated annually for drug-related offenses has grown from 40,000 to 450,000, resulting in an incarcerated population with high rates of reported drug use. An estimated 80% of incarcerated individuals have a history of substance abuse, whereas as many as 20% of state prisoners report a history of injection drug use (Rich et al., 2005).

While injection drug use in correctional facilities is documented to be a problem, qualitative research into the HIV risks faced by inmates is lacking. The harm normally associated with drug addiction and injection drug use is exacerbated in prison. Studies examining the prevalence of medical illnesses in prison show that infectious diseases constitute the most prevalent major disease category among inmates (Baillargeon et al., 2000). Prevalence rates of HIV among male inmates have been recorded at between 6% and 8.5%, and one study of incarcerated women in New York found an 18.8% rate of HIV infection (Weisfuse et al., 1991).

The absence of adequate methadone maintenance programs, the difficult living conditions, the lack of personal space, the lack of social and interpersonal support, the violence and abuse, and the availability of drugs often increase the perceived need to use substances within the prison (Hughes, 2001), thus facilitating the spread of HIV and hepatitis C in the community (Laurence, 2005). The absence of needle exchange programs in prisons has resulted in patterns of needle sharing among large numbers of persons. Continual reuse of syringes poses serious health hazards; bleach distribution is an inadequate solution (Small et al., 2005). Depriving prisoners of the means to protect themselves from HIV infection and failing to provide prisoners living with HIV with care, treatment, and support equivalent to that available in the community at large offend international human rights norms (Dubler et al., 1990; Betteridge, 2004; Jurgens, 2004).

It is estimated that 3%–11% of prison inmates have co-occurring mental health disorders and substance abuse disorders (Teplin, 1990; Edens et al., 1997).

Patients with psychiatric disorders are more likely to engage in behaviors that increase their risk of HIV infection because of their limited impulse control, difficulties in establishing stable social and sexual relationships, limited knowledge about HIV-related risk factors, increased susceptibility to coercion, and co-morbid alcohol and drug use. These same characteristics often lead to incarceration, making the prevalence of psychiatric disorders among inmates particularly high. Studies evaluating psychiatric disorders in prisons indicate that HIV-infected inmates exhibit consistently higher rates of psychiatric disorders than their uninfected counterparts. These associations persist across all psychiatric disorders and across demographic factors (Baillargeon et al., 2003).

Dual-diagnosis treatment programs have been developed in state and federal prisons. Many of these have evolved from existing substance abuse treatment programs and approaches. Dual-diagnosis treatment in prisons includes an extended assessment period, orientation and motivational activities, psychoeducational groups, cognitive-behavioral interventions such as restructuring of "criminal thinking errors," self-help groups, medication monitoring, relapse prevention, and transition into institution or community-based aftercare facilities (Edens et al., 1997).

Drug Treatment in Prison

The current policy for the management and treatment of addictions in prisons is highly controversial. The first needle exchange program within a prison was started in 1992 in Switzerland. All European evaluations of these programs have been favorable. Drug use decreased or remained stable over time, and syringe sharing declined dramatically. No new cases of HIV, hepatitis B, or hepatitis C were reported. The evaluations found no reports of serious unintended negative events, such as initiation of injection or use of needles as weapons (Dolan et al., 2003a).

Methadone has been widely used for over 35 years to treat opiate-dependent individuals. Short-term detoxification with methadone is rarely successful and often is followed by a rapid relapse to heroin use. The aim of methadone maintenance treatment is to sta-bilize opiate-dependent individuals in the long term; it has been shown to significantly reduce opiate use and its associated risks (Bellin et al., 1999). This long-term stabilization and continuous contact with medical providers greatly improve the individual's quality of life and have significant social advantages (Rich et al., 2005). In U.S. prisons, methadone treatment is currently confined to treatment of pregnant individuals, treatment of methadone withdrawal (for those in community methadone maintenance treatment), and detoxification of opiate-dependent inmates. Despite the high risk of relapse to drug use and overdose in the period immediately following release from correctional facilities, only occasionally are opiate-dependent inmates referred to methadone programs upon release (Dolan and Wodak, 1996; Dolan et al., 2003b; Rich et al., 2005). Programs enhancing the linkage between prison and community treatment have been developed in recent years. These programs show that transitional linkage to methadone maintenance treatment is feasible and extremely important in combating the cycle of drug relapse, related risk behavior, and criminality among the incarcerated, opiate-dependent population (Rich et al., 2005).

Sexual Behavior in Prison

Risk of HIV infection in prison is mainly from needle sharing. Unprotected sexual intercourse is another high-risk behavior that is common practice in prisons. Unprotected sexual activity can be secondary to sexual deprivation, be disinhibition related to drug use, or result from exchange of sex for drugs among inmates. In addition, in the U.S. federal penitentiary system, conjugal visits are prohibited, leading to further sexual deprivation among inmates who would otherwise have a source of sexual satisfaction in a monogamous relationship.

There is evidence of condom use among inmates, but most research has tended to focus on adolescent populations (Kingree et al., 2000; Castrucci and Martin, 2002; Nagamune and Bellis, 2002). Most studies focus on issues related to inmates' access to condoms while incarcerated. Very few studies target sexual behaviors of adult male inmates in the United States. In recent studies, both marijuana and cocaine were found to be significant predictors of not using a condom during sex prior to incarceration. Education level appears to be another predictor of the reported frequency of sexual intercourse (Braithwaite and Stephens, 2005). These data can be extremely helpful for the development of health education curricula for inmate populations.

Maltreatment, Discrimination, and Quarantine of HIV-Seropositive Individuals in Correctional Facilities

The correctional facility setting tends to magnify the stigma and discrimination that persons with HIV and AIDS may experience in the community at large. In the 25 years since the onset of the AIDS epidemic, some of the most overt stigma and discrimination have diminished as a result of campaigns targeting the general public and educating about risk behaviors. While obvious evidence of stigma may be lower than in the past, recent surveys uncovered persisting attitudes of fear, judgment, and mistrust toward individuals living with HIV (Herek et al., 2002). It is understandable, therefore, that many individuals with HIV fear the consequences of stigma when their diagnosis becomes known to others.

Patients with HIV and AIDS report discrimination not only from the community but also from treatment providers. Many individuals report experiencing coerced testing; others were refused treatment after disclosing their HIV status; others reported delays in the provision of health care services (Gruskin, 2004; Schuster et al., 2005). Such fears are likely to have detrimental effects on these individuals and persons at risk for HIV (Bird et al., 2004). They will also affect the success of programs and policies intended to prevent HIV transmission. Thus, eradicating AIDS stigma remains an important public health goal for effectively combating HIV (Cohen, 1990; Searight and Bound, 1994; Alonzo et al., 1995; Annas, 1998; Gostin and Webber, 1998; Gostin et al., 1999; Herek et al., 2002; Schuster et al., 2005).

In the correctional system, individuals living with HIV and individuals living with psychiatric conditions are forced to endure great discrimination. Mentally ill inmates are often denied reductions in sentences, parole opportunities, placement in less restrictive facilities, and opportunities to participate in sentence-reducing programs because of their status as psychiatric patients or their need for psychotropic medications (Miller and Metzner, 1994). HIV-positive inmates are often isolated and denied appropriate specialized medical treatment. The effect of this kind of discrimination is very severe, since compliance to a strict medication schedule is necessary for HAART to be effective. These two vulnerable populations face even more discrimination in other countries where education about psychiatric conditions and HIV is limited. In some countries patients with HIV have been quarantined or sanctioned to mandatory sanatoriums (Baldwin et al., 1996; Hansen and Groce, 2003). Both underdeveloped and developed countries continue to need educational policies addressing discrimination of both psychiatric and HIV-positive populations that remain vulnerable in our societies (Merati et al., 2005).

CONCLUSION

Having a clear understanding of both the problems and the opportunities for improvement in special settings may lead to decreased HIV transmission and to improvement in the quality of the lives of persons with HIV and AIDS.

References

Alonzo AA, and Reynolds NR (1995). Stigma, HIV and AIDS: an exploration and elaboration of a stigma trajectory. *Soc Sci Med* 41:303–315.

American Psychiatric Association (2000). Practice guideline for the treatment of patients with HIV/AIDS. Work Group on HIV/AIDS. *Am J Psychiatry* 157: 1–62.

Annas GJ (1998). Protecting patients from discrimination—the Americans with Disabilities Act and HIV infection. *N Engl J Med* 339:1255–1259.

Ashman JJ, Conviser R, and Pounds MB (2002). Associations between HIV-positive individuals' receipt of ancillary services and medical care receipt and retention. *AIDS Care* 14:109–118.

Baillargeon J, Black SA, Pulvino J, and Dunn K (2000). The disease profile of Texas prison inmates. *Ann Epidemiol* 10:74–80.

Baillargeon J, Ducate S, Pulvino J, Bradshaw P, Murray O, and Olvera R (2003). The association of psychiatric disorders and HIV infection in the correctional setting. *Ann Epidemiol* 13:606–612.

Baldwin JA, Bowen AM, and Trotter RR (1996). Factors contributing to retention of not-in treatment drug users in an HIV/AIDS outreach prevention project. *Drugs Soc* 9:19–35.

Basu S, Smith-Rohrberg D, Bruce RD, and Altice FL (2006). Models for integrating buprenorphine therapy into the primary HIV care setting. *Clin Infect Dis* 42(5):716–721.

Batki SL (1990). Drug abuse, psychiatric disorders, and AIDS: dual and triple diagnosis. *West J Med* 152: 547–552.

Bellin E, Wesson J, Tomasino V, Nolan J, Glick AJ, and Oquendo S (1999). High dose methadone reduces criminal recidivism in opiate addicts. *Addict Res* 7:19–29.

Betteridge G (2004). Prisoners' health and human rights in the HIV/AIDS epidemic. *HIV AIDS Policy Law Rev* 9:96–99.

Bird ST, Bogart LM, and Delahanty DL (2004). Health-related correlates of perceived discrimination in HIV care. *AIDS Patient Care STDS* 18:19–26.

Blustein J, Schultz B, Knickman J, Kator M, Richardson H, and McBride L (1992). AIDS and long-term care: the use of services in an institutional setting. *AIDS Public Policy J* 7:32–41.

Bosworth HB, Calhoun PS, Stechuchak KM, and Butterfield MI (2004). Use of psychiatric and medical health care by veterans with severe mental illness. *Psychiatr Serv* 55:708–710.

Bozzette SA, Berry SH, Duan N, Frankel MR, Leibowitz AA, Lefkowitz D, Emmons CA, Senterfitt JW, Berk ML, Morton SC, and Shapiro MF (1998). The care of HIV-infected adults in the United States: HIV cost and services utilization study consortium. *N Engl J Med* 339:1897–1904.

Braithwaite R, and Stephens T (2005). Use of protective barriers and unprotected sex among adult male prison inmates prior to incarceration. *Int J STD AIDS* 16:224–226.

Braucht GN, Reichardt CS, Geissler LJ, Bormann CA, Kwiatkowski CF, and Kirby MW (1995). Effective services for homeless substance abusers. *J Addict Dis* 14:87–109.

Brugal MT, Domingo-Salvany A, Puig R, Barrio G, Garcia de Olalla P, and de la Fuente L (2005). Evaluating the impact of methadone maintenance programmes on mortality due to overdose and aids in a cohort of heroin users in Spain. *Addiction* 100:981–989.

Brunette MF, Drake RE, Marsh BJ, Torrey WC, and Rosenberg SD (2003). Responding to blood-borne infections among persons with severe mental illness. *Psychiatr Serv* 54:860–865.

Buchanan RJ, Wang S, and Huang C (2001). Analyses of nursing home residents with HIV and dementia using the minimum data set. *J Acquir Immune Defic Syndr* 26:246–255.

Budin J, Boslaugh S, Beckett E, and Winiarski MG (2004). Utilization of psychiatric services integrated with primary care by persons of color with HIV in the inner city. *Commun Ment Health J* 40:365–378.

Burnam MA, Morton SC, McGlynn EA, Petersen LP, Stecher BM, Hayes C, and Vaccaro JV (1995). An experimental evaluation of residential and nonresidential treatment for dually diagnosed homeless adults. *J Addict Dis* 14:111–134.

Carroll JF, McGovern JJ, McGinley JJ, Torres JC, Walker JR, Pagan ES, and Biafora FA (2000). A program evaluation study of a nursing home operated as a modified therapeutic community for chemically dependent persons with AIDS. *J Subst Abuse Treat* 18:373–386.

Castrucci BC, and Martin SL (2002). The association between substance use and risky sexual behaviors among incarcerated adolescents. *Maternal Child Health J* 6:43–47.

[CDC] Centers for Disease Control and Prevention (2003). Prevention and control of infections with hepatitis viruses in correctional settings. *MMWR Recomm Rep* 52:1–36.

[CDC] Centers for Disease Control and Prevention (2006) Epidemiology of HIV/AIDS—United States, 1981–2005. *MMWR Morb Mortal Wkly Rep* 55(21): 589–592.

Clarke S, Keenan E, Ryan M, Barry M, and Mulcahy F (2002). Directly observed antiretroviral therapy for injection drug users with HIV infection. *AIDS Read* 12:305–316.

Cohen MA (1990). Biopsychosocial approach to the human immunodeficiency virus epidemic. A clinician's primer. *Gen Hosp Psychiatry* 12:98–123.

Cohen MA (1992). Biopsychosocial aspects of the HIV epidemic. In GP Wormser (ed.), *AIDS and Other Manifestations of HIV Infection*, second edition (pp. 349–371). New York: Raven Press.

Cohen MA (1998). Psychiatric care in an AIDS nursing home. *Psychosomatics* 39:154–161.

Cohen MA (1999). Psychodynamic psychotherapy in an AIDS nursing home. *J Am Acad Psychoanal* 27: 121–133.

Cohen MA, Alfonso CA, Hoffman RG, Milau V, and Carrera G (2001). The impact of PTSD on treatment adherence in persons with HIV infection. *Gen Hosp Psychiatry* 23:294–296.

Cohn SE, Berk ML, Berry SH, Duan N, Frankel MR, Klein JD, McKinney MM, Rastegar A, Smith S, Shapiro MF, and Bozzette SA (2001). The care of HIV-infected adults in rural areas of the United States. *J Acquir Immune Defic Syndr* 28:385–392.

Conway B, Prasad J, Reynolds R, Farley J, Jones M, Jutha S, Smith N, Mead A, and DeVlaming S (2004). Directly observed therapy for the management of HIV-infected patients in a methadone program. *Clin Infect Dis* 38:S402–S408.

Cooper JR (1989). Methadone treatment and acquired immunodeficiency syndrome. *JAMA* 262:1664–1668.

Cournos F, McKinnon K, and Sullivan G (2005). Schizophrenia and comorbid human immunodeficiency virus or hepatitis C virus. *J Clin Psychiatry* 66:27–33.

Cunningham CO, Sohler NL, McCoy K, Heller D, and Selwyn PA (2005). Health care access and utilization patterns in unstably housed HIV-infected individuals in New York City. *AIDS Patient Care STDS* 19:690–695.

Dolan KA, and Wodak A (1996). An international review of methadone provision in prisons. *Addict Res* 4:85–97.

Dolan K, Kimber J, Fry C, Fitzgerald J, McDonald D, and Frautmann F (2000). Drug consumption facilities in Europe and the establishment of supervised injecting centres in Australia. *Drug Alcohol Rev* 19:337–346.

Dolan K, Rutter S, and Wodak AD (2003a). Prison-based syringe exchange programmes: a review of international research and development. *Addiction* 98:153–158.

Dolan KA, Shearer JD, MacDonald M, Mattick RP, Hall W, and Wodak AD (2003b). A randomized controlled trial of methadone maintenance treatment versus wait list control in an Australian prison. *Drug Alcohol Depend* 72:59–65.

Dore GJ, Correll PK, Li Y, Kaldor JM, Cooper DA, and Brew BJ (1999). Changes to AIDS dementia complex in the era of highly active antiretroviral therapy. *AIDS* 13:1249–1253.

Dubler NN, Bergmann CM, and Frankel ME (1990). New York State AIDS Advisory Council. Ad Hoc Committee on AIDS in correctional facilities management of HIV infection in New York State prisons. *Columbia Human Rights Law Rev* 21:363–400.

Edens JF, Peters RH, and Hiulls HA (1997). Treating prison inmates with co-occuring disorders: an integrative review of existing programs. *Behav Sci Law* 15:439–457.

Friedmann PD, Alexander JA, Jin L, and D'Aunno TA (1999). On-site primary care and mental health services in outpatient drug abuse treatment units. *J Behav Health Serv Res* 26:80–94.

Gaughan DM, Hughes MD, Oleske JM, Malee K, Gore CA, and Nachman S (2004). Psychiatric hospitalizations among children and youths with human immunodeficiency virus infection. *Pediatrics* 113: e544–e551.

Gentry D, Fogarty TE, and Lehrman S (1994). Providing long-term care for persons with AIDS: results from a survey of nursing homes in the United States. *AIDS Patient Care* 8:130–137.

Goldberg RW (2005). Supported medical care: a multifaceted approach to helping HIV/hepatitis C virus co-infected adults with serious mental illness. *AIDS* 19:S215–S220.

Gomez MF, Klein DA, Sand S, Marconi M, and O'Dowd MA (1999). Delivering mental health care to HIV-positive individuals: a comparison of two models. *Psychosomatics* 40:321–324.

Gostin LO, Feldblum C, and Webber DW (1999). Disability discrimination in America: HIV/AIDS and other health conditions. *JAMA* 281:745–752.

Goulet JL, Molde S, Constantino J, Gaughan D, and Selwyn PA (2000). Psychiatric comorbidity and the long-term care of people with AIDS. *J Urban Health* 77:213–221.

Gourevitch MN, Alcabes P, Wasserman WC, and Arno PS (1998). Cost-effectiveness of directly observed chemoprophylaxis of tuberculosis among drug users at high risk for tuberculosis. *Int J Tuberc Lung Dis* 2:531–540.

Grau LE, Bluthenthal RN, Marshall P, Singer M, and Heimer R (2005). Psychosocial and behavioral differences among drug injectors who use and do not use syringe exchange programs. *AIDS Behav* 9(4): 495–505.

Gruer L, Wilson P, Scott R, Elliott L, Macleod J, Harden K, Forrester E, Hinshelwood S, McNulty H, and Silk P (1997). General practitioner centered scheme for treatment of opiate-dependent drug injectors in Glasgow. *BMJ* 314:1730–1735.

Gruskin S (2004). Bangkok 2004. Current issues and concerns in HIV testing: a health and human rights approach. *HIV AIDS Policy Law Rev* 9:99–103.

Hansagi H, Allebeck P, Edhag O, and Magnusson G (1990). Frequency of emergency department attendances as a predictor of mortality: nine-year follow-up of a population-based cohort. *J Public Health Med* 12:39–44.

Hansen H, and Groce N (2003). Human immunodeficiency virus and quarantine in Cuba *JAMA* 290:2875.

Harris SK, Samples CL, Keenan PM, Fox DJ, Melchiono MW, Woods ER; Boston HAPPENS program (2003). Outreach, mental health, and case management services: can they help to retain HIV-positive and at-risk youth and young adults in care? *Matern Child Health J* 7:205–218.

Hartel DM, and Schoenbaum EE (1998). Methadone treatment protects against HIV infection: two decades of experience in the Bronx, New York City. *Public Health Rep* 113:107–115.

Herek GM, Capitanio JP, and Widaman KF (2002). HIV-related stigma and knowledge in the United States: prevalence and trends, 1991–1999. *Am J Public Health* 92:371–377.

Hoover DR, Sambamoorthi U, Walkup JT, and Crystal S (2004). Mental illness and length of inpatient stay for Medicaid recipients with AIDS. *Health Serv Res* 39:1319–1339.

Hughes RA (2001). Assessing the influence of need to inject and drug withdrawal on drug injectors' perceptions of HIV risk behavior. *J Psychoact Drugs* 33:185–189.

Joyce GF, Chan KS, Orlando M, and Burnam MA (2005). Mental health status and use of general medical services for persons with human immunodeficiency virus. *Med Care* 43:834–839.

Jurgens R (2004). Dublin Declaration on HIV/AIDS in prisons launched. *Can HIV/AIDS Policy Law Rev* 9:40.

Kagay CR, Porco TC, Liechty CA, Charlebois E, Clark R, Guzman D, Moss AR, and Bangsberg DR (2004). Modeling the impact of modified directly observed antiretroviral therapy on HIV suppression and resistance, disease progression, and death. *Clin Infect Dis* 38:S414–S420.

Kaplan EH, and Heimer R (1994). A circulation theory of needle exchange. *AIDS* 8:567–574.

Kerr T, Palepu A, Barness G, Walsh J, Hogg R, Montaner J, Tyndall M, and Wood E (2004). Psychosocial determinants of adherence to highly active antiretroviral therapy among injection drug users in Vancouver. *Antivir Ther* 9:407–414.

Kerr T, Tyndall M, Li K, Montaner J, and Wood E (2005). Safer injection facility use and syringe sharing in injection drug users. *Lancet* 366:316–318.

Kingree JB, Braithwaite R, and Woodring T (2000). Unprotected sex as a function of alcohol and marijuana use among adolescent detainees. *J Adolesc Health* 27:179–185.

Klinkenberg WD, and Sacks S (2004). HIV/AIDS treatment adherence, health outcomes and cost study group: mental disorders and drug abuse in persons living with HIV/AIDS. *AIDS Care* 16:S22–S42.

Knowlton AR, Hua W, and Latkin C (2005). Social support networks and medical service use among HIV-positive injection drug users: implication to intervention. *AIDS Care* 17:479–492.

Laurence J (2005). The role of prisons in dissemination of HIV and hepatitis. *AIDS Read* 15:54–55.

Leserman J, Whetten K, Lowe K, Stangl D, Swartz MS, and Thielman NM (2005). How trauma, recent stressful events, and PTSD affect functional health status and health utilization in HIV-infected patients in the south. *Psychosom Med* 67:500–507.

Lin YG, Melchiono MW, Huba GJ, and Woods ER (1998). Evaluation of a linked service model of care for HIV-positive, homeless and at-risk youths. *AIDS Patient Care STDS* 12:787–796.

Lucas GM, Weidle PJ, Hader S, and Moore RD (2004). Directly administered antiretroviral therapy in an urban methadone maintenance clinic: a nonrandomized comparative study. *Clin Infect Dis* 38:S409–S413.

Lundgren L, Chassler D, Ben-Ami L, Purington T, and Schilling R (2005). Factors associated with emergency room use among injection drug users of African-American, Hispanic and White-European background. *Am J Addict* 14:268–280.

Lyketsos CG, Fishman M, and Treisman G (1995). Psychiatric issues and emergencies in HIV infection. *Emerg Med Clin North Am* 13:163–177.

Macalino GE, Mitty JA, Bazerman LB, Singh K, McKenzie M, and Flanigan T (2004). Modified directly observed therapy for the treatment of HIV-seropositive substance users: lessons learned from a pilot study. *Clin Infect Dis* 38:S393–S397.

Magnus M, Schmidt N, Kirkhart K, Schieffelin C, Fuchs N, Brown B, and Kissinger PJ (2001). Association between ancillary services and clinical and behavioral outcomes among HIV-infected women. *AIDS Patient Care STDS* 15:137–145.

McCance-Katz EF, Gourevitch MN, Arnsten J, Sarlo J, Rainey P, and Jatlow P (2002). Modified directly observed therapy (MDOT) for injection drug users with HIV disease. *Am J Addict* 11:271–278.

McGovern JJ, Guida F, and Corey P (2002). Improved health and self-esteem among patients with AIDS in a therapeutic community nursing program. *J Subst Abuse Treat* 23:437–440.

Meyer I, Empfield M, Engel D, and Cournos F (1995). Characteristics of HIV-positive chronically mentally ill inpatients. *Psychiatr Q* 66:201–207.

Miller NS, Sheppard LM, Colenda CC, and Magen J (2001). Why physicians are unprepared to treat patients who have alcohol and drug related disorders. *Acad Med* 76:410–418.

Miller RD, and Metzner JL (1994). Psychiatric stigma in correctional facilities. *Bull Am Acad Psychiatry Law* 22:621–628.

Mitty J, Stone V, Sands M, Macalino G, and Flanigan T (2002). Directly observed therapy for the treatment of people with human immunodeficiency virus infection: a work in progress. *Clin Infect Dis* 34:984–990.

Nagamune N, and Bellis JM (2002). Decisional balance of condom use and depressed mood among incarcerated male adolescents. *Acta Med Okayama* 56:287–294.

NIH (1998). NIH Consensus Development Panel on Effective Medical Treatment of Opiate Addiction: effective medical treatment of opiate addiction. *JAMA* 280:1936–1943.

O'Connor PG, Oliveto AH, Shi JM, Triffleman EG, Carroll KM, Kosten TR, Rounsaville BJ, Pakes JA, and Schottenfeld RS (1998). A randomized trial of buprenorphine maintenance for heroin dependence in a primary care clinic for substance users versus a methadone clinic. *Am J Med* 105:100–105.

Okin RL, Boccellari A, Azocar F, Shumway M, O'Brien K, Gelb A, Kohn M, Harding P, and Wachsmuth C (2000). The effects of clinical case management on hospital service use among ER frequent users. *Am J Emerg Med* 18:603–608.

Palepu A, Strathdee SA, Hogg RS, Anis AH, Rae S, Cornelisse PG, Patrick DM, O'Shaughnessy MV, and Schechter MT (1999). The social determinants of emergency department and hospital use by injection drug users in Canada. *J Urban Health* 76:409–418.

Paxton S, Gonzales G, Uppakaew K, Abraham KK, Okta S, Green C, Nair KS, Merati TP, Thephthien B, Marin M, and Quesada A (2005). AIDS-related discrimination in Asia. *AIDS Care* 17:413–424.

Pearson WS, and Hueston WJ (2004). Treatment of HIV/AIDS in the nursing home: variations in rural and urban long-term care settings. *South Med J* 97:338–341.

Rahav M, Rivera JJ, Nuttbrock L, Nuttbrock L, Ng-Mak D, Sturz EL, Link BG, Struening EL, Pepper B, and Gross B (1995). Characteristics and treatment of homeless, mentally ill, chemical-abusing men. *J Psychoactive Drugs* 27:93–103.

Reindollar RW (1999). Hepatitis C and the correctional population. *Am J Med* 107:100S–103S.

Rich JD, Boutwell AE, Shield DC, Key RG, McKenzie M, Clarke JG, and Friedmann PD (2005). Attitudes and practices regarding the use of methadone in US state and federal prisons. *J Urban Health* 82:411–419.

Rosenheck RA, and Dennis D (2001). Time-limited assertive community treatment for homeless persons with severe mental illness. *Arch Gen Psychiatry* 58: 1073–1080.

Rosenheck R, and Lam JA (1997). Homeless mentally ill clients' and providers' perceptions of service needs and clients' use of services. *Psychiatr Serv* 48:381–386.

Rothbard AB, Metraux S, and Blank MB (2003). Cost of care for Medicaid recipients with serious mental illness and HIV infection or AIDS. *Psychiatr Serv* 54:1240–1246.

Sacks M, Burton W, Dermatis H, Looser-Ott S, and Perry S (1995). HIV-related cases among 2,094 admissions to a psychiatric hospital. *Psychiatr Serv* 46:131–135.

Schaedle R, McGrew JH, Bond GR, and Epstein I (2002). A comparison of experts' perspectives on assertive community treatment and intensive case management. *Psychiatr Serv* 53:207–210.

Scheft H, and Fontenette DC (2005). Psychiatric barriers to readiness for treatment for hepatitis C virus (HCV) infection among injection drug users: clinical experience of an addiction psychiatrist in the HIV-HCV coinfection clinic of a public health hospital. *Clin Infect Dis* 40:S292–S296.

Schuster MA, Collins R, Cunningham WE, Morton SC, Zierler S, Wong M, Tu W, and Kanouse DE (2005). Perceived discrimination in clinical care in a nationally representative sample of HIV-infected adults receiving health care. *J Gen Intern Med* 20:807–813.

Searight HR, and Pound P (1994) The HIV-positive psychiatric patient and the duty to protect: ethical and legal issues. *Psychiatry Med* 24:259–270.

Selwyn PA, Goulet JL, Molde S, Constantino J, Fennie KP, Wetherill P, Gaughan DM, Brett-Smith H, and Kennedy C (2000). HIV as a chronic disease: implications for long-term care at an AIDS-dedicated skilled nursing facility. *J Urban Health* 77:187–203.

Sherer R, Stieglitz K, Narra J, Jasek J, Green L, Moore B, Shott S, and Cohen M (2002). HIV multidisciplinary teams work: support services improve access to and retention in HIV primary care. *AIDS Care* 14:S31–S44.

Shin JK, Newman LS, Gebbie KM, and Fillmore HH (2002). Quality of care measurement in nursing home AIDS care: a pilot study. *J Assoc Nurses AIDS Care* 13:70–76.

Small W, Kain S, Laliberte N, Schechter MT, O'Shaughnessy MV, and Spittal PM (2005). Incarceration, addiction and harm reduction: inmates experience injecting drugs in prison. *Subst Use Misuse* 40:831–843.

Stoskopf CH, Kim YK, and Glover SH (2001). Dual diagnosis: HIV and mental illness, a population-based study. *Community Ment Health J* 37:469–479.

Swartz MS, Swanson JW, Hannon MJ, Bosworth HS, Osher FC, Essock SM, and Rosenberg SD (2003). Five-site health and risk study research committee: regular sources of medical care among persons with severe mental illness at risk of hepatitis C infection. *Psychiatr Serv* 54:854–859.

Taylor LE (2005). Delivering care to injection drug users coinfected with HIV and hepatitis C virus. *Clin Infect Dis* 40:S355–S361.

Teplin L (1990). The prevalence of severe mental disorders among male urban jail detainees: comparison with the Epidemiologic Catchment Area program. *Am J Public Health* 80:663–669.

Thompson AS, Blankenship KM, Selwyn PA, Khoshnood K, Lopez M, Balacos K, and Altice FL (1998). Evaluation of an innovative program to address the health and social service needs of drug-using women with or at risk for HIV infection. *J Community Health* 23:419–440.

Turner BJ, Laine C, Lin YT, and Lynch K (2005). Barriers and facilitators to primary care or human immunodeficiency virus clinics providing methadone or buprenorphine for the management of opioid dependence. *Arch Intern Med* 165:1769–1776.

[USDHHS] U.S. Department of Health and Human Services (2005). http://hab.hrsa.gov/special/bup_index.htm accessed April 13, 2007.

Weinrich M, and Stuart M (2000). Provision of methadone treatment in primary care medical practices. *JAMA* 283:1343–1348.

Weisfuse IB, Greenberg BL, Makki HA, Thomas P. Rooney WC, and Rautenberg EL (1991). HIV-1 infection among New York City inmates. *AIDS* 5(9):1133–1138.

Wiener PK, Schwartz MA, and O'Connell RA (1994). Characteristics of HIV-infected patients in an inpatient psychiatric setting. *Psychosomatics* 35: 59–65.

Willenbring ML (2005). Integrating care for patients with infectious, psychiatric and substance use disorders: concepts and approaches. *AIDS* 19:S227–S237.

Witbeck G, Hornfield S, and Dalack GW (2000). Emergency room outreach to chronically addicted individuals. a pilot study. *J Subst Abuse Treat* 19: 39–43.

Wood E, Kerr T, Montaner JS, Strathdee SA, Wodak A, Hankins CA, Schechter MT, and Tyndall MW (2004). Rationale for evaluating North America's first medically supervised safer injecting facility. *Lancet Infect Dis* 4:301–306.

Woods ER, Samples CL, Melchiono MW, Keenan PM, Fox DJ, Chase LH, Tierney S, Price VA, Paradise JE, O'Brien RF, Mansfield CJ, Brooke RA, Allen D, and Goodman E (1998). Boston HAPPENS program: a model of health care for HIV-positive, homeless, and at-risk youth. *J Adolesc Health* 23: 37–48.

Woods ER, Samples CL, Melchiono MW, Keenan PM, Fox DJ, Chase LH, Burns MA, Price VA, Paradise J, O'Brien R, Claytor RA, Brooke R, and Goodman E (2000). Needs and use of services by HIV-positive compared to at-risk youth, including gender differences. *Eval Program Plan* 23:187–198.

Woods ER, Samples CL, Melchiono MW, Keenan PM, Fox DJ, and Harris SK (2002). Boston HAPPENS Program Collaborators: Initiation of services in the Boston HAPPENS program: human immunodeficiency virus–positive, homeless, and at-risk youth can access services. *AIDS Patient Care STDS* 16: 497–510.

Woods ER, Samples CL, Melchiono MW, and Harris SK (2003). Boston HAPPENS program: HIV-positive, homeless and at-risk youth can access care through youth oriented HIV services. *Semin Pediatr Infect Dis* 14:43–53.

Wright NM, and Tompkins CN (2004). Supervised injecting centres. *BMJ* 328:100–102.

Young AS, Sullivan G, Bogart LM, Koegel P, and Kanouse DE (2005). Needs for services reported by adults with severe mental illness and HIV. *Psychiatr Serv* 56:99–101.

Zaric GS, Barnett PG, and Brandeau ML (2000). HIV transmission and the cost-effectiveness of methadone maintenance. *Am J Public Health* 90:1100–1111.

Chapter 32

Psychopharmacologic Treatment Issues in AIDS Psychiatry

Kelly L. Cozza, Scott G. Williams, and Gary H. Wynn

HIV/AIDS patients are often prescribed a plethora of medications, all requiring special attention to pharmacokinetics and pharmacodynamics. This chapter will briefly highlight the available literature on the effectiveness of psychotropics for patients with HIV. A more complete review of antiretrovirals and their interactions with psychotropics and select other medications will follow. Finally, clinical issues pertaining to the prescribing of psychotropics and monitoring of patients on medications who live with HIV will be discussed, highlighted with case examples.

PSYCHOTROPIC USE AND EFFECTIVENESS IN HIV

Antidepressants

Treatment of depression in patients with HIV in many ways mirrors the treatment of non-HIV-infected patients. However, there are important differences that

should be highlighted. Treatment of HIV itself can improve depressive symptoms, and highly active antiretroviral therapy (HAART) has been associated with a decrease in severity of depression (Brechtl et al., 2001). In addition, patients with HIV are more susceptible to drug–drug interactions and may be more sensitive to side effects, making treatment similar to that for the geriatric population (Goldstein and Goodnick, 1998). Treatment is important not just for emotional well-being but also for physical well-being, since comorbid mood disorders increase the risk of nonadherence to medical care (DiMatteo et al., 2000). We review the available literature on antidepressants below. Although not supported by multiple, well-controlled clinical trials, all have been found to be clinically effective, though not systematically studied. Many clinicians advocate, therefore, that the selection of an antidepressant be based on its side effect profile, comorbid symptomatology, and the potential for drug–drug interactions. A brief review of medication trials involving antidepressant use in the setting of HIV follows.

Tricyclic Antidepressants

Tricyclic antidepressants (TCAs) were among the first psychotropics studied in HIV. Prior to the advent of HAART, imipramine was found to be effective in multiple studies of HIV-positive patients without the diagnosis of AIDS (Manning et al., 1990; Rabkin and Harrison, 1990; Rabkin et al., 1994a). There was a high rate of discontinuation, mostly because of side effects or increased pill burden. Markowitz and colleagues compared various forms of psychotherapy to a combination of supportive psychotherapy with imipramine and found that patients had significantly greater improvement in symptoms with imipramine than with supportive psychotherapy or cognitive-behavioral therapy alone. There was a slight but not statistically significant improvement over interpersonal psychotherapy (Markowitz et al., 1998). Desipramine was shown to be as effective as amitriptyline in homosexual men with AIDS, and side effects were not appreciably different (Fernandez et al., 1988). While many clinicians avoid TCAs for fear of anticholinergic side effects, tachycardia and hypotension, and toxicity in overdose, this class remains effective especially in regions that do not have access to selective serotonin reuptake inhibitors (SSRIs) (Razali and Hasanah, 1999). In addition, it is possible to use TCA side effects to clinical advantage, especially in patients who have diarrhea, weight loss, or insomnia or who have a comorbid pain disorder. Despite the potential for toxicity due to drug–drug interactions, therapeutic drug monitoring (TDM) and clinical observation allow for safe use in combination with HIV medications.

Fluoxetine

Since fluoxetine is the oldest SSRI, there is a considerable set of data to support its use in HIV patients, both for depressive symptoms and for decreasing cocaine cravings (Levine et al., 1990; Batki et al., 1993; Cazzullo et al., 1998). Early data comparing efficacy to imipramine showed comparable results and greater tolerability (Rabkin et al., 1994b). In 1997 Ferrando and colleagues performed a small, 6-week open-label trial using fluoxetine, sertraline, and paroxetine. All of the medications improved depressive symptoms but the power was not great enough to detect any difference among the SSRIs. Interestingly, there was a statistically significant improvement in somatic symptoms. This is an important point because many of the

presenting somatic symptoms such as weight loss, fatigue, decreased libido, gastrointestinal upset, musculoskeletal complaints and even cardiopulmonary symptoms were often attributed to the HIV illness. The study showed a roughly 70%–80% improvement in each category of somatic symptoms, further illustrating the fact that affective disorders can exacerbate the perception of underlying disease processes. The most common side effects reported and the reasons for discontinuation included agitation, anxiety, and insomnia (Ferrando et al., 1997). Fluoxetine was also found to be synergistic with psychotherapy and there was a significant improvement in symptoms when fluoxetine was combined with psychotherapy, compared with psychotherapy alone (Zisook et al., 1998).

The first large double-blind, placebo-controlled trial involving an SSRI compared fluoxetine to placebo (Rabkin et al., 1999) and found fluoxetine to be more effective than placebo, despite a large placebo effect. Fluoxetine, because of its long half-life and active metabolite, may be useful in patients who have difficulty remembering to take their medication on a daily basis. Its slight anorexic properties may not benefit some patients. Fluoxetine's propensity for drug interactions is of clinical importance and is discussed in the section Drug Interactions with Highly Active Antiretroviral Therapy below.

Paroxetine

A small open-label study in 1997 was the first to show the benefit of paroxetine in HIV patients with depression or adjustment disorder (Grassi et al., 1997). Elliot and colleagues (1998) showed equivalent efficacy in a randomized, placebo-controlled trial comparing paroxetine and imipramine. Paroxetine was better tolerated, but there was a significant attrition rate from both medications and placebo, and the sample size was small. Paroxetine may be useful in patients with insomnia since it is one of the more sedating SSRIs. In addition, there are in vitro data to suggest that paroxetine may also have antiviral activity and may work synergistically with HAART (Kristiansen and Hansen, 2000). Paroxetine's significant withdrawal syndrome (autonomic instability and flu-like symptoms) may be problematic for nonadherent patients. Paroxetine's drug interaction profile is clinically significant, and is discussed in the section Drug Interactions with Highly Active Antiretroviral Therapy below.

Sertraline

Sertraline has an advantageous side effect profile compared with that of other antidepressants, and it is very safe in overdose (Hansen et al., 2005). The first study of sertraline in HIV patients with depression was a small, open-label trial conducted in 1994. The results were quite impressive, showing a 70% response rate with a dropout rate of 18%. Sertraline was not shown to have any effect on CD4 count or natural killer cell count (Rabkin et al., 1994c). Sertraline was also shown to be effective in a case report of an HIV-positive man with trichotillomania (Rahman and Gregory, 1995).

Citalopram and Escitalopram

Citalopram and escitalopram are the most selective antidepressants for the serotonin receptor and have few reported drug–drug interactions. They are very commonly used in treating HIV patients, although they have not been studied well in the HIV population. Two studies in 2004 both demonstrated good efficacy. One study observed the effect of citalopram on 20 HIV-infected patients with comorbid chronic hepatitis C receiving interferon alpha who had moderate to severe interferon-related depressive symptoms. Among patients started on citalopram, 95% responded and there were no reported drug–drug interactions or adverse events (Laguno et al., 2004). In a 6-week, open-label study of citalopram use in 14 Hispanic and 6 non-Hispanic patients, 50% responded to treatment and 10% discontinued because of adverse effects. There were no statistically significant differences between the two ethnic groups (Currier et al., 2004). These two drugs both have very favorable drug-interaction profiles and few side effects, which speaks to their current clinical popularity.

Fluvoxamine

Fluvoxamine has not been well tolerated in patients with HIV and is not recommended for routine use. The only published study had a 63% discontinuation rate due to insomnia, gastrointestinal disturbance, anorexia, behavioral changes, and sedation (Grassi et al., 1995). It is unclear why HIV-infected patients have a much higher rate of side effects than that in the general population, but drug–drug interactions likely play a large role. Fluvoxamine is extensively metabolized by the liver through multiple pathways and inhibits many of the enzymes responsible for metabolizing antiretrovirals.

Reboxetine

Reboxetine is the first medication in a new class of antidepressants termed norepinephrine reuptake inhibitors (NARI). Currently unavailable in the United States, the NARI data from Europe suggest efficacy in patients without medical comorbidity. There is also one small, open-label study from Brazil that suggests good efficacy in patients with HIV (Carvalhal et al., 2003). As yet it is unclear whether this drug will gain U.S. Food and Drug Administration (FDA) approval, but it may have a role in treating HIV patients since it is not metabolized by P450 enzymes and may have a lower potential for drug–drug interactions.

Serotonin and Norepinephrine Reuptake Inhibitors (Venlafaxine, Duloxetine)

Serotonin and norepinephrine reuptake inhibitors (SNRIs) may have a role in treating HIV depression as they have shown effectiveness for somatic symptoms (Barkin and Barkin, 2005). They have not, however, been systematically studied in the setting of HIV. Their clinically relevant drug–drug interactions are listed in the section Drug Interaction with Highly Active Antiretroviral Therapy below.

Atypical Antidepressants (Nefazodone, Mirtazapine, Trazodone, Bupropion)

Nefazodone and mirtazapine have not been well studied but small, open-label trials have demonstrated effectiveness, and side effects were not significant. Potential drug–drug interactions are a concern, especially with nefazodone, and will be described below (Elliott et al., 1999; Elliott and Roy-Byrne, 2000). Mirtazapine may also have a niche in the treatment of AIDS wasting syndrome as it can reduce nausea through 5HT$_3$ blockade and promote weight gain through its antihistaminergic effects. Trazodone may be an attractive antidepressant for HIV patients with depression and anxiety, especially when the clinician is fearful of prescribing potentially addictive benzodiazepines. One study found that trazodone was slightly more effective than the benzodiazepine clorazepate for HIV patients with adjustment disorder. Though this study failed to achieve statistical significance, it highlights trazodone's properties of sedation and its ability to reduce anxiety without the abuse or dependence risks of benzodiazepines (De Wit et al., 1999). A 6-week open-label trial of bupropion in 20 HIV-positive patients with major depression showed relatively good efficacy, with 60% of patients responding, while 25% of patients dropped out because of intolerable side effects. No changes in the CD4 count or drug toxicity were noted (Currier et al., 2003). While bupropion may be effective, its use is limited because of the potential for drug interactions with antiretrovirals (Hesse et al., 2001). However, in vivo data are scarce, and some feel that the significance of the putative drug–drug interactions has been overstated (Park-Wyllie and Antoniou, 2003). Caution should also be taken when treating patients with central nervous system (CNS) pathology such as opportunistic infections or metastasis because of bupropion's propensity to lower the seizure threshold.

Stimulants

Although the above data suggest that most of the currently available antidepressant medications have good clinical efficacy with respect to mood state, many patients continue to experience fatigue and generalized low energy, especially those with advanced HIV or AIDS (Wagner et al., 1997). Early reviews of the data with stimulants in depressed patients without medical comorbidity did not suggest a statistically significant response, largely because of a profound placebo effect. However, when looking at subpopulations with medical illness, there was significant benefit to the use of psychostimulants (Satel and Nelson, 1989). In addition to their use for fatigue and depression in the medically ill, stimulants may be necessary in patients with comorbid attention-deficit hyperactivity disorders.

Dextroamphetamine

Dextroamphetamine has been reported as being effective for fatigue and depression since the late 1980s. Early case reports touted its quick onset of action and positive effects on concentration and cognition (Fernandez et al., 1988). In 1997 Wagner and colleagues conducted a small open-label trial of dextroamphetamine in 24 men with depression, low energy, a CD-4 count <200, and an AIDS-defining illness. There was a 75% response rate according to intention-to-treat

analysis. Results were seen as quickly as 2 to 3 days after starting treatment. Only two patients discontinued the study because of adverse effects with "overstimulation" as the most common adverse side effect. In a follow-up to this open-label study, performed by the same group, 23 men with HIV, depression, and fatigue were enrolled. The study consisted of a 2-week randomized, placebo-controlled phase followed by 6 weeks of continued treatment for responders. After 8 weeks, the trial was converted to open label and continued for the remainder of the 6-month study period. Using intention-to-treat analysis, the investigators found that 73% of patients responded and there was no evidence of tolerance, abuse, or dependence (Wagner and Rabkin, 2000).

Methylphenidate

There are few high-quality data to analyze the efficacy of methylphenidate in HIV patients. An n-of-1 trial was conducted in 1992 on a patient with HIV, depression, and mild dementia. The study was conducted in three 2-week phases (placebo, methylphenidate, placebo). There was a significant response in Hamilton Rating Scale for Depression (HAM-D) scores during the active drug phase, and cognition improved (White et al., 1992). Methylphenidate was also used in an open-label trial with dextroamphetamine and both medications demonstrated significant improvement (Holmes et al., 1989). When compared with desipramine, methylphenidate showed equal efficacy. Interestingly, methylphenidate did not produce antidepressant effects any faster than desipramine and was very well tolerated in this study (Fernandez et al., 1995).

Non-Amphetamine-Based Stimulants (Atomoxetine, Modafinil)

Because of the abuse potential inherent in amphetamine-based products, newer stimulants have been developed that were initially targeted at children with attention deficit hyperactivity disorder (e.g., atomoxetine) and for patients with sleep disorders such as narcolepsy (e.g., modafinil). To date, there is no trial documenting the effects of atomoxetine in patients with HIV. There is one open-label trial by Rabkin and colleagues (2004) that showed promising results using modafinil to treat fatigue in HIV. In this study, patients also had affective improvement, but there was no placebo to compare the magnitude of the effect. There was no significant effect on CD4 count or viral load, and the treatment was very well tolerated (Rabkin et al., 2004).

Mood Stabilizers

Lithium

The treatment of bipolar disorder in HIV-positive patients and AIDS mania is similar to that for the general population. The mainstay of bipolar treatment remains lithium, either alone or in combination with other antiepileptic mood stabilizers. Lithium has also been used with some success for antidepressant augmentation in the general population (Stein and Bernadt, 1993). There have been no studies to support its use in depressed patients with HIV. In addition to its mood-stabilizing effects, lithium may also improve the course of HIV infection through granulopoesis and cytokine mediation, which may improve the body's immune response (Parenti et al., 1988). In addition, animal studies have shown a neuroprotective effect on the hippocampus from HIV-gp120 (Everall et al. 2002). There is also a possible neurotrophic effect of lithium salt, which might slow the progression of AIDS dementia (Harvey et al., 2002). An early human study conducted before the development of HAART showed poor tolerability of lithium and had a high dropout rate. The potential benefits described through in vitro and animal studies were not seen, and viral titers increased throughout the 8-week period (Parenti et al., 1988). There has not been a published trial comparing the effects of lithium to placebo in HIV care. The evidence for its use in HIV-positive and AIDS patients remains largely anecdotal.

Lithium's common side effects, which include fatigue and slowed cognition, weight gain, and skin changes, may pose significant burdens to medically ill patients. Symptoms of lithium toxicity (nausea, vomiting, diarrhea, confusion, etc.) may mimic symptoms common in AIDS. Lithium use also requires adequate electrolyte balance, which may be difficult to obtain in patients with AIDS who have diarrhea, nausea and vomiting, and general debility. Patients with HIV-associated nephropathy may also be poor candidates for lithium treatment (Cohen and Alfonso, 2004). Starting lithium after there has been significant neurological damage as evidence by MRI findings predicts poor tolerability. Despite these obstacles, lithium has a fa-

vorable drug–drug interaction, profile and for some manic patients it is the only mood stabilizer that is effective. Careful monitoring for toxicity is essential.

Anticonvulsants

Despite the possible protective effects of lithium, one case series suggests that if a combination of lithium and conventional neuroleptics is not effective for bipolar disorder, treatment with anticonvulsants may be an alternative. Clinically, anticonvulsants are used often in HIV patients. Valproic acid, carbamazepine, and phenytoin were used in a series of 11 patients with good results (Halman et al., 1993). This study also suggested that pretreatment MRI abnormalities or late-stage immunosuppression is related to poor tolerability of lithium. The most common MRI abnormalities were T2 signal enhancements or generalized atrophy, but ring-enhancing lesions suggestive of toxoplasmosis or lymphoma were also present. Even with these MRI findings, the anticonvulsants were all well tolerated. This small study was not powered to infer any additional hypotheses with regard to relative efficacy of the anticonvulsants

In addition to the mood-stabilizing effects of anticonvulsants, some have also shown efficacy in the treatment of HIV neuropathy. Carbamazepine and phenytoin have been studied in treatment of trigeminal neuralgia and diabetic peripheral neuropathy, but not HIV-associated neuropathy. Carbamezapine's potential for leukopenia and its anticholinergic effects limit its use in patients with HIV. Gabapentin was studied initially in 2000 during an open-label trial of 19 HIV-positive patients. Pain was significantly improved, independent of whether neurotoxic antiretroviral therapy was used (La Spina et al., 2001). Hahn and colleagues (2004) studied gabapentin in 26 patients and concluded that it was effective when compared with placebo in controlling neuropathic pain. It was very well tolerated up to 3600 mg/day, with somnolence being the most common side effect.

Lamotrigine was shown to be superior to placebo in a small, randomized trial, but adverse events did limit its use in a small number of patients (Simpson et al., 2000). Of the adverse reactions, rash was the most common and potentially the most serious. No patients developed Stevens-Johnson syndrome, and all dermatologic manifestations resolved with discontinuation of the study drug. A larger trial by the same group showed that lamotrigine was effective in treating pain among patients receiving neurotoxic antiretroviral therapy. However, there was no change, compared to placebo, for patients who were not receiving neurotoxic antiretroviral therapy. The authors postulated that different mechanisms of neuropathy in these patients might account for the lack of therapeutic response (Simpson et al., 2003). Lamotrigine has also been studied for treatment of cocaine dependence owing to its indirect inhibition of glutamate release and has shown promise in preliminary trials (Margolin et al., 1998).

There is a theoretical possibility of valproic acid increasing HIV replication (Moog et al., 1996), though in vivo studies have not confirmed this threat (Maggi and Halman, 2001). In addition, valproic acid has multiple drug–drug interactions that are difficult to reliably predict (see below). Caution should be used with all anticonvulsants, as there are special considerations in this population of patients. All drugs with a narrow therapeutic index will require more frequent monitoring because of the great potential for toxicity and drug–drug interactions, as discussed below.

Neuroleptics

Conventional Neuroleptics

Several small trials have demonstrated efficacy of conventional neuroleptics. In a study of 13 male patients with history of psychosis prior to infection with HIV, thioridazine and haloperidol were used in an open-label trial. There was a modest improvement in positive symptoms but no improvement of negative symptoms. There was also a high rate of extrapyramidal side effects (Sewell et al., 1994). Patients with HIV seem to be exquisitely vulnerable to side effects of conventional neuroleptics (Ramachandran et al., 1997), which may be heightened by drug–drug interactions with ritonavir (see below). Molindone has been used with HIV patients with few side effects (Fernandez and Levy, 1993). Breitbart and colleagues (1996) designed a three-arm study to determine the relative efficacy of haloperidol, chlorpromazine, and lorazepam in hospitalized patients with delirium. To ensure informed consent, patients were enrolled upon admission to the hospital prior to developing delirium, resulting in a small number of subjects in the active study. Because only a small number of patients (30/244) developed delirium, the study was not powered to determine any subtle differences between the medications. Haloperidol and chlorpromazine had roughly equivalent efficacy.

Atypical Neuroleptics

Clozapine, the first "atypical" neuroleptic, was found to be effective in relieving psychotic symptoms and drug-induced Parkinson's in a small open-label trial (Lera and Zirulinik, 1999). In a small nursing home population, risperidone was well tolerated and effective in six of nine patients with AIDS dementia and behavioral disturbances. Doses ranged from 0.5 mg daily to 1 mg twice daily (Belzie, 1996). In a larger case series, 12 manic and 9 schizophreniform HIV patients were treated with risperidone at doses comparable to that seen in the general population. Of the 21 patients treated, 20 responded and 13 became symptom-free after 2–12 weeks of treatment. No serious adverse events were reported, drowsiness was the most common side effect, and there were no reported hematologic effects (Singh et al., 1997). Aripiprazole was found to work in combination with lorazepam in a patient with catatonia and psychosis (Alisky, 2004). It has also been hypothesized that atypical neuroleptics, because of their effects at the 5HT2A receptor, may actually provide prophylaxis or treatment against progressive multifocal leukoencephalopathy (Huffman and Fricchione, 2005). Additional data are anecdotal or presented as case reports (Lodge et al., 1998; Maha and Goetz, 1998; Meyer et al., 1998; Zilikis et al., 1998; Altschuler and Kast, 2005). No studies comparing neuroleptics in HIV subjects have been found in the literature.

As with conventional neuroleptics, it is important to remember that HIV-infected patients may be more susceptible to extrapyramidal symptoms and may even have abnormal movements prior to therapy with dopamine antagonists, given that HIV can attack the basal ganglia (Nath et al., 1987). Importantly, risperidone has a greater propensity to cause extrapyramidal side effects than most other atypicals in the general population. Although there have been no large controlled studies on risperidone use in patients with HIV, in clinical practice, persons with HIV/AIDS are prone to difficulties with risperidone. In addition, risperidone is more vulnerable to drug–drug interactions with potent metabolic inhibitors such as ritonavir (see below), which may raise serum levels of risperidone, placing the patient at greater risk of side effects and tardive dyskinesia.

Anxiolytics

Benzodiazepines

Benzodiazepines are prescribed for relatively mild to moderate cases of anxiety. They are also used as a sleep aid, to treat delirium, as an adjunct in psychosis or even for acute mania (Budman and Vandersall, 1990). Some investigators postulate that advanced dementia, including HIV-related dementia, might actually be a form of catatonia responsive to benzodiazepines (see the case report cited above of ariprazole and lorazepam [Alisky, 2004]). The only benzodiazepine that has been studied specifically in HIV-positive patients is lorazepam. As detailed previously, Breitbart and colleagues (1996) compared lorazepam to the neuroleptics haloperidol and chlorpromazine in treating delirium, and benzodiazepine use was shown to be ineffective. In fact, adverse side effects caused an early termination of this treatment arm. There are no clinical trials evaluating the commonly used agents diazepam, clonazepam, alprazolam, midazolam, or temezepam in HIV-infected patients, but literature on their use in other medically ill populations suggests that they are efficacious if used wisely (Fernandez and Levy, 1991). Diazepam may also have the added benefit of inhibiting HIV-1 expression. In vitro studies have shown that diazepam, through its binding to human microglial cells, may inhibit the expression of HIV-1 p24 antigen, thus potentially mitigating AIDS dementia (Lokensgard et al., 1997).

HIV-infected patients may be very sensitive to the effects of benzodiazepines, leading to confusion, cognitive impairment, disinhibition, and frank delirium (Uldall and Berghuis, 1997). Long-acting formulations with active metabolites should be avoided to limit the possibility of disinhibition, amnesia, and delirium. There are also significant drug–drug interactions that may occur with some benzodiazepines and antiretrovirals (particularly the triazolobenzodiazepines and protease inhibitors), and this will be discussed below.

Nonbenzodiazepine Anxiolytics

Buspirone has the theoretical advantage of having a slow onset of action and thus reducing the "rush" associated with benzodiazepines. There may even be the side effect of curbing the ideation for drug-seeking behavior in some susceptible patients (Batki, 1990). It

also has immunomodulatory effects and may influence some immune reconstitution (Eugen-Olsen et al., 2000). However, buspirone has the potential for confusion related to its dopaminergic effects, and drug–drug interactions, particularly with protease inhibitors and efavirenz, limit its use. Thus, some clinicians advocate using buspirone in patients not taking HAART who may have substance abuse problems (Fernandez and Levy, 1994).

Substance Abuse Medications

Methadone

Methadone has long been the standard maintenance therapy for opiate drug abuse. In a review of 28 clinical studies, methadone therapy has been shown to decrease the risk of transmission of HIV through the reduction of injection drug use and sharing of injection drug paraphernalia (Gowing et al., 2006). It has been associated with an increase in the likelihood of using antiretroviral therapy (Wood et al., 2005). Methadone has been shown to decrease the number of reports of multiple sex partners and the practice of exchanging drugs for money (Stark et al., 1996). Methadone may also decrease the risk for heroin overdose. A large study in Spain (Brugal et al., 2005) concluded that the relative risk of overdose for patients not receiving methadone treatment was 7.1 times the risk for patients receiving methadone. Because of the comorbidity of heroin and cocaine dependence, Grabowski and colleagues (2004) combined methadone with d-amphetamine to assess whether agonist therapy for cocaine use was effective. Methadone with d-amphetamine showed a greater reduction in cocaine use than that with methadone and placebo. All individuals reduced their use of opiates. A similar study by the same group compared methadone with antagonist therapy with risperidone and found that, while opiate use decreased, cocaine use did not decrease. They concluded that methadone is effective for treating opiate dependence, and amphetamine is a useful replacement for treating cocaine dependence, but risperidone is not effective (Grabowski et al., 2004).

Buprenorphine

Buprenorphine, a partial mu-opioid agonist, is a newer treatment for opioid dependence and has been less well studied. It has been shown to be very effective worldwide in the opioid-dependent population but its efficacy in preventing HIV risk behavior and transmission has not been well studied. A 12-week trial combining buprenorphine, bupropion, and psychotherapy showed some benefit over standard treatment with methadone in HIV-positive patients with opioid and cocaine dependency. The small sample size and short duration of treatment coupled with no data on long-term follow-up make it difficult to generalize this treatment approach (Avants et al., 1998). A more recent randomized trial has demonstrated a decrease in HIV risk behaviors, but there was no significant improvement in its ability to suppress heroin use over that with methadone treatment (Mattick et al., 2003). Another consideration when using buprenorphine is drug–drug interactions, since buprenorphine is metabolized via the 3A4 pathway and susceptible to interactions with all protease inhibitors and efavirenz. This set of interactions is discussed in more detail below.

Naltrexone

Naltrexone, an opiate antagonist, has a variety of roles in the treatment of opiate and cocaine dependence. It has been used successfully for induction to "reset" the patient's receptor profile, and has also been used for maintenance therapy (Krupitsky et al., 2004). Currently there are no specific trials studying naltrexone use exclusively in HIV-positive patients. Since adherence and pill burden are issues in HIV care, the newly developed long-acting depot formulation of naltrexone may be promising (Hulse et al., 2004). In addition, naltrexone and a related compound, methylnaltrexone, have been shown to reverse opioid-mediated enhancement of HIV infection within macrophages (Ho et al., 2003). This "side effect" of naltrexone therapy may prove to be clinically important as HIV-infected patients continue to live longer with their disease.

Disulfiram

Although there are no studies of disulfiram treatment in HIV patients, a drug safety trial has shown no negative immunomodulatory effects and concluded that the use of disulfiram should not enhance disease progression (Hording et al., 1990). The potential for hepatotoxicity, particularly in HIV patients also infected with hepatitis B and C, has not been formally studied and requires monitoring (Forns et al., 1994). Continuous alcohol ingestion may carry a greater risk

of morbidity than disulfiram use; further study in HIV patients is needed (Kulig and Beresford, 2005).

BRIEF REVIEW OF DRUG INTERACTION PRINCIPLES

Pharmacodynamic interactions are those that occur at the intended receptor site of a medication. They are exemplified by the serotonin syndrome (sweating, autonomic dysfunction, etc.), as can be seen with monoamine oxidase inhibitors (MAOIs) and SSRIs because of the additive effect on monoamines. Most of these interactions are intuitive and easily predictable. Pharmacokinetic interactions are less intuitive and include issues of absorption, distribution, metabolism, and excretion. Many HAART drugs are affected by timing with food or buffers (see Tables 32.2 and 32.3 below), and these are also relatively predictable. Metabolic interactions are a bit more complex, as they are affected by issues of metabolic inhibition, induction, and pharmacogenetics or by the particular metabolic enzymes a patient is born with. For a complete explanation of pharmacokinetic interactions, the reader is referred elsewhere (Cozza et al., 2003). We present briefly the concepts of metabolic inhibition and induction below.

Figure 32.1 presents what happens to serum levels of drug A when a potent inhibitor of drug A's metabolic enzyme (usually in the gut wall or the liver) is present. Inhibition of metabolism is immediate and generally causes the serum level of the parent drug to increase. If that parent drug (for example, a tricyclic antidepressant) has a narrow therapeutic window, then toxicity may result. Inhibition slows the metabolism of a drug dependent on the inhibited enzyme. Inhibition may occur at P450 enzymes in the liver and gut wall (phase I metabolism) or during phase II metabolism (glucuronidation [UGTs], sulfation [SULTs], methylation, etc.) in the liver. P450 enzymes that metabolize current medications include 3A4, 2D6, 1A2, 2C9, 2C19, 2E1, and 2B6, among others. 3A4 and 2D6 are commonly affected by HAART and psychotropics. Table 32.1 presents many of the most common inhibitors of 3A4 and 2D6, as well as the drugs with narrow therapeutic windows that are dependent on those enzymes for metabolism.

Figure 32.2 presents what happens to drug A when a potent inducer of drug A's metabolic enzymes is introduced. Induction of metabolism actually increases the number of sites available for metabolism.

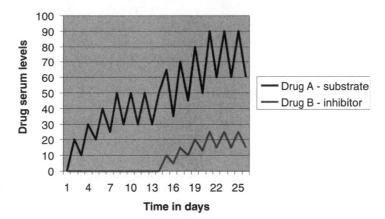

FIGURE 32.1. Drug–drug interaction—inhibition. Drug A develops steady-state concentrations after 4 1/2 lives. Its peak levels are 50 and trough levels 30 at steady state. Drug B is introduced sometime later after drug A is in steady-state concentrations. Drug B develops its own steady state after 4 1/2 lives. Drug B, however, is a competitive inhibitor of the enzyme(s) that drug A uses for its metabolism. Drug A develops a new steady state, with peak levels at 90 and trough levels at 60. Adapted with permission from Cozza KL, Armstrong SC, and Oesterheld JR. *Concise Guide to Drug Interaction Principles for Medical Practice: Cytochrome P450s, UGTs, P-Glycoproteins*, second edition. Copyright (2003), American Psychiatric Press, Inc.

This process is not immediate and can take up to 2 weeks to occur. When more enzymes are available, more drug is metabolized, and the net effect is a lowering of available parent drug, or more rapid metabolism. An inducer may cause the level of a drug dependent on that enzyme to drop below the level needed for clinical effectiveness. Table 32.1 presents many of the most common inducers of 3A4, as well as some of the medications with narrow therapeutic windows dependent on those enzymes for metabolism.

BRIEF REVIEW OF HIGHLY ACTIVE ANTIRETROVIRAL THERAPY

The advancement of HAART for HIV/AIDS is among the most rapid of any disease therapy. From the early days of single-drug zidovudine (AZT) administration to the current multiple drug regimen with new classes of medications, treatments are complex and require near-constant review to remain current. At the time of publication, HAART includes protease inhibitors, nucleotide analogue reverse transcriptase inhibitors (NRTIs), nonnucleoside reverse transcriptase inhibi-

tors (NNRTIs), and fusion inhibitors. These four classes of medications have helped transform HIV/AIDS from being a fatal disease to a more manageable chronic illness. To select adequate psychopharmacological therapies and to become helpful consultants to HIV specialists one needs an understanding of the components of HAART, including drug interactions, pill burdens, and special idiosyncrasies. We present a brief review below.

Protease Inhibitors

Protease inhibitors currently constitute the largest class of HIV/AIDS medications. These medications act at the latest stage of the HIV replication cycle of any of the four classes. During the replication cycle, the virus co-opts the host cell's replication process to make lengthy viral protein precursors, which are cleaved by "HIV protease" into active particles. These active particles are then packaged into virions and bud out of the cell. Protease inhibitors stop the HIV protease from cleaving the protein precursors into active viral particles.

Protease inhibitors, like all HIV therapies, have significant side effects that warrant monitoring in

TABLE 32.1. Common Substrates, Inhibitors and Inducers of Cytochrome P450 Isoenzymes 2D6 and 3A4

P450 Enzyme	Common Substrates*	Common Inhibitors	Common Inducers
2D6	Antiarrhythmics Tricyclic antidepressants Tramadol Typical antipsychotics Metoprolol	**Bupropion** **Fluoxetine** **Paroxetine** **Ritonavir** **Quinidine**	Pan-inducers[†] possibly
3A4	Antitarrythmics β-blockers Carbamazepine Calcium channel blockers Cyclosporine Oral contraceptives Protease inhibitors Statins Triazolobenzodiazepines[‡] Zolpidem	**Atanazanavir** **Cimetidine** **Clarithromycin** Delavirdine Diltiazem **Efavirenz** **Erythromycin** **Grapefruit Juice** **Indinivir** **Itraconazole** **Ketoconazole** **Nefazodone** **Ritonavir** **Tipranavir**	**Carbamazepine** Efavirenz Nevirapine Oxcarbazepine **Pan-inducers**[†] **Ritonavir** St. John's wort

All drugs in bold type are potent in their inhibition or induction.

*A substrate is a drug that must utilize the enzyme for metabolism.

[†]Carbamazepine, phenobarbital, phenytoin, rifamycins.

[‡]Alprazolam, midazolam, triazolam.

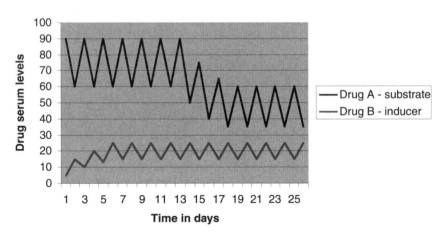

FIGURE 32.2. Drug–drug interaction—induction. Drug A is in steady state, having been introduced sometime before this graph, with peak levels of 90 and trough levels of 60. Drug B is started on day 1, and develops steady state after 4 1/2 lives. After 2 weeks, levels of drug A decrease, as drug B has gradually induced the enzyme(s) involved in metabolizing drug A. Drug A now has a steady state, with peak levels at 60 and trough levels at 35. Adapted with permission from Cozza KL, Armstrong SC, and Oesterheld JR. *Concise Guide to Drug Interaction Principles for Medical Practice: Cytochrome P450s, UGTs, P-Glycoproteins*, second edition. Copyright (2003), American Psychiatric Press, Inc.

combination with patient education. The side effects common to the entire class include gastrointestinal disruption, dysfunction of lipid and glucose metabolism, sexual dysfunction, and hepatic toxicity.

Gastrointestinal side effects are wide ranging in nature, occurring during both initiation and alteration of therapy, and are frequently the cause of drug discontinuation (d'Arminio et al., 2000). The most frequent of these gastrointestinal symptoms are nausea, vomiting, and diarrhea, which can occur in up to 75% of patients (Duran et al., 2001).

Lipodystrophy, hyperglycemia, and hyperlipidemia can occur with administration of any protease inhibitor. The fat redistribution associated with lipodystrophy, particularly to the neck and abdomen area, is frequently resistant to treatment and may not resolve after the discontinuation of protease inhibitor therapy. Protease inhibitor therapy also causes hyperglycemia and hyperlipidemia by suppressing a breakdown of regulatory mechanism in adipose tissue (Hui, 2003). Discontinuation of therapy can result in resolution.

Among HAART therapy components, protease inhibitors carry the highest risk of sexual dysfunction. Some studies show rates as high as 70%, though the physiologic mechanism for decreased libido, erectile dysfunction, or delayed ejaculation is still under investigation (Lallemand et al., 2002). Treatment for sexual dysfunction should be tailored to the individual; medication therapy such as sildenafil should be administered with care because of a potential drug–drug interaction at 3A4.

All protease inhibitors can cause elevated liver-associated enzymes. Roughly one-third of patients receiving protease inhibitors will experience some elevation during regimen initiation or adjustment, but most are mild and transient in nature (Lana et al., 2001). Coinfection with hepatitis B or C as well as heavy alcohol use greatly increases the risk of potential liver injury.

Protease inhibitors are primarily metabolized at 3A4 with some minor involvement by 2D6 for ritonavir and 2C19 for nelfinavir. Enzymatic inhibition by protease inhibitors also occurs primarily at 3A4. Of all the protease inhibitor, ritonavir causes the most varied and potent inhibition (a "pan-inhibitor") and requires the most monitoring when used in combination with other medications. Table 32.2 delineates protease inhibitor metabolism, inhibition, and induction.

Nucleoside Reverse Transcriptase Inhibitors

The NRTIs are "defective" nucleotide analogues that prevent the formation of a phosphodiesterase bond, thereby inhibiting strand synthesis and viral replication (Hoggard et al., 2000). As a class, these medications are safe and effective and in general do not interact with the P450 system. NRTIs have several significant side effects, including mitochondrial toxicity, ototoxicity, and hematopoietic toxicity. The most common severe manifestations of mitochondrial toxicity include neuropathy, myopathy, lactic acidosis, hepatic steatosis, pancreatitis, and lipodystrophy (Moyle, 2000). Hematopoietic toxicity can negatively affect any of the three major cell lines causing anemia, neutropenia, or thrombocytopenia. Notable side effects outside of those applicable to the entire class include a potentially fatal hypersensitivity reaction in up to 5% of patients on abacavir (Clay, 2002). Definitive therapy consists of discontinuation of abacavir, as rechallenge has been associated with significant worsening of symptoms.

Nonnucleoside Reverse Transcriptase Inhibitors

Currently three NNRTIs are available for use (delavirdine, efavirenz, and nevirapine). Though different in chemical structure, these three are similar in mechanism of action, side effects, and in some aspects of metabolism (Table 32.3).

The NNRTIs act by binding directly and noncompetitively to HIV reverse transcriptase causing a conformational change, which results in decreased affinity for nucleoside binding. This decreased affinity results in a blockage of complementary DNA elongation (De Clercq, 1998). This mechanism of action has a relatively potent antiviral effect and, when combined with their tolerability, makes NNRTIs a favorable choice in a HAART regimen.

Most frequently, rash, elevation of liver-associated enzymes, and lipodystrophy are the side effects associated with NNRTIs. Unlike abacavir, the rash associated with NNRTIs is usually mild in nature and does not always require discontinuation. The elevation of liver-associated enzymes is most often asymptomatic and usually requires no intervention outside of periodic monitoring. Lipodystrophy frequently causes discontinuation of therapy and does not always resolve after discontinuation of therapy (Dieterich et al., 2004).

TABLE 32.2. Protease Inhibitors

Drug Name	Metabolism Site	Enzyme(s) Inhibited	Enzyme(s) Induced	Drug and Food Interactions	Side Effects and Toxicities	Contraindicated Medications
Protease inhibitors (common features)				All inhibit CYP 3A4 metabolism and may affect drugs metabolized at CYP 3A4 (e.g., use lower doses of sildenafil with all PIs) All metabolized at CYP and may lose effectiveness with CYP 3A4 inducers Possibly P-glycoprotein substrate and inducer	Gastrointestinal Headaches Hepatitis Lipodystrophy Risk for bleeding Sexual dysfunction	Antiarrhythmics Ergots "Pan-inducers"[b] Pimozide Statins dependent on 3A4[g] St. John's wort Triazolobenzodiazapines[a]
Amprenavir (Agenerase)	3A4	3A4[d]	Possible 3A4	Discontinue vitamin E supplement due to high content in formulation Do not take with high-fat meal	Lactic acidosis Perioral paresthesias Peripheral paresthesias Stevens-Johnson syndrome	Bepridil
Atazanavir (Reyataz)	P450, likely 3A4	3A4, 1A2, 2C9, UGT1A1	None known	Take with light meal or high-fat meal to increase bioavailability and reduce pharmacokinetic variability	Direct (unconjugated) hyperbilirubinemia (especially in overdose) Lactic acidosis Prolonged PR interval on ECG (especially in overdose)	Bepridil Irinotecan Proton-pump inhibitors
Indinavir (Crixivan)	3A4	3A4	None known	Do not take with high-fat or high-protein meals Grapefruit juice decreases indinavir levels	Potential for cross-sensitivity in sulfa-sensitive patients Altered sense of taste Chelitis Dry eyes, mouth, skin Hyperbilirubinemia Nephrolithiasis Paronychia Rash Neutropenia Leukocytoclastic vasculitis;	See "Common Features"
Lopinavir/ritonavir (Kaletra)	3A4	Lopinavir: 3A4,[d] 2D6[f]	Lopinavir: glucuronidation (phase II)	Take with food	Pancreatitis	Same as ritonavir

Drug	Metabolized	Inhibits	Induces	Common features	Side effects	Contraindicated drugs
Nelfinavir (Viracept)	3A4, 2C19	3A4,[e] 1A2, 2B6[d,f]	Possibly 2C9	Take with food	Diarrhea (most severe of PIs) Nephrolithiasis	Amiodarone Quinidine
Ritonavir (Norvir)	3A4, 2D6	**3A4, 2D6, 2C9, 2C19, 2B6[f]**	**3A4**, 1A2,[d] 2C9,[d] 2C19	See Protease Inhibitors (common features)	Pancreatitis Altered sense of taste	Amiodarone Bepridil Clozapine Estradiol Flecainide Lovastatin Meperidine Methadone Propafenone Quinidine
Saquinavir (Fortovase)	3A4	3A4[e]	None known	Take with food	Altered sense of taste	
Tipranavir (Aptivus)	3A4	**3A4**, 1A2, 2C9, 2C19 2D6	None known	Usually administered with ritonavir 200 mg Take with food Contains sulfonamide, beware of sulfa allergy	See "Common Features" and ritonavir	See ritonavir Amiodarone Bepridil Flecainide Propafenone Quinidine

[a] Alprazolam (Xanax); midazolam (Versed); triazolam (Halcion).

[b] Pan-inducers: drugs that induce many if not all CYP P450 enzymes and include barbiturates, carbamazepine, ethanol, phenytoin, and rifamycins.

[c] Potent inhibitors or inducers are in bold type.

[d] Moderate inhibition or induction.

[e] Mild inhibition.

[f] Inhibited in vitro.

[g] Statins dependent on 3A4 include all but pravastatin and rosuvastatin (minor 3A4 metabolism).

Source: From Wynn GH, Zapor MJ, Smith BH, et al. Antiretrovirals, Part 1: Overview, history, and focus on protease inhibitors. *Psychosomatics*, 45:262–270. Copyright (2004), with permission from American Psychiatric Publishing.

TABLE 32.3. Nucleotide Analogue Reverse Transcriptase Inhibitors (NRTIs) and Nonnucleoside Reverse Transcriptase Inhibitors (NNRTIs)

Drug Name	Metabolism Site	Enzyme(s) Inhibited[a]	Enzyme(s) Induced	Drug and Food Interactions	Side Effects and Toxicities	Contraindicated Medications
Common features					Hepatomegaly with steatosis, Lactic acidosis, Lipodystrophy, Myopathy, Pancreatitis, Peripheral neuropathy	
NRTIs						
Abacavir (Ziagen)	Alcohol dehydrogenase, glucuronyl transferase	None known	None known	With or without food	Abacavir hypersensitivity reaction (rechallenge is contraindicated)	
Didanosine (ddI, Videx)	Purine nucleoside phosphorylase	None known	None known	Take on an empty stomach; Do not crush or chew EC tablets	Optic neuritis and retinal depigmentation, Pancreatitis, Peripheral neuropathy	Allopurinol, Dapsone[f], Delavirdine, Ganciclovir, Itraconazole[f], Ketoconazole[f], Methadone, Pyrimethamine[f], Quinolones[g], Ribavirin, Stavudine, Tenofovir, Tetracyclines[g], Trimethoprim/sulfamethoxazole
Emtricitabine (Emtriva)	Full recovery in urine and feces	None known	None known	None	Discontinuation in hepatitis B virus–infected persons may exacerbate hepatitis	
Lamivudine (3TC, Epivir)	Minimal metabolism	None known	None known	With or without food	Generally well tolerated	Ribavirin, Trimethoprim/sulfamethoxazole, Zalcitabine[h]

468

Stavudine (d4T, Zerit)	Not yet known	None known	With or without food	Peripheral neuropathy (increased risk with didanosine)	Didanosine Ribavirin Trimethoprim/sulfamethoxazole Zidovudine[j]
Tenofovir (Viread)	Renal	1A2[d]	High-fat meals increase bioavailability	Nausea	Atazanavir Didanosine[j]
Zalcitabine (ddC, Hivid)	Renal	None known	Do not take with antacids	Pancreatitis Peripheral neuropathy Stomatitis	Antacids[k] Didanosine Doxorubicin Lamivudine Metoclopramide[k] Ribavirin Stavudine
Zidovudine (AZT, Retrovir)	UGT 2B7, CYP P450 b5	None known	With or without food	Anemia Granulocytopenia Headache Gastrointestinal complaints Pancytopenia	Atovaquone[l] Fluconazole[l] Ganciclovir[n] Methadone Rifampin[m] Ritonavir[m] Valproic acid[l]
NNRTIs Common features				Rash Asymptomatic elevation of liver associated enzymes Fat redistribution	See "Common Features"
Delavirdine (Rescriptor)	3A4, 2D6,[d] 2C9,[e] 2C19[e]	3A4, 2C9,[d] 2D6,[d] 2C19[d]	None known	With or without food	See "Common Features"	Atorvastatin Calcium channel blockers Ergots Lovastatin Pimozide Triazolobenzodiazepines St. John's wort Phenobarbital Phenytoin Rifampin

(continued)

TABLE 32.3. (continued)

Drug Name	Metabolism Site	Enzyme(s) Inhibited[a]	Enzyme(s) Induced	Drug and Food Interactions	Side Effects and Toxicities	Contraindicated Medications
Efavirenz (Sustiva)	3A4, 2B6	**3A4**, 2C9,[d] 2C19,[d] 2D6,[d] 1A2[d]	3A4,[b] 2B6[c]	Take on an empty stomach, preferably at bed time	CNS (insomnia, vivid dreams, depression, euphoria, confusion, agitation, amnesia, hallucinations, stupor, altered cognition)	Atorvastatin Carbamazepine Ergots Lovastatin Pimozide Phenobarbital Phenytoin Rifampin St. John's wort
Nevirapine (Viramune)	3A4, 2B6	None known	3A4,[b] 2B6[b]	High-fat meals increase bioavailability	Hepatotoxicity	Antiarrythmics Beta-blockers Cyclosporine Protease inhibitors St. John's wort Tacrolimus
Fusion Inhibitor						
Enfuvirtide (Fuzeon)	Likely hepatic and renal peptidases (not P450)	None known	None known	Subcutaneous injection	Injection site reactions	None known

[a]Potent inhibitors or inducers are in bold type.
[b]Moderate inhibition or induction.
[c]Mild inhibition.
[d]Inhibited in vitro.
[e]Minor pathway.
[f]Drug that requires an acidic pH for absorption and thus should not be co-administered with didanosine, which is buffered with an antacid.
[g]Antibiotic that would be chelated by didanosine's buffered formulation.
[h]Lamivudine and zalcitabine may inhibit each other's intracellular phosphorylation, worsening toxicity, and should not be co-administered.
[i]Zidovudine may inhibit the intracellular phosphorylation of stavudine, worsening toxicity, and should not be co-administered.
[j]Take tenofovir 2 hours before or 1 hour after didanosine.
[k]Decreases absorption of zalcitabine.
[l]Increases zidovudine levels and toxicity.
[m]Decreases zidovudine levels.
[n]Increases hematologic toxicity.

Source: From Zapor MJ, Cozza KL, Wynn GH, et al. Antiretrovirals, Part II: Focus on non-protease inhibitor antiretrovirals (NRTIs, NNRTIs, and fusion inhibitors). *Psychosomatics,* 45:524–535. Copyright (2004), with permission from American Psychiatric Publishing.

All NNRTIs are primarily metabolized at 3A4 with minor contribution by 2B6 for efavirenz and nevirapine. Cytochromes 2D6, 2C9, and 2C19 play a small role in delavirdine's metabolism. Efavirenz and nevirapine are multienzyme inhibitors whereas nevirapine has not shown any enzymatic inhibition. Efavirenz and delavirdine both inhibit 3A4 potently with mild in vitro inhibition of 2C9, 2D6, and 2C19. In addition, efavirenz weakly inhibits 1A2 (Smith et al., 2001; von Moltke et al., 2001).

Both efavirenz and delavirdine induce 3A4 and 2B6. Although efavirenz initially inhibits 3A4 in vitro, clinical evidence shows that over time efavirenz becomes a potent inducer (Clarke et al., 2001; Mouly et al., 2002). This initial inhibition followed by long-term induction necessitates close monitoring of any co-administered medication using 3A4 for metabolism.

Cell Membrane Fusion Inhibitors

The most recent addition in the fight against HIV/AIDS is the class of cell membrane fusion inhibitors such as enfuvirtide. Fusion inhibitors prevent the fusion of virions to host cells by preventing a necessary conformational change. Enfuvirtide is a synthetic peptide derived from viral membrane protein. The most noted side effect with enfuvirtide is a local injection-site reaction. Studies thus far have shown no P450 interactions (Zhang et al., 2004). Overall, enfuvirtide has been shown to be a safe, well-tolerated medication with limited side effects or drug–drug interactions.

DRUG INTERACTIONS WITH HIGHLY ACTIVE ANTIRETROVIRAL TREATMENT

A full review of the drug interactions of psychotropics in the medically ill would be too detailed for this text, and the reader is referred elsewhere (Cozza et al., 2003, 2006; Sandson et al., 2005). We provide selected tables for illustration here. A brief discussion of specific interactions between psychotropics and selected other medications and HAART is presented with case examples. We review the metabolism of psychotropics in table format below, which includes potential drug–drug interactions with HAART. At the time of this publication, a reliable and complete source of information on drug interactions with HAART may be found at www.HIV-druginteractions.org.

Psychotropics

In some clinical settings, more than 50% of HIV patients seeking medical care have a comorbid psychiatric disorder or substance use disorder (Treisman et al., 2001). It is imperative that psychiatrists who treat HIV-infected patients become part of the multidisciplinary treatment team and assist in medication management. An understanding of the drug–drug interactions between HAART and psychotropics prevents morbidity, supports adherence, and improves quality of life (Yun et al., 2005). We present some significant examples of interactions between HAART and psychotropics below. Most interactions may be predicted by using the tables provided (Table 32.4, Table 32.5, Table 32.6, Table 32.7).

SSRIs

Patients taking fluoxetine with ritonavir may develop serotonin syndrome, a constellation of symptoms including mental status changes, diarrhea, and myoclonus (DeSilva et al., 2001). Theoretically, the same may be true with other SSRIs, but there have been no clinical reports to date. SSRIs are mostly metabolized at 2D6 and 3A4, which are both inhibited by ritonavir. No cases of SSRI withdrawal syndrome have been reported with prolonged ritonavir or efavirenz use.

Tricyclic Antidepressants

Tricyclic antidepressants have a narrow therapeutic window and significant cardiotoxicity in overdose. All tricyclics utilize 2D6 as well as 3A4 and others for metabolism. Potent pan-inhibitors like ritonavir may lead to tricyclic toxicity (Abbott Laboratories, 1995; Bertz et al., 1996) (see case summary below).

Case 1: Tricyclic Antidepressants and HAART

A 37-year-old HIV positive man with severe depression was started on nortriptyline, reaching serum levels of 87 ng/dl with some improvement in symptoms. His infectious disease clinician started him on ritonavir and saquinavir, and his primary psychiatrist told him to get a repeat TCA serum level checked in 5–7 days. The patient returned 1 month later complaining of worsened sleep, irritability, depressed mood, hopelessness, and suicidal ideation. The TCA level was 203 ng/dl. In this

TABLE 32.4. Antidepressants

Drug Name	Metabolized	Inhibits	Potential Drug–Drug Interaction with HAART
SSRIs			
Citalopram (Celexa)	3A4, 2C19, 2D6, and renal	2D6[a]	Protease inhibitors[k] Delavirdine Efavirenz
Escitalopram (Lexapro)	3A4, 2C19, 2D6	2D6[b]	Protease inhibitors[k] Delavirdine Efavirenz
Fluoxetine[e] (Prozac)	2D6, 2C9, 2C19, 3A4	**2D6, 2C19,** 2B6,[c] 2C9,[c] 3A4,[c] 1A2[d]	Protease inhibitors[l] Delavirdine Efavirenz
Fluvoxamine[e] (Luvox)	1A2, 2D6	**1A2, 2C19,** 2B6,[c] 2C9,[c] 3A4,[c] 2D6[d]	Efavirenz Tenofovir[m]
Paroxetine (Paxil)	2D6	**2D6, 2B6,** 2C19,[c] 1A2[d]	
Sertraline (Zoloft)	2D6, 3A4, 2C9, 2C19, 2B6	2D6,[c] 2B6,[c] 3A4,[c] UGTs,[c] 1A2,[d] 2C19[f]	Protease inhibitors[l] Delavirdine Efavirenz Zidovudine[n]
Atypical Antidepressants			
Buproprion (Wellbutrin/Zyban)	2B6, 1A2, 2C9, 2E1, 3A4	**2D6**	Protease inhibitors[l] Delavirdine Efavirenz Tenofovir[m]
Duloxetine (Cymbalta)	2D6, 1A2	2D6[c]	Tenofovir[m]
Mirtazepine (Remeron)	1A2, 2D6, 3A4	None known	Tenofovir[m]
Nefazodone (Serzone)	3A4, 2D6	**3A4,** 2D6[g]	Protease inhibitors[k,o] Delavirdine Efavirenz
Trazodone (Deseryl)	3A4, 2D6	None known	Protease inhibitors[k] Delavirdine Efavirenz
Venlafaxine (Effexor)	2D6, 3A4	2D6[d]	Protease inhibitors[l] Delavirdine Efavirenz
Tricyclics			
Amitriptyline (Elavil)	2C19, 2D6, 3A4, UGT 1A4	2C19,[h] 2D6[h]	Protease inhibitors[l] Delavirdine Efavirenz
Clomipramine (Anafranil)	2C19, 2D6, 3A4	2D6[h]	Protease inhibitors[l] Delavirdine Efavirenz
Doxepin (Adapin, Sinequan)	1A2, 2D6, 3A4, UGT 1A3/4	None known	Protease inhibitors[l] Delavirdine Efavirenz Tenofovir[m]
Imipramine (Tofranil)	2C19, 1A2, 2D6, 3A4, UGT 1A3/4	2C19,[h] 2D6[h]	Protease inhibitors[l] Delavirdine Efavirenz Tenofovir[m]

(continued)

TABLE 32.4. *(continued)*

Drug Name	Metabolized	Inhibits	Potential Drug–Drug Interaction with HAART
Trimipramine (Surmontil)	2C19, 2D6, 3A4	None known	Protease inhibitors[l] Delavirdine Efavirenz
Desipramine (Norpramin)	2D6, 3A4, UGTs	2D6[h]	Protease inhibitors[l] Delavirdine Efavirenz
Nortriptyline (Pamelor)	2D6, 3A4, UGTs	2D6[h]	Protease inhibitors[l] Delavirdine Efavirenz
Protriptyline (Vivactil)	2D6[i]	2D6[j]	Protease inhibitors[l] Delavirdine Efavirenz

Primary route of metabolism listed first. Bold type indicates potent inhibition at that cytochrome or UGT.

[a]May inhibit 2D6 moderately at 40+ mg/day.

[b]Moderate inhibition of 2D6 at starting doses.

[c]Moderate inhibition.

[d]Mild inhibition.

[e]"Pan-inhibitor."

[f]Moderate to potent inhibition in vitro.

[g]Weak inhibition.

[h]Mild to moderate inhibition.

[i]Possible site of metabolism.

[j]Possible mild inhibition.

[k]Most likely of the protease inhibitors to cause increased drug levels are ritonavir, atazanavir, and indinavir, due to potent 3A4 inhibition.

[l]Most likely of the protease inhibitors to cause increased drug levels is ritonavir due to "pan-inhibition."

[m]Potential interaction due to induction of CYP 1A2 by tenofovir.

[n]May increase zidovudine levels due to inhibition of UGTs.

[o]Nefazodone's potent 3A4 inhibition will likely cause an increase in protease inhibitor levels.

Source: Adapted from Cozza KL, Armstrong SC, Oesterheld JR, and Sandson N (2006). Psychotropic drug interactions in psychosomatic medicine. In M Blumenfield and JJ Strain (eds.), *Psychosomatic Medicine*, with permission from Philadelphia: Lippincott Williams and Wilkins.

case, ritonavir's potent inhibition of 2D6, 3A4, 2C9, and 2C19 raised nortriptyline levels (metabolized in part by 2D6 and others) beyond the therapeutic window.

Bupropion

Bupropion is primarily metabolized by the minor P450 enzyme 2B6 (Hesse et al., 2001). Nelfinavir, ritonavir, and efavirenz are all inhibitors of this enzyme. Since bupropion has the potential to lower the seizure threshold at high doses, there is a potential for bupropion to become toxic when co-administered with 2B6 inhibitors. HIV patients with a previous history of seizures, or who are severely immunocompromised and at risk for secondary seizures are not candidates for these combinations. A recent case series (Park-Wyllie and Antoniou, 2003) in which concomitant use of these agents occurred for as long as 2 years found no recorded episodes of seizures. Although encouraging, no pharmacokinetic data were available and none of the patients were on high-dose ritonavir. Further pharmacokinetic study is needed. Careful monitoring using lower doses of bupropion (preferably of the longer-acting formulation) and careful informed consent and

TABLE 32.5. Mood Stabilizers

Drug Name	Metabolized	Inhibits/Induces	Potential Drug–Drug Interaction with HAART
Carbamazepine (CBZ, Tegretol)	3A4, 2C9, UGTs	Induces **3A4, 1A2, 2C9, UGT1A4** Inhibits 2C19	Protease inhibitors[b,c] Delavirdine Efavirenz Zidovudine[e]
Gabapentin (Neurontin)	Not metabolized	None	None known
Lamotrigine (Lamictal)	UGT 1A4	Induces UGTs[a]	Zidovudine[e]
Levitiracetam (Keppra)	One-third metabolized by noncytochromal hydrolysis	None	None known
Lithium	Renal	None	None known
Oxcarbazepine (Trileptal)	Noncytochromal metabolism	Induces 3A4,[a] 3A5,[a] UGTs[a] Inhibits 2C19[a]	Zidovudine[e]
Tiagabine (Gabitril)	3A4, UGTs	None	Protease inhibitors[b] Delavirdine Efavirenz
Topiramate (Topamax)	Renal, P450, UGTs	Induces 3A4,[a] UGTs[a] Inhibits 2C19[a]	Protease inhibitors[d]
Valproic acid (VPA, Depakote, Depakene)	UGT 1A6, UGT 1A8, UGT 2B7, 2C9, 2A6	Inhibits UGT 1A8, UGT 2B15, 2C9, epoxide hydroxylase	None known
Vigabatrin (Sabril)	None	None	None known
Zonisamide (Zonegran)	Acetylation, UGTs, 3A4, 3A5	Induces 3A4[a]	Protease inhibitors[b,d] Delavirdine Efavirenz

Primary route of metabolism listed first. Bold type indicates potent inhibition or induction at that cytochrome or UGT.

[a]Moderate.

[b]Most likely of the protease inhibitors to cause increased drug levels are ritonavir, atazanavir, and indinavir.

[c]Carbamazepine's potent induction of 3A4 will likely reduce available protease inhibitor levels.

[d]Induction of 3A4 may reduce available protease inhibitor levels.

[e]May decrease zidovudine levels due to induction of UGTs.

Source: Adapted from Cozza KL, Armstrong SC, Oesterheld JR, and Sandson N (2006). Psychotropic drug interactions in psychosomatic medicine. In M Blumenfield and JJ Strain (eds.), *Psychosomatic Medicine*, with permission from Philadelphia: Lippincott Williams and Wilkins.

warning about the potential for seizures would be prudent with this combination of medications.

Trazodone

In a single-dose, blinded, four-way crossover study of healthy volunteers, Greenblatt and colleagues (2003) found that ritonavir significantly increased trazodone plasma concentration, which in turn increased sedation and fatigue and impaired performance on the digit-symbol substitution test.

Triazolobenzodiazepines

The triazolobenzodiazepines alprazolam, triazolam, and midazolam are all dependent on 3A4 for metabolism. All protease inhibitors inhibit the metabolism of these medications. Merry and colleagues (1997) reported a case of prolonged sedation for bronchoscopy with a protease inhibitor and midazolam combination. A 32-year-old man with HIV infection underwent an initial bronchoscopy with midazolam while taking zidovudine and lamivudine.

TABLE 32.6. Classic and Novel Antipsychotics

Drug Name	Metabolized	Inhibits/Induces	Potential Drug–Drug Interaction with HAART
Classic Antipsychotics			
Fluphenazine (Prolixin)	2D6, 1A2	Inhibits 2D6[a]	Tenofovir[d]
Haloperidol (Haldol)	3A4, glucuronidation, 1A2, 2D6	Inhibits **3A4, 2D6** Induces 3A4[a]	Protease inhibitors[c] Delavirdine Efavirenz Tenofovir[d]
Mesoridazine (Serentil)	2D6, 1A2, 2C19, FMO3	Inhibits 2D6[a]	Tenofovir[d]
Thioridazine (Mellaril)	2D6, 1A2, 2C19, FMO3	Inhibits 2D6[a]	Tenofovir[d]
Molindone (Moban)	2D6 and phase 2	None	
Perphenazine (Trilafon)	2D6, 3A4, 1A2, 2C19	Inhibits **2D6**	Tenofovir[d]
Pimozide (Orap)	3A4, 1A2	Inhibits **2D6, 3A4**	Protease inhibitors[c] Delavirdine Efavirenz Tenofovir[d]
Novel Antipsychotics			
Aripiprazole (Abilify)	2D6, 3A4	None known	Protease inhibitors[c] Delavirdine Efavirenz
Clozapine (Clozaril)	1A2, 3A4, 2D6, 2C19, UGT 1A3, UGT 1A4	Inhibits 2D6[a]	Tenofovir[d]
Olanzapine (Zyprexa)	UGT 1A4, 1A2, 2D6, FMO3	None	Tenofovir[d]
Quetiapine (Seroquel)	3A4, sulfoxidation, oxidation, P-gP substrate	None	Protease inhibitors[c] Delavirdine Efavirenz
Risperidone (Risperdal)	2D6, 3A4	Inhibits 2D6,[b] 3A4[b]	Protease inhibitors[c] Delavirdine Efavirenz
Ziprasidone (Geodon)	Aldehyde oxidase, 3A4, 1A2	None	Protease inhibitors[c] Delavirdine Efavirenz Tenofovir[d]

Primary route of metabolism listed first. Bold type indicates potent inhibition or induction at that cytochrome or UGT.

[a]Moderate.

[b]Mildly.

[c]Most likely of the protease inhibitors to cause increased drug levels are ritonavir, atazanavir, and indinavir.

[d]Potential interaction due to induction of CYP 1A2 by tenofovir.

Source: Adapted from Cozza KL, Armstrong SC, Oesterheld JR, and Sandson N (2006). Psychotropic drug interactions in psychosomatic medicine. In M Blumenfield and JJ Strain (eds.), *Psychosomatic Medicine*, with permission from Philadelphia: Lippincott Williams and Wilkins.

At a later date, saquinavir was added. A second bronchoscopy with the same dose of midazolam necessitated the addition of flumazenil for prolonged sedation, and the patient remained cognitively impaired for more than 5 hours. Ritonavir's interaction with alprazolam and triazolam has proven to be more complex. Short-term use of ritonavir has been show to potently inhibit metabolism of these drugs, resulting in enhanced sedation and impairment (Greenblatt et al., 2000). After using ritonavir for more than

TABLE 32.7. Sedative-Hypnotics

Drug Name	Metabolized	Inhibits/Induces	Potential Drug–Drug Interaction with HAART
Triazolobenzodiazepines			
Alprazolam Midazolam Triazolam	3A4, glucuronidation	None known	Protease inhibitors[a] Delavirdine Efavirenz
Benzodiazepines			
Clonazepam (Klonopin)	Acetylation, 3A4	None known	Protease inhibitors[a] Delavirdine Efavirenz
Diazepam (Valium)	2C19, 3A4, 2B6, 2C9, glucuronidation	None known	Protease inhibitors[a] Delavirdine Efavirenz
Flunitrazepam (Rohypnol)	2C19, 3A4	Inhibits UGT 1A1, UGT 1A3, UGT 2B7	Protease inhibitors[a] Delavirdine Efavirenz Zidovudine[c]
Lorazepam (Ativan)	UGT 2B7, glucuronidation	None known	None known
Oxazapem (Serax)	S-oxazepam—UGT 2B15 R-oxazepam—UGT 1A9, UGT 2B7	None known	None known
Temazepam (Restoril)	UGT 2B7, glucuronidation, 2C19, 3A4	None known	Protease inhibitors[a] Delavirdine Efavirenz
Non-benzodiazepines			
Barbiturates	2C9, 2C19, 2E1	"pan-inducer"	
Buspirone (Buspar)	3A4	None known	Protease inhibitors[a] Delavirdine Efavirenz
Diphenhydramine (Benadryl)	2D6	**2D6**	
Zaleplon (Sonata)	3A4, aldehyde oxidase, 1A2, 2D6	None known	Protease inhibitors[a] Delavirdine Efavirenz Tenofovir[b]
Zolpidem (Ambien)	3A4, 1A2, 2C9, 2C19, 2D6	None known	Protease inhibitors[a] Delavirdine Efavirenz Tenofovir[b]
Zopiclone (Zimovane)	3A4, 2C9	None known	Protease inhibitors[a] Delavirdine Efavirenz
Eszopiclone (Lunesta)	3A4, 2C9	None known	Protease inhibitors[a] Delavirdine Efavirenz

Primary route of metabolism listed first. Bold type indicates potent inhibition or induction at that cytochrome or UGT.

[a]Most likely of the protease inhibitors to cause increased drug levels are ritonavir, atazanavir, and indinavir.

[b]Potential interaction due to induction of CYP 1A2 by tenofovir.

[c]Flunitrazepam may increase zidovudine levels due to inhibition of UGT 2B7.

Source: Adapted from Cozza KL, Armstrong SC, Oesterheld JR, and Sandson N (2006). Psychotropic drug interactions in psychosomatic medicine. In M Blumenfield and JJ Strain (eds.), *Psychosomatic Medicine*, with permission from Philadelphia: Lippincott Williams and Wilkins.

a few days, the clearance of the benzodiazepines increases enough to effect a slight net 3A4 induction by ritonavir.

Case 2: Zolpidem and HAART

A 28-year-old man with mild depression and insomnia on ritonavir-containing HAART had been stable on sertraline 50 mg for months. He had worsened sleep while visiting family and took his mother's zolpidem 5 mg one time. He was difficult to arouse for 18 hours that night and the next day. Because zolpidem is dependent on 3A4 for metabolism, ritonavir's potent inhibition of 3A4 led to elevated serum levels of zolpidem and prolonged effect.

Buspirone

Buspirone is metabolized at 3A4. Clay and Adams (2003) reported a case of pseudo-parkinsonism in a 54-year-old HIV-positive patient after ritonavir was added to his high-dose buspirone (70 mg/day). They successfully treated his adverse reaction by reducing the buspirone dose, discontinuing the ritonavir and replacing it with amprenavir. In review of this case, it may have been sufficient to reduce the dose of buspirone and monitor the patient until ritonavir began inducing the metabolism of buspirone, when the dose could then be titrated back up.

Antipsychotics

Pimozide, generally used in the treatment of tic disorders, has risks for arrhythmias, seizures, and blood disorders. Pimozide is metabolized primarily at 3A4, and therefore must never be co-administered with protease inhibitors or NNRTIs (Abbott Laboratories, 1995). Most antipsychotics are partially metabolized at 2D6 (ziprasidone and pimozide being notable exceptions), and those that are would be susceptible to inhibition by ritonavir, which has been reported to lead to worsened side effects, including extrapyramidal symptoms (Kelly et al., 2002) and possibly tardive dyskinesia. Antipsychotics dependent on 1A2 may be susceptible to reduced serum levels and hence effectiveness when co-administered with the mixed inhibitor-inducers ritonavir or ritonavir/lopinavir (Penzak et al., 2002).

Antiepileptics and Mood Stabilizers

Most older antiepileptics are pan-inducers of multiple P450 enzymes. Phenytoin, phenobarbital, carbamazepine, and oxcarbazepine induce metabolism at 3A4 (Armstrong and Cozza, 2000), and therefore may reduce the serum levels of protease inhibitors and NNRTIs, resulting in lowered serum levels and viral resistance. The newer antiepileptics that are not inducers of 3A4 may be better first choices for patients on HAART who require seizure treatment. For mood stabilization, lithium has the fewest pharmacokinetics interactions with HAART, although side effects may limit its use in patients with HIV. Ritonavir may induce the metabolism of lamotrigine and valproic acid, lowering serum levels (Back, 2006). Careful attention to viral load, disease progression, and therapeutic drug monitoring of antiepileptics is prudent whenever prescribing antiretrovirals with anticonvulsants. We review the commonly used antiepileptics in psychiatry below. The reader is referred elsewhere for a more complete review of antiepileptics in general (Hachad et al., 2002; Cozza et al., 2003; LaRoche and Helmers, 2004).

Carbamazepine

Carbamazepine (CBZ) is a potent pan-inducer at 3A4, and also induces 1A2 and 2C19. It has the potential to reduce serum levels of all the protease inhibitors and NNRTIs. CBZ is metabolized at many P450 enzymes, yet is subject to inhibition by pan-inhibitors such as ritonavir. Kato and colleagues (2000) revealed the immediate nature of ritonavir's pharmacokinetic inhibition with their report of vomiting, vertigo, and elevated liver enzymes with increased serum concentrations of CBZ within 12 hours of the first dose of ritonavir.

Valproic Acid

Valproic acid is highly protein bound and is involved in many interactions because of protein-binding displacement. This agent is also extensively metabolized in the liver to 50 or more metabolites (Pisani, 1992). When valproic acid's metabolic enzymes are induced, the production of a toxic metabolite, 4-ene-valproic acid, may be increased. Levels of this toxic metabolite are not measured in routine valproic acid laboratory tests. The risk factors for valproic acid–induced hepatotoxicity are male gender, age less than 2 years, neurological disease (other than seizures), and concomitant treatment with a P450-inducing medication. There have been reports of valproic acid–induced hepatotoxicity with co-administration of P450 inducers like nevirapine (Cozza et al., 2000). Ritonavir, efavirenz, and lopinavir may also have complicated drug–drug interactions with valproic acid. There is some debate in the literature about valproate acid potentially increasing viral replication (Maggi and Halman, 2001; Romanelli and Pomeroy, 2003), which may limit its usefulness even more.

Opiates

Protease inhibitors inhibit methadone N-demethylation and buprenorphine N-dealkylation in vitro, which, at least upon initial co-administration in humans, may lead to respiratory compromise secondary to opiate toxicity (Iribarne et al., 1998). Clinically, drug–drug interactions with methadone and HAART are more complex. Geltko and Erickson (2000) reported that a patient taking methadone experienced withdrawal symptoms within 7 days of starting ritonavir and was noted to have decreased methadone plasma levels, most likely due to eventual 3A4 induction by ritonavir. Efavirenz is another mixed inhibitor and inducer of 3A4. Boffito and colleagues (2002) described three patients who required 66%, 1%, and 3% increase in methadone dosage after 3–7 days of efavirenz co-administration. Another study described efavirenz co-administration in 11 patients on methadone therapy that resulted in >50% decrease in methadone AUC after only 24 hours of efavirenz administration. By day 8 of efavirenz therapy, 9 patients suffered withdrawal symptoms (Clarke et al., 2001). The NNRTI nevirapine is a 3A4 inducer (Boehringer Ingelheim Pharmaceuticals, 2002) and may reduce the plasma AUC of nelfinavir, indinavir, and saquinavir. In recent postmarketing surveillance, nevirapine was found to induce methadone metabolism, causing methadone withdrawal in some patients and necessitating an increase in methadone dosage (Altice et al., 1999). Interestingly, there are prospective, open-label studies in opiate-dependent HIV patients on methadone maintenance therapy who were co-administered ritonavir/saquinavir (Gerber et al., 2001) and amprenavir (Hendrix et al., 2004) that revealed decreased total methadone and active metabolite plasma levels, yet subjects did not report withdrawal symptoms or re-

quire increases in methadone dose. In summary, whenever opiate-dependent HIV-positive patients are introduced to HAART or experience changes in HAART, monitoring for opiate toxicity or withdrawal is necessary.

Selected Nonpsychotropics

Ergots

Ergots are metabolized at 3A4, and co-administration with 3A4-inhibiting HAART medications may lead to frank ergotism. Vila et al. (2001) reported that after 5 days of co-administration of an ergot-containing antimigraine drug with newly administered ritonavir, a patient developed pain, claudication, paresthesia, coldness, and cyanosis of both lower limbs. This is one of many reported cases of serious ergotism associated with ritonavir.

Glucocorticoids

Some ritonavir interactions may take longer to become apparent. There have been case reports of patients taking ritonavir who developed Cushing's syndrome after many months of inhaled fluticasone due to ritonavir's inhibition of 3A4 metabolism of the corticosteroid (Clevenbergh et al., 2002; Gupta and Dube, 2002). Although metabolic inhibition of 3A4 was immediate, the pharmacodynamic effects of the higher concentrations of substrate became apparent over time. Other glucocorticoids such as prednisilone may also have elevated serum levels when co-administered with ritonavir (Abbott Laboratories, 1995; Roche Pharmaceuticals, 2003/2004). Dexamethasone is a 3A4 inducer and may decrease saquinavir and other protease inhibitor levels.

Oral Contraceptives

Oral contraceptives (OCPs) are dependent on 3A4, 2C9, glucuronidation, and sulfation for metabolism. Most protease inhibitors and efavirenz inhibit 3A4 and place patients at risk for increased side effects (headache, breast tenderness, weight gain, etc.) (Bristol-Myers Squibb, 2004). Ritonavir, being both an inhibitor and inducer of 3A4, has been found in effect to reduce the AUC and C_{max} of ethinyl estradiol (EE) (Ouellet et al., 1998; Piscitelli et al., 2000), placing patients at risk for breakthrough bleeding and pregnancy. Lopinavir, which induces glucuronidation, and the 3A4-inducing NNRTI nelfinivir have also been reported to do the same. Women of childbearing age taking OCPs who are placed on HAART need to be warned to use barrier methods of contraception. Higher-dose preparations of OCPs may also be an option, but these recommendations have not been thoroughly studied with HAART (Cozza et al., 2003).

Statins

Slowed or inhibited metabolism of the statins can lead to toxicity (muscle breakdown and rhabdomyolysis). Only pravastatin and rosuvastatin have minimal or non-P450 metabolic pathways. All other statins are dependent on 3A4 for their metabolism. All protease inhibitors, efavirenz, and delavirdine inhibit 3A4. Efavirenz and nevirapine induce 3A4 metabolism. Protease inhibitors given with simvastatin in healthy volunteers raised simvastatin levels 30-fold (Fichtenbaum et al., 2002). In a retrospective cohort study of 3448 persons receiving protease inhibitors, one of every five persons on a protease inhibitor and on a statin (N = 200) was on a contraindicated combination (Hulgan et al., 2005). In a review of 2110 claims of persons on HAART from a database of private insurance holders (MarketScan, 1999–2000; Hellinger and Encinosa, 2005), 2% had "inappropriate statin drug combination" (IDC), and those with an IDC had a higher number of claims and 39% higher costs than those without an IDC. Those on an IDC were 17 times more likely to have myopathy, polyneuropathy, or myositis. One-half of those cases with an IDC involved simvastatin. Those patients on simvastatin and protease inhibitors had claims for muscle damage. Efavirenz-induced metabolism of simvastatin, atorvastatin, and even pravastatin lowered effectiveness (patients developed an increase in low-density lipoprotein (LDL) with a simvastatin-efavirenz combination) (Gerber et al., 2005).

Case 3: Statins and HAART

A 65-year-old man with HIV, hypertension, hyperlipidemia, and anxious depression was taking simvastatin (Zocor), citalopram, nortriptyline, lisinopril, and diltiazem for years with an indinavir-containing HAART regimen. His HAART was changed to an efavirenz-containing regimen because of PI-induced "buffalo hump" and increasing viral load. Once on efavirenz/lamivudine/

stavudine regimen, his appearance improved and his viral load was reduced initially. After 2 months, he had an increase in LDL and total cholesterol after years of being stable on simvastatin. The drug–drug interaction here involves efavirenz, which is a 3A4 inducer, leading to increased metabolism of simvastatin. The change to pravastatin brought lipids back under control.

Case 4: Beta-Blockers and HAART

A 35-year-old man had a history of alcohol abuse, minor depression, and newly diagnosed HIV and hypertension. His primary care physician, while awaiting HIV-related laboratory results, started the patient on metoprolol for blood pressure. Three days later a psychiatry resident started paroxetine for depression. On the following day, the patient felt dizzy and fell; his blood pressure at the time was 80/60. The infectious disease team wanted to start a ritonavir-containing regimen the same day, and asked the attending psychiatrist and primary physician to review the medications to allow HAART selection. Metoprolol is dependent on 2D6 for metabolism. Paroxetine is a potent inhibitor of 2D6, as is ritonavir. Both of these agents will inhibit the metabolism of metoprolol, enhancing its beta-blocking effects. Several alternatives include selecting a beta-blocker that is not dependent on 2D6 (or choosing an antihypertensive agent from another class, like a diuretic), or selecting an SSRI and protease inhibitor that do not potently inhibit 2D6.

SUMMARY

The prescribing of psychotropics or any other class of medications to HIV-positive patients taking HAART is a complicated undertaking. An understanding of the potential drug–drug interactions is essential and is helpful to the multidisciplinary team. Knowing that the potential exists for an interaction allows for either more careful monitoring (as in the case of tricyclic antidepressants) or the choice of alternative treatments or precautions (such as barrier contraceptive methods).

Protease inhibitors are the most difficult antiretrovirals in terms of drug–drug interactions. All protease inhibitors are metabolized at 3A4 and are susceptible to inhibition and, more importantly, induction (i.e., lowered serum levels leading to viral resistance to HAART). All protease inhibitors are inhibitors of 3A4 and can increase levels of medications dependent on 3A4 for metabolism (this is especially important for drugs with potential toxicity or narrow therapeutic windows). Ritonavir is a pan-inhibitor of multiple enzymes and an inducer of 3A4. This induction can lower serum levels of OCPs, immunosuppressants, and other medications. Efavirenz is also a mixed inhibitor and inducer of 3A4, and nevirapine is an inducer of 3A4.

Memorization of the potent inhibitors and inducers of the P450 enzymes 2D6 and 3A4 most likely encountered in practice and the medications with narrow therapeutic windows that are dependent on those enzymes for metabolism will aid in careful pharmacotherapy.

ACKNOWLEDGMENTS The opinions and assertions contained herein are the private views of the individual authors and are not to be construed as official or as reflecting the views of the Department of the Army or the Department of Defense of the United States of America.

References

Abbott Laboratories (1995). Norvir prescribing information.

Alisky JM (2004). Is the immobility of advanced dementia a form of lorazepam-responsive catatonia? *Am J Alzheimers Dis Other Demen* 19(4):213–214.

Altice FL, Friedland GH, and Cooney EL. (1999). Nevirapine induced opiate withdrawal among injection drug users with HIV infection receiving methadone. *AIDS* 13(8):957–962.

Altschuler EL, and Kast RE (2005). The atypical antipsychotic agents ziprasidone, risperdone and olanzapine as treatment for and prophylaxis against progressive multifocal leukoencephalopathy. *Med Hypotheses* 65(3):585–586.

Armstrong SC, and Cozza KL (2000). Consultation-liaison psychiatry drug–drug interactions update. *Psychosomatics* 41(6):541–543.

Avants SK, Margolin A, DePhilippis D, and Kosten TR (1998). A comprehensive pharmacologic-psychosocial treatment program for HIV-seropositive cocaine- and opioid-dependent patients. Preliminary findings. *J Subst Abuse Treat* 15(3):261–265.

Back D (2006). HIV drug interactions. Retrieved June 19, 2006, from www.HIV-druginteractions.org.

Barkin RL, and Barkin S (2005). The role of venlafaxine and duloxetine in the treatment of depression with decremental changes in somatic symptoms of pain, chronic pain, and the pharmacokinetics and clinical considerations of duloxetine pharmacotherapy. *Am J Ther* 12(5):431–438.

Batki SL (1990). Buspirone in drug users with AIDS or AIDS-related complex. *J Clin Psychopharmacol* 10(3 Suppl.):111S–115S.

Batki SL, Manfredi LB, Jacob P 3rd, and Jones RT (1993). Fluoxetine for cocaine dependence in methadone maintenance: quantitative plasma and urine cocaine/benzoylecgonine concentrations. *J Clin Psychopharmacol* 13(4):243–250.

Belzie LR (1996). Risperidone for AIDS-associated dementia: a case series. *AIDS Patient Care STDS* 10(4):246–249.

Bertz RJ, Cao G, and Cavanaugh JH (1996). Abstract mo.B.1201. Effect of ritonavir on the pharmacokinetics of desipramine. Presented at the 11th International Conference on AIDS, Vancouver, Canada.

Boehringer Ingelheim Pharmaceuticals (2002). Nevirapine prescribing information.

Boffito M, Rossati A, Reynolds HE, Hoggard PG, Back DJ, and Di Perri G (2002). Undefined duration of opiate withdrawal induced by efavirenz in drug users with HIV infection and undergoing chronic methadone treatment. *AIDS Res Hum Retroviruses* 18(5):341–342.

Brechtl JR, Breitbart W, Galietta M, Krivo S, and Rosenfeld B (2001). The use of highly active antiretroviral therapy (HAART) in patients with advanced HIV infection: impact on medical, palliative care, and quality of life outcomes. *J Pain Symptom Manage* 21(1):41–51.

Breitbart W, Marotta R, Platt MM, Weisman H, Derevenco M, Grau C, Corbera K, Raymond S, Lund S, and Jacobsen P (1996). A double-blind trial of haloperidol, chlorpromazine, and lorazepam in the treatment of delirium in hospitalized AIDS patients. *Am J Psychiatry* 153(2):231–237.

Bristol-Myers Squibb Pharmaceuticals Ltd. (2004). Sustiva: summary of product characteristics.

Brugal MT, Domingo-Salvany A, Puig R, Barrio G, Garcia de Olalla P, and de la Fuente L (2005). Evaluating the impact of methadone maintenance programmes on mortality due to overdose and AIDS in a cohort of heroin users in Spain. *Addiction* 100(7):981–989.

Budman CL, and Vandersall TA (1990). Clonazepam treatment of acute mania in an AIDS patient. *J Clin Psychiatry* 51(5):212.

Carvalhal AS, de Abreu PB, Spode A, Correa J, and Kapczinski F (2003). An open trial of reboxetine in HIV-seropositive outpatients with major depressive disorder. *J Clin Psychiatry* 64(4):421–424.

Cazzullo CL, Bessone E, Bertrando P, Pedrazzoli L, and Cusini M (1998). Treatment of depression in HIV-infected patients. *J Psychiatry Neurosci* 23(5): 293–297.

Clarke SM, Mulcahy FM, Tjia J, Reynolds HE, Gibbons SE, Barry MG, and Back DJ. (2001). The pharmacokinetics of methadone in HIV-positive patients receiving the non-nucleoside reverse transcriptase inhibitor efavirenz. *Br J Clin Pharmacol* 51(3):213–217.

Clay PG (2002). The abacavir hypersensitivity reaction: a review. *Clin Ther* 24(10):1502–1514.

Clay PG, and Adams MM (2003). Pseudo-Parkinson disease secondary to ritonavir–buspirone interaction. *Ann Pharmacother* 37(2):202–205.

Clevenbergh P, Corcostegui M, Gerard D, Hieronimus S, Mondain V, Chichmanian RM, Sadoul JL, and Dellamonica P (2002). Iatrogenic Cushing's syndrome in an HIV-infected patient treated with inhaled corticosteroids (fluticasone propionate) and low dose ritonavir enhanced PI containing regimen. *J Infect* 44(3):194–195.

Cohen MA, and Alfonso CA (2004). AIDS psychiatry: psychiatric and palliative care, and pain management. In GP Wormser (ed.), *AIDS and Other Manifestations of HIV Infection* (pp. 537–576). New York: Elsevier.

Cozza KL, Armstrong SC, and Oesterheld JR (2003). *Concise Guide to Drug Interaction Principles for Medical Practice: Cytochrome P450s, UGTs, P-glycoproteins*, second edition. Washington, DC: American Psychiatric Publishing.

Cozza KL, Armstrong SC, Oesterheld JR, and Sandson N (2006). Psychotropic drug interactions in psychosomatic medicine. In M Blumenfield and JJ Strain (eds.), *Psychosomatic Medicine*. Philadelphia: Lippincott Williams and Wilkins.

Cozza KL, Swanton EJ, and Humphreys CW (2000). Hepatotoxicity with combination of valproic acid, ritonavir, and nevirapine: a case report. *Psychosomatics* 41(5):452–453.

Currier MB, Molina G, and Kato M (2003). A prospective trial of sustained-release bupropion for depression in HIV-seropositive and AIDS patients. *Psychosomatics* 44(2):120–125.

Currier MB, Molina G, and Kato M (2004). Citalopram treatment of major depressive disorder in Hispanic HIV and AIDS patients: a prospective study. *Psychosomatics* 45(3):210–216.

d'Arminio Monforte A, Lepri AC, Rezza G, Pezzotti P, Antinori A, Phillips AN, Angarano G, Colangeli V, De Luca A, Ippolito G, Caggese L, Soscia F, Filice G, Gritti F, Narciso P, Tirelli U, and Moroni M (2000). Insights into the reasons for discontinuation of the first highly active antiretroviral therapy (HAART) regimen in a cohort of antiretroviral naive patients. I.Co.N.A. Study group. Italian cohort of antiretroviral-naive patients. *AIDS* 14(5):499–507.

De Clercq E (1998). The role of non-nucleoside reverse transcriptase inhibitors (NNRTIs) in the therapy of HIV-1 infection. *Antiviral Res* 38(3):153–179.

DeSilva KE, Le Flore DB, Marston BJ, and Rimland D (2001). Serotonin syndrome in HIV-infected individuals receiving antiretroviral therapy and fluoxetine. *AIDS* 15(10):1281–1285.

De Wit S, Cremers L, Hirsch D, Zulian C, Clumeck N, and Kormoss N (1999). Efficacy and safety of trazodone versus clorazepate in the treatment of HIV-positive subjects with adjustment disorders: A pilot study. *J Int Med Res* 27(5):223–232.

Dieterich DT, Robinson PA, Love J, and Stern JO (2004). Drug-induced liver injury associated with the use of nonnucleoside reverse-transcriptase inhibitors. *Clin Infect Dis* 38(Suppl. 2):S80–S89.

DiMatteo MR, Lepper HS, and Croghan TW (2000). Depression is a risk factor for noncompliance with medical treatment: meta-analysis of the effects of anxiety and depression on patient adherence. *Arch Intern Med* 160(14):2101–2107.

Duran S, Spire B, Raffi F, Walter V, Bouhour D, Journot V, Cailleton V, Leport C, and Moatti JP (2001). Self-reported symptoms after initiation of a protease inhibitor in HIV-infected patients and their impact on adherence to HAART. *HIV Clin Trials* 2(1):38–45.

Elliott AJ, and Roy-Byrne PP (2000). Mirtazapine for depression in patients with human immunodeficiency virus. *J Clin Psychopharmacol* 20(2):265–267.

Elliott AJ, Uldall KK, Bergam K, Russo J, Claypoole K, and Roy-Byrne PP (1998). Randomized, placebo-controlled trial of paroxetine versus imipramine in depressed HIV-positive outpatients. *Am J Psychiatry* 155(3):367–372.

Elliott AJ, Russo J, Bergam K, Claypoole K, Uldall KK, and Roy-Byrne PP (1999). Antidepressant efficacy in HIV-seropositive outpatients with major depressive disorder: an open trial of nefazodone. *J Clin Psychiatry* 60(4):226–231.

Eugen-Olsen J, Benfield T, Axen TE, Parner J, Iversen J, Pedersen C, and Nielsen JO (2000). Effect of the serotonin receptor agonist, buspirone, on immune function in HIV-infected individuals: a six-month randomized, double-blind, placebo-controlled trial. *HIV Clin Trials* 1(1):20–26.

Everall IP, Bell C, Mallory M, Langford D, Adame A, Rockestein E, and Masliah E (2002). Lithium ameliorates HIV-gp120-mediated neurotoxicity. *Mol Cell Neurosci* 21(3):493–501.

Fernandez F, and Levy JK (1991). Benzodiazepines in the medically ill. In PP Roy-Byrne and D Cowlet (eds.), *Benzodiazepines in Clinical Practice: Risks and Benefits* (pp. 179–200). Washington, DC: American Psychiatric Press.

Fernandez F, and Levy JK (1993). The use of molindone in the treatment of psychotic and delirious patients infected with the human immunodeficiency virus. Case reports. *Gen Hosp Psychiatry* 15(1):31–35.

Fernandez F, and Levy JK (1994). Psychopharmacology in HIV spectrum disorders. *Psychiatr Clin North Am* 17(1):135–148.

Fernandez F, Levy JK, and Galizzi H (1988). Response of HIV-related depression to psychostimulants: case reports. *Hosp Community Psychiatry* 39(6):628–631.

Fernandez F, Levy JK, Samley HR, Pirozzolo FJ, Lachar D, Crowley J, Adams S, Ross B, and Ruiz P (1995).

Effects of methylphenidate in HIV-related depression: a comparative trial with desipramine. *Int J Psychiatry Med* 25(1):53–67.

Ferrando SJ, Goldman JD, and Charness WE (1997). Selective serotonin reuptake inhibitor treatment of depression in symptomatic HIV infection and AIDS. Improvements in affective and somatic symptoms. *Gen Hosp Psychiatry* 19(2):89–97.

Fichtenbaum CJ, Gerber JG, Rosenkranz SL, Segal Y, Aberg JA, Blaschke T, Alston B, Fang F, Kosel B, and Aweeka F (2002). Pharmacokinetic interactions between protease inhibitors and statins in HIV seronegative volunteers: ACTG study a5047. *AIDS* 16(4):569–577.

Forns X, Caballeria J, Bruguera M, Salmeron J.M, Vilella A, Mas A, Pares A, and Rodes L (1994). Disulfiram-induced hepatitis. Report of four cases and review of the literature. *J Hepatol* 21(5):853–857.

Geletko SM, and Erickson AD (2000). Decreased methadone effect after ritonavir initiation. *Pharmacotherapy* 20(1):93–94.

Gerber JG, Rosenkranz S, Segal Y, Aberg J, D'Amico R, Mildvan D, Gulick R, Hughes V, Flexner C, Aweeka F, Hsu A, and Gal J (2001). Effect of ritonavir/saquinavir on stereoselective pharmacokinetics of methadone: results of AIDS clinical trials group (ACTG) 401. *J Acquir Immune Defic Syndr* 27(2):153–160.

Gerber JG, Rosenkranz SL, Fichtenbaum CJ, Vega JM, Yang A, Alston BL, Brobst SW, Segal Y, and Aberg JA (2005). Effect of efavirenz on the pharmacokinetics of simvastatin, atorvastatin, and pravastatin: results of AIDS clinical trials group 5108 study. *J Acquir Immune Defic Syndr* 39(3):307–312.

Goldstein BJ, and Goodnick PJ (1998). Selective serotonin reuptake inhibitors in the treatment of affective disorders—III. Tolerability, safety and pharmacoeconomics. *J Psychopharmacol* 12(3 Suppl. B): S55–S87.

Gowing LR, Farrell M, Bornemann R, Sullivan LE, and Ali RL (2006). Brief report: methadone treatment of injecting opioid users for prevention of HIV infection. *J Gen Intern Med* 21(2):193–195.

Grabowski J, Rhoades H, Stotts A, Cowan K, Kopecky C, Dougherty A, Moeller FG, Hassan S, and Schmitz J (2004). Agonist-like or antagonist-like treatment for cocaine dependence with methadone for heroin dependence: two double-blind randomized clinical trials. *Neuropsychopharmacology* 29(5):969–981.

Grassi B, Gambini O, and Scarone S (1995). Notes on the use of fluvoxamine as treatment of depression in HIV-1-infected subjects. *Pharmacopsychiatry* 28(3):93–94.

Grassi B, Gambini O, Garghentini G, Lazzarin A, and Scarone S (1997). Efficacy of paroxetine for the treatment of depression in the context of HIV infection. *Pharmacopsychiatry* 30(2):70–71.

Greenblatt DJ, von Moltke LL, Harmatz JS, Durol AL, Daily JP, Graf JA, Mertzanis P, Hoffman JL, and Shader RI (2000). Alprazolam–ritonavir interaction: implications for product labeling. *Clin Pharmacol Ther* 67(4):335–341.

Greenblatt DJ, von Moltke LL, Harmatz JS, Fogelman SM, Chen G, Graf JA, Mertzanis P, Byron S, Culm KE, Granda BW, Daily JP, and Shader RI (2003). Short-term exposure to low-dose ritonavir impairs clearance and enhances adverse effects of trazodone. *J Clin Pharmacol* 43(4):414–422.

Gupta SK, and Dube MP (2002). Exogenous Cushing syndrome mimicking human immunodeficiency virus lipodystrophy. *Clin Infect Dis* 35(6):E69–E71.

Hachad H, Ragueneau-Majlessi I, and Levy RH (2002). New antiepileptic drugs: review on drug interactions. *Ther Drug Monit* 24(1):91–103.

Hahn K, Arendt G, Braun JS, von Giesen HJ, Husstedt IW, Maschke M, Straube ME, and Schiekle E. (2004). A placebo-controlled trial of gabapentin for painful HIV-associated sensory neuropathies. *J Neurol* 251(10):1260–1266.

Halman MH, Worth JL, Sanders KM, Renshaw PF, and Murray GB (1993). Anticonvulsant use in the treatment of manic syndromes in patients with HIV-1 infection. *J Neuropsychiatry Clin Neurosci* 5(4): 430–434.

Hansen RA, Gartlehner G, Lohr KN, Gaynes BN, and Carey TS (2005). Efficacy and safety of second-generation antidepressants in the treatment of major depressive disorder. *Ann Intern Med* 143(6):415–426.

Harvey BH, Meyer CL, Gallichio VS, and Manji HK (2002). Lithium salts in AIDS and AIDS-related dementia. *Psychopharmacol Bull* 36(1):5–26.

Hellinger FJ, and Encinosa WE (2005). Inappropriate drug combinations among privately insured patients with HIV disease. *Med Care* 43(9 Suppl.): III53–III62.

Hendrix CW, Wakeford J, Wire MB, Lou Y, Bigelow GE, Martinez E, Christopher J, Fuchs EJ, and Snidow JW (2004). Pharmacokinetics and pharmacodynamics of methadone enantiomers after coadministration with amprenavir in opioid-dependent subjects. *Pharmacotherapy* 24(9):1110–1121.

Hesse LM, von Moltke LL, Shader RI, and Greenblatt DJ (2001). Ritonavir, efavirenz, and nelfinavir inhibit cyp2b6 activity in vitro: potential drug interactions with bupropion. *Drug Metab Dispos* 29(2): 100–102.

Ho WZ, Guo CJ, Yuan CS, Douglas SD, and Moss J (2003). Methylnaltrexone antagonizes opioid-mediated enhancement of HIV infection of human blood mononuclear phagocytes. *J Pharmacol Exp Ther* 307(3):1158–1162.

Hoggard PG, Sales SD, Kewn S, Sunderland D, Khoo SH, Hart CA, and Back DJ (2000). Correlation between intracellular pharmacological activation of nucleoside analogues and HIV suppression in vitro. *Antivir Chem Chemother* 11(6):353–358.

Holmes VF, Fernandez F, and Levy JK (1989). Psychostimulant response in AIDS-related complex patients. *J Clin Psychiatry* 50(1):5–8.

Hording M, Gotzsche PC, Bygbjerg IC, Christensen LD, and Faber V (1990). Lack of immunomodulating effect of disulfiram on HIV positive patients. *Int J Immunopharmacol* 12(2):145–147.

Huffman JC, and Fricchione GL (2005). Catatonia and psychosis in a patient with AIDS: treatment with lorazepam and aripiprazole. *J Clin Psychopharmacol* 25(5):508–510.

Hui DY (2003). Effects of HIV protease inhibitor therapy on lipid metabolism. *Prog Lipid Res* 42(2):81–92.

Hulgan T, Sterling TR, Daugherty J, Arbogast PG, Raffanti S, and Ray W (2005). Prescribing of contraindicated protease inhibitor and statin combinations among HIV-infected persons. *J Acquir Immune Defic Syndr* 38(3):277–282.

Hulse GK, Arnold-Reed DE, O'Neil G, Chan CT, and Hansson RC (2004). Achieving long-term continuous blood naltrexone and 6-beta-naltrexol coverage following sequential naltrexone implants. *Addict Biol* 9(1):67–72.

Iribarne C, Berthou F, Carlhant D, Dreano Y, Picart D, Lohezic F, and Riche C (1998). Inhibition of methadone and buprenorphine n-dealkylations by three HIV-1 protease inhibitors. *Drug Metab Dispos* 26(3):257–260.

Kato Y, Fujii T, Mizoguchi N, Takata N, Ueda K, Feldman MD, and Kayser SR (2000). Potential interaction between ritonavir and carbamazepine. *Pharmacotherapy* 20(7):851 854.

Kelly DV, Beique LC, and Bowmer MI (2002). Extrapyramidal symptoms with ritonavir/indinavir plus risperidone. *Ann Pharmacother* 36(5):827–830.

Kristiansen JE, and Hansen JB (2000). Inhibition of HIV replication by neuroleptic agents and their potential use in HIV infected patients with AIDS related dementia. *Int J Antimicrob Agents* 14(3):209–213.

Krupitsky EM, Zvartau EE, Masalov DV, Tsoi MV, Burakov AM, Egorova VY, Didenko TY, Romanova TN, Ivanova EB, Bespalov AY, Verbitskaya EV, Neznanov NG, Grinenko AY, O'Brien CP, and Woody GE (2004). Naltrexone for heroin dependence treatment in St. Petersburg, Russia. *J Subst Abuse Treat* 26(4):285–294.

Kulig CC, and Beresford T P (2005). Hepatitis C in alcohol dependence: drinking versus disulfiram. *J Addict Dis* 24(2):77–89.

La Spina I, Porazzi D, Maggiolo F, Bottura P, and Suter F (2001). Gabapentin in painful HIV-related neuropathy: a report of 19 patients, preliminary observations. *Eur J Neurol* 8(1):71–75.

Laguno M, Blanch J, Murillas J, Blanco JL, Leon A, Lonca M, Larrousse M. Biglia A, Martinez E, Garcia F, Miro JM, de Pablo J, Gatell JM, and Mallolas J (2004). Depressive symptoms after initiation of interferon therapy in human immunodeficiency virus-infected patients with chronic hepatitis C. *Antivir Ther* 9(6):905–909.

Lallemand F, Salhi Y, Linard F, Giami A, and Rozenbaum W (2002). Sexual dysfunction in 156 ambulatory HIV-infected men receiving highly active antiretroviral therapy combinations with and without protease inhibitors. *J Acquir Immune Defic Syndr* 30(2):187–190.

Lana R, Nunez M, Mendoza JL, and Soriano V (2001). Rate and risk factors of liver toxicity in patients receiving antiretroviral therapy [in Spanish]. *Med Clin (Barc)* 117(16):607–610.

LaRoche SM, and Helmers SL (2004). The new antiepileptic drugs: scientific review. *JAMA* 291(5):605–614.

Lera G, and Zirulnik J (1999). Pilot study with clozapine in patients with HIV-associated psychosis and drug-induced parkinsonism. *Mov Disord* 14(1):128–131.

Levine S, Anderson D, Bystritsky A, and Baron D (1990). A report of eight HIV-seropositive patients with major depression responding to fluoxetine. *J Acquir Immune Defic Syndr* 3(11):1074–1077.

Lodge P, Tanner M, and McKeogh MM (1998). Risperidone in the management of agitation in HIV dementia. *Palliat Med* 12(3):206–207.

Lokensgard JR, Gekker G, Hu S, Arthur AF, Chao CC, and Peterson PK (1997). Diazepam-mediated inhibition of human immunodeficiency virus type 1 expression in human brain cells. *Antimicrob Agents Chemother* 41(11):2566–2569.

Maggi JD, and Halman MH (2001). The effect of divalproex sodium on viral load: a retrospective review of HIV-positive patients with manic syndromes. *Can J Psychiatry* 46(4):359–362.

Maha A, and Goetz K (1998). Risperidone for the treatment of delusional disorder due to HIV disease. *J Neuropsychiatry Clin Neurosci* 10(1):111.

Manning D, Jacobsberg L, and Erhart S (1990). The efficacy of imipramine in the treatment of HIV-related depression. Presented at the VI International Conference on AIDS, San Francisco.

Margolin A, Avants SK, DePhilippis D, and Kosten TR (1998). A preliminary investigation of lamotrigine for cocaine abuse in HIV-seropositive patients. *Am J Drug Alcohol Abuse* 24(1):85–101.

Marketscan (1999–2000). http://www.medstatmarketscan.com/. Ann Arbor, MI: Thomson Medstat.

Markowitz JC, Kocsis JH, Fishman B, Spielman LA, Jacobsberg LB, Frances AJ, Klerman GL, and Perry SW (1998). Treatment of depressive symptoms in human immunodeficiency virus–positive patients. *Arch Gen Psychiatry* 55(5):452–457.

Mattick RP, Ali R, White JM, O'Brien S, Wolk S, and Danz C (2003). Buprenorphine versus methadone maintenance therapy: a randomized double-blind trial with 405 opioid-dependent patients. *Addiction* 98(4): 441–452.

Merry C, Mulcahy F, Barry M, Gibbons S, and Back D (1997). Saquinavir interaction with midazolam: pharmacokinetic considerations when prescribing protease inhibitors for patients with HIV disease. *AIDS* 11(2):268–269.

Meyer JM, Marsh J, and Simpson G (1998). Differential sensitivities to risperidone and olanzapine in a human immunodeficiency virus patient. *Biol Psychiatry* 44(8):791–794.

Moog C, Kuntz-Simon G, Caussin-Schwemling C, and Obert G (1996). Sodium valproate, an anticonvulsant drug, stimulates human immunodeficiency virus type 1 replication independently of glutathione levels. *J Gen Virol* 77(Pt. 9):1993–1999.

Mouly S, Lown KS, Kornhauser D, Joseph JL, Fiske WD, Benedek IH, and Watkins PB (2002). Hepatic but not intestinal CYP3A4 displays dose-dependent induction by efavirenz in humans. *Clin Pharmacol Ther* 72(1):1–9.

Moyle G (2000). Clinical manifestations and management of antiretroviral nucleoside analog-related mitochondrial toxicity. *Clin Ther* 22(8):911–936; discussion 898.

Nath A, Jankovic J, and Pettigrew LC (1987). Movement disorders and AIDS. *Neurology* 37(1):37–41.

Ouellet D, Hsu A, Qian J, Locke CS, Eason CJ, Cavanaugh JH, Leonard JM, and Granneman GR (1998). Effect of ritonavir on the pharmacokinetics of ethinyl oestradiol in healthy female volunteers. *Br J Clin Pharmacol* 46(2):111–116.

Parenti DM, Simon GL, Scheib RG, Meyer WA 3rd, Sztein MB, Paxton H, DiGiola RA, and Schulof RS (1988). Effect of lithium carbonate in HIV-infected patients with immune dysfunction. *J Acquir Immune Defic Syndr* 1(2):119–124.

Park-Wyllie LY, and Antoniou T (2003). Concurrent use of bupropion with CYP2B6 inhibitors, nelfinavir, ritonavir and efavirenz: a case series. *AIDS* 17(4): 638–640.

Penzak SR, Hon YY, Lawhorn WD, Shirley KL, Spratlin V, and Jann MW (2002). Influence of ritonavir on olanzapine pharmacokinetics in healthy volunteers. *J Clin Psychopharmacol* 22(4):366–370.

Pisani F (1992). Influence of co-medication on the metabolism of valproate. *Pharm Weekbl Sci* 14(3A): 108–113.

Piscitelli SC, Kress DR, Bertz RJ, Pau A, and Davey R (2000). The effect of ritonavir on the pharmacokinetics of meperidine and normeperidine. *Pharmacotherapy* 20(5):549–553.

Rabkin JG, and Harrison WM (1990). Effect of imipramine on depression and immune status in a sample of men with HIV infection. *Am J Psychiatry* 147(4):495–497.

Rabkin JG, Rabkin R, Harrison W, and Wagner G (1994a). Effect of imipramine on mood and enumerative measures of immune status in depressed patients with HIV illness. *Am J Psychiatry* 151(4):516–523.

Rabkin JG, Rabkin R, and Wagner G (1994b). Effects of fluoxetine on mood and immune status in depressed patients with HIV illness. *J Clin Psychiatry* 55(3):92–97.

Rabkin JG, Wagner G, and Rabkin R (1994c). Effects of sertraline on mood and immune status in patients with major depression and HIV illness: an open trial. *J Clin Psychiatry* 55(10):433–439.

Rabkin JG, Wagner GJ, and Rabkin R (1999). Fluoxetine treatment for depression in patients with HIV and AIDS: a randomized, placebo-controlled trial. *Am J Psychiatry* 156(1):101–107.

Rabkin JG, McElhiney MC, Rabkin R, and Ferrando SJ (2004). Modafinil treatment for fatigue in HIV+ patients: a pilot study. *J Clin Psychiatry* 65(12): 1688–1695.

Rahman MA, and Gregory R (1995). Trichotillomania associated with HIV infection and response to sertraline. *Psychosomatics* 36(4):417–418.

Ramachandran G, Glickman L, Levenson J, and Rao C (1997). Incidence of extrapyramidal syndromes in AIDS patients and a comparison group of medically ill patients. *J Neuropsychiatry Clin Neurosci* 9(4):579–583.

Razali SM, and Hasanah CI (1999). Cost-effectiveness of cyclic antidepressants in a developing country. *Aust N Z J Psychiatry* 33(2):283–284.

Roche Pharmaceuticals (2003/2004). Fortovase/invirase prescribing information.

Romanelli F, and Pomeroy C (2003). Concurrent use of antiretrovirals and anticonvulsants in human immunodeficiency virus (HIV) seropositive patients. *Curr Pharm Des* 9(18):1433–1439.

Sandson NB, Armstrong SC, and Cozza KL (2005). An overview of psychotropic drug–drug interactions. *Psychosomatics* 46:464–494.

Satel SL, and Nelson JC (1989). Stimulants in the treatment of depression: a critical overview. *J Clin Psychiatry* 50(7):241–249.

Sewell DD, Jeste DV, McAdams LA, Bailey A, Harris MJ, Atkinson JH, Chandler JL, McCutchan JA, and Grant I (1994). Neuroleptic treatment of HIV-associated psychosis. HNRC group. *Neuropsychopharmacology* 10(4):223–229.

Simpson DM, Olney R, McArthur JC, Khan A, Godbold J, and Ebel-Frommer K (2000). A placebo-controlled trial of lamotrigine for painful HIV-associated neuropathy. *Neurology* 54(11): 2115–2119.

Simpson DM, McArthur JC, Olney R, Clifford D, So Y, Ross D, Baird BJ, Barrett P, and Hammer AE (2003). Lamotrigine for HIV-associated painful sensory neuropathies: a placebo-controlled trial. *Neurology* 60(9):1508–1514.

Singh AN, Golledge H, and Catalan J (1997). Treatment of HIV-related psychotic disorders with risperidone: a series of 21 cases. *J Psychosom Res* 42(5):489–493.

Smith PF, DiCenzo R, and Morse GD (2001). Clinical pharmacokinetics of non-nucleoside reverse transcriptase inhibitors. *Clin Pharmacokinet* 40(12): 893–905.

Stark K, Muller R, Bienzle U, and Guggenmoos-Holzmann I (1996). Methadone maintenance treatment and HIV risk-taking behaviour among injecting drug users in Berlin. *J Epidemiol Community Health* 50(5):534–537.

Stein G, and Bernadt M (1993). Lithium augmentation therapy in tricyclic-resistant depression. A controlled trial using lithium in low and normal doses. *Br J Psychiatry* 162:634–640.

Treisman GJ, Angelino AF, and Hutton HE (2001). Psychiatric issues in the management of patients with HIV infection. *JAMA* 286(22):2857–2864.

Uldall KK, and Berghuis JP (1997). Delirium in AIDS patients: recognition and medication factors. *AIDS Patient Care STDS* 11(6):435–441.

Vila A, Mykeitiuk A, Bonvehi P, Temporiti E, Uruena A, and Herrera F (2001). *Scand J Infect Dis* 33(10): 788–789.

Vocci FJ, Acri J, and Elkashef A (2005). Medication development for addictive disorders: the state of the science. *Am J Psychiatry* 162(8):1432–1440.

von Moltke LL, Greenblatt DJ, Granda BW, Giancarlo GM, Duan SX, Daily JP, Hamatz JS, and Shader RI (2001). Inhibition of human cytochrome p450 isoforms by nonnucleoside reverse transcriptase inhibitors. *J Clin Pharmacol* 41(1):85–91.

Wagner GJ, and Rabkin R (2000). Effects of dextroamphetamine on depression and fatigue in men with HIV: a double-blind, placebo-controlled trial. *J Clin Psychiatry* 61(6):436–440.

Wagner GJ, Rabkin JG, and Rabkin R (1997). Dextroamphetamine as a treatment for depression and low energy in AIDS patients: a pilot study. *J Psychosom Res* 42(4):407–411.

White JC, Christensen JF, and Singer CM (1992). Methylphenidate as a treatment for depression in acquired immunodeficiency syndrome: an n-of-1 trial. *J Clin Psychiatry* 53(5):153–156.

Wood E, Hogg RS, Kerr T, Palepu A, Zhang R, and Montaner JS (2005). Impact of accessing methadone on the time to initiating HIV treatment among antiretroviral-naive HIV-infected injection drug users. *AIDS* 19(8):837–839.

Yun LW, Maravi M, Kobayashi JS, Barton PL, and Davidson AJ (2005). Antidepressant treatment improves adherence to antiretroviral therapy among depressed HIV-infected patients. *J Acquir Immune Defic Syndr* 38(4):432–438.

Zhang X, Lalezari JP, Badley AD, Dorr A, Kolis SJ, Kinchelow T, and Patel IH. (2004). Assessment of drug–drug interaction potential of enfuvirtide in human immunodeficiency virus type 1–infected patients. *Clin Pharmacol Ther* 75(6):558–568.

Zilikis N, Nimatoudis I, Kiosses V, and Ierodiakonou C (1998). Treatment with risperidone of an acute psychotic episode in a patient with AIDS. *Gen Hosp Psychiatry* 20(6):384–385.

Zisook S, Peterkin J, Goggin KJ, Sledge P, Atkinson JH, and Grant I (1998). Treatment of major depression in HIV-seropositive men. HIV Neurobehavioral Research Center Group. *J Clin Psychiatry* 59(5): 217–224.

Part IX

AIDS Psychiatry and Comorbid Medical Conditions

Chapter 33

Hepatitis C and HIV Coinfection

Silvia Hafliger

Chronic monoinfection with hepatitis C virus (HCV) is currently a major pandemic that leads to great suffering among patients and families. It is a major cause for decreased quality of life, as well as increased mortality due to end-stage liver disease and hepatocellular carcinoma. In 1999, the World Health Organization (WHO) reported that four million Americans had been exposed to the virus and 170 million people were infected worldwide. Two million seven-hundred thousand Americans have progressed to chronic infection and over 200,000 Americans live with cirrhosis; this number is expected to increase to 375,000 by 2015. Worldwide, 7.8 million people have cirrhosis due to HCV and 13.8 million will suffer from cirrhosis by 2015 (Everson, 2005).

Chronic HCV coinfection is prevalent and HCV-related liver disease is a leading cause of death among persons with HIV and AIDS (Salmon-Ceron et al., 2005; Weber et al., 2006). Thirty percent of persons with HIV are coinfected with hepatitis C. In coinfected individuals, the rate of progression to cirrhosis

is accelerated. Normal progression to end-stage liver disease takes 20–30 years, but in coinfected patients this time frame is reduced to 6–10 years. Hepatocellular carcinoma, a feared complication of HCV infection, occurs at an earlier age: 42 years versus 62 years in monoinfected patients, and within 18 years of infection versus 28 years in the monoinfected cohort (Chun and Sherman, 2005).

Hepatitis C infection is highly relevant to psychiatry; it is a neurotrophic virus causing alterations in subcortical brain structures. One-third of patients with HCV score in the impaired range on more than two of neuropsychological measures without evidence of clinical liver disease and prior to treatment with interferon/ribavirin (Hilsabeck et al., 2005). Coinfected patients are facing a triple neuropsychiatric burden: there are viral alterations in subcortical brain areas, in addition to damage caused by hyperammonemia and basilar manganese deposition due to persistent hepatic encephalopathy.

As with HIV, HCV is primarily a psychiatric and behavioral epidemic. Close to 80% of intravenous drug users are infected with HCV. The psychiatric comorbidity is high, with 30% of infected patients meeting criteria for depression and dysthymia, 18% to 26% for anxiety disorders including posttraumatic stress disorder (PTSD), and 6% for bipolar illness (Hilsabeck et al., 2005).

Psychiatric support is essential for patients undergoing treatment with interferon and ribavirin. Neuropsychiatric complications can be as high as 50%. Abstinence from alcohol, illicit drugs, and nicotine can slow the progression to cirrhosis and decrease the need for liver transplant. In the United States, the main cause of end-stage liver disease resulting in a need for liver transplant is HCV-related cirrhosis. Liver transplant is not a cure for hepatitis C since HCV infection post-transplant is universal, with up to 20% of patients 5 years post-transplant developing recurrent cirrhosis. Patients suffering with liver disease are frequently disenfranchised. Being stigmatized, they struggle with issues of poverty, lack of insurance, shame, and guilt. Because non-response to interferon treatment can affect up to 50% of patients, a sense of hopelessness and despair is common among persons with HCV.

VIRAL CHARACTERISTICS

Hepatitis C is a single-stranded RNA virus belonging to the *Flaviridiae* family. It does not integrate into the human genome. An outer protein envelope surrounds a nucleocapsid core protein and RNA genome of 9000 nucleotide base pairs, encoding a 3000 amino acid polyprotein. After translation, the polypeptide is cleaved by at least two viral proteases into structural (envelope and core protein) and nonstructural proteins (RNA polymerase and helicase).

It is one of the most antigenetically diverse viruses; there are six genotypes recognized and up to 50 subtypes. Genotype 1 is most common in the United States and the most treatment resistant. Genotypes 2 and 3 are more responsive to interferon treatment, with an expectant 80% cure rate compared to 40% for genotype 1.

Coinfected patients have a lower response rate to treatment with interferon; only 20%–35% are able to attain a negative viral load after 6 months of completing treatment. Nucleotide sequence change following infection leads to the development of quasispecies,

which can evade the immune system. There is currently no vaccine available.

The virus was discovered in 1989. Commercial testing became available in 1991. Prior to 1989, infection with HCV was known as non-A non-B hepatitis (Crone and Gabriel, 2003).

PREVALENCE AND MODE OF TRANSMISSION

Hepatitis C is a blood-borne virus with predominant parenteral transmission (Koziel and Peters, 2007). The prevalence in the general population is about 2%. Intravenous drug use accounts for the majority of infection, with close to 80% of injection drug users testing positive for the hepatitis C antibody. Five percent of infections occur from nosocomial exposure such as sharing of toothbrushes, razors, body piercing, and tattoos. Ten percent of patients receiving transfusion prior to 1991 were infected with HCV. Patients on hemodialysis have a rate of infection of approximately 9% secondary to nosocomial spread (Fabrizi et al., 2002). In the United States, coinfection with HIV and HCV is most prevalent among persons with hemophilia or injection drug use with rates of coinfection of 70% to 95% (Alter, 2006).

Mother–infant transmission is less than 8% in monoinfected patients but up to 15% in coinfected mothers. Sexual transmission is usually less than 5% but increases with sexual promiscuity (20 or more lifetime sexual partners). The prevalence of HCV among alcohol-dependent patients is reported to be close to 10%. African Americans have higher prevalence: 3.2% versus Caucasians or Hispanics. The viral load is usually higher and the response to treatment is lower (Pyrsopoulos and Lennox, 2005).

Up to 30% of HIV-positive patients are HCV positive, which accounts for 250,000–300,000 coinfected individuals in the United States.

DIAGNOSIS

It is imperative for physicians to have a high index of suspicion of HCV infection. All HIV-positive patients need to be tested for HCV, as well as all patients with a history of substance abuse whether past or current.

Enzyme immune assay testing for the antibody to core protein 100/22c is usually reactive 4–10 weeks after exposure. False-positive reactions are seen in autoimmune hepatitis and false-negative reactions in immunosuppressed or dialysis patients. If a patient tests positive, the follow-up consists of quantitative polymerase chain reaction (PCR) for viral load as well as genotyping. The results are usually in the range of several hundred thousand to millions. Coinfected patients have higher serum RNA levels.

Liver function tests are not reliable. Thirty percent of patients are asymptomatic and have normal liver function tests (LFT); 50% are asymptomatic with minimal LFT elevations two to four times the upper limit of normal. ALT is a more sensitive indicator of hepatocellular injury. Only 20% of patients are symptomatic with malaise, right upper quadrant tenderness, and elevated liver enzymes. Fluctuations in viral load and liver enzymes are common. Hepatitis C causes immune-mediated hepatic cellular destruction and progressive scarring in 20% of infected patients. A liver biopsy is the gold standard to predict progression to fibrosis.

Grade reflects inflammatory changes and is rated 0–4. Stage describes the level of fibrosis, 0–4. It usually takes 12 years to progress from stages 1 to 3, and 18 months from stages 3 to 4. Since coinfected patients progress at a much faster rate, it is prudent to add one level to the reported biopsy results. Treatment is indicated if there is evidence of fibrosis, high inflammatory activity, or high viral load (Jacobson, 2001; Koziel and Peters, 2007).

DISEASE PROGRESSION

In contrast to acute hepatitis B, where 95% of immunocompetent patients are able to clear the virus, 80% of HCV-infected patients become chronic carriers, and 20% of these chronically infected patients progress to cirrhosis. Older age at the time of infection, male gender, immunosuppression, coinfection with hepatitis B, HIV, or schistosomiasis, nonalcoholic steatohepatitis (fatty liver disease/diabetes), and alcohol intake are associated with faster progression to cirrhosis.

The natural history of HCV spans decades and is usually silent. There are no classic symptoms such as chest pain or shortness of breath as in cardiovascular disease. Eighty percent of liver parenchyma is replaced by scar tissue before symptoms appear.

Three mechanisms have been proposed to explain HCV-mediated liver damage: direct cytotoxicity,

immune-mediated hepatocyte destruction, or viral-induced autoimmunity. There is growing evidence for sensitized T cell–mediated destruction of hepatocytes.

Catastrophic bleeding from esophageal varices, sudden onset of ascites, spontaneous bacterial peritonitis, and hepatic encephalopathy or coincidental diagnosis of hepatocellular cancer may be among the first symptoms of decompensated liver disease. Extrahepatic manifestations of HCV disease can present as mixed cryogloulinemia, a systemic vasculitis involving vital organs, kidney, skin, and the central nervous system (CNS). The vasculitis is caused by immune complex deposition on endothelium of small and medium-sized blood vessels. Membranoproliferative glomerulonephritis leads to chronic renal failure and dialysis in some HCV-infected patients. Skin involvement consists of porphyria cutanea tarda. Type 2 diabetes has a higher prevalence in HCV patients as well as thyroid abnormalities, both hypo- and hyperthyroidism.

Patients with cirrhosis have a 5% yearly risk of developing hepatocellular carcinoma. If the cancer is confined to the liver and is less than 5 cm in size, these patients can be treated with transplant. Chemoembolization or radiofrequency ablations are measures to contain the cancer but are not curative.

Like HIV, HCV is a neurotrophic virus. It enters the CNS via infected monocytes akin to the "Trojan horse mechanism." The CNS is a site of active replication, which is postulated to occur in microglial cells (Laskus et al., 2002). The cerebral choline-to-creatine ratio is elevated in basal ganglia and white matter, suggestive of minor cell damage. Alterations in neuroendocrine, neurotransmitters, inflammatory cytokines, or immune response to viral protein within the CNS are believed to cause the frontal- subcortical dysfunction (Forton et al., 2003). Coinfection leads to a greater neuropsychiatric burden.

TREATMENT

Psychiatrists can play a major role in helping patients make treatment decisions, assisting them through the year-long treatment of chemotherapy with interferon alpha and ribavirin. The goal is collaboration with medical colleagues to ensure that patients take 80% of the interferon/ribavirin dose 80% of the time.

Three potential virologic responses to therapy are described. *Non-responders* have no reduction in viral load after initiation of therapy. *Relapsers* have an initial response to therapy with a decrease in viral load but then an increase in viral load occurs within 6 months or more of ending treatment. *Sustained viral responders* (SVRs) have a long-term response to therapy and a nondetectable viral load 6 months or more after terminating treatment.

Weekly injection of pegylated interferon alpha in combination with daily oral ribavirin is the current standard of care, but new treatments with protease inhibitors are now in phase 3 studies.

Cells of the immune system, in response to viral infections, normally produce interferon. Injection of high doses of interferon is essentially an augmentation of the immune response. Interferon is believed to have antiviral, antiproliferative, and immunoregulatory properties. Seventy percent of interferon is hepatically metabolized. It can inhibit cytochrome P450 1A2.

Ribavirin is a nucleoside analogue; it inhibits RNA polymerase and depletes intracellular GTP. Ribavirin does not have antiviral properties when taken alone and only works synergistically with interferon. It is metabolized both hepatically and renally, and has a long half-life of over 200 hours. It is teratogenic, thus birth control is essential.

Significant drug toxicity can occur when zidovudine and ribavirin are administered in combination. Together, zidovudine and ribavirin can cause pancreatitis and lactic acidosis. Stavudine-induced lactic acidosis has been noted in treatment with interferon and ribavirin.

All coinfected patients should be considered candidates for treatment with interferon/ribavirin, because of the rapid progression to cirrhosis and higher risk of liver toxicity after starting antiretroviral therapy. Response to interferon depends on CD4 count and treatment should be initiated with a CD4 count of 350. If CD4 count is less than 200, treatment risks outweigh benefits. Evidence of hepatic decompensation, history of active alcohol or drug use, current psychiatric illness, or history of neuropsychiatric complications are relative contraindications (Soriano et al., 2004; Wagner and Ryan, 2005).

Side effects seen early in treatment are flu-like symptoms—myalgia, chills, fever, headache, loss of appetite, nausea, and diarrhea. As treatment progresses, bone marrow suppression with anemia, neutropenia, and thrombocytopenia can occur. Hematological complications are a frequent reason for dose reduction or additional supportive treatment with erythropoietin (Epogen). Ribavirin is associated with hemolytic anemia. Thyroid dysfunction (hypo- and hyperthyroidism) and hair loss have been noted. Weakness, fatigue, anorexia, and weight loss can be overwhelming. The impact of hair loss and weight loss can be especially disturbing to individuals with HIV who feel that they can no longer hide their illness and fear the consequences of HIV stigma.

NEUROPSYCHIATRIC SIDE EFFECTS OF TREATMENT

At least 20%–40% of patients without any psychiatric history or reported symptoms at the beginning of interferon therapy develop neuropsychiatric side effects, usually after 4–6 weeks of treatment. Mood disturbance, irritability, tearfulness, rage, and anhedonia are predominant symptoms. Insomnia, increased anxiety, decreased frustration tolerance, and mania/hypomania have been noted as well. Suicidal ideation and suicide attempts have been reported but are rare (Onyike et al., 2004). Psychosis (auditory hallucinations and paranoid delusions) in the absence of delirium has been noted in coinfected patients (Hoffman et al., 2003). Cognitive dysfunction, mainly impaired short-term memory, generalized slowing, decreased attention span, and reduced executive skills, occurs the longer the treatment progresses.

Fatigue is a universal complaint in about 90% of interferon-treated patients. A history of traumatic brain injury or neurological illness decreases brain reserve and makes patients more vulnerable to interferon- and ribavirin-induced side effects.

Patients who are currently symptomatic with a mood or anxiety disorder need to be stabilized first. A history of severe depression or previous neuropsychiatric side effects to interferon may point to vulnerability for developing interferon-induced mood and cognitive disorder. In this group of patients, prophylactic treatment with a selective serotonin reuptake inhibitor (SSRI) may be indicated. Coinfected patients are at greater risk to develop neuropsychiatric side effects during treatment with interferon/ribavirin.

Diagnosis and treatment of interferon-induced mood disorder is critical HCV treatment (Trask et al., 2001; Loftus and Hauser, 2003; Ondria, 1999; Raison et al., 2005). Fatigue and depression are prevalent and are major factors in discontinuation of interferon treatment (Trask et al., 2001).

Sustained viral response is lower in patients with alcohol consumption. Every effort should be undertaken to keep patients abstinent from alcohol and illicit drug use (Zhang et al., 2003; Hafliger, 2005b).

Neuropathophysiology of Interferon-Induced Mood Disorder

Interferon causes a dysregulation in the neuroendocrine, neurotransmitter, and cytokine pathways. Interferon stimulates interleukin-1 (IL-1) release, which is responsible for fever, sleep disturbance, and neuroendocrine dysfunction. IL-2 causes an increase in corticotrophin releasing hormone (CRH) and hyperactivity in the hypothalamic–pituitary–adrenal (HPA) axis, as does IL-6. Tumor necrosis factor alpha stimulates fever, as well as CRH (Trask et al., 2001).

Serotonin dysregulation seems to underlie the observed mood changes—mainly irritability, tearfulness, and anger. Interferon induces tryptophan dioxygenase and indolamine dioxygenase enzymes, catalyzing the destruction of tryptophan, thereby lowering serotonin levels. Opioid and dopamine dysregulation may be responsible for the cognitive changes, mental slowing, and decreased attention and memory loss (Lerner et al., 1999; Dieperink, 2000).

Treatment of Cytokine-Induced Mood and Cognitive Disorder

Mood and anxiety symptoms respond well to treatment with serotonergic antidepressants (Gleason et al., 2002). All serotonergic antidepressants are equally effective. Musselman and colleagues (2001) conducted a pivotal study showing that prophylactic treatment with paroxetine (Paxil) in melanoma patients, who were receiving high doses of intravenous interferon, decreased the rate of depression to 11% in the paroxetine-treated group, versus 45% in the placebo group.

Prophylactic treatment with an SSRI may be indicated if a patient reports prior severe episodes of mood disorder or interferon-induced depression. Unlike the treatment response time for major depressive disorder, where the average response to an antidepressant may take up to 4–6 weeks, interferon-induced mood disorder responds quickly. Improvement in symptoms is seen as early as 2 weeks. As treatment with interferon progresses, the dose of antidepressant generally needs to be increased. Upon completion of interferon therapy, antidepressants should be continued for approximately 3 more months and then slowly tapered. It can take up to 6 months for the effects of interferon and ribavirin to clear. Patients need to be supported and reminded of this, as they are generally eager to feel "normal" again.

If symptoms do not improve, physicians should have a high index of suspicion of bipolar disorder, as interferon and antidepressants are known to induce a switch into mania. Should mania/hypomania develop, treatment with valproic acid (Depakote), or atypical antipsychotics such a quetiapine (Seroquel) or olanzapine (Zyprexa), is indicated. The dose of interferon may have to be lowered until mood symptoms are stabilized (Crone et al., 2004). Treatment with atypical antipsychotics is also indicated in patients who develop interferon-induced psychosis (Hoffman et al., 2003).

Fatigue and cognitive dysfunction are the least amenable to treatment. Fatigue may be secondary to anemia and treatment with erythropoietin (Epogen) may be beneficial. Aerobic exercise of a minimum of 20 minutes a day may decrease fatigue. Modafinil (Provigil) has been shown to decrease fatigue in coinfected patients undergoing HCV treatment.

Cognitive dysfunction, which may be secondary to prefrontal cortical hypometabolism, may respond to low-dose methylphenidate (Schwartz et al., 2002). Patients who clear the virus may nevertheless have ongoing mood and cognitive dysfunction. Fatigue and chronic neuromuscular pain syndromes have been noted. Some investigators speculate that interferon-induced immune system abnormalities persist, as some patients are unable to "switch off" the CRH/HPA dysregulation.

Alternative therapies include milk thistle (*Silybum marianum*) at 200–400 mg doses. Milk thistle decreases inflammatory changes in the liver, but does not reduce the viral load. S-adensosylmethionine (SAMe), with both antioxidant and mood-elevating properties, may be a safe alternative for patients reluctant to use an antidepressant.

SUBSTANCE ABUSE AND HEPATITIS C/HIV

Alcohol consumption in HCV-positive patients increases viremia and progression to fibrosis and cancer. Every effort must be made to assist patients with abstinence. Alcohol compromises effect of interferon, as the SVR is only 20% in patients consuming more than 70 g of alcohol a day, compared to 54% SVR in nondrinkers.

Interferon and ribavirin can be used in patients maintained on methadone. The methadone dose generally needs to be increased as treatment progresses because of increased neuromuscular pain secondary to interferon. Active use of heroin or cocaine leads to poor treatment adherence, a higher discontinuation rate, and a much lower SVR than that of abstinent patients. THC use has helped some patients tolerate interferon-induced nausea, anorexia, and pain (Fireman, 2003; Sylvestre, 2003).

HEPATIC ENCEPHALOPATHY

Hepatic encephalopathy (HE) is the most common neuropsychiatric condition seen in patients with liver disease or portosystemic shunting. It causes enormous suffering to patients and families, with dysfunction at work, in driving, or in carrying out simple activities of daily living.

Hepatic encephalopathy is classified as type A, associated with acute liver failure; type B, seen in portal-systemic bypass; and type C, associated with cirrhosis.

Type C is further classified as episodic, persistent, or minimal HE. Most patients with hepatitis C fall into type C classification. The spectrum of HE can be as subtle as minor personality changes to frank delirium or coma.

Stage I of HE generally presents with personality changes, irritability, and mental rigidity. Patients report mental slowing or "brain fog;" there is perseveration and decreased short-term memory. Alteration in sleep–wake cycle, with fatigue and sleepiness during the day and inability to sleep at night, is an early and sensitive indicator. Patients may present with treatment-resistant depression, anhedonia. Insight and judgment are impaired. Motor abnormalities include clumsiness, tremor, decreased fine motor control, and asterixis.

In stage II of HE there is worsening of lethargy, disorientation to time, inappropriate behavior, asterixis, and abnormal reflexes.

Stage III of HE is characterized by deepening of lethargy. Patients are difficult to arouse and have marked confusion, incomprehensible speech, disorientation to time and place, and abnormal reflexes.

In stage IV HE patients are in a coma and have a positive Babinski reflex and decerebrate posture.

Precipitating Factors

The most common factors are gastrointestinal bleeding, uremia, dehydration, and infection (cellulitis, spontaneous bacterial peritonitis [SBP]). Use of psychoactive medication such as zolpidem, opioids, and benzodiazepines can likewise precipitate HE. Hypoxemia, hyperkalemia, constipation, and dietary indiscretion (high protein intake) are other factors that can worsen HE.

Pathophysiology

Although the exact pathophysiology of HE has not been fully elucidated, ammonia seems to take a central role. Ammonia, a nitrogenous product generated by colonic bacteria, is converted in the liver to urea and glutamine, which are subsequently eliminated via the kidneys. In liver cirrhosis this detoxification is impaired, resulting in hyperammonemia. Muscle and brain take up ammonia and convert it to glutamine.

Astrocytes play a major role in maintaining and regulating the ionic content of the CNS microenvironment and neurotransmission, as well as maintaining integrity of the blood–brain barrier. Astrocytes are responsible for regulating ammonia homeostasis in the brain. The astrocytic enzyme, glutamine synthetase, utilizes ammonia to convert glutamate to glutamine. Excess intracellular glutamine leads to astrocytes swelling (Alzheimer type II astrocytes), causing impairment in diverse neurotransmitter systems, especially glutaminergic and GABAergic neurotransmission. Glutamate released by presynaptic neurons is taken up by astrocytes. However, swollen astrocytes have decreased uptake ability, causing excess postsynaptic NMDA receptor activation by glutamate, stimulating production of nitric oxide, and accelerating neuronal cell death. Ammonia alters gene expression of peripheral benzodiazepine receptors, glutamine and glutamate transporters, and MAO-A. It alters the blood–brain barrier, reduces metabolic rates of glucose and oxygen, and generates reactive oxygen species. Serotonin homeostasis is impaired in HE, leading to alteration in circadian rhythm, temperature regulation, motor function, and personality changes.

Manganese levels are elevated in cirrhotic patients because of decreased hepatobiliary excretion. Manganese accumulates in the basal ganglia, altering dopamine neurotransmission. Patients with end-stage liver disease resemble Parkinson patients in their increased manifestation of extrapyramidal symptoms, tremor, shuffling gait, masked faces, and increased sensitivity to neuroleptic medication with potent dopamine D2 receptor antagonism. Manganese accumulation is the cause of hyperintensities seen on T1-weighted MRI in cirrhotic patients. The degree of hyperintensity does not correlate with the severity of HE.

Diagnosis

A careful mental status and neurological exam is key in establishing a diagnosis of HE. A family member may be the best source to obtain the patient's history. Subtle personality changes, alteration in sleep–wake patterns, mental slowing, and inattention are early signs, frequently missed by examiners and often not recognized by patients.

Asterixis or "liver flap" is elicited by asking the patient to extend upper extremities, open fingers, and retroflex the wrists. Patients with metabolic encephalopathy are unable to maintain this position. Asterixis can also be spontaneous in severe HE.

Evaluation of handwriting is another simple diagnostic test that can be performed even by family members. Patients lose fine motor skills, handwriting becomes illegible, and use of space is impaired. Extrapyramidal symptoms, such as tremor, rigidity, and ataxia, may be seen.

Ammonia levels are not helpful and frequently are abnormally high, due to venous blood sampling and lack of cold environment, thereby causing in situ generation of ammonia. Ammonia levels are of clinical use only in acute liver failure, where levels of over 200 predict development of brain edema and cerebral herniation.

Neuropsychological tests of diagnostic help may include Trailmaking A and B, digit symbol, and block design tests. The EEG may be nonspecific and show general background slowing or there may be a characteristic evolution of theta stage (4- to 7-Hz waves) followed by triphasic stage and subsequent delta stage, random, nonrhythmic slowing (Lockwood, 2001). Neuroimaging such as CT scan and MRI are useful to exclude other causes of mental status changes.

Treatment and Prevention of Hepatic Encephalopathy

Families and patients need to be educated about signs and symptoms of this often confusing and frightening presentation of delirium. Families need to intervene with activities such as driving. They need to assist the patient in managing finances and other activities of daily living. Families need to monitor medication compliance, especially intake of lactulose. Finally, families should be informed that the main goal of treatment is to reduce generation of ammonia by colonic bacteria.

Lactulose is a nonabsorbable disaccharide, which is used by bacteria as an energy source instead of protein or purine, thereby reducing ammonia production. It induces osmotic diarrhea. As a result, the patient should have two to three daily bowel movements.

Poorly absorbed antibiotics such as neomycin and metronidazole, may help by altering the bowel flora or decreasing ammonia-producing bacteria. Another approach involves improvement in hepatic elimination of ammonia, by providing zinc and L-carnitine supplementation. Zinc is a cofactor in the urea cycle. Dietary changes should include decreased intake in animal protein, increased use of plant protein, soy, and dairy or increased intake of branched-chain amino acids. In addition, avoidance of psychoactive medications, especially hypnotics such as Ambien, benzodiazepines, and opioids, is essential. Correction of dehydration and electrolyte imbalance, especially hypokalemia and hyponatremia, is essential. Treatment of infections, cellulitis, and spontaneous bacterial peritonitis and evaluation for gastrointestinal bleeding are equally important (Weissenborn, 2003; Blei, 2005; Stewart and Cerhan, 2005; Crone et al., 2006).

LIVER TRANSPLANT

Brief History of Organ Transplantation

The first successful kidney transplantation between monozygotic twin brothers occurred in 1954 at the Brigham Hospital in Boston. In 1959, the antimetabolite 6-mercaptopurine was introduced and found to have immunosuppressant actions. Azathioprine (Imuran), a derivative of 6-mercaptopurine, was first used by Calne in 1963 to prevent rejection of kidney grafts. In 1968 Dr. Thomas Starzl performed the first successful liver transplant. He is considered to be the pioneer of liver transplantation. During these early years, 1-year survival was 25%. In 2005, there were 5437 liver transplants with 80%–90% 1-year survival.

Cyclosporine, isolated from a soil fungus, showed immunosuppressive actions. It was first used in humans in 1978 and was approved by the U.S. Food and Drug Administration (FDA) in 1983. The introduction of cyclosporine ushered in a new area of solid organ transplantation as it took transplantation out of experimental medicine and made it an acceptable treatment modality for end-stage organ failure.

Infection with HIV was initially a contraindication for transplant. With the introduction of HAART, however, and consequent improved survival and decreased incidence of opportunistic infections, transplantation has become a treatment option for some HIV-infected patients. A multicenter National Institutes of Health study is currently in progress to evaluate prognosis, complications, and long-term survival in coinfected patients (Roland and Stock, 2006).

Organ Procurement

The United Network for Organ Sharing (UNOS), a private, nonprofit organization, is responsible for allocation of organs within the United States. Each year there are at least 20,000 potential deceased donors, but of these only 10%–20% are able to donate organs. Even if there is a signed donor card, families have the final veto power. Organs come from brain-dead patients. Non-heart-beating donors are patients taken off life support after families have given consent. Five to 10 minutes after the patient dies, the liver and kidney can be obtained. Living donation is a possibility for liver (60% of liver is donated in adult-to-adult donation), kidney, and lung.

Currently, there are over 18,000 people waiting for a new liver. A new name is added to the transplant list every 16 minutes and 11 people die waiting each day. The demand for organs greatly outnumbers the supply.

Organ Allocation

In order to provide fair access to organs, patients are now stratified according to their health status and probability of death. Introduced in 2002, The MELD system (Model of End Stage Liver Disease) uses a mathematical formula to predict death within 3 months. It replaced the Child-Turcotte-Pugh score and eliminated time on the wait list as a factor in obtaining an organ.

Total bilirubin, creatinine, and INR (coagulation time) are used to calculate the MELD score, a number between 6 and 40. A higher MELD score increases risk of dying without a liver transplant. There is no universal sharing of livers. Some geographic areas in the United States have few people on the wait list and more available organs; the Northeast, New York, Massachusetts, and California have the longest waiting lists. The greater waiting time and higher MELD score needed to receive a liver cause severe suffering, stress, and anxiety for families and patients. Patients in acute liver failure from acetaminophen (Tylenol) overdose, medication toxicity, or acute viral decompensation from hepatitis A/B are given priority over patients listed with cirrhosis. The mortality of coinfected patients is greater than that of monoinfected patients on the wait list.

Transplant Selection Process

Because of the scarcity of organs and to ensure long-term survival after transplant, a multidisciplinary transplant team carefully evaluates patients and his or her care team (family and friends). The transplant team includes a hepatologist, cardiologist, surgeon, transplant coordinator (nurse practitioner), social worker, financial coordinator, and/or psychiatrist or psychologist.

Patients are screened for cardiac and pulmonary disease, cancer, and end-organ manifestation of diabetes. They must demonstrate an understanding of their illness, understand the risk and benefits, show good compliance with current medical treatment, and have adequate social support, means of paying for food, rent, medications, and medical care. Patients must have comorbid illnesses under control, including diabetes, depression, and substance abuse. The HIV viral load should be undetectable and the CD4 count above 200, and there should be no drug resistance to HAART.

Patients and families must understand that transplantation is a treatment and not a cure—hepatitis C universally recurs. Immunosuppression brings risk of infection, increased skin and blood cancers (lymphoma), neurotoxicity, and peripheral neuropathy, thus patients have to agree to life-long compliance with immunosuppression, blood work, and medical care. Transplantation does not allow for mistakes, as failure to take immunosuppression leads to rejection of the organ and death. Patients must be committed to maintain healthy life-style changes such as weight control and abstinence from nicotine, alcohol, and illicit drugs. Although a transplant can restore a patient to full health, it does not magically improve life (Levenson and Olbrisch, 2000).

Assessment of Psychiatric Disorders

Alcohol dependence has a lifetime prevalence of 7% to 10%. Of persons with alcohol dependence, 10% to 15% will develop liver cirrhosis and only 6% will proceed to liver transplant. Twenty to 40% of all liver transplants are for alcoholic cirrhosis, the second most common indication after hepatitis C. Persons with alcohol-induced cirrhosis generally do as well as other transplant patients, with the same 1-year survival rate of 80% to 90%. Relapse to some drinking occurs in about 20% to 30% of patients post-transplant (DiMartini and Trzepacz, 2000; DiMartini et al., 2001).

Most transplant centers have a 6-month waiting period after cessation of drinking before accepting an alcohol-dependent patient and require documented alcohol rehabilitation in addition to AA attendance. Patients and families must understand that addiction is a brain disease, not "cured" by transplantation. Patients must have a plan in place to deal with cravings or potential relapses both before and after transplant (Beresford, 1994).

A cocaine abuse history should be of great concern to the treating physician. Cocaine abuse history places patients at higher risk for relapse than any other drug abuse before or after transplant. Ideally, patients with a cocaine abuse history should demonstrate a year of abstinence before being considered transplant candidates.

Patients in a methadone program who have demonstrated abstinence from heroin are accepted at most transplant centers. It is unethical to discontinue methadone, as this will lead to relapse in close to 80% of patients. As the liver disease progresses, the methadone dosage may need to be lowered to diminish worsening of hepatic encephalopathy (Koch and Banys, 2001).

Abstinence from nicotine is strongly encouraged, as patients post-transplant are at higher risk for cancers, including lung and oropharyngeal cancers. There is an increased risk of cardiovascular complications post-transplant due to immunosuppression-induced hypercholesteremia or triglyceremia and hypertension.

Marijuana use is not acceptable because of the high risk of pulmonary infection with aspergillus post-transplant and the risk of worsening of hepatic encephalopathy.

If patients are diagnosed with a psychiatric illness such as dysthymia, depression, bipolar illness, or schizophrenia, they are encouraged to obtain treatment in their community. Patients with personality disorders are especially challenging and can create chaos in a transplant team because of splitting and projective identification. Patients with borderline personality disorder have greater difficulty coping with the medical demands in the post-transplant period and have higher rates of noncompliance and graft failure (Shapiro et al., 1995).

The psychiatric interview focuses on a patient's history of compliance with medical care and life-style changes. The patient and family have to demonstrate an understanding about diagnosis, risks, and benefits of transplantation.

Social support both before and after transplant is crucial, as hepatic encephalopathy greatly diminishes a patient's ability to comply with the rigorous demands of the evaluation process and complicated post-transplant care. Lack of a supportive network of friends and family is a potential contraindication for transplant. However, there are no absolute psychiatric contraindication for transplantation other than active substance abuse and untreated psychosis. It is the responsibility of the psychosocial team "to build a ramp" so that each patient has a chance of success.

Post-Transplant Psychiatric Issues

Delirium is the most common encountered psychiatric condition in the early post-transplant period. Etiology of the delirium is multifactorial, i.e., steroids, infection, rejection, and toxic levels of immunosuppressant.

The treatment of choice is an atypical neuroleptic, such as olanzapine or quetiapine, as these patients are especially vulnerable to extrapyramidal symptoms, due to potent D2 antagonism of first-generation neuroleptics such as haloperidol (Hafliger, 2005a).

Living with Immunosuppression

Allograft rejection is an example of cell-mediated immunity involving T lymphocytes, macrophages, dendritic cells, antigen-presenting cells, and natural killer cells. All immunosuppressant medications modulate and interfere with T-cell activation, differentiation, receptor binding, or cytokine release (Vierling, 1999).

Most patients will be on at least two or three immunosuppressants for the rest of their lives. Higher doses are used in the early postoperative period. Depending on the graft function, medication tapering occurs within 6 months. All patients will initially be on steroids and two anti-rejection drugs. Steroids are tapered early because of the multi-organ side effects. At the same time, it is important to achieve a balance between rejection and risk of infection.

HIV-coinfected patients are particularly sensitive to toxicity of immunosuppression drugs. Drug levels of immunosuppression medication need to be carefully monitored to avoid over-immunosuppression, which will accelerate HCV progression. Inhibition of P450 3A4 enzymes by HAART, especially protease inhibitors, will dramatically increase levels of Prograf and cyclosporine.

Cyclosporine (Sandimmune, Neoral) Cyclosporine is a lipophilic cyclic polypeptide isolated from soil fungus *Tolycladium inflatum Gams*. It inhibits cellular immunity by prevention of expression of IL-2 and other cytokines by helper T lymphocytes, thus impairing proliferation. Its metabolism is hepatic and involves cytochrome P450 3A4. Toxic trough levels are above 300 ng/ml. Adverse drug reactions are common and include nephrotoxicity, hypertension (renal vasoconstriction), electrolyte abnormalities (hyperkalemia, hypoglycemia), gingival hyperplasia, hirsutism, nausea, and diarrhea. Neuropsychiatric side effects include tremor, especially of hands, restlessness, insomnia, anxiety, headaches, delirium, seizures, toxic leukoencephalopathy, and cortical blindness (Strouse et al., 1998; Filley and Kleinschmidt-DeMasters, 2001).

Drug interactions involve P450 3A4 cytochromes. Inhibitors of 3A4 of particular importance are erythromycin, cimetidine, ketoconazole, clarithromycin, paroxetine (weak), fluvoxamine (Luvox), and grapefruit juice. Inducers to be aware of are phenobarbital, phenytoin (Dilantin), modafinil, St. John's wort, rifampin, and carbamazepine(Tegretol).

Tacrolimus (Prograf) Tacrolimus is a fungal macrolide antibiotic. It also interferes with transcription of IL-2, thus preventing T-helper cell differentiation. It is more potent than cyclosporine and is hepatically metabolized by P450 3A4. Therapeutic levels range between 5 and 15 ng/ml. Drug–drug interactions involve the P450 3A4 cytochrome system. Adverse reactions are similar to those of cyclosporine, but neuropsychiatric complications are higher.

Mycophenolate Mofetil (Cellcept) Mycophenolate is a fermentation product of several *Penicillium* species.

The active drug, mycophenolic acid, noncompetitively and reversibly inhibits inosine monophosphate dehydrogenase, the rate-limiting enzyme for the de novo pathway of purine synthesis. T- and B-lymphocyte proliferation is impaired. It is a cousin of azathioprine (Imuran) with less myelotoxic effects. There currently is no drug level monitoring. Metabolism is via hepatic glucuronidation. Side effects are mostly gastrointestinal with diarrhea and nausea, leukopenia (2%), and sepsis. There is an increased risk of developing lymphoproliferative disease or other malignancies.

Sirolimus (Rapamycin) Rapamycin is one of the newest medications approved by the FDA to prevent organ rejection. It is similar to tacrolimus, as it is also a macrolide antibiotic, produced by *Streptomyces hygroscoicus*. Rapamycin inhibits transduction of cytokine IL-2, thus interfering with T- and B-cell proliferation at a later stage in the cell cycle. It is 100 times more potent than cyclosporine and is metabolized via cytochrome P450 3A4. Adverse effects include thrombocytopenia, hypercholesteremia, and poor wound healing. This drug is brain and renal sparing. There have not been any reports of neurotoxicity.

Prednisone Corticosteroids in combination with azathioprine provided the cornerstone of immunosuppression in the early 1960s and 1970s. Steroids are potent anti-inflammatory drugs that prevent the release of inflammatory mediators by macrophages, i.e., IL-1. Production of prostaglandins and leukotrienes is decreased and eosinophil and mast-cell migration is impaired. Steroids form complexes with cytosolic receptors and, after entering the nucleus, prevent transcription of IL-1, -2, -3, and -6 as well as of tumor necrosis factor alpha and interferon gamma. Nearly every cell expresses receptors for glucocorticoids, which accounts for the profound effect on multiple organs. Glucocorticoids bind to albumin and only a free steroid is able to bind with cytosolic receptors. Bioavailability is therefore increased during hypoalbuminemia and reduced during pregnancy. Systemic side effects of steroids include osteoporosis, avascular necrosis, cataracts, diabetes mellitus, cushingoid features, and weight gain due to appetite stimulation.

Neuropsychiatric effects are many, and symptoms are in the spectrum of mood disorders, including depression and mania, anxiety symptoms such as irritability or restlessness and insomnia, and delirium. Treatment of neuropsychiatric side effects includes atypical neuroleptics for delirium or mania, an SSRI or SNRI for depression, and clonazepam for anxiety and restlessness. Impaired cognition, with decreased short-term memory and concentration, has been observed as well. Cognitive side effects improve with lowering of the steroid dose. Steroid withdrawal presents with dysphoria and anxiety and resolves over time, frequently without treatment (Beresford, 2001; Wijdicks, 2001).

Advances in Transplantation

Because of the shortage of organs and increased mortality on the waiting list, adult-to-adult living donation became a treatment option in 1996. The right lobe is donated (60%), with 80% organ regeneration occurring within 6–8 weeks in the donor. Living liver donation carries a 10-fold greater morbidity than that of kidney donation. There is a 0.4% risk of mortality, with at least two reported donor deaths in the United States and one donor-liver transplant death. Worldwide, three to nine donors have died. Biliary tract (strictures and leaks) and wound infections are the most common complications in the donor, followed by prolonged incisional pain, body image changes, incisional hernias, and possible depression and posttraumatic stress symptoms. Donors face an enormously difficult task in balancing altruism with self-preservation. Recipients of living donation deal with feelings of guilt and indebtedness (Russell and Jacob, 1993; Trotter et al., 2002).

PRACTICAL PSYCHOPHARMACOLOGY FOR PATIENTS WITH LIVER DISEASE

Basic Liver Anatomy

The liver has a dual blood supply, in which nutrient-rich, venous blood draining the intestine enters the liver via the portal vein, and oxygenated blood enters via the hepatic artery. The basic structural unit is the liver lobule, which consists of hepatocytes arranged in a hexagonal pattern. Portal and arterial blood percolates from the portal triad to the central vein. The central veins coalesce to form hepatic veins, which exit the liver and empty into the inferior vena cava and heart. Phase I metabolism, or oxidation and hy-

droxylation, occurs mainly pericentrally. Phase II metabolism, or glucuronidation, takes place in the periportal region.

Pharmacokinetics

Most psychotropic drugs are weak bases and lipophilic, and are absorbed in the alkaline environment of the small intestine. When patients have gastroparesis, gastritis, or delayed emptying, due to anticholinergic drugs, there is decreased drug absorption. Most psychotropic drugs are absorbed by passive diffusion. With vascular congestion seen in portal hypertension or cytomegalovirus enteritis, there is decreased drug absorption.

First Pass or Presystemic Elimination

Cytochrome P450 3A4 enzymes are found in the small intestine and can be inhibited by grapefruit juice, cimetidine, erythromycin, and ketoconazole. Drugs metabolized by 3A4 will therefore be absorbed in higher concentrations. High-clearance drugs are rate limited by hepatic blood flow, as with tricyclic antidepressants (TCAs), haloperidol, meperidine, morphine, beta-blockers, and verapamil. If there is decreased hepatic perfusion as seen in portal systemic shunting or intrahepatic shunting, there will be increased bioavailability of high-clearance drugs. Low-clearance drugs are rate limited by enzyme saturation, as with benzodiazepines, digoxin, and acetaminophen (Tylenol). Cirrhosis leads to decreased enzyme concentration and therefore higher drug concentrations.

Volume of Distribution

Dehydration, loss of muscle mass, aging, means less volume of distribution and higher serum drug concentration. Obesity, ascites, edema leads to increase in volume of distribution, therefore decreased drug concentration.

Protein Binding

Most psychoactive drugs are protein bound except for lithium, gabapentin (Neurontin), and pregabalin. At the receptor site only the free unbound drug is active. Decreased plasma protein, i.e., low albumin as seen in malnutrition, cirrhosis, and older age, will lead to higher drug activity. This result is important to consider when prescribing TCAs, fluoxetine (Prozac), and valproic acid. Endogenous inhibitors of albumin binding are also often seen in renal disease, which will lead to higher drug concentration at receptor sites.

Metabolism

Phase I metabolism renders a compound more hydrophilic and polar via hydroxylation or oxidation. These reactions are carried out by the P450 cytochromes. Acute liver injury seen in alcoholic hepatitis or acute viral hepatitis damages the pericentral area and thus affects phase I reactions the most. Diazepam (Valium), chlordiazepoxide (Librium), and chlorpromazine (Thorazine) depend on phase I metabolism and should be avoided in the setting of acute liver injury. The pericentral area is more susceptible to acute damage because of decreased availability of oxygen and accumulation of free radicals from oxidation and hydroxylation reactions. Phase II reactions are conjugation reactions and occur in highest concentration in the periportal regions. Any process that leads to bile duct injury, e.g., primary biliary cirrhosis, will interfere with these processes, causing higher drug concentration. Glucuronidation reactions are preserved in acute and chronic liver damage (Trzepacz et al., 1993a, 1993b; Crone et al., 2006).

Most patients with liver disease are undermedicated because of fear of causing further liver damage. It is far more important to treat the underlying psychiatric illness, as untreated psychopathology leads to worsening of suffering and interferes with patient's ability to withstand the rigorous transplant process. HCV does far more damage to the liver than any psychiatric medication.

When treating a patient with cirrhosis, the physician should always "start low and go slow"(the maxim for geriatric patients), and follow the patient closely. Drugs with a short half-life and less protein binding are recommended. Selective serotonin inhibitors such as citalopram (Celexa), sertraline (Zoloft), or venlafaxine (Effexor) are preferable choices. When treating transplant candidates, the physician may not want to use 3A4 inhibitors, since all immunosuppressant drugs are metabolized by 3A4. Medication should be chosen on the basis of clinical presentation and side-effect profile. Benzodiazepines and opioids should be avoided because these medications can worsen hepatic encephalopathy. Atypical neuroleptics are preferred over typical neuroleptics, as there are less par-

kinsonian side effects. Mood stabilizers, such as valproic acid and lamotrigine, have been safely used in pre- and post-transplant patients with HCV.

CONCLUSION

Persons with HIV and hepatitis C have the burdens of two complex and severe medical illnesses, both with multiorgan and multisystem involvement, including profound psychiatric complications. An integrated team approach and the skills of a psychosomatic medicine psychiatrist can help alleviate suffering and promote adherence to care.

References

Alter MJ (2006). Epidemiology of viral hepatitis and HIV coinfection. *J Hepatol* 44:Suppl:S109–S113.

Beresford T (1994). Overt and covert alcoholism. In M Lucey, R Merion, and T Beresford (eds.), *Liver Transplantation: The Alcoholic Patient.* Cambridge, UK: Cambridge University Press.

Beresford T (2001). Neuropsychiatric complications of liver and other solid organ transplantation. *Liver Transplant* 7(11 Suppl. 1):S36–S45.

Blei TA (2005). Hepatic encephalopathy, clinical gastroenterology and hepatology. In WM Weinstein, C Hawkey, and J Bosch (eds.), *Clinical Gastroenterology and Hepatology* (pp. 735–743). Philadelphia: Mosby.

Crone CC, and Gabriel GM (2003). Comprehensive review of hepatitis C for psychiatrists: risks, screening, diagnosis, treatment, and interferon-based therapy complications. *J Psychiatr Pract* 9:93–100.

Crone CC, Gabriel GM, and Wise TN (2004). Managing the neuropsychiatric side effects of interferon-based therapy for hepatitis C. *Cleve Clin J Med* 71: S27–S32.

Crone CC, Gabriel GM, and DiMartini A (2006). An overview of psychiatric issues in liver disease for the consultation-liaison psychiatrist. *Psychosomatics* 47: 188–205.

Chun S, and Sherman KE (2005). Treatment of hepatitis C virus/HIV coinfection. *Clin Liver Dis* 9:525–534.

Dieperink E (2000). Neuropsychiatric symptoms associated with hepatitis C and interferon alpha: a review. *Am J Psychiatry* 157:867–875.

DiMartini A, Day N, Dew MA, Lane T, Fitzgerald MG, et al. (2001). Alcohol use following liver transplantation. *Psychosomatics* 42:55–62.

DiMartini A, and Trzepacz P (2000). Alcoholism and organ transplantation. In P Trzepacz and A DiMartini (eds.), *The Transplant Patient* (pp. 214–238). Cambridge, UK: Cambridge University Press.

Everson GT (2005). Treatment of hepatitis C in patients who have decompensated cirrhosis. *Clin Liver Dis* 9:473–486.

Fabrizi F, Poordad FF, and Martin P (2002). Hepatitis C infection and the patient with end-stage renal disease. *Hepatology* 36:3–10.

Filley CM, and Kleinschmidt-DeMasters BK (2001). Toxic leukoencephalopathy. *N Engl J Med* 345: 425–432.

Fireman M (2003). Hepatitis C treatment and substance use disorders. *Psychiatr Ann* 33:402–408.

Forton DM, Taylor-Robinson SD, and Thomas HC (2003). Cerebral dysfunction in chronic hepatitis C infection. *J Viral Hepatitis* 10:81–86.

Gleason OC, Yates WR, Isbell MD, and Philipsen MA (2002). Open-label trial of citalopram for major depression in patients with hepatitis C. *J Clin Psychiatry* 63:194–198.

Hafliger S (2005a). A primer on solid organ transplant psychiatry. In A Wyszynski and B Wyszynski (eds.), *Manual of Psychiatric Care for the Medically Ill* (pp. 205–219). Washington, DC: American Psychiatric Publishing.

Hafliger S (2005b). The patient with hepatitis C. In A Wyszynski and B Wyszynski (eds.) *Manual of Psychiatric Care for the Medically Ill* (pp. 201–204). Washington, DC: American Psychiatric Publishing.

Hilsabeck RC, Castellon SA, and Hinkin CH (2005). Neuropsychological aspects of coinfection with HIV and hepatitis C virus. *Clin Infect Dis* 41:S38–S44.

Hoffman RG, Cohen MA, Alfonso CA, Weiss JJ, Jones S, Keller M, et al. (2003). Treatment of interferon-induced psychosis in patients with comorbid hepatitis C and HIV. *Psychosomatics* 44:417–420.

Jacobson I (2001). Managing chronic hepatitis C infection. *Hosp Physician* 37:34–41.

Koziel MJ, and Peters MG (2007). Viral hepatitis in HIV infection. *N Engl J Med* 356:1445–1454.

Koch M, and Banys P (2001). Liver transplantation in opioid dependence. *JAMA* 285:1056–1058.

Laskus T, Radkowski M, Bednarska A, Wilkinson J, Adair D, Nowicki M, et al. (2002). Detection and analysis of hepatitis C virus sequences in cerebrospinal fluid. *J Virol* 76:10064–10068.

Lerner DM, Stoudemire A, and Rosenstein DL (1999). Neuropsychiatric toxicity associated with cytokine therapies. *Psychosomatics* 40:428–435.

Levenson J, and Olbrisch M (2000). Psychosocial screening and selection of candidates for organ transplantation. In P Trzepacz and A DiMartini (eds.), *The Transplant Patient* (pp. 21–41). Cambridge, UK: Cambridge University Press.

Lockwood AH (2001). Hepatic encephalopathy. In A Aminoff (ed.), *Neurology and General Medicine* (pp. 233–246). New York: Churchill Livingstone.

Loftis J, and Hauser P (2003). Co-management of depression and HCV treatment. *Psychiatr Ann* 33: 385–391.

Musselman DL, Lawson DH, Gumnick JF, Manatunga AK, Penna S, Goodkin RS, et al. (2001). Paroxetine for the prevention of depression induced by high dose interferon alpha. *N Engl J Med* 344:961–965.

Ondria G (1999). Five cases of interferon alpha induced depression treated with antidepressant therapy. *Psychosomatics* 40:510–512.

Onyike CU, Bonner JO, Lyketsos CG, and Treisman GJ (2004). Mania during treatment of chronic hepatitis C with pegylated interferon and ribavarin *Am J Psychiatry* 161:429–435.

Pyrsopoulos N, and Jeffers L (2005). Chronic hepatitis C in African Americans. *Clin Liver Dis* 9(3):427–438.

Raison CL, Borisov AS, Broadwell SD, Capuron L, Woolwine BJ, Jacobson IM, et al. (2005). Depression during pegylated interferon-alpha plus ribavirin therapy: prevalence and prediction. *J Clin Psychiatry* 66:41–48.

Roland ME, and Stock PG (2006). Liver transplantation in HIV-infected recipients. *Semin Liver Dis* 26(3): 273–284.

Russell S, and Jacob RG (1993). Living-related organ donation: the donor's dilemma. *Patient Educ Couns* 21:89–99.

Shapiro P, Williams DL, Foray AT, Gelman IS, Wukich N, and Sciacca R (1995). Psychosocial evaluation and prediction of compliance problems and morbidity after heart transplantation. *Transplantation* 60:1462–1466.

Schwartz AL, Thompson JA, and Masood N (2002). Interferon-induced fatigue in patients with melanoma: a pilot study of exercise and methylphenidate. *Oncol Nurs Forum* 29:E85–E90.

Stewart CA, and Cerhan J (2005). Hepatic encephalopathy: a dynamic or static condition. *Metabol Brain Dis* 20(3):193–204.

Soriano V, Puoti M, Sulkowski M, et al. (2004). Care of patients with hepatitis C and HIV co-infection. *AIDS* 18(1):1–12.

Strouse TB, El-Saden SM, Glaser N, Bonds C, Ayars N, and Busuttil R (1998). Immunosuppressant neurotoxicity in liver transplant recipients. *Psychosomatics* 39(2):124–133.

Sylvestre DL (2003). Injection drug use and hepatitis C: from transmission to treatment. *Psychiatr Ann* 33(6): 377–382.

Trask P, Esper P, Riba M, and Redman B (2000). Psychiatric side effects of interferon therapy: prevalence, proposed mechanisms, and future directions. *Clin Oncol* 18(11):2316–2326.

Trotter JF, Wachs M, Everson G, and Kam I (2002). Adult-to-adult transplantation of the right hepatic lobe from a living donor. *N Engl J Med* 346(14): 1074–1082.

Trzepacz PT, DiMartini A, and Tringali R (1993a). Psychopharmacologic issues in organ transplantation. Part I: Pharmacokinetics in organ failure and psychiatric aspects of immunosuppressants and anti-infectious agents. *Psychosomatics* 34(3):199–207.

Trzepacz PT, DiMartini A, and Tringali R (1993b). Psychopharmacologic issues in organ transplantation. Part 2: Psychopharmacologic medications. *Psychosomatics* 34(4):290–298.

Vierling J (1999). Immunology of acute and chronic hepatic allograft rejection. *Liver Transplant Surg* 5:S1–S20.

Wagner GJ, and Ryan GW (2005). Hepatitis C virus treatment decision-making in the context of HIV co-infection: the role of medical, behavioral and mental health factors in assessing treatment readiness *AIDS* 19(S3):S190–S198.

Weissenborn K (2003). Clinical features of hepatic encephalopathy. In D Zakim and TD Boyer (eds.), *Zakim and Boyer's Hepatology*, fourth edition (pp. 431–444). Philadelphia: WB Saunders.

Wijdicks E (2001). Neurotoxicity of immunosuppressive drugs. *Liver Transplant* 7:937–942.

World Health Organization (1999). Weekly Epidemiological Record. No. 49, 10 December 1999, WHO; Hepatitis C Fact Sheet No.164. October 2000. Available at http://www.who.int/inf-fs/en/fact164.html. Accessed May 4, 2007.

Zhang T, Li Y, Lai JP, Douglas SD, Metzger DS, O'Brien CP, and Ho WZ (2003). Alcohol potentiates hepatitis C virus replicon expression *Hepatology* 38(1):57–65.

Chapter 34

HIV-Associated Nephropathy, End-Stage Renal Disease, Dialysis, and Kidney Transplant

Jonathan Winston, Harold W. Goforth, Norman B. Levy, and Mary Ann Cohen

Persons with AIDS are often overwhelmed by the stigma, discrimination, and rejection associated with having this illness. In addition, they may have to cope with prevalent comorbid conditions, such as chronic kidney disease and end-stage renal disease (ESRD). The causes of ESRD may be multifactorial, but HIV-associated nephropathy is the single most common cause of kidney disease in black patients with HIV. Persons with AIDS are now living longer and healthier lives and are also becoming infected at older ages. They may develop concomitant illnesses that can also lead to ESRD, such as diabetes, hypertension, and a variety of other primary renal diseases. Similar to AIDS itself, ESRD is associated with a high prevalence of psychiatric comorbidity and a high rate of suicide. This chapter reviews the common causes of kidney disease in HIV, the approach to their diagnosis and treatment, and special issues relating to patient with end stage renal failure.

Kidney disease is a major public health problem. Approximately 325,000 people in the United States currently require hemodialysis as part of the End Stage Renal Disease (ESRD) Program, and 100,000 new patients begin treatment each year. Predictions are that 600,000 people will require maintenance dialysis by the end of the decade (U.S. Renal Data System, 2005). Kidney disease in the United States falls disproportionately on the ethnic minority community. African Americans account for 10% of the general population but more than 30% of the population with ESRD. Kidney disease is the ninth leading cause of death in the United States and the seventh leading cause for Black Americans (National Center for Statistics, 2005). The higher disease burden among blacks is a consequence of genetic factors that alter the susceptibility to kidney disease and of health care disparities along racial and socioeconomic lines. In HIV infection, the same associations exist between race and kidney disease. An estimated 10%–15% of patients with HIV infection have chronically impaired kidney function, a clinical syndrome now termed chronic kidney disease. Older age, black race, preexisting hypertension or diabetes, a prior AIDS-defining illness, injection drug use, and hepatitis C virus (HCV) coinfection are frequent predisposing causes (Gardner et al., 2003; Gupta et al., 2004; Szczech et al., 2004).

HIV-ASSOCIATED NEPHROPATHY

Although a wide spectrum of kidney diseases occur in association with HIV, HIV-associated nephropathy (HIVAN) remains the single most common cause of chronic kidney disease (Ross and Klotman, 2004). It is defined morphologically by collapse of the glomerular capillary tuft, glomerulosclerosis, and microcystic tubulointerstitial disease. Its association with black race is a striking clinical characteristic. Biopsy studies in North America, Europe, and Asia confirm that well over 90% of affected patients are of African descent. This racial predilection accounts for differences in prevalence reported from various centers. HIVAN is second only to sickle cell–associated renal disease in its racial clustering toward blacks. HIVAN is now the third leading cause of ESRD in blacks between the age of 20 and 64 years old, more common than lupus nephritis, polycystic disease, or primary glomerulonephritis (U.S. Renal Data System, 2005). A better understanding of the pathogenesis and genetic basis for HIVAN promises to uncover more information about renal susceptibility genes in African Americans.

The characteristic clinical presentation of HIVAN is heavy proteinuria, often in the nephrotic range, with varying degrees of renal insufficiency. Prior to the highly active antiretroviral therapy (HAART) era, the clinical course of HIVAN was marked by progression to renal failure requiring dialysis within weeks to months. The natural history has changed dramatically, however; now patients who are receiving antiviral therapy have a more indolent course and can have only mild to moderate proteinuria and a stable but impaired glomular filtration rate (GFR). Several studies demonstrate a slower progression to ESRD with HAART (Cosgrove et al., 2002; Szczech et al., 2002). Fewer cases of fulminant renal failure have been observed in the HAART era (Lucas et al., 2004). Several well-described case reports provide unequivocal evidence that HAART can reverse the structural and functional abnormalities in HIVAN, particularly when therapy is initiated early in the course of disease before glomerulosclerosis has been established (Wali et al., 1998; Winston et al., 2001). Antiretroviral therapy eliminates new rounds of renal cell infection, which interrupts the disease process. Compliance with antiretroviral therapy, therefore, has important implications for the outcome of kidney disease.

It is important to realize that patients are often asymptomatic during the early stages of kidney disease. Therefore, annual screening for kidney disease is recommended in high-risk HIV-1-infected patients— persons with hypertension, diabetes, or HCV coinfection as well as African Americans (Gupta et al., 2005). Patients in whom kidney disease is detected should undergo a comprehensive evaluation for the cause of the disease, and this may include a kidney biopsy. Willingness to adhere to an antiviral regimen will have important implications for the outcome of HIVAN.

HIV-associated nephropathy accounts for approximately 800–900 incident cases of ESRD each year. The number of new patients with HIV-ESRD has stabilized and has not decreased, in contrast to the decline in AIDS-associated mortality and opportunistic infections. This stabilization is likely due to the increased pool of patients at risk for kidney disease, as more patients (black patients in this instance) are living with AIDS. A mathematical model has quantified the dynamics of new ESRD cases arising from the risk pool before and after the widespread use of effective antiretrovirals. HAART is responsible for at least a 30% reduction in new ESRD cases from HIVAN. Looking to the future, without a dramatic decrease in the number of cases of HIV infection in the black community, the beneficial effect of HAART to slow the progression of kidney disease will be offset by an ever-growing risk pool, and the number of new cases of ESRD may soon rise (Schwartz et al., 2005).

OTHER CHRONIC KIDNEY DISEASES IN HIV

The pathogenesis, natural history, and therapy of other renal diseases commonly associated with HIV are less well defined because of the relatively small number of patients at any one center and the lack of joint collaborative studies or randomized controlled trials. Coinfection with HCV is associated with renal disease, at least in observational studies, but its role is unclear. HCV infection could be a marker for high-risk behavior such as injection drug use, it could directly affect kidney function, or its effects could be indirect and through abnormal liver function. Antibodies to HCV induce immune-complex glomerular disease (Johnson et al., 1994; Stokes et al., 1997). Antiviral therapy with interferon alpha and ribavirin is the treatment of choice for hepatitis C and membrano-proliferative glomerulonephritis (MPGN). Improved kidney function has been reported in single cases and small cohorts. Most often treatment is indicated for the liver disease, with or without cryoglobulinemia, and in this setting it is realistic to anticipate that kidney function will improve if therapy effectively eradicates the virus. A more difficult decision arises when antiviral therapy is ineffective but the kidney disease is especially active, as defined by the extent of inflammation on kidney biopsy or progressively falling GFR. Treatment options in these cases are based on case reports and include steroids, plasma exchange, and, more recently, rituxamab, a human-mouse chimeric monoclonal antibody to CD20 that selectively targets B cells. These approaches require careful monitoring and would be most risky in coinfected patients with low CD4 counts and/or high HIV viral loads (Kamar et al., 2006).

THERAPY FOR KIDNEY DISEASE IN HIV

The availability of treatment modalities for persons with kidney disease can be limiting and varies greatly regionally. Kidney disease is a chronic and progressive illness. Commonly used medications include antiretrovirals, ACE inhibitors, corticosteroids or even other immunosuppressants. However, these medications, which enjoy common usage in Western nations, are difficult to access in developing countries, making it more likely that patients there with early kidney disease will continue to progress in their illness to end-stage organ failure. It is unclear whether populations in developing countries sustain the same risk as that of African Americans in the United States, although some degree of increased risk similar that seen in the United States is accepted at this point (Behar et al., 2006; Gerntholtz et al., 2006; Han et al., 2006).

Use of HAART has reduced the incidence of HIV nephropathy, but access to HAART therapy has been a long-standing difficulty in developing nations. The effect of HAART on reducing the incidence of HIV nephropathy and preventing a serious end-stage organ disease merely reinforces the need for access to HAART around the world.

ADVANCED KIDNEY DISEASE AND END STAGE RENAL FAILURE

Patients with more advanced kidney disease often present with constitutional symptoms such as fatigue and anorexia. Although these symptoms may be due to uremia, they can be confused with symptoms attributable to the underlying HIV infection. Patients progressing to end-stage renal failure remain a special clinical challenge. Treatment must be initiated to control lipid abnormalities, Ca/PO4 metabolism, and anemia. Hypertension must also be treated as kidney function deteriorates, and the therapeutic focus should shift to preparation for renal replacement therapy. Proper planning for hemodialysis, peritoneal dialysis, or kidney transplantation should be made well in advance of uremic symptoms. Kidney transplantation is a viable option in selected patients. Its safety and efficacy is currently under study through a cooperative research program sponsored by the National Institute of Allergy and Infectious Diseases (NIAID) (http://spitfire.emmes.com/study/htr/index.html). Criteria for transplantation include undetectable viral RNA for at least 3 months, CD4 cells >200/μl, and no history of an opportunistic infection or neoplasm.

In those patients who are likely to start hemodialysis, an arteriovenous (AV) fistula (AVF) should be created months before an anticipated start date. This can be especially difficult in injection drug-using patients, because they often lack appropriate veins for fistula construction and medical follow-up is often inconsistent. Venous mapping and close collaboration with vascular surgeons can increase the success rate of fistula creation. Fistulae are far superior to polytetra-fluoroethylene (PTFE, Gore-Tex) grafts or percutaneous dialysis catheters because of lower thrombosis and infection rates. The long-term prognosis of patients with HIV on dialysis is determined by the stage of AIDS. These patients must also be aggressively treated with effective antiretroviral therapy. One- and two-year survival for incident ESRD patients has improved dramatically in the HAART era, and 1-year survival now approaches 80% (Ahuja, 2002). Survival on dialysis should continue to improve with newer antiviral drug therapies.

DIALYSIS AND HIV INFECTION

Implementation of renal replacement therapy is also prohibited by a lack of sustainable funding. Hemodialysis has been noted to be the preferred modality in most countries except Mexico, which employs widespread use of chronic ambulatory peritoneal dialysis (CAPD). Dialysis in the developing world is further complicated by high rates of HBV and HCV infections, and aluminum toxicity remains problematic. Under-dialysis remains common, and almost half of patients in the developing world receive less than 12 hours of dialysis weekly, provided over one or two sessions. Few are offered erythropoietin therapy and thus require repeated blood transfusions (Barsoum, 2002).

In a recent retrospective review of HIV-seropositive patients on peritoneal dialysis (PD), Khanna and colleagues (2005) found that HIV seropositivity was an independent predictor of mortality in PD patients; however, survival average in HIV patients remained encouragingly high at 12.5 years, in contrast to the 15 years associated with HIV-seronegative patients. HIV-seropositive patients were also more likely to be hospitalized or develop peritonitis than their seronegative counterparts. The use of HAART and higher CD4 counts at the time of dialysis initiation were associated with improved survivability, though, and these data indicate that long-term survival of HIV-seropositive patients is possible through use of PD with attention to maintaining HAART adherence and treatment of peritonitis. Although there are no long-term studies on survival of HIV-positive persons on hemodialysis, this treatment is widely used in this population. Particular areas of concern in hemodialysis include maintenance and maturation of the AV fistula. Preliminary evidence suggests that HIV patients do not suffer from clinically significantly higher AVF failure rates than those of their seronegative counterparts (Schild et al., 2004).

KIDNEY TRANSPLANTATION AND HIV

In recent years, an increasing number of HIV-seropositive patients have undergone solid organ transplantation, with good success and without significant differences in survival from that of HIV-negative pa-tients in preliminary studies (Abbott et al., 2004; Kumar et al., 2005). Similar results have been noted among liver transplant recipients (Ragni et al., 2003). Careful monitoring of transplant recipients is necessary to ensure good outcome, including timely availability of drug levels and attention to potential interactions between HIV protease inhibitors and immunosuppressive agents, especially the calcineurin inhibitors (cyclosporine, tacrolimus, sirolimus) (Mueller et al., 2006).

The logistics of solid organ transplantation pose special challenges in developing countries, as evidenced by Kenya's experience, where it was reported that 65% of dialysis patients died prior to successful transplantation, and another 14% were discharged from dialysis for conservative management. Only two patients (3%) received transplants, and both were unsuccessful and required ongoing dialysis. The authors note that potential contributing factors to this transplant experience included selection of only critically ill patients for transplant, shortages of trained staff, overdependence on AV shunts for dialysis access, recurrent shortages of essential equipment and reagents, and poor centralization of patient management (McLigeyo et al., 1988). Similar problems, including lack of access to dialysis technology, delayed referral to a nephrologists, and increased illness acuity resulting in high rates of early death, were noted more recently in Tunisia and Nigeria (Abderrahim et al., 2001; Anochie and Eke, 2005), although these issues continue to plague most of Sub-Saharan Africa.

The use of non-ideal organ transplantation in HIV patients has been controversial, and the advantages of increasing the number of potentially available organs must be weighed against the risks of transplanting non-ideal organs (e.g., hepatitis B–infected donors). Mueller and colleagues (1996) have reported at least one successful such case, and note that medications used to treat HIV such as lamivudine can also be used to treat hepatitis B, which may have contributed to a favorable outcome. Further studies are required on this topic.

PALLIATIVE CARE

Patients with HIV on chronic dialysis lead challenging but often rewarding lives. It has been noted, however, that an increasing number of ESRD patients are choosing to withdraw from dialysis prior to death. The percentage of patients choosing to withdraw from dialysis rose from 8.4% in 1988–1990 to 17.8% in 1990–1995 (Leggat et al., 1997). Such data necessitate a close relationship between nephrology, psychiatry, and palliative care teams to ensure maximal quality of life in end-stage patients. Withdrawal of care is a complex decision even when medically, legally, and ethically justifiable, and often is experienced through a combination of ambivalence, changes in decisions, and needed time to process the decision on an emotional level (Cohen et al., 2000; Neely and Roxe, 2000). Family dynamics and support play a large role, and such decisions impact an entire group of people, rather than a singular patient. Psychosomatic medicine psychiatrists can often be beneficial during this time by providing support and attempting to allay the natural anxieties experienced by the patient, family, and other medical caregivers during times of crisis and of complex decision-making. More comprehensive approaches to palliative and end-of-life care are presented in Chapters 30, 39, and 40 of this book.

PSYCHIATRIC DISORDERS AND DISTRESS ASSOCIATED WITH RENAL DISEASE

A great burden is placed on patients in their testing positive for HIV, and a similar, heavy burden is faced by those requiring dialysis. When an individual faces both the dependency and loss of function required by dialysis in addition to the distress associated with HIV, including that from chronic illness, potential discrimination, and other psychosocial stressors, the situation can evolve into an overwhelming one, even to the most resilient individuals. One of the more dramatic aspects of dialysis is the patient's dependence on the dialysis machine, a procedure that requires large amounts of time and a large number of specialized personnel to give the treatment. This dependence is unrelenting until renal transplant is performed, making patient cooperation and adjustment a priority if it is to be a successful bridge to transplantation. People who are very independent do not do well on dialysis, although some tailoring of the procedure may be possible to make it more palatable for them, including use of modalities emphasizing self-care such as home dialysis, peritoneal dialysis, or early renal transplantation (Reichsman and Levy, 1972).

Work-related difficulties are common to both HIV patients and dialysis patients, and both groups suffer a marked reduction in their ability to continue the work they performed prior to their illness, with rates of underemployment or unemployment approaching two-thirds for dialysis patients. Thus, the impact of these combined illnesses on the ability of patients to remain productive in their previous work environment should not be underestimated (Cohen et al., 2000). Losses include work, school, and housework-related responsibilities. The absence of existential gains provided by these venues can significantly increase distress levels in an already challenging group, with further loss of self-esteem, gender identity, sexual function, and perceived freedom.

The distress experienced by patients undergoing dialysis is further increased by apparent physical changes. Chronic dermatological changes in dialysis patients include skin discoloration, scars secondary to hemodialysis access operations, and artificially created AV fistulas. Women often lose their menstrual cycle and are unable to become pregnant, and men have diminished sexual function with reduced sperm counts. Uremia has also been noted to have a direct impact upon sexual function (Procci et al., 1981). All of these factors may affect not only the self-esteem of the patient but also their very concept of sexual role identity (Levy, 2000, 1973).

Among the greatest stresses that persons with ESRD on dialysis endure is that of a special diet, which requires a significant restriction in fluid intake to minimize the risk of peripheral and pulmonary edema that may follow excess fluid intake during renal failure. Drinking water or other beverages that most members of the general population take for granted is impossible; cracked ice is used to quench thirst. Similarly, protein intake is restricted severely, and persons with ESRD must often avoid dairy and fruit intake to avoid sodium, phosphates, and potassium, respectively. Thus, diets become artificial and difficult to follow outside of strictly controlled environments such as the patient's own home. The prospect of eating a "normal meal" at a restaurant is difficult if not impossible, leading further to isolation of the individual (Valderrqabano et al., 2001).

The actual procedure of being dialyzed is traumatic and anxiety provoking for most individuals. Peritoneal dialysis may be more benign in this respect because it involves only the transport of dialysate fluid, but patients undergoing hemodialysis witness their blood leaving their bodies, being sent into the hemodialyzer, and returned. Patients may be aware that a leak in the equipment can result in considerable blood loss, and they often experience significant hypotension during the procedure. If severe, this may lead to complications including stroke and death.

PSYCHOLOGICAL COMPLICATIONS IN DIALYSIS OF HIV PATIENTS

The most common psychological problem seen in people with medical or surgical illness is depression or the combination of anxiety and depression (O'Donnell and Chung, 1997; Kimmel et al., 1993); mood disorders are further discussed in Chapter 9. Persons on dialysis appear to have a higher incidence of suicide than that of both the general population and others with different chronic medical illnesses (Abram et al., 1975; Cutter et al., 1971; Haenel et al., 1980). Therefore, clinicians need to be aware of the potential for self-injurious behavior in these patients, who have two illnesses, each of which is associated with a high suicide incidence (Lyketsos and Federman, 1995).

Patients who are HIV positive and suffer end-stage renal failure are also predisposed to becoming delirious during treatment; delirium in HIV is more fully addressed in Chapter 10. Causes of delirium in this population are varied; many individuals with HIV-related nephropathy are mildly azotemic at baseline that may progress to a mild chronic delirium. Also, hemodialysis predisposes many patients to dysequilibrium syndrome, which is a mild, time-limited delirium caused by a relatively rapid change in fluid and electrolytes. Delirium is also seen in the not uncommon complications of secondary and tertiary hyperparathyroidism.

The importance of delirium is that it may have primary and secondary psychological sequelae (Trzepacz and Meagher, 2005), such as a worsening of the premorbid psychological characteristics of patients as well as increased rates of secondary anxiety and depression.

Treatment of Psychological Problems in HIV Patients on Dialysis

The accepted and ideal treatment of depression and anxiety is with antidepressants and psychotherapy. This topic is covered more extensively in Chapter 9. In this population, sexual dysfunction appears to play a large role in the maintenance and onset of distress, and some patients respond by withdrawing from intimacy altogether, resulting in increased isolation and poor self-coping (Levy, 1973). The treatment of sexual dysfunction in this population can often restore the ability to be intimate, with high rates of success. Sildenafil (Viagra) and allied medications tend to be 60% to 80% effective in reversing or reducing impotence; more permanent solutions include penile implants. Other modalities of treatment such as the Masters and Johnson techniques and their modifications involve less risk. In any case, it is important to keep in mind that sexual dysfunction is common in this population but is amenable to effective treatment (Abram et al. 1973).

Two major considerations in the pharmacology of renal failure are to avoid using a drug that is entirely eliminated by the kidney or one that is a small molecule that will be dialyzed (Levy et al., 2006). Pharmacokinetics is also significantly affected in renal failure, and the aspect that requires our greatest attention is the effect of renal failure on protein binding (Brater, 1999). Most drugs, especially the psychotropics, bind primarily to albumin, and the free portion serves as the active component. In renal failure there is decrease in available circulating protein, and thus, a decrease in binding capacity. Therefore, the rule of thumb is that the maximum dose of a medication used for a patient in renal failure should be no more than two-thirds of the maximum dose used for a patient with normal kidney function. Fortunately, virtually all psychiatrically active medications are fat-soluble, pass the blood–brain barrier, are metabolized by the liver, and are excreted in bile.

Concerning the use of anxiolytics, although lorazepam is ordinarily eliminated by the kidney, in kidney failure this medication is detoxified by the liver and excreted in bile. Further discussion of treatment in this complex medical population can be found in Chapter 33.

Renal Transplant

Solid organ transplantation has been noted to be among the triumphs of modern medicine and stands alongside the advances in treatment of HIV disease as one of the major advances in medical technology. The increase in organ transplantation, however, is limited to the number of available organs, which has not increased in proportion to the demand for new organs (Belle et al., 1996). The psychosomatic medicine psychiatrist is frequently called upon to perform pre-transplant evaluations to assess for psychiatric stability prior to organ placement and provide ongoing psychiatric care post-transplantation in the context of common affective disorders and neuropsychiatric syndromes that occur in this complex set of individuals. In this respect, transplantation psychiatry approaches the complexity commonly encountered in HIV psychiatry. The needs of HIV-seropositive patients with concurrent transplantation needs are highly complex. Frequently these patients are subject to not only the psychosocial strain of transplantation but also significant psychosocial stressors associated with HIV seropositivity.

Donor organ resources remain a problem, with the need of organs being much greater than the number of organs available (Surman, 1989). Transplant selection committees frequently serve as the gatekeeper for transplantation patients, orchestrating the selection of appropriate candidates on the basis of ethical, psychosocial, and biomedical factors (Freeman et al., 1992; Orentlicher, 1996). Skotzko and Strouse (2005) have remarked that psychosocial assessment should promote fairness and avoid discrimination. However, there are frequent implicit or explicit conflicts between the needs of the patient and the transplant program, so it often falls to the transplantation psychiatrist to advocate for the needs of the patient according to the principles of fairness and equal access.

Selection of transplant recipients with concurrent HIV is especially complex, given the perceived terminal quality of this illness among many medical practitioners. In fact, as noted in other portions of this chapter, the long-term survival of HIV patients with kidney transplants is favorable, even though it may be somewhat less than that of HIV-seronegative controls. Thus, the AIDS psychiatrist can serve as a potent advocate for those individuals who are otherwise good candidates medically and psychosocially and who have demonstrated good adherence to HAART.

Ironically, persons with HIV and AIDS have already proven their capacity to maintain a complex pharmacological regimen in the face of chronic medical illness, so they may, in fact, be better candidates for transplant than individuals who have no such medical adherence history and may suffer higher graft loss rates (DeLong et al., 1989; Schweizer et al., 1990; Rodriguez et al., 1991). This proven history must be balanced against the fact that high numbers of prescribed medications correlate with increased risk for nonadherence (Kiley et al., 1993). In general, it can be asserted that HIV-seropositive individuals with good control of their underlying HIV disease can be acceptable transplant candidates.

HIV-seropositive transplantations are complex psychiatrically, and these patients must deal with adjustment issues related to not only HIV status but also transplant status and the ever-present possibility of graft rejection. Patients requiring a second transplant may be obtunded and incapable of medical decision-making, reinforcing the role of surrogate decision makers for these individuals as for non-transplant HIV patients. Other common psychotherapeutic issues involve expectations for the future, death and dying, acceptance of another serious illness, and overall quality of life.

Psychopharmacological considerations are also complex in this patient group; transplant patients and HIV patients often do not tolerate tricyclic use, which necessitates use of newer agents with potentially less data. Also, neurotoxicity associated with cyclosporine-derived compounds is not infrequent and may present as syndromes mimicking neuropsychiatric illness such as toxicity, delirium, and seizures (Estol et al., 1989a; Estol et al., 1989b; Kershner and Wang-Cheng, 1989; Coleman and Norman, 1990; Burkhalter et al., 1994). The practitioner's differential diagnosis is confounded, as these patients suffer from both an immunosuppressive disease and pharmacological immunosuppression, so a full assessment of any presenting symptom is required prior to preemptive therapy.

CONCLUSIONS

In summary, the goal of HIV psychiatrists in addressing HIV transplant candidates is to provide preoperative assessment and post-transplant treatment and support designed to return these patients to a reasonable quality of life. Paris and colleagues (1993) have listed six predictors for return to employment: feeling able to work, having no risk of losing health insurance, longer length of time since transplant, education, maintenance of disability income, and relatively short periods of disability. For any transplant patient these factors are obviously complicated by the presence of another chronic illness such as HIV, for which distress rates are high, derived from complex factors, and underrecognized by most practitioners. AIDS psychiatrists can provide support to persons with HIV/AIDS and comorbid chronic renal disease at every stage of illness, from prevention to end stage. Initial involvement with an integrated and comprehensive approach to care can help prevent HIV-associated nephropathy by encouraging adherence and treating comorbid psychiatric illness. Psychiatric care can provide support for patients as well as for their families and caregivers. The AIDS psychiatrist can help alleviate distress, encourage behavior change and adherence, work with HIV clinicians and nephrologists to help reverse the ravages of HIVAN, provide assessments prior to dialysis and transplant, provide psychotherapy during dialysis and post-transplant, and continue to work with palliative psychiatry staff at the end of life.

References

Abbott KC, Swanson SJ, Agodoa LY, and Kimmel PL (2004). Human immunodeficiency virus infection and kidney transplantation in the era of highly active antiretroviral therapy and modern immunosuppression. *J Am Soc Nephrol* 15:1633–1639.

Abderrahim E, Zouaghi K, Hedri H, Ben Abdallah T, Ben Hamida F, Kaaroud H, Goucha R, Ben Abdallah N, Khiari K, El Younsi F, Ben Moussa F, Kheder A, and Ben Maiz H (2001). Renal replacement therapy for end stage renal disease. Experience of a Tunisian hospital centre. *Diabetes Metab* 27:584–590.

Abram HS, Hester LR, and Epstein GM (1973). Sexual functioning in patients with chronic renal failure. *J Nerv Ment Dis* 166:220–226.

Abram HS, Moore GL, and Westerfelt BS (1975). Suicidal behavior in chronic dialysis patients. *Am J Psychiatry* 127:1199–1204.

Ahuja TS, Grady J, and Khan S (2002). Changing trends in the survival of dialysis patients with human immunodeficiency virus in the United States. *J Am Soc Nephrol* 13:1889–1893.

Anochie IC, and Eke FU (2005). Acute renal failure in Nigerian children: Port Harcourt experience. *Pediatr Nephrol* 20:1610–1614.

Barsoum RS (2002). Overview: end-stage renal disease in the developing world. *Artif Organs* 26:737–746.

Behar DM, Shlush LI, Maor C, Lorber M, and Skorecki K (2006). Absence of HIV associated nephropathy in Ethiopians. *Am J Kidney Dis* 47:88–94.

Belle SH, Beringer KC, and Detre DM (1996). Recent findings concerning liver transplantation in the United States. *Clin Transplant* 10:15–29.

Brater DC (1999). Drug dosing in renal failure. In HR Brady and CS Wilcox (eds.), *Therapy in Nephrology and Hypertension: A Companion to Brenner and Rector's The Kidney*, fifth edition (pp. 641–653) Philadelphia: WB Saunders.

Burkhalter EL, Starzl TE, and Van Thiel DH (1994). Severe neurological complications following orthotopic liver transplant in patients receiving FK-506 and prednisone. *J Hepatol* 21:572–577.

Cohen LM, McCue J, and Germain M (2000). Denying the dying: advance directives and dialysis discontinuation. *Psychosomatics* 41:195–203.

Cohen LM, Levy NB, Tessier EG, and Germain MJ (2005). Renal disease. In JL Levenson (ed.), *Textbook of Psychosomatic Medicine* (pp. 483–493). Washington, DC: American Psychiatric Publishing.

Coleman AE, and Norman DJ (1990). OKT3 encephalopathy. *Ann Neurol* 128:837–838.

Cosgrove CJ, Abu-Alfa AK, and Perazella MA (2002). Observations on HIV-associated renal disease in the era of highly active antiretroviral therapy. *Am J Med Sci* 323:102–106.

Cutter F, Abram HS, Moore GL (1971). Chronic dialysis patients: suicide incidence rates. *Am J Psychiatry* 128:495–497.

DeLong P, Trollinger JH, Fox N, et al. (1989). Noncompliance in renal transplant recipients: methods for recognition and intervention. *Transplant Proc* 21:2982–3984.

Estol CJ, Faris AA, Martinez AJ, and Ahdab-Barmada M (1989a). Central pontine myelinolysis after liver transplantation. *Neurology* 39:493–498.

Estol CJ, Lopez O, Brenner RP, and Martinez AJ (1989b). Seizures after liver transplantation: a clinicopathologic study. *Neurology* 39:1297–1301.

Freeman A, Davies L, Libb JW, et al. (1992). Assessment of transplant candidates and prediction of outcome. In J Craven and G Rodin (eds.), *Psychiatric Aspects of Organ Transplantation* (pp. 9–19). Oxford, England: Oxford University Press.

Gardner LI, Holmberg SD, Williamson JM, et al. (2003). Development of proteinuria or elevated serum creatinine and mortality in HIV-infected women. *J Acquir Immune Defic Syndr* 32:203–209.

Gerntholtz TE, Goetsch SJW, and Katz I (2006). HIV related nephropathy: a South African perspective. *Kidney Int* 69:1885–1891.

Gupta SK, Mamlin BW, Johnson CS, et al. (2004). Prevalence of proteinuria and the development of chronic kidney disease in HIV-infected patients. *Clin Nephrol* 61:1–6.

Gupta SK, Eustace JA, Winston JA, et al. (2005). Guidelines for the management of chronic kidney disease in HIV-infected patients: recommendations of the HIV Medicine Association of the Infectious Diseases Society of America. *Clin Infect Dis* 40:1559–1585.

Haenel T, Brunner F, and Battegay R (1980). Renal dialysis and suicide: occurrence in Switzerland and in Europe. *Compr Psychiatry* 21:140–145.

Han TM, Naicker S, Ramdial PK, and Assounga AG (2006). A cross-sectional study of HIV seropositive patients with varying degrees of proteinuria in South Africa. *Kidney Int* 69:2243–2250.

Johnson RJ, Willson R, Yamabe H, et al. (1994). Renal manifestations of hepatitis C virus infection. *Kidney Int* 46:1255–1263.

Kamar N, Rostaing L, and Alric L (2006). Treatment of hepatitis C virus–related glomerulonephritis. *Kidney Int* 69:436–439.

Kershner P, and Wang-Cheng R (1989). Psychiatric side effects of steroid therapy. *Psychosomatics* 30:135–139.

Khanna R, Tachopoulou OA, Fein PA, Chattopadhyay J, and Avram MM (2005). Survival experience of peritoneal dialysis patients with human immunodeficiency virus: a 17-year retrospective study. *Adv Perit Dial* 21:159–163.

Kiley DJ, Lam CS, and Pollak R (1993). A study of treatment compliance following kidney transplantation. *Transplantation* 55:51–56.

Kimmel PL, Weihs K, and Peterson RA (1993). Survival in hemodialysis patients: the role of depression. *J Am Soc Nephrol* 3:12–27.

Kumar MS, Sierka DR, Damask AM, Fyfe B, McAlack RF, Heifets M, Moritz MJ, Alvarez D, and Kumar A (2005). Safety and success of kidney transplantation and concomitant immunosuppression in HIV-positive patients. *Kidney Int* 67:1622–1629.

Leggat JE, Bloembergen WE, Levine G, Hulbert-Shearon TE, and Port FK (1997). An analysis of risk factors for withdrawal from dialysis before death. *J Am Soc Nephrol* 8:1755–1763.

Levy NB (1973). Sexual adjustment to hemodialysis and renal transplantation: national survey by questionnaire: preliminary report. *Trans Am Soc Artif Intern Organs* 19:138–142.

Levy NB (2000). Psychiatric considerations in primary medical care of the patient in renal failure. *Adv Ren Replace Ther* 7:231–238.

Levy NB, Cohen LM, and Tessier EG (2006). Renal disease. In M Blumenfield and JJ Strain (eds.), *Psychosomatic Medicine* (pp. 157–175). Philadelphia: Lippincott Williams & Wilkins.

Lucas GM, Eustace JA, Sozio S, Mentari EK, Appiah KA, and Moore RD (2004). Highly active antiretroviral therapy and the incidence of HIV-1-associated nephropathy: a 12-year cohort study. *AIDS* 18:541–546.

Lyketsos CG, and Federman EB (1995). Psychiatric disorders and HIV infection: impact of one on the other. *Epidimiol Rev* 17:152–164.

McLigeyo SO, Otieno LS, Kinuthia DM, Ongeri SK, Mwongera FK, and Wairagu SG (1998). Problems with a renal replacement programme in a developing country. *Postgrad Med J* 64:783–786.

Mueller NJ, Furrer H, Kaiser L, Hirschel B, Cavassini M, Fellay J, Chave JP, Wuethrich RP, Weber M, Muellhaupt B, Candinas D, Reichen J, Giostra E, Mentha G, Halkic N, Hirsch HH, Weber R, and Swiss HIV Cohort Study (2006). HIV and solid organ transplantation: the Swiss experience. *Swiss Med Wkly* 136:194.

National Center for Health Statistics (2005). *United States, 2005, With Chartbook on Trends in the Health of Americans.* Hyattsville, MD: U.S. Government Printing Office.

Neely KJ, and Roxe DM (2000). Palliative care/hospice and the withdrawal of dialysis. *J Palliat Med* 3:57–67.

O'Donnell K, and Chung Y (1997). The diagnosis of major depression in end-stage renal disease. *Psychother Psychosom* 66:38–43.

Orentlicher D (1996). Psychosocial assessment of organ transplant candidates and the Americans with Disabilities Act. *Gen Hosp Psychiatry* 18:5S–12S.

Paris W, Woodbury A, Thompson S, Levick M, Nothegger S, Arbuckle P, Hutkin-Slade L, and Cooper DK (1993). Returning to work after heart transplantation. *J Heart Lung Transplant* 12:46–53.

Procci WR, Goldstein DA, and Adelstein J (1981). Sexual function in the male with uremia: a reappraisal. *Kidney Int* 19:317–323.

Ragni MV, Belle SH, Im K, Neff G, Roland M, Stock P, Heaton N, Human A, and Fung JF (2003). Survival of human immunodeficiency virus–infected liver transplant recipients. *J Infect Dis* 188:1412–1420.

Reichsman F, and Levy NB (1972). Adaptation to hemodialysis: a four-year study of 25 patients. *Arch Intern Med* 138:859–865.

Rodriguez A, Diaz M, Colon A, and Santiago-Delpin EA (1991). Psychosocial profile of noncompliant transplant patients. *Transplant Proc* 23:1807–1809.

Ross MJ, and Klotman PE (2004). HIV-associated nephropathy. *AIDS* 18:1089–1099.

Schild AF, Prieto J, Glenn M, Livingstone J, Alfieri K, and Raines J (2004). Maturation and failure rates in a large series of arteriovenous dialysis access fistulas. *Vasc Endovasc Surg* 38:449–453.

Schwartz EJ, Szczech LA, Ross MJ, et al. (2005). Highly active antiretroviral therapy and the epidemic of HIV+ end-stage renal disease. *J Am Soc Nephrol* 16:2412–2420.

Schweizer RT, Rovelli M, Palmeri D, Vossler E, Hull D, and Bartus S (1990). Noncompliance in organ transplant recipients. *Transplantation* 49:374–377.

Skotzko CE, and Strouse TB (2005). Solid organ tranplantation. In JT Levenson (ed.), *The American Psychiatric Publishing Textbook of Consultation-Liaison Psychiatry,* second edition (pp. 623–654). Washington DC: American Psychiatric Publishing.

Stokes MB, Chawla H, Brody RI, et al. (1997). Immune complex glomerulonephritis in patients coinfected with human immunodeficiency virus and hepatitis C virus. *Am J Kidney Dis* 29:514–525.

Surman OS (1989). Psychiatric aspects of organ transplantation. *Am J Psychiatry* 146:972–982.

Szczech LA, Edwards LJ, Sanders LL, van der Horst C, Bartlet JA, Heald AE, and Svetkey LP (2002). Protease inhibitors are associated with a slowed progression of HIV-related renal diseases. *Clin Nephrol* 57:336–341.

Szczech LA, Hoover DR, Feldman JG, et al. (2004). Association between renal disease and outcomes among HIV-infected women receiving or not receiving antiretroviral therapy. *Clin Infect Dis* 39:1199–1206.

Trzepacz PT and Meagher DJ (2005). Delirium. In JL Levenson (ed.), *The American Psychiatric Publishing Textbook of Psychosomatic Medicine* (pp. 91–130). Washington, DC: American Psychiatric Publishing.

U.S. Renal Data System (2005). *USRDS 2005 Annual Data Report: Atlas of End-Stage Renal Disease in the United States*. Bethesda, MD: National Institutes of Health, National Institute of Diabetes and Digestive and Kidney Diseases.

Valderrqabano E, Jofre R, and Lopez-Gomez JM (2001). Quality of life in end-stage renal disease patients. *Am J Kidney Dis* 38:443–464.

Wali RK, Drachenberg CI, Papadimitriou JC, Keay S, and Ramos E (1998). HIV-1-associated nephropathy and response to highly active antiretroviral therapy [letter]. *Lancet* 352:783–784.

Winston JA, Bruggeman LA, Ross MD, et al. (2001). Nephropathy and establishment of a renal reservoir of HIV type 1 during primary infection. *N Engl J Med* 344:1979–1984.

Chapter 35

Endocrine Comorbidities
in Persons with HIV

Jocelyn Soffer, Joseph Z. Lux,
and Michael P. Mullen

Human immunodeficiency virus (HIV) and the acquired immunodeficiency syndrome (AIDS) have been associated with a wide spectrum of endocrine abnormalities that underscore the complex relationships between immunological, endocrinological, and psychological systems. Endocrine changes associated with HIV infection occur through multiple mechanisms, including direct cytopathologic effects, intercurrent illness, and pharmacotherapies used to treat the virus. Some of these changes may not be specific to HIV, but rather represent the body's response to any severe illness; others may be HIV specific yet not have clear clinical significance. As treatments for HIV improve, however, and the population of HIV-infected individuals increases and ages, even subtle changes in endocrine function may carry increasingly important consequences for morbidity, mortality, and quality of life. This chapter will review HIV-associated changes in the function of the hypothalamic–pituitary axis, adrenal glands, thyroid, gonads, and bone and mineral metab-

olism, and consider the psychosocial implications of such endocrinopathies.

ADRENAL GLAND IN HIV INFECTION

Altered Hypothalamic–Pituitary–Adrenal Axis: Pathophysiology and Assessment of Adrenal Function

Many studies have demonstrated alterations in adrenal function in patients with HIV and AIDS. Associated infections and tumors, as well as direct invasion of the adrenal glands by the virus, partly explain these changes. Patients are also commonly prescribed drugs that alter steroid synthesis or metabolism; for example, ketoconazole decreases steroid synthesis, megesterol acetate suppresses pituitary secretion of corticotropin, and rifampin increases p450 activity, leading to increased metabolism of cortisol. The altered cytokine milieu in immune deficiency states may also affect the hypothalamic–pituitary–adrenal (HPA) axis. Tumor necrosis factor alpha (TNF-α), for example, found in increased levels in HIV patients, impairs corticotrophin-releasing hormone (CRH)-stimulated release of adrenocorticotropin hormone (ACTH) and cortisol.

Alterations at all levels of the HPA axis have been described in patients with HIV. With the traditional 250 μg ACTH stimulation test to detect adrenal response, many studies have revealed subnormal peak cortisol responses in patients with HIV (Membreno et al., 1987; Merenich et al., 1990; Raffi et al., 1991), although some have demonstrated normal responses (Findling et al., 1994). Azar and Melby (1993) examined patients with advanced HIV (CD4 < 500) but without signs of adrenal or pituitary insufficiency. In response to CRH stimulation, 25% displayed normal ACTH but decreased cortisol response (suggesting reduced adrenal reserve), while 25% showed both impaired ACTH and cortisol production (suggesting reduced pituitary reserve). Other studies have similarly demonstrated decreased responses of both ACTH and cortisol to CRH stimulation (Biglino et al., 1995; Lortholary et al., 1996).

In the late 1980s, many postmortem studies demonstrated high rates of adrenal involvement in patients dying from AIDS (Welch et al., 1984; Laulund et al., 1986). Cytomegalovirus (CMV) was the most common associated infectious agent, found in the adrenal glands in 33%–88% of cases (Glasgow et al., 1985, Pulakhandam and Dincsoy, 1990; Marik et al., 2002). Less common agents observed in autopsy studies included *Cryptococcus*, *Toxoplasma*, *Histoplasma*, *Mycobacteria*, and neoplasms such as lymphoma and Kaposi's sarcoma. Recent autopsy studies (including a series of 128 patients who died of AIDS) have continued to demonstrate high rates of adrenal abnormalities, with compromise or inflammation of the adrenal glands observed in nearly 100% of cases, approximately half involving CMV infection (Duch et al., 1998; Rodrigues et al., 2002).

Clinical symptoms of adrenal insufficiency in patients with HIV, in contrast, are much less commonly observed, probably because more than 80% to 90% of the adrenal glands must be destroyed before symptoms appear, whereas adrenal cortical necrosis observed in autopsy studies rarely exceeds 60%–70% (Sellmeyer and Grunfeld, 1996; Mayo et al., 2002). In fact, despite the association of HIV with adrenal dysfunction and blunted stress responses discussed above, most studies have found normal or more commonly elevated basal cortisol levels in patients with HIV infection (Villette et al., 1990; Biglino et al., 1995; Sellmeyer and Grunfeld, 1996; Christeff et al., 1997). Serum cortisol typically increases as disease progresses, negatively correlating with CD4 counts (Lortholary et al., 1996).

Multiple factors could explain the hypercortisolism commonly observed in patients with HIV infection, including comorbid depression and severe psychosocial stress, both of which are associated with increased levels of cortisol. More specifically, increased levels of cytokines present during HIV infection may stimulate cortisol production by the adrenal glands. Biglino and others (1995) demonstrated a correlation between cortisol and levels of interleukin-6 (IL-6) and IL-1β. They suggested that observed blunting of pituitary and adrenal responses to CRH stimulation occurs as compensation for chronic cytokine-induced adrenal stimulation.

Changes in steroid carrier proteins and steroid receptor binding might contribute to altered hormone metabolism. Studies have demonstrated decreased binding of corticosteroid-binding globulin (CBG) to cortisol in HIV patients compared to that in controls, despite an increased number of binding sites (Martin et al., 1992). A phenomenon of glucocorticoid resistance has also been described in patients with HIV that could further explain the paradoxical combination of increased serum cortisol and clinical symptoms of adrenal insufficiency. Norbiato and others (1992) demonstrated a decreased affinity of glucocorticoid receptors for glucocorticoids in AIDS patients, despite an increase in receptor density.

Finally, there appears to be a shift in adrenal steroid metabolism from androgenic pathways to those of cortisol production. Villette and others (1990) found significantly higher 24-hour cortisol levels in patients with HIV than those in control subjects, but decreases in dehydroepiandrosterone (DHEA), DHEA-sulfate (DHEA-S), and ACTH. With advancing HIV infection, cortisol levels typically increase, while DHEA and DHEA-S levels decrease (Findling et al., 1994; Clerici et al., 1997), in some cases correlating with CD4 cell counts (Wisniewski et al., 1993; Christeff et al., 1997). The ratio of DHEA to cortisol declines significantly in patients with more advanced clinical illness. Although most studies have been conducted with men, studies of women with AIDS have also demonstrated a correlation between CD4 cell counts and DHEA-to-cortisol ratios (Grinspoon et al., 2001).

Despite the clear evidence for alterations in the HPA axis in this population, the prevalence and clinical significance of such abnormalities remain controversial, in part because of methodological difficulties in assessing adrenal function. The diagnosis of adrenal insufficiency from stimulation testing depends both on the dose of ACTH used and the laboratory cutoffs for a "normal" cortisol stress response. Some investigators have claimed that the supraphysiologic 250 µg dose of ACTH masks some adrenal dysfunction; low-dose stimulation testing (e.g., 1 or 10 µg) increases sensitivity (Marik et al., 2002) but might result in false positives. Stolarczyk and others (1998) found that AIDS patients both with and without symptoms had a decreased cortisol response compared to comparably sick HIV-negative patients and healthy controls, despite achieving "normal" cortisol values on stimulation testing.

These complexities are highlighted by the frequent lack of correlation between symptoms and detection of laboratory abnormalities (Bhansali et al., 2000; Eledrisi and Verghese, 2001). In a study of 104 patients using a 10 µg ACTH stimulation test in which nearly one-third of patients had clinical signs of adrenal insufficiency, only 5% responded abnormally, with an additional 16% demonstrating borderline responses, and no reliable correlation with disease symptoms (Gonzalez-Gonzalez et al., 2001). In another study of 63 patients with advanced AIDS, 19% had abnormally low levels of stimulated cortisol, suggesting a need for supplementation, but no associated opportunistic diseases, signs, or symptoms (Wolff et al., 2001).

Despite these methodological difficulties, most clinicians would agree that adrenal insufficiency is relatively common in advanced AIDS patients, especially those positive for CMV, and that function be evaluated in all severely ill patients with AIDS (Hoshino et al., 2002). Normal findings on adrenal stimulation in the presence of clinical signs and symptoms of insufficiency should be interpreted with caution. Finally, glucocorticoid replacement is crucial for all patients with a diagnosis of adrenal insufficiency, and should be considered and increased in AIDS patients during times of febrile illness or worsening infection.

Fewer studies have examined mineralocorticoid response during HIV infection. Some studies report lower levels of basal aldosterone than those in controls, including one of asymptomatic patients newly diagnosed with HIV (Merenich et al., 1990). There are only a few isolated case reports of primary aldosteronism in HIV infection (Fradley et al., 2005). The clinical significance of possibly altered mineralocorticoid function remains uncertain.

Psychosocial Implications

There can be considerable overlap between symptoms of HIV itself, adrenal insufficiency, and psychiatric illness, including fatigue, anorexia, nausea, vomiting, and orthostatic hypotension. Some patients report a sensation of heavy and weak muscles, dizziness, and tachycardia, which may be confused with a depressive or anxiety disorder. Patients with adrenal insufficiency have been misdiagnosed with hypochondriasis, conversion disorder, and anorexia nervosa (Starkman, 2003). When signs more specific to adrenal insufficiency are present, such as salt craving, hyponatremia, or, in the case of primary adrenal insufficiency, increased skin pigmentation, the diagnosis is more easily made.

Associated behavioral changes in patients with adrenal insufficiency may include lethargy, apathy, irritability, crying, and impaired sleep. Cognitive difficulties have also been reported, including decreased concentration, decreased memory, and episodic confusion (Starkman, 2003). Impaired thought process can worsen to frank psychosis during an adrenal crisis (Starkman, 2003).

As discussed earlier, most patients with HIV do not exhibit signs of adrenal insufficiency but rather are marked by increased levels of circulating cortisol. These patients do not generally present with features of Cushing's syndrome either, however, which may have different neuropsychiatric manifestations. The clinical significance of hypercortisolemia seen in most HIV patients, then, remains unclear, being associated with classical manifestations of neither Cushing's syndrome nor adrenal insufficiency.

DHEA and DHEA-S are not only adrenal androgens but also centrally acting neurosteroids whose levels decrease with chronic stress and illness (in contrast to cortisol, which tends to rise). Decreased ratios of DHEA and DHEA-S to cortisol have been reported in many conditions including aging, depression, and dementia (Wolkowitz et al., 2003) in addition to HIV infection. Given that DHEA and DHEA-S have been shown to have memory-enhancing (Roberts et al.,

1987) and antidepressant-like effects in animals (Reddy et al., 1998), it is not surprising that low levels of these neurosteroids have been reported in patients with depression, psychosocial stress, and functional limitations (Berr et al., 1996; Yaffe et al., 1998). In one study of post-menopausal women, DHEA-S levels were inversely associated with depressed mood, independently of age, physical activity, or weight change (Barrett-Connor et al., 1999). In a controlled study of depressed patients, salivary levels of DHEA were lower than those in controls, with a negative correlation found between morning readings and the severity of depression (Michael et al., 2000). The evening salivary cortisol was elevated in the depressed population.

The indications for replacement of DHEA, however, remain controversial. In one study of women with adrenal insufficiency, replacement of DHEA improved overall well-being, depression and anxiety, and satisfaction with both mental and physical aspects of sexuality (Arlt et al., 1999). In another study of patients with Addison's disease, replacement with DHEA significantly enhanced self-esteem, mood, and fatigue, with a tendency toward improved overall well-being, but did not affect cognitive or sexual function (Hunt et al., 2000). To date, however, there are limited studies specifically addressing the psychosocial implications of adrenal dysfunction in persons with HIV and no clear guidelines for how and under what circumstances to replace DHEA in men or women with HIV.

In the subpopulation of HIV-positive patients who abuse substances, in some cases by injection drug use, there may be associated endocrine changes that mimic or exacerbate those seen in HIV infection. A high prevalence of adrenal dysfunction has been described in opiate-dependent patients (Tennant et al., 1991). Hypercortisolism occurs after abrupt withdrawal of heroin in addicts (Cami et al., 1992). In rat studies, chronic exposure to morphine causes naltrexone-preventable increases in corticobinding globulin that lowers the amount of free active cortisol (Nock et al., 1997). In a study of heroin and cocaine users, higher cortisol levels were associated with depressive symptoms, particularly in women (Wisniewski et al., 2006), with gender differences being most pronounced in women who were both infected with HIV and injection drug users (Wisniewski et al., 2005).

Some investigators have examined the hypothesis that stress management interventions would help counter some of the HPA dysfunction observed in patients with HIV, given that high levels of stress and mood disturbances might contribute to high levels of cortisol (Mulder et al., 1995). A cognitive-behavioral stress management (CBSM) intervention consisting of 10 weekly group sessions demonstrated post-treatment decreases in depression, anxiety, and general psychological distress, compared to a wait-list comparison group (Antoni et al., 2000a). The treatment group had lower levels of urinary cortisol, with improved mood paralleling cortisol decreases in urine. Furthermore, at 6- to 12-month follow-up, the CBSM group had improved immunological parameters, including increased transitional naïve T cells (Antoni et al., 2002) and cytotoxic T cells (Antoni et al., 2000b). Interestingly, only mood changes during the training period predicted such delayed immune status changes; there was no association with post-intervention mood changes, medication status, or health behaviors (Antoni et al., 2005).

THYROID GLAND IN HIV INFECTION

Abnormalities in Thyroid Function Tests and Pathophysiology

Patients with HIV and AIDS often manifest abnormalities in thyroid function tests that are distinct from those seen in other nonthyroidal illness. Such changes are usually subclinical, however, with elevated thyroid-stimulating hormone (TSH) but normal free T4 (FT4). Changes in the hypothalamic–pituitary–thyroid axis have been reported even early in the course of infection, one study finding 8% prevalence of subclinical hypothyroidism in 40 asymptomatic, untreated patients newly diagnosed with HIV (Merenich et al., 1990). Another study found 16% of patients with HIV in various stages of illness to have low T3 and/or T4 (Raffi et al., 1991). More recent studies have demonstrated approximately 7% rates of subclinical hypothyroidism in patients with HIV (Beltran et al. 2003), with rates of overt hypothyroidism ranging between 2% and 9%.

The clinical significance of such changes remains uncertain. In many cases, alterations of thyroid function tests (TFTs) are asymptomatic, especially in patients with early disease. Most weight-stable patients with HIV maintain overall normal thyroid function (Sellmeyer and Grunfeld, 1996; Koutkia et al., 2002). Grunfeld and colleagues (1993) found that asymptomatic HIV patients with stable weight had normal

T3 levels, while those with more advanced AIDS but stable weight had 19% and 30% decreases in levels of T3 and FT3, respectively. In AIDS patients with active secondary infections, anorexia, and short-term weight loss, abnormalities in T3 and FT3 were more marked, with declines of 45% and 50%. In this study, TSH was increased but still within normal limits in the patients with AIDS.

The alterations of TFTs in AIDS patients seem to be different from those changes observed in the phenomenon of the "euthyroid sick syndrome," commonly seen in non-HIV-related, nonthyroidal illness. In studies of HIV patients, reverse T3 (rT3) is decreased (Grunfeld et al., 1993; Hommes et al., 1993), whereas in the euthyroid sick syndrome rT3 is usually increased. The clinical significance of this change remains unclear (Sellmeyer and Grunfeld, 1996). Furthermore, T3 levels are often normal in patients with HIV (Olivieri et al., 1993), in contrast to the euthyroid sick syndrome in which T3 is typically decreased. Hommes and others (1993) found lower FT4 and higher mean TSH, both at baseline and as peak response to TRH simulation, despite normal T3 and T4, concluding that there is hypothyroid-like regulation of the pituitary–thyroid axis in HIV infection that differs from that in the euthyroid sick syndrome.

Patients with HIV demonstrate increases in thyroid-binding globulin (TBG) (Grunfeld et al., 1993; Hommes et al., 1993, Olivieri et al., 1993), which can also be seen in other severe illnesses. In patients with HIV, increased TBG has been associated with progressive HIV infection, inversely correlating with CD4 count. While this has no clear clinical significance, some investigators have suggested the utility of TBG as a prognostic marker. In advanced infection, high levels of TBG could cause decreases in T3, proposed to be beneficial by conserving (already limited) energy expenditure; serum T3 itself has been proposed as a prognostic marker for AIDS (Lambert, 1994). Increased TBG can also cause decreases in free T4 levels.

In summary, what may be unique to thyroid alterations in patients with HIV as compared to other major illnesses is the combination of normal T3, decreased rT3, and increased TBG. In advanced illness, however, T3 levels typically decline, and some patients exhibit overt hypothyroidism with decreased fT4 levels.

While the pathophysiology of alterations in thyroid function remains unclear, it has in some cases been related to associated infections and tumors, particularly in the early literature. There have been isolated case reports of *Pneumocystis* infection of the thyroid gland (Ragni et al., 1991; Guttler et al., 1993). Clinically, many of these cases presented with symptoms or signs of hypothyroidism (Ragni et al., 1991; Spitzer et al., 1991; McCarty et al., 1992) and/or as a neck mass or thyroid goiter (Battan et al., 1991; Ragni et al., 1991). One group of authors reported a case of a thyroid goiter associated with mild hyperthyroidism (Drucker et al., 1990). Other cases of Kaposi's sarcoma invading the thyroid gland and causing clinical hypothyroidism (Mollison et al., 1991) or a palpable thyroid mass (Krauth and Katz, 1987) have been reported. Autopsy studies have also found CMV inclusions in the thyroid follicles of patients dying of AIDS (Frank et al., 1987), in addition to other infections.

Medications prescribed for patients with HIV may have an impact on thyroid function. IFN-α has been associated with thyroid dysfunction, possibly through an autoimmune mechanism. Medications that induce hepatic p450 enzyme systems, such as rifampin and ketoconazole, increase excretion of thyroid hormones. Patients on thyroid replacement may thus need higher doses, while those with normal thyroid function may have decreases in T4 (usually with normal or even increased T3 and no change in TSH) (Sellmeyer and Grunfeld, 1996).

While highly active antiretroviral therapy (HAART) has generally not been implicated in causing thyroid dysfunction, there have been recent reports of autoimmune thyroid disease developing in association with immune reconstitution. Five patients were described who presented with Graves disease within 2 years of starting HAART (Gilquin et al., 1998; Jubault et al., 2000). In all cases the diagnosis occurred several months after viral RNA levels became undetectable and after a significant rise in CD4 counts. In a recent multicenter study in England tracking all patients starting on HAART, there were 17 new cases of autoimmune thyroid disease, the majority with Graves disease, for an estimated prevalence of 3% for females and 0.2% for males (Chen et al., 2005). There have been other isolated reports of thyroid dysfunction with antiretroviral therapy, including one study in which receipt of stavudine was associated with hypothyroidism (Beltran et al., 2003).

Psychosocial Implications

True clinical hypothyroidism can cause multiple neuropsychiatric symptoms and signs of which the psychiatrist should be aware, most commonly cognitive dysfunction and depression. Severe forms can be manifested by psychotic and delusional symptoms, including visual and auditory hallucinations. Cognitive changes can include inattentiveness, slowed thought process, and impaired memory; mood changes can include anxiety, irritability, and emotional lability in addition to other depressive symptoms (Bauer et al., 2003). While these changes are not specific to patients with HIV, the presence of other HIV-associated medical and psychiatric comorbidities increases the challenge and complexity of identifying and treating such symptoms.

In most cases, hypothyroidism-associated behavioral changes remit after treatment and restoration to euthyroid status. The clinical significance of subclinical hypothyroidism commonly observed in patients with HIV remains uncertain. Treatment of hypothyroidism should be avoided unless clearly indicated, as replacement can increase HIV-related weight loss, although one study suggested that patients given thyroid hormones in pharmacological doses had improvements in weight gain, energy, endurance, and well-being (Derry, 1995).

GONADAL FUNCTION IN HIV INFECTION

Hypogonadism in Men with HIV

Hypotestosteronemia has been one of the most prevalent endocrine abnormalities observed in patients with HIV. Testosterone is important for the maintenance of normal bone health, muscle mass, strength, energy level, and general sense of well-being. Testosterone levels decrease routinely in healthy men starting in the fourth decade of life. As the population infected with HIV ages due to HAART-related decreases in mortality, normal declining testosterone levels will be compounded by HIV-associated decreases in testosterone.

Early studies documented approximately 50% of men with AIDS to have hypogonadism (Dobs et al., 1988). In a recent study of androgen levels in older men (ages 49–81) with or at risk for acquiring HIV infection, 54% had total testosterone levels below 300 ng/dl (Klein et al., 2005). Factors encountered at high rates in some psychiatric subpopulations were significantly associated with low total testosterone and low free androgen indices, including injection drug use, hepatitis C virus (HCV) infection, high body

mass index (BMI), and use of psychotropic medications. High viral load (>10,000) correlated with low total testosterone levels (<200 ng/dl). Low testosterone was associated with typical symptoms of low libido, difficulty sleeping, loss of concentration, impaired memory, poorer subjective health, and other symptoms of depression.

Many of the early studies suggested that decreases in testosterone were related to stage of HIV illness or CD4 count, with hypogonadism following later than the earlier lowering of adrenal androgens seen in HIV infection. In one study, testosterone was decreased only in HIV patients with advanced infection, in contrast to DHEA and DHEA-S, which were significantly decreased at all stages of infection (Villette et al., 1990). In a prospective study of 98 patients with various stages of infection, 29% of men with AIDS had hypotestosteronemia, assessed by total testosterone levels (Raffi et al., 1991). Deficiency was correlated with the degree of illness, including weight loss and low CD4+ cell count. In another study of clinically asymptomatic HIV-positive homosexual men, total testosterone was decreased only in patients with CD4 levels less than 200 (Laudat et al., 1995). Testosterone not bound to sex hormone–binding globulin (SHBG) was decreased in all groups and correlated with CD4 cell count, supporting the idea that hypogonadism worsens as CD4 lymphocytes decrease.

The prevalence of hypogonadism is felt to be lower but still significant in the era of HAART. More recent studies have failed to demonstrate an association with CD4 cell count or HIV viral load (Grinspoon et al., 1996; Rietschel et al., 2000). In one study of patients with HIV-associated wasting, most of whom were receiving HAART, free testosterone levels were low in 19% of patients with AIDS wasting (81% of whom complained of decreased libido) (Rietschel et al., 2000). Other HAART era studies have similarly demonstrated approximately 20% rates of hypogonadism (Crum et al., 2005).

Elevated levels of SHBG are commonly seen in all stages of HIV infection and can affect total testosterone levels (Laudat et al., 1995). In one study, HIV-positive patients had sex steroid–binding protein concentrations 39%–51% above those of controls (Martin et al., 1992). In the Rietschel study, the mean total testosterone was actually greater than that of healthy control subjects, which may be explained by the observed increase in levels of SHBG. This highlights the importance of correctly assessing for hypotestosteronemia; most clinicians agree that bioavailable or free testosterone is the best laboratory measure of androgen deficiency (Mylonakis et al., 2001).

The relationship between weight loss or wasting and hypogonadism remains unclear, with relevant studies yielding inconsistent results. Grinspoon and others (1996) demonstrated that loss of lean body and muscle mass as well as functional decline in exercise capacity correlate with androgen levels in hypogonadal men with AIDS-associated wasting. In another study, serum testosterone and free testosterone correlated with weight change (Arver et al., 1999). Dobs and others (1996) found that testosterone levels declined early in the course of HIV infection with weight loss that eventually led to wasting. Rietschel and others (2000), in contrast, found that hypogonadism was not associated with weight.

Most cases of androgen deficiency in patients with HIV result from secondary hypogonadism (pituitary or hypothalamic failure), with reduced or inappropriately normal gonadotropin levels despite low testosterone levels. This may be due to effects of severe illness on the hypothalamic–pituitary–gonadal (HPG) axis, or to associated infections or malignancies compromising pituitary or hypothalamic function. In these cases, other markers of pituitary function including TSH and prolactin should be tested, with any abnormal findings prompting MRI evaluation of the hypothalamus and pituitary.

Other cases of hypogonadism in HIV infection are primary, approximately 20% in one survey (Arver et al., 1999), caused by abnormal production of testosterone by testicular Leydig cells. This may be due to associated opportunistic infections, malignancies of the testes, or cytokine-related decreased testicular functioning (Mylonakis et al., 2000; Crum et al., 2005). Shifting of adrenal steroids from androgen production to cortisol, as described earlier, can also contribute to decreased levels of testosterone.

In many studies, infectious and other pathologic changes in the testes were demonstrated in patients with HIV, as well as decreased spermatogenesis. Testicular pathologic changes and functioning of the HPG axis were assessed in a study of 84 homosexual men, 56 with HIV infection (Salehian et al., 1999). While testosterone, luteinizing hormone (LH), and follicle-stimulating hormone (FSH) were similar among all patients at baseline, testosterone significantly decreased during the 4-year study period only in the HIV-positive group. This group was further divided into progressors (to AIDS) and nonprogressors, with only the former demonstrating increases in LH and FSH. Forty-eight percent of patients with AIDS had hypogonadism, and all five AIDS patients on whom autopsy was performed had wall thickening of the seminiferous tubules and decreased spermatogenesis.

Breast enlargement due to true gynecomastia, the proliferation of glandular ducts and periductal stroma in men, occurs in approximately 1% of adult men in the general population, although male breast enlargement involving fat tissue is more common. There have been few large studies of gynecomastia in men with HIV. One recent study evaluated 2275 patients for breast enlargement at HIV referral centers, finding 40 (1.8%) with sonographically confirmed gynecomastia (Biglia et al., 2004). When compared with matched HIV-positive controls, gynecomastia was independently associated with hypogonadism (as well as with lipoatrophy and hepatitis C).

There have been inconsistent reports linking hypogonadism with antiretroviral therapy. One study found HAART to be associated with low libido, erectile dysfunction (ED), and increased estradiol levels in HIV-infected men (Lamba et al., 2004). HIV-negative or unknown-status gay and bisexual men were compared to a group of HIV-infected men. An increased incidence of low libido (48%) and ED (25%) was found in those on HAART compared to that in HIV-infected men not taking HAART (26% for each) and in the control group (2% and 10%, respectively). Other studies, however, have failed to demonstrate any association with antiretroviral treatment. In one study of patients with HIV, most of whom were receiving HAART, free testosterone levels were low in 19% of patients with AIDS wasting, 81% of whom complained of decreased libido (Rietschel et al., 2000). There was no association with weight, CD4 count, or any class of antiviral medications.

Besides antiretrovirals, other medications commonly used by patients with HIV might have an impact on the HPG axis. Ketoconazole inhibits gonadal production of steroids. Megestrol acetate (a progestational agent), glucocorticoids, and anabolic steroids can all reduce secretion of gonadotropins (Mylonakis et al., 2001). Antipsychotics can elevate prolactin to varying degrees. Patients on methadone replacement (and those using heroin) have been found to have lower gonadotropin and testosterone levels (Celani et al., 1984).

There are many available forms of testosterone replacement today, including intramuscular injection, transdermal patch, and gel. Injections of depot forms are commonly used for androgen replacement but are complicated by the difficulty of achieving steady states. Peak supraphysiological testosterone levels occur in the first day or two after injection, in some cases adversely affecting mood (Mylonakis et al., 2001), while levels may decline to subtherapeutic levels before the next injection.

The patch and gel forms of testosterone replacement have become more popular and are generally thought to be equally effective, although some data indicate lower efficacy for symptomatic HIV-associated hypogonadism. One multicenter, randomized, double-blind, placebo-controlled trial demonstrated that while hypogonadal men with AIDS and weight loss were able to correct testosterone levels by using a transscrotal testosterone patch, this method of replacement did not improve weight or quality of life (Dobs et al., 1999). The patch can be associated with dermatologic reactions, while the gel is usually well tolerated. In general, testosterone supplementation is fairly safe but should be avoided in patients with polycythemia or prostate cancer and used cautiously in patients with prostrate enlargement.

Hypogonadism in Women with HIV

Hypogonadism in women with HIV has been much less well studied. Amenorrhea has been observed in up to 20% of women with HIV, with increased prevalence of 38% in women with AIDS wasting (Grinspoon et al., 1997). Testosterone circulates at levels approximately 10% of that in men, half produced from the ovaries and half from the adrenal glands. Ideally, androgen levels should be measured during the early follicular phase, but normal ranges have not been well standardized (Mylonakis et al., 2001). Limited studies have indicated hypoandrogenic states to be present in women with HIV at similar rates to those observed in men, with a similar pattern of increased SHBG levels. Total and free testosterone levels are significantly lower in HIV-infected women than those in healthy controls, with approximately 58% scoring below the normal tenth percentile (Sinha-Hikim et al., 1998). In contrast to men with AIDS wasting, women lose fat mass disproportionately to lean mass (Grinspoon et al., 1997).

One study of ovarian and adrenal function in 13 HIV-infected women with wasting demonstrated significantly lower baseline levels of testosterone, free

testosterone, adrostenedione, DHEA, and DHEA-S when matched with healthy controls (Grinspoon et al., 2001). ACTH stimulation resulted in increased cortisol response and decreased DHEA response. DHEA-to-cortisol ratios correlated with CD4 count. This finding supports a similar shunting mechanism of adrenal steroid metabolism observed in men. In contrast to decreased adrenal production of steroids, ovarian androgen responsivity to hCG stimulation was intact in this population of HIV-positive women (Grinspoon et al., 2001).

Treatment options for hypogonadism in women are still limited. Oral contraceptives or isolated estrogen or progesterone preparations have traditionally been used for replacement. A pilot study for a transdermal test of testosterone replacement in women showed promising results, but more research is needed (Miller et al., 1998).

Psychosocial Implications

The diagnosis of hypogonadism can present a challenge, as many symptoms are nonspecific and overlap with those of depression or chronic illness. These include fatigue, decreased energy, depressed affect, and poor self-image (Mylonakis et al., 2001). More specific symptoms can include decreased male-pattern hair, testicular atrophy, decreased libido, and gynecomastia (Crum et al., 2005). In some early studies of antidepressants for the treatment of depression in men with HIV, patients reported improved mood but residual diminished libido and low energy. Since then, considerable evidence has amassed supporting the beneficial effect of testosterone supplementation on mood and energy level in patients with HIV and depression.

Many studies have documented the positive effects of testosterone replacement on mood in non-HIV populations with hypogonadism. Wang and others (2000) demonstrated that a transdermal testosterone gel treatment improved sexual function and mood parameters, increased lean body mass, and decreased fat mass in hypogonadal men, with mood improvement sustained during a 36-month follow-up study (Wang et al., 2004).

Several studies have yielded similar findings in HIV-positive patients. Grinspoon and others (2000) found that hypogonadal patients with HIV scored significantly higher on the Beck Depression Inventory, with an inverse correlation between Beck score and both free and total testosterone levels, even when controlling for weight, viral load, CD4 count, and antidepressant use. With testosterone supplementation Beck scores decreased significantly compared to control scores. Rabkin and others (2000) investigated testosterone therapy for HIV patients with hypogonadal symptoms of low libido, depressed mood, low energy, and decreased muscle mass in a double-blind, placebo-controlled trial, finding improved libido in 74% of testosterone-treated patients, in contrast with 19% of placebo-treated patients. Of completers with fatigue at baseline, 59% of testosterone-treated patients and 25% of those receiving placebo reported improved energy; of completers with depression at baseline, 58% of the treated group and 14% of the placebo group reported improved mood. Improvements were maintained for up to 18 weeks during a subsequent open-label treatment phase.

Other studies have demonstrated the benefits of testosterone for fatigue in HIV-positive patients. In a double-blind, placebo-controlled study of testosterone versus fluoxetine in HIV/AIDS patients with Axis I mood disorders, testosterone was superior to both fluoxetine and placebo in improving fatigue (Rabkin et al., 2004). Wagner and others (1998) assessed the effects of biweekly intramuscular injections of testosterone on fatigue in an open 12-week trial of 72 HIV-positive men with low libido and at least one associated symptom of depressed mood, fatigue, or weight loss. In this study, 79% of completers responded favorably with increased energy levels and quality of life scores. Of the 26 patients who completed the study and had depression at baseline, 62% reported improvement in both mood and energy (while 31% reported no improvement in either).

BONE AND MINERAL METABOLISM IN HIV INFECTION

Prevalence and Pathophysiology of Bone Disease

In recent years, an extensive body of literature has emerged demonstrating the high prevalence of changes in bone and mineral metabolism in patients with HIV. These are likely due to multiple etiologies, including direct interactions of the virus with bone and marrow cells, as well as indirect effects through immune system activation and altered cytokine production. Increased levels of cytokines such as tumor necrosis factor and IL-6 are associated with osteoclast activation and thus bone resorption. Associated illness and adverse effects of drugs used to treat HIV may also contribute to altered bone metabolism. Decreased physical activity, hypogonadism, and malabsorption of calcium and vitamin D, all common in patients with HIV infection, might additionally lead to decreases in bone mineral density (BMD). In the subpopulation of HIV patients who are on methadone or using heroin, effects may be more pronounced, as opiates can contribute to lowered BMD (Pedrazzoni et al., 1993).

Paton and others first demonstrated such decreases in BMD in HIV patients, although in this study significant differences from those in control subjects were minimal (Paton et al., 1997). Since then, many studies have shown a higher prevalence of osteopenia and osteoporosis in patients with HIV compared to control subjects, with rates ranging from 46% (Mondy et al., 2003) to 89% (Knobel et al., 2001). Many of these studies differentiate between more mild *osteopenia*, with rates ranging from 44% to 68%, and *osteoporosis*, with observed rates ranging from 3% to 21% (Tebas et al., 2000; Carr et al., 2001; Knobel et al., 2001; Gold et al., 2002; Amiel et al., 2004). Most of these studies focus on men with HIV, but a few have examined bone density in women. One large study found a similar high prevalence of low BMD in women with HIV, 62% and 14% with osteopenia and osteoporosis, respectively (Teichmann et al., 2003).

Many factors have been postulated to cause lowered BMD and have been examined in various studies. Decreased weight and BMI, observed in many patients with HIV, have been shown to reliably correlate with low BMD (Knobel et al., 2001; Gold et al., 2002; Mondy et al., 2003; Amiel et al., 2004), including a history of significant weight loss or severe wasting (Mondy et al., 2003) and lower weight prior to starting HAART (Carr et al., 2001). Studies have yielded conflicting data on the relationship between length of disease or severity of HIV and osteopenia. Some studies have failed to demonstrate an association of BMD with CD4 count, viral load, or duration of disease (Knobel et al., 2001; Teichmann et al., 2003). Other studies have shown a significant association between duration of infection and reduced BMD (Gold et al., 2002; Bruera et al., 2003; Mondy et al., 2003), and one longitudinal study demonstrated that as CD4 counts improved, BMD actually increased (Mondy et al., 2003).

Increased production of lactate (Carr et al., 2001) and an uncoupling of bone resorption and formation (Amiel et al., 2004) have also been suggested to contribute to lowered BMD. This latter mechanism was noted in one study in which bone resorption was increased and bone formation decreased in HIV patients (Aukrust et al., 1999). There were similar findings in another study demonstrating decreased formation markers and increased bone resorption markers in HIV patients (Teichmann et al., 2000).

Irregularities in vitamin D metabolism, parathyroid hormone (PTH), and calcium have also been examined. Dysfunction of the PTH axis in patients with HIV has been described, including reports of impaired PTH release, possibly mechanistically related to a common protein in PTH cells and CD4 cells (Hellman et al., 1994). Hypocalcemia when observed in HIV patients is usually mild, although severe hypocalcemia can be associated with medications, for example, foscarnet (used to treat CMV) (Thomas and Doherty, 2003). Associated infections and malignancies may result in hypercalcemia in a small percentage of cases.

A recent study demonstrated vitamin D deficiency in 86% of HIV patients (Garcia Aparicio et al., 2006). Some studies have shown decreased PTH and decreased 1,25-hydroxyvitamin D levels compared to those in healthy age-matched controls, in addition to increased urinary calcium and decreased serum osteocalcin (Teichman et al., 2003). In a more recent study, while 1,25-hydroxyvitamin D was significantly decreased in the HIV group, there were no significant differences in 25-hydroxyvitamin D, PTH, calcium, osteocalcin, or phosphorus (Dolan et al., 2004). This finding supports a previous hypothesis that a specific defect in the hydroxylation of 1-α-vitamin D to the more bioactive 1,25 form contributes to the vitamin D deficiency observed in HIV patients (Haug et al., 1998). Some investigators have suggested this to be a possible treatment effect of protease inhibitors (PIs), with in vitro demonstrations of PIs inhibiting α-1-hydroxylation of vitamin D (Cozzolino et al., 2003). The clinical significance of such data must be questioned, however, in view of the extensive literature failing to demonstrate an association with HAART (see below).

Earlier studies indicated that altered BMD observed in patients with HIV might result partially from treatment effects, with particular implication of PIs and nonnucleoside reverse transcription inhibitors (NNRTIs). Tebas and others (2000) found increased

rates of osteoporosis (21%) in HIV patients on HAART including a PI, compared to HIV-positive patients not receiving a PI (11%) and HIV-negative controls (6%). Since then, however, multiple further studies have failed to show specific associations with treatment (Bruera et al., 2003; Amiel et al., 2004; Garcia Aparicio et al., 2006). Knobel and others (2001) found no association with the use of any type of HAART or duration of treatment, and other studies have similarly demonstrated a lack of association between osteopenia and any antiretroviral class (Carr et al., 2001; Mondy et al., 2003). Gold and others (2002) failed to find an effect of PIs on BMD, and one study demonstrated an increase of BMD in patients treated with indinavir (Nolan et al., 2001). Similarly, in the longitudinal follow-up component of Mondy's study, BMD increased with HAART, correlating with improved CD4 counts.

Several studies have indicated the efficacy of bisphosphonates for the treatment of osteopenia and osteoporosis in the HIV population. Appropriate calcium and vitamin D supplementation should be provided as well. In an open-label randomized pilot trial of alendronate plus calcium and vitamin D in HIV-infected persons on HAART with osteopenia or osteoporosis, lumbar spine BMD was increased at 48 weeks compared to that in subjects given vitamin D and calcium alone (Mondy et al., 2005). This is in keeping with findings of previous studies (Guaraldi et al., 2004). The convenience of once-weekly dosing of alendronate may appeal to patients. An open-label randomized study demonstrated significant reduction of osteoporosis after 96 weeks, from 96% in controls (receiving dietary counseling only) to 27% in patients receiving weekly alendronate (plus dietary counseling) (Negredo et al., 2005). Interestingly, improved BMD was seen in the lumbar spine in the first year and in the femur during the second year, highlighting the importance of long-term treatment. Recent studies, however, have raised the specter of risks of osteonecrosis of the jaw in association with bisphosphonate use (Woo et al., 2006). Further research will be important to determine the safety and efficacy of treatment modalities for osteoporosis.

Psychosocial Implications

Kumano (2005) recently described three hypothetical relationships between stress and osteoporosis. Stress might induce specific physiologic changes that cause or exacerbate a lowering of BMD and might additionally cause behavioral changes that affect eating, exercise, and sleep habits, thus impacting bone health. Osteoporosis and associated health consequences can cause anxiety, depression, loss of social roles and functioning, and isolation and thus increase stress itself. It is unclear to what extent data bear out each of these relationships in patients with HIV.

Mood disorders such as major depression, in some cases associated with high levels of cortisol, have been reported to increase the risk of developing osteoporosis. One study examined psychoaffective and psychodynamic aspects in patients with osteoporosis, finding increased rates of anxiety, depression, and alexithymia (Zonis De Zukerfeld et al., 2003). There was also association of osteoporosis with early traumatic life events, decreased support networks, and lower reported quality of life. Both psychosocial support and specific intervention programs can improve independence and the quality of life in patients with osteoporosis (Bayles et al., 2000). There is a paucity of literature specifically addressing the psychosocial implications of osteoporosis in patients with HIV.

CONCLUSION

A wide range of endocrine abnormalities commonly accompany and complicate HIV infection, many of which have implications for psychiatrists and other mental health professionals working with this population. Such changes can include decreased thyroid function, adrenal insufficiency, hypercortisolism, hypogonadism, and decreased bone mineral density. Because many new HIV infections occur in intravenous drug users, it should be borne in mind that abuse of substances, and opiates in particular, can itself cause endocrine dysfunction contributing to or mimicking effects seen with HIV infection (Cooper et al., 2003).

These illnesses may cause considerable suffering and impact a patient's quality of life. Endocrinopathies are great mimickers of psychiatric disorders, manifesting in some cases as disturbance of mood, sleep, appetite, thought process, energy level, or general sense of well-being. Endocrinopathies may present insidiously or abruptly, in either case with potentially tragic consequences when misdiagnosed as psychopathology. Prompt recognition of reversible alterations in endocrine function is essential to prevent unnecessary morbidity and mortality. An understanding of the complex interactions between endocrine and psychological systems may improve recognition and treatment of endocrinopathies, diminish suffering, and enhance quality of life and longevity in persons with HIV and AIDS.

References

Amiel C, Ostertag A, Slama L, Baudoin C, N'Guyen T, Lajeunie E, Neit-Ngeilh L, Rozenbaum W, and De Vernejoul MC (2004). BMD is reduced in HIV-infected men irrespective of treatment. *J Bone Mineral Res* 19(3):402–409.

Antoni MH, Cruess S, Cruess DG, Kumar M, Lutgendorf S, Ironson G, Dettmer E, Williams J, Klimas N, Fletcher MA, and Schneiderman N (2000a). Cognitive-behavioral stress management reduces distress and 24-hour urinary free cortisol output among symptomatic HIV-infected gay men. *Ann Behav Med* 22(1):29–37.

Antoni MH, Cruess S, Lutgendorf S, Kumar M, Ironson G, Klimas N, Fletcher MA, and Schneiderman N (2000b). Cognitive-behavioral stress management intervention effects on anxiety, 24-hr urinary norepinephrine output, and T-cytotoxic/suppressor cells over time among sympomatic HIV-infected gay men. *J Consult Clin Psychol* 68(1):31–45.

Antoni MH, Cruess DG, Klimas N, Maher K, Cruess S, Kumar M, Lutgendorf S, Ironson G, Schneiderman N, and Fletcher MA (2002). Stress management and immune system reconstitution in symptomatic HIV-infected gay men over time: effects on transitional naive T cells (CD4(+)CD45RA(+)CD29(+)). *Am J Psychiatry* 159(1):143–145.

Antoni MH, Cruess DG, Klimas N, Carrico AW, Maher K, Cruess S, Lechner SC, Kumar M, Lutgendorf S, Ironson G, Fletcher MA, and Schneiderman N (2005). Increases in a marker of immune system reconstitution are predated by decreases in 24-h urinary cortisol output and depressed mood during a 10-week stress management intervention in symptomatic HIV-infected men. *J Pscyhosom Res* 58:3–13.

Arlt W, Callies F, van Vlijmen JC, Koehler I, Reincke M, Bidlingmaier M, Huebler D, Oettel M, Ernst M, Schulte HM, and Allolio B (1999). Dehydroepiandrosterone replacement in women with adrenal insufficiency. *N Engl J Med* 341(14):1013–1020.

Arver S, Sinha-Hikim I, Beall G, Guerrero M, Shen R, and Bhasin S (1999). Serum dihydrotestosterone and testosterone concentrations in human immunodeficiency virus–infected men with and without weight loss. *J Androl* 20(5):611–618.

Aukrust P, Haug CJ, Ueland T, Lien E, Muller F, Espevik T, Bollerslev J, and Froland SS (1999). Decreased bone formative and enhanced resorptive markers in human immunodeficiency virus infection: indication of normalization of the bone-remodeling process during highly active antiretroviral therapy. *J Clin Endocrinol Metab* 84(1):145–150.

Azar ST, and Melby JC (1993). Hypothalamic-pituitary-adrenal function in non-AIDS patients with advanced HIV infection. *Am J Med Sci* 305(5):321–325.

Barrett-Connor E, von Muhlen D, Laughlin GA, and Kripke A (1999). Endogenous levels of dehydroepiandrosterone sulfate, but not other sex hormones, are associated with depressed mood in older women: the Rancho Bernardo Study. *J Am Geriatr Soc* 47(6): 685–691.

Battan R, Mariuz P, Raviglione MC, Sabatini MT, Mullen MP, and Poretsky L (1991). *Pneumocystis carinii* infection of the thyroid in a hypothyroid patient with AIDS: diagnosis by fine needle aspiration biopsy. *J Clin Endocrinol Metab* 72(3):724–726.

Bauer M, Szuba MP, and Whybrow PC (2003). Psychiatric and behavioral manifestations of hyperthyroidism and hypothyroidism. In OM Wolkowitz and AJ Rothschild (eds.), *Psychoneuroendocrinology: The Scientific Basis of Clinical Practice* (pp. 419–444). Arlington VA: American Psychiatric Publishing.

Bayles CM, Cochran K, and Anderson C (2000). The psychosocial aspects of osteoporosis in women. *Nurs Clin North Am* 35(1):279–286.

Beltran S, Lescure FX, Desailloud R, Douadi Y, Smail A, El Esper I, Arlot S, Schmit JL; Thyroid and VIH Group (2003). Increased prevalence of hypothyroidism among human immunodeficiency virus–infected patients: a need for screening. *Clin Infect Dis* 37:579–583.

Berr C, Lafont S, Debuire B, Dartigues JF, and Baulieu EE (1996). Relationships of dehydroepiandrosterone sulfate in the elderly with functional, psychological, and mental status, and short-term mortality: a French community-based study. *Proc Natl Acad Sci U S A* 93(23):13410–13415.

Bhansali A, Dash RJ, Sud A, Bhadada S, Sehgal S, and Sharma BR (2000). A preliminary report on basal and stimulated plasma cortisol in patients with acquired immunodeficiency syndrome. *Indian J Med Res* 11:173–177.

Bhasin S, Singh AB, and Javanbakht M (2001). Neuroendocrine abnormalities associated with HIV infection. *Endocrinol Metab Clin North Am* 30(3):749–764.

Biglia A, Blanco JL, Martinez E, Domingo P, Casamitjana R, Sambeat M, Milinkovic A, Garcia M, Laguno M, Leon A, Larrousse M, Lonca M, Mallolas J, and Gatell JM (2004). Gynecomastia among HIV-infected patients is associated with hypogonadism: a case–control study. *Clin Infect Dis* 39:1514–1519.

Biglino A, Limone P, Forno B, Pollona A, Cariti G, Molinatti GM, and Gioannini P (1995). Altered adrenocorticotropin and cortisol response to corticotropin-releasing hormone in HIV-1 infection. *Eur J Endocrinol* 133(2):173–179.

Bruera D, Luna N, David DO, Bergoglio LM, and Zamudio J (2003). Decreased bone mineral density in HIV-infected patients is independent of antiretroviral therapy. *AIDS* 17(13):1917–1923.

Cami J, Gilabert M, San L, and de la Torre R (1992). Hypercortisolism after opioid discontinuation in rapid detoxification of heroin addicts. *Br J Addict* 87(8):1145–1151.

Carr A, Miller J, Eisman JA, and Cooper DA (2001). Osteopenia in HIV-infected men: association with asymptomatic lactic acidemia and lower weight pre-antiretroviral therapy. *AIDS* 15(6):703–709.

Celani MF, Carani C, Montanini V, Baraghini GF, Zini D, Simoni M, Ferretti C, and Marrama P (1984). Further studies on the effects of heroin addiction on the hypothalamic-pituitary-gonadal function in man. *Pharmacol Res Commun* 16(12): 1193–1203.

Chen F, Day SL, Metcalfe RA, Sethi G, Kapembwa MS, Brook MG, Churchill D, de Ruiter A, Robinson S, Lacey CJ, and Weetman AP (2005). Characteristics of autoimmune thyroid disease occurring as a late complication of immune reconstitution in patients with advanced human immunodeficiency virus (HIV) disease. *Medicine* 84(2):98–106.

Christeff N, Gherbi N, Mammes O, Dalle MT, Gharakhanian S, Lortholary O, Melchior JC, and Nunez EA (1997). Serum cortisol and DHEA concentrations during HIV infection. *Psychoneuroendocrinology* 22(Suppl. 1):S11–S118.

Clerici M, Trabattoni D, Piconi S, Fusi ML, Ruzzante S, Clerici C, and Villa ML (1997). A possible role for the cortisol/anticortisols imbalance in the progression of human immunodeficiency virus. *Psychoneuroendocrinology* 22(Suppl. 1):S27–S31.

Cooper OB, Brown TT, Dobs AS (2003). Opiate drug use: a potential contributor to the endocrine and metabolic complications in human immunodeficiency virus disease. *Clin Infect Dis* 37(Suppl 2): S132–S136.

Cozzolino M, Vidal M, Arcidiacono MV, Tebas P, Yarasheski KE, and Dusso AS (2003). HIV-protease inhibitors impair vitamin D bioactivation to 1,25-dihydroxyvitamin D. *AIDS* 17(4):513–520.

Crum NF, Furtek KJ, Olson PE, Amling CL, and Wallace MR (2005). A review of hypogonadism and erectile dysfunction among HIV-infected men during the pre- and post-HAART ears: diagnosis, pathogenesis, and management. *AIDS Patient Care STDS* 19(10):655–671.

Derry DM (1995). Thyroid therapy in HIV-infected patients. *Med Hypotheses* 45(2):121–124.

Dobs AS, Dempsey MA, Ladenson PW, and Polk BF (1988). Endocrine disorders in men infected with human immunodeficiency virus. *Am J Med* 84(3 Pt. 2):611–616.

Dobs AS, Few WL 3rd, Blackman MR, Harman SM, Hoover DR, and Graham NM (1996). Serum hormones in men with human immunodeficiency virus–associated wasting. *J Clin Endocrinol Metab* 81(11):4108–4112.

Dobs AS, Cofrancesco J, Nolten WE, Danoff A, Anderson R, Hamilton CD, Feinberg J, Seekins D,

Yangco B, and Rhame F (1999). The use of a trans-scrotal testosterone delivery system in the treatment of patients with weight loss related to human immunodeficiency virus infection. *Am J Med* 107(2): 126–132.

Dolan SE, Huang JS, Killilea KM, Sullivan MP, Aliabadi N, and Grinspoon S (2004). Reduced bone density in HIV-infected women. *AIDS* 18(3):475–483.

Drucker DJ, Bailey D, and Rotstein L (1990). Thyroiditis as the presenting manifestation of disseminated extrapulmonary *Pneumocystis carinii* infection. *J Clin Endocrinol Metab* 71(6):1663–1665.

Duch FM, Repele CA, Spadaro F, dos Reis MA, Rodrigues DB, Ferraz ML, and Teixeira Vde P (1998). Adrenal gland morphological alterations in the acquired immunodeficiency syndrome. *Rev Soc Bras Med Trop* 31(3):257–261.

Eledrisi MS, and Verghese AC (2001). Adrenal insufficiency in HIV infection: a review and recommendations. *Am J Med Sci* 321(2):137–144.

Findling JW, Buggy BP, Gilson IH, Brummitt CF, Bernstein BM, and Raff H (1994). Longitudinal evaluation of adrenocortical function in patients infected with the human immunodeficiency virus. *J Clin Endocrinol Metab* 79(4):1091–1096.

Fradley M, Liu J, and Atta MG (2005). Primary aldosteronism with HIV infection: important considerations when using the aldosterone:renin ratio to screen this unique population. *Am J Ther* 12(4): 368–374.

Frank TS, LiVolsi VA, and Connor AM (1987). Cytomegalovirus infection of the thyroid in immunocompromised adults. *Yale J Biol Med* 60(1):1–8.

Garcia Aparicio AM, Munoz Fernandez S, Gonzalez J, Arribas JR, Pena JM, Vazquez JJ, Martinez ME, Coya J, and Martin Mola E (2006). Abnormalities in the bone mineral metabolism in HIV-infected patients. *Clin Rheumatol* 25(4):537–539.

Gilquin J, Viard JP, Jubault V, Sert C, and Kazatchkine MD (1998). Delayed occurrence of Graves' disease after immune restoration with HAART. Highly active antiretroviral therapy. *Lancet* 352(9144):1907–1908.

Glasgow BJ, Steinsapir KD, Anders K, and Layfield LJ (1985). Adrenal pathology in the acquired immune deficiency syndrome. *Am J Clin Pathol* 84(5):594–597.

Gold J, Pocock N, and Li Y (2002). Bone mineral density abnormalities in patients with HIV infection. *J Acquir Immune Defic Syndr* 30(1):131–132.

Gonzalez-Gonzalez JG, de la Garza-Hernandez NE, Garza-Moran RA, Rivera-Morales IM, Montes-Villarreal J, Valenzuela-Rendon J, and Villarreal-Perez JZ (2001). Prevalence of abnormal adrenocortical function in HIV infection by low-dose cosyntropin test. *Int J STD AIDS* 12(12):804–810.

Grinspoon S, Corcoran C, Lee K, Burrows B, Hubbard J, Katznelson L, Walsh M, Guccione A, Cannan J, Heller H, Basgoz N, and Klibanski A (1996). Loss of lean body and muscle mass correlates with androgen levels in hypogonadal men with acquired immunodeficiency syndrome and wasting. *J Clin Endocrinol Metab* 81(11):4051–4058.

Grinspoon S, Corcoran C, Miller K, Biller BM, Askari H, Wang E, Hubbard J, Anderson EJ, Basgoz N, Heller HM, and Klibanski A (1997). Body composition and endocrine function in women with acquired immunodeficiency syndrome wasting. *J Clin Endocrinol Metab* 82(5):1332–1337.

Grinspoon S, Corcoran C, Stanley T, Baaj A, Basgoz N, and Klibanski A (2000). Effects of hypogonadism and testosterone administration on depression indices in HIV-infected men. *J Clin Endocrinol Metab* 85:60–65.

Grinspoon S, Corcoran C, Stanley T, Rabe J, and Wilkie S (2001). Mechanisms of androgen deficiency in human immunodeficiency virus–infected women with the wasting syndrome. *J Clin Endocrinol Metabol* 86(9):4120–4126.

Grunfeld C, Pang M, Doerrler W, Jensen P, Shimizu L, Feingold KR, and Cavalieri RR (1993). Indices of thyroid function and weight loss in human immunodeficiency virus infection and the acquired immunodeficiency syndrome. *Metabolism* 42(10): 1270–1276.

Guaraldi G, Orlando G, Madeddu G, Vescini F, Ventura P, Campostrini S, Mura MS, Parise N, Caudarella R, and Esposito R (2004). Alendronate reduces bone resorption in HIV-associated osteopenia/osteoporosis. *HIV Clin Trials* 5(5):269–277.

Guttler R, Singer PA, Axline SG, Greaves TS, and McGill JJ (1993). *Pneumocystis carinii* thyroiditis. Report of three cases and review of the literature. *Arch Intern Med* 153(3):393–396.

Haug CJ, Aukrust P, Haug E, Morkrid L, Muller F, and Froland SS (1998). Severe deficiency of 1,25-dihydroxyvitamin D3 in human immunodeficiency virus infection: association with immunological hyperactivity and only minor changes in calcium homeostasis. *J Clin Endocrinol Metab* 83(11):3832–3838.

Hellman P, Albert J, Gidlund M, Klareskog L, Rastad J, Akerstrom G, and Juhlin C (1994). Impaired parathyroid hormone release in human immunodeficiency virus infection. *AIDS Res Hum Retroviruses* 10(4):391–394.

Hommes MJ, Romijn JA, Endert E, Adriaanse R, Brabant G, Eeftinck Schattenkerk JK, Wiersinga WM, and Sauerwein HP (1993). Hypothyroid-like regulation of the pituitary-thyroid axis in stable human immunodeficiency virus infection. *Metabolism* 42(5):556–561.

Hoshino Y, Yamashita N, Nakamura T, and Iwamoto A (2002). Prospective examination of adrenocortical function in advanced AIDS patients. *Endocr J* 49(6): 641–647.

Hunt PJ, Gurnell EM, Huppert FA, Richards C, Prevost AT, Wass JA, Herbert J, and Chatterjee VK (2000).

Improvement in mood and fatigue after dehydroe-piandrosterone replacement in Addison's disease in a randomized, double blind trial. *J Clin Endocrinol Metab* 85(12):4650–4656.

Jubault V, Penfornis A, Schillo F, Hoen B, Izembart M, Timsit J, Kazatchkine MD, Gilquin J, and Viard JP (2000). Sequential occurrence of thyroid autoanti-bodies and Grave's disease after immune restoration in severely immunocompromised human immuno-deficiency virus-1-infected patients. *J Clin Endocri-nol Metab* 85:4254–4257.

Klein RS, Yungtai L, Santoro N, and Dobs AS (2005). Androgen levels in older men who have or who are at risk of acquiring HIV infection. *Clin Infect Dis* 41:1794–1803.

Knobel H, Guelar A, Vallecillo G, Nogues X, and Diez A (2001). Osteopenia in HIV-infected patients: is it the disease or is it the treatment? *AIDS* 15(6):807–808.

Koutkia P, Mylonakis E, and Levin RM (2002). Human immunodeficiency virus infection and the thyroid. *Thyroid* 12(7):577–582.

Krauth PH, and Katz JF (1987). Kaposi's sarcoma involving the thyroid in a patient with AIDS. *Clin Nucl Med* 12(11):848–849.

Kumano H (2005). Osteoporosis and stress. *Clin Calcium* 15(9):1544–1547.

Lambert M (1994). Thyroid dysfunction in HIV infec-tion. *Baillieres Clin Endocrinol Metab* 8(4):825–835.

Lamda H, Goldmeier D, Mackie NE, and Scullard G (2004). Antiretroviral therapy is associated with sex-ual dysfnction and with increased serum oestradiol levels in men. *Int J STD AIDS* 15:234–237.

Laudat A, Blum L, Guechot J, Picard O, Cabane J, Imbert JC, and Giboudeau J (1995). Changes in systemic gonadal and adrenal steroids in asymptom-atic human immunodeficiency virus–infected men: relationship with the CD4 cell counts. *Eur J Endo-crinol* 133(4):418–424.

Laulund S, Visfeldt J, and Klinken L (1986). Patho-anatomical studies in patients dying of AIDS. *Acta Pathol Microbiol Immunol Scand* A 94(3):201–221.

Lortholary O, Christeff N, Casassus P, Thobie N, Veyssier P, Trogoff B, Torri O, Brauner M, Nunez EA, and Guillevin L (1996). Hypothalamo-pituitary-adrenal function in human immunodeficiency virus–infected men. *J Clin Endocrinol Metab* 81(2):791–796.

Marik PE, Kiminoyo K, and Zaloga GP (2002). Adrenal insufficiency in critically ill patients with human immunodeficiency virus. *Crit Care Med* 30(6):1267–1273.

Martin ME, Benassayag C, Amiel C, Canton P, and Nunez EA (1992). Alterations in the concentra-tions and binding properties of sex steroid binding protein and corticosteroid-binding globulin in HIV+ patients. *J Endocrinol Invest* 15(8):597–603.

Mayo J, Collazos J, Martinez E, and Ibarra S (2002). Adrenal function in the human immunodeficiency virus–infected patient. *Arch Intern Med* 162(10):1095–1098.

McCarty M, Coker R, and Claydon E (1992). Case report: disseminated *Pneumocystis carinii* infection in a patient with the acquired immune deficiency syndrome causing thyroid gland calcification and hypothyroidism. *Clin Radiol* 45(3):209–210.

Membreno L, Irony I, Dere W, Klein R, Biglieri EG, and Cobb E (1987). Adrenocortical function in ac-quired immunodeficiency syndrome. *J Clin Endo-crinol Metab* 65(3):482–487.

Merenich JA, McDermott MT, Asp AA, Harrison SM, and Kidd GS (1990). Evidence of endocrine in-volvement early in the course of human immuno-deficiency virus infection. *J Clin Endocrinol Metab* 70(3):566–571.

Michael A, Jenaway A, Paykel ES, and Herbert J (2000). Altered salivary dehydroepiandrosterone levels in major depression in adults. *Biol Psychiatry* 48(10):989–995.

Miller K, Corcoran C, Armstrong C, Caramelli K, Anderson E, Cotton D, Basgoz N, Hirschhorn L, Tuomala R, Schoenfeld D, Daugherty C, Mazer N, and Grinspoon S (1998). Transdermal testos-terone administration in women with acquired immunodeficiency syndrome wasting: a pilot study. *J Clin Endocrinol Metab* 83(8):2717–2725.

Mollison LC, MijchA, McBride G, and Dwyer B (1991). Hypothyroidism due to destruction of the thyroid by Kaposi's sarcoma. *Rev Infect Dis* 13(5):826–827.

Mondy K, Yarasheski K, Powderly WG, Whyte M, Clax-ton S, DeMarco D, Hoffmann M, Tebas P (2003). Longitudinal evolution of bone mineral density and bone markers in human immunodeficiency virus-infected individuals. *Clin Infect Dis* 36(4):482–490.

Mondy K, Powderly WG, Claxton SA, Yarasheski KH, Royal M, Stoneman JS, Hoffmann ME, and Tebas P (2005). Alendronate, vitamin D, and calcium for the treatment of osteopenia/osteoporosis associated with HIV infection. *J Acquir Immune Defic Syndr* 38(4):426–431.

Mulder CL, Antoni MH, Emmelkamp PM, Veugelers PJ, Sandfort TG, van de Vijver FA, and de Vries MJ (1995). Psychosocial group intervention and the rate of decline of immunological parameters in asymptomatic HIV-infected homosexual men. *Psy-chother Psychosom* 63(3–4):185–192.

Mylonakis E, Koutkia P, and Grinspoon S (2001). Diagnosis and treatment of androgen deficiency in human immunodeficiency virus–infected men and women. *Clin Infect Dis* 33:857–864.

Negredo E, Martinez-Lopez E, Paredes R, Rosales J, Perez-Alvarez N, Holgado S, Gel S, del Rio L, Tena X, Rey-Joly C, and Clotet B (I2005). Reversal of HIV-1-associated osteoporosis with once-weekly alendronate. *AIDS* 19(3):343–345.

Nock B, Wich M, and Cicero TJ (1997). Chronic expo-sure to morphine increases corticosteroid-binding globulin. *J Pharmacol Exp Ther* 282(3):1262–1268.

Nolan D, Upton R, McKinnon E, John M, James I, Adler B, Roff G, Vasikaran S, and Mallal S (2001). Stable or increasing bone mineral density in HIV-infected patients treated with nelfinavir or indinavir. *AIDS* 15(10):1275–1280.

Norbiato G, Bevilacqua M, Vago T, Baldi G, Chebat E, Bertora P, Moroni M, Galli M, and Oldenburg N (1992). Cortisol resistance in acquired immunodeficiency syndrome. *J Clin Endocrinol Metab* 74(3): 608–613.

Olivieri A, Sorcini M, Battisti P, Fazzini C, Gilardi E, Sun Y, Medda E, Grandolfo M, Tossini G, Natili S, et al. (1993). Thyroid hypofunction related with the progression of human immunodeficiency virus infection. *J Endocrinol Invest* 16(6):407–413.

Paton NI, Macallan DC, Griffin GE, and Pazianas M (1997). Bone mineral density in patients with human immunodeficiency virus infection. *Calcif Tissue Int* 61(1):30–32.

Pedrazzoni M, Vescovi PP, Maninetti L, Michelini M, Zaniboni G, Pioli G, Costi D, Alfano FS, and Passeri M (1993). Effects of chronic heroin abuse on bone and mineral metabolism. *Acta Endocrinol (Copenh)* 129(1):42–45.

Pulakhandam U, and Dincsoy HP (1990). Cytomegaloviral adrenalitis and adrenal insufficiency in AIDS. *Am J Clin Pathol* 93(5):651–656.

Rabkin JG, Wagner GJ, and Rabkin R (2000). A double-blind, placebo-controlled trial of testosterone therapy for HIV-positive men with hypogonadal symptoms. *Arch Gen Psychiatry* 57:141–147.

Rabkin JG, Wagner GJ, McElhiney MC, Rabkin R, and Lin SH (2004). Testosterone versus fluoxetine for depression and fatigue in HIV/AIDS: a placebo-controlled trial. *J Clin Psychopharmacol* 24:379–385.

Raffi F, Brisseau JM, Planchon B, Remi JP, Barrier JH, and Grolleau JY (1991). Endocrine function in 98 HIV-infected patients: a prospective study. *AIDS* 5(6):729–733.

Ragni MV, Dekker A, DeRubertis FR, Watson CG, Skolnick ML, Goold SD, Finikiotis MW, Doshi S, and Myers DJ (1991). *Pneumocystis carinii* infection presenting as necrotizing thyroiditis and hypothyroidism. *Am J Clin Pathol* 95(4):489–493.

Reddy DS, Kaur G, and Kulkarni SK (1998). Sigma (sigma1) receptor mediated anti-depressant-like effects of neurosteroids in the Porsolt forced swim test. *Neuroreport* 9(13):3069–3073.

Rietschel P, Corcoran C, Stanley T, Basgoz N, Klibanski A, and Grinspoon S (2000). Prevalence of hypogonadism among men with weight loss related to human immunodeficiency virus who were receiving highly active antiretroviral therapy. *Clin Infect Dis* 31:1240–1244.

Roberts E, Bologa L, Flood JF, and Smith GE (1987). Effects of dehydroepiandrosterone and its sulfate on brain tissue in culture and on memory in mice. *Brain Res* 406(1–2):357–362.

Rodrigues D, Reis M, Teixeira V, Silva-Vergara M, Filho DC, Adad S, and Lazo J (2002). Pathologic findings in the adrenal glands of autopsied patients with acquired immunodeficiency syndrome. *Pathol Res Pract* 198(1):25–30.

Salehian B, Jacobson D, Swerdloff RS, and Abbasian M (1999). Testicular pathologic changes and the pituitary–testicular axis during human immunodeficiency virus infection. *Endocr Pract* 5(1):1–9.

Sellmeyer DE, and Grunfeld C (1996). Endocrine and metabolic disturbances in human immunodeficiency virus infection and the acquired immune deficiency syndrome. *Endocr Rev* 17(5):518–532.

Sinha-Hikim I, Arver S, Beall G, Shen R, Guerrero M, Sattler F, Shikuma C, Nelson JC, Landgren BM, Mazer NA, and Bhasin S (1998). The use of a sensitive equilibrium dialysis method for the measurement of free testosterone levels in healthy, cycling women and in human immunodeficiency virus–infected women. *J Clin Endocrinol Metab* 83(4): 1312–1318.

Spitzer RD, Chan JC, Marks JB, Valme BR, and McKenzie JM (1991). Case report: hypothyroidism due to *Pneumocystis carinii* thyroiditis in a patient with acquired immunodeficiency syndrome. *Am J Med Sci* 302(2):98–100.

Starkman MN (2003). Psychiatric manifestations of hyperadrenocorticism and hypoadrenocorticism (Cushing's and Addison's diseases). In OM Wolkowitz and AJ Rothschild (eds.), *Psychoneuroendocrinology: The Scientific Basis of Clinical Practice* (pp. 165–188). Arlington VA: American Psychiatric Publishing.

Stolarczyk R, Rubio SI, Smolyar D, Young IS, and Poretsky L (1998). Twenty-four-hour urinary free cortisol in patients with acquired immunodeficiency syndrome. *Metabolism* 47(6): 690–694.

Tebas P, Powderly WG, Claxton S, Marin D, Tantisiriwat W, Teitelbaum SL, and Yarasheski KE (2000). Accelerated bone mineral loss in HIV-infected patients receiving potent antiretroviral therapy. *AIDS* 14(4):F63–F67.

Teichmann J, Stephan E, Discher T, Lange U, Federlin K, Stracke H, Friese G, Lohmeyer J, and Bretzel RG (2000). Changes in calciotropic hormones and biochemical markers of bone metabolism in patients with human immunodeficiency virus infection. *Metabolism* 49(9):1134–1139.

Teichmann J, Stephan E, Lange U, Discher T, Friese G, Lohmeyer J, Stracke H, and Bretzel RG (2003). Osteopenia in HIV-infected women prior to highly active antiretroviral therapy. *J Infect* 46(4):221–227.

Tennant F, Shannon JA, Nork JG, Sagherian A, and Berman M (1991). Abnormal adrenal gland metabolism in opioid addicts: implications for clinical treatment. *J Psychoactive Drugs* 23(2):135–149.

Thomas J, and Doherty SM (2003). HIV infection—a risk factor for osteoporosis. *J Acquir Immune Defic Syndr* 33(3):281–291.

Villette JM, Bourin P, Doinel C, Mansour I, Fiet J, Boudou P, Dreux C, Roue R, Debord M, and Levi F (1990). Circadian variations in plasma levels of hypophyseal, adrenocortical and testicular hormones in men infected with human immunodeficiency *J Endocrinol Metab* 70(3):572–577.

Wagner GJ, Rabkin JG, and Rabkin R (1998). Testosterone as a treatment for fatigue in HIV+ men. *Gen Hosp Psychiatry* 20:209–213.

Wang C, Swerdloff RS, Iranmanesh A, Dobs A, Snyder PJ, Cunningham G, Matsumoto AM, Weber T, and Berman N (2000). Transdermal testosterone gel improves sexual function, mood, muscle strength, and body composition parameters in hypogonadal men. *J Clin Endocrinol Metab* 85:2839–2853.

Wang C, Cunningham G, Dobs A, Iranmanesh A, Matsumoto AM, Snyder PJ, Weber T, Berman N, Hull L, and Swerdloff RS (2004). Long-term testosterone gel (AndroGel) treatment maintains beneficial effects on sexual functioning and mood, lean and fat mass, and bone mineral density in hypogonadal men. *J Clin Endocrinol Metab* 89:2085–2098.

Welch K, Finkbeiner W, Alpers CE, Blumenfeld W, Davis RL, Smuckler EA, and Beckstead JH (1984). Autopsy findings in the acquired immune deficiency syndrome. *JAMA* 252(9):1152–1159.

Wisniewski TL, Hilton CW, Morse EV, and Svec F (1993). The relationship of serum DHEA-S and cortisol levels to measures of immune function in human immunodeficiency virus–related illness. *Am J Med Sci* 305(2):79–83.

Wisniewski AB, Apel S, Selnes OA, Nath A, McArthur JC, and Dobs AS (2005). Depressive symptoms, quality of life, and neuropsychological performance in HIV/AIDS: the impact of gender and injection drug use. *J Neurovirol* 11(2):138–143.

Wisniewski AB, Brown TT, John M, Cofranceso J Jr, Golub ET, Ricketts EP, Wand G, and Dobs AS (2006). Cortisol levels and depression in men and women using heroin and cocaine. *Psychoneuroendocrinology* 31(2):250–255.

Wolff FH, Nhuch C, Cadore LP, Glitz CL, Lhullier F, and Furlanetto TW (2001). Low-dose adrenocorticotropin test in patients with the acquired immunodeficiency syndrome. *Braz J Infect Dis* 5(2):53–59.

Wolkowitz OM, Kramer JH, Reus VI, Costa MM, Yaffe K, Walton P, Raskind M, Peskind E, Newhouse P, Sack D, De Souza E, Sadowsky C, and Roberts E (2003). DHEA treatment of Alzheimer's disease: a randomized, double-blind, placebo-controlled study. *Neurology* 60(7):1071–1076.

Woo SB, Hellstein JW, and Kalmar JR (2006). Systematic review: bisphosphonates and osteonecrosis of the jaws. *Ann Intern Med* 144(10):753–761.

Yaffe K, Ettinger B, Pressman A, Seeley D, Whooley M, Schaefer C, and Cummings S (1998). Neuropsychiatric function and dehydroepiandrosterone sulfate in elderly women: a prospective study. *Biol Psychiatry* 43(9):694–700.

Zonis De Zukerfeld R, Ingratta R, Sanchez Negrete G, Matusevich A, and Intebi C (2003–2004). Psychosocial aspects in osteoporosis [in Spanish]. *Vertex* 14(54):253–259.

Chapter 36

Lipodystrophy, Metabolic Disorders, and Cardiovascular Disorders in Persons with HIV

Joseph Z. Lux and Michael P. Mullen

HIV-associated lipodystrophy is a syndrome of fat redistribution associated with antiretroviral therapy. Although many of the complications occur most commonly with protease inhibitors, lipodystrophy is associated with all antiretroviral classes. Lipodystrophy is associated with a number of changes in fat redistribution including central and dorsocervical fat accumulation, limb and facial subcutaneous fat atrophy, and associated metabolic complications such as insulin resistance and diabetes, lactic acidosis, osteopenia, and dyslipidemia. The presentation is heterogeneous; patients may develop one or a number of these complications. There has also been increasing attention paid to potential effects on cardiovascular risk and events. In the combination antiretroviral era, HIV infection has become a chronic disease. Living with a chronic medical illness may increase psychological stress (Lipowski, 1970). As a result of surviving so much longer, persons with HIV and AIDS also experience high levels of stress associated with HIV and AIDS, its treatments, stigma, and comorbid illnesses and may have increased levels of distress as well as decreased quality of life.

Despite substantial research in the medical literature, the definition of lipodystrophy has remained ambiguous. Prevalence rates have largely been determined by patient self-report, physical examination, signs of insulin resistance and dyslipidemia, radiographic imaging, and body anthropometry. A study by the HIV Lipodystrophy Case Study Group sought to clarify the definition (Carr et al., 2003). Using patients identified as lipodystrophic by both patient and physician agreement, a clinical model was devised using 10 variables: age, gender, duration of HIV infection, HIV disease stage, waist-to-hip ratio, anion gap, serum high-density-lipoprotein (HDL) cholesterol concentration, trunk-to-peripheral fat ratio, percentage leg fat, and intraabdominal-to-extraabdominal fat ratio. The model, which used anthropometry, DEXA scans, CT fat measurements, and laboratory testing, had 79% sensitivity and 80% specificity for the diagnosis of lipodystrophy.

A number of cross-sectional studies have measured the prevalence of lipodystrophy-associated body changes in patients receiving antiretroviral therapy. In one study, physicians assessed 1348 patients, predominantly male, for the presence of lipodystrophy (Miller et al., 2003). Lipodystrophy prevalence was 53%. Of the total population, 27% reported both peripheral fat loss and central fat accumulation, 20% experienced peripheral fat loss only, and 6% had central fat accumulation only. The prevalence of lipodystrophy was 62% in protease inhibitor-experienced patients, 32% in other antiretroviral-experienced patients, and 21% in antiretroviral-naive patients. Lipodystrophy was significantly associated with older age, advanced disease, undetectable HIV viral load levels, the use of protease inhibitors, and a longer exposure to nucleoside reverse transcriptase inhibitors (NRTIs). These data suggest that HIV viral suppression, especially with protease inhibitors, may predispose patients to lipodystrophy, although all HIV-infected patients are potentially at risk.

Although both fat accumulation and loss occur in HIV-infected individuals, it has remained unclear if these two manifestations of lipodystrophy represent different components of the same process. The Study of Fat Redistribution and Metabolic Change in HIV Infection [FRAM] compared HIV-infected and HIV-negative men and confirmed their reports of changes in fat distribution by physical examination and magnetic resonance imaging (FRAM, 2005). Peripheral fat loss in HIV-infected individuals was not associated with central fat accumulation, which suggests that lipohypertrophy and lipoatrophy are different syndromes.

Other studies have reported on the prevalence of body fat redistribution in HIV-infected women and gender-related differences. One study reported an increased risk for any type of lipodystrophy, with a relative hazard of 1.87 in women compared with that for men (Martinez et al., 2001). A second study supported this observation, with 29.5% of the men and 41.9% of the women being diagnosed with fat redistribution (Galli et al., 2003). After adjusting for various risks through a logistic regression analysis, the prevalence remained different between the two groups, with men having a 0.47 adjusted risk, compared to women presenting with any type of fat redistribution. Men had a lower risk of lipohypertrophy, whereas there was no difference between men and women in the risk of developing only lipoatrophy. This concerning prevalence of lipodystrophy in women has even wider implications as fat accumulation in women has been associated with increased metabolic and inflammatory markers of cardiac risk (Dolan et al., 2005).

The pathogenesis of lipodystrophy is complex. The postulated mechanisms include increased expression of tumor necrosis factor alpha, dysfunction of the sterol regulatory element–binding protein 1 (SREBP-1) and decreased adipocyte differentiation factor peroxisome proliferator-activated receptor gamma (PPAR-gamma) expression (Bastard et al., 2002), impaired SREBP1 nuclear localization and adipocyte differentiation in patients on protease inhibitors (Caron et al., 2003), reduced estrogen receptor expression (Barzon et al., 2005), and depletion of mitochondrial DNA by NRTIs (Birkus et al., 2002).

The optimal management of lipodystrophy is still unclear. Expert guidelines have been published to assist clinicians in managing antiretroviral-associated metabolic complications (Schambelan et al., 2002). The three main approaches are initiation of antiretroviral therapy later to postpone the metabolic side effects, switching to a less metabolically toxic agent, and continuation of the current treatment but treating the metabolic effect. There appears to be no association between dietary fat intake and changes in fat distribution (Batterham et al., 2000). Exercise may ameliorate truncal adiposity, but it may also worsen peripheral lipoatrophy (Driscoll et al., 2004). Thiazolinedones, such as rosiglitazone, are PPARG-gamma agonists that treat type-2 diabetes and have also been studied for the treatment of lipoatrophy. The results have been mixed, with some studies showing improvement in lipoatrophy (Arioglu et al., 2000; Hadigan et al., 2004) but other trials showing no effect (Sutinen et al., 2003; Carr et al., 2004). Recombinant human growth hormone can be efficacious in HIV-associated fat accumulation syndromes, but it may worsen insulin resistance and peripheral lipoatrophy (Engelson et al., 2002; Burgess and Wanke, 2005).

The impact of switching antiretroviral medications, particularly protease inhibitors and thymidine analogues such as stavudine, has been studied. Although switching from a protease inhibitor may improve lipodystrophy (Barreiro et al., 2000), switching from a thymidine analogue appears to be the intervention that most consistently improves peripheral fat loss (Carr et al., 2002; McComsey et al., 2004).

Plastic surgery is a tested option for patients with lipodystrophy. Liposuction for central accumulation and treatment of buffalo hump can be helpful (Gervasoni et al., 2004), although reaccumulation may occur. Facial lipoatrophy can be particularly psychologically disabling, and filler injections have been used in this situation. Polylactic acid injections, which have been approved by the U.S. Food and Drug Association (FDA) for this indication, have been satisfying for patients with minimal adverse effects (Burgess and Quiroga, 2005). Unfortunately, plastic surgery is generally considered cosmetic by private health insurance companies as well as by Medicaid and Medicare and is therefore not reimbursed. As a result, for those without significant financial means, surgical correction is not a feasible option for patients who suffer the consequences of disfigurement from lipodystrophy.

LACTIC ACIDOSIS

Lactic acidosis is a potentially life-threatening metabolic complication associated with lipodystrophy. Antiretroviral nucleoside therapy is associated with mitochondrial dysfunction. Mitochondrial pathology is associated with hyperlactatemia, lactic acidosis, lipoatrophy, hepatic steatosis, peripheral neuropathy, neuromuscular weakness, pancreatitis, and myopathies (McComsey and Lonergan, 2004). Asymptomatic hyperlactatemia is common in patients taking antiretrovirals, but lactic acidosis is infrequent (Boubaker et al., 2001; John et al., 2001; Imhof et al., 2005). Mild hyperlactatemia diagnosed in HIV-infected individuals has a low positive predictive value for progression to symptomatic lactic acidosis (Brinkman, 2001). Clinical symptoms with severe lactatemia include fatigue, dyspnea, tachycardia, abdominal pain, weight loss, and peripheral neuropathy (Carr et al., 2000; Gerard et al., 2000; Falco et al., 2002; Imhof et al., 2005).

In one prospective study following 1566 HIV-infected individuals, both treatment-naive patients and patients on antiretroviral treatment developed hyperlactatemia (lactate >2.4 mmol/l), with 11% of the antiretroviral-naive patients, 35% of the patients beginning antiretrovirals during the study period, and 48% of the patients receiving antiretrovirals at the beginning of the study developing an elevated lactate level (Imhof et al., 2005). Although lactatemia developed in all groups, even those never treated with antiretroviral therapy, the more severe cases occurred uncommonly and only in those patients on treatment with antiretroviral agents. Severe hyperlactatemia (>5.0 mmol/l) was recorded in 2.6% of patients,

all on antiretroviral therapy. The four patients diagnosed with lactic acidosis were all receiving treatment with stavudine and didanosine.

The mechanism of NRTI-associated lactic acidosis is likely related to mitochondrial toxicity. Nucleoside analogues may affect the mitochondrial respiratory chain function and redox status by depleting enzymatic activity encoded by mitochondrial DNA (Brivet et al., 2000). The more potent NRTI inhibitors of mitochondrial synthesis, in decreasing order, are zalcitabine, didanosine, stavudine, and zidovudine (Birkus et al., 2002). Other nucleoside/nucleotide reverse transcriptase inhibitors such as lamivudine, abacavir, and tenofovir are less potent inhibitors of mitochondrial synthesis (Birkus et al., 2002). Administration with essential cofactors, including thiamine, riboflavin, L-carnitine, prostaglandin E, and coenzyme Q, that are thought to improve mitochondrial function for mitochondrial illnesses have been used to treat nucleoside-associated lactic acidosis with promising but still unproven benefit (Falco et al., 2002).

DIABETES

Hyperglycemia is increasingly seen in HIV-infected patients, particularly those on protease inhibitor therapies (Dube et al., 1997). Lipodystrophy is associated with insulin resistance and the development of diabetes. Advanced HIV illness may itself predispose patients to insulin resistance. In HIV antiretroviral-naive patients, a lower CD4 count is associated with increased insulin resistance (El-Sadr et al., 2005). The incidence of diabetes among HIV-infected individuals receiving antiretrovirals ranges between 1% and 7% (Carr et al., 1999; Palacios et al., 2003), with a higher percentage, in one study 16%, developing impaired glucose tolerance (Carr et al., 1999). Risk factors for development of diabetes include obesity, duration of treatment on protease inhibitors, and lipodystrophy (Palacios et al., 2003).

Different protease inhibitors appear to pose different risks. While atazanavir appears to have minimal or no effect on insulin sensitivity, indinavir causes a substantial decline in glucose disposal with just one dose (Hruz et al., 2002; Noor et al., 2002), and lopinavir/ritonavir worsened glucose tolerance after a 4-week trial (Lee et al., 2004). Amprenavir-treated patients exhibited a trend toward insulin resistance after

48 weeks (Dube et al., 2002). Other antiretroviral classes may also be a factor in developing insulin resistance and glucose tolerance. Cumulative NRTI therapy, in particular stavudine, is associated with increased insulin levels (Brown et al., 2005).

The pathogenesis of protease inhibitor–mediated insulin resistance is complex and includes impaired function of the glucose transporters, notably GLUT4 (Murata et al., 2002), and impaired pancreatic beta-cell function (Dube et al., 2001). Increased rates of lipolysis and free fatty acid levels may worsen insulin resistance (Hadigan et al., 2002). An association exists between soluble type 2 tumor necrosis factor alpha receptor and HIV patients with insulin resistance. Higher receptor levels in those with lipodystrophy and insulin resistance suggest an inflammatory contribution (Mynarcik et al., 2000).

Strategies to address glucose intolerance, insulin resistance, and diabetes include lifestyle changes, change in antiretroviral treatment, and treatment with insulin-sensitizing medications. Exercise may improve hyperinsulinemia (Driscoll et al., 2004). Metformin therapy reduces insulin resistance in HIV-infected patients with lipodystrophy and impaired glucose metabolism (Hadigan et al., 2000). The strategy of switching from a protease inhibitor–based regimen to nevirapine is useful in lowering glucose and insulin resistance (Martinez et al., 1999). However, the use of switch strategies must be approached cautiously. One study that switched patients' treatment from a protease inhibitor–based regimen to nevirapine, efavirenz, or abacavir showed a trend of virological failure for patients switched to abacavir (Martinez et al., 2003).

HYPERLIPIDEMIA

Changes in lipid metabolism occur in HIV-infected individuals. One study showed that HIV seroconversion resulted in marked decreases in HDL cholesterol, low-density lipoprotein (LDL) cholesterol, and total cholesterol levels, with a pattern of increases in total and LDL cholesterol after initiation of combination antiretroviral therapy (Riddler et al., 2003). In a study of 419 antiretroviral-naive patients, an AIDS diagnosis was associated with higher levels of total cholesterol, very-low-density lipoprotein (VLDL) cholesterol, and triglycerides (El-Sadr et al., 2005). Elevated HIV RNA levels were associated with lower concentrations of HDL cholesterol and LDL cholesterol, and higher levels of VLDL cholesterol and triglycerides.

The protease inhibitor class is particularly associated with dyslipidemia. In one population-based cohort, increased cholesterol or triglyceride concentrations were associated with protease inhibitor use by an adjusted odds ratio of 7.17 (Heath et al., 2002). The effects, however, can vary widely between protease inhibitors. Changes in lipid levels are significantly less in patients treated with atazanvir than those in patients receiving nelfinavir (Wood et al., 2004).

A number of studies have been conducted to assess strategies for minimizing antiretroviral-associated lipid abnormalities. The nucleotide reverse transcriptase inhibitor tenofovir SR had a more favorable lipid panel than that of stavudine when used in combination with lamivudine and efavirenz (Gallant et al., 2004). The substitution of nevirapine for a protease inhibitor increased HDL cholesterol and decreased total, LDL, and VLDL cholesterol (Negredo et al., 2002). There is a role for dietary interventions; increased total protein, animal protein and *trans* fat intake, as well as reduced soluble fiber intake worsen the lipid profile in patients with lipodystrophy on protease inhibitor therapy (Shah et al., 2005).

A number of mechanisms have been postulated to explain antiretroviral-associated dyslipidemia. Protease inhibitors may induce the expression of genes responsible for lipid biosynthesis by increasing levels of activated sterol regulatory element-binding protein in the nucleus (Riddle et al., 2001). There is an association between the accumulation of lipoparticles that are important components of lipid synthesis and catabolism and the hypertriglyceridemia associated with protease inhibitors (Bonnet et al., 2001). Certain lipoprotein polymorphisms may predispose individuals to protease inhibitor–associated dyslipidemia (Fauvel et al., 2001).

Treatment recommendations have been published for the evaluation and management of dyslipidemia in HIV-infected adults that build on the treatment recommendations for dyslipidemia in the general adult population (Expert Panel, 2001; Dube et al., 2003). Consideration should be given to obtaining baseline and follow-up lipid profiles, assessing for coronary heart disease risk factors, counseling for modifiable risk factors, and changing antiretroviral therapy or beginning lipid-lowering agents as necessary.

CARDIOVASCULAR RISK

Many of the metabolic abnormalities associated with lipodystrophy are coronary risk factors in non-HIV-infected individuals. Overall mortality has decreased since the advent of protease inhibitors, but there have been concerns that cardiovascular risk and events may have risen at the same time. Treatment with antiretrovirals overall appears to lower the total death rate (Bozzette et al., 2003) but predisposes patients, especially those being treated with protease inhibitors, to cardiovascular risk factors such as dyslipidemia and insulin resistance. A significant number of HIV patients also smoke, which increases their cardiovascular risk (Shah et al., 2005).

A number of studies have tried to assess the future risk of cardiovascular disease in HIV-infected patients taking protease inhibitors by measuring surrogate markers of increased coronary risk. Carotid intima-media thickness, a marker of atherosclerosis, was initially observed at higher levels and progressed more quickly in an HIV-infected protease inhibitor–experienced population compared to age-matched controls (Hsue et al., 2004b). A cross-sectional study measuring flow-mediated vasodilatation found evidence of endothelial dysfunction in HIV-infected patients treated with protease inhibitors (Stein et al., 2001).

A series of large, well-designed epidemiological studies have revealed conflicting results on the relationship between the rate of coronary events in the HIV-infected population and use of antiretroviral therapy. An analysis of the French Hospital Database on HIV noted an association between the length of exposure to protease inhibitor therapy and the incidence of myocardial infarction (Mary-Krause et al., 2003). Patients exposed to at least 30 months of therapy with a protease inhibitor had approximately three times the risk of an age-matched control group of men in the general population. The multi-cohort Data Collection on Adverse Events of Anti-HIV Drugs Study Group (DAD) found that the incidence of myocardial infarction increased with longer exposure to combination antiretroviral therapy, with a relative risk of 1.26 per year (Friis-Moller et al., 2003).

Other studies that support this association between antiretroviral therapy and coronary events point toward reasons for optimism. A study conducted by the Centers for Disease Control and Prevention that no-ted an elevated rate of myocardial infarctions in an HIV-infected cohort later observed that the myocardial infarction rate subsequently went down as protease inhibitor use declined and statin therapy use increased in frequency (Holmberg et al., 2002, 2004).

In contrast, other studies have not shown an association between antiretroviral therapy and coronary events. An observational study using the Kaiser Permanente Data Base compared hospitalization rates of HIV-positive and HIV-negative members (Klein et al., 2002). The study found no association between antiretroviral exposure and coronary heart disease hospitalization rate, but did find an overall coronary heart disease hospitalization rate that was significantly higher for HIV-infected individuals than that for HIV-negative members. A retrospective analysis of patients receiving care for HIV infection through the Veterans Affairs medical system reported both a decrease in total rate of death and incidence of cardiovascular and cerebrovascular events between the years 1995 and 2001 (Bozzette et al., 2003). The use of antiretroviral medications was associated with an overall decreased hazard of death. There was no association between antiretroviral therapy and cardiovascular or cerebrovascular events.

There can be no final judgment on this issue, as studies have produced disparate results. Nevertheless, there is a significant amount of data suggesting an increased risk of coronary risk and events in HIV-infected patients, particularly those treated with protease inhibitors. Compounding this concern is recent evidence that patients with HIV infection treated for acute coronary events are at high risk for coronary artery restenosis and stent thrombosis (Matetzky et al., 2003; Hsue et al., 2004a). Until more data can resolve the issue, the ambiguity and the fact that the HIV population is aging, predisposing them to greater cardiovascular risk, as well as the evidence that a number of the metabolic side effects of antiretroviral therapy are known risk factors for cardiovascular disease in HIV-negative patients suggest the need for continued vigilance.

PSYCHOLOGICAL EFFECTS

The visible effects of lipodystrophy and its association with HIV infection lead to a range of psychological issues. In a population of homosexual men in

Amsterdam, lipodystrophy was associated with a decrease in sexual activity, enjoyment of sex, and confidence in relationships (Dukers et al., 2001). A qualitative study conducted with patients recruited from a clinic in London, many of whom had facial atrophy and peripheral wasting, revealed symptoms related to poor body image and self-imposed social isolation (Power et al., 2003). Individuals changed their diet, exercised more, used steroids, and underwent plastic surgery in attempts to improve the signs of lipodsytrophy. Those patients with a history of more serious HIV-related illness or with partners accepted lipodystrophy with less psychological distress. A study in Spain measured the impact of lipodystrophy on psychosocial functioning and quality of life and observed considerable impairment (Blanch et al., 2004). The development of lipodystrophy influenced dressing style for 65% of patients, stimulated attempts to solve problems due to these body changes for 54%, and induced feelings of shame for 49% of patients. In a study of Singapore HIV-infected individuals, mainly men, 85% of affected patients stated that others had noticed changes, 36% reported anxiety or unhappiness from the changes, and 23% reported that the changes had affected their work or social life (Paton et al., 2002). Surprisingly, less than 1% of these patients considered discontinuation of antiretroviral treatment, in contrast to French and Italian studies in which medication-adherent patients with lipodystrophy were at higher risk of subsequent adherence failure (Duran et al., 2001; Ammassari et al., 2002).

Another commonly expressed concern among patients is that as the signs of lipodystrophy become more recognizable, they may serve to "out" people as HIV positive in an unwanted manner. The emergence of Kaposi's sarcoma earlier in the epidemic created an analogous scenario (Persson, 2005).

Patients may be willing to trade years of life for quality of life. In one study conducted in the United States, patients, many of whom were well-educated male homosexuals, believed that the quality-of-life effects with lipodystrophy were substantial enough that they would warrant trading years of life or taking a risk of death to avoid the syndrome (Lenert et al., 2002).

However, other research indicates that lipodystrophy does not necessarily worsen patients' quality of life. In a German study consisting mostly of male homosexuals, the presence of lipodystrophy did not affect patients' feelings of health and well-being (Oette et al., 2002). A second study in the Toronto, Canada,

area concluded that lipodystrophy may cause a worsening body image but otherwise demonstrated few effects on mental health or quality of life (Burgoyne et al., 2005). In a third study conducted in Spain, generally lipodystrophy did not appear to influence quality of life, although homosexual patients and those undergoing psychiatric treatment showed greater psychological impairment (Blanch et al., 2002).

In summary, the balance of the data suggests that patients with lipodystrophy are at risk for increased social and psychological distress. Clinicians who treat patients with HIV infection should focus not only on the physical issues related to lipodystrophy but also on any associated issues of anxiety, depression, social isolation, altered body image, or medication nonadherence. There should be a low threshold for referral to mental health professionals with experience in treating HIV-infected individuals.

References

Ammassari A, Antinori A, Cozzi-Lepri A, Trotta MP, Nasti G, Ridolfo AL, Mazzotta F, Wu AW, d'Arminio Monforte A, Galli M; AdICoNA and the LipoICoNA Study Groups (2002). Relationship between HAART adherence and adipose tissue alterations. *J Acquir Immune Defic Syndr* 31:S140–S144.

Arioglu E, Duncan-Morin J, Sebring N, Rother KI, Gottlieb N, Lieberman J, Herion D, Kleiner D, Reynolds J, Premkumar A, Sumner AE, Hoofnagle J, Reitman ML, and Taylor SI (2000). Efficacy and safety of troglitazone in the treatment of lipodystrophy syndromes. *Ann Intern Med* 133:263–274.

Barreiro P, Soriano V, Blanco F, Casimiro C, de la Cruz JJ, and Gonzalez-Lahoz J (2000). Risks and benefits of replacing protease inhibitors by nevirapine in HIV-infected subjects under long-term successful triple combination therapy. *AIDS* 14:807–812.

Barzon L, Zamboni, M, Pacenti M, Milan G, Bosello O, Federspil G, Palu G, and Vettor R (2005). Do oestrogen receptors play a role in the pathogenesis of HIV-associated lipodsytrophy? *AIDS* 19:531–533.

Bastard JP, Caron M, Vidal H, Jan V, Auclair M, Vigouroux C, Luboinski J, Laville M, Maachi M, Girard PM, Rozenbaum W, Levan P, and Capeau J (2002). Association between altered expression of adipogenic factor SREBP1 in lipoatrophic adipose tissue from HIV-1-infected patients and abnormal adipocyte differentiation and insulin resistance. *Lancet* 359:1026–1031.

Batterham MJ, Garsia R, and Greenop PA (2000). Dietary intake, serum lipids, insulin resistance, and body composition in the era of highly active antiretroviral therapy 'Diet FRS Study.' *AIDS* 14:1839–1843.

Birkus G, Hitchcock MJM, and Cihlar T (2002). Assessment of mitochondrial toxicity in human cells treated with tenofovir: comparison with other nucleoside reverse transcriptase inhibitors. *Antimicrob Agents Chemother* 46:716–723.

Blanch J, Rousaud A, Martinez E, De Lazzari E, Peri JM, Milinkovic A, Perez-Cuevas JB, Blanco JL, and Gatell JM (2002). Impact of lipodystrophy on the quality of life of HIV-1 infected patients. *J Acquir Immune Defic Syndr* 31:404–407.

Blanch J, Rousaud A, Martinez E, De Lazzari E, Milinkovic A, Peri JM, Blanco JL, Jaen J, Navarro V, Massana G, and Gatell JM (2004). Factors associated with severe impact of lipodystrophy on the quality of life of patients infected with HIV-1. *Clin Infect Dis* 38:1464–1470.

Bonnet E, Ruidavets JB, Tuech J, Ferrieres J, Collet X, Fauvel J, Massip P, and Perret B (2001). Apoprotein C-III and E-containing lipoparticles are markedly increased in HIV-infected patients treated with protease inhibitors: association with the development of lipodystrophy. *J Clin Endocrinol Metab* 86:296–302.

Boubaker K, Flepp M, Sudre P, Furrer H, Haensel A, Hirschel B, Boggian K, Chave JP, Bernasconi E, Egger M, Opravil M, Rickenbach M, Francioli P, and Telenti A; Swiss HIV Cohort Study (2001). Hyperlactatemia and antiretroviral therapy: the Swiss HIV cohort study. *Clin Infect Dis* 33:1931–1937.

Bozzette SA, Ake CF, Tam HK, Chang SW, and Louis TA (2003). Cardiovascular and cerebrovascular events in patients treated for human immunodeficiency virus infection. *N Engl J Med* 348:702–710.

Brinkman K (2001). Management of hyperlactatemia: no need for routine lactate measurements. *AIDS* 15:795–797.

Brivet FG, Nion I, Megarbane B, Slama A, Brivet M, Rustin P, and Munnich A (2000). Fatal lactic acidosis and liver steatosis associated with didanosine and stavudine treatment: a respiratory chain dysfunction? *J Hepatol* 32:364–365.

Brown TT, Li X, Cole SR, Kingsley LA, Palella FJ, Riddler SA, Chmiel JS, Visscher BR, Margolick JB, and Dobs AS (2005). Cumulative exposure to nucleoside analogue reverse transcriptase inhibitors is associated with insulin resistance markers in the Multicenter AIDS Cohort Study. *AIDS* 19:1375–1383.

Burgess CM, and Quiroga RM (2005). Assessment of the safety and efficacy of poly-L-lactic acid for the treatment of HIV-associated facial lipoatrophy. *J Am Acad Dermatol* 52:233–239.

Burgess E, and Wanke C (2005). Use of recombinant human growth hormone in HIV-associated lipodystrophy. *Curr Opin Infect Dis* 18:17–24.

Burgoyne R, Collins E, Wagner C, Abbey S, Halman M, Nur M, and Walmsley S (2005). The relationship between lipodystrophy-associated body changes and measures of quality of life and mental health for HIV-positive adults. *Qual Life Res* 14:981–990.

Caron M, Auclair M, Sterlingot H, Kornprobst M, and Capeau J (2003). Some HIV protease inhibitors alter lamin A/C maturation and stability, SREBP-1 nuclear localization and adipocyte differentiation. *AIDS* 17:2437–2444.

Carr A, Samaras K, Thorisdottir A, Kaufman GR, Chisholm DJ, and Cooper DA (1999). Diagnosis, prediction, and natural course of HIV-1 protease-inhibitor-associated lipodystrophy, hyperlipidaemia, and diabetes mellitus: a cohort study. *Lancet* 353:2093–2099.

Carr A, Miller J, Law M, and Cooper DA (2000). A syndrome of lipoatrophy, lactic acidaemia, and liver dysfunction associated with HIV nucleoside analogue therapy: contribution to protease inhibitor–related lipodystrophy syndrome. *AIDS* 14:F25–F32.

Carr A, Workman C, Smith DE, Hoy J, Hudson J, Doong N, Martin A, Amin J, Freund J, Law M, and Cooper DA (2002). Mitochondrial Toxicity (MITOX) Study Group: abacavir substitution for nucleoside analogs in patients treated with HIV lipoatrophy: a randomized trial. *JAMA* 288:207–215.

Carr A, Emery S, Law M, Puls R, Lundgren JD, and Powderly WG (2003). HIV Lipodystrophy Case Definition Study Group: an objective case definition of lipodystrophy in HIV-infected adults: a case–control study. *Lancet* 361:726–735.

Carr A, Workman C, Carey D, Rogers G, Martin A, Baker D, Wand H, Law M, Samaras K. Emery S, Cooper DA; Rosey investigators (2004). No effect of rosiglitazone for treatment of HIV-1 lipoatrophy: randomised, double-blind, placebo-controlled trial. *Lancet* 363:429–438.

Dolan SE, Hadigan C, Killilea K, Sullivan M, Hemphill L, Lees RS, Schoenfeld D, and Grinspoon S (2005). Increased cardiovascular disease risk indices in HIV-infected women. *J Acquir Immune Defic Syndr* 39:44–54.

Driscoll SD, Meininger GE, Ljungquist K, Hadigan C, Torriani M, Klibanski A, Frontera WR, and Grinspoon S (2004). Differential effects of metformin and exercise on muscle adiposity and metabolic indices in human immunodeficiency virus–infected patients. *J Clin Endocrinol Metab* 89:2171–2178.

Dube MP, Johnson DL, Currier JS, and Leedom JM (1997). Protease inhibitor–associated hyperglycaemia. *Lancet* 350:713–714.

Dube MP, Edmondson-Melancon H, Qian D, Aqeel R, Johnson D, and Buchanan TA (2001). Prospective evaluation of the effect of initiating indinavir-based therapy on insulin sensitivity and B-cell function in HIV-infected patients. *J Acquir Immune Defic Syndr* 27:130–134.

Dube MP, Qian D, Edmondson-Melancon H, Sattler FR, Goodwin D, Martinez C, Williams V, Johnson D, and Buchanan TA (2002). Prospective, intensive study of metabolic changes associated with 48 weeks of amprenavir-based antiretroviral therapy. *Clin Infect Dis* 35:475–481.

Dube MP, Stein JH, Aberg JA, Fichtenbaum CJ, Gerber JG, Tashima KT, Henry WK, Currier JS, Sprecher D, and Glesby MJ; Adult AIDS Clinical Trials Group Cardiovascular Subcommittee (2003). Guidelines for the evaluation and management of dyslipidemia in human immunodeficiency virus (HIV)–infected adults receiving antiretroviral therapy: recommendations of the HIV Medicine Association of the Infectious Disease Society of America and the Adult AIDS Clinical Trials Group. *Clin Infect Dis* 37:613–627.

Dukers NHTM, Stolte IG, Albrecht N, Coutinho RA, and de Wit JBF (2001). The impact of experiencing lipodystrophy on the sexual behavior and well-being among HIV-infected homosexual men. *AIDS* 15:812–813.

Duran S, Saves M, Spire B, Cailleton V, Sobel A, Carrieri P, Salmon D, Moatti JP, Leport C; APROCO Study Group (2001). Failure to maintain long-term adherence to highly active antiretroviral therapy: the role of lipodystrophy. *AIDS* 15:2441–2444.

El-Sadr WM, Mullin CM, Carr A, Gibert C, Rappoport C, Visnegarwala, Grunfeld C, and Raghavan SS (2005). Effects of HIV disease on lipid, glucose, and insulin levels: results from a large antiretroviral-naive cohort. *HIV Med* 6:114–121.

Engelson, ES, Glesby MJ, Mendez D, Albu JB, Wang J, Heymsfield SB, and Kotler DP (2002). Effect of recombinant human growth hormone in the treatment of visceral fat accumulation in HIV infection. *J Acquir Immune Defic Syndr* 30:379–391.

Expert Panel on Detection, Evaluation, and Treatment of High Blood Cholesterol in Adults (2001). Executive summary of the third report of the National Cholesterol Education Program (NCEP) Expert Panel on Detection, Evaluation, and Treatment of High Blood Cholesterol in Adults (Adult Treatment Panel III). *JAMA* 285:2486–2497.

Falco V, Rodriguez D, Ribera E, Martinez E, Miro JM, Domingo P, Diazaraque R, Arribas JR, Gonzalez-Garcia JJ, Montero F, Sanchez L, and Pahissa A (2002). Severe nucleoside-associated lactic acidosis in human immunodeficiency virus–infected patients: report of 12 cases and review of the literature. *Clin Infect Dis* 34:838–846.

Fauvel J, Bonnet E, Ruidavets JB, Ferrieres J, Toffoletti A, Massip P, Chap H, and Perret B (2001). An interaction between apo C-III variants and protease inhibitors contributes to high triglyceride/low HDL levels in treated HIV patients. *AIDS* 15:2397–2406.

Friis-Moller N, Sabin CA, Weber R, d'Arminio Monforte A, El-Sadr WM, Reiss P, Thiebaut R, Morfeldt L, De Wit S, Pradier C, Calvo G, Law MG, Kirk O, Phillips AN, and Lundgren JD (2003). Data Collection on Adverse Events of Anti-HIV Drugs (DAD) Study Group: combination antiretroviral therapy and the risk of myocardial infarction. *N Engl J Med* 349:1993–2003.

[FRAM] Study of Fat Redistribution and Metabolic Changes in HIV Infection (FRAM) (2005). Fat distribution in men with HIV infection. *J Acquir Immune Defic Syndr* 40:121–131.

Gallant JE, Staszewski S, Pozniak AL, DeJesus E, Suleiman JMAH, Miller MD, Coakley DF, Lu B, Toole JJ, and Cheng AK (2004). The 903 Study Group: efficacy and safety of tenofovir DF vs. stavudine in combination therapy in antiretroviral-naive patients: a 3-year randomized trial. *JAMA* 292:191–201.

Galli M, Veglia F, Angarano G, Santambrogio S, Meneghini E, Gritti F, Cargnel A, Mazzotta F, and Lazzarin A (2003). Gender differences in antiretroviral drug–related adipose tissue alterations: women are at higher risk than men and develop particular lipodystrophy patterns. *J Acquir Immune Defic Syndr* 34:58–61.

Gerard Y, Maulin L, Yazdanpanah Y, de la Tribonniere X, Amiel C, Maurage CA, Robin S, Sablonniere B, Dhennain C, and Mouton Y (2000). Symptomatic hyperlactataemia:an emerging complication of antiretroviral therapy. *AIDS* 14:2723–2730.

Gervasoni C, Ridolfo AL, Vaccarezza M, Fedeli P, Morelli P, Rovati L, and Galli M (2004). Long-term efficacy of the surgical treatment of buffalo hump in patients continuing antiretroviral therapy. *AIDS* 18:574–576.

Hadigan C, Corcoran C, Basgoz N, Davis B, Sax P, and Grinspoon S (2000). Metformin in the treatment of HIV lipodystrophy syndrome: a randomized controlled trial. *JAMA* 284:472–477.

Hadigan C, Borgonha S, Rabe J, Young V, and Grinspoon S (2002). Increased rates of lipolysis among human immunodeficiency virus–infected men receiving highly active antiretroviral therapy. *Metabolism* 51:1143–1147.

Hadigan C, Yawetz S, Thomas A, Havers F, Sax PE, and Grinspoon S (2004). Metabolic effects of rosiglitazone in HIV lipodystrophy: a randomized, controlled trial. *Ann Intern Med* 140:786–794.

Heath KV, Hogg RS, Singer J, Chan KJ, O'Shaughnessy MV, and Montaner JS (2002). Antiretroviral treatment patterns and incident HIV-associated morphologic and lipid abnormalities in a population-based cohort. *J Acquir Immune Defic Syndr* 30:440–447.

Holmberg SD, Moorman AC, Williamson JM, Tong TC, Ward DJ, Wood KC, Greenberg AE, and Janssen RS (2002). HIV Outpatient Study (HOPS) Investigators: protease inhibitors and cardiovascular outcome in patients with HIV-1. *Lancet* 360:1747–1748.

Holmberg SD, Moorman AC, and Greenberg AE (2004). Trends in rates of myocardial infarction among patients with HIV. *N Engl J Med* 350:730–731.

Hruz PW, Murata H, Qiu H, and Mueckler M (2002). Indinavir induces acute and reversible peripheral insulin resistance in rats. *Diabetes* 51:937–942.

Hsue PY, Giri K, Erickson S, MacGregor JS, Younes N, Shergill A, and Waters DD (2004). Clinical features of acute coronary syndromes in patients with human immunodeficiency virus infection. *Circulation* 109:316–319.

Hsue PY, Lo JC, Franklin A, Bolger AF, Martin JN, Deeks SG, and Waters DD (2004). Progression of atherosclerosis as assessed by carotid intima-media thickness in patients with HIV infection. *Circulation* 109:1603–1608.

Imhof A, Ledergerber B, Gunthard HF, Haupts S, and Weber R (2005). Swiss HIV Cohort Study: risk factors for and outcome of hyperlactatemia in HIV-infected persons: is there a need for routine lactate monitoring? *Clin Infect Dis* 41:721–728.

John M, Moore CB, James IR, Nolan D, Upton RP, McKinnon EJ, and Mallal SA (2001). Chronic hyperlactatemia in HIV-infected patients taking antiretroviral therapy. *AIDS* 15:717–723.

Klein D, Hurley LB, Quesenberry CP Jr, and Sidney S (2002). Do protease inhibitors increase the risk for coronary heart disease in patients with HIV-1 infection? *J Acquir Immune Defic Syndr* 30:471–477.

Lee GA, Seneviratne T, Noor MA, Lo JC, Schwarz JM, Aweeka FT, Mulligan K, Schambelan M, and Grunfeld C (2004). The metabolic effects of lopinavir/ritonavir in HIV-negative women. *AIDS* 18:641–649.

Lenert LA, Feddersen M, Sturley A, and Lee D (2002). Adverse effects of medications and trade-offs between length of life and quality of life in human immunodeficiency virus infection. *Am J Med* 113:229–232.

Lipowski ZJ (1970). Physical illness, the individual and the coping processes. *Psychiatry Med* 1:91–102.

Martinez E, Conget I, Lozano L, Casamitjana R, and Gatell JM (1999). Reversion of metabolic abnormalities after switching from HIV-1 protease inhibitors to nevirapine. *AIDS* 13:805–810.

Martinez E, Mocroft A, Garcia-Viejo MA, Perez-Cuevas JB, Blanco JL, Mallolas J, Bianchi L, Conget I, Blanch J, Phillips A, and Gatell JM (2001). Risk of lipodystrophy in HIV-1-infected patients treated with protease inhibitors: a prospective cohort study. *Lancet* 357:592–598.

Martinez E, Arnaiz JA, Podzamczer D, Dalmau D, Ribera E, Domingo P, Knobel H, Riera M, Pedrol E, Force L, Llibre JM, Segura F, Richart C, Cortes C, Javaloyas M, Aranda M, Cruceta A, de Lazzari E, and Gatell JM (2003). Nevirapine, Efavirenz, and Abacavir (NEFA) Study Team: substitution of nevirapine, efavirenz, or abacavir for protease inhibitors in patients with human immunodeficiency virus infection. *N Engl J Med* 349:1036–1046.

Mary-Krause M, Cotte L, Simon A, Partisani M, and Costagliola D (2003). Clinical Epidemiology Group from the French Hospital Database: increased risk of myocardial infarction with duration of protease inhibitor therapy in HIV-infected men. *AIDS* 17:2479–2486.

Matetzky S, Domingo M, Kar S, Noc M, Shah P, Kaul S, Daar E, and Cercek B (2003). Acute myocardial infarction in human immunodeficiency virus–infected patients. *Arch Intern Med* 163:457–460.

McComsey G, and Lonergan JT (2004). Mitochondrial dysfunction: patient monitoring and toxicity management. *J Acquir Immune Defic Syndr* 37:S30–S35.

McComsey GA, Ward DJ, Hessenthaler SM, Sension MG, Shalit P, Lonergan JT, Fisher RL, Williams VC, and Hernandez JE (2004). Trial to Assess the Regression of Hyperlactatemia and to Evaluate the Regression of Established Lipodystrophy in HIV-1-Positive Subjects (TARHEEL; ESS40010) Study Team: Iimprovement in lipoatrophy associated with highly active antiretroviral therapy in human immunodeficiency virus–infected patients switched from stavudine to abacavir or zidovudine: the results of the TARHEEL study. *Clin Infect Dis* 38:263–270.

Miller J, Carr A, Emery S, Law M, Mallal S, Baker D, Smith D, Kaldor J, and Cooper DA (2003). HIV lipodystrophy: prevalence, severity and correlates of risk in Australia. *HIV Med* 4:293–301.

Murata H, Hruz PW, and Mueckler M (2002). Indinavir inhibits the glucose transporter isoform Glut4 at physiologic concentrations. *AIDS* 16:859–863.

Mynarcik DC, McNurlan MA, Steigbigel RT, Fuhrer J, and Gelato MC (2000). Association of severe insulin resistance with both loss of limb fat and elevated serum tumor necrosis factor receptor levels in HIV lipodystrophy. *J Acquir Immune Defic Syndr* 25:312–321.

Negredo E, Ribalta J, Paredes R, Ferre R, Sirera G, Ruiz L, Salazar J, Reiss P, Masana L, and Clotet B (2002). Reversal of atherogenic lipoprotein profile in HIV-1 infected patients with lipodystrophy after replacing protease inhibitors by nevirapine. *AIDS* 16:1383–1389.

Noor MA, Seneviratne T, Aweeka FT, Lo JC, Schwarz JM, Mulligan K, Schambelan M, and Grunfeld C (2002). Indinavir acutely inhibits insulin-stimulated glucose disposal in humans: a randomized, placebo-controlled study. *AIDS* 16:F1–F8.

Oette M, Juretzko P, Kroidl A, Sagir A, Wettstein M, Siegrist J, and Haussinger D (2002). Lipodystrophy syndrome and self-assessment of well-being and physical appearance in HIV-positive patients. *AIDS Patient Care STDS* 16:413–417.

Palacios R, Santos J, Ruiz J, Gonzalez M, and Marquez M (2003). Factors associated with the development of diabetes mellitus in HIV-infected patients on antiretroviral therapy: a case-control study. *AIDS* 17:933–935.

Paton NI, Earnest A, Ng YM, Karim F, and Aboulhab J (2002). Lipodystrophy in a cohort of human immunodeficiency virus–infected Asian patients: prevalence, associated factors, and psychological impact. *Clin Infect Dis* 35:1244–1249.

Persson A (2005). Facing HIV: body shape change and the (in)visibility of illness. *Med Anthropol* 24:237–264.

Power R, Tate HL, McGill SM, and Taylor C (2003). A qualitative study of the psychosocial implications of lipodystrophy syndrome on HIV positive individuals. *Sex Transm Infect* 79:137–141.

Riddle TM, Kuhel DG, Woollett LA, Fichtenbaum J, and Hui DY (2001). HIV protease inhibitor induces fatty acid and sterol biosynthesis in liver and adipose tissues due to the accumulation of activated sterol regulatory element-binding proteins in the nucleus. *J Biol Chem* 276:37514–37519.

Riddler SA, Smit E, Cole SR, Li R, Chmiel JS, Dobs A, Palella F, Visscher B, Evans R, and Kingsley LA (2003). Impact of HIV infection and HAART on serum lipids in men. *JAMA* 289:2978–2982.

Schambelan M, Benson CA, Carr A, Currier JS, Dube MP, Gerber JG, Grinspoon SK, Grunfeld C, Kotler DP, Mulligan K, Powderly WG, and Saag MS (2002). Management of metabolic complications associated with antiretroviral therapy for HIV–1 infection: recommendations of an International AIDS Society–USA panel. *J Acquir Immune Defic Syndr* 31:257–275.

Shah M, Tierney K, Adams-Huet B, Boonyavarakul A, Jacob K, Quittner C, Dinges WL, Peterson D, and Garg A (2005). The role of diet, exercise, and smoking in dyslipidaemia in HIV-infected patients with lipodystrophy. *HIV Med* 6:291–298.

Stein JH, Klein MA, Bellehumeur JL, McBride PE, Wiebe DA, Otvos JD, and Sosman JM (2001). Use of human immunodeficiency virus-1 protease inhibitors is associated with atherogenic lipoprotein changes and endothelial dysfunction. *Circulation* 104:257–262.

Sutinen J, Hakkinen AM, Westerbacka J, Seppala-Lindroos A, Vehkavaara S, Halavaara J, Jarvinen A, Ristola M, and Yki-Jarvinen H (2003). Rosiglitazone in the treatment of HAART associated lipodystrophy—a randomized double-blind placebo-controlled study. *Antivir Ther* 8:199–207.

Wood R, Phanuphak P, Cahn P, Pokrovskiy V, Rozenbaum W, Pantaleo G, Sension M, Murphy R, Mancini M, Kelleher T, and Giordano M (2004) Long-term efficacy and safety of atazanavir with stavudine and lamivudine in patients previously treated with nelfinavir or atazanavir. *J Acquir Immune Defic Syndr* 36:684–692.

Chapter 37

Overview of HIV-Associated Comorbidities

Michael P. Mullen and Joseph Z. Lux

Since the introduction of effective antiretroviral therapy, the incidence of HIV-related opportunistic infections has been significantly reduced and patients are living longer. The frequency of pulmonary, gastrointestinal, hepatic, hematologic, cardiac, dermatologic, renal, and neoplastic manifestations are still very significant and in some areas appear to be increasing.

This review is not intended to provide a lengthy discourse on each topic addressed, but an overview that will provide the reader with a working knowledge of HIV-associated comorbidities.

PULMONARY MANIFESTATIONS OF HIV INFECTION

The spectrum and incidence of AIDS-related pulmonary opportunistic infections have changed significantly over the past 25 years since the first description of gay men with *Pneumocystis jiroveci* (*P. carinii*) in New York City and San Francisco in 1981 (Gottlieb et al., 1981; Masur et al., 1981). Effective combination antiretroviral therapy and prophylaxis with agents targeted against these infections have largely been responsible for the decrease in their incidence. In the Center for Disease Control and Prevention's HIV Outpatient Study (HOPS), which has followed large numbers of HIV-infected patients since 1993, there was a reduction in overall pulmonary mortality and morbidity between 1994 and 2003. This has been largely attributed to the introduction of antiretroviral therapy and prophylaxis (Palella et al., 1998).

Despite these advances, there are still significant amounts of these infections seen in inner-city hospitals in undiagnosed, nonadherent, or drug-resistant HIV-infected individuals. In addition, in the developing world the epidemic still remains largely untargeted. The most commonly associated infections will be reviewed here with references for more extensive discussion.

Pneumocystis jiroveci (carinii)

Pneumocystis still remains the most common AIDS-associated opportunistic infection in the United States (Jones et al., 1999). The CD4 lymphocyte count has been found to be a good predictor for risk of infection, since 80%–90% of infections are associated with a CD4 count of less than 200 cells/mm^3 (Masur et al., 1988). Patients can present with a wide array of pulmonary symptomatology, from mild dyspnea on exertion to rapidly progressive respiratory failure. In general, patients have fever, nonproductive cough, hypoxemia, elevated serum lactate dehydrogenase (LDH), and bilateral interstitial infiltrates on chest X-ray (Hoover et al., 1993).

A diagnosis of Pneumocystis carinii pneumonia (PCP) requires the detection of organisms in sputum or bronchoalveolar lavage fluid. Bronchoalveolar lavage has a sensitivity of 95%–99%, which makes transbronchial or open lung biopsy rarely necessary (Ognibene et al., 1984). Early diagnosis may prevent hospitalization and progression to respiratory failure (Brenner et al., 1987; Benfield et al., 2001).

Trimethoprim-sulfamethoxazole is the treatment of choice unless the patient has demonstrated a severe hypersensitivity to sulfa in the past. Desensitization to trimethoprim-sulfamethoxazole under controlled conditions can be considered in those patients who have had a mild reaction in the past (Gluckstein and Ruskin, 1995). Corticosteroids should be added for patients with moderate to severe hypoxemia (Gagnon et al., 1990). Alternative agents include pentamidine, clindamycin-primaquine, atovaquone, trimethoprim-dapsone, and trimetrexate. (Leoung et al., 1986; Medina et al., 1990; Hughes et al., 1993; Sattler et al., 1994; Toma et al., 1998). Resistance to sulfonamides has been reported, but there is no clear association with treatment failure (Kazanjian et al., 2000). The mortality rate of untreated PCP is 100%. Severe disease requiring ventilator support is associated with a worse prognosis.

PCP is clearly a preventable disease, and the need for prophylaxis for patients with a CD4 lymphocyte count of less than 200 cells/per cubic mml cannot be overemphasized. As in treatment, the preferred regimen for prophylaxis is trimethoprim-sulfamethoxazole (Kovacs et al., 2001). Controversy still remains as to when to initiate antiretroviral therapy in the setting of acute PCP. In addition to drug toxicity, the major concern is immune reconstitution inflammatory syndrome (IRIS), which has been associated with worsening respiratory failure (Wislez et al., 2001).

Other HIV-Related Respiratory Illnesses

Retrospective and prospective multicentered trials have shown that HIV-infected individuals have an increased rate of both upper and lower respiratory infections compared to that in uninfected controls (Wolff and O'Donnell, 2001). Infections and other related respiratory illnesses that can occur at any CD4 lymphocyte count include sinusitis, bacterial pneumonia and bronchitis, Mycobacterium tuberculosis pneumonia, bronchogenic carcinoma, non-Hodgkins lymphoma, and nonspecific interstitial pneumonitis.

As in the general population, the most frequent cause of bacterial pneumonia in HIV-infected patients is Streptococcus pneumoniae (Boyton, 2005). Other bacteria such as Haemophilus influenzae, Staphylococcus aureus, Klebsiella pneumoniae, and Rhodococcus equi can also be associated. When CD4 counts approach 200 cells/mm^3 and below, PCP, Cryptococcus neoformans pneumonia, bacterial pneumonia with bacteremia or sepsis, and extrapulmonary or disseminated Mycobactrium tuberculosis need to be considered. At CD4 counts fewer than 100 cells/mm^3, bacterial pneumonia due to Pseudomonas aeruginosa, Toxoplasma gondii pneumonia, and pulmonary Kaposi's sarcoma are more frequently seen. In advanced AIDS, with CD4 counts less than 50 cells/mm^3, disseminated endemic fungal diseases with pneumonia, such as histoplasmosis and coccididomycosis, disseminated viral infections, i.e., cytomegalovirus, and disseminated atypical Mycobacterium infection with pneumonia need to be considered (Boyton, 2005).

Mycobacterium Tuberculosis

Although the incidence of acute tuberculosis is decreasing in the United States, worldwide Mycobacterium tuberculosis infection is the leading cause of mortality in persons infected with HIV. Of the estimated 40 million persons living with HIV, approximately one-third are coinfected (Raviglione et al., 1995). The extensive spread of HIV has had a direct effect on increasing outbreaks of tuberculosis.

Similarly, tuberculosis has an adverse effect on HIV progression, accounting for one-third of all AIDS deaths (Dye et al., 1999). Patients with active tuberculosis have been found to have significant increases in HIV replication leading to increases in opportunistic infections (Jones et al., 1993).

The incidence of tuberculosis in HIV-infected patients has declined steadily with prolonged use of antiretroviral therapy, and patients on effective antiretroviral therapy with acute tuberculosis have been shown to have prolonged survival (Giardi et al., 2001). In the United States most cases were thought to be due to a reactivation of latent infection, but with the progression to AIDS and declining CD4 count primary infection becomes more likely. In fact, in one study done in New York City, DNA fingerprinting showed primary infection to be the cause of new infection in 40% of patients (Small and Fujiwara, 2001). The mean CD4 count at tuberculosis presentation is approximately $200–400$ cells/mm^3. The course of acute tuberculosis appears to behave similarly in HIV-infected and noninfected individuals when the CD4 count is above 300 cells/mm^3. The typical presentation is pulmonary with fever, weight loss, night sweats, apical infiltrates that can cavitate. As the CD4 count declines below 200 cells/mm^3, the presentation can be more atypical, making the diagnosis more difficult. In patients with AIDS and severe immunodeficiency, extrapulmonary tuberculosis becomes more likely (Jones et al., 1993).

Tuberculosis skin testing (PPD) should be performed on all individuals with HIV infection, regardless of whether a diagnosis of active tuberculosis is suspected. A 5 mm or greater area of induration is considered to be positive; however, in acute tuberculosis the PPD skin test is often falsely negative. Since an AFB positive smear is seen in approximately 60% of HIV-infected patients with culture-proven tuberculosis and isolation of the organism can take up to 6 weeks, a high index of suspicion must be maintained and empiric treatment started in all truly suspected cases (CDC, 2000). Initial therapy for tuberculosis includes four highly active drugs—isoniazid, rifampin, pyrazinamide, and ethambutol. Pyridoxine should be added to prevent isoniazid-induced peripheral neuropathy. Treatment for the initial 2 months should include all four agents. Ethambutol can be discontinued if the organism is shown to be sensitive to the other three agents.

Isoniazid and rifampin should be continued for the final 4 months. For patients who cannot tolerate pyrazinamide, a 9- to 12-month regimen of isoniazid and rifampin is recommended. In general, the response to therapy is similar in both HIV-infected and negative individuals (CDC, 2003).

A paradoxical worsening of symptomatology can occur with initial treatment; this is thought to be due to immune reconstitution. Treatment should not be interrupted, but a short course of steroids may be necessary to ameliorate the worsening symptoms (Navas et al., 2002). In general, it is necessary to treat both HIV and *Mycobacterium* tuberculosis simultaneously. Significant drug interactions often make this difficult. Rifampin is a potent p450 inhibitor, which interacts with many of the antiretroviral agents, therefore consultation with an experienced HIV provider should be sought to ensure the proper regimen selection.

Drug-resistant tuberculosis in HIV infection is an ongoing issue and therapy should be based on sensitivity testing and infectious disease staff consultation. Preventive therapy for the treatment of latent tuberculosis infection is essential to stop the development of active tuberculosis, since this occurs at a rate of 5% to 10% per year in HIV-infected individuals (Jasmer et al., 2002). The current recommendation for HIV-infected PPD-positive patients is to receive daily isoniazid and pyridoxine for 9 months.

GASTROINTESTINAL MANIFESTATIONS OF HIV INFECTION

Gastrointestinal complaints associated with HIV infection are almost universal. From the time of acute seroconversion through the diagnosis of AIDS, diarrhea stands out as the most frequent gastrointestinal complaint. Added to the list are nausea, vomiting, dysphagia, odonyphagia, wasting, abdominal pain, gastrointestinal bleeding, jaundice, and anorectal ulceration. Disorders can be secondary to opportunistic infection, chronic coinfection with hepatitis B or C, malignancies, drug toxicities, and HIV itself. It is clear that the degree of immunosuppression as manifested by the CD4 count reflects the prevalence of gastrointestinal symptoms (May et al., 1993). In addition, effective antiretroviral therapy and chemoprophylaxis against the most common opportunistic pathogens, such as *Mycobacterium avium* and cytomegalovirus

(CMV), has changed the spectrum of gastrointestinal disorders in patients with HIV infection.

Esophagitis

Candida albicans is the most common cause of esophagitis in patients with AIDS. Although the majority of patients with *Candida* esophagitis have oral candida or thrush, the absence of thrush does not preclude the diagnosis (Wilcox et al., 1995). Empiric therapy with fluconozole is indicated in patients with esophageal complaints and thrush, reserving endoscopy for treatment failures (Wilcox et al., 1996). Other infectious causes of esophagitis in AIDS are CMV, herpes simplex virus (HSV), and idiopathic esophageal ulceration (IEU) (Wilcox, 1992). Unlike *Candida* esophagitis, odonyphagia is a more common complaint than dysphagia in IEU (Raufman, 1988). HIV-associated IEU can be seen at the time of acute seroconversion, but, like CMV, it is more commonly seen with a CD4 lymphocyte count of fewer than 100 cells/mm^3 (Kotler et al., 1992). Less common infections reported to cause esophagitis in AIDS patients are *Mycobacterium avium* intracellulare (MAI), *Bartonella henselae, Cryptosporidim, Histoplasma capsulatum*, Epstein-Barr virus, and human papilloma virus (Monkemuller and Wilcox, 1999). HIV-related malignancies, such as, non-Hodgkin's lymphoma and Kaposi's sarcoma, and gastroesophageal reflux disease also need to be considered when a patients presents with esophageal symptoms.

Diarrhea

As mentioned previously, diarrhea remains the most common gastrointestinal complaint among patients with HIV disease. The etiology of diarrhea is often multifactorial. A thorough history including travel should be elicited from all HIV patients presenting with diarrhea. The patient's symptoms may help in localizing the area of bowel most affected. Symptoms of crampy abdominal pain with bloating and voluminous, watery diarrhea suggest small bowel enteritis with pathogens such as *Cryptosporidium* and *Giardia*. Proctitis may indicate CMV or HSV infection.

A wide array of viruses, bacteria, fungi, and parasites has been implicated in the etiology of diarrhea (Smith et al., 1992). The degree of immunodeficiency makes certain pathogens and refractory disease more likely. Prior to effective antiretroviral therapy and che-

moprophylaxis, infections such as CMV, *Cryptosporidium, Microsporidia*, and disseminated MAI were more commonly seen and were associated with severe recalcitrant disease (Connolly et al., 1988; Asmuth et al., 1994; Gordin et al., 1997). In addition, unusual presentations with bacteremia of the usual pathogens that cause diarrhea in the normal host, such as *Salmonella, Campylobacter*, and *Shigella* may be seen (Smith et al., 1985; Molina et al., 1995). *Clostridium difficile*–associated diarrhea has also been shown to be more frequent in patients with AIDS, which most likely reflects the increased use of antimicrobial agents and stays in hospital (Hutin et al., 1993). Certain antiretroviral agents are commonly associated with diarrhea, specifically nelfinavir, lopinavir/ritonavir, saquinavir, and didanosine (buffered formulation). More often than not, despite extensive workups with multiple stool cultures and repeated endoscopies with multiple tissue biopsies, an etiologic agent is not isolated. In this clinical scenario, empiric therapy with antimicrobial and antiparasitic agents is indicated. When the diarrhea is unremitting, antidiarrheal agents should be considered to prevent dehydration.

Patients with HIV disease may also complain of abdominal pain, hematemesis, hematochezia, jaundice, and anorectal pain. The possible etiologies are numerous, including both opportunistic and nonopportunistic disorders, malignancies, and drug-related toxicities. A detailed history and physical exam with appropriate workup will usually reveal the cause of the disorder.

Hepatobiliary Disease

Hepatic disease in HIV infection is a significant cause of morbidity and mortality. Most patients with AIDS will have some evidence of liver dysfunction. Like gastrointestinal disorders they tend to occur later in the course of HIV infection, reflecting increasing immunosuppression (Cappell, 1991). A wide array of opportunistic infections including MAI, CMV, HSV, *Mycobacterium* tuberculosis, *Bartonella hensalae, Pneumocystis*, disseminated fungal disease, and HIV-associated malignancies, such as Kaposi's sarcoma and non-Hodgkin's lymphoma, have all been shown to involve the liver (Perkocha et al., 1990; Bonacini, 1992).

Hepatotoxicity can also be due to antiretroviral therapy, idiosyncratic or immunoallergic mechanisms, or direct cytotoxicity due to underlying liver disease.

Chronic coinfection with hepatitis B virus (HBV) is more common with HIV seropositivity. Only 5% of HIV-negative individuals with acute hepatitis B will go on to develop chronic disease, whereas in coinfection 50% or more will have evidence of chronic HBV replication. There is an increased risk of chronic active hepatitis progressing to cirrhosis and the development of hepatocellular carcinoma with HIV infection. In addition, HIV-infected individuals who are immune to HBV, as evidenced by hepatitis B surface antibody positivity, may with increasing immunosuppression go on to lose antibody and again become hepatitis B surface-antigen positive with antigenemia (Lazizi et al., 1988). There is no clear evidence whether HBV has a negative effect on HIV progression.

Several HIV antiretroviral agents (epivir, emtrivir, tenofovir) have been shown to be effective in decreasing the HBV DNA in the blood with eventual development of hepatitis B surface antibody. Initiating HIV antiretroviral therapy in patients with chronic HBV may be associated with flares of hepatitis B due to immunoreconstitution syndrome. There is an increase in highly active antiretroviral therapy (HARRT)-related hepatotoxicity in patients with chronic hepatitis B (Ogedegbe and Sulkowski, 2003).

Hepatitis C virus (HCV) is more frequently associated with chronic infection, since only approximately 15% of individuals clear virus from the blood after acute infection (Alter et al., 1992). Coinfection with HIV is associated with an increased rate of the development of cirrhosis and hepatocellular carcinoma. Hepatitis C does not appear to accelerate HIV progression, nor does it respond to antiretroviral therapy (Sulkowski et al., 2002). Caution must be used in selecting HIV antiretroviral agents, because of the risk of hepatotoxicity. Liver biopsy should be strongly considered to determine the degree of fibrosis and to aid in selection of patients for hepatitis C therapy (Saadeh et al., 2001).

Pegylated interferon and ribavirin for 48 weeks is the currently available therapy that has shown the best results. Most patients in the United States are genotype 1, which has a less than optimal response to therapy with a sustained virologic response (SVR) of under 30% (Toriani et al., 2004). In general, those with genotypes 2 and 3 have a better response to therapy. All patients should be considered for therapy; it must be said, however, that the multiple drug-related side effects encountered on therapy often make this a difficult option. All patients who are considered for therapy should be

under the care of an experienced provider. The neuropsychiatric effects of interferon are of major concern and are discussed in further detail in Chapter 33.

All coinfected patients should limit alcohol and hepatotoxic agents. The HAV and HBV vaccine should be offered to all seronegative patients. Another gastrointestinal syndrome, AIDS cholangiopathy, has been seen largely in patients with advanced disease. Patients present with right upper quadrant pain, jaundice, and hepatomegaly. The alkaline phosphatase level in the blood is often quite elevated. All clinical syndromes can be diagnosed by endoscopic retrograde cholangiopancreatography (ERCP). Although there is no clear causal relationship, *Cryptosporidium*, *Microsporidia*, CMV, and *Cyclospora* have all been associated. If possible, the offending pathogens should be treated, although often the treatment requires biliary stenting. In general, the prognosis is poor (Ko et al., 2003).

HEMATOLOGIC MANIFESTATIONS OF HIV INFECTION

Hematologic disorders have long been associated with HIV infection. These disorders are widely recognized and are the cause of significant morbidity and mortality. In fact, anemia, the most commonly associated abnormality, has been shown to have a negative effect on survival (Moore et al., 1998). The most common cause of anemia is HIV infection of marrow progenitor cells, and increasing levels of tumor necrosis factor leading to ineffective erythropoiesis (Zhang et al., 1995). In general, the incidence of anemia has a direct correlation with the degree of immunosuppression, and improvement is generally seen with immune recovery secondary to effective antiretroviral therapy (Huang et al., 2000). Some other causes of anemia in HIV infection are infiltration of the bone marrow by tumor or opportunistic infections.

Infections more commonly associated with anemia are *Mycobacterium avium* complex (MAC), tuberculosis, CMV, and histoplasmosis. The most frequently associated tumors are lymphomas and Kaposi's sarcoma (Coyle, 1997). Parvovirus B 19 has been reported to selectively infect erythroid precursors leading to severe anemia (Abkowitz et al., 1997).

Nutritional deficiencies need also to be considered. Vitamin B12 deficiency has been reported to occur in up to 20% of HIV-infected patients (Evans et al., 2000). Iron deficiency anemia is usually associated with blood loss from the gastrointestinal tract. In addition, drug-induced marrow suppression, such as that seen with the nucleoside analogue reverse transcriptase inhibitor zidovudine (AZT), always needs to be considered. Management consists of treatment of the underlying cause with the appropriate agents and, when applicable, dose adjustment of drug therapy.

Erythropoietin can be of benefit in many patients with refractory HIV-associated anemia. Neutropenia is seen in HIV infection and is most often due to chronic infection, bone marrow failure, or drug toxicity (Sloand, 2005). Thrombocytopenia can be seen at any stage of HIV infection (Sullivan et al., 1997). Although HIV and drug-related toxicity can directly affect platelet production, immune destruction of platelets is the most common cause (ITP). Treatment consists of effective antiretroviral therapy and the removal of any causative agent. ITP may require steroids, intravenous gamma globulin, and at times splenectomy (Oksenhendler et al., 1993). Thrombotic thrombocytopenic purpura has been reported to occur in HIV infection but the association is less clear. Patients present with hemolytic anemia, thrombocytopenia, renal insufficiency, fever, and change in mental status. The prognosis is usually poor. The standard treatment is plasmaphoresis (Sloand, 2005).

DERMATOLOGIC DISORDERS ASSOCIATED WITH HIV INFECTION

Dermatologic conditions are clearly associated with HIV infection. In fact, greater that 90% of HIV-infected individuals will have a dermatologic complaint at some time in the course of their illness (Coldiron and Bergstresser, 1989). Disorders of the skin and mucous membranes were described in the first reported cases of AIDS (Friedman-Kien et al., 1982). As with other HIV-associated conditions, these manifestations worsen as the degree of immunosuppression increases. These disorders can be secondary to viral, bacterial, or fungal infections. In addition, cutaneous drug eruptions and malignancies need to be included.

In acute HIV seroconversion, rash is seen in greater than 70% of patients. It is usually maculopapular and involves the face and trunk. It can involve the palms and soles, similar to secondary syphilis. Oral candidiasis, usually seen in more advanced immunosuppression, can also be seen in acute seroconversion (Kahn and Walker, 1998).

Oral hairy leukoplakia is an HIV-associated disorder localized to the oral mucosa and consists of whitish plaques on the lateral border of the tongue. It is often confused with oral candidiasis, but it cannot be removed by scraping. It is associated with a low CD4 lymphocyte count and generally resolves with immune recovery (Greenspan et al., 1987).

Seborrheic dermatitis is the most common cutaneous manifestation associated with HIV infection. It tends to be localized to the face with involvement of the eyebrows and nasolabial fold. It can be very severe with worsening immunodeficiency and is often recalcitrant to treatment. Topical steroids and antifungal agents are the treatment of choice (Tschachler et al., 1996).

Pruritus is a common complaint in HIV infection and is generally a more significant issue in advanced disease. The etiology includes primary association with HIV disease and adverse cutaneous drug eruptions. A chronic dermatosis associated with severe pruritus is eosinophilic folliculitis, usually seen with advanced disease; eosinophilia is commonly seen (Milazzo et al., 1999). It can also occur with the initiation of effective antiretroviral therapy as a result of immune reconstitution syndrome. Lesions tend to resolve as the CD4 lymphocyte count improves (Bonacini, 2000). Bacterial folliculitis is most commonly associated with *Staphylococcus aureus* infection, however, there have been increasing reports of a new, more virulent, methicillin-resistant strain that has a propensity to develop into abscesses that, in addition to antimicrobial coverage, require incision and drainage (Mathews et al., 2005).

Other bacterial agents that have been associated with cutaneous infections in the HIV population are *Bartonella* (bacillary angiomatosis), tuberculosis, and MAC (Tappero et al., 1995; Rigopoulos et al., 2004). Secondary syphilis, which is known to occur with increased frequency in HIV infected individuals, can present with a diffuse maculopapular rash involving the palms and soles (Hutchinson et al., 1994).

Viral infections with cutaneous manifestation include *Molluscum contagiosum*, HPV, common warts, HSV-1 and -2, *Varicella zoster* (shingles), CMV, Epstein-Barr virus, and HHV-8 (Kaposi's sarcoma) (Tappero et al., 1995). Since cutaneous fungal infections are seen more frequently with compromised immunity, it is not surprising that they would be common in HIV infection. Dermatophytes and, to a lesser degree, *Candida*, infect the skin, hair, and nails (Elewski and Sullivan, 1994). Because these infections tend to be chronic and recurrent they are a frequent source of distress. Treatment response to systemic and topical agents is suboptimal. Improvement is seen with antiretroviral therapy and immune recovery.

A hyperkeratotic form of scabies (Norwegian) is seen more frequently in severely immunocompromised HIV individuals. Patients can present with disseminated, crusted, popular, or eczematoid lesions that are highly contagious (Portu et al., 1996).

Lastly, no discussion of cutaneous manifestations of HIV disease would be complete without a description of cutaneous drug eruptions. HIV-infected individuals seem to be at increased risk for adverse drug reactions, and this risk increases with advancing immunosuppression (Coopman et al., 1993). Trimethoprim-sulfamethoxazole, the agent of choice to treat *Pneumocystis jiroveci* (*carinii*) pneumonia, has been shown in its intravenous form to cause an erythematous rash that is usually associated with fever. In general, this reaction occurs 10 to 14 days after starting therapy (Roudier et al., 1994). The oral preparation is also associated with increased skin reactions that may be due to a toxic drug metabolite. If this drug is gradually initiated into the patient's regimen, there is an approximately 50% decrease in adverse reaction (Para et al., 2000). Although rare, a mild rash can progress to life-threatening Stevens-Johnson syndrome (SJS) and toxic epidermal necrolysis (TEN). These reactions are seen more commonly with sulfonamides.

The nonnucleoside reverse transcriptase inhibitors (nevirapine, delavirdine, and efaverenz) have been reported to be associated with this type of hypersensitivity reaction, with nevirapine having the highest incidence (Warren et al., 1998). Abacavir, a nucleoside analogue reverse transcriptase inhibitor, is associated with a severe hypersensitivity reaction, in which a maculopapular or urticarial skin rash can be part of the constellation of symptoms. These reactions are rare in African-American patients and appear to be associated with a genetic link or susceptibility.

Patients should be instructed to immediately contact their provider at the first sign of any reaction. If the drug is discontinued, then the patient should never be rechallenged with this agent, since fatalities are known to occur (Hewitt, 2002).

HIV-ASSOCIATED OPHTHALMOLOGIC DISEASE

Prior to the development of effective antiretroviral therapy, HIV-associated ocular complications were very common. In fact, CMV retinitis was the most common ocular infection in patients with AIDS, affecting an estimated 20%–45% of patients (Holland et al., 1983). Patients required life-long therapy and had a mean survival after diagnosis of 6–10 months (Hoover et al., 1993). Multiple trials have shown that intravenous ganciclovir, foscarnet, cidofovir, oral ganciclovir, and local intravitreal ganciclovir implant are all effective. Studies have shown that the time to relapse is longest with the implant (Martin et al., 1999).

Currently, largely because of effective antiretroviral therapy, new cases of CMV retinitis are rare, with a decline in incidence of 80% (Goldberg et al., 2005). Patients with a history of CMV retinitis who have had a successful response to antiretroviral therapy with increasing CD4 lymphocyte count can safely discontinue maintenance therapy with close observation for recurrence (MacDonald et al., 2000). A new ocular inflammatory syndrome associated with immune recovery in patients with CMV retinitis is immune recovery uveitis (IRU). The pathogenesis is though to be secondary to an immune response to CMV present in the retina (Jacobson et al., 1997). This syndrome needs to be anticipated and recognized early, since it can result in a substantial loss of vision.

Other ocular diseases that were seen prior to effective antiretroviral therapy were acute retinal necrosis secondary to herpes zoster virus (HZV) and HSV, toxoplasmosis retinochoroiditis, *Pneumocystis jiroveci* (*carinii*) choroididtis, syphilitic retinitis, tuberculosis choroididtis, cryptococcal choroididtis, and ocular lymphomas (Moraes, 2002).

Although the incidence of ocular complications of HIV infection has decreased considerably, it is important for all HIV providers to have a working knowledge of these disorders because the long-term sequelae can be devastating. In addition, in the developing world, where the majority of HIV infection resides and effective antiretroviral therapy is not readily available, these ocular complications will continue to be seen with increasing numbers. Patients with HIV and compromised immune systems should be instructed to alert their provider to any change in visual acuity and should undergo an annual regular ophthalmologic exam performed by an experienced ophthalmologist. Those individuals with persistent CD4 lymphocyte counts below 50 cells/mm^3 should be seen more frequently, and chemoprophylaxis for CMV should be considered in certain selected individuals.

HIV AND MALIGNANCIES

It is a well-known fact that defects in cell-mediated immunity have been associated with the development of certain tumors. This has been reported in congenital immunodeficiency disorders, transplant recipients on chronic immunosuppressive medication, and in patients with autoimmune disorders (Penn, 1975; Frizzera et al., 1980). Hence it was no surprise that there would be such an association with HIV infection. The initial reports of Kaposi's sarcoma (KS), a rare vascular tumor, and *Pneumocystis carinii* pneumonia in gay men in San Francisco and New York City in 1981 initiated the beginning of what is now known as the AIDS epidemic (Friedman-Kien et al., 1982). Subsequently, it was noted that there were increasing reports of non-Hodgkin's lymphoma (NHL) and, later, invasive cervical carcinoma in this population, placing these diagnoses in the category of AIDS-defining illnesses (CDC, 1985). In addition, over the years of the epidemic there have been other associated malignancies that are not considered AIDS defining but have been reported with some increased frequency, such as Hodgkin's disease, lung cancer, anogenital carcinomas, testicular cancers, gastric cancers, hepatomas, and multiple myeloma (Remick, 1996). Other cofactors may influence the development of these tumors, including tobacco, alcohol, and coinfection with hepatitis B, hepatitis C, and HPV, where the association with HIV and immunosuppression is less clear.

With the development of antiretroviral therapy, the incidence of KS has had such a significant decline that in developed countries it is a rare diagnosis (Hengge et al., 2002). Although less dramatic, the incidence of NHL has also shown a decrease since the development of effective antiretroviral therapy (Grulich and Vajdic, 2005; Wood and Harrington, 2005).

Kaposi's Sarcoma

Kaposi first described KS in 1812. Classical KS is usually seen in men of Mediterranean or Eastern European ancestry. It is normally localized to the skin of the lower extremity and it has a chronic, indolent course. In rare cases, it disseminates to other organs. In HIV infection KS has a varied course. It can be localized to the skin, but often has a progressively invasive course, with visceral dissemination being not unusual. With cutaneous involvement it can produce significant disfigurement. Visceral involvement can have associated odonyphagia, hypoxia and hemoptysis, gastrointestinal bleeding, and sepsis (Schwartz, 2004).

As mentioned previously, although KS still causes a significant amount of morbidity and even mortality in the developing world, the incidence of KS in the United States has been dramatically reduced since the introduction of potent antiretroviral therapy (Hengge et al., 2002). The Multi-Centered AIDS Cohort Study (MACS) showed a clear decline in the incidence of KS in 1995–1997, which paralleled the introduction of antiretroviral therapy (Jacobson et al., 1999).

The consensus is that this decline in incidence is most likely due to improved immunity, which in turn influences the host response to the causative agent, human herpes virus 8 (HHV-8). HHV-8 has been found in all types of KS, including classic, African and endemic, transplant-associated, and AIDS-related KS (Chang et al., 1994). In addition to antiretroviral therapy there are varied treatment options available, including intralesional chemotherapy, radiation therapy, laser therapy, and systemic chemotherapy (Schwartz, 2004). Treatment needs to be individualized according to the severity of the disease and is often associated with drug toxicities from the complexity of interactions between antiretroviral therapy and chemotherapy. Treatment needs to be done in conjunction with an oncologist who has had experience in treating KS in HIV-infected individuals.

Non-Hodgkin's Lymphoma

Among HIV-infected individuals, the first cases of NHL began to be reported in gay men in 1982. With increasing reports it soon became apparent that there was an association (Ziegler et al., 1984). We now know that for patients with an AIDS diagnosis, the risk of developing lymphoma is greater than 200 times that of the general population (Beral et al., 1991; Rabkin et al., 1991). Risk of NHL in people with HIV infection is independently predicted by the degree and duration of immunodeficiency and chronic B-cell stimulation (Grulich et al., 2001). The etiology is poorly understood, but it is most likely multifactorial. Epstein-Barr virus, HHV-8, and immune dysregulation all may play a role in HIV-associated NHL (Krause, 2005).

Similar to KS in HIV disease, the lymphomas can present in various stages. High-grade diffuse, large-cell or Burkitt's-like lymphomas are seen in over 70% of reported cases, although recently there appears to be an increase in low-grade B-cell and T-cell lymphomas (Biggar, 2001).

AIDS lymphoma is more likely to be symptomatic and disseminated at presentation. The lymphomas that develop in the AIDS population are similar to those found in other immunodeficient states. Unlike HIV-associated central nervous system (CNS) lymphomas, for which there is clear evidence that the incidence is declining, there remains controversy as to whether the incidence of NHL has increased or decreased since the advent of potent antiretroviral therapy (Bower, 2001). Both the Multicenter AIDS Cohort Study and the Swiss HIV Cohort Study have shown no difference in the incidence of NHL after the introduction of potent antiretroviral therapy (Jacobson et al., 1999; Ledergerber et al., 1999), however, as mentioned previously, there are other studies that support a decline in incidence.

In any case, prior to use of antiretroviral therapy the prognosis for HIV-related NHL was bleak; the median survival despite chemotherapy was 5–8 months (Bower, 2001). Since that time there has been a dramatic improvement in outcomes. Although it may be difficult to integrate antiretroviral therapy with systemic chemotherapy because of the level of toxicity, this combination is generally considered appropriate. Because of the complexity of treatment, a team approach is clearly warranted.

Cervical Carcinoma and Anal Carcinoma

In 1993 invasive cervical carcinoma was added to the case definition of AIDS, as there were early reports of aggressive cervical carcinoma with a mean survival of 10 months in a group of HIV-infected women (Maiman et al., 1990). Despite these reports, invasive cervical carcinoma in AIDS remains a rare diagnosis. Human papilloma viral infection (HPV), which is sexually transmitted, is a risk factor for both cervical and anal carcinoma. HIV infection has clearly been shown to increase the risk for the development of HPV-associated neoplasia. This association can be seen throughout the anogenital tract, including cervix, anus, penis, vulva, and skin.

In HIV-infected men who have sex with men (MSM) the incidence of anal squamous cell carcinoma is rising (Palefsky et al., 1998). In one study, 93% of HIV-positive MSM and 61% of HIV-negative MSM had anal HPV infection. The more oncogenic genotypes (HPV-16 and HPV-18) were more commonly associated with HIV infection (Pfister, 1996). High-grade dysplasia is also more frequent in HIV-positive men with low CD4 counts. Unfortunately, HIV-positive men have a poor prognosis, because they frequently present with advanced disease. Therefore, it is important for clinicians to screen for dysplasia with periodic anal Papanicolaou smears. It is unclear what impact potent antiretroviral therapy will have on the incidence of anogenital carcinoma, but it appears that those patients with dysplasia on therapy do better (Palefsky et al., 2001).

Other Cancers

Although Hodgkin's disease is not an AIDS-defining illness, it has been reported with increase frequency in HIV. The risk for an HIV-infected individual of developing Hodgkin's disease is 8–10 times higher than that of the general population (Hessol et al., 1992). It tends to have a more aggressive histologic cell type with widely disseminated extranodal disease (Levine, 1996). The diagnosis is often difficult to make. Prior to potent antiretroviral therapy the response to treatment was poor. It appears that the response to therapy is related to degree of immunosuppression and CD4 count.

There have been isolated reports of the increase of certain other cancers in HIV-infected individuals, but these are complex associations, where other risk factors may play a more significant role than HIV infection itself. The U.S. National Cancer Institute published data in 2003 that these cancers are not more common in people with HIV who are living longer in developed countries with access to HIV medication, despite studies reporting opposite findings (Mbulaiteye et al., 2003). In the HIV Outpatient Study (HOPS), reported in 2004, four cancers were seen with increasing frequency among individuals with HIV compared to that of the general population: anorectal cancer, Hodgkin's disease, melanoma, and lung cancer. The study adjusted for age, race, smoking, and gender. The researchers reported that those individuals who did develop cancer had a lower nadir CD4 (Patel et al., 2004). Despite the debate, patients with HIV infection should be screened regularly for the development of any neoplastic process. In addition, at each encounter every HIV provider should emphasize the importance of lifestyle modifications that may alter the development of cancer.

CONCLUSIONS

The intent of this chapter is to provide the reader with a working knowledge of the complexities associated with the medical comorbidities associated with HIV infection. When persons with HIV and AIDS have access and adherence to medical care and treatment with potent antiretroviral therapy, they can live longer lives. For persons with HIV and AIDS to live healthier and longer lives, it is also important for clinicians to encourage adherence to a healthy lifestyle with exercise, safe sex, a well-balanced diet, and stress reduction. The avoidance of illicit drug use, excessive alcohol, and tobacco should be emphasized at every encounter.

References

Abkowitz JL, Brown KE, Wood RW, et al. (1997). Clinical relevance of parvovirus B19 as a cause of anemia in patients with human immunodeficiency virus infection. *J Infect Dis* 176(1):269–273.

Alter MJ, Margolis HS, Krawczynski K, et al. (1992). The natural history of community acquired hepatitis C in the United States. *N Engl J Med* 327: 1899–1905.

Asmuth DM, DeGirolami PC, Federman M, et al. (1994). Clinical features of microsporidiosis in patients with AIDS. *Clin Infect Dis* 18:819–825.

Baughman RD, Dohn MN, and Frame PT (1994). The continuing utility of bronchoalveolar lavage to diagnose opportunistic infection in AIDS patients. *Am J Med* 97(6):515–522.

Benfield TL, Helweg-Larsen J, Bang D, et al. (2001). Prognostic markers of short-term mortality in AIDS-associated *Pneumocystis carinii* pneumonia. *Chest* 119:844–851.

Beral V, Peterman T, Berkalman R, et al. (1991). AIDS associated non-Hodgkin's lymphoma. *Lancet* 337: 805–809.

Biggar RJ (2001). AIDS related cancers in the era of highly active antiretroviral therapy. *Oncology* 15: 439–444.

Biggar RJ, and Rabkin CS (1992). The epidemiology of acquired immunodeficiency syndrome–related lymphomas. *Curr Opin Oncol* 4:883–893.

Bonacini M (1992). Hepatobiliary complications in patients with human immunodeficiency virus infection. *Am J Med* 92(4):404–411.

Bonacini M (2000). Prutitus in patients with chronic human immunodeficiency virus, hepatitis B and C virus infections. *Dig Liver Dis* 32(7):621–625.

Bower M (2001). Acquired immunodeficiency syndrome related systemic non-Hodgkin's lymphoma. *Br J Haematol* 112(4):863–873.

Boyton RJ (2005). Infectious lung complications in patients with HIV/AIDS. *Curr Opin Pulm Med* 11: 203–207.

Brenner M, Ognibenc FP, Lack EE, et al. (1987). Prognostic factors and life expectancy of patients with acquired immunodeficiency syndrome and *Pneumocystis carinii* pneumonia. *Am Rev Respir Dis* 136:1199–1206.

Cappell MS (1991). Hepatobiliary manifestations of the acquired immune deficiency syndrome. *Am J Gastroenterol* 86(1):1–15.

[CDC] Centers for Disease Control and Prevention (1985). Centers for Disease Control revision of the case definition of acquired immunodeficiency syndrome for national reporting–United States. *MMWR Morb Mortal Wkly Rep* 4:373–374.

[CDC] Centers for Disease Control and Prevention (2002). Targeted tuberculin testing and treatment of latent tuberculosis. *MMWR Morb Mortal Wkly Rep* 49(RR-6):1–54.

[CDC] Centers for Disease Control and Prevention (2003). Treatment of tuberculosis. American Thoracic Society, CDC, and Infectious Diseases Society of America. *MMWR Morb Mortal Wkly Rep* 52(RR-11):1–77.

Chang Y, Cesarman E, Pessin MS, et al. (1994). Identification of herpesvirus-like DNA sequences in AIDS-associated Kaposi's sarcoma. *Science* 266: 1865–1869.

Coldiron BM, and Bergstresser PR (1989). Prevalence and clinical spectrum of skin disease in patients infected with human immunodeficiency virus. *Arch Dermatol* 125(3):357–361.

Connolly GM, Dryden MS, Shanson DC, et al. (1988). Cryptosporidial diarrhea in AIDS and its treatment. *Gut* 29:593–597.

Coopman SA, Johnson RA, Platt R, and Gazzard BG (1993). Cutaneous disease and drug reactions in HIV infection. *N Engl J Med* 328(23):1670–1674.

Coyle TE (1997). Hematologic complications of human immunodeficiency virus infection in the acquired immunodeficiency syndrome. *Med Clin North Am* 81(2):449–470.

Dye C, Scheele S, Dolin P, et al. (1999). Consensus statement. Global burden of tuberculosis: estimated incidence, prevalence, and mortality by country.

WHO Global Surveillance and Monitoring Project. *JAMA* 282(7):677–686.

Elewski BE, and Sullivan J (1994). Dermatophytes as opportunistic pathogens. *J Am Acad Dermatol* 30(6): 1021–1022.

Evans RH, and Scadden DT (2000). Haematological aspects of HIV infection. *Ballieres Clin Haematol* 13:215.

Friedman-Kien A, Laubenstein LJ, Rubinstein P, et al. (1982). Disseminated Kaposi's sarcoma in homosexual men. *Ann Intern Med* 96:693–700.

Frizzera G, Rosa J, Denher L, et al. (1980). Lymphoreticular disorders in primary immunodeficiency. New findings based on up to date histologic classification of 35 cases. *Cancer* 46:692–699.

Gagnon S, Botta AM, Fischl MA, et al. (1990). Corticosteroids as adjunctive therapy for severe *Pneumocystis carinii* pneumonia in acquired immunodeficiency syndrome: a double-blind placebo controlled trial. *N Engl J Med* 323:1144–1150.

Gluckstein D, and Ruskin J (1995). Rapid oral desensitization to trimethoprim-sulfamethoxazole: use in prophylaxis for *Pneumocystis carinii* pneumonia in patients with AIDS who were previously intolerant to TMP-SMZ. *Clin Infect Dis* 20(4):849–853.

Goldberg DE, Smithen LM, Angelilli A, et al. (2005). HIV-associated retinopathy in the HAART era. *Retina* 25(5):633–649.

Gordin FM, Cohn DL, Sullam PM, et al. (1997). Early manifestations of disseminated *Mycobacterium avium* complex disease: a prospective evaluation. *J Infect Dis* 176(1):126–132.

Gottlieb MS, Schroff R, Schanker HM, et al. (1981). *Pneumocystis carinii* pneumonia and mucosal candidiasis in previously healthy homosexual men: evidence of an acquired cellular immunodeficiency. *N Engl J Med* 305:1425–1431.

Greenspan D, Greenspan JS, Hearst NG, et al. (1987). Relation of oral hairy leukoplakia to infection with human immunodeficiency virus and risk of development of AIDS. *J Infect Dis* 155(3):475–481.

Grulich AE, and Vajdic CM (2005). The epidemiology of non-Hodgkin lymphoma. *Pathology* 37(6):409–419.

Grulich AE, Li Y, McDonald AM, et al. (2001). Decreasing rate of Kaposi's sarcoma and non-Hodgkin's lymphoma in the era of potent combination anti-retroviral therapy. *AIDS* 15(5):629–633.

Hengge UR, Ruzicka T, Tyring SK, et al. (2002). Update on Kaposi's sarcoma and other HHV-8 associated diseases. Part 1: Epidemiology, environmental predispositions, clinical manifestations, and therapy. *Lancet Infect Dis* 2(5):281–292.

Hessol NA, Katz MH, Liu JY, et al. (1992). Increased incidence of Hodgkin disease in homosexual men with HIV infection. *Ann Intern Med* 117:309–311.

Hewitt RG (2002). Abacavir hypersensitivity reaction. *Clin Infect Dis.* 34(8):1137–1142.

Holland GN, Pepose TS, Petit TH, et al. (1983). Acquired immune deficiency syndrome: ocular manifestations. *Ophthalmology* 96:1092–1099.

Hoover Dr, Saah J, Bacellar H, et al. (1993). Clinical manifestations of AIDS in the era of pneumocystis prophylaxis. Multicenter AIDS Cohort Study. *N Engl J Med* 329:1922–1926.

Huang SS, Barbour JD, Deeks SG, et al. (2000). Reversal of human immunodeficiency virus type-1 associated hematosuppression by effective antiretroviral therapy. *Clin Infect Dis* 30(3):504–510.

Hughes W, Leoung G, Kramer F, et al. (1993). Comparison of atovaquone (566C80) with trimethoprim-sulfamethoxazole to treat *Pneumocystis carinii* pneumonia in patients with AIDS. *N Engl J Med* 328 (21):1521–1527.

Hutchinson CM, Hook EW III, Shepherd M, et al. (1994). Altered clinical presentation and manifestations of early syphilis in patients with human immunodeficiency virus infection. *Ann Intern Med* 121(2):94–100.

Hutin Y, Molina JM, Casin I, et al. (1993). Risk factors for *Clostridium difficile*–associated diarrhea in HIV-infected patients. *AIDS* 7(11):1441–1447.

Jacobson LP, Yamashita TE, Detel SR, et al. (1999). Impact of potent antiretroviral therapy on the incidence of Kaposi's sarcoma and non-Hodgkins lymphoma among HIV infected individuals. *J Acquir Immune Defic Syndr* 21(Suppl.):S34–S48.

Jacobson MA, Zegans M, Pavian PR, et al. (1997). Cytomegalovirus retinitis after initiatiation of highly active antiretroviral therapy. *Lancet* 349:1443–1445.

Jasmer RM, and Nahid P (2002). Clinical Practice. Latent tuberculosis infection. *N Engl J Med* 347(23): 1860–1866.

Jones BE, Young SM, Antoniskis D, et al. (1993). Relationship of the manifestations of tuberculosis to CD4 counts in patients with human immunodeficiency virus infection. *Am Rev Respir Dis* 148: 1292–1297.

Jones JL, Hanson DC, Dworkin MS, et al. (1999). Surveillance for AIDS-defining opportunistic illnesses, 1992–1997. *MMWR CDC Surveill Summ* 48:1–22.

Kahn JO, and Walker BD (1998). Acute human immunodeficiency virus type 1 infection. *N Engl J Med* 339(1):33–39.

Kazanjian P, Armstrong W, Hossler PA, et al. (2000). *Pneumocystis carinii* mutations are associated with duration of sulfur or sulfone prophylaxis exposure in AIDS patients. *J Infect Dis.* 182(2):551–557.

Ko WF, Cello TP, Rogers SJ, et al. (2003). Prognostic factors for the survival of patients with AIDS cholangiopathy. *Am J Gastroenterol* 10:2111–2112.

Kotler DP, Reka S, Orenstein JM, et al. (1992). Chronic idiopathic esophageal ulcerations in acquired immunodeficiency syndrome. Characterization and treatment with corticosteroids. *J Clin Gastroenterol* 15(4):284–290.

Kovacs JA, Gill VJ, Meshnick S, et al. (2001). New insights into transmission, diagnosis, and drug treatment of *Pneumocystis carinii* pneumonia. *JAMA* 286(19):2450–2460.

Krause J (2005). AIDS related non-Hodgkins lymphoma. *Microsc Res Tech* 68:168–175.

Lazizi Y, Grangeot-Keros L, and Delfraissy JF (1988). Reappearance of hepatitis B virus in immune patients infected with HIV-1. *J Infect Dis* 158:666–667.

Ledergerber B, Telenti A, and Eggu M (1999). Risk of HIV related Kaposi's sarcoma and non-Hodgkins lymphoma with potent antiretroviral therapy. Swiss Cohort Study. *BMJ* 319:23–24.

Leoung GS, Mills JS, Hopewell PC, et al. (1986). Dapsone-trimethoprim for *Pneumocystis carinii* pneumonia in acquired immunodeficiency syndrome. *Ann Intern Med* 105(1):45–48.

Levine AM (1996). HIV associated Hodgkin's disease. Biologic and clinical aspects. *Hematol Oncol Clin North Am* 10:1135–1148.

MacDonald JC, Karoravellas MP, Torriani FJ, et al. (2000). Highly active antiretroviral therapy-related immune recovery in AIDS patients with cytomegalovirus retinitis. *Ophthalmology* 107:877–883.

Maiman M, Fruchter RG, Serur E, et al. (1990). Human immunodeficiency virus infection and cervical neoplasia. *Gynecol Oncol* 38:377–382.

Martin DF, Kuppermann BD, Woltz RA, et al. (1999). Oral ganciclovir for patients with cytomegalovirus retinitis treated with ganciclovir implants. Roche Ganciclovir Study. *N Engl J Med* 340(14):1063–1070.

Masur H, Michelis MA, Greene J, et al. (1981). An outbreak of community-acquired *Pneumocystis carinii* pneumonia. Initial manifestation of cellular immune dysfunction. *N Engl J Med* 305:1431–1438.

Masur H, Ognibene FP, Yarchoan R, et al. (1988). CD4 counts as predictors of opportunistic pneumonias in human immunodeficiency virus (HIV) infection. *Ann Intern Med* 111:222–231.

Mathews WC, Caperna JC, Barber RE, et al. (2005). Incidence of and risk factors for clinically significant methicillin-resistant *Staphylococcus aureus* infection in a cohort of HIV infected adults. *J Acquir Immune Defic Syndr* 40(2):155–160.

May GR, Gill MJ, Church DL, et al. (1993). Gastrointestinal symptoms in ambulatory infected patients. *Dig Dis Sci* 138:1388–1394.

Mbulaiteye SM, Biggar RJ, Goedert JJ, et al. (2003). Immune deficiency and risk of malignancy among people with AIDS. *J Acquir Immune Defic Syndr* 32:527–533.

Medina I, Mills J, Leoung G, et al. (1990). Oral therapy for *Pneumocystis carinii* pneumonia in acquired immunodeficiency syndrome. A controlled trial of trimethoprim-sulfamethoxazole versus trimethoprim-dapsone. *N Engl J Med* 323(12):776–782.

Milazzo F, Piconi S, Trabottoni D, et al. (1999). Intractable pruritus in HIV infection; immunology and characterization. *Allergy* 54(3):266–272.

Molina JM, Castin I, Hausfater P, et al. (1995). *Campylobacter* infections in HIV-infected patients. Clinical and bacteriologic features. *AIDS* 9:881–885.

Monkemuller KE, and Wilcox CM (1999). Diagnosis and treatment of esophageal ulcers in AIDS. *Semin Gastroenterol* 10(3):85–92.

Moore RD, Keruly TC, and Chaisson RE (1998). Anemia and survival in HIV infection. *J Acquir Immune Defic Syndr Hum Retrovirol* 19(1):29–33.

Moraes HV (2002). Ocular manifestations of HIV/AIDS. *Curr Opin Ophthalmol* 6:397–403.

Navas E, and Martin-Davilla P (2002). Paradoxical reactions of tuberculosis in patients with the acquired immunodeficiency syndrome who are treated with highly active antiretrovireal therapy. *Arch Intern Med* 162:197–199.

Ogedegbe AO, and Sulkowski MS (2003). Antiretroviral-associated liver injury. *Clin Liver Dis* 7:475–499.

Ognibene FP, Shelhamer J, Gill V, et al. (1984). The diagnosis of *Pneumocystis carinii* pneumonia in patients with the acquired immunodeficiency syndrome using subsegmental bronchoalveolar lavage. *Am Rev Respir Dis* 129:929.

Oksenhendler E, Bierling P, Chevret S, et al. (1993). Splenectomy is safe and effective in HIV-related immune thrombocytopenia. *Blood* 82:29–32.

Palefsky JM, Holly EA, Ralston ML, et al. (1998). Prevalence and risk factors for human papillomavirus infection of the anal canal in human immunodeficiency virus (HIV) positive and HIV negative homosexual men. *J Infect Dis* 177:361–367.

Palefsky JM, Holly EA, Ralston M, et al. (2001). Effect of highly active antiretroviral therapy on the natural history of anal squamous interepithelial and anal human papilloma viral infections. *J Acquir Immune Defic Syndr* 28:422–428.

Palella FJ, Delaney KM, Moorman AC, et al. (1998). Declining morbidity and mortality among patients with advanced human immunodeficiency virus infection. HIV Outpatient Study Investigators. *N Engl J Med* 338:853–860.

Para MF, Finkelstein D, Becker S, et al. (2000). Reduced toxicity with gradual initiation of trimethoprim-sulfamethoxazole as primary prophylaxis for *Pneumocystis carinii* pneumonia: AIDS Clinical Trials Group 268. *J Acquir Immune Defic Syndr.* 24(4):337–343.

Penn I (1975). The incidence of malignancies in transplant recipients. *Transplant Proc* 7(2):323–326.

Perkocha L, Geaghans S, and Yen T (1990). Clinical and pathologic features of bacillary peliosis hepatitis in association with human immunodeficiency virus infection. *N Engl J Med* 323:1581–1586.

Pfister H (1996). The role of human papillomavirus in anogenital cancer. *Obstet Gynecol Clin North Am* 23:579–595.

Portu JJ, Santamaria JM, Zubero Z, et al. (1996). Atypical scabies in HIV-positive patients. *J Am Acad Dermatol* 34(5 Pt.2):915–917.

Rabkin CS, Biggar RJ, and Horm JW (1991). Increasing incidence of cancers associated with the human immunodeficiency virus epidemic. *Int J Cancer* 47: 692–696.

Raufman JP (1988). Odonophagia/dysphagia in AIDS. *Gastroenterol Clin North Am* 17(3):599–614.

Raviglione MC, Snider DE, and Kochi A (1995). Global epidemiology of tuberculosis: morbidity and mortality of a worldwide epidemic. *JAMA* 273(3):220–226.

Remick S (1996). Non-AIDS defining cancers. *Hematol Oncol Clin North Am* 10:1203–1213.

Rigopoulos D, Paparizos V, and Katsambas A (2004). Cutaneous markers of HIV infection. *Clin Dermatol* 22(6):487–498.

Roudier C, Caumes E, Rogeaux O, et al. (1994). Adverse cutaneous reactions to trimethoprim-sulfamethoxazole in patients with the acquired immune deficiency syndrome and *Pneumocystis carinii* pneumonia. *Arch Dermatol* 130(11):1383–1386.

Saadeh S, Cammell G, Carey WD, et al. (2001). The role of liver biopsy in chronic hepatitis C. *Hepatology* 33:196–200.

Sattler FR, Frame P, Davis R, et al. (1994). Trimetrexate with leucovorin vs. trimethoprim-sulfamethoxazole for moderate to severe episodes of *Pneumocystis carinii* pneumonia in patients with AIDS. *J Infect Dis* 170(1):165–172.

Schwartz RA (2004). Kaposi's sarcoma: an update. *J Surg Oncol* 87(3):146–151.

Sloand E (2005). Hematologic complications of HIV infection. *AIDS Rev* 7(4):187–196.

Small PM, and Fujiwara PI (2001). Treatment of tuberculosis in the United States. *N Engl J Med* 345: 189–200.

Smith PD, Macher AM, Bookman MA, et al. (1985). *Salmonella typhimurium* enteritis and bacteremia in the acquired immune deficiency syndrome. *Ann Intern Med* 102:207–209.

Smith PD, Quinn TC, Strober V, et al. (1992). Gastrointestinal infections in AIDS. *Ann Intern Med* 116:63–77.

Sulkowski MS, Moore RD, Mehta SH, et al. (2002). Hepatitis C and progression of HIV disease. *JAMA* 288(2):199–206.

Sullivan PS, Hanson DC, Chu SY, et al. (1997). Surveillance for thrombocytopenia in persons infected with HIV: reults from the multistate Adult and Adolescent Spectrum of Disease Project. *J Acquir Immune Defic Syndr Human Retrovirol* 14(4):374–379.

Tappero JW, Perkins BA, Wenger JD, et al. (1995). Cutaneous manifestations of opportunistic infections in patients infected with human immunodeficiency virus. *Clin Microbiol Rev* 8(3):440–450.

Toma E, Thorme A, Singer J, et al. (1998). Clindamycin with primaquine vs. trimethoprim-sulfamethoxazole for mild and moderately severe *Pneumocystis carinii* pneumonia in patients with AIDS: a multicenter double-blind randomized trial (CTN004). CTN-PCP Study Group. *Clin Infect Dis* 3:524–530.

Toriani FJ, Rodriguez-Torres M, Rockstroh JK, et al. (2004). Peginteferon alpha-2a plus ribavirin for chronic hepatitis C virus infection in HIV-infected patients. *N Engl J Med* 351(5):438–450.

Tschachler E, Bergstresser PR, and Stingl G (1996). HIV related skin disorders. *Lancet* 348(9028):659–663.

Warren KJ, Boxwell DE, Kim NY, et al. (1998). Nevirapine-associated Stevens-Johnson syndrome. *Lancet* 351(9102):567.

Wilcox CM (1992). Esophageal disease in the acquired immune deficiency syndrome: etiology, diagnosis, and management. *Am J Med* 92:412–421.

Wilcox CM, Straub RF, and Clark WS (1995). Prospective evaluation of oropharyngeal findings in HIV-infected patients with esophageal ulcers. *Am J Gastroenterol* 90(11):1938–1941.

Wilcox CM, Alexander LN, Clark WS, and Thompson SE III (1996). Fluconozole compared with endoscopy for human immunodeficiency virus infected patients with esophageal symptoms. *Gastroenterology* 110(6):1803–1809.

Wislez M, Bergot F, Antoine M, et al. (2001). Acute respiratory failure following HAART introduction in patients treated for *Pneumocystis carinii* pneumonia. *Am J Respir Crit Care Med* 164(5):847–851.

Wolff AJ, and O'Donnell AE (2001). Pulmonary manifestations of HIV infection in the era of highly active antiretroviral therapy. *Chest* 120:1888–1893.

Wood C, and Harington W (2005). AIDS and associated malignancies. *Cell Res* 15:947–952.

Zhang Y, Harada A, Bluethmann H, et al. (1995). Tumor necrosis factor (TNF) is a physiologic regulator of hematopoietic cells. *Blood* 86(8):2930–2937.

Ziegler JL, Beckstead JA, Volberding PA, et al. (1984). Non-Hodgkins lymphoma in 90 homosexual men. Relation to generalized adenopathy and the acquired immunodeficiency syndrome. *N Engl J Med* 311(9):565–570.

Part X

Ethical and Health Policy
Aspects of AIDS Psychiatry

Chapter 38

Burnout, Occupational Hazards, and Health Care Workers with HIV

Asher D. Aladjem and Frances Wallach

Burnout as a phenomenon relates to work and occupational psychological distress (Maslach et al., 2001). Because burnout is multifactorial, research has focused on two general categories of contributory factors: those in the individual and those related to the work environment. These factors are summarized in Table 38.1.

BURNOUT IN THE CARE OF PERSONS WITH HIV AND AIDS

Research on burnout in AIDS-related work was initially in literature on nurse professionals; only recently has it been applied to medicine, dentistry, public health, health education, and social work. The close association between burnout and work differentiates it from more general emotional states such as depression that may pervade every aspect of life. When the focus is on work-related distress, it leaves the separation of work-related distress from the rest of one's life

ill defined. As a result, other sources of distress may be minimized or overlooked and the boundary with psychiatric diagnoses remains blurred. Even though the distress may be only work related, it clearly has implications for other areas of the caregiver's life.

Although we refer to burnout as a phenomenon that has particular etiologies, a particular course, and specific treatments, the concept is not of an illness and any attempt to medicalize and/or pathologize such a phenomenon may not yield the desired outcome. Burnout has not been added to the *Diagnostic and Statistical Manual of Mental Disorders* as a diagnosis and has been relatively ignored by the psychiatric literature in AIDS-related work (Felton, 1994).

The AIDS epidemic began in the early 1980s and forced significant changes in the understanding and management of an illness in the context of behavior, social acceptance, personal and social responsibility, and disease management. The enormous challenge of HIV/AIDS-related work can lead to the onset of symptomatic disorders in some susceptible providers.

TABLE 38.1. Factors Contributing to Burnout

Individual Factors	Work-Related Factors
Meaning of one's work, dealing with conflicting values	Work or case load and/or responsibilities, excessive paperwork
Balance between work and family and other areas of life	Bereavement overload and unresolved grief
Fit between clinician's interests and goals and how they integrate at the work environment	Lack of rewards and devaluation of contribution, lack of resources
External/internal cognitive/behavior, coping styles, and skills	External locus of control leading to diminished job control by the individual; "responsibility without power"
Overidentification with clients	Increasing number of patients with character disorders
Difficulties discussing patient's condition with his or her family	Failure of pain control
Poor communication among hospital staff and/or providers	Witnessing physical deterioration of patients

Research to date has failed to produce a comprehensive picture of the ways in which the demands of HIV/AIDS-related work differ from those of other fields in the health care delivery system, such as geriatrics, oncology, intensive care, or hospice care. The changing environment of the HIV/AIDS pandemic continues to present new challenges and struggles and to demand responses that are flexible and modifiable. As new knowledge is integrated and the resources available remain vulnerable, constant vigilance is required to ensure responsible allocation of resources to care for persons with AIDS.

In a speech at the UN General Assembly High Level Meeting on AIDS on June 2, 2006, the Executive Director of UNAIDS stressed that what is currently needed is "a response that is embedded in social change and the need to address the fundamental drivers of this crisis, including the low status of women, sexual violence, homophobia and AIDS-related stigma and discrimination." He continued: "Not only is there room for everybody, but also a need for everybody," referring to retention of providers and recruitment of individuals to work in health care of HIV-infected people and the fight against AIDS.

Recognizing all the challenges and not diminishing or trivializing their contributions, health care providers continue to have lifelong, satisfying work experience, managing work-related stressors in this environment in an effective manner. While most studies on stress and burnout in AIDS health care have focused on the negative and difficult aspects of this work, these aspects are by no means universal phenomena. Health care providers' involvement with HIV/AIDS covers the whole spectrum of the disease and infection; this is clearly not a homogeneous group of providers. As the impact of HIV/AIDS has grown, more services have become available to comprehensively treat persons with AIDS. Caregivers include outpatient providers, inpatient providers, acute care and chronic care providers, hospice care, including home hospice providers, and others. Service organizations employ individuals from many different types of occupational categories, including health educators, HIV pre- and post-test counselors, nurses, primary care physicians, infectious disease specialists, pediatricians, and other medical and surgical specialists. All of these professionals work together to provide care for persons with AIDS and its diverse and complex presentations. The more extended circle of providers includes laboratory technicians, psychiatrists, psychologists, and other mental health providers, substance abuse treatment providers, dentists, social workers, case managers, and many dedicated volunteers.

Some clinicians' involvement with AIDS-related work may be very brief but very intense and emotional, while other clinicians may have to care for patients on a long-term basis. Ongoing care entails providing treatment and follow-up, monitoring adherence with antiviral treatment. Furthermore, clinicians may be forced to observe patients' decline in health, despite all efforts and treatments available. Others may be providers in acute care hospitals, palliative care, and/or long-term health care facilities including hospice care.

Among prisoners there are high rates of HIV infection; prison staff and health care workers are required to care for inmates with HIV/AIDS under increased pressure and levels of stress (D'Aniello, 1994). Issues regarding prisoners with HIV and AIDS are explored in depth in Chapter 5 and are also addressed in Chapter 31 of this textbook. Likewise, home care has expanded since AIDS has become a chronic illness. Caregivers in each of these environments face different challenges and stressors and have different risks and rates of reported burnout. The occurrence of burnout has a negative impact on work satisfaction and has been seen in large part as the problem of the individual suffering from it. The organizational context in which clinicians practice is a very important variable in the experience of burnout, but research in this field has been hampered by the absence of instruments to measure organizational factors. Those who focus on the negative impact that HIV disease has had on society will add the risk of burning out as another negative consequence of working with HIV/AIDS. Numerous stressors have been reported in the literature as specific aspects of AIDS-related health care delivery and are summarized in Table 38.2.

Early in the epidemic, "national experts" claimed that health care providers were not likely to be infected by the HIV on the job as long as they followed safety guidelines and used universal precautions (Wallack, 1989). These claims were met with a significant degree of mistrust. Despite these safety pronouncements, the real and/or perceived occupational hazard and its management remain serious concerns to providers.

OCCUPATIONAL HAZARDS

Over two decades ago, William Haddon commented that "the notion of an accident is descriptive, not

TABLE 38.2. Stressors in AIDS-related Health Care Delivery

Patient-Related Stressors	Health Care Worker–Related Stressors	Systemic Stressors	Societal Stressors
High mortality rates	Unresolved personal losses	High caseload	Social stigma and sense of professional isolation
Increasing number of patients with character disorders	Unrealistic goals for patient outcomes	Optimal levels of infection control and fear of contagion	Caring for patients living nontraditional and different styles that clinicians are unfamiliar with
Homophobia and issues of human sexuality	Uncertainty about treatment	Ensuring the availability of support services required for comprehensive care of HIV complications	Homophobia and issues of human sexuality
Issues of substance abuse	Maintaining professional competence in HIV care		Ethical and legal dilemmas
Lack of supports and unmet needs assumed by providers	Inadequacy in treating patients suffering, psychosocial, and neuropsychiatric symptoms		Issues of substance abuse

etiological" (Haddon, 1980). He developed the notion that the phenomenon of trauma must be based not on descriptive categorizations but on etiologic ones. Most of the literature on needle sticks in health care workers, however, fits into the former, not the latter category. Occupational exposure to blood-borne pathogens is a major concern among health care workers in many different settings (Gerberding, 2003). Health care workers are one of the few occupational groups who remain at risk for infection from blood-borne pathogens (Sepkowitz, 1996), despite the use of universal and standard precautions and the introduction of needle safety products. The primary blood-borne pathogens of concern are HIV, hepatitis B (HBV), and hepatitis C (HCV). Other potentially infectious, blood-borne agents to which workers may be exposed, albeit at a lower risk, include malaria, syphilis, babesiosis, brucellosis, leptospirosis, arboviral infections, relapsing fever, Creutzfeldt-Jacob disease, HTLV-I and -II, and viral hemorrhagic fevers (OSHA, 1999). Because of the relative rarity of these diseases in the United States, the focus has been primarily on the risks of HIV, HBV, and HCV infections.

An exposure may involve a percutaneous injury, mucous membrane, or non-intact skin contact or prolonged and extensive skin contact with blood, tissue, or infectious body fluids. Potentially infectious body fluids in addition to blood include semen, vaginal secretions, breast milk, cerebral spinal fluid, or other body fluid contaminated with visible blood. Under special circumstances laboratory specimens and unfixed tissues are also considered infectious.

The risks of transmission of HIV vary with the type and severity of the exposure. In prospective studies, the average risk of HIV transmission after a percutaneous injury with HIV-infected blood is estimated at 0.3% (95% confidence interval [CI] 0.2%–0.5%) (Bell, 1997). After a mucous membrane exposure the risk is approximately 0.09% (CI = 0.006%–0.5%) (Bell, 1997). The risk of transmission through a bite or following exposure to fluids other than blood has not been quantified, but is believed to be considerably lower than that for blood exposures.

Because the specific information about a source and an exposure vary on a case-by-case basis, the actual risk to a given "exposed" individual will also vary. In an often-quoted retrospective case–control study involving health care workers who had percutaneous exposures, an increased risk of HIV transmission was associated with the following four factors: (1) a hollow-

bore needle visibly contaminated with the source patient's blood; (2) a procedure involving placement of a needle directly into a vein or artery; (3) a deep "stick" injury; and (4) terminal AIDS illness in the source (CDC, 1996). This last factor is believed to be a surrogate marker for a high viral load in the source patient. This same retrospective study found that zidovudine (AZT) monotherapy was able to reduce the risk of HIV transmission by about 80% (CDC, 1996).

Once an exposure has occurred the exposed area should be immediately washed with soap and water. In the case of mucous membrane exposures, the region involved should be flushed with water.

All health care institutions are required to maintain a policy and standard operating procedure for dealing with employee exposures. Updated recommendations for post-exposure prophylaxis have been developed by the Centers for Disease Control (CDC, 2005). Although these recommendations will vary from one institution to another, the overall goal of evaluating the incident and, if necessary, providing the exposed person with post-exposure prophylaxis (PEP) within a 2- to 4-hour window is the gold standard (Tables 38.3 and 38.4).

The selection of a particular medication regimen for HIV PEP must balance the risk for infection against the potential toxicities of the antiretroviral agents used. Given the complexities of choosing and caring for a person taking PEP, whenever possible, consultation with a physician who has experience with antiretroviral agents is recommended. If an infectious physician is not available, the National Clinician's Post-Exposure Prophylaxis Hotline (PEP line), telephone number 888–448–4911, is operational 24 hours a day.

Hepatitis B and C viruses can also be transmitted through blood and body fluids. The risk of an HCV-negative employee acquiring HCV from a patient with chronic hepatitis following a percutaneous injury is approximately 10-fold greater than the risk of becoming HIV infected from the same needle stick, or 3% (CDC, 2001). Unfortunately, there is no established regimen for prevention of HCV transmission. There are, however, anecdotal case reports of eradication of early HCV infection with the administration of pegylated alpha interferon and ribavirin.

Hepatitis B virus remains the most infectious of the three viruses transmissible by blood and body fluids. A non-immune person who sustains a percutaneous injury from a patient with chronic, active hepatitis B (hepB Sag+ Eag+) runs a risk of acquiring hepatitis B

TABLE 38.3. Recommended HIV Postexposure Prophylaxis (PEP) for Percutaneous Injuries

Exposure type	Infection Status of Source				
	HIV-Positive, Class 1[*]	HIV-Positive, Class 2[*]	Source of Unknown HIV Status[†]	Unknown Source[§]	HIV Negative
Less severe[¶]	Recommend basic 2-drug PEP	Recommend expanded ≥ 3-drug PEP	Generally, no PEP warranted; however, consider basic 2-drug PEP[**] for source with HIV risk factors[††]	Generally, no PEP warranted; however, consider basic 2-drug PEP[**] in settings in which exposure to HIV-infected persons is likely	No PEP warranted
More severe[§§]	Recommend expanded 3-drug PEP	Recommend expanded ≥ -drug PEP	Generally, no PEP warranted; however, consider basic 2-drug PEP[**] for source with HIV risk factors[††]	Generally, no PEP warranted; however, consider basic 2-drug PEP[**] in settings in which exposure to HIV-infected persons is likely	No PEP warranted

[*]HIV-positive, class 1—asymptomatic HIV infection or known low viral load (e.g., <1500 ribonucleic acid copies/ml). HIV-positive, class 2—symptomatic HIV infection, acquired immunodeficiency syndrome, acute seroconversion, or known high viral load. If drug resistance is a concern, obtain expert consultation. Initiation of PEP should not be delayed pending expert consultation, and, because expert consultation alone cannot substitute for face-to-face counseling, resources should be available to provide immediate evaluation and follow-up care for all exposures.

[†]For example, deceased source person with no samples available for HIV testing.

[§]For example, a needle from a sharps disposal container.

[¶]For example, solid needle or superficial injury.

[**]The recommendation "consider PEP" indicates that PEP is optional; a decision to initiate PEP should be based on a discussion between the exposed person and the treating clinician regarding the risks versus benefits of PEP.

[††]If PEP is offered and administered and the source is later determined to be HIV negative, PEP should be discontinued.

[§§]For example, large-bore hollow needle, deep puncture, visible blood on device, or needle used in patents artery or vein.

Source: From the Centers for Disease Control and Prevention. Morbidity and Mortality Weekly Report, Sept. 30, 2005, 54(RR09): 1–17.

as high as 33% (CDC, 2001). Non-immune employees exposed to the hepatitis B virus should be given HBIG along with the first dose of the hepatitis B vaccine at the time of the exposure.

Hepatitis B, however, is a vaccine-preventable illness. The Centers for Disease Control and Prevention recommends that all category A employees (those with patient or body fluids contact) who are not hepatitis B immune undergo hepatitis B vaccination at the time of their initial employment with a standard three-dose vaccination series. Approximately 90%–95% of people vaccinated with the full series will develop protective immunity to hepatitis B virus.

Exposure prevention remains the primary strategy for reducing occupational blood-borne pathogen in-fections in the health care setting. Examples of this include standard glove precautions for patient contact, and safer needle and phlebotomy devices to reduce percutaneous injuries.

In summary, although blood and body fluid exposures remain a significant concern, much progress has been made in the prevention of acquisition of hepatitis B, hepatitis C, and HIV in the health care environment.

VULNERABILITY TO BURNOUT

A cross-sectional survey of 103 HIV/AIDS and 100 oncology staff in nine treatment sites in London aimed

TABLE 38.4. Recommended HIV Postexposure Prophylaxis (PEP) for Mucous Membrane Exposures and Nonintact Skin[*] Exposures

Exposure Type	Infection Status of Source				
	HIV-Positive, Class 1[†]	HIV-Positive, Class 2[†]	Source of Unknown HIV Status[§]	Unknown Source[¶]	HIV Negative
Small volume[**]	Consider basic 2-drug PEP[††]	Recommend basic 2-drug PEP	Generally, no PEP warranted[§§]	Generally, no PEP warranted	No PEP warranted
Large volume[¶¶]	Recommend basic 2-drug PEP	Recommend expanded ≥ 3-drug PEP	Generally, no PEP warranted; however, consider basic 2-drug PEP[††] for source with HIV risk factors[§§]	Generally, no PEP warranted; however, consider basic 2-drug PEP[††] in settings in which exposure to HIV-infected persons is likely	No PEP warranted

[*]For skin exposures, follow-up is indicated only if evidence exists of compromised skin integrity (e.g., dermatitis, abrasion, or open wound).

[†]HIV-positive, class 1—asymptomatic HIV infection or known low viral load (e.g., <1500 ribonucleic acid copies/mL). HIV-positive, class 2—symptomatic HIV infection, AIDS, acute seroconversion, or known high viral load. If drug resistance is a concern, obtain expert consultation. Initiation of PEP should not be delayed pending expert consultation, and, because expert consultation alone cannot substitute for face-to-face counseling, resources should be available to provide immediate evaluation and follow-up care for all exposures.

[§]For example, deceased source person with no samples available for HIV testing.

[¶]For example, splash from inappropriately disposed blood.

[**]For example, a few drops.

[††]The recommendation "consider PEP" indicates that PEP is optional; a decision to initiate PEP should be based on a discussion between the exposed person and the treating clinician regarding the risks versus benefits of PEP.

[§§]If PEP is offered and administered and the source is later determined to be HIV negative, PEP should be discontinued.

[¶¶]For example, a major blood splash.

Source: From the Centers for Disease Control and Prevention. *Morbidity and Mortality Weekly Report*, Sept. 30, 2005, 54(RR09): 1–17.

to identify ways in which stress affected the domestic and social lives of such staff (Miller and Gillies, 1996). Of all staff members, one-third of those without a long-term emotional relationship stated that they felt their work-related issues interfered with their developing and maintaining relationships. Most participants reported spending a considerable amount of time discussing work with partners. Work-related issues caused conflict for just under half of the total sample. Thirty-nine percent reported that their partners complained regularly about their commitment to work, and 25% overall reported their relationship had suffered as a result of their work in HIV or oncology.

Bennett and colleagues (1991) found that oncology nurses suffered burnout with greater frequency than that of AIDS nurses, although AIDS nurses showed greater intensity of burnout after adjustment for frequency of burnout. Men were as likely to suffer burnout as women, and age significantly influenced burnout inversely (Bennett et al., 1991).

Bianchi and colleagues (1997) found that among doctors and nurses on a pediatric service in Rome, there was a correlation between experience and time on the job and lower rates of emotional exhaustion. Clinicians with less than a year on the job showed a higher degree of physical and emotional exhaustion, suffered from a high density of stress factors, and set up a large number of defensive strategies. Clinicians at work for 1 to 3 years showed a moderate degree of physical, emotional, and mental exhaustion, did not suffer from particular stress factors, and perceived a high level of social support from colleagues. Those with more than 3 years experience did not suffer from particular physical or emotional exhaustion and experienced medium levels.

While feeling the action of various daily stressors, they did not use the social support offered at work.

Aiken and Sloane (1997) surveyed 820 nurses working with AIDS patients. Nurses who worked in dedicated or specialized units or in "magnet" hospitals known to possess organizational characteristics attractive to nurses exhibited lower levels of emotional exhaustion than those among nurses working in general, scattered-bed medical units. These differences persisted after nurse characteristics were statistically controlled, but they were accounted for in part by controlling for the amount of the organizational support that nurses perceived was present at the work place.

In a study by Mueller (1997) of a sample of 144 social workers providing care for HIV/AIDS clients, the predictors of burnout included measures of social support, caregiver values, characteristics of the work setting, the nature of the work with HIV/AIDS clients, and demographic factors. Study data demonstrated that burnout was significantly and inversely related to social support received from co-workers, supervisors, the caregiver's age, education level, income, caseload size, and years of work with AIDS clients. Burnout was significantly and positively associated with the number of recent caregiver client deaths and the proportion of caseload that was comprised of HIV/AIDS clients. Total burnout was not related to spouse support, caregiver's gender, sexual orientation, HIV serostatus, or theoretical orientation.

Demmer (2002) surveyed the motivations, stressors, and rewards of 180 workers employed in nine AIDS service organizations in New York City. The sample consisted of social service workers (56%), administrative workers (22%), health care workers (18%), and other workers (4%). Forty-two percent of the workers had been working in the AIDS field for 5 years or more years. The two main reasons for choosing this line of work were a desire to help others, followed by having experienced the loss of a loved one to AIDS. Overall, respondents rated their level of stressors in their job as moderate. The main category of stress was lack of support. The most important individual stressors were societal attitudes towards AIDS, salary, client deaths, and administrative duties. The most highly valued reward factor associated with AIDS caregivers was "personal effectiveness." Nurses in AIDS care experiencing high levels of stress in their workplace were significantly more likely to use wishful thinking, planful problem solving, and avoidance as coping strategies, whereas stress originating from

patient care was more likely to be dealt with by using positive assessment and acceptance (Kalichman et al., 2000).

Des Jarlais (1990) reported that caregivers who had worked previously in the area of drug abuse treatment went from working in a drug abuse treatment program to working in an AIDS program without a conscious choice in the matter. Part of the strain in burnout in this group came from the sense that the needs created by the epidemic had completely taken over one's professional life, not having had the opportunity to make a professional choice.

MENTAL HEALTH CONSULTANTS

Mental health consultants are important members of the treating teams and their contributions are significant. However, there have been no large studies of occupational distress in mental health providers working with HIV illness in medical or psychiatric settings.

In one study, consultants who felt insufficiently trained in communication and management skills were at higher risk for burnout, although job satisfaction was found to protect consultants' mental health against the adverse effects of job related stress (Ramirez at al., 1996). In another study, while some psychiatrists conveyed nonjudgmental attitudes about homosexuality, they were, along with family physicians, the least comfortable with the infectious aspects of AIDS (Frierson and Lippman, 1987).

The stress of a consultant is much reduced when, as members of the team, they are confident that the treatment recommendations are going to be valued, implemented, and integrated into the overall care of the patient. Psychotherapists experience burnout at a rate of about 2%–6%; institutionally based and inexperienced therapists seem most at risk for burnout. Farber (1990) described three types of burned-out therapists: those who in response to frustration work increasingly harder, those who in response to frustration give up entirely, and those who perform their job unthinkingly.

Burnout Measures

The Maslach Burnout Inventory (MBI) has been established as a credible measure of burnout and focuses on the personal experience of work (Lee and Ashforth, 1990, Enzmann et al. 1995). It measures dimensions that include exhaustion–energy;

depersonalization–involvement; and inefficacy–accomplishment. The MBI was tested to see if it could be translated to other languages, while preserving its psychometric properties; issues of theoretical flaws and cultural bias need further validation (Enzmann et al., 1995).

Other tools have been used in an attempt to measure and quantify burnout. These include Coping Orientation to Problem Experience (COPE) and the State Trait Anxiety Inventory (STAI). Burnout may include symptoms of depression, anxiety, posttraumatic stress disorder (PTSD), and personality disorders. These boundaries are sometimes blurred, as in efforts to distinguish between depression and demoralization syndrome and burnout using anhedonia or the ability of the individual to experience pleasure. Individuals suffering from depression cannot experience pleasure, whereas individuals suffering from burnout or demoralization should be able to experience pleasure. This is distinction is made by self-reporting and is open to a wide range of understanding and interpretations (see Table 38.5).

The expansion in the terminology used to label job-related distress may be due in part to an attempt to avoid the stigma of mental illness, labeling clinically relevant symptoms with more socially acceptable, politically correct, current concepts. The clear intent is to stay away from the better-known entity of psychiatric diagnoses (for example, depression), as these diagnoses are still feared and stigmatized.

Responsible and accurate reporting of burnout is necessary to avoid negative, further stigmatizing, and frightening implications that may turn people away from gravitating toward the field of HIV/AIDS health care delivery. A study by Van Servellen and Leake (1993), conducted in Los Angeles, examined burnout among nurses working on AIDS special care units (SCUs), oncology SCUs, medical intensive care

TABLE 38.5. Symptoms of Burnout

Exhaustion
A sense of being physically run down
Cynicism, irritability, and negativity
Exploding easily at seemingly trivial things
Anger at those making demands
Ineffectiveness
Sleeping problems, headache and stomach symptoms, and other psychical complaints
Weight loss or gain
Anxiety

units, and general medical units and measured the extent to which delivery method, patient diagnosis, or other key personal and work-related characteristic were associated with the level of distress in these nurses. A sample of 237 nurses from 18 units in seven hospitals was surveyed, using the MBI. This study showed no significant differences in burnout scores across nurse samples representing variations in patient diagnosis and delivery method, and all nurses had similar level of distress.

A study done by Catalan and colleagues (1996) compared serious disease, psychological stress, and work-related burnout in staff working with AIDS patients and with cancer patients. Seventy nurses and 41 doctors were compared through a self-reported method of assessment, using the MBI, General Health Questionnaire (GHQ), and the Social Adjustment Scale-Modified (SAS-M). One-third of the staff had substantial levels of psychological morbidity and about a fifth had significant levels of work-related stress. The study confirmed the existence of stress but found no difference in stress between AIDS and cancer-related work.

Clinicians' reactions to stressors are both positive and negative and should be mobilized to enable them to continue in a constructive fashion within their professional and personal lives. People do their best when they believe in what they are doing and when they can maintain their pride, integrity, and self-respect. The best reward is receiving recognition for the things one likes to do. If an individual reaches the best fit in terms of their professional preparation and level of personal maturity, introspection, and goals, they should be able to deal with challenges, such as working in the field of HIV/AIDS, and feel a sense of personal reward and professional accomplishment. There is a significant reward even if and when a patient dies, in the awareness of having provided the patient with the best care. Burnout is more likely when there is a mismatch between the nature of the job and the character of the person who does the job.

When a disease is as stigmatized and feared as AIDS, it is not always effortless to maintain a sense of pride, and clinicians may suffer attitudes toward them that are similar to those directed toward the disease. Consequently the clinician may experience a sense of isolation, distance, and trepidation or apprehension. Visintini and colleagues (1996) studied the role played by psychological stress and sociodemographic factors as predictors of burnout in nurses, administering the AIDS Impact Scale (AIS) and the MBI to nurses in the

AIDS field. The sample was composed of 410 nurses from 19 departments for the treatment of infectious diseases. A low level of burnout was indicated by MBI scores, but a small proportion had a high level of burnout with no significant association between sociodemographic variables and the MBI scales. There was a significant correlation between low burnout rate and the emotional involvement of nurses in their relationships with patients. The results suggest that an empathically involved relationship appears to protect against burnout, in contrast to a frustrating relationship. Moreover, nurses tolerated stress better if they received supportive social rewards.

HIV/AIDS health care providers consist of a very diverse group of physicians and other professionals who care for very diverse patient populations. The nature of HIV infection is that it affects patients as individuals and as groups identified by behavior and not by gender, age, race, or ethnicity. Many HIV/AIDS service providers have experienced the loss of not only numerous clients but also colleagues and community members, leading to "bereavement overload." For these individuals the rewards outweigh the stressors and the level of job satisfaction is very high. The most highly valued reward factor is "personal effectiveness." Burnout among these dedicated individuals weakens their response and contributes to increased strain on the HIV/AIDS care system. The challenge of workload and mastery and management of it have become very evident with HIV/AIDS (Bennett et al., 1994; Bennett et al., 1996). The sense of the immensity of the task and the insufficient tools to cover the need is one of the biggest demoralizing factors in this epidemic.

EVOLVING MENTAL HEALTH ROLES

The role of psychiatrists and other mental health professionals in addressing burnout in HIV caregivers gradually evolved over the past quarter century. During the early phase of the AIDS pandemic and with the development of HIV testing in 1985, young individuals were dying from an illness that progressed rapidly (Frierson and Lippmann, 1987). Most available treatments were inadequate to stop or even slow the course of illness. Ignorance associated with fear and prejudice dominated that stage. During the initial period of AZT treatment, there was a shift from hopelessness to testing and engaging patients and staff in treatment. When

better treatment became available, highly active antiretroviral therapy (HAART), compliance and adherence, and availability of medications became the focus. The most overwhelming experience for physicians now at this fast-changing phase is the stress of keeping up with the new and current body of knowledge and the anxiety about drug–drug interactions and extreme compliance with diverse regimens. Making treatment decisions based on patient's behavior becomes as important as empirical treatment of an infection. Clinicians again may have to observe patients as their disease progresses or even as they die from their disease, because they did not comply with possibly effective and long-term treatments. Clinicians can benefit from the support of psychiatrists and other mental health professionals in order to cope better with the stressors of this complex and rapidly evolving illness (Grossman and Silverstein, 1993; Killeen, 1993).

From a public health perspective, routine HIV testing is the recommended approach. This approach will identify individuals who have never suspected HIV infection and will require focused medical and psychological interventions.

ADDRESSING BURNOUT

When burnout is recognized and diagnosed, specific institutional and/or individual strategies need to be used. Institutional planning for addressing burnout can be conceptualized as prevention, recognition, and treatment, with the goals of longevity in the field and retention of committed workers who stay healthy and derive satisfaction from their work. These strategies include administrative policies, a philosophical framework, mechanisms for reward, and educational goals and objectives. These can be achieved by comprehensive orientation for new employees and refresher courses for employees already on the job, effective forums for conflict resolution and shared decision making, effective vertical communication, and the fostering of collaborative models, as opposed to aggressive, personally competitive styles.

Shifting in funding and costs is indicative of a very fast-paced change in the HIV/AIDS health care delivery system. Inpatient virology, tuberculosis, and dedicated AIDS units are being downsized or closed because of length-of-stay issues and the reduced need for long-term, inpatient treatment of HIV/AIDS-related conditions. These changes could lead to anxiety about job loss and to the end of some very resilient and productive careers.

A large source of satisfaction after 25 years in the field is derived from recognizing the monumental achievements in social and clinical aspects of the HIV epidemic. Individually, nurses, doctors, and other professionals face the constant challenge of adapting to new and evolving work environments. Insight and individual coping styles can be supported and enhanced by shared values. This can help balance the institutional–individual fit.

Coping has been described as "constantly changing cognitive and behavioral efforts to manage specific external and/or internal demands that are appraised as taxing or exceeding the resources of the person" (Lazarus and Folkman, 1984). Strategies for coping in a stressful work environment apply to coping in the HIV/AIDS workplace.

CORRELATION WITH RELIGION AND SPIRITUALITY

Religion and the healing powers of spirituality have not been described as central strategies in the fight against AIDS. From the very first manifestation of the epidemic, moral judgment was attached to the "forbidden behavior" and the "sins" involved in contracting AIDS. Promiscuity, homosexuality, and the sharing of needles have all been unacceptable for most organized religions. Most involvement of religious organizations has been in taking care of the dying. It is obvious that nuns, ministers, priests, and chaplains find strength in prayer and in selected passages from the scriptures, but for most of the secular public and health care providers, these rituals are very foreign and are often overlooked as an option.

Spirituality, as distinct from religion, has helped workers in finding meaning in their work and value in their contributions and their own experience. Resilience among many workers has been achieved through maintenance of a sense of coherence. Spirituality gives people meaning and purpose in life. It can be achieved through participation in a religion, but can be much broader than that, such as involvement in family, humanism, or the arts. Keeping alive the spirit of the far-too-many fatalities and continuing a relationship with the deceased have become a very effective mode for survivors, significant others, and HIV/AIDS health care providers to value, respect, and cherish their lives.

December 1st was designated Annual World's AIDS Day to increase global awareness of AIDS and to pay tribute to the people who lost their battle to the disease. An institutional memorial service, described by Tiamson and colleagues (1998), serves as a model to help providers with closure and renewal. The AIDS Memorial Quilt Project was one of the most powerful images of the AIDS epidemic. Tens of thousands of colorful individual panels full of stories of diverse life experiences of men, women, and children were combined together on display to concretize the magnitude of the loss. They have become another avenue to channel the overwhelming sense of loss of people and the immeasurable life potential. A letter written by loved ones and a favorite memory accompany each individual panel, made in a way that the individual would have liked as a memorial.

CONCLUSION

The number of AIDS cases and death toll increase every day. This number includes new infections, large numbers of patients who continue to struggle with the disease on a daily basis, and the overwhelming number of patients who have lost their fight to the epidemic. The public health perspective has helped clarify that the goal of providing treatment to entire populations is the only safe, long-term approach. To accomplish this monumental task, an organized direction for recruitment and training is needed to assist retention, and sustain resilience in the field HIV/AIDS health care delivery.

References

Aiken LH, and Sloane DM (1997). Effects of organizational innovations in AIDS care on burnout among urban hospital nurses. *Work Occup* 24:453–477.
Bell DM (1997). Occupational risk of human immunodeficiency virus infection in healthcare workers: an overview. *Am J Med* 102(5B):9–15.
Bennett L, Michie P, and Kippaz S (1991). Quantitative analysis of burnout and its associated factors in AIDS nursing. *AIDS Care* 3:181–192.
Bennett L, Kelaher M, and Ross MW (1994). Quality of life in health care professionals: burnout and its associated factors in HIV/AIDS related care. *Psychol Health* 9:273–283.
Bennett L, Ross MW, and Sunderland R (1996). The relationship between recognition, rewards and burnout in AIDS caring. *AIDS Care* 8:145–153.

Bianchi A, Ferrari V, Soccorsi R, and Tatarelli R (1997). The burnout syndrome in a pediatrics department: pilot project. *New Trends Exp Clin Psychiatry* 13: 193–208.

Catalan J, Burgess A, Pergami A, Hulme N, Gazzard, B, and Phillips R (1996). The psychological impact on staff of caring for people with serious diseases: the case of HIV infection and oncology. *J Psychosom Res* 40:425–435.

[CDC] Centers for Disease Control and Prevention (1996). Update: provisional Public Health Service recommendations for chemoprophylaxis after occupational exposure to HIV. *MMWR Morb Mortal Wkly Rep* 45(22):468–480.

[CDC] Centers for Disease Control and Prevention (2001). Update: U.S. Public Health Service guidelines for the management of occupational exposures to HBV, HCV, and HIV and recommendations for post-exposure prophylaxis. *MMWR Morb Mortal Wkly Rep* 50(No RR11):1–52.

[CDC] Centers for Disease Control and Prevention (2005). Updated U.S. Public Health Service guidelines for the management of occupational exposures to HIV. Recommendations for post-exposure prophylaxis. *MMWR Morb Mortal Wkly Rep* 54 (RR09):1–17.

D'Aniello M (1994). Psychological and methodological problems of prison doctors facing the spreading of AIDS/HIV. *Int Med J* 1:29–31.

Demmer C (2002). Stressors and rewards for workers in AIDS service organizations. *AIDS Patient Care STDS* 16:179–187.

Des Jarlais DC (1990). Stages in the response of drug abuse treatment system to AIDS epidemic in New York City. *J Drug Issues* 20:335–347.

Enzman D, Schaufeli W, and Girault, N (1995). The validity of the Maslach Burnout Inventory in three national samples. In L Bennett, D Miller D, and M Ross (eds.), *Health Workers and AIDS: Research, Intervention and Current Issues in Burnout and Response* (pp. 131–150). Amsterdam: Harwood Academic Publishers.

Farber BA (1990). Burnout in psychotherapists: incidence, types, and trends. *Psychother Private Pract* 8:35–44.

Felton JS (1998). Burnout as a clinical entity—its importance in health care workers [review]. *Occup Med (Oxford)* 48:237–250.

Frierson RL, and Lippmann SB (1987). Stresses on physicians treating AIDS. *Am Fam Physician* 35: 153–159.

Gerberding JL (2003). Occupational exposure to HIV in health care settings. *N Engl J Med* 348:826–833.

Grossman AH, and Silverstein C (1993). Facilitating support groups for professionals working with people with AIDS. *Soc Work* 38:144–151.

Haddon W (1980). Advances in the epidemiology of injuries as a basis for public policy. *Public Health Rep* 95(5):411–421.

Kalichman SC, Gueritault-Chalvin V, and Demi A (2000). Sources of occupational stress and coping strategies among nurses working in AIDS care. *J Assoc Nurses AIDS Care* 11(3):31–37.

Killeen ME (1993). Getting through our grief. For caregivers of persons with AIDS. *Am J Hospice Palliat Care* 10:18–9, 23–24.

Lazarus RS, and Folkman S (1984). *Stress Appraisal and Coping.* New York: Springer.

Lee R, and Ashforth B (1990). On the meaning of Maslach's three dimensions of burnout. *J Appl Psychol* 75(6):743–747.

Maslach C, Schaufeli WB, and Leiter MP (2001). Job burnout. *Annu Rev Psychol* 52:397–422.

Miller D, and Gillies P (1996). Is there life after work? Experiences of HIV and oncology health staff. *AIDS Care* 8:167–182

Mueller KP (1997). The relationship between social support and burnout among social work caregivers of HIV/AIDS clients. *Dissertation Abstracts International Section A: Humanities and Social Sciences* Vol. A, p. 3683.

Nesbitt WH, Ross MW, Sunderland RH, and Shelp E (1996). Prediction of grief and HIV/AIDS-related burnout in volunteers. *AIDS Care* 8(2):137–143.

[OSHA] Occupational Safety and Health Administration (1999). OSHA Directives, CPL 2–2. 44D (11/05/99). Enforcement Procedures for the Occupational Exposures to Bloodborne Pathogens.

Pleck JH, O'Donnell L, O'Donnell C, and Snarey J (1998). AIDS phobia, contact with AIDS, and AIDS-related job stress in hospital workers. *J Homosex* 15:41–54.

Ramirez AJ, Graham J, Richards MA, Cull A, and Gregory WM (1996). Mental health of hospital consultants: the effect of stress and satisfaction at work. *Lancet* 16:724–728.

Sepkowitz KA (1996). Occupationally acquired infections in health care workers. Part II *Ann Intern Med* 125(11):917–928.

Silverman DC (1993). Psychosocial impact of HIV-related care giving on health providers: a review and recommendations for the role of psychiatry. *Am J Psychiatry* 150:705–712.

Tiamson ML, McArdie R, Girolamer T, and Horowitz HW (1998). The institutional memorial service: a strategy to prevent burnout in HIV healthcare workers. *Gen Hospital Psychiatry* 20(2):124–126.

Van Servellen G, and Leake B (1993). Burn-out in hospital nurses: a comparison of acquired immunodeficiency syndrome, oncology, general medical, and intensive care unit nurse samples. *J Prof Nurs* 9(3):169–177.

Visintini R, Campnini E, Fossati A, Bagnato M, Novella A, and Maffei C (1996). Psychological stress in nurses' relationships with HIV-infected patients: the risk of burnout syndrome. *AIDS Care* 8(2):183–194.

Wallack JJ (1989). AIDS anxiety among health care professionals. *Commun Psychiatry* 40:507–510.

Chapter 39

End-of-Life Issues

Rebecca W. Brendel and Mary Ann Cohen

As a result of medical advances, people with AIDS are living longer and healthier lives. Nonetheless, between 2000 and 2004, AIDS accounted for more than 500,000 deaths in the United States, or between 15,000 and 18,000 deaths per year (CDC, 2004). Although the number of AIDS deaths per year has declined, the number of annual deaths among young adult and minority populations has remained relatively constant (Selwyn and Rivard, 2003). End-of-life treatment, therefore, remains a critical area in the care of patients with AIDS, who often exhibit a complex array of biological, psychological, and social factors contributing to their clinical presentations.

In addition to increasing the significance of end-of-life care, potent antiretroviral therapy and competent medical care have led to an increase in the number of individuals with HIV/AIDS living with the burdens of a chronic illness. Therefore, to adequately address the mental and physical burdens of HIV/AIDS, the concept of AIDS palliative care can no longer be limited strictly to end-of-life care. Instead, AIDS palliative care has grown, and must continue to expand, to incorporate the alleviation of suffering and the provision of comfort care at every stage of the illness (Grady et al., 2001; Selwyn and Rivard, 2003; Cohen and Alfonso, 2004; Selwyn, 2005a, 2005b).

The issues involved with care of persons with AIDS who are dying are complex and multidimensional and are addressed in several chapters in this text. These include Chapter 30, on palliative and spiritual care, as well as Chapters 28 and 29, for discussions of social work and nursing support.

This chapter begins by addressing general principles of end-of-life care and their application to the dying patient with AIDS. It then focuses on common presenting medical and psychiatric symptoms in AIDS patients at the end of life and strategies for their management and palliation. It concludes with a consideration of major ethical and legal considerations at the end of life.

TREATMENT GOALS AT THE END OF LIFE

Notwithstanding the numerous advances in medical and palliative care since the 1970s, the central goal of treatment at the end of life remains, as Saunders (1978) described it then, to keep patients feeling like themselves as long as possible. This principle continues in today's definition of hospice care as "total care of patients whose disease is not responsive to curative treatments" (WHO, 1990). Hospice care aims to minimize the burdens of illness and to maximize quality of life, with the ultimate aim of supporting the highest level of physical ability possible, facilitating the continuation of social relationships, and helping patients achieve the greatest mental and emotional capacity possible.

A terminally ill individual is eligible for hospice when his or her life expectancy is 6 months or less, under Medicare guidelines. Hospice services may be provided in a patient's home, or in a residential or long-term care facility. Historically, the average patient has enrolled in hospice 1 month prior to death and the vast majority of patients enrolled in hospice have had a diagnosis of cancer, although the proportion with cancer is dropping (Haupt, 1998a, 1998b; Christakis and Iwashyna, 2000; National Hospice and Palliative Care Organization, 2005). While hospice care is not the only means of providing care for the dying patient, its multidisciplinary approach incorporating medical and nursing care, spiritual and family support, pain management, and respite services may assist patients in completing important end-of-life tasks and experiencing a comfortable death.

The end of life is an important opportunity for resolving "unfinished business" (Kübler-Ross, 1969). Kübler-Ross, in her ground-breaking 1969 treatise on dying, identified the end-of-life as a time for reconciliation, conflict resolution with loved ones, and pursuit of remaining hopes. In addition, she described the now classic psychological stages of dying, which may occur in any order: denial and isolation, anger, bargaining, guilt and depression, and acceptance. Overall, the five goals for "appropriate death" have been identified as freedom from pain, operating as effectively as possible within the constraints of disability, satisfaction of remaining wishes, recognition and resolution of residual conflict, and yielding of control to trusted individuals (Hackett and Weisman, 1962).

Psychiatrists and other mental health professionals are in a unique position to assist patients in the real-ization of end-of-life goals because of their abilities to understand personality styles and traits, and to engage with patients to modulate and alter maladaptive responses to illness and to dying (Cassem and Brendel, 2004; Kim and Greenberg, 2004). In addition, the abilities to appreciate both the medical aspects of disease and to understand the highly subjective and individual factors that contribute to the personal significance of illness offer the psychiatrist a pivotal role in the treatment of medically ill and dying patients (Cassem and Brendel, 2004; Kim and Greenberg, 2004).

THE DYING PATIENT WITH AIDS

Dying patients with AIDS face the same set of challenges and opportunities at the end of life, introduced above, as those of other dying patients. However, in addition, there are added features of AIDS that distinguish individuals dying from AIDS from other populations at the end of life and that may limit the applicability of hospice interventions, which have evolved predominantly on the basis of needs and characteristics of cancer patients (Grady et al., 2001). Demographic and ethnic factors, concerns about discrimination and pain management, and the changing success rates of HIV treatment are several often-identified factors that contribute to the challenge of developing a treatment model that adequately addresses the end-of-life needs of AIDS patients (Grady et al., 2001; Selwyn and Rivard, 2003; Beck and Worth, 2004). Recent research has suggested that palliative and hospice care for terminally ill AIDS patients is associated with better pain and symptom management as well as improvements in insight, anxiety, and spiritual well-being (Harding et al., 2005). As a result, it is critical to understand the unique characteristics of AIDS patients in order to provide competent and compassionate care to as many individuals with HIV/AIDS as possible.

Age

The life expectancy of Americans is approximately 77 years, and the average age of all hospice enrollees is approximately 79 years (Christakis and Iwashyna, 2000; CDC, 2005). As a result, end-of-life care is often targeted at the needs of a geriatric population and the physical needs and psychological conflicts of this age group. In comparison, the age of death for AIDS patients is significantly lower, with more than two-thirds of patients who died of AIDS in 2004 dying before the age of 50 and less than 10% dying at age 60 or above (CDC, 2004). Similarly, the average age in traditional nursing homes is 65–85 while in AIDS nursing homes the average age is 41 (Cohen, 1998a). Some end-of-life concerns are common across all age groups, such as coping with loss, concerns about progressive disability, reconciling remaining conflicts, and obtaining adequate pain management. For the patient with AIDS, however, the end-of-life agenda may be less about realizing the accomplishments of a life lived, often thought of as the task at death, and more about reconciling feelings regarding unrealized goals and expectations. These concerns often include issues of remorse, longing for missed opportunities, and concerns about ongoing childcare and guardianship—all issues with psychological and practical urgency (Beck and Worth, 2004; Kutzen, 2004). Psychodynamic psychotherapy and development of attainable goals have been used to resolve the conflicts of young persons with AIDS who are coming to terms with lost opportunities at the end of life (Cohen, 1999). However, physicians are often described as hesitant to introduce end-of-life discussions and hospice care for patients. Physicians have a tendency to be overly optimistic about their patients' prognoses and reluctant to ruin patients' hopes with a poor prognosis, and they tend to employ aggressive medical therapy until the very end of life (Grady et al., 2001).

Race

Although African Americans account for a minority of the U.S. population, African Americans account for the majority of HIV/AIDS diagnoses (CDC, 2006). For example, in 2003, the most recent year for which data were available, a survey of 33 states showed that African Americans accounted for approximately 13% of the population and for 51% of HIV/AIDS diagnoses (CDC, 2006). Overall, African Americans and other minorities, however, are less likely to enroll in hospice or use palliative care (Crawley et al., 2000). Specifically, African Americans represent less than 10% of patients in hospice, whereas whites represent more than 80% (Crawley et al., 2000).

Research has shown that underutilization of end-of-life care is clearly associated with lack of insurance (Krakauer et al., 2002). In addition to access to and funding for care, however, there are other cultural factors, supported by varying amounts of data, that contribute to the disparity between white Americans and minorities in the use of end-of-life care (Crawley et al., 2000; Krakauer et al., 2002; Perkins et al., 2002). These factors include ethnic differences in preferences for life-sustaining care, mistrust of the medical establishment, and differences in spiritual, religious, and cultural attitudes toward death and disability.

In general, African Americans are more likely to want aggressive, life-sustaining care than whites and other minorities, and more likely to request CPR even after a diagnosis of terminal illness (Caralis et al., 1993; Garrett et al., 1993; O'Brien et al., 1995; Phillips et al., 1996; Krakauer et al., 2002). Also, although empirical evidence is still being gathered, African Americans are more likely to mistrust the medical establishment, and this mistrust may be heightened in situations where HIV/AIDS is involved (Crawley, 2000; Krakauer et al., 2002; Perkins et al., 2002; Bogart and Thorburn, 2005). Recent research on attitudes of African Americans has shown that between 1% and 59% of those surveyed either agreed or strongly agreed with conspiracy theories about HIV/AIDS (Bogart and Thorburn, 2005). For example, while only 1%–2% of individuals surveyed agreed somewhat or strongly with the conspiracy theory that "doctors put HIV into condoms," more than 16% of respondents agreed somewhat or strongly that "AIDS was created by the government to control the black population," and nearly 60% of respondents agreed somewhat or strongly that "a lot of information about AIDS is being held back from the public" (Bogart and Thorburn, 2005). A 2006 study also supported a high prevalence of belief in a conspiracy theory of HIV/AIDS among African Americans (Ross et al. 2006). Yet, at the same time, in the 2005 study, more than three-quarters of respondents strongly or somewhat agreed that "Medical and public health institutions are trying to stop the spread of HIV in black communities," indicating that views about HIV/AIDS in the African-American community are complex and require further study (Bogart and Thorburn, 2005). Finally, spiritual and religious beliefs among African Americans may make them more likely to accept suffering and functional impairment than other ethnic and cultural groups (Crawley, 2000; Krakauer et al., 2002).

Cultural competency and attention to the specific beliefs and needs of minority populations are especially critical in addressing the end-of-life needs of patients with AIDS, given the disproportionate effect of HIV/AIDS on minority populations. In addition, it is important that focus not be solely on African Americans. For example, another recent study of conspiracy beliefs about HIV/AIDS suggested that conspiracy beliefs may also exist with relatively high prevalence in Latino communities (Ross et al., 2006). Attention to the patient's life circumstances, relationships, religion, and faith can help forge an alliance with the dying patient in the hope of facilitating support and working through complicating factors (Crawley et al., 2000; Cassem and Brendel, 2004).

Substance Abuse

Freedom from pain is a central principle in end-of-life care. In general, pain in HIV/AIDS patients is undertreated, and, in particular, patients with active addiction and addiction histories are more likely to be undertreated for pain than other patients (Breitbart et al., 1997, 1999; Gilson and Joranson, 2002; Cohen and Alfonso, 2004; Harding et al., 2005; Selwyn, 2005a, 2005b). Psychiatrists are often asked to evaluate patients who require larger-than-expected doses of pain medication because of concerns about the presence of a substance use disorder and concerns of misuse of pain medication by patients with known underlying substance use disorders (Cassem and Brendel, 2004). Physicians have implicit and explicit negative reactions to patients with substance use disorders who request pain medications, fearing that these patients are abusing prescribed narcotics and that the prescribing physician will be subject to legal sanction for prescribing controlled substances to an addict (Breitbart et al., 1999; Gilson and Joranson, 2002).

Because injection drug use is a major risk behavior associated with HIV infection, patients dying of AIDS often suffer from concomitant substance use disorders. In addition, other drug and alcohol use may be overrepresented in HIV-infected individuals because of the tendency of these substances to increase the risk of unsafe sexual practices through effects on perception and behavior, including impulsivity, disinhibition, altered cognition, and impaired judgment (Beck and Worth, 2004). As a result, treating the patient with end-stage AIDS often means treating a patient with a substance use disorder, either active or in some phase of remission. Adequate treatment of the dying AIDS patient requires the clinician to separate management

of the patient's addiction from adequate management of the patient's pain and to treat both effectively (Beck and Worth, 2004; Renner and Gastfriend, 2004).

Fear of Discrimination

A dying person may feel shame for his or her actions and may also feel disowned by society because of chronic illness or prior behaviors (Cassem and Brendel, 2004). Patients with HIV/AIDS are no exception and may be more vulnerable to humiliation and shame from the stigma associated with HIV. Also, historically HIV has disproportionately affected vulnerable and disenfranchised populations, including minorities, intravenous drug users, the poor, women, the incarcerated and convicted criminals, and homosexual men (Linder et al., 2002a, 2002b; Beck and Worth, 2004; CDC 2006) These factors may have a negative impact on HIV/AIDS patients' use of end-of-life care resources through a reluctance to seek assistance, limited availability of and access to care, and other factors (Kutzen, 2004). Attention to these barriers and the internal experience of patients' dying of AIDS can result in these patients achieving meaningful treatment and community supports as well as a sense of being respected as human beings (Beck and Worth, 2004; Cassem and Brendel, 2004).

Course of Illness

Since the introduction of highly active antiretroviral therapy (HAART), HIV is no longer an infection that causes a linear progression to a most certain death as CD4 cell counts wane; AIDS has become a chronic illness (Selwyn, 2005a, 2005b). In addition, in the era of effective treatments for even late-stage disease, there are few data about the prognostic factors that are associated with morbidity in late-stage AIDS (Selwyn, 2005a, 2005b; Shen et al., 2005). In an era of rapidly advancing medical therapy, the absence of prognostic data can translate into a reluctance to address end-of-life care needs in favor of continued aggressive therapy (Grady et al., 2001).

One recent study of more than 200 late-stage AIDS patients in a specialized New York HIV palliative care program found that the only statistically significant predictors of mortality in late-stage AIDS were age above 65 and total impairment in activities of daily living (ADLs); further research is required to assist in prognostication (Shen et al., 2005). Such study may elucidate critical prognostic factors to improve the accuracy of patients' prognosis. However, even in the absence of these data, it is critical that focus on aggressive treatment does not eclipse the alleviation of suffering, provision of palliative care, attention to closure, completion of unfinished business, reconciliation, and other end-of-life tasks. Specifically, palliative care means providing comfort at every stage of HIV infection and must not be forgotten, even when aggressive treatment is also being provided.

SYMPTOMATIC MANAGEMENT OF THE DYING PATIENT WITH AIDS

Patients with late-stage AIDS generally have a high symptom burden that spans across the biological, psychological, and social spectrum (Cohen, 1998b; Cohen and Alfonso, 2004; Selwyn, 2005a). Effectively addressing the significant symptomatology of these patients is a complex and critical task. However, without adequate palliation of symptoms, patients with AIDS are deprived of a comfortable, dignified, and meaningful death, and of the opportunity to complete unfinished business. The foundation of treatment remains the same as for all patients at the end of life—to maximize functioning and minimize disease burdens in order to help patients feel like themselves for as long as possible. The following discussion focuses on common symptoms and major areas of focus.

Biological Symptoms

One of the five most common fears of dying patients is that death will cause physical pain, injury, or suffocation (Reddick et al., 2004). Even in the patient who is most certain to die, physical symptoms require attention and investigation to their underlying cause. A reversible cause of a distressing or debilitating symptom may be discovered, and treatment of that cause could lead to improvement in, if not eradication of, the symptom. That being said, the absence of a clear underlying cause of a symptom should not be interpreted as evidence that the patient's symptom is not "real." This situation is especially true in the case of pain.

Patients with HIV/AIDS commonly experience pain of multiple types and etiologies. Common etiologies of pain in the AIDS patient include opportunistic infections, virus-related neurotoxicity, medication toxicity, other medical and traumatic conditions, and nonspecific symptoms (Selwyn, 2005a). Pain experienced by AIDS patients includes multiple types of neuropathy, headache, and visceral and somatic pain; depending on the type of pain, varying classes of medications may be more or less helpful (Cohen and Alfonso 1998, 2004; Selwyn, 2005a). Taking a clear history of the pain is critical to an effective treatment strategy. Careful assessment of pain is especially critical in patients with substance abuse because these patients are at particular risk for undertreatment of pain (Breitbart et al. 1997, 1999; Cohen and Alfonso, 1998, 2004; Gilson and Joranson, 2002; Harding et al., 2005; Selwyn 2005a).

Other distressing physical symptoms at the end of life include itching and persistent hiccups, both potential sources of significant distress. Topical and low-dose systemic doxepin or antihistamine may alleviate itching, and antipsychotic medication is often helpful for hiccups (Cohen and Alfonso, 2004). Treatment of constitutional symptoms such as fatigue, weakness, anorexia, fevers, and sweats also improves quality of life. In this regard, corticosteroids, stimulants, nonsteroidal anti-inflammatory agents, and hormone therapies may alleviate symptoms (Selwyn, 2005a). AIDS patients frequently suffer from gastrointestinal disturbance, and efforts to reduce nausea, vomiting, and diarrhea may contribute significantly to greater comfort, dignity, and functional ability. Many different pharmacologic agents may be employed in the management of gastrointestinal symptoms, including dopamine agonists, prokinetic agents, benzodiazepines, serotonin antagonists, and acid-reducing drugs, and corticosteroids for nausea and vomiting, and antimotility and other preparations for diarrhea.

Dyspnea is another particularly distressing symptom for dying patients, and individuals with HIV are no exception. Dyspnea is associated with intense anxiety and fear of death by asphyxiation (Cohen and Alfonso, 2004). Treatment interventions include oxygen, morphine, relaxation, and use of a fan.

The person dying of AIDS is likely to suffer from psychiatric comorbidity, with the most common diagnoses being dementia, substance abuse, and delirium (Cohen, 1998a, 1998b). In addition to cognitive disorders and substance use disorders, adjustment disorder, major depression, and other mood disorders with depressive and manic symptoms are common (Cohen 1998a, 1998b). Given the distress and limits on functioning associated with these psychiatric diagnoses, aggressive treatment is critical to the goal of compassionate care (Cassem and Brendel, 2004).

Psychological Considerations

The complexity of HIV/AIDS leads individuals with HIV/AIDS to suffer from high levels of distress associated with symptoms, medical and psychiatric illness, discrimination and stigma, social factors, and financial stressors (Cohen and Weisman, 1986; Cohen 1987, 1990, 1992; Cohen and Alfonso, 1998). One study showed that more than two-thirds of patients in an HIV-clinic waiting room sample reported distress; these patients also had high rates of anxiety (70%) and depression (46%), highlighting the need for attention to both biological and psychological interventions for distress (Cohen et al., 2002).

Dying patients may be reluctant to talk about death because they do not want to burden others. At the same time, most people are very reluctant to let dying patients express themselves (Cassem and Brendel, 2004). As a result, it is possible for the patient and others, including family, friends, and caregivers, to enter into a "collusion of silence." Communication is essential, however, for the dying person to address lingering fears, hopes, and concerns—many of which are associated with high degrees of existential anxiety (Cassem and Brendel, 2004; Cohen and Alfonso, 2004). Anxious patients are often not consciously aware of what frightens them about death, and the process of exploring fear with others is critical to reduction in anxiety (Reddick et al., 2004).

Attention to spirituality is also critical in alleviating distress, as many individuals have a strong personal sense of faith that may be helpful in coping with a terminal illness. (Cassem and Brendel, 2004) Exploring an individual's sense of faith and spirituality is another opportunity to understand what factors may be contributing to anxiety or other subjective distress. Working with chaplains or religious figures close to the individual may provide care and consolation (Cohen and Alfonso, 2004). In addition, religious persons often belong to a community that can offer support.

Social Factors

As the burden of disease and illness increases, the dying patient's functional abilities necessarily decline. A decline in functional ability often leads to isolation and fears of dying alone. Patients with HIV/AIDS may be more vulnerable to isolation because of reluctance to disclose their HIV status and because of the nature of the illness. For example, because HIV is a communicable disease, a spouse or loved one might also be ill and unavailable to care for and attend to the dying patient (Kutzen, 2004). Home visits by care providers, family, and friends may alleviate these fears and provide an opportunity for reflection and closure.

Even if an individual has few or no readily identifiable social contacts or supports, avenues exist to assist the dying person in forging supportive social connections. For example, support groups, community groups, religious organizations, and hospice programs may provide much-needed social connections and support. Regular visits by physicians, visits by children, family cohesion and integration, cheerfulness, equanimity, competence, and concern are all factors that dying patients and their families have identified as essential features in the care of dying patients (Cassem and Brendel, 2004). Finally, AIDS patients often feel lonely, stigmatized, contaminated, and abandoned. Holding hands with a patient dying of AIDS is an important step in reducing stigma and feelings of isolation, and may help the patient die feeling less lonely and more appreciated and treated as a human being.

FINAL CONSIDERATIONS AT THE END OF LIFE

Advances in medical technology allow physicians to sustain life even in the setting of irreversible and devastating illness. The complex ethical, legal, and emotional aspects of end-of-life care have led many decisions about end-of-life care to end in courtrooms, and as a result some clear principles have emerged. Perhaps the most important principle of autonomy resulting from attention to difficult issues at the end of life is the right of competent patients to refuse treatment, even if the treatment refused would be life sustaining. The patient's will is supreme, but patients may not demand interventions that are medically futile even if life would be prolonged in the short run (Cassem and Brendel, 2004; Reddick et al., 2004).

However, a complicating dimension occurs when patients rely on physicians to prognosticate and recommend the amount and form of treatment in the face of life-threatening or likely terminal illness. In these situations, although life could be prolonged, additional questions must be addressed before aggressive treatment is recommended. Specifically, would the treatment be more burdensome than beneficial? Are there less invasive alternatives? What are the patient's wishes and views about death? What outstanding hopes and business does the patient wish to accomplish? How does the patient hope to die? At home? In a hospital? Elsewhere? It is critically important for caregivers to be honest and forthright with patients about their clinical conditions and to allow patients to make their own decisions about death and dying rather than for caregivers to implicitly or explicitly impose their own views. The ability of caregivers to share knowledge about hospice and palliative care resources is critical to help patients achieve their desired last goals and wishes.

Finally, while patient autonomy is broad relative to decisions surrounding death, there are limits on a patient's ability to control the mode and manner of death. Patients may express wishes to have their physicians end their lives. Active killing, even out of mercy, is euthanasia and is illegal in all 50 states. On the other hand, physician-assisted suicide is now legal in Oregon, after multiple legal challenges, several of which have reached the U.S. Supreme Court. Under the Oregon Death With Dignity Act, physicians in Oregon are authorized to write prescriptions for lethal medications to patients who request to die and meet the state's other legal requirements. While Oregon has sanctioned this practice, the American Medical Association and, by incorporation, the American Psychiatric Association are opposed to the practice of physician-assisted suicide. Notwithstanding, at the time of this writing, laws authorizing physician-assisted suicide were in planning in several other states.

As the legal and organizational issues continue to unfold, it is critical for individual physicians to explore desires for death with all dying patients. Sound clinical and ethical practice requires the physician to assist the terminally ill patient in the complex and often simultaneous processes of grieving and celebrating, reconciliation of conflict and completion of unfinished business, achievement of last hopes and acceptance of unrealized goals—all while alleviating suffering and maximizing autonomy and personhood until the last possible moment.

In summary, end-of-life care is a critical dimension in the care of the patient with AIDS, and is an important opportunity to assist patients to die a meaningful, peaceful, and comfortable death. At the same time, significant work remains to ensure that end-of-life care for AIDS patients takes into account the distinct and complex challenges of this population to adequately address their substantial and continuing needs. Overall, good end-of-life care builds on the foundation of compassionate and competent care throughout all stages of HIV infection. The unique characteristics of the AIDS patient require caregivers to alleviate suffering and to provide a nurturing environment so that the AIDS patient may die a meaningful death.

References

Beck BJ, and Worth JL (2004). Patients with HIV infection and AIDS. In TA Stern, GL Fricchione, NH Cassem, MS Jellinek, and JF Rosenbaum (eds.), *Massachusetts General Hospital Handbook of General Hospital Psychiatry*, fifth edition (pp. 671–695). Philadelphia: Mosby.

Bogart LM, and Thorburn S (2005). Are HIV/AIDS conspiracy beliefs a barrier to HIV prevention among African Americans? *J Acquir Immune Defic Syndr* 38:213–218.

Breitbart W, Rosenfeld B, Passik S, Kaim M, Funesti-Esch J, and Stein K (1997). A comparison of pain report and adequacy of analgesic therapy in ambulatory AIDS patients with and without a history of substance abuse. *Pain* 72:235–243.

Breitbart W, Kaim M, and Rosenfeld B (1999). Clinicians' perception of barriers to pain management in AIDS. *J Pain Symptom Manage* 18:203–212.

Caralis PV, Davis B, Wright K, and Marcial E (1993). The influence of ethnicity and race on attitudes toward advance directives, life-prolonging treatments, and euthanasia. *J Clin Ethics* 4:155–165.

Cassem NH, and Brendel RW (2004). End of life issues: principles of care and ethics. In TA Stern, GL Fricchione, NH Cassem, MS Jellinek, and JF Rosenbaum (eds.), *Massachusetts General Hospital Handbook of General Hospital Psychiatry*, fifth edition (pp. 365–387). Philadelphia: Mosby.

[CDC] Centers for Disease Control and Prevention (2004). HIV/AIDS Surveillance Report, 2004, Vol. 16. Atlanta: U.S. Department of Health and Human Services, Centers for Disease Control and Prevention.

[CDC] Centers for Disease Control and Prevention (2005). Deaths: preliminary data for 2003. *Natl Vital Stat Rep* 53:1–48.

[CDC] Centers for Disease Control and Prevention (2006). Racial/ethnic disparities in diagnoses of HIV/AIDS—33 states, 2001–2004. *MMWR Morb Mortal Wkly Rep* 55:121–125.

Christakis NA, and Iwashyna TJ (2000). Impact of individual and market factors on the timing of initiation of hospice terminal care. *Med Care* 38:528–524.

Cohen MA (1987). Psychiatric aspects of AIDS: a bio-psychosocial approach. In GP Wormser, RE Stahl, and EJ Bottone (eds.), *AIDS-Acquired Immune Deficiency Syndrome and Other Manifestations of HIV Infection* (pp. 579–622). Park Ridge, NJ: Noyes Publishers.

Cohen MA (1990). A biopsychosocial approach to the HIV epidemic. *General Hospital Psychiatry* 12:98–123.

Cohen MA (1992). Biopsychosocial aspects of the HIV epidemic. In GP Wormser (ed.), *AIDS and Other Manifestations of HIV Infection*, second edition (pp. 349–371). New York: Raven Press.

Cohen MA (1998a). Psychiatric care in an AIDS nursing home. *Psychosomatics* 39:154–161.

Cohen MA (1998b). Psychiatric care for patients with AIDS in a long-term care setting. *Dir Psychiatry* 18:365–383.

Cohen MA (1999). Psychodynamic psychotherapy in an AIDS nursing home. *J Am Acad Psychoanal* 27:121–133.

Cohen MA, and Alfonso CA (1998). Psychiatric care and pain management in persons with HIV infection. In GP Wormser (ed.), *AIDS and Other Manifestations of HIV Infection*, third edition (pp. 475–503). Philadephia: Lippincott-Raven.

Cohen MA, and Alfonso CA (2004). AIDS psychiatry: psychiatric and palliative care, and pain management. In GP Wormser (ed.), *AIDS and Other Manisfestations of HIV Infection*, fourth edition (pp. 537–576). San Diego: Elsevier.

Cohen MA, and Weisman H (1986). A biopsychosocial approach to AIDS. *Psychosomatics* 27:245–249.

Cohen, MA, Hoffman, RG, Cromwell C, Schmeidler J, Ebrahim F, Carrera G, Endorf F, Alfonso CA, and Jacobson JM (2002). The prevalence of distress in persons with human immunodeficiency virus infection. *Psychosomatics* 43:10–15.

Crawley V, Payne R, Bolden J, Payne T, Washington P, and Williams S (2000). Palliative and end-of-life care in the African American community [commentary]. *JAMA* 284:2518–2521.

Garrett JM, Harris RP, Norburn JK, Patrick DL, and Danis M (1993). Life-sustaining treatments during terminal illness: who wants what? *J Gen Intern Med* 8:361–368.

Gilson AM, and Joranson DE (2002). U.S. policies relevant to the prescribing of opioid analgesics for the treatment of pain in patients with addictive disease. *Clin J Pain* 18:S91–S98.

Grady PA, Knebel AR, and Draper A (2001). End-of-life issues in AIDS: the research perspective. *J R Soc Med* 94:479–482.

Hackett TP, and Weisman AD (1962). The treatment of the dying. *Curr Psychiatr Ther* 2:121–126.

Harding R, Karus D, Easterbrook P,.Ravies VH, Higginson IJ, and Marconi K (2005). Does palliative care improve outcomes for patients with HIV/AIDS? A systematic review of the evidence. *Sex Transm Infect* 81:5–14.

Haupt B (1998a). An overview of home health and hospice care patients: 1996 National Home and Hospice Care Survey. *Adv Data* 1998(297):1–35.

Haupt B (1998b). Characteristics of hospice care users: data from the 1996 National Home and Hospice Care Survey. *Adv Data* 1998(299):1–16.

Kim HG, and Greenberg DB (2004). Coping with medical illness. In TA Stern and JB Herman (eds.), *Massachusetts General Hospital Psychiatry Update and Board Preparation*, second edition (pp. 511–516). New York: McGraw-Hill.

Krakauer EL, Crenner C, and Fox K (2002). Barriers to optimum end-of-life care for minority patients. *J Am Geriatr Soc* 50:182–190.

Kübler-Ross E (1969). *On Death and Dying*. New York: Macmillan.

Kutzen HS (2004). Integration of palliative care into primary care for human immunodeficiecy virus-infected patients. *Am J Med Sci* 328:37–47.

Linder JF, Enders SR, Craig E, Richardson J, and Meyers FJ (2002a). Hospice care for the incarcerated in the United States: an introduction. *J Palliat Med* 5:549–552.

Linder JF, Knauf K, Enders SR, and Meyers FJ (2002b). Prison hospice and pastoral care services in California. *J Palliat Med* 5:903–908.

National Hospice and Palliative Care Organization, NHPCO's facts and figures – 2005 findings, Available at http://www.nhpco.org/files/public/2005-facts-and-figures.pdf, accesed on February 21, 2007.

O'Brien LA, Grisso JA, Maislin G, LaPann K, Krotki KP, Greco PJ, Siegert EA, and Evans LK (1995). Nursing home residents' preferences for life-sustaining treatments, *JAMA* 274:1775–1779.

Perkins HS, Geppert CM, Gonzales A, Cortez JD, and Hazuda HP (2002). Cross-cultural similarities and differences in attitudes about advance care planning. *J Gen Intern Med* 17:48–57.

Phillips RS, Wenger NS, Teno J, Oye RK, Younger S, Califf R, Lavde P, Desbiens N, Connors AF Jr, and Lynn J (1996). Choices of seriously ill patients about cardiopulmonary resuscitation: correlates and outcomes. *Am J Med* 100:128–137.

Reddick B, Brendel RW, and Cassem NH (2004). Treatment decisions at the end of life. In TA Stern and JB Herman (eds.), *Massachusetts General Hospital Psychiatry Update and Board Preparation*, second edition (pp. 517–521). New York: McGraw Hill.

Renner JA Jr, and Gastfriend DR (2004) Drug-addicted patients. In TA Stern, GL Fricchione, NH Cassem, MS Jellinek, and JF Rosenbaum (eds.), *Massachusetts General Hospital Handbook of General Hospital Psychiatry*, fifth edition (pp. 217–229). Philadelphia: Mosby.

Ross MW, Essien EJ, and Torres I (2006). Conspiracy beliefs about the origin of HIV/AIDS in four racial/ethnic groups. *J Acquir Immune Defic Syndr* 41:342–344.

Saunders C (ed.) (1978). *The Management of Terminal Illness*. Chicago: Year Book.

Selwyn PA (2005a). Palliative care for patients with human immunodeficiency virus/acquired immune deficiency syndrome. *J Palliat Med* 8:1248–1268.

Selwyn PA (2005b). Why should we care about palliative care for AIDS in the era of antiretroviral therapy? *Sex Transm Infect* 81:2–3.

Selwyn PA, and Rivard M (2003). Palliative care for AIDS: challenges and opportunities in the era of highly active anti-retroviral therapy. *J Palliat Med* 6:475–487.

Shen JM, Blank A, and Selwyn PA (2005). Predictors of mortality for patients with advanced disease in an HIV palliative care program. *J Acquir Immune Defic Syndr* 40:445–447.

[WHO] World Health Organization (1990). *Cancer Pain Relief and Palliative Care: Report of a WHO Expert Committee*. Geneva: World Health Organization.

Chapter 40

Ethical Issues, Advance Directives, and Surrogate Decision-Making

Rebecca Brendel and Mary Ann Cohen

The doctor–patient relationship is the cornerstone of all psychiatric treatment and requires the physician to act in the patient's interest and put the patient's needs first. As early as 430 BC, the Hippocratic Oath (Hippocrates, translated by Chadwick and Mann, 1983) outlined many of the elements of this relationship that continue today, including helping the sick, doing no harm, and maintaining confidentiality. These early principles are today supplemented by principles of ethics promulgated by professional organizations such as the American Medical and Psychiatric Associations and by legal mandates on the state and federal levels (Brendel and Brendel, 2005).

Although many of the fundamental principles of ethics guiding the doctor–patient relationship and medical practice are centuries old, ethical dilemmas often arise in the course of treating patients. These conflicts may emerge when the fundamental principles of the individual doctor–patient relationship are challenged by competing societal interests or by factors within the individual doctor–patient relationship

itself. Treating patients with HIV/AIDS is no exception. For example, the infectious nature of HIV/AIDS raises many questions regarding physicians' obligations to report new cases of HIV/AIDS to state agencies and other individuals who may be at risk, and the principle of informed consent may be challenged when a patient's mental status no longer allows him or her to make autonomous decisions. This chapter focuses on issues of autonomy, decision-making, and confidentiality, as well as additional selected ethical issues that arise in the course of treating patients with HIV/AIDS.

CONFIDENTIALITY

Confidentiality is one of the basic cornerstones of the doctor–patient relationship. All physicians and psychiatrists in particular are required to maintain strict confidentiality in the interest of promoting the trusting disclosure of information to promote treatment (Brendel, 2005). In addition, persons with HIV and

AIDS may be more concerned about the protection of confidentiality because of concerns about discrimination and stigma associated with the illness. However, confidentiality issues increasingly come into conflict with other societal interests and necessities, and are magnified in the care of persons with HIV and AIDS.

As such, there is special protection for HIV-related information, but at the same time there continue to be many exceptions to the traditional concept of strict doctor–patient confidentiality. This section will provide a discussion of some of the main considerations regarding topics related to protection for and limitations on confidentiality in the setting of treating patients with HIV/AIDS.

Special Protection for HIV-Related Information

Because of concerns about stigma and discrimination when the first tests became available to detect the HIV virus in the mid 1980s, many states passed laws granting special protection to HIV-related health information. Although laws vary from state to state, types of laws that emerged included a subset requiring written informed consent for HIV testing and another subset requiring specific, written informed consent for release of HIV-related records to third parties. For example, Connecticut requires either written consent or oral consent documented in the medical chart for "HIV-related tests" (CONN. GEN. STAT. § 19a-582) and Georgia requires written consent to release "AIDS Confidential Information" (GA. CODE ANN. 24-9 § 47 and 31-22 § 9.1).

Mandated Reporting of Cases

Although informed consent is generally required for the release of HIV-related information, the government also has an interest in tracking and following cases of HIV to monitor and address this serious infectious illness. The precedent for monitoring cases of infectious and sexually transmitted illnesses has a long history (Gostin and Hodge, 1998). HIV is no exception. Different states have different requirements for who must report HIV status and to whom. It is important for physicians to know the applicable laws in the jurisdiction(s) in which they practice in order to comply with the legal requirements.

Knowledge of the applicable standards is critical to providing ethical care. Specifically, if a state requires a report of HIV seropositivity with a patient's name, the patient should be notified *prior* to testing so that the patient may give full informed consent to the testing. For example, New York State requires this type of reporting (New York State Department of Health, 2003). Where there are exceptions to confidentiality, the trust inherent in the doctor–patient relationship is best preserved by advance disclosure on the limits of confidentiality.

However, even with a physician's advance disclosure of the limits on confidentiality of HIV test results, patients may ask their physicians not to disclose their HIV status. While it is critical for physicians to be aware of the law in the jurisdictions in which they practice, the cornerstone of managing difficult situations remains sound clinical care and judgment. Although the clinician's final course of action may be dictated by law, the best approach is to explore the patient's concerns and to engage in an open discussion to help the patient come to his or her own decision that is consistent with the provider's legal mandate. In this regard, other resources such as social supports, clergy, mental health clinicians, and other trusted individuals may be critically important to helping the patient make what would otherwise be a legally mandated disclosure by the physician.

Contact Notification and Duty to Warn

The general default is that physicians must safeguard information related to patients' HIV status and may not release it without consent, except in limited circumstances such as mandated reporting. But what happens when a physician becomes aware that a patient either has exposed or continues to expose another person or persons to HIV? The first approach to either situation should be discussion with the patient in an effort to persuade the patient to disclose the risk to potentially affected person(s). However, patients may be reluctant, leaving the physician in a difficult ethical and legal situation.

Nearly 20 years ago, the Council on Ethics and Judicial Affairs of the American Medical Association (AMA) called for the drafting of specific laws that balanced the protection of confidential patient information with the need to provide a method of warning unsuspecting sexual partners of HIV-positive individuals. Specific issues that were highlighted included the need to provide physicians with protection from liability for failure to warn at-risk contacts, to establish clear standards for when a physician should inform public health authorities, and to provide clear guidelines for public health authorities who may need to trace the at-risk contacts (AMA, 1987). However, physicians in these situations are still often left without legal direction. Currently, the AMA is continuing to address confidentiality and ethical issues raised by HIV-positive individuals who do not inform their partners or change their behavior (AMA, 2003b). In addition, because some states impose a duty to warn on mental health professionals that is not required of general medical practitioners, psychiatrists may face an even more complex ethical–legal dilemma about how to handle such situations.

For example, Massachusetts law expressly prohibits the release of HIV information and records without written consent, but also requires mental health providers to warn third parties in certain situations in which a patient has expressed an explicit threat to kill or inflict "serious bodily injury" upon a reasonably identified victim or victims (MASS. GEN. LAWS (M.G.L.) Ch. 111 § 70F 2005; M.G.L. Ch. 123 § 36B 2005). The following vignette is illustrative of the ethical dilemma of beneficence versus maleficence that physicians are faced with regarding disclosure of HIV information. Mr. A was admitted to a medicine floor for treatment of an HIV-related illness and disclosed to his medical team that he was having unprotected vaginal intercourse with his girlfriend and that he had not informed her of his HIV serostatus. He vehemently insisted that he did not want his physicians to inform his girlfriend that he was HIV positive and used the confidentiality statute as the basis for his request. When the team requested a psychiatric consultation to assist in managing this patient's challenging behavior toward the medical staff, the issue of which statute prevailed, i.e., the duty to warn or the confidentiality statute, emerged given the conflicting obligations on the psychiatrist as a mental health provider. Ultimately, the person at risk discovered her partner's HIV status through other sources, but this case illustrates the complexity and practical necessity of contact notification.

States vary in how the law handles contact notification. In New York, for example, physicians have an obligation to report contacts to public health officials (New York State Department of Health, 2000). Furthermore, in cases where a patient does not notify contacts, public health officials will (New York State Department of Health, 2000). However, not all states have these channels and some states, such as Massachusetts, collect HIV infection data without patient names. As a result, it is critical for physicians to be aware of requirements in the jurisdictions in which they practice, and also to be aware of legal and medical resources to consult should ethically and legally challenging situations arise. The AMA position supports continuing work on the state level to address these complex and competing issues of contact notification and confidentiality (AMA, 2003b).

Health Insurance Portability and Accountability Act

In 2003, privacy regulations established by the Health Insurance Portability and Accountability Act (HIPAA) went into effect (Schouten and Brendel, 2004). These broad regulations affect the management of health information by providers and other entities such as health plans. Although HIPAA is generally thought of as increasing privacy for medical record information, its effect is actually to increase the number of situations in which patient medical information may be shared without the patient's express, written, and informed consent (Brendel and Bryan, 2004). Specifically, HIPAA permits the disclosure of otherwise protected private health information for treatment, payment, and health care operations purposes without specific consent, so long as the patient has signed a privacy notice (Brendel and Bryan, 2004).

However, HIPAA is not the final determinant of what medical information can be released without specific consent. HIPAA explicitly states that specific state and federal laws that are more protective of patient privacy than HIPAA itself should prevail. In the case of patients with HIV/AIDS, state laws that require specific, written, informed consent prior to the release of HIV/AIDS records prevail over HIPAA and must be followed. In addition, federal legislation offers an added degree of protection over what HIPAA requires for substance abuse treatment records, a provision that also arises frequently in treating patients with HIV/AIDS. Specifically, written and specific consent is required for the release of these records (Brendel and Bryan, 2004). Finally, psychotherapy records may also have added protections that require specific, written consent for their release, but these records must either meet narrowly defined criteria under HIPAA or be protected by state laws that supersede HIPAA regulations (Brendel and Bryan, 2004).

It is critical for physicians to be aware of the relevant law in the jurisdiction(s) in which they practice in order to treat patient information confidentially within the confines of the law.

AUTONOMY

Like confidentiality, autonomy is another fundamental principle of the doctor–patient relationship. Within the doctor–patient relationship, decision-making authority rests with the patient so long as the patient has the mental and physical faculties to make decisions and express them. The physician may not decide on a patient's course of treatment based on what the physician believes is in the patient's best interest unless it is the will of the patient (Cassem and Brendel, 2004; Reddick et al., 2004).

But, what happens when a patient can no longer make autonomous decisions? In that case, ethical care requires that a substitute decision maker be found to make decisions according to what the patient would have wanted. Advance directives are legal instruments that either describe a patient's wishes or appoint a substitute decision maker for the future if the patient should become incapacitated. There are several different types of advance directives, which are introduced below. In addition, the final part of this section will describe ethical and legal considerations in cases where no advance directive exists and a patient becomes unable to make autonomous decisions.

Advance Directives

The Patient Self-Determination Act of 1990 is a federal law that requires hospitals, nursing facilities, and other agencies that provide health care to provide written information about patient autonomy and the right to have an advance directive, to document if a patient has an advance directive, and to provide education for staff and the community about advance directives (Patient Self-Determination Act, 42 U.S.C. 1395 cc(a) (1990); 60 C.F.R. 123 at 33294 (1995)). Notwithstanding the efforts to promote the use of advance directives in the interest of patient autonomy, many individuals, especially young people, still do not fashion advance directives.

It is important to note that the most common types of advance directives, including health care proxies and durable power of attorney for health care, do not

come into effect unless or until the individual who has executed the document becomes unable to make his or her own decisions. In other words, substitute decision makers appointed under these mechanisms do not become the patient's substitute decision maker until such time, if it should occur, that the patient him- or herself becomes unable to make his or her own decisions, i.e., becomes incapacitated. This feature of an advance directive may be misinterpreted by health care providers. For example, at times, when an individual provides his or her treating physicians with a health care proxy upon arrival at a hospital, some physicians may assume that a surrogate decision maker must be involved. Alternatively, a potential surrogate decision maker under a health care proxy may demand access to a patient's health information or to be involved in a patient's care. The critical feature of health care proxies and durable power of attorneys for health care is that they do not take effect until the patient him- or herself becomes incapacitated, if ever. As such, so long as the patient is competent, physicians should not automatically include those listed on documents as potential surrogate decision makers in discussions of care without the patient's express permission. In addition, so long as the patient is able to make his or her own decisions, potential surrogate decision makers have no right to information or to make decisions for that patient.

Advance directives may take two general forms. Instructional advance directives give information about a patient's wishes in the event of incapacity. An example of an instructional advance directive is a living will, a document that is often used to express a patient's wishes to limit potential treatments should he or she become incapacitated. Examples of living wills include directions to avoid "extraordinary measures," prolonged intubation or artificial nutrition and hydration, and resuscitation when there is little or no expectation of "meaningful recovery." While living wills and instructional advance directives were an early measure aimed at promoting patients' wishes, these instruments are limited because they require interpretation and can never practically be fashioned for every level of disability or every possible medical situation. For example, how are "extraordinary measures" to be interpreted? What is "meaningful recovery" in a patient who has experienced progressive HIV-associated dementia? And what if the HIV-associated dementia reverses with potent antiretroviral therapy?

That being said, instructional advance directives may be an especially valuable tool for persons with

AIDS who have no family, friends, or significant others that they trust. For example, homeless intravenous drug users with severe mental illness may be alienated from family and friends and may also feel that they cannot trust anyone to make such decisions. At times this isolation may change with psychiatric treatment and efforts at networking but this may not always work. Therefore, the instructional advance directives allow the individual's wishes to be made clearer, even in the absence of an available surrogate decision maker.

The second broad type of advance directives is used to appoint a substitute decision maker. These advance directives are characterized by a springing clause—that is, they are crafted in advance to take effect in the event of an individual's incapacity. These advance directives generally take the form of a durable power of attorney for health care, or a health care proxy. These forms of advance directives appoint an individual and/or substitute individuals to make health care decisions for a patient should the patient become incapacitated in the future. They grant no authority to make decisions for the patient until such a time, if ever, that the individual becomes unable to make his or her own decisions.

This feature of advanced directives is especially important for persons with AIDS who may not have disclosed information about their HIV status to potential surrogate decision makers or to other loved ones. Although this level of concern about disclosure is not common, it does occur and must be honored. While most patients do disclose their HIV status to their surrogate decision-makers, the possibility that they have not suggests that physicians need to ask about this. It is also important to ensure that the surrogate decision-maker is aware that he or she has been appointed and to encourage the patient to discuss advance directives with the surrogate.

The specific requirements for executing these documents vary from state to state. Though a witness or witnesses or notarization may be required, these advance directives do not require judicial action. Physicians should be aware of the requirements in each state in order to provide information and support to patients on executing a legally binding advance directive. If a patient executes one of these types of advance directives in one state and travels to another, the document should be honored by the state to which the patient has traveled.

Some states also allow for a directional component in the health care proxy that specifies broad principles guiding the designated decision-maker. For example, the directional component may give decision-making authority to an individual but bar that individual from authorizing intubation or artificial nutrition and hydration. Even if the state does not permit a directional component, other tools are available to accompany the proxy or power of attorney document to help the future substitute decision-maker faithfully execute the standard of making the decision that the patient would have made, if he or she were able or, in other words, had capacity to do so. In situations where a patient has an advanced directive, the clinical determination of a patient's ability to make decisions is generally made by the patient's treating physicians. This type of clinical determination is referred to as a capacity determination. On the other hand, if formal legal proceedings for guardianship or other purposes are required, a judge would make a formal determination of an individual's ability to make decisions. A formal, or judicial, determination of decision-making ability is referred to as competency. Psychiatrists may be asked to assess an individual's decision-making ability or capacity when the primary physicians treating the patient are uncertain and need assistance in making the determination. They may also be involved in working with a patient who is becoming progressively ill and must face the inevitable possibility that he or she may not be able to make autonomous decisions for much longer. The role of psychiatrists as persons with HIV and AIDS approach the end of life is further discussed in Chapter 39, on end-of-life issues. One issue that may be forgotten is ascertaining that the person who is designated by the health care proxy as the substitute decision-maker actually is aware of his or her role as health care agent. Furthermore, it is very important to ensure that the health care agent has participated or is participating in a dialogue with the individual (or principal) in order to really understand what his or her wishes are.

Other Mechanisms

What happens when a patient becomes incapacitated and there is no advance directive? From a clinical and ethical standpoint, this is the worst-case scenario because it often requires guesswork as to who is in the best position to make decisions for the patient and exercise the patient's autonomy. Some states, such as Illinois, have statutory law about determining substitute decision makers (755 ILL. COMP. STAT. 40 (2005)).

In the situation where there is no advance directive, these laws allow for the determination of a substitute decision maker without court involvement according to a hierarchy of relationships.

In Illinois, this statutory hierarchy gives the highest priority to the patient's guardian, followed by spouse, adult child, and then parent. It continues along other progressively lesser blood relations to the lowest two priorities of a close friend and finally the guardian of the estate. These types of laws may be particularly problematic in the setting of HIV/AIDS where even long-time same-sex partners may only have the legal status of a "close friend," leaving them out of the decision-making should other family members be able and willing to act on behalf of the patient.

In states that do not have substitute decision-maker statutes, the decision about who acts on behalf of the patient may be ad hoc. If family is at the bedside and agreeable, the process of finding a substitute decision maker is often informal. If there is family dissention, however, a formal process of guardianship that requires a judicial hearing may be necessary. In addition, in situations where family or other suitable individuals cannot be located to act on behalf of the patient, formal guardianship proceedings are required.

While the legal requirements governing advance directives vary from jurisdiction to jurisdiction, the core ethical principle governing determination of the substitute decision maker remains that of autonomy. Even when the patient is no longer able to make and/ or express his or her preferences, it is critical that his or her humanity and dignity are respected by finding the best possible individual to act on his or her behalf.

OTHER CONSIDERATIONS

While issues of autonomy and confidentiality have tended to be most prominent in the context of HIV/ AIDS, additional ethical challenges frequently arise from other principles and clinical situations. Ethical concerns have emerged over a new method of home rapid HIV-testing, routine HIV-testing, possible workplace exposures to HIV/AIDS, and physician obligations to treat HIV patients. These issues are explored briefly below. Further details about routine testing and occupational exposures are found in Chapters 41 and 38 of this text.

Home Testing

As seen above, ethical issues often arise in the course of treating patients with HIV/AIDS when a balancing of individual and societal considerations occurs. Another topic that has raised ongoing ethical concerns is the issue of home HIV testing kits (Wright and Katz, 2006). Before home blood collection kits that allowed samples to be sent to labs for anonymous testing were first approved by the U.S. Food and Drug Administration (FDA) in 1996, there was significant debate about the pros and cons of making home tests available over the counter, with a significant amount of concern focused on the impact of inaccurate results and the potential for an increase in the risk of suicide of HIV-positive individuals (Wright and Katz, 2006). These concerns ultimately paled in comparison to the effect that the anonymous home collection system had on the rate of HIV testing; during the first year of availability nearly 175,000 tests were submitted to the manufacturers for testing, with a 97% rate of calling for results (Branson, 1998). Nearly half of those who tested positive for HIV had not been previously tested (Branson, 1998).

Now, in the setting of the release of a rapid home test using oral fluid to test for HIV, the debate over risks and benefits of home HIV testing modalities has resurfaced. An important consideration in bringing the test to the over-the-counter market is that it would improve access to anonymous HIV testing in the United States, where it is estimated that 250,000 HIV-positive people are unaware of their HIV status (Marks et al., 2005; Wright and Katz, 2006). In addition, a recent meta-analysis of self-report concluded that the prevalence of unprotected anal and vaginal intercourse is substantially reduced after people become aware they are HIV positive (Marks et al., 2005). On the other hand, unlike the collection kits, which required users to call for results and to interact with counselors when receiving the results, this proposed oral fluid test would eliminate that step. The absence of any contact to discuss the test results again raises concerns about the psychological effects of a positive result. Data to support or refute this concern are limited, although there is clear evidence that the rate of suicide among HIV-seropositive individuals and individuals with AIDS is higher than the base rate of suicide in the general population (Starace and Sherr, 1998). Finally, bypassing post-test counseling might lead to an important opportunity for risk reduction being missed;

specifically, a 2004 study showed that brief counseling emphasizing the negative consequences of unprotected sex can reduce risk behaviors in sexually active HIV-positive patients (Richardson et al., 2004).

Routine Testing

Routine HIV-testing would enable more persons who do not know that they are HIV-positive to gain access to medical care and awareness of their status. Similar to concerns raised by home HIV-testing, the need for pre- and post-test counseling cannot be forgotten and may overtax the health care system leading to less counseling availability. Furthermore, concerns arise over eventual changes in policy and elimination of specific written informed HIV consent requirements. Once again, ethical issues arise about exceptionalism and balancing individual and societal concerns.

Workplace Exposures

Although informed consent is generally required for HIV testing by law, and although informed consent is an important ethical foundation of the doctor–patient relationship, what happens when a physician or other health care worker has a high-risk exposure to blood, such as a needle stick? Do ethical principles allow or even require that the source individual of the blood be tested for HIV, even if the source does not consent? Availability of prophylaxis may make this a less critical question than it was 10 years ago, given the high efficacy of HIV prophylaxis after a needle stick. However, it is still important for physicians to be aware of the laws in the jurisdictions in which they practice regarding testing of the source after an exposure and to know whom to contact for support and assistance. Courts have upheld laws about involuntary testing of sources in other situations. For example, a California law provides for involuntary AIDS testing of a person who assaults a peace officer (*Johnetta v. Municipal Court* [Cal. App. 1990]) The California Court of Appeals more recently interpreted this law to allow for mandatory HIV testing of an individual whose sweat made contact with an officer during an assault (*People v. Hall* [Cal. App. 2002]).

Physician Obligations

From a legal standpoint, the doctor–patient relationship is a contract, and either party can decide to enter into a doctor–patient relationship and/or to end it at any time, so long as certain safeguard criteria such as a referral are met if the physician terminates the relationship. Exceptions to this general rule exist, for example, in the case of an emergency, where failure to accept a patient could be deadly. The American Medical Association's Principles of Medical Ethics echo this standard (AMA, 2001). In addition, with largely the same emergency exceptions, ethical principles also posit that physicians may determine that they will not perform certain services for personal, religious, or other reasons. One example is abortion.

But what happens when a physician refuses to treat all patients with a particular infectious illness, such as HIV? Such a practice would result in discrimination at the individual provider level, but could also lead to problems of access if it occurs on a broader scale. According to the American Medical Association, refusal to treat a patient "based solely on his or her seropositivity" is impermissible and unethical. In addition, since 1847, the American Medical Association has maintained that "when an epidemic prevails, a physician must continue his labors without regard to the risk to his own health" (AMA 1987, 1998).

On the other hand, what happens when a physician is HIV positive? What is the physician's obligation to his or her patients? For the past nearly 20 years, the AMA Council on Ethical and Judicial Affairs (CEJA) has maintained that "patients are entitled to expect that their physicians will not increase their exposure to the risk of contracting an infectious disease, even minimally" (AMA, 1987). As such, disclosure of HIV/AIDS status is not considered a remedy. Specifically, if there is no risk of transmission, disclosure of HIV status to patients "will serve no rational purpose" and if there is a risk of transmission, "the physician should not engage in the activity" (AMA, 1987). Finally, while the 1987 CEJA report recommended that seropositive physicians consult colleagues to determine if a proposed activity poses any risk to patients, the American Medical Association has more recently recommended local review committees to address the question of risk to potential patients treated by a seropositive physician (AMA, 1987, 2003a).

CONCLUSION

Treating patients with HIV/AIDS raises many issues in which the traditional tenets of the doctor–patient relationship may come into conflict with other societal concerns or with particularities of a specific treatment relationship. It is important for physicians to be aware of the basic ethical and legal principles surrounding practice in their own jurisdiction, and even more critical that practitioners are aware of resources to assist them in managing the care of complex patients.

References

[AMA] American Medical Association Council on Ethical and Judicial Affairs (1987). Ethical issues involved in the growing AIDS crisis, Report A–I-87, American Medical Association 1987–1988. Retrieved April 9, 2006, from www.ama-assn.org.

[AMA] American Medical Association (1998). Policy E-9.131: HIV-Infected Patients and Physicians, American Medical Association 1998. Retrieved May 8, 2006, from www.ama-assn.org.

[AMA] American Medical Association (2001). Principles of Medical Ethics, American Medical Association 2001. Retrieved May 6, 2006, from www.ama-assn.org.

[AMA] American Medical Association (2003a). Policy H-20-912: Guidance for HIV-Infected Physicians and other Health Care Workers, American Medical Association 2003. Retrieved May 8, 2006, from www.ama-assn.org.

[AMA] American Medical Association (2003b). Policy H-20-915: HIV/AIDS Reporting, Confidentiality, and Notification, American Medical Association 2003. Retrieved April 9, 2006, from www.ama-assn.org.

Branson BM (1998). Home sample collection tests for HIV infection. JAMA 280(19):1699–1701.

Brendel RW (2005). An approach to forensic issues. In TA Stern (ed.), The Ten-Minute Guide to Psychiatric Diagnosis and Treatment (pp. 399–412). New York: Professional Publishing Group.

Brendel RW, and Brendel DH (2005). Professionalism and the doctor–patient relationship in psychiatry. In TA Stern TA (ed.), The Ten-Minute Guide to Psychiatric Diagnosis and Treatment (pp. 1–7). New York: Professional Publishing Group.

Brendel RW, and Bryan E (2004). HIPAA for psychiatrists. Harv Rev Psychiatry 12(3):177–183.

Cassem NH, and Brendel RW (2004). End of life issues: principles of care and ethics. In TA Stern, GL Fricchione, NH Cassem, MS Jellinek, and JF Rosenbaum (eds.), Massachusetts General Hospital Handbook of General Hospital Psychiatry, fifth edition (pp. 365–387). Philadelphia: Mosby.

CONN. GEN. STAT. § 19a-582 (2006). Retrieved April 16, 2006, from www.cga.ct.gov.

Gostin LO, and Hodge JG (1998). Piercing the veil of secrecy in HIV/AIDS and other sexually transmitted diseases: theories of privacy and disclosure in partner notification. Duke J Gender Law Policy 5(9): 9–88.

Hippocrates (1983). The Oath. Translated by J Chadwick and WN Mann. In GER Lloyd (ed.), Hippocratic Writings (p. 67). London: Penguin Books.

755 ILL. COMP. STAT. 40 (2005).

Johnetta v. The Municipal Court for the San Francisco Judicial District of the City and County of San Francisco and San Francisco Sheriff's Department, 218 Cal. App. 3d 1255 (1990).

Marks G, Crepaz N, Senterfitt JW, and Janssen RS (2005). Meta-analysis of high-risk sexual behavior in persons aware and unaware they are infected with HIV in the United States: implications for HIV prevention programs. J Acquir Immune Defic Syndr 39(4):446–453.

MASS. GEN. LAWS Ch. 111 § 70F (2005). Retrieved March 26, 2006, from www.mass.gov/legis/laws/mgl.

MASS. GEN. LAWS Ch. 123 § 1 (2005). Retrieved March 26, 2006, from www.mass.gov/legis/laws/mgl.

MASS. GEN. LAWS Ch. 123 § 36B (2005). Retrieved March 26, 2006, from www.mass.gov/legis/laws/mgl.

New York State Department of Health AIDS Institute (2003). Identification and ambulatory care of HIV-exposed and -infected adolescents, Appendix B–summary, HIV reporting and partner notification. Retrieved April 16, 2006, from www.hivguidelines .org.

New York State Department of Health (2000). HIV reporting and partner notification questions and answers, NYSDOH 2000. Retireved March 26, 2006, from www.health.state.ny.us.

GA. CODE ANN. ch. 24-9 §47 (2005). Retrieved April 16, 2006, from www.legis.state.ga.us.

GA. CODE ANN. ch. 31-22 § 9.1 (2005). Retrieved April 16, 2006, from www.legis.state.ga.us.

Patient Self Determination Act, 42 U.S.C. 1395 cc(a) (1990).

Patient Self Determination Act, Final Regulations, 60 C.F.R. 123 at 33294 (1995).

People v. Hall, 101 Cal. App. 4th 1009 (2002).

Reddick B, Brendel RW, and Cassem NH (2004). Treatment decisions at the end of life. In TA Stern and JB Herman (eds.), Massachusetts General Hospital Psychiatry Update and Board Preparation, second edition (pp. 517–521). New York: McGraw Hill.

Richardson JL, Milam J, McCutchan A, Stoyanoff S, Bolan R, Weiss J, Kemper C, Larsen RA, Hollander H, Weismuller P, Chou C, and Marks G (2004). Effect of brief safer-sex counseling by medical providers to HIV-1 seropositive patients: a multi-clinic assessment. AIDS 18(8):1179–1186.

Schouten R, and Brendel RW (2004). Legal aspects of consultation. In TA Stern, GL Fricchione, NH Cassem, MS Jellinek, and JF Rosenbaum (eds.), Massachusetts General Hospital Handbook of General Hospital Psychiatry, fifth edition (pp. 349–364). Philadelphia: Mosby.

Starace F, and Sherr L (1998). Suicidal behaviours, euthanasia and AIDS. AIDS 12(4):339–347.

Wright AA, and Katz IT (2006). Home testing for HIV. N Engl J Med 354(5):437–440.

Chapter 41

Health Services and Policy Issues in AIDS Psychiatry

James T. Walkup and Stephen Crystal

Two salient developments of the past 25 years have been the advent of the HIV/AIDS epidemic and the growth of health services research (HSR) from modest roots to a substantial enterprise. The developments have co-evolved, since today's HSR grew out of efforts to grapple with issues of cost, equity, and the organization of care that have also been challenged in new ways by the HIV/AIDS epidemic. Many health services researchers have been drawn to the study of HIV/AIDS care, which has presented in new and concentrated forms a range of systemic issues for the health care system, including racial and ethnic disparities in health care and the impact of stigma; the complexities of caring for patients with co-occurring medical, substance abuse, and psychiatric conditions; the factors influencing adherence to demanding medical regimens; and numerous others.

Health services research draws on sociology and economics, but is defined as much by a set of concerns as by a disciplinary perspective. The most prominent single model is the behavioral model (e.g., Andersen et al., 2000). Multiple versions exist, but the basic components specify that utilization is influenced by predisposing factors, such as sociodemographic characteristics; enabling factors, such as a person's ability to pay, or a community's store of accessible services; and need factors. For example, studies of receipt of highly active antiretroviral therapy (HAART) have examined the influence of predisposing factors, such as race (Palacio et al., 2002), gender (Giordano et al., 2003) or injection drug use (IDU) status (Gebo et al., 2005); enabling factors such as insurance status (Bhattacharya et al., 2003); and measures of need including clinical indicators like disease stage, CD4 counts, and viral load (Gebo et al., 2005), as well as patient self-report measures. Some versions of the model also add context variables, such as provider or organizational characteristics. For example, just after HAART was introduced, research found that patients were more likely to receive potent antiretrovirals if they were cared for by physicians who were more experienced in HIV care (Kitahata et al., 2000).

The Andersen model helps a policy maker examine claims that a group is "underserved," or is "high utilizing," and operationalize the implied "compared to what?" question. Implicit in the model is the value-based assumption that health care ought typically to correspond to need rather than other characteristics of patients. HSR concerned with cost tends to look for subgroups with unusually high utilization, examining whether costly services being used are unneeded, or if the need could have been prevented. HSR concerned about equity tends to look for evidence that use of appropriate services varies in relation to predisposing or enabling factors, rather than need, when these classes of factors are considered concurrently. (Such departures from need-based care can be considered an operational definition of "inequitable access.") In such analyses, definitions of need are particularly important. Results may vary, for example, under alternative measures of need based on the view of the patient, of clinicians, or of evidence-based guidelines.

The challenges of HIV have highlighted problems in the U.S. health care delivery system that have long occupied health service researchers. In this chapter, we focus primarily on research in the United States as we review recent work on financing, service fragmentation, and difficulties integrating different sectors of care, as well as problems related to the functioning of medicine in a complex, stratified society. The one significant exception is our attention to research on syringe exchange programs in Canada.

FINANCING

The HIV Cost and Services Utilization Study (HCSUS) found that in the mid- to late 1990s, most people living with HIV or AIDS (PLWHA) were uninsured (20%) or covered by a public insurance program, such as Medicaid (44%) or Medicare (6%); a similar payment distribution probably holds today. The proportion with private insurance is estimated to be less than half that found in the general population (31% vs. 73%) (Kaiser Family Foundation, 2004). Some care is also available through various safety net programs, such as free clinics, state psychiatric hospitals, or services paid for through the Ryan White Comprehensive AIDS Resources Emergency (CARE) Act. The burden of public payers has been impacted by illness-related work disability, which can deprive

patients of employment-based coverage; the increasing concentration of HIV in poor communities; and the high cost of care, particularly pharmaceuticals.

A recurrent issue has been the impact of insurance status on receipt of appropriate HIV care. Several studies suggest that the most significant gaps are between the uninsured and the insured, not between those with coverage from private versus public insurance (Shapiro et al., 1999; Cunningham et al., 2000; Smith and Kirking, 2001; Keruly et al., 2002; Knowlton et al., 2001; Goldstein et al., 2005). This rough equivalence between private and public insurance has been challenged, however. Criticizing prior work for not adjusting for possible unobserved associations between health status and coverage, Bhattacharya and others (2003) concluded that private (versus public) insurance was associated with lower mortality, partly attributable to better access to HAART. Private insurance has also been associated with lower rates of unmet need for care for some specific symptoms (Kilbourne et al., 2002).

FRAGMENTATION OF CARE

The epidemiology of HIV has highlighted fragmentation in the delivery system. Extensive comorbidity is found with two conditions that have historically been served by different delivery systems that are not well integrated with general medicine, substance abuse and psychiatric illness (Bing et al., 2001). HCSUS data indicate more than three of five adults under care for HIV have used mental health or substance abuse services in the prior 6 months (Burnam et al., 2001). HIV rates are elevated among psychiatric patients in various settings, sometimes dramatically (Cournos and McKinnon, 1997) and, among those with HIV, patients with severe mental illness (SMI) are overrepresented in relation to population prevalence (Walkup et al., 1999; Blank et al., 2002).

Case management, integration of services across sectors, and the creation of specialty services are all strategies to counter fragmentation. Randomized trials indicate that strong integration strategies, such as on-site medical care for methadone patients, are significantly more likely to ensure receipt of care (92%) than referral contracting (35%) (Umbricht-Schneiter et al., 1994), and integration of methadone maintenance with primary care and case management decreases progression to AIDS (Webber et al., 1998). Yet extensive integration can be costly and may require sacrifice of some agency autonomy.

Problems have sometimes been encountered when top-down efforts to develop innovative specialty services are diverted from their original intent by unanticipated clinical needs. For example, specialty sites intended to serve seriously ill psychiatric patients with HIV have filled with difficult-to-treat PLWHA with anxiety or depression, rather than those with more severe mental illness (Sullivan et al., 1999). Similarly, a long-term care facility for people with AIDS in New York City found that residents with a lifetime history of severe psychiatric illness were less likely to die or be discharged, which means that, over time, they occupy an ever-growing proportion of total beds (Goulet et al., 2000).

DISPARITIES IN HIV CARE

Evidence regarding antiretroviral care and race presents a mixed picture, both in the pre-HAART era and, more recently, in access to HAART. Palacio et al. (2002) reviewed 26 studies published on race and antiretroviral use and concluded that the weight of the evidence suggests some non-white disadvantage. Two studies using HCSUS data found disadvantage for African Americans in receipt of protease inhibitor and nonnucleoside reverse transcriptase inhibitor (NNRTI) therapies by December 1996 (Shapiro et al., 1999; Andersen et al., 2000). A third study, covering 1996–1998, found this disadvantage in some models, but not others (Cunningham et al., 2000).

Differential access to financial coverage for health care contributes to disparities, but disparities also exist when this factor is controlled for (e.g., among those with a single payer source such as Medicaid) (Crystal et al., in press). Using Medicaid claims files, our group found evidence for race differences in the pre-HAART period (Crystal et al., 1995). Some disparities were also identified in the HAART era (Sambamoorthi et al., 2001), but these appear to have narrowed over time. Cunningham and colleagues (2005) did not find race disparities in mortality in adjusted models, but did find that socioeconomic characteristics such as wealth, education, and employment substantially impact mortality risk. End-of life care may differ by race. Using 1991–1998 Medicaid claims, our group found

that African Americans were more likely to die in the hospital rather than at home, and were less likely to receive pain medication (Sambamoorthi et al., 2000).

Whether race differences in care reflect differences in system access can be further evaluated with research on veterans or military personnel, where few or no differences in coverage exist. McGinnis and colleagues (2003) found no race differences in clinical management or adherence. White veterans with HIV had lower mortality, perhaps due to differences in illness severity and comorbidities. In the HAART era, Silverberg and colleagues (2006) found no race differences among military seroconverters in relative hazards of AIDS and death. Giordano and colleagues (2006) found no race-related effects on mortality in a group of veterans with HIV, either in the 30 days after initial hospitalization or in subsequent survival (during the 4-year study window).

MULTI-NEED PSYCHIATRIC PATIENTS AND CARE DELIVERY

In predicting the impact of psychiatric comorbidity on HIV care, two alternative scenarios have been suggested. Poorer and less consistent HIV treatment might occur, either because psychiatric symptoms interfere or because the provider's need to attend to some conditions leaves others neglected, a kind of "clinical crowd-out" effect (Redlemeier et al., 1998). Conversely, patients with chronic mental health conditions might receive more consistent HIV care if they are more connected than others to the health care system and better socialized into patient roles (cf. Walkup et al., 2001). Each scenario is clinically plausible, and psychiatric conditions probably exert multiple different effects on HIV care, some diagnosis specific; the balance of effects is an empirical question. The first scenario may strike some clinicians as more intuitive. However, it has not always been supported empirically. Despite shortcomings, HIV care patterns among the dually or multiply diagnosed are better than might be expected, given that people with a SMI are highly stigmatized (Phelan et al., 2000) and often receive substandard medical care (Druss et al., 2002).

Evidence from surveys (Bogart et al., 2000) and chart review studies (Fairfield et al., 1999) suggested that physicians might be reluctant to initiate antiretroviral care for such patients. However, in several

studies of antiretroviral use among Medicaid beneficiaries, in both the pre-HAART and HAART eras,
we did not find patients with SMI were less likely
to receive antiretrovirals. These studies used a data-
set created by a de-identified linking of the New
Jersey HIV/AIDS Registry with Medicaid claims. We
also found that, in the pre-HAART era, patients with
schizophrenia maintained higher levels of persistent
use of antiretrovirals than other patients (Walkup
et al., 2001), and in the HAART era, their persistence
was not significantly less than those without a serious
mental illness (Walkup et al., 2004). (Major mood
disorders did not hamper access to HAART, but did
affect adherence.)

Electronic monitoring of adherence with a small
group of patients with schizophrenia (n = 47) added
further evidence regarding adherence, which was
found to correlate with recent mental health appointments (Wagner et al., 2003). Retrospective data on a
group of patients treated in urban clinic with integrated psychiatric care between 1996 and 2002 found
that HAART-naïve psychiatric patients in treatment
were more likely to commence it to stay on it for 6
months or more, and to survive than were their counterparts without a psychiatric diagnosis (Himelhoch
et al., 2004). Bogart and colleagues (2006) found that
a majority of SMI patients with HIV recruited from
Los Angeles mental health clinics were on HAART
and were receiving close monitoring of CD4 counts
and viral load.

This tendency of treatments to cluster, and to be
associated with positive outcomes, may reflect various influences, including both selection effects and
direct effects of one or another element of treatment
(e.g., impact of antidepressants on cognition or energy
level). Several studies have found that, although mood
disorders are associated with compromised antiretroviral adherence (Walkup et al., 2004), depression
treatment has been associated with a higher probability of antiretroviral treatment among patients with
depression (Sambamoorthi et al., 2000; Tegger et al.,
2007) and with adherence to antiretrovirals (Turner
et al., 2003) and HAART (Yun et al., 2005), although
evidence for this last association has been criticized
(Wilson and Jacobson, 2006). More research is needed on the impact of different forms of psychiatric
comorbidity on HIV care, including the various roles
of intervening factors such as patients' adherence,
patient socialization, increased provider surveillance,
and stigma.

DIRECT OBSERVED THERAPY

Some subgroups of patients with HIV and comorbid
mental health and substance abuse problems are
likely to be perceived as particularly poor risks for
HAART therapy. In such instances, as with individuals expected to be nonadherent to treatments for tuberculosis, direct observed therapy (DOT) is potentially a conceptually appealing alternative, though
challenging to operationalize. The trend toward simpler HAART regimens, including those with once-
daily dosing, may increase interest in this alternative.
Indeed, interest in DOT has recently increased, and a
2004 supplement to *Clinical Infectious Diseases* was
devoted to it (Mitty and Flanigan, 2004).

However, research on multiply diagnosed individuals suggests several reasons for caution in this
regard. First, as noted, even severe mental illness is
not necessarily associated with poorer adherence to
HAART regimens. Thus, it is not obvious which patients are in fact at greater risk of nonadherence.
Second, in contrast to time-limited situations such
as tuberculosis treatment, HAART treatment is a
lifetime undertaking. DOT strategies are no "magic
bullet" for the adherence challenges for such situations, and it remains necessary to develop a therapeutic partnership with multiply diagnosed patients
and provide support and reinforcement for their own
self-management capabilities. Indeed, today's advocates are at pains to deemphasize social control implications of DOT, stressing the need to modify and
tailor it to reflect both patient needs and, to the extent
possible, preferences. Articles are now more apt to refer to modified DOT, abbreviated as MDOT, or to directly administered antiretroviral therapy, or DAART.

Finally, careful monitoring of such programs is
needed. It is often not possible to observe every antiviral dose. However, given the demanding nature of
HIV therapy, half-measures could be worse than none
from the perspective of causing development of resistant HIV virus (Kagay et al., 2004). Partial improvements in adherence could potentially move patients
from a low level of adherence unlikely either to provide
viral suppression or to create the highest level of risk of
viral resistance, to a higher (but still inadequate) level
with higher risk of viral resistance. Altice and colleagues (2004) report on the results of a DAART intervention, concluding that DAART programs should
ideally provide daily monitoring of once-daily dosing, and that DAART should incorporate enhanced

elements such as convenience, flexibility, confidentiality, cues and reminders, responsive pharmacy and medical services, and specialized training for staff.

ADDICTION SERVICES, SYRINGE EXCHANGE, AND PUBLIC POLICY

In the abstract, the accumulation of evidence supporting syringe exchange programs (SEPs) ought to have provided a textbook illustration of the value for policy making of research in addiction medicine and health services. For a decade and a half, one or another official panel or commission reviewed the evidence and issued reports, each finding significant evidence of benefit. Experts now credit SEPs with a major role in stemming, then reversing, the HIV epidemic among injection drug users in New York City. Survey-based national estimates indicate that in 2002 U.S. SEPs distributed almost 25 million syringes (CDC, 2005). Yet the SEP story has been anything but a textbook technology transfer from researchers to providers.

Commentaries, including reflections by key participants, describe how efforts to promote SEP quickly became entangled with conflicts associated with the war on drugs (Des Jarlais and Friedman, 1998; Vlahov et al., 2001). In 1998, when research was sufficient to convince Department of Health and Human Services Secretary Donna Shalala to take official notice, a last-minute effort by the Director of the Office of National Drug Control Policy, "drug czar" Barry McCaffrey was able to convince President Clinton not to allow federal funding of SEPs, according to the *Washington Post* (Harris and Goldstein, 1998, cited in Vlahov et al., 2001).

Political controversy over SEP has been abetted by disputes about research findings themselves (e.g., Des Jarlais, 2000; Moss 2000a, 2000b). SEP users in Vancouver (Strathdee et al., 1997) were found more likely, not less likely, to have HIV, and, in Montreal, to seroconvert (Burneau et al., 1997). These results figured prominently in a 2004 letter criticizing SEPs sent to NIH director Zerhouni from Congressman Mark Souder (Harm Reduction Coalition, 2004).

Questions posed by the Vancouver and Montreal results have been given serious attention by researchers (Bastos and Strathdee, 2000; Gibson et al., 2001). The possibility has been acknowledged that SEPs, like any intervention, could produce unintended negative consequences. For example, it is conceivable that SEPs might facilitate new needle sharing networks, for

example, but the evidence indicates that this does not appear to be the case (Schechter et al., 1999; Junge et al., 2000). Instead, selection bias has been credited with influencing the lack of beneficial effect of the Vancouver and Montreal programs, since more high-risk intravenous drug users may gravitate to SEPs. Hahn et al. (1997) and Schoenbaum et al. (1996) reported on data collection begun prior to SEP introduction and each found evidence that intravenous drug users with high risks were attracted to SEP use.

A recent review identified 45 studies between 1989 and 2002 with SEP as an intervention and outcome variables of IDU risk behavior, HIV seroconversion, or HIV seroprevalence (Wodak and Cooney, 2006). Of the 10 studies looking at either of these latter two outcomes, six found SEP protective, two found no effect, and two found negative associations with SEP use. Reviews have also noted the possibility of a "dilution" effect (Gibson et al., 2001). That is, if SEP research is conducted in a community where syringes are legally available elsewhere, the SEP effect is likely to be weaker than it would be in a place without alternatives. When studies conducted in sites with legal access are removed from the group of studies using risk behavior or seroconversion as outcomes, the remaining studies all show a positive association. Des Jarlais's measured judgment in 2000 still holds today, that "as part of a larger HIV prevention program, needle exchange usually, but not always, leads to low rates of HIV transmission among injection drug users" (p. 1393).

SEP delivery systems make a difference. SEPs differ in how they interpret "exchange," for example. Some use a strict one-for-one approach; some are willing to add a few extra syringes; and a third group does not limit syringes based on the number exchanged. In a study of 23 SEPs in California, clients in this last (i.e., no-limit) group had lower odds of reusing syringes (Kral et al., 2004), but did not differ in needle sharing. Similar findings emerged in a three-city study (Bluthenthal et al., 2004); however, once SEPs are up and running, simply increasing the cap on number of syringes—as happened twice in Connecticut—seems to have had only limited impact on syringe-related risks (Heimer et al., 2002).

HIV TESTING CONTROVERSIES

Knowledge that one is HIV positive is a necessary condition for other HIV-related services, and increasing the proportion of PLWHA who know their serostatus is a major Centers for Disease Control and Prevention (CDC) objective. Levels of CDC prevention funding appear to impact odds of testing (Linas et al., 2006), and aggressive outreach has produced impressive results in some high-risk groups, such as men who have sex with men (MSM), more than 90% of whom reported lifetime testing in a recent study (CDC, 2006a).

Concerns about poor identification of HIV among patients with severe mental illness led some policymakers in the 1990s to consider mandatory inpatient testing (Walkup et al., 2002), but rates of voluntary testing seem generally comparable to those of other groups across a range of settings (Blumberg et al., 2003; Goldberg et al., 2005; Meade and Sikkema, 2005). Even in inpatient settings, where reports indicate the greatest need for improvements (Walkup et al., 2000; Pirl et al., 2005), analysts point to the need for research and funding to improve outcomes, rather than legal changes in testing policy (Walkup et al., 2002).

A wealth of research suggests that risk factor testing has failed to reach many of the patients most likely to benefit. In one high-risk community sample, a majority of never-tested heterosexual men and women reported that they had not been offered an HIV test— 81% of men, and 65% of women (Bond et al., 2005). Other studies suggest continuing failure to attain adequate testing rates in high-risk populations (Rust et al., 2003; Liddicoat et al., 2004). Studies have found that testing may often occur late in disease progress (e.g., Bozzette et al., 1998; Samet et al., 1998). In 2002, more than one-third (39%) of those with a positive test received an AIDS diagnosis within a year (CDC, 2002). In a June 2006 editorial appearing in the *American Journal of Public Health*, critics of risk-focused approaches called for "less targeting, more testing" (Koo et al., 2006, p. 962).

The CDC has developed guidelines that emphasize routine testing in medical settings (CDC, 2006b). Feasibility of new testing services has been investigated (Walensky et al., 2002; Walensky et al., 2005). Using simulation models, Paltiel and colleagues (2005) concluded that adding voluntary testing every 3 to 5 years would be cost effective both in high-risk populations with a 3.0% prevalence and in lower-risk populations with a 1.0% prevalence. Increased testing has implications for prevention as well, since approximately half of new cases of HIV are attributable

to the 25% of people with HIV unaware of their status (Marks et al., 2006).

HIV STIGMA AND DISCRIMINATION IN CARE

In HCSUS data from 1996–1997, 26% of patients reported perceiving at least one type of discrimination (Schuster et al., 2005). Longer life spans produced by treatment changes raise new issues, for example, the re-examination of practices regarding organ transplantation and assisted reproduction. The medical basis of opposition to transplantation, built largely on the patient's poor prognosis, is now questioned, and attention has focused on questions about allocation of a scarce resource to a person with HIV. Sometimes this argument is examined directly; sometimes the more indirect point is made that transplants to PLWHA might undermine public willingness to donate organs (Roland et al., 2003).

Increasingly, as well, with longer survival and more-effective prevention of perinatal transmission, PLWHA now consider planned pregnancy, and may desire both conventional fertility services and special technologies to minimize viral transmission to partner or child. Through interviews conducted in 1998, Chen and colleagues (2001) found that a significant minority of adult PLWHA said they desired children in the future, and a majority of these said they wanted more than one. (Presumably these figures have, if anything, increased.) Yet significant barriers preventing access to such services remain for PLWHA (Stern et al., 2002; Gurmankin et al., 2005; Sauer, 2006).

CONCLUSION

Many structural characteristics important for good HIV care are not well developed in the U.S. health care system—need-focused financing, integration, organizational flexibility, collaboration, and accessibility. Yet despite the many built-in constraints faced by patients, doctors, and advocates, important achievements have been produced by the combination of perseverance with a willingness to rethink directions when necessary.

We have seen that, under the right circumstances, adequate care can be delivered to patients with multiple medical and psychosocial needs, and public health values can exert substantial influence in the face of political opposition. Yet some of the most difficult work lies ahead, as strategies must be developed to improve outreach and ease of access for the many PLWHA who do not know they are ill or are poorly linked to service systems, integrate into multiple settings the prevention services needed to bring down incidence rates, and, in the face of political and fiscal challenges, provide the evidence needed to demonstrate the value of effective service delivery strategies. These challenges will require both focus and flexibility, but the record so far provides grounds for optimism.

ACKNOWLEDGMENTS   Preparation of this chapter was supported with funding from National Institute of Mental Health grant R01 MH058984, and Agency for Health Care Research and Quality grants U18 HS016097 and R24 HS011825.

References

Altice FL, Mezger JA, Hodges J, Bruce RD, Marinovich A, Walton M, Springer SA, and Friedland GH (2004). Developing a directly administered antiretroviral therapy intervention for HIV-infected drug users: implications for program replication. *Clin Infect Dis* 38(Suppl 5):S376–S387.

Andersen R, Bozzette S, Shapiro M, St. Clair, Morton S, Crystal S, Goldman N, Wenger A, Gifford A, Leibowitz A, Asch S, Berry S, Nakazono T, Heslin K, and Cunningham W (2000). Access of vulnerable groups to antiretroviral therapy among persons in care for HIV disease in the United States. *Health Serv Res* 35:389–416.

Bastos FI, and Strathdee SA (2000). Evaluating effectiveness of syringe exchange programmes: current issues and future prospects. *Soc Sci Med* 51:1771–1782.

Bhattacharya J, Goldman D, and Sood N (2003). The link between public and private insurance and HIV-related mortality. *J Health Econ* 22:1105–1122.

Bing EG, Burnam MA, Longshore D, Fleishman JA, Sherbourne CD, London AS, Turner BJ, Eggan F, Beckman R, Vitiello B, Morton SC, Orlando M, Bozzette SA, Ortiz-Barron L, and Shapiro M (2001). Psychiatric disorders and drug use among human immunodeficiency virus–infected adults in the United States. *Arch Gen Psychiatry* 58:721–728.

Blank M, Mandell D, Linda Aiken L, and Hadley T (2002). Co-occurrence of HIV and serious mental illness among Medicaid recipients. *Psychiatr Serv* 53:868–873.

Blumberg SJ, and Dickey WC (2003). Prevalence of HIV risk behaviors, risk perceptions, and testing among US adults with mental disorders. *J Acquir Immune Defic Syndr* 32:77–79.

Bluthenthal RN, Malik MR, Grau LE, Singer M, Marshall P, Heimer R, for the Diffusion of Benefit through Syringe Exchange Study Team (2004). Sterile syringe access conditions and variations in HIV risk among drug injectors in three cities. *Addiction* 99:1136–1146.

Bogart LM, Kelly JA, Catz SL, and Sosman JM (2000). Impact of medical and nonmedical factors on physician decision making for HIV/AIDS antiretroviral treatment. *J Acquir Immune Defic Syndr* 23:396–404.

Bogart LM, Fremont AM, Young AS, Pantoja P, Chinman M, Morton S, Koegel P, Sullivan G, and Kanouse DE (2006). Patterns of HIV care for patient with serious mental illness. *AIDS Patient Care STDS* 20:175–182.

Bond L, Lauby J, and Batson H (2005). HIV testing the role of individual- and structural-level barriers and facilitators. *AIDS Care* 17:125–140.

Bozzette SA, Berry SH, Duan N, Frankel MR, Leibowitz, AA, Lefkowitz D, Emmons CA, Senterfitt JW, Berk ML, Morton SC, and Shapiro MF (1998). The care of HIV-infected adults in the United States. HIV Cost and Services Utilization Study Consortium. *N Engl J Med* 339:1897–1904.

Burnam MA, Bing EG, Morton SC, Sherbourne C, Fleishman JA, London AS, Vitiello B, Stein M, Bozzette SA, and Shapiro MF (2001). Use of mental health and substance abuse treatment services among adults with HIV in the United States. *Arch Gen Psychiatry* 58:729–736.

Burneau J, Lamothe F, Franco E, Lachance N, Desy M, Soto J, and Vincelette J (1997). High rates of HIV infection among injection drug users participating in needle exchange programs in Montreal: results of a cohort study. *Am J Epidemiol* 146:994–1002.

[CDC] Centers for Disease Control and Prevention (2002). *HIV/AIDS Surveillance Report, 2002*, Vol. 14, pp. 1–50. Retrieved August 8, 2006, from http://www.cdc.gov/hiv/topics/surveillance/resources/reports/2002report/pdf/2002SurveillanceReport.pdf.

[CDC] Centers for Disease Control and Prevention (2005). Update: syringe exchange programs—United States, 2002. *MMWR Morb Mortal Wkly Rep* 54: 673–676.

[CDC] Centers for Disease Control and Prevention (2006a). Human immunodeficiency virus (HIV) risk, prevention, and testing behaviors—United States, national HIV behavioral surveillance system: men who have sex with men. *MMWR Morb Mortal Wkly Rep* 55:1–16.

[CDC] Centers for Disease Control and Prevention (2006b). Revised recommendations for HIV testing of adults, adolescents, and pregnant women in health care settings. *MMWR Morb Mortal Wkly Rep* 55:1–17.

Chen JL, Philips KA, Kanouse DE, Collins RL, and Miu A (2001). Fertility desires and intentions of HIV-positive men and women. *Fam Plann Perspect* 33:144–152, 165.

Cournos F, and McKinnon K (1997). HIV seroprevalence among people with severe mental illness in the United States: a critical review. *Clin Psychol Rev* 17:259–269.

Crystal S, Akincigil A, Bilder S, Walkup J. Studying Prescription Drug Use and Outcomes with Medicaid Claims Data: Strengths, Limitations, and Strategies. In press, *Medical Care*.

Crystal S, Sambamoorthi U, and Merzel C (1995). The diffusion of innovation in AIDS treatment: zidovudine use in two New Jersey cohorts. *Health Serv Res* 30:593–614.

Cunningham WE, Markson LE, Andersen RM, Crystal SH, Fleishman JA, Golin C, Gifford A, Liu HH, Nakazono TT, Morton S, Bozzette SA, Shapiro MF, and Wenger NS (2000). Prevalence and predictors of highly active antiretroviral therapy use in patients with HIV infection in the United States. HCSUS Consortium. HIV Cost and Services Utilization. *J Acquir Immune Defic Syndr* 25:115–123.

Cunningham, WE, Hays, RD, Duan, N, Andersen, R, Nakazono, TT, Bozzette SA, and Shapiro MF (2005). The effect of socioeconomic status on the survival of people receiving care for HIV infection in the United States. *J Health Care Poor Underserved* 16:655–676.

Des Jarlais DC (2000). Research, politics, and needle exchange. *Am J Public Health* 90:1392–1394.

Des Jarlais DC, and Friedman SR (1998). Fifteen years of research on preventing HIV infection among injecting drug users: what we have learned, what we have done, what we have not done. *Public Health Rep* 113(Suppl. 1):182–188.

Druss BG, Rosenheck RA, Desai MM, and Perlin JB (2002). Quality of preventive medical care for patients with mental disorders. *Med Care* 40:129–136.

Fairfield KM, Libman H, Davis RB, and Eisenberg DM (1999). Delays in protease inhibitor use in clinical practice. *J Gen Intern Med* 14:395–401.

Gebo KA, Fleishman JA, Conviser R, Reilly ED, Korthuis PT, Moore RD, Hellinger J, Keiser P, Rubin HR, Crane L, Hellinger FJ, and Mathews WC (2005). Racial and gender disparities in receipt of highly active antiretroviral therapy persist in a multistate sample of HIV patients in 2001. *J Acquir Immune Defic Syndr* 38:96–103.

Gibson DR, Flynn NM, and Perales D (2001). Effectiveness of syringe exchange programs in reducing HIV risk behavior and HIV seroconversion among injecting drug users. *AIDS* 15:1329–1341.

Giordano TP, White AC Jr, Sajja P, Graviss EA, Arduino RC, Adu-Oppong A, Lahart CJ, and Visnegarwala F (2003). Factors associated with the use of highly active antiretroviral therapy in patients newly entering care in an urban clinic. *J Acquir Immune Defic Syndr* 32:399–405.

Giordano TP, Morgan RO, Kramer JR, Suarez-Almazer ME, and El-Serag HB (2006). Is there a race-based disparity in the survival of veterans with HIV? *J Gen Intern Med* 21:613–617.

Goldberg RW, Himelhoch S, Kreyenbuhl J, Dickerson FB, Hackman A, Fang LJ, Brown CH, Wohlheiter KA, and Dixon LB (2005). Predictors of HIV and hepatitis testing and related service utilization among individuals with serous mental illness. *Psychosomatics* 46:573–577.

Goldstein RB, Rotheram-Borus MJ, Johnson MO, Weinhardt LS, Remien RH, Lightfoot M, Catz SL, Gore-Felton C, Kirshenbaum S, and Morin SF (2005). Insurance coverage, usual source of care, receipt of clinically indicated care for comorbid conditions among adults living with human immunodeficiency virus. *Med Care* 43:401–410.

Goulet JL, Molde S, Constantino J, Gaughan D, and Selwyn PA (2000). Psychiatric comorbidity and the long-term care of people with AIDS. *J Urban Health* 77:213–221.

Gurmankin AD, Caplan AL, and Braverman AM (2005). Screening practices and beliefs of assisted reproductive technology programs. *Fertil Steril* 83:61–67.

Hahn JA, Vranizan KM, and Moss AR (1997). Who uses needle exchange? A study of injection drug users in treatment in San Francisco, 1989–1990. *J Acquir Immune Defic Syndr Hum Retrovirol* 15:157–164.

Harm Reduction Coalition (2004). Congressional attack on harm reduction. Retrieved August 8, 2006, from http://hepcproject.typepad.com/hep_c_project/2004/05/congressional_a.html.

Harris JF, and Goldstein A (1998). Puncturing an AIDS initiative; at last minute, White House political fears killed needle funding. *Washing Post* April 23, A1.

Heimer R, Clair S, Teng W, Grau LE, Khoshnood K, and Singer M (2002). Effects of increasing syringe availability on syringe-exchange use and HIV risk: Connecticut, 1990–2001. *J Urban Health* 79:556–570.

Himelhoch S, Moore RD, Treisman G, and Gebo KA (2004). Does the presence of a current psychiatric disorder in AIDS patients affect the initiation of antiretroviral treatment and duration of therapy? *J Acquir Immune Defic Syndr* 37:1457–1463.

Junge B, Valente T, Latkin C, Riley E, and Vlahov D (2000). Syringe exchange not associated with social network formation: results from Baltimore. *AIDS* 14:423–426.

Kagay CR, Porco TC, Liechty CA, Charlebois E, Clark R, Guzman D, Moss AR, and Bangsberg DR (2004). Modeling the impact of modified directly observed antiretroviral therapy on HIV suppression and resistance, disease progression, and death. *Clin Infect Dis* 38(Suppl. 5):S414–S420.

Kaiser Family Foundation (2004). Financing HIV/AIDS care: a quilt with many holes. Retrieved August 8,

2006, from http://www.kff.org/hivaids/loader.cfm?url=/commonspot/security/getfile.cfm&PageID=13374.

Keruly JC, Conviser R, and Moore RD (2002). Association of medical insurance and other factors with receipt of antiretroviral therapy. *Am J Public Health* 92:852–857.

Kilbourne AM, Andersen RM, Asch S, Nakazono T, Crystal S, Stein M, Gifford AL, Bing EG, Bozzette SA, Shapiro MF, and Cunningham WE (2002). Response to symptoms among a US national probability sample of adults infected with human immunodeficiency virus. *Med Care Res Rev* 59: 36–58.

Kitahata MM, Van Rompaey SE, and Shields AW (2000). Physician experience in the care of HIV-infected persons is associated with earlier adoption of new antiretroviral therapy. *J Acquir Immune Defic Syndr* 24:106–114.

Knowlton AR, Hoover DR, Chung SE, Celentano DD, Vlahov D, and Latkin CA (2001). Access to medical care and service utilization among injection drug users with HIV/AIDS. *Drug Alcohol Dep* 64:55–62.

Koo DJ, Begier EM, Henn MH, Sepkowitz KA, and Kellerman SE (2006). HIV counseling and testing: less targeting, more testing. *Am J Public Health* 96:962–964.

Kral AH, Anderson R, Flynn NM, and Bluthenthal RN (2004). Injection risk behaviors among clients of syringe exchange programs with different syringe dispensation policies. *J Acquir Immune Defic Syndr* 37:1307–1312.

Liddicoat RV, Horton NJ, Urban R, Maier E, Christiansen D, and Samet JH (2004). Assessing missed opportunities for HIV testing in medical settings. *J Gen Intern Med* 19:349–356.

Linas BP, Zheng H, Losina E, Walensky RP, and Freedberg KA (2006). Assessing the impact of federal HIV prevention spending on HIV testing and awareness. *Am J Public Health* 196:1038–1043.

Marks G, Crepaz N, and Janssen RS (2006). Estimating sexual transmission of HIV from persons aware and unaware that they are infected with the virus in the USA. *AIDS* 20:1447–1450.

McGinnis KA, Fine MJ, Sharma RK, Skanderson M, Wagner JH, Rodriguez-Barradas MC, Rabeneck L, and Justice AC (2003). Understanding racial disparities in HIV using data from the veterans aging cohort 3-site study and VA administrative data. *Am J Public Health* 93:1728–1733.

Meade CS, and Sikkema KJ (2005). Voluntary HIV testing among adults with severe mental illness: frequency and associated factors. *AIDS Behav* 9:465–473.

Mitty JA, and Flanigan TP (2004). Community-based interventions for marginalized populations. *Clin Infect Dis* 38(Suppl. 5):S373–S375.

Moss AR (2000a). Epidemiology and the politics of needle exchange. *Am J Public Health* 90:1385–1387.

Moss AR (2000b). "For God's sake, don't show this letter to the president…". *Am J Public Health* 90:1395–1396.

Palacio H, Kahn JG, Richards TA, and Morin SF (2002). Effect of race and/or ethnicity in use of antiretrovirals and prophylaxis for opportunistic infection: a review of the literature. *Public Health Rep* 117:233–251.

Paltiel AD, Weinstein MC, Kimmel AD, Seage GR III, Losina E, Zhang H, Freedberg KA, and Walensky RP (2005). Expanded screening for HIV in the United States—an analysis of cost-effectiveness. *N Engl J Med* 352:586–595.

Phelan JC, Link BG, Stueve A, and Pescosolido BA (2000). Public conceptions of mental illness in 1950 and 1996: what is mental illness and is it to be feared? *J Health Soc Behav* 41:188–207.

Pirl WF, Greer JA, Weissquarber C, and Safren SA (2005). Screening for infectious diseases among patients in a state psychiatric hospital. *Psychiatr Serv* 56:1614–1616.

Redlemeier DA, Tan SH, and Booth GL (1998). The treatment of unrelated disorders in patients with chronic medical diseases. *N Engl J Med* 338:1516–1520.

Roland ME, Adey D, Carlson LL, and Terrault NA (2003). Kidney and liver transplantation in HIV-infected patients: case presentations and review. *AIDS Patient Care STDS* 17:501–507.

Rust G, Minor P, Jordan N, Mayberry R, and Satcher D (2003). Do clinicians screen Medicaid patients for syphilis or HIV when they diagnose other sexually transmitted diseases? *Sex Transm Dis* 30:723–727.

Sambamoorthi U, Walkup J, McSpiritt E, Warner L, Castle N, and Crystal S (2000). Racial differences in end-of-life care for patients with AIDS. *AIDS Public Policy J* 15:136–148.

Sambamoorthi U, Moynihan PJ, McSpiritt E, and Crystal S (2001). Use of protease inhibitors and non-nucleoside reverse transcriptase inhibitors among Medicaid beneficiaries with AIDS. *Am J Public Health* 91:1474–1481.

Samet JH, Freedberg KA, Stein MD, Lewis R, Savetsky J, Sullivan L, Levenson SM, and Hingson R (1998). Trillion virion delay: time from testing positive for HIV to presentation for primary care. *Arch Intern Med* 158:734–740.

Sauer MV (2006). American physicians remain slow to embrace the reproductive needs of human immunodeficiency virus–infected patients. *Fertil Steril* 85:295–297.

Schechter MT, Strathdee SA, Cornelisse PG, Currie S, Patrick DM, Rekart ML, and O'Shaughnessy MV (1999). Do needle exchange programmes increase the spread of HIV among injection drug users? An investigation of the Vancouver outbreak. *AIDS* 13: F45–F51.

Schoenbaum EE, Hartel DM, and Gourevitch MN (1996). Needle exchange use among a cohort of injecting drug users. *AIDS* 10:1729–1734.

Schuster MA, Collins R, Cunningham WE, Morton SC, Zierler S, Wong M, Tu W, and Kanouse DE (2005). Perceived discrimination in clinical care in a nationally representative sample of HIV-infected adults receiving health care. *J Gen Intern Med* 20:807–813.

Shapiro M, Morton S, McCaffrey D, Senterfitt JW, Fleishman JA, Perlman JF, Athey LA, Keesey JW, Goldman DP, Berry SH, and Bozzette SA (1999). Variations in the care of HIV-infected adults in the United States: results from the HIV Cost and Services Utilization Study. *JAMA* 281:2305–2315.

Silverberg MJ, Wegner SA, Milazzo MJ, McKaig RG, Williams CF, Agan BK, Armstrong AW, Gange SJ, Hawkes C, O'connell RJ, Ahuja SK, Dolan MJ, for the Tri-Service AIDS Clinical Consortium Natural History Study Group (2006). Effectiveness of highly active antiretroviral therapy by race/ethnicity. *AIDS* 20:1531–1538.

Smith SR, and Kirking DM (2001). The effect of insurance coverage changes on drug utilization in HIV disease. *J Acquir Immune Defic Syndr* 28:140–149.

Stern JE, Cramer CP, Garrod A, and Green RM (2002). Attitudes on access to services at assisted reproductive technology clinics: comparisons with clinic policy. *Fertil Steril* 77:537–541.

Strathdee SA, Patrick DM, Currie SL, Cornelisse PG, Rekart ML, Montaner JS, Schechter MT, and O'Shaughnessy MV (1997). Needle exchange is not enough: lessons from the Vancouver injecting drug use study. *AIDS* 11:F59–F65.

Sullivan G, Koegel P, Kanouse D, Cournos F, McKinnon K, Young A, and Bean D (1999). HIV and people with serious mental illness: the public sector's role in reducing HIV risk and improving care. *Psychiatr Serv* 50:648–652.

Tegger M, Uldall K, Tapia K, Holte S, Crane H, and Kitahata M (2007) Depression treatment decreases delay in HAART initiation among depressed HIV-infected patients. Presented at: 2nd International Conference on HIV Treatment Adherence; 2007; Jersey City, New Jersey, USA.

Turner BJ, Laine C, Cosler L, and Hauck WW (2003). Relationship of gender, depression, and health care delivery with antiretroviral adherence in HIV-infected drug users. *J Gen Intern Med* 18:248–257.

Umbricht-Schneiter A, Ginn DH, Pabst KM, and Bigelow GE (1994). Providing medical care to methadone clinic patients: referral vs. on-site care. *Am J Public Health* 84:207–210.

Vlahov D, Safaien M, Lai S, Strathdee SA, Johnson L, Sterling T, and Celentano DD (2001). Sexual and drug risk-related behaviours after initiating highly active antiretroviral therapy among injection drug users. *AIDS* 15:2311–2316.

Wagner GJ, Kanouse DE, Koegel P, and Sullivan G (2003). Adherence to HIV antiretrovirals among persons with serious mental illness. *AIDS Patient Care STDS* 17:179–186.

Walensky RP, Losina E, Steger-Craven KA, and Freedberg KA (2002). Identifying undiagnosed human immunodeficiency virus: the yield of routine, voluntary inpatient testing. *Arch Intern Med* 162:887–892.

Walensky RP, Losina E, Malatesta L, Barton GE, O'Connor CA, Skolnik PR, Hall JM, McGuire JF, and Freedberg KA (2005). Effective HIV case identification through routine HIV screening at urgent care centers in Massachusetts. *Am J Public Health* 95:71–73.

Walkup J, Crystal S, and Sambamoorthi U (1999). Schizophrenia and major affective disorder among Medicaid recipients with HIV/AIDS in New Jersey. *Am J Public Health* 89:1101–1103.

Walkup J, McAlpine DD, Olfson M, Boyer C, and Hansell S (2000). Recent HIV testing among general hospital inpatients with schizophrenia: findings from four New York City sites. *Psychiatr Q* 71:177–193.

Walkup J, Sambamoorthi U, and Crystal S (2001). Incidence and consistency of antiretroviral use among HIV-infected Medicaid beneficiaries with schizophrenia. *J Clin Psychiatry* 62:174–178.

Walkup J, Satriano J, Barry D, Sadler P, and Cournos F (2002). HIV testing policy and serious mental illness. *Am J Public Health* 92:1931–1940.

Walkup J, Sambamoorthi U, and Crystal S (2004). Use of newer antiretroviral treatments among HIV-infected Medicaid beneficiaries with serious mental illness. *J Clin Psychiatry* 65:1180–1189.

Webber MP, Schoenbaum EE, Gourevitch MN, Buono D, Chang CJ, and Klein RS (1998). Temporal trends in the progression of human immunodeficiency virus disease in a cohort of drug users. *Epidemiology* 9:613–617.

Wilson IB and Jacobson D (2006). Regarding "Antidepressant treatment improves adherence to antiretroviral therapy among depressed HIV-infected patients." *J Acquir Immune Defic Syndr* 41:254–255.

Wodak A, and Cooney A (2006). Do needle syringe programs reduce HIV infection among injecting drug users: a comprehensive review of the international evidence. *Subst Use Misuse* 41:777–813.

Yun LW, Maravi M, Kobayashi JS, Barton PL, and Davidson AJ (2005). Antidepressant treatment improves adherence to antiretroviral therapy among depressed HIV-infected patients. *J Acquir Immune Defic Syndr* 38:432–438.

Index